CROWLEY'S

AN INTRODUCTION TO

HUMAN DISEASE

Pathology and Pathophysiology Correlations

TENTH EDITION

Emily G. Reisner, PhD

Faculty, Physician's Assistant Program
Duke University
Durham, NC

Howard M. Reisner, PhD

Professor of Pathology
University of North Carolina
Chapel Hill, NC
Associate Professor of Pathology
Campbell University School of Osteopathic Medicine
Lillington, NC

JONES & BARTLETT
LEARNING

World Headquarters
Jones & Bartlett Learning
5 Wall Street
Burlington, MA 01803
978-443-5000
info@jblearning.com
www.jblearning.com

Jones & Bartlett Learning books and products are available through most bookstores and online booksellers. To contact Jones & Bartlett Learning directly, call 800-832-0034, fax 978-443-8000, or visit our website, www.jblearning.com.

Substantial discounts on bulk quantities of Jones & Bartlett Learning publications are available to corporations, professional associations, and other qualified organizations. For details and specific discount information, contact the special sales department at Jones & Bartlett Learning via the above contact information or send an email to specialsales@jblearning.com.

09938-6

Production Credits

General Manager: Eduardo Moura
VP, Executive Publisher: David D. Cella
Publisher: Cathy L. Esperti
Editorial Assistant: Carter McAlister
Associate Director of Production: Julie C. Bolduc
Senior Production Editor: Leah Corrigan
Director of Marketing: Andrea DeFronzo
VP, Manufacturing and Inventory Control: Therese Connell
Composition: Cenveo® Publisher Services
Project Management: Cenveo Publisher Services
Cover Design: Kristin E. Parker
Rights & Media Specialist: Jamey O'Quinn
Media Development Editor: Troy Liston
Cover Image: © CDC/Dr. Dudman, Dr. Kaplan
Printing and Binding: RR Donnelley
Cover Printing: RR Donnelley

Library of Congress Cataloging-in-Publication Data

Names: Reisner, Emily G., author. | Reisner, Howard M., author. | Crowley, Leonard V., 1926- Introduction to human disease. Preceded by (work): Title: Crowley's an introduction to human disease: pathology and pathophysiology correlations / Emily G. Reisner, Howard M. Reisner.
Other titles: Introduction to human disease
Description: Tenth edition. | Burlington, MA: Jones & Bartlett Learning, [2017] | Preceded by An introduction to human disease / Leonard V. Crowley. 9th ed. c2013. | Includes bibliographical references and index.
Identifiers: LCCN 2016010951 | ISBN 9781284050233 (casebound: alk. paper)
Subjects: | MESH: Disease | Pathology
Classification: LCC RB112 | NLM QZ 4 | DDC 616.07—dc23 LC record available at http://lccn.loc.gov/2016010951

6048

Printed in the United States of America
20 19 18 17 16   10 9 8 7 6 5 4 3 2 1

This Tenth Edition is dedicated to the memory of Dr. Leonard V. Crowley, without whom there would be no book.

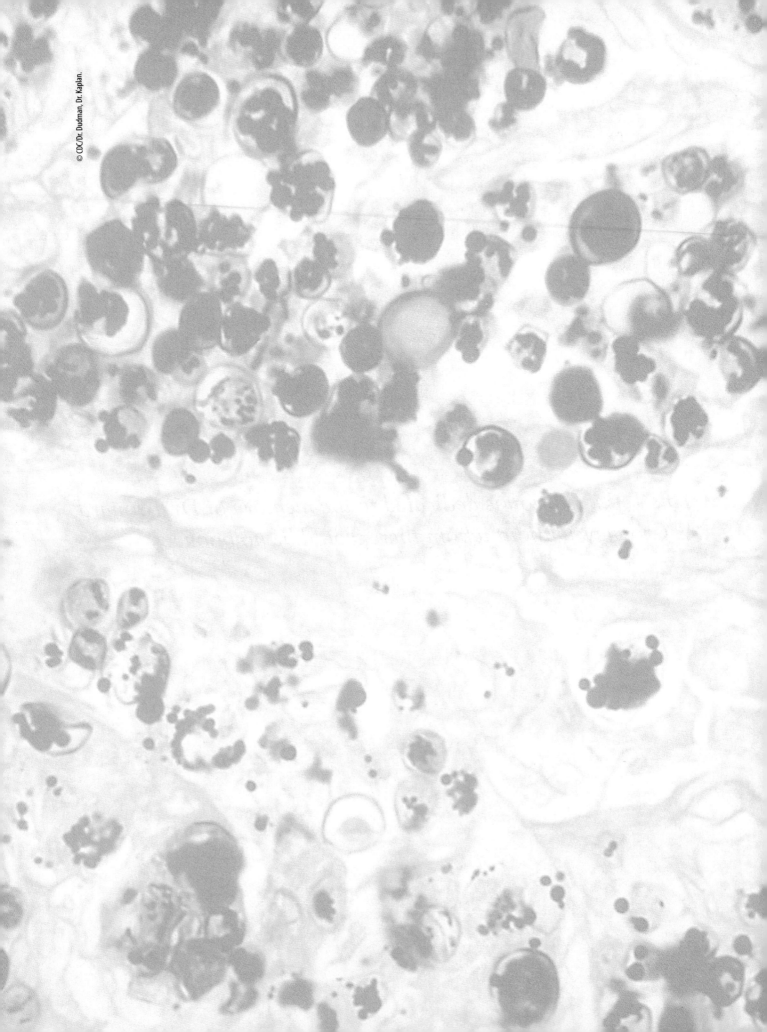

Brief Contents

Contents

3 GENES, DNA, CHROMOSOMES, AND CELL DIVISION 47

4 CONGENITAL AND HEREDITARY DISEASES 67

5   INFLAMMATION AND REPAIR   93

6   IMMUNITY, HYPERSENSITIVITY, ALLERGY, AND AUTOIMMUNE DISEASES   107

18 PRENATAL DEVELOPMENT AND CONDITIONS ASSOCIATED WITH PREGNANCY 465

21   THE LIVER AND THE BILIARY SYSTEM

22   THE PANCREAS AND DIABETES MELLITUS

23   **THE GASTROINTESTINAL TRACT**   **605**

Preface

In recent years, increased emphasis has been placed on how changes in the genome are expressed as disease. This information now has a larger role in both diagnosis and therapy, which is reflected in the text for this edition. We have preserved Dr. Crowley's organization from the *Ninth Edition*, starting with six general chapters followed by chapters on organ systems and their diseases, but in this *Tenth Edition* we have provided more information on the cellular and molecular roots of disease.

The Audience

How did we visualize the reader of this work? The authors hope that any individual interested in the health sciences who wishes to understand the nature of disease would find the text of interest. Specifically, we hope that the text would allow a beginning student of the health sciences who has a working knowledge of biology to equip themselves with the concepts and vocabulary for more specialized areas of study in any of the health related fields. To do this we have taken particular care to present recent information relating to the therapy and molecular diagnosis of disease.

New to This Edition

Throughout this new edition, extensive updates have been made.

Chapter 1

- Expanded principles of diagnosis, including additional material on taking a history, performing a physical diagnosis, and selecting a diagnostic test
- Updated information on clinical laboratory testing and imaging techniques
- Introduction of concepts including evidence-based and patient-centered medicine
- Addition of new testing procedures, such as virtual colonoscopy and single-photon computed tomography (SPECT)
- Updated with new figures
- Case presentation added
- Expansion of definition list
- Update of reference list

Chapter 2

- Added information on cell–cell signaling
- Added/updated information on cell injury and cell death
- Added information on Hayflick limit for cell division
- Case presentation added
- Expansion of definition list
- Update of reference list

Chapter 3

- Information on genes and DNA moved from previous edition Chapter 2 and integrated into presentation of genetics
- Information added on pedigree analysis and inheritance patterns

- Information on the HLA system moved to Chapter 5
- Information added regarding definition of race
- Case presentation added
- More than doubled the number of definitions
- Update of reference list

Chapter 4 (was Chapter 9 in the previous edition)

- Reorganized to better integrate with Chapter 3
- Presentation on fetal testing updated
- Material added on HIV infection in the mother
- Cases reviewed and updated
- New figures
- Number of definitions increased
- Update of reference list

Chapter 5 (was Chapter 4 in the previous edition)

- Material and terminology modernized; chapter linked to Chapter 6 on immunology
- Case presentation added
- Number of definitions more that doubled
- Figures replaced
- Update of reference list

Chapter 6 (was Chapter 5 in the previous edition)

- Eighty percent rewritten to focus on the most recent information on the development of adaptive immunity
- Material added on immunodeficiency
- Number of definitions increased
- New figures added
- New case added
- Update of reference list

Chapter 7 (was Chapter 10 in the previous edition)

- Extensively rewritten to focus on principles of neoplastic process in general rather than results of the process in specific organs; neoplasia presentations are now in the specific organ chapters
- Added two additional figures to illustrate critical points; updated other figures and tables

- Expanded presentation of oncogenes and tumor suppressor genes
- Updated presentation on immunotherapy and anticancer drugs
- Case presentation added; original short cases deleted
- Update of reference list

Chapter 8 (was Chapter 6 in the previous edition)

- Material added on hemorrhagic fevers, including Ebola
- Material added on molecular testing for microorganisms
- Material added on aspergillosis
- Number of definitions increased
- New figures added
- New case about measles added
- Update of reference list

Chapter 9 (was Chapter 7 in the previous edition)

- Chapter renamed to better reflect material
- Material added on Chagas disease, leishmaniasis, strongyloidiasis, and trichomoniasis
- Case presentation added; original short cases deleted
- Figures replaced
- Update of reference list

Chapter 10 (was Chapter 8 in the previous edition)

- Chapter renamed to better reflect material
- Chapter reorganized to improve presentation
- Material on Ebola transmission control added
- HIV material updated
- Case presentation added; original short cases deleted
- Figures replaced
- Update of reference list

Chapter 11 (was Chapter 13 in the previous edition)

- Completely rewritten; now focused on the heart and associated diseases
- Material on vascular disease moved to Chapter 12

- Updated terminology
- Expanded definition list
- Replaced figures
- New case
- Update of reference list

Chapter 12 (was Chapter 13 in the previous edition)

- Completely rewritten; now focused on the vasculature and associated diseases
- Section on risks for atherosclerosis updated and completely rewritten
- Updated terminology
- Expanded definition list
- Replaced figures
- New case
- Update of reference list

Chapter 13

- Material on leukemia and lymphoma added and updated (This chapter contains all information on these systems, including neoplasms, which were previously split between Chapters 10 and Chapter 14.)
- Material on thalassemia was expanded
- Consolidation of all material on diseases of hematopoietic tissue
- Presentation on stem cell therapy updated
- Case presentation added; original short case deleted
- Update of definitions
- Update of reference list

Chapter 14

- Major rewrite of primary and secondary hemostasis to bring up-to-date with current concepts
- Material added on molecular mechanisms of Coumadin
- Enhanced presentation of coagulation diagnostic tests
- Case presentation added; original short cases deleted
- Update of definitions
- Figures replaced
- Update of reference list

Chapter 15

- Tuberculosis information updated
- Lung cancer information updated

- Information on MERS added
- Case presentation added; original short cases deleted
- Figures replaced
- Update of reference list

Chapter 16

- Material added on molecular diagnosis of breast cancer
- Material updated to reflect most recent American Cancer Society diagnosis and treatment guidelines
- Case presentation added; original short cases deleted
- Figures replaced
- Update of reference list

Chapter 17

- Material added on the anatomy of the female reproductive tract and the menstrual cycle
- Material added on polycystic ovary disease (PECOS)
- Expanded presentation of uterine cancer
- Terminology updated for presentation of HPV and cancer
- Case presentation added; original short cases deleted
- Update of reference list

Chapter 18

- Condensed and updated presentation of red cell system incompatibilities
- Updated presentation of preeclampsia and eclampsia
- New case
- Additional definitions
- Revised figures
- Update of reference list

Chapter 19 (incorporates material from previous edition Chapters 19 and 24)

- Material on body water management integrated from Chapter 24
- Expanded and revised section on glomerular injury
- Material on transplantation updated
- New case added with two diagnoses
- Update of definitions
- Update of illustrations
- Update of reference list

Chapter 20

- Material added on developmental abnormalities of the ureter and penis
- Material updated on adenocarcinoma of the prostate
- Case presentation added; original short cases deleted
- Figures replaced
- Update of reference list

Chapter 21

- Chapter reorganized
- Material updated
- Case presentation added; original short cases deleted
- Figures replaced
- Update of reference list

Chapter 22

- Chapter reorganized
- Material updated, especially in regard to genetics of diabetes and metabolic syndrome
- Two case presentations added; original cases deleted
- Figures added
- Update of reference list

Chapter 23

- Chapter reorganized
- Material updated, especially in regard to addition of discussions of cholera and colorectal cancer
- Case presentation added on gluten sensitivity; original cases deleted
- Figures reviewed and replaced
- Update of reference list

Chapter 24 (was Chapter 25 in the previous edition)

- Material added on multiple endocrine neoplasia (MEN)
- Thyroid neoplasia presentation updated
- Case presentation added on short stature and growth hormone deficiency; original cases deleted
- Figures reviewed and replaced
- Update of reference list

Chapter 25

- Material added on rabies and brain cancer
- Peripheral neuritis presentation updated
- Material on Creutzfeldt-Jakob syndrome corrected
- Presentation on structure and function condensed
- Case presentation added; original cases deleted
- Update of definition list
- Figures reviewed and replaced
- Update of reference list

Chapter 26

- Discussion of rheumatoid arthritis updated
- Presentation of tumors of bone added
- Case presentation added
- Figures reviewed and replaced; figures describing skeleton and muscle structure added, along with others
- Definition list expanded
- Update of reference list

About the Authors

Howard Reisner and Emily Reisner met in graduate school and hold PhDs from Case Western Reserve University in Cleveland, Ohio. Howard is Professor of Pathology at the University of North Carolina in Chapel Hill and Associate Professor of Pathology at the Campbell University School of Medicine. Emily has been a laboratory director at Duke University Medical Center and Director of Medical Writing in the pharmaceutical industry. She currently teaches medical writing for the physician's assistant program at Duke University. Both are authors or editors of numerous books on pathology and have been involved in programs for teaching pathology in the Allied Health field.

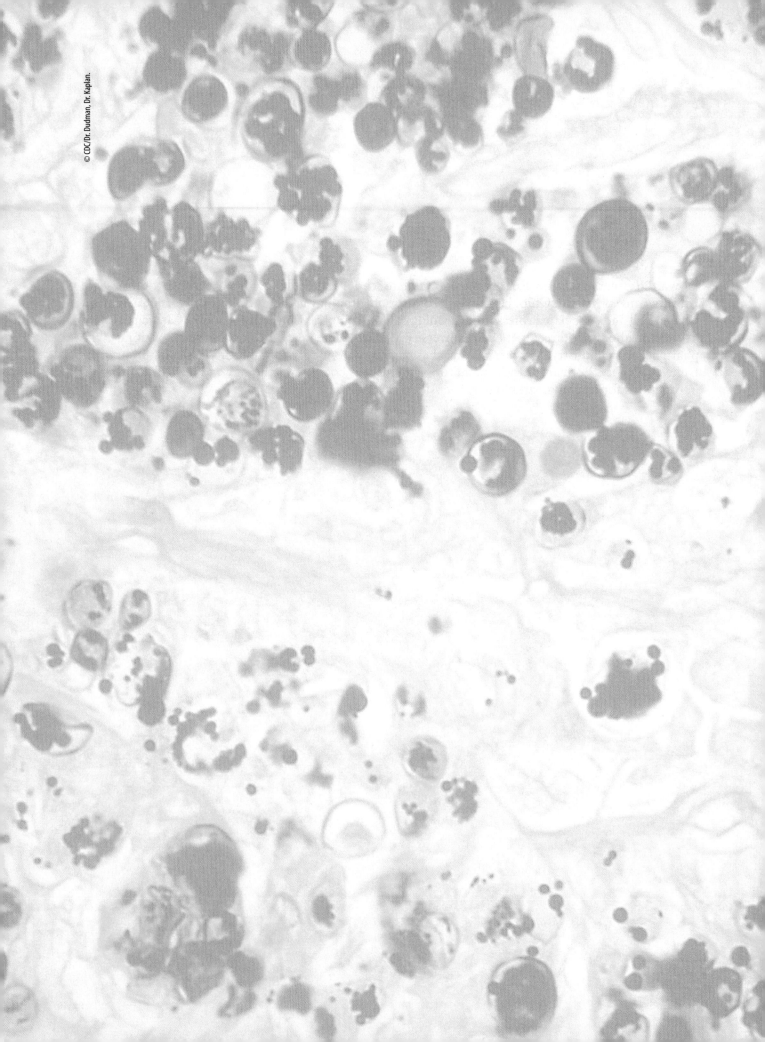

Acknowledgments

The authors would like to thank the team at Jones & Bartlett Learning for their support throughout this project: Cathy Esperti, publisher; Carter McAlister, editorial assistant; Leah Corrigan, senior production editor; Troy Liston, media development editor; and Jamey O'Quinn, rights and media specialist. We would also like to thank Apoorva Goel, project manager at Cenveo Publisher Services.

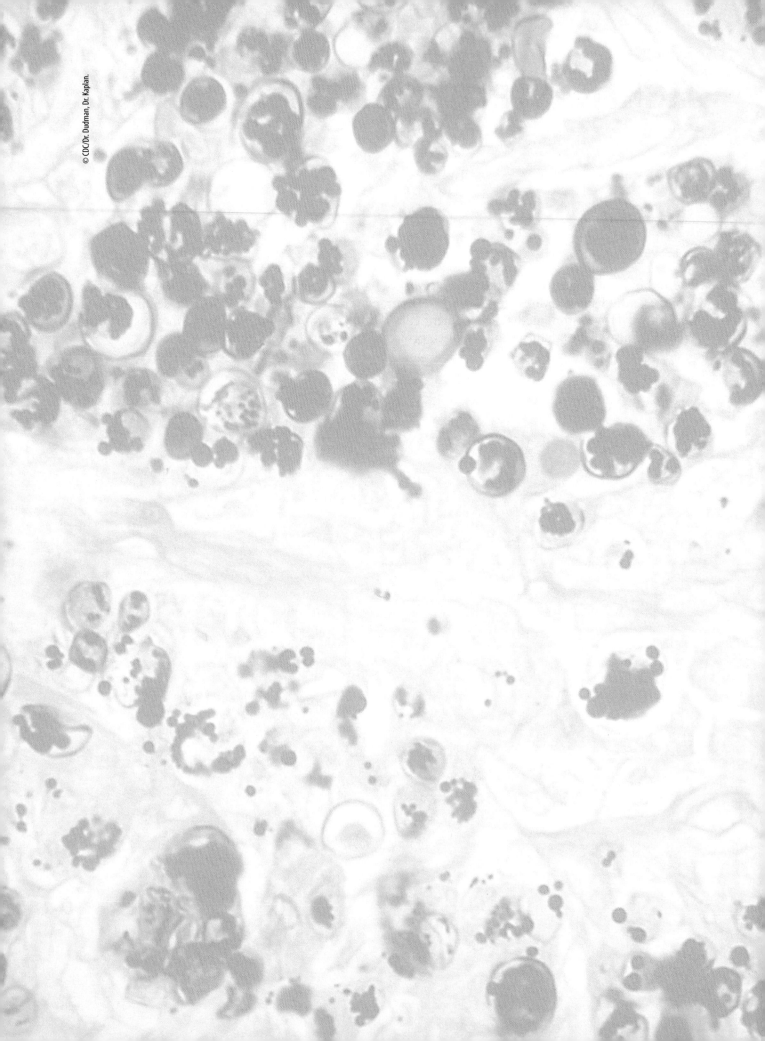

Reviewers

Jones & Bartlett Learning and the authors would like to thank the following people for reviewing the *Ninth Edition* and providing feedback for updating this edition.

Carol J. Bunge, RN, BSN, MHA
Molina Healthcare

Julian Wade Farrior, PhD
Gwynedd Mercy College

Reid Fisher, EdD, ATC
University of the Incarnate Word

Susan Hay, BS, MA
Adjunct Instructor
Department of Clinical Research and Leadership
School of Medicine and Health Sciences
George Washington University

Marilyn Hughes, RHIA, CCS
Health Information Management
University of Mississippi Medical Center
Health Information Technology Instructor
Hinds Community College

Robert N. Phalen, PhD
Associate Professor
University of Houston, Clear Lake

Michele M. Suhie, PhD, MT (ASCP),
ACSM/NPAS-PAPHS
Coordinator, Geriatric Health and Wellness
Program
College of Health Professions
Sacred Heart University

Jessica M. Goodman, PT, DPT
Gateway Community College

Danyel Anderson, MPH, MT (ASCP), MLT
Program Clinical Coordinator
Ozarks Technical Community College

Zach Frank, PT, DPT, MS
Assistant Professor
Washburn University

Suzanne Moore
Manchester Community College

Zada T. Wicker, MBA, RHIT, CCS, CCS-P
Brunswick Community College

Penny Taylor, RN, MSN/ED, MSU
Department of Nursing
Montana State University–Northern

Will Walker, PhD
Associate Professor of Kinesiology
East Texas Baptist University

Joseph F. Stano
Springfield College

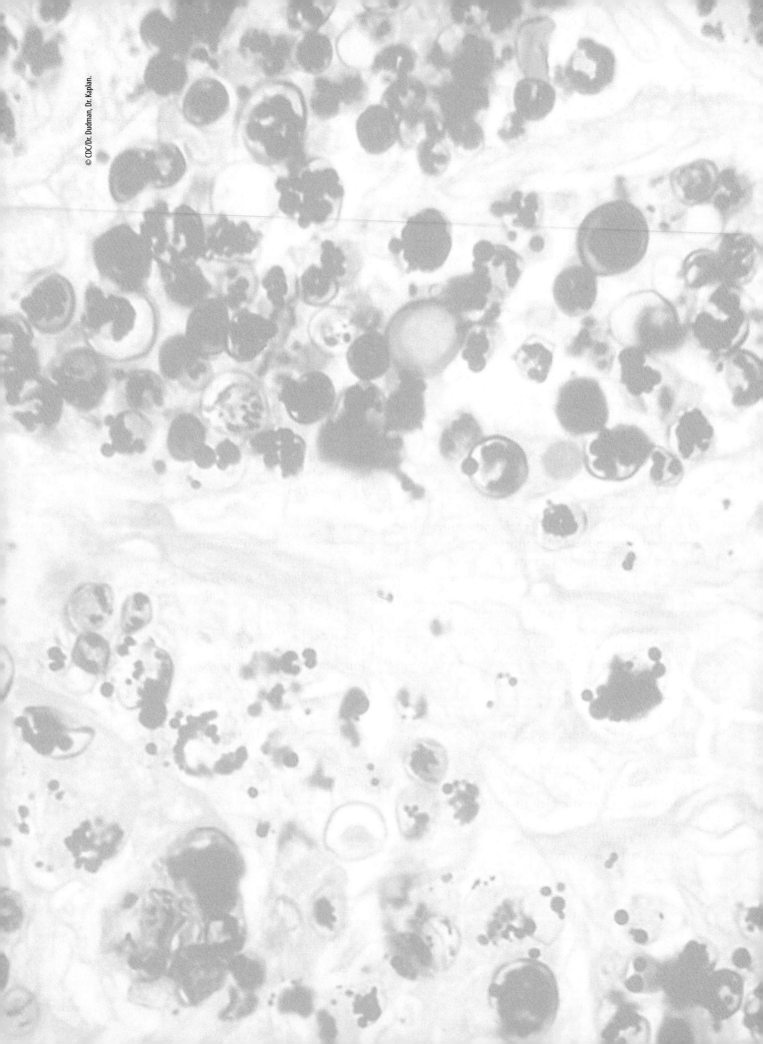

A Visual Walkthrough

Various learning features are included to enhance the usefulness of this product.

LEARNING OBJECTIVES

Learning objectives provide students with expected outcomes for each chapter as well as a checklist for measuring comprehension.

LEARNING OBJECTIVES

1. Explain the basic anatomic and physiologic principles of ventilation and gas exchange.
2. Describe the physiological basis and use of pulmonary function tests.
3. Describe the causes, clinical effects, complications, and treatment of pneumothorax and atelectasis.
4. Describe the clinical symptoms, complications, and treatment of pneumonia.
5. Describe the histologic characteristics of a tuberculous infection. Explain the possible outcome of an infection. Describe methods of diagnosis and treatment.
6. Differentiate between bronchitis and bronchiectasis.
7. List the anatomic and physiologic derangements in cl obstructive lung disease. Explain its pathogenesis. De clinical manifestations and methods of treatment.
8. Describe the pathogenesis and manifestations of bro asthma and respiratory distress syndrome.
9. Explain the causes and effects of pulmonary fibrosis. the special problems associated with asbestosis.
10. List the major types of lung carcinoma. Describe the c manifestations of lung carcinoma and explain the pri treatment.

EXTENSIVE GLOSSARY

The extensive glossary proves useful to students who may not have had a course in medical terminology. It also serves as a convenient reference for students who want to quickly review a particular term. Words appearing in the glossary are set in boldface type in the text and set off in the margin for easy reference.

Introduction

Transmission of genetic information was initially studied through the analysis of the inheritance of detectable traits (phenotypic traits) from parent through successive generations of offspring using patterns of inheritance. These phenotypic traits are now understood as the expression of the genotype of the individual; that is, the genes that are the functional manifestation of the chemical code of the DNA organized in chromosomes in the nucleus of the cell. The human genome contains about

Phenotype Collection of inherited/phenotypic traits detectable in an individual.

Phenotypic traits Characteristics apparent in the individual.

EXTENSIVE ART PROGRAM

The extensive art program with a number of new photos and revised illustrations has been updated and enhanced to support the new focus on the cellular and molecular roots of disease, as well as to provide additional visual support for student comprehension.

FIGURE 2-1 Structure of a typical cell. Note that the cell is divided into two compartments, the nuclear and cytoplasmic. The cytoplasm contains a variety of structures called organelles.

Labels: Plasma membrane, Mitochondrion, Centriole, Vacuole, Lysosome, Nuclear membrane, Nucleolus, Chromatin, Nucleus, Ribosomes, Glycogen, Golgi apparatus, Intermediate filament, Microtubule, Cytoplasm, Smooth endoplasmic reticulum, Rough endoplasmic reticulum, Microfilaments

ANIMATIONS

Animations come with new, unused purchases of this book. Animations add visual clarity to key concepts and competencies.

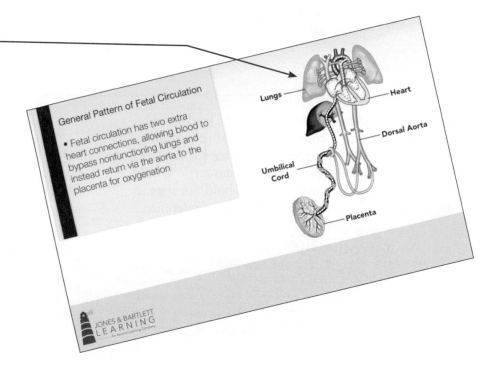

General Pattern of Fetal Circulation
• Fetal circulation has two extra heart connections, allowing blood to bypass nonfunctioning lungs and instead return via the aorta to the placenta for oxygenation

Labels: Lungs, Heart, Dorsal Aorta, Umbilical Cord, Placenta

JONES & BARTLETT LEARNING
An Ascend Learning Company

CASE STUDIES

Case studies in each chapter provide an opportunity for the student to apply the concepts presented in the text to a medical setting. The cases range from common diseases likely to be encountered by the student to more uncommon conditions, both of which serve to teach specific information that expands on what is presented in the chapter. For this reason, the cases are integral to the information we hope to impart.

CASE 10-1

The patient, an eighteen-year-old female, is seen at the emergency room of a local hospital complaining of severe abdominal pain, vaginal bleeding, and delay in her expected menstrual period. She notes that she had unprotected vaginal intercourse about seven weeks prior and is concerned about a sexually transmitted disease. She experienced coitarche (initial sexual intercourse) at age fifteen and has been sexually active since that time with a variety of partners. She states that usually barrier protection was used by the male (condoms) but they did sometimes "forget." She notes that she has been seen in a venereal disease clinic several times in the past and was diagnosed with both gonorrhea and chlamydia infections for which she received antibiotic therapy "several times." A rapid pregnancy test is ordered, which is positive. Transvaginal ultrasound detects signs of an ectopic pregnancy (the fetuses is implanted in a site other than the uterus) located in the fallopian tube (oviduct), a so-called tubal pregnancy. She suffers a decrease in blood pressure with hemorrhage (hemorrhagic shock) and is rushed to surgery. At surgery blood is found in the abdominal cavity (hemoperitoneum) and an 8 cm left mass was found that encompassed both the left fallopian tube and ovary. The mass contained a nonviable fetus judged to be of eight weeks gestational age (FIGURE 10-10). Both the left ovary and fallopian tube were removed (salpingo-oophorectomy). The contralateral fallopian tube and ovary showed numerous adhesions that distorted their anatomy and were considered to be consistent with long-standing pelvic inflammatory disease. Recovery was complicated by ongoing infections, but she eventually recovered.

REVIEW QUESTIONS AND A DETAILED OUTLINE SUMMARY

Review questions and a detailed outline summary are provided for each chapter and provide students with a means to measure their learning.

QUESTIONS FOR REVIEW

1. Why do spontaneous abortions occur? What are the consequences of prolonged retention of a dead fetus within the uterine cavity?
2. What is an ectopic pregnancy? What factors predispose to development of an ectopic pregnancy in the fallopian tube? What are the consequences of a tubal pregnancy?
3. What is the difference between a hydatidiform mole and a choriocarcinoma?
4. In infants with hemolytic disease, why does jaundice increase after delivery? Why does anemia become more severe after delivery?
5. How does the physician make a diagnosis of hemolytic disease? How is the disease treated?
6. What structures contribute to the formation of the placenta? What are the main functions of the placenta?
7. Describe some of the important abnormalities of the placenta and umbilical cord that may have an unfavorable effect on pregnancy.
8. What is the source of amnionic fluid? What factors regulate the total volume of amnionic fluid?
9. What are the possible causes and the significance of polyhydramnios? of oligohydramnios?

SUPPLEMENTARY READINGS

Supplementary readings were selected to provide an opportunity for the student to dig deeper. We have tried to emphasize information sources that review and expand on the text although in some cases we have suggested more research-based material that we think is of specific interest. Such papers may be a challenge to some readers, but we hope they will encourage the learner. When possible we have tried to include authoritative sources and freely available material, much of which is web-based. We hope this text will interest and encourage anyone interested in pursuing a health-related career to continue in what is an area of critical importance to our society.

SUPPLEMENTARY READINGS

Loeffler, A. G., and Hart, M. N. 2015. *Introduction to Human Disease.* 6th ed. Burlington, MA: Jones & Bartlett Learning.
- ▶ Those interested in the detailed study of male reproductive disease should consult a work on human pathology aimed at the undergraduate medical curriculum. However, a good place to start at a less advanced level is by reading Chapter 16 in this book.

Simmons, M. N., Berglund, R. K., and Jones, S. J. 2011. A practical guide to prostate cancer diagnosis and management. *Cleveland Clinic Journal of Medicine* 78:321–31.

Ilic, D., Neuberger, I. D., Djulbegovic, M., and Dahm, P. 2013. Screening for prostate cancer (Review). Wiley Online Library. The Cochrane Collaboration. doi: 10.1002/14651858.CD004720.pub3

Hayes, J. H., and Barry, M. J. 2014. Screening for prostate cancer with prostate-specific antigen test. A review of current literature. *JAMA* 311:1143–49.
- ▶ One of the more controversial areas in urology is the appropriate role of prostate cancer screening. The first reference represents a conservative point of view for both diagnosis and therapy. The second entry provides a book-length review (see pages 1–9 for a brief review aimed at nontechnical readers). Both the second and third entries provide exhaustive of the literature with results that suggest little or no benefit for most groups of men (as measured in reduced deaths as a result of prostate cancer) using current approaches to screening.

Case Studies

Chapter	Case Study
1	Appendicitis
2	Steatosis or Alcoholic Fatty Liver Disease
3	Hemophilia B
4	Congenital Cytomegalovirus Infection
5	Wound Infection
6	IgA Deficiency
7	Colon Cancer
8	Measles
9	Chagas Disease
10	Tubal Pregnancy
11	Sudden Cardiac Death
12	Kawasaki Disease
13	Acute Lymphoblastic Leukemia
14	Hemolytic Uremic Syndrome
15	Childhood Asthma
16	Fat Necrosis
17	Polycystic Ovary Syndrome
18	Potter Sequence
19	Minimal Change Disease
20	Testicular Cancer
21	Tylenol Overdose
22	Diabetes Cases (2)
23	Celiac Disease
24	Isolated GH Deficiency
25	Meningitis
26	Duchenne Muscular Dystrophy

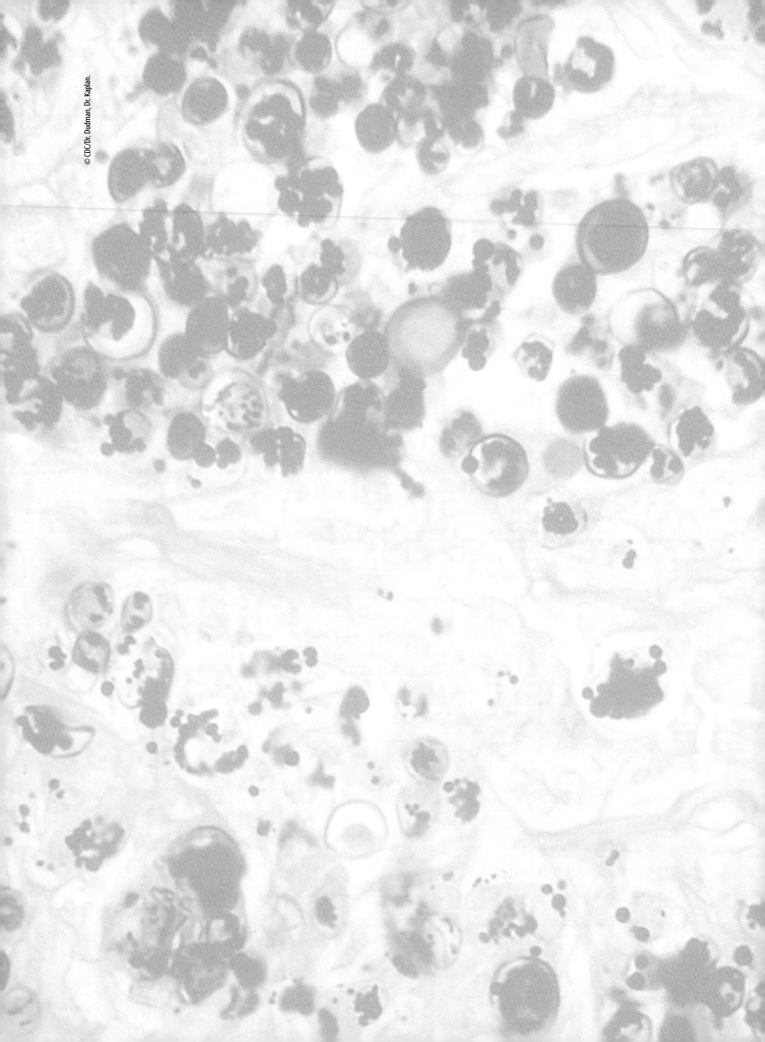

Teaching and Learning Aids

Instructor Resources Include:

- Testbank
- Slides in PowerPoint Format
- Answers to Student Workbook
- Animations
  - Chromosomes -> DNA
  - Mitosis Stages A–F
  - Meiosis
  - Gametogenesis
  - Phagocytosis
  - Formation of Antigen Binding Regions in T and B Cells
  - How Antibodies Work in Host Defense
  - Pathogenesis of an Allergy
  - Replication Cycle of HIV
  - Blood Flow in the Heart
  - Fetal Circulation
  - Development of Gametes and Fertilization
  - Maturation of Ovum
  - TIPS Procedure
  - Rotary Twist of Sigmoid Colon

Student Resources Include:

- Writable workbook exercises
- Student practice activities and assessments

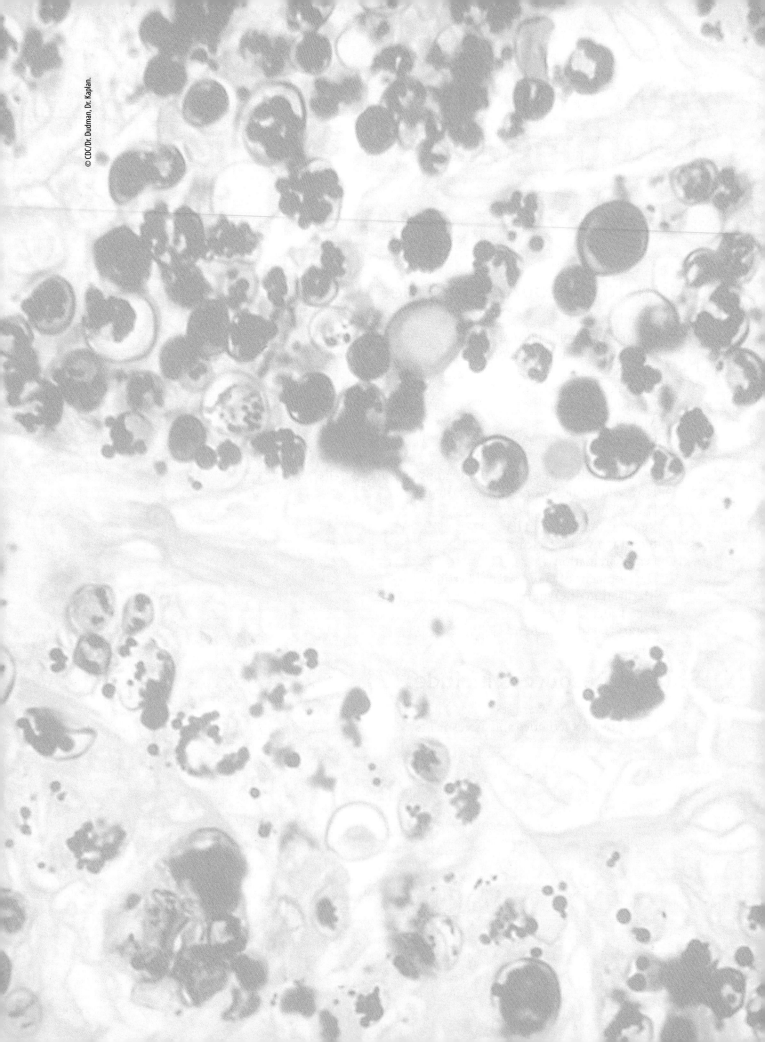

General Concepts of Disease: Principles of Diagnosis

LEARNING OBJECTIVES

1. Define the common terms used to describe disease including, but not limited to, lesions, symptomatic and asymptomatic disease, etiology, and pathogenesis.

2. List the major categories of human disease.

3. Outline the approach a practitioner uses to make a diagnosis and decide on a patient's treatment.

4. Describe the various types of diagnostic tests and procedures that can help the practitioner make a diagnosis.

5. Compare and contrast the different imaging techniques described.

What Is Disease?

Disease, in its broadest sense, is any compromise to the normal function of the body and the systems of which it is composed. However, it is best to consider health and illness as two extremes of a continuum. At one extreme is severe, disabling, or life-threatening illness with corresponding effects on our physical and emotional well-being. At the other extreme is ideal, perfectly good health, a state of physical and mental well-being wished for but rarely attained. Between these two extremes are many gradations of health and disease, ranging from mild or short-term illness that limits activities to some extent to moderate good health that falls short of the ideal state. The midpoint in this continuum, one in which one is neither ill nor in ideal good health, is where most of us are likely to fall. Who does not suffer from an occasional cold, sprain, upset stomach, or headache? As we get older, our average position in the continuum begins to shift. Disease is no longer occasional but becomes chronic as we suffer from degenerative conditions, which are part of the inevitable process of aging.

> **Disease** Any disturbance of the structure or function of the body.

How Do We Know We Are Sick?

How do you know you are sick? This seems an obvious question. Sometimes you do know and sometimes you don't. The subjective manifestations of disease, called

Symptoms Subjective manifestations of disease.

Lesion Any structural abnormality or pathologic change.

Trauma Injury caused by a physical extrinsic agent.

Pathogen Causative agent of disease.

Inflammation An early defensive reaction by the body to insult.

Pathologist Person who studies the structural and functional changes in the body caused by disease.

Etiology The cause, especially the cause of a disease.

Pathogenesis Manner in which a disease develops.

Gross examination Study of diseased organ with the naked eye.

Histologic examination Study of disease using a microscope to examine tissue.

Immunological techniques Techniques using antibody or antigen preparations, usually with chemical labels.

Laboratory medicine Study of the composition of body fluids to diagnose disease.

Mnemonics Aides to memory.

Idiopathic Disease of unknown origin.

Iatrogenic Disease resulting from a medical intervention.

Clinician Physician having direct contact with patients.

Signs Physical findings of disease.

Asymptomatic Disease without symptoms.

symptoms, may be related to apparent **lesions** such as structural abnormalities like a broken bone or a painful swelling. Often, symptoms are the result of the body's reaction to injury, which may be the result of **trauma** or infection by **pathogens**. Symptoms such as fever, muscle aches, and pain are part of the process of **inflammation**, an early defensive reaction by the body to insult (discussed in the presentation on inflammation).

Pathologists study the **etiology** (cause) and **pathogenesis** (progression or "natural history") of disease by evaluating lesions at the level of organs, the tissues that comprise the organs, the cells that form the tissues, and the molecules of which the cells are composed. The pathologist may observe the diseased tissue with the naked eye (**gross examination**) or with the aid of a microscope (**histologic examination**). Histologic examination may be supplemented by the use of special methods of identifying normal or abnormal tissue components using biochemical or **immunological techniques** (see the discussion of immunology). It is increasingly common for pathologists to study the molecules of which the tissue is composed using the techniques of molecular biology. In addition, pathologists working in the area of **laboratory medicine** study the composition of our body fluids (blood and urine, for example) to look for markers of disease.

Classifications of Disease

Pathologists interested in etiology classify diseases into several large categories. Although these categories are broad, this helps in understanding how a disease is likely to progress and how it will affect the patient. There are several alternative systems but medical students (who appreciate **mnemonics**) often use the term VINDICATE'M as a scheme:

> Vascular
> Infectious (or Inflammatory)
> Neoplastic
> Degenerative (or Deficiency)
> Idiopathic (or Iatrogenic)
> Congenital
> Allergic (or Autoimmune)
> Traumatic
> Endocrine (or Environmental)
> Metabolic

With the exceptions of **idiopathic** (of unknown origin) and **iatrogenic** (physician caused), most of these terms will be familiar and discussed in detail in subsequent chapters. Although the above scheme is useful, many diseases fit in multiple categories or fit poorly in any.

Principles of Diagnosis

The first physician to see the patient and to diagnose the disease is the **clinician** (the generalist physician, or specialist in a particular area of medicine or surgery) who is expert in detecting and evaluating the objective manifestations of disease, the **signs** or physical findings. However, a disease may cause the affected individual no discomfort or disability (an **asymptomatic** disease). Because disease is most often asymptomatic in its early stages, it may progress to the point where it causes subjective symptoms, abnormal physical findings, and is more difficult, impossible, or costly to treat. Therefore, early detection of disease, even before it is brought to the attention of the clinician, is of great importance to the public and is a major concern of the specialist in **public health** who might design **screening** systems for early diagnosis.

Determination of the nature and cause of a patient's illness by a physician or other health practitioner is called a **diagnosis**. It is based on the practitioner's evaluation of the patient's history, subjective symptoms, the physical findings (signs), and the results of various laboratory tests, together with other appropriate diagnostic procedures. Many diagnostic procedures are **noninvasive** (requiring no physical invasion of the body, its openings, or cavities). A common example of such noninvasive diagnostic testing is the use of imaging technology (x-rays or ultrasound, for example). Sometimes diagnosis requires an **invasive** procedure. Such procedures may be relatively minor and have little discomfort associated with them. Common examples are drawing blood, obtaining a **Pap smear** (to collect a sample of cervical cells), or sampling fluid and cells from a surface accessible lesion with a very fine needle (**fine needle aspiration**). Somewhat more invasive are a variety of endoscopic procedures in which a tube (generally flexible) is passed into a body opening such as the esophagus or anus (as is done in the case of **colonoscopy**). Laparoscopic procedures involving the introduction of devices into body cavities or obtaining samples of internal organs (liver, kidney, and lungs, for example) by the use of sampling devices guided by imaging technology are yet more invasive, but much safer and potentially less costly than a surgical procedure.

The effort to reach a diagnosis may be minimal and require nothing more than evaluation of the patient's history and a physical examination, or it may require multiple diagnostic procedures and the intervention of several diagnostic specialists and extensive testing. Whatever the case, when the clinician has reached a diagnosis, he or she can then offer a **prognosis**, an opinion concerning the eventual outcome of the disease. A course of therapy (possibly in consultation with therapeutic specialists, e.g., physical therapists) may also be instituted. The foundation for the process of obtaining a diagnosis is the history and a physical examination.

THE HISTORY

The clinical history is a critical initial step in the evaluation. As is the case in any interaction between individuals, this requires the physician to establish a relationship with the patient that facilitates the accurate verbal transmission of information. This is a two-way street. The patient must feel enabled to present his or her history both fully and accurately. The physician must be able to elicit such information and accurately interpret it without prejudgment or bias (either scientific or social). This is often called a **patient-centered approach** to the history. Acquiring such interviewing skill is an early and essential part of the training of a medical student. To facilitate obtaining and recording an accurate, organized, patient history, a standard approach is generally used on an initial encounter, although it may be modified on subsequent visits. This approach consists of several parts:

1. *Chief complaint*: This introduction to the history seeks to establish why the patient has sought medical attention. Most often this is elicited in the patient's own words. It may be followed up by a brief survey of any additional problems currently being experienced by the patient.
2. *History of the current illness*: The physician develops a chronological framework of the patient's illness from first symptoms to the present. This part of the history establishes the "when, where, and how" of the chief complaint, that is, the source of the symptoms experienced.
3. *Past medical history*: To establish the patient's general state of health, information about past illnesses and medical interventions, medications, allergies, immunizations, reproductive history, and participation in health maintenance programs is recorded.

Public health Area of medicine concerned with the health of populations.

Screening Examining a large asymptomatic population for signs of future disease.

Diagnosis The determination of the nature and cause of a patient's illness.

Noninvasive testing Diagnostic procedure requiring no physical invasion of the body.

Invasive Test requiring a physical invasion of the body.

Pap smear A study of cells from the cervix. Commonly used as a screening test for cancer.

Fine needle aspiration Sampling fluid and cells from a surface accessible lesion.

Colonoscopy Examination of the colon with an endoscopic procedure.

Prognosis The probable outcome of a disease or disorder, the outlook for recovery.

Patient-centered approach Interviewing technique empowering the patient to provide a candid and complete medical history.

3a. *The family health history*: This part of the history provides background information about potential environmental or genetic aspects pertinent to the patient's complaint, the health status of the entire living family, and historical information about deceased relatives. Family history is important in diagnosing many common chronic diseases such as diabetes and heart disease.

3b. *The psychosocial and sexual history*: The patient's education and life experiences (including personal relationships, employment), and in females the gynecological/reproductive history, may provide important information to the diagnostician. Questions are asked about potentially addictive behaviors such the use of alcohol, tobacco products, and recreational drugs.

4. *The review of systems*: This is often considered to be the center of the patient–physician encounter and consists of a body system–oriented, head to toe-review of all presenting symptoms in an organized manner. The review may disclose additional symptoms not initially reported by the patient that are important to the diagnosis. A physician investigating the presenting symptom of back pain may elicit the additional symptom of pain on urination during the review, which suggests potential urinary tract disease. The experienced physician often will undertake this review as part of the physical examination.

THE PHYSICAL EXAMINATION

The physical examination is a system-based examination of the patient in an ordered manner. The practitioner places particular emphasis on the part of the body affected by the illness, such as the ears, throat, chest, and lungs in the case of a potential respiratory infection. However, particularly in a first encounter, all body systems are examined. For example, respiratory symptoms may be associated with a range of etiologies affecting multiple body systems (e.g., allergic diseases). Any abnormalities detected on the physical examination are correlated with the clinical history. At this point, the practitioner begins to construct a hypothesis regarding diseases or conditions that best fit with the clinical findings. Often, more than one diagnosis must be considered, and such consideration is likely to be altered by the results of laboratory and other diagnostic tests. In a **differential diagnosis**, the practitioner must consider a number of diseases that are characterized by the patient's symptoms. For example, respiratory symptoms might, based on patient history, suggest a seasonal allergy. Simple blood-based tests can aid in establishing such a diagnosis. A suggestion of renal problems in the patient could point to a serious, multisystem disease involving blood vessels (a vascular disease). Additional laboratory tests and potentially invasive procedures to sample patient tissue would be needed to support such a diagnosis.

In difficult cases, the clinician may also obtain the opinion of a medical consultant (a physician with special training and experience in the type of medical problem presented by the patient). For a respiratory disease, a pathologist experienced in tissue-based diagnosis or a **radiologist** expert in the analysis of x-ray and other visualization data produced by physical methods might be consulted. The wise physician always maintains a probabilistic approach in constructing the diagnosis. Given the patient's history, the most likely diagnosis is considered first (a respiratory infection) followed by alternatives (a seasonal allergy) and far less likely (but potentially life-threatening) multisystem vascular disease. In testing the diagnostic hypothesis, the clinician uses a variety of tests and procedures and considers the usefulness of possible results of the tests in the clinical reasoning process.

Differential diagnosis Consideration of the different diseases possible given the patient's symptoms.

Radiologist Physician expert in the use and analysis of imaging techniques and results.

Diagnostic Tests and Procedures

Today a huge number of tests and procedures are available to the physician, with more than 60,000 medical and surgical procedures recognized in the standard coding system used in the United States (ICD-10-PCS). One major medical center lists more than 1,300 laboratory tests that are available to its staff. How does the clinician choose from this massive array? Medical procedures carry a degree of risk, ranging from trivial to potentially serious. Diagnostic tests and procedures also vary in the amount of information they provide in relation to a potential diagnosis. For example, colonoscopy provides no information in the case of respiratory symptoms, but it may lead to a definitive diagnosis in the case of possible bleeding from the rectum. Tests and procedures differ in complexity and cost. Colonoscopy costs thousands of dollars at a major medical center, whereas determination of fecal blood (i.e., blood in stool) is trivial in cost. In a period of increased concern about the economic aspects of health care, cost must also be considered.

Choosing a Diagnostic Test

A diagnostic test can be defined in terms of a set of characteristics that help the clinician judge the usefulness of the procedure in diagnosing a specific disease. A perfect test would always be positive in a patient who has the disease in question and always negative in one who does not. Such a test does not exist. Instead, tests are classified by the terms *sensitivity* and *specificity*. **Sensitivity** refers to the percentage of patients classified as positive by a test who *do* have the disease. A test with a high sensitivity will miss few people with the disease (have a low rate of **false negatives**). The obverse of sensitivity is **specificity**. Specificity refers to the percentage of patients without the disease who are classified as negative by the test. Tests with a high specificity will have a low rate of **false positives**. The clinician attempts to choose a test with as high a sensitivity and specificity as possible for the diagnosis in question. Unfortunately, highly sensitive tests tend to have lower specificity (misdiagnosing people as having a disease they do not have; i.e., having a higher rate of false positives). "Missing" a disease is obviously harmful, leading to a delay in therapy and potentially a more severe illness. However, a false positive result, assuming a patient has a disease he or she does not, may also lead to anxiety, discomfort, and unneeded therapy.

Choice of tests also depends on the patient population. For example, a patient in a clinic who is suspected of having a disease (based on prior clinical information) is much less likely to yield a false negative result than an individual chosen at random off the street. A physician who is considering an invasive, painful, or costly mode of therapy might choose to use a test with high specificity to exclude a false positive result. However, the case is different when choosing screening assays to be applied to a population in which the diagnostic target is a relatively uncommon but potentially serious (possibly fatal) illness where early diagnosis might effect a cure. If we choose a highly sensitive test (so as not to miss the uncommon affected person), the test is likely to lack specificity, increasing the number of individuals incorrectly suspected of having the disease. If there is an acceptable confirmatory test, or if the therapy is relatively harmless, such a test might be considered for use in screening. However, if the only confirmatory test (or therapy) requires a risky procedure (such a surgery), the test would be unacceptable. This is a very real problem. For example, a number of noninvasive tests have been proposed to screen for ovarian cancer because undiagnosed and untreated ovarian cancer is fatal. However, the currently available tests lack specificity and would expose an appreciable number of nonaffected women to invasive diagnostic procedures (although undoubtedly the test would lead to

Sensitivity Classification of diagnostic tests in regard to percentage of patients classified as positive by a test who do have the disease.

False negative Negative test result which should be positive.

Specificity Classification of diagnostic tests in regard to the percentage of patients without the disease who are classified as negative by the test.

False positive Positive test result which should be negative.

early diagnosis in some). So decisions in screening assay use are difficult and often lead to controversy—even among experts. The recent discussion about the utility of mammography as a screening test for breast cancer (discussed in greater detail in the presentation of breast tissue) is an example of how complex such decisions are.

In summary, the clinician makes a risk/benefit/cost determination in choosing diagnostic procedures. What set of tests will yield the greatest information with the least risk and cost to the patient? At times this can be a very difficult determination in which the clinician is guided by the findings of the clinical epidemiologist. Such determinations are part of **evidence-based medicine**, which seeks to define risk/benefit/cost ratios based on prior rigorous investigations. Going hand in hand with evidence-based medicine is **patient-centered medicine**, in which patients have a central role in decisions about their care. Patients are fully informed about the possible risks and benefits so that they can make informed decisions as to whether or not to consent to the procedure or ask to consider alternative approaches.

> **Evidence-based medicine** Definition of treatment plan, risks/benefits/costs based on prior rigorous investigation.
>
> **Patient-centered medicine** Practice of medicine encouraging patients to have a role in decision making.

Classification of Diagnostic Tests and Procedures

Diagnostic tests and procedures can be classified into several major categories:

1. Clinical laboratory tests: including biochemical, immunological, and molecular-based tests; determination of gases in the blood; analysis of blood cells; and microbiological analysis.
2. Imaging techniques including x-ray, ultrasound, computerized tomography (CT), magnetic resonance imaging (MRI), or positron emission tomography (PET scans), and measurement of the distribution of radioisotopes (also called radionuclides).
3. Cytologic and histologic examination of cells and tissues removed from the patient.
4. Endoscopy.
5. Tests that measure the electrical activity in portions of the body.

There is often overlap among these categories. For example, endoscopy may provide a sample that will be examined histologically or cultured in the clinical laboratory to detect an infectious agent. Some endoscopic procedures are done using radiographic guidance. Another way of classifying tests is by the medical specialty responsible for providing them. Clinical laboratory medicine, a division of pathology, is responsible for the broad range of clinical laboratory tests. Anatomic pathology provides tissue and cell-based analysis and the autopsy service. Radiology is responsible for essentially all image-based techniques but also provides a number of therapeutic procedures. Endoscopy covers a broad range of procedures that may be performed by specific medical specialists (gastroenterologists perform colonoscopy, e.g., cardiologists are responsible for a number of intravascular procedures such as placing stents to open blocked blood vessels supplying the heart). Other endoscopic procedures are performed by the surgical specialties. For example, examination of the urinary tract is the purview of urologists.

CLINICAL LABORATORY TESTS

Laboratory medicine is the area of pathology that provides and interprets diagnostic testing related to patient care. Clinical laboratory tests serve not only to aid in diagnosing disease but also in searching for occult (unrecognized) disease, establishing the severity of disease, and monitoring its progression and treatment. In laboratory medicine, basic analytical science meets medical science, and it is often the place where a new aspect of biomedicine is "translated" into patient care. Hence, analytical aspects of biochemistry, immunology, microbiology, physiology, and molecular biology are used in the clinical laboratory.

The role of the clinical laboratory and the tests it provides often are not obvious to the patient, who might simply donate several tubes of blood or a urine sample as part of a visit to the physician. However, it has been estimated that 60 to 70 percent of medical diagnoses rely on clinical tests. Almost 7 billion clinical tests are performed each year in the United States, and a major medical center may perform more than 6 million tests a year. In general, such tests are a "good buy." Less than 5 percent of health care dollars are spent on laboratory tests.

Given the large number of available tests it is difficult to summarize the many uses of clinical tests. FIGURE 1-1 provides an example of a standard set of laboratory tests along with normal ranges for the results.

Results that are "out of range" are flagged as either low or high, and it is up to the physician to determine the significance of the results. Determining the concentration of various constituents in the blood and urine is of major importance in evaluating the function of organ systems. For example, the concentration of a substance in the

Patient Name: DOE, MARY   **Patient MRNO: 0000012345**

Order Number: C6140101
Collection Date: 2009-06-14 at 0400

Source:
Site:

Date Completed	Test Name	Result	Flag	Units	Range
		Individual Test(s)			
2009-06-14	SODIUM	129	L	MMOL/L	135-145
2009-06-14	POTOSSIUM	4.2		MMOL/L	3.5-5.0
2009-06-14	CHLORIDE	97	L	MMOL/L	98-107
2009-06-14	CO_2	25		MMOL/L	22-30
2009-06-14	UREA NITROGEN	26	H	MG/DL	7-21
2009-06-14	CREATININE	0.82		MG/DL	0.60-1.00
2009-06-14	EST. GFR (MDRD)	>= 60		mL/min/1.73m2	>=60
2009-06-14	ANION GAP	7	L	MMOL/L	9-15
2009-06-14	BUN/CREAT RATIO	32			UNDEFINED
2009-06-14	GLUCOSE, RANDOM	108		MG/DL	65-179
2009-06-14	MAGNESIUM	1.7		MG/DL	1.6-2.2
2009-06-14	PHOSPHORUS	3.5		MG/DL	2.4-4.5
		CBC+PLATELETS			
2009-06-14	CBC+PLATELETS	:			
2009-06-14	WBC	11.7	H	×10 9th/L	4.5-11.0
2009-06-14	RBC	3.80	L	×10 12th/L	4.00-5.20
2009-06-14	HGB	11.9	L	G/DL	12.0-16.0
2009-06-14	HCT	33.1	L	%	36.0-46.0
2009-06-14	MCV	87		FL	80-100
2009-06-14	MCH	31		PG	26-34
2009-06-14	MCHC	36		G/DL	31-37
2009-06-14	RDW	13.1		%	12.0-15.0
2009-06-14	MPV	7.2		FL	7.0-10.0
2009-06-14	PLATELET COUNT	247		×10 9th/L	150-440

FIGURE 1-1 Example of a laboratory report.

Courtesy of Dr. Catherine Hammett-Stabler, Department of Pathology and Laboratory Medicine, University of North Carolina at Chapel Hill.

blood called urea is elevated if the kidneys are not functioning properly because this constituent is normally excreted by the kidneys. The concentrations of hemoglobin and the quantity of red cells are reduced in patients with anemia. Sometimes the enzyme level in the blood is elevated because (a) enzymes are leaking from damaged cells in the diseased or injured organs ("liver function tests" are an example), (b) enzyme synthesis is increased as a result of disease, or (c) excretion of enzymes is impaired because disease has caused failure of normal excretory pathways.

Clinical laboratory tests also are used to evaluate the specific functions of organs. Pulmonary function tests measure the rate and efficiency with which air moves in and out of the lungs. Determinations of the concentration of oxygen and carbon dioxide in the blood also can indicate pulmonary function by evaluating how efficiently the lungs oxygenate the blood and eliminate carbon dioxide. A simple device (pulse oximeter) applied to the finger can determine the amount of oxygen carried by hemoglobin in circulating blood as another measure of pulmonary function. This is an example of a **point-of-care test**, which can be performed outside of the laboratory in the physician's office or at a patient's bedside. Of increasing importance are tests to detect and measure concentrations of substances that are likely to be produced by tumors growing within the body. Serial analyses of these substances can be used to monitor the response of certain tumors to treatment. Microbiologic tests detect the presence of disease-producing organisms in urine, blood, bronchial secretions, and feces. These tests also can determine the responsiveness of the organisms to antibiotics. Serologic tests detect and measure the presence of antibodies as an indication of response to infectious agents and can evaluate the suitability of blood for transfusion or organs for transplantation into a patient.

IMAGING TECHNIQUES

Imaging technology enables the physician (and specifically the radiologist, the expert in obtaining and interpreting the results of imaging studies) to produce a view of the body and its organ systems previously available only to the surgeon (or to the anatomist or pathologist postmortem). Imaging technology permits anatomic investigation of the living patient, most often with little or no risk and minimal discomfort. The earliest and still an important use of imaging technology is the production of two-dimensional projected images of interior organ systems, **x-rays** or **radiographs**. However, modern computer technology now allows three-dimensional reconstruction of body systems (tomography) either using x-rays as an imaging source (**computed tomographic [CT] scans**) or by using the magnetic properties of certain body constituents (most often ^{1}H in body water). To the physicist this property is called nuclear magnetic resonance; to the physician such studies are termed **magnetic resonance imaging (MRI)**. Of growing importance is the use of ultrasound to image accessible areas of the body. The technique depends on the differences in acoustical properties of tissue, so the movement and velocity of blood in vessels (Doppler ultrasound) is easily studied; images of the developing fetus can also safely be produced.

X-Ray Examination

X-ray examinations are conducted in many ways, but the basic principle is the same. X-rays (electromagnetic radiation akin to visible light or radio waves, but much higher in energy) are produced in a vacuum tube by the impact of electrons on a tungsten target. The x-rays pass through the area of interest and are detected most commonly by a digital detecting device (formerly photographic film). X-rays are absorbed to a variable degree depending on the density of the tissue they pass through. Tissues

---

Point-of-care test Laboratory test that can be performed at the patient's bedside or in the physician's office.

Radiograph/x-ray An image taken with x-rays.

Computed tomographic (CT) scan An x-ray technique producing detailed cross-sectional images of the body by means of x-ray tube and detectors connected to a computer. Sometimes called a CAT scan.

Magnetic resonance imaging (MRI) A diagnostic procedure that yields computer-generated images based on the movement of hydrogen atoms in tissues subjected to a strong magnetic field.

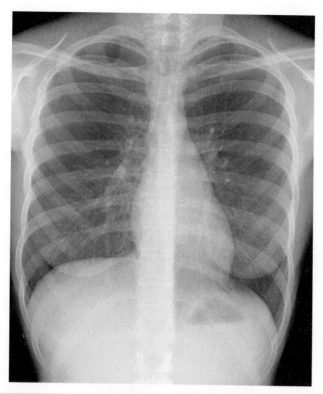

FIGURE 1-2 Chest x-ray (normal). Normal chest x-ray shows white bones and dark lung fields. The heart (*center of image*) and organs below the diaphragm (*bottom third of image*) are also white because of the density of the soft tissue through which the x-rays pass.

Courtesy of Dr. Donald Yandow, Department of Radiology, University of Wisconsin School of Medicine and Public Health.

of low density, such as the air-filled lungs, transmit most of the x-rays and appear black on the image. Tissues of high density, such as bone, absorb most of the rays and appear white on the image. Tissues of intermediate densities appear in varying shades of gray. The two-dimensional image produced is called a radiograph, or sometimes a "plain film" (**FIGURE 1-2**).

Special terminology is used for particular radiographic studies. For example, a specialized radiographic study of the breast is called a mammogram.

The lining of some internal organ systems, such as the digestive and urinary tract, have little contrast. To aid in their examination, a nontoxic radiopaque substance (a contrast medium) designed to coat the lining (mucosa) of the organ systems may be used to outline the area of interest. For example, barium contrast media may be swallowed or given as an enema to outline portions of the gastrointestinal tract. Irregularities in the column of barium may represent constrictions in a portion of the GI tract. After the bulk of contrast material either passes through or is expelled from the tract, the remainder coats the surface of the tract and outlines details of the internal surface such as tumors, erosions, or ulcers for detection (**FIGURE 1-3**).

Other soluble radiopaque substances can be injected into the circulation to aid in detecting irregularities or blockages in the vascular system and to study the renal and urinary system as the material is excreted from the kidney and passes through the bladder and remainder of the urinary tract (an intravenous pyelogram [IVP]) (**FIGURE 1-4**). The movement of contrast agents in portions of the body also can be studied in "real time" or be recorded as a movie using a technique known as fluoroscopy.

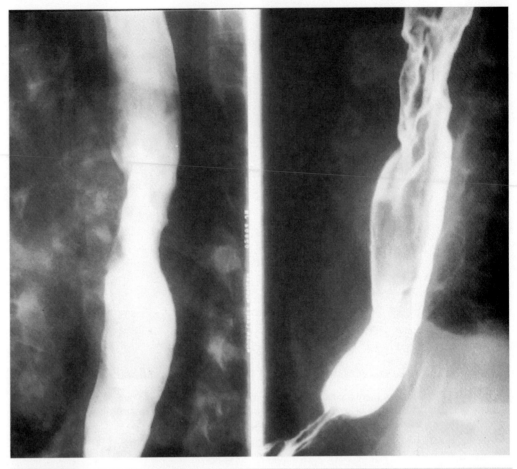

FIGURE 1-3 Barium contrast swallow study of the esophagus. X-ray of barium column in the esophagus showing narrowed area (*center of left image*) suggestive of an esophageal tumor (*left*). Following passage of the bulk of the barium, a coating of contrast medium outlines the mucosa, demonstrating irregularity and constriction as a result of esophageal cancer (*right*).

Image courtesy of Dr. David Warshauer, Department of Radiology, University of North Carolina at Chapel Hill.

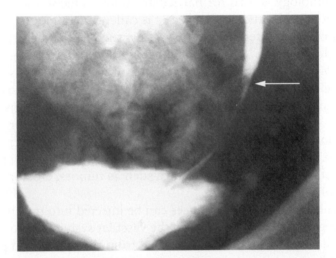

FIGURE 1-4 Intravenous pyelogram (IVP). Contrast media fills the bladder at the bottom of the image and the proximal (closer to the kidney) portion of the right ureter (*top of image*). A stone (*white arrow*) is lodged in the ureter, causing dilation of the ureter above the stone and preventing the filling of the ureter below. The dye in the bladder has come from the urine passing through the opposite ureter (not shown).

Computed Tomographic Scans

A computed tomographic scan (CT scan) produces a continuous series of x-ray images of the body by rotating the x-ray tube around the patient as the patient is moved past the x-ray source. The x-ray tube rotates on a toroidal (doughnut-shaped) frame linked to an array of sensitive radiation detectors that rotate around and encircle the patient, who is moving through the center of the frame. As the x-ray tube and detector array move around the patient, the radiation detectors record the amount of radiation passing through the body (**FIGURE 1-5**).

The data from the radiation detectors is fed into a computer, which reconstructs the information into a three-dimensional image comprised of a series of voxels (the three-dimensional equivalent of the two-dimensional pixels on a computer monitor), each representing the x-ray density of a small volumetric area of the patient's body. Most often the image is displayed as a series of transverse cross-sections of the patient's anatomy (with the patient prone on his or her back with feet toward the viewer). However, the computer is just as capable of presenting information as a series of slices in any orientation (sagittal: head to foot dividing the body into a series of left to right slices; coronal: head to foot dividing the body into a series of front to back slices). Abnormalities of internal organs that cannot be identified by means of standard x-ray examinations can often be discovered with CT scans because the geometry of an organ and the relationship of one organ to another can be seen while scanning through an entire region of the body. For example, **FIGURE 1-6** shows a lung tumor that might not have been obvious on a plain film.

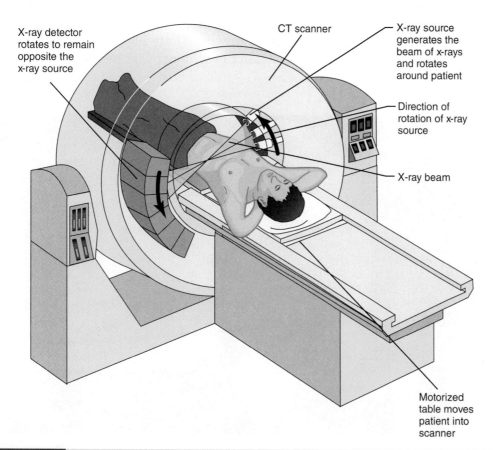

X-ray detector rotates to remain opposite the x-ray source

CT scanner

X-ray source generates the beam of x-rays and rotates around patient

Direction of rotation of x-ray source

X-ray beam

Motorized table moves patient into scanner

FIGURE 1-5 Computed tomographic (CT) scan. The patient lies on a table that is gradually advanced into the scanner. The x-ray tube mounted in the scanner rotates around patient, and radiation detectors also rotate so that detectors remain opposite the x-ray source. Data from radiation detectors generate computer-reconstructed images of the patient's body at multiple levels.

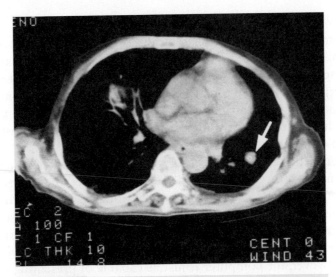

FIGURE 1-6 CT scan of chest. Mediastinum and heart appear white in the center of the scan, with less-dense lungs on either side. A lung tumor (*arrow*) appears as a white nodule in the lung.

Courtesy of Leonard V. Crowley, MD, Century College.

Virtual colonoscopy
A high resolution contrast CT image of the colon. May be substituted for colonoscopy in special cases.

Modern computational techniques allow entire organ systems to be reconstructed as three-dimensional images, which can be examined in great detail. In the technique of **virtual colonoscopy**, the surface mucosa of the entire colon can be reconstructed and "flown through" by the radiologist sitting at a computer who examines it for lesions such as polyps and other mucosal growths. The technique can substitute for endoscopy in patients for whom an invasive procedure might have additional risks (**FIGURE 1-7**).

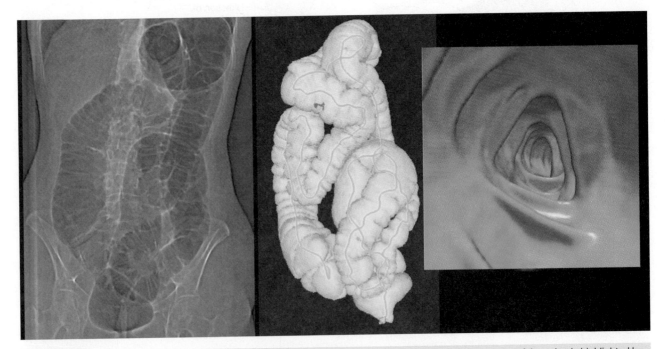

FIGURE 1-7 Virtual colonoscopy. A high resolution contrast CT image of the colon is produced. The mucosa of the colon is highlighted by the contrast medium (*left*). A computer reconstruction of the entire colon in three dimensions is produced. The green line traces the center of the colon (*center*). The radiologist can "fly through" the colon and examine the mucosal surface of the interior (*right*).

Courtesy of Dr. David Warshauer, Department of Radiology, University of North Carolina at Chapel Hill.

Magnetic Resonance Imaging

Magnetic resonance imaging (MRI) produces computer-constructed images of various organs and tissues somewhat like CT scans. The device consists of a strong superconducting magnet capable of developing a extremely powerful magnetic field (greater than 50,000 times that of the Earth), coils that can transmit and receive radio frequency (RF) waves, and a computer that receives impulses from the scanner and forms them into images that can be interpreted. The MRI scanner with the enclosed magnet and coils appears somewhat similar to an elongated, tubular CT scanner. The patient lies on a table that is gradually moved into the scanner, as is done in CT. The physical principles of MRI, however, are different from those of CT scanning. MRI scans, in contrast to the radio density used in CT, most often depend on the response of hydrogen protons (positively charged particles in the nucleus around which electrons rotate) contained within the body's water molecules. Hydrogen protons behave as if they are spinning rapidly about an axis. When subjected to a strong magnetic field, the protons become aligned in the direction of the magnetic field. After a pulse of RF waves, the protons are temporarily dislodged from their orientation. As they return to their original orientation, they emit a signal (resonance) that can be measured and used to produce the computer-constructed images. Body tissues, which have a high water content, are a rich source of protons capable of excitation. The intensity of the signals produced is related to the varying water content (and hence hydrogen ion content) of body tissues and the strength and duration of the RF pulse plus the geometry of the applied magnetic gradient. The many combinations of RF pulse and magnetic gradients are termed MRI sequences and are chosen for particular imaging applications. For example, "T2 weighted MRI" is particularly useful in detecting regions in the brain and spinal cord where myelin sheaths of nerve fibers have been damaged, as in a neurologic disease called multiple sclerosis (described in the discussion on the nervous system) (**FIGURE 1-8** and **FIGURE 1-9**).

Because an MRI does not use ionizing radiation, the patient does not receive radiation exposure. An MRI does expose the patient to strong magnetic and RF fields, but this appears safe provided the patient does not have implanted or embedded

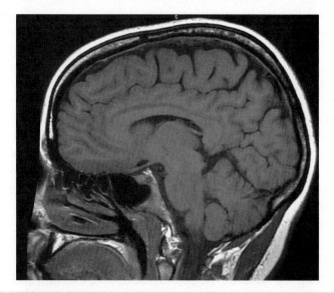

FIGURE 1-8 MRI normal brain in sagittal view. The nose is on the left. Notice how clearly the fissures and folds over the surface of the brain can be seen as well as the distinction between the different neural elements of which the brain is comprised.

Courtesy of Dr. Patrick Turski, Department of Radiology-MRI, University of Wisconsin School of Medicine and Public Health.

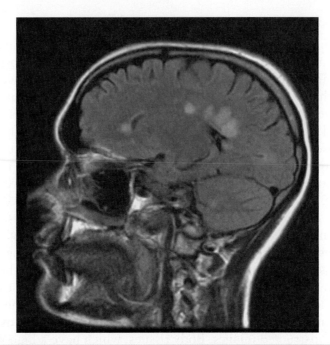

FIGURE 1-9 MRI of brain from a patient with multiple sclerosis in sagittal view (as in Figure 1-8). Multiple plaques (light areas) where neurons have lost their myelin coating are visible.

Courtesy of Dr. Patrick Turski, Department of Radiology-MRI, University of Wisconsin School of Medicine and Public Health.

ferromagnetic material that might interact with the powerful magnetic field. Recent advances in the use of special contrast agents for MRI have greatly expanded the utility of the technique.

IMAGING TECHNOLOGY TO DETECT SPECIFIC MOLECULES AND PROCESSES

There is great interest in using imaging technology to detect specific chemical constituents or metabolic activity in regions of the body. For example, Alzheimer's disease, a degenerative dementia most often associated with aging, is associated with accumulation of an abnormal protein component beta-amyloid (Aβ) in areas of the brain. Definitive diagnosis of this disease previously required obtaining brain tissue (most often postmortem) for analysis. Modern imaging technology can now detect and localize both changes in brain metabolism and the specific abnormal protein associated with Alzheimer's disease and provide early, noninvasive diagnoses. This technology depends on the ability to detect and localize radiolabeled compounds injected into the patient. The location and distribution of the radiation emitting compounds can be mapped within the body to produce a planar (two-dimensional) image using a gamma camera or to produce tomographic (three-dimensional) images using single-photon computed tomography (SPECT), or PET technology used with positron emitting tracers.

Radioisotope Studies Using Gamma Emitters

Using specially designed radiation detectors, the uptake location and excretion of the labeled substance can be mapped. The ability of the thyroid gland to concentrate and utilize radioactive iodine is used as a measure of thyroid function and, more importantly, can be used to detect tumors within the thyroid gland. Ventilation/perfusion (V/Q) lung scans measure the distribution of an inhaled radioactive gas (Xenon-133)

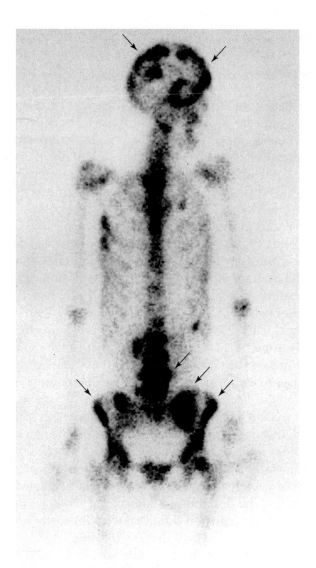

FIGURE 1-10 Radioisotope bone scan of head, chest, and pelvis. Dark areas (*arrows*) indicate the concentration of radioisotope around tumor deposits in bone.

Courtesy of Leonard V. Crowley, MD, Century College.

to locate obstructions to the airways and combine it with a radiolabeled albumin injected into the circulation to measure pulmonary blood flow and to detect possible blood clots lodged within the lung (pulmonary emboli).

Phosphorus-containing isotopes are concentrated in the skeletal system. If there are deposits of tumor in bone, the isotopes are concentrated around the tumor deposits and can be easily identified (**FIGURE 1-10**).

Radioactive materials injected intravenously also can be used to evaluate blood flow to the heart muscle and to identify areas of damaged heart muscle. Three-dimensional tomographic techniques using SPECT or PET provide much better localization of tracers and are supplanting the use of planar gamma cameras in many radioisotope localization studies.

Positron Emission Tomography

Related to radioisotope studies using compounds labeled with gamma ray emitters is the technique of **positron emission tomography (PET),** or simply PET scans. PET

Positron emission tomography (PET scan)
Imaging using positron emitting radiolabels.

imaging uses a special class of radiolabel that emits positrons. Almost all positron emitting radio tracers are very short lived and are produced at the imaging site using a cyclotron, which limits the technology to major medical centers. Positrons are subatomic particles that have the same mass as electrons but carry a positive charge. They are formed when atoms such as carbon, oxygen, or nitrogen are bombarded in a cyclotron with high-energy particles to produce a short-lived positron emitting radio tracer. For example, one of the most commonly used positron emitting radio tracers is fludeoyglucose ^{18}F (^{18}F-FDG), which has a half life of under two hours and is made by initially bombarding oxygen isotope ^{18}O enriched water with protons to produce the positron emitting ^{18}F, which must be incorporated into the glucose-like molecule on site. A positron escaping from the nucleus collides with a negatively charged electron in a nearby atom, simultaneously producing two gamma rays emitted 180 degrees apart. The PET scanner registers this very weak but nearly simultaneous pair of pulses while ignoring nonpaired background radiation. The scanner uses this information to build a tomographic view of the distribution of the radio tracer. To further localize the source, the patient may also be CT scanned at the same time and the two images combined.

One of the most widely used applications of PET is to study the metabolic activity of areas of the body using ^{18}F-FDG, a compound that is metabolized like glucose in the patient. This provides information on the metabolic activities of the organ or tissue being studied, the site within an organ where the compound is being metabolized, and the blood flow to the organ being studied. One can detect and measure changes in brain functions associated with various neurologic diseases such as strokes, brain tumors, Alzheimer's disease, Parkinson's disease, and some hereditary degenerative diseases of the nervous system. The method may also be used to evaluate changes in blood flow and metabolism in the heart muscle after a heart attack. Malignant tumors (cancer) often have higher metabolic rates than benign tumors (or normal tissue). Hence, mapping the distribution and rate of ^{18}F-FDG metabolism may be used to detect and evaluate potential occult cancers (metastases) spread within the body and to follow the effectiveness of therapy (**FIGURE 1-11**).

Even more exciting is the ability to synthesize PET radio tracers, which can bind to and localize specific abnormal molecules such as the abnormal Aβ found in Alzheimer brains.

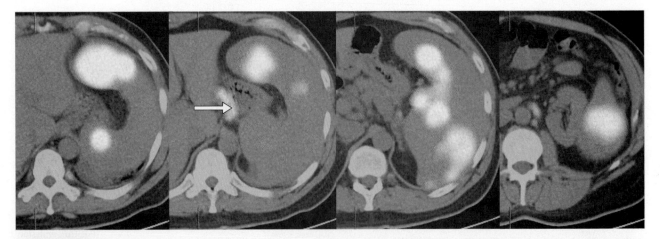

FIGURE 1-11 Combined PET scan and CT. Color represents PET scan results indicating distribution of ^{18}F-FDG metabolism in spleen (large organ on right of images) of a patient with lymphoma (cancer of lymphocytes). The PET scan has detected the spread of the cancer to adjacent lymph nodes (*arrow in second image*).

Image courtesy of Dr. David Warshauer, Department of Radiology, University of North Carolina at Chapel Hill.

ULTRASOUND

Unlike the imaging techniques that depend on detection of electromagnetic radiation as part of the imaging process, ultrasound is a technique for mapping the reflected echoes produced by high-frequency sound waves transmitted into the body. Echoes are reflected wherever there is a change in the density of the tissue. The reflected waves are recorded on a detector, and visual images are produced, generally on a small monitor. Unlike the complex equipment needed for CT or PET scans, ultrasound devices commonly use a single handheld transducer to produce the ultrasound and record the reflected echoes. The transducers may be moved over any external area of the body (using a water soluble gel to couple the ultrasound to the area of study) to produce a real-time image of internal organs under and within range of the acoustical beam as the transducer is moved. Although there are limits to the depth of penetration of ultrasound from the body surface (and hence to what internal areas of the body can be imaged), ultrasound transducers are small enough to be introduced into the rectum (to image the prostate in males), the vagina (for gynecological investigations in females), and the esophagus (to image abdominal organs such as the pancreas). This method is widely used to study the uterus during pregnancy because it does not require the use of potentially harmful radiation and poses no risk to the fetus (**FIGURE 1-12**).

The technique can be used to determine the position of the placenta and the fetus within the uterus; it also can identify some fetal abnormalities and detect twin pregnancies. Ultrasound is also often used to examine the cardiovascular system. When used for this purpose, the procedure is usually called an **echocardiogram**. An echocardiogram can detect the structure and function of the heart valves as well as determine abnormal communications between adjacent cardiac chambers. Abnormal blood flow patterns characteristic of congenital or acquired valvular heart disease or other abnormalities in cardiac function can be detected in real time as the heart

Echocardiogram An examination of the cardiovascular system using ultrasound.

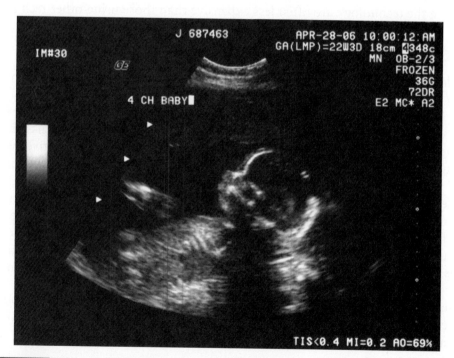

FIGURE 1-12 Ultrasound examination of a twenty-two-week-old fetus.

Courtesy of Belinda Thresher.

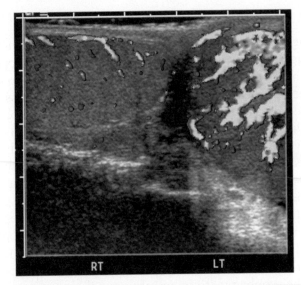

FIGURE 1-13 Doppler ultrasound examination of a testicular mass. Left testes (LT) shows an excess of blood vessels suggestive of testicular cancer. Blue indicates blood flowing toward and red indicates flow away from the transducer placed in contact with the scrotum.

Image courtesy of Dr. David Warshauer, Department of Radiology, University of North Carolina at Chapel Hill.

beats. Doppler ultrasound can determine both the direction and velocity of blood as it moves through the heart and other organs and can detect irregularities in flow. Doppler flow images are "color coded" to show flow direction in relation to the transducer (**FIGURE 1-13**).

Ultrasound has replaced many radiology procedures because ultrasound avoids radiation, is most often not invasive (or only minimally so), and is easily performed in a doctor's office. Ultrasound devices are relatively small and inexpensive, and studies using the technology are often less expensive than those using other techniques.

CYTOLOGIC AND HISTOLOGIC EXAMINATIONS

Cytology studies the characteristics of individual cells or small groups of cells that are either shed or sampled from body organs. Such cells may be naturally cast off into body fluids and secretions or may be removed by brushes, spatulas, or similar tools. For example, the Pap (Papanicolaou) smear mentioned previously (discussed more fully in the presentations of Neoplastic Disease and the Female Reproductive System) uses such a device to obtain cells dislodged from the surface of the cervix and uterine canal to screen for cancer or early precursors to this disease. Similar approaches can be used to obtain bronchial cells and cells from the bladder. Cell samples may be obtained using very fine needles and a syringe to aspirate surface accessible lesions. Such fine needle aspirations (FNAs) are often painless and rapid, requiring no anesthesia. Cytological examination of blood and bone marrow (**FIGURE 1-14**) is critical in the diagnosis of hematologic (blood-related) diseases and is often performed to diagnose neoplastic disease in blood cell precursors found in the marrow.

Such studies are carried out by hematopathologists, who use microscopes and flow cytometers that can quickly evaluate thousands of cells for multiple parameters such as size, internal contents, and surface characteristics as they flow past a series of detectors.

Histology examines the structure of organs and the tissues and groups of cells of which they are composed. The pathologist uses histopathology to recognize changes

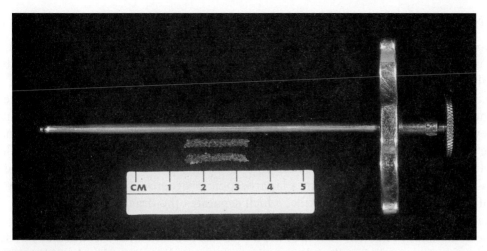

FIGURE 1-14 Two samples of bone marrow (*adjacent to scale*) obtained from a pelvic bone by means of a specially designed needle (*upper part* of photograph).

Courtesy of Leonard V. Crowley, MD, Century College.

in tissue that are indicative of, or help to characterize, disease. The tissue may be obtained as part of a surgical procedure (a surgical specimen) either to confirm a diagnosis or to evaluate the adequacy of the surgical procedure, or the tissue may be removed from the target organ for the specific purpose of histopathological examination (a **biopsy** specimen).

Samples of tissue can be obtained from any part of the body. Gastroscopes, bronchoscopes, and other instruments used for endoscopic examination, for example, are constructed so that specimens for biopsy can be obtained while the internal organs are being examined. Biopsy specimens also can be taken directly from internal organs such as the liver or kidney by inserting a thin needle through the skin directly into the organ to produce a biopsy core. This is often done using ultrasound or other imaging techniques for guidance.

TESTS OF ELECTRICAL ACTIVITY

Several different tests measure the electrical impulses associated with various bodily functions and activities. These include the **electrocardiogram (ECG)**, the **electroencephalogram (EEG)**, and the **electromyogram (EMG)**. The most widely used of these tests is the ECG. Electrodes attached to the arms, legs, and chest are used to measure the serial changes in the electrical activity of the heart during the various phases of the cardiac cycle. The ECG also identifies disturbances in the heart rate or rhythm and identifies abnormal conduction of impulses through the heart. Heart muscle injury, such as occurs after a heart attack, also can be recognized by means of characteristic abnormalities in the cardiogram. The EEG measures the electrical activity of the brain by means of small electrodes attached to different areas in the scalp. Abnormalities of cerebral structure or function may cause altered brain wave patterns that are detected by this examination. The EMG measures the electrical activity of skeletal muscle during contraction and at rest. Abnormal electrical activity is often encountered in various inflammatory or degenerative diseases involving the skeletal muscles and the nerves that control them. The test is performed by inserting a needle into the muscle that is being studied. The speed at which a nerve conducts impulses also can be measured by means of electrodes taped to the surface of the skin over the nerve being tested.

Biopsy Removal of a small sample of tissue for examination and diagnosis by a pathologist.

Electrocardiogram (ECG)/ electroencephalogram (EEG)/electromyogram (EMG) Tests using the electrical impulses of the body to measure activity in the heart, brain, and nervous systems.

ENDOSCOPY AND LAPAROSCOPY

An **endoscopy**, or endoscopic examination (*endo* = within + *skopeo* = examine), is an examination of the interior of the body by means of various types of flexible tubular instruments, all of similar design, that are named according to the part of the body they are designed to examine. These instruments have an optical system and light source and contain ports through which either sampling or therapeutic devices can be guided to the site under investigation. In addition, gas or liquid may be passed through the scope to help visualize the area studied. An instrument called a **laparoscope** is used to visualize the abdominal and pelvic organs in the procedure called *laparoscopy*. To perform a laparoscopic procedure, the peritoneal cavity is inflated first with carbon dioxide, which separates the organs so that they can be visualized more easily. Then the laparoscope is inserted through a small incision in the abdominal wall, often in or near the umbilicus. Modern laparoscopes may be used to perform surgical as well as diagnostic procedures. For example, appendectomies and gall bladder removal often are performed using laparoscopic surgical techniques (as opposed to "open" surgery).

TREATMENT

After the diagnosis has been established, a course of treatment is initiated. A **specific treatment** is used when the cause and nature of the disease is known. For example, an antibiotic may be given to a patient who has an infection that is responsive to the antibiotic, or insulin may be given to a patient with diabetes. **Symptomatic treatment** is designed to relieve symptoms associated with the disease but may or may not influence the course of the underlying condition. Examples are the treatment of fever, pain, and cough by means of appropriate medications. There may be overlap between different treatment regimens. Tumors may be treated to relieve pain caused by pressure to organs, but such therapy, in shrinking tumor bulk, may also prolong the life of the patient. Often, the clinician must be content with treating the debilitating manifestations of the disease, perhaps prolonging life, without being able to offer a lasting cure.

When dealing with patients who have long-standing chronic diseases such as chronic heart, kidney, or lung disease, or some types of cancer, the physician may be assisted by a disease-management team composed of a group of people with special skills useful in the care and treatment of patients with these diseases. The team may contain dieticians, nurse clinicians, physician assistants, respiratory therapists, physiotherapists, pharmacists, and social workers, who bring their own special skills to help physicians care for and patients cope with chronic illnesses. Of course, no discussion of treatment would be complete without mention of the financial counselors who can help patients cope with the burden of health care costs.

Endoscopy An examination of the interior of the body by means of various lighted tubular instruments. Method may also be used to obtain tissue samples.

Laparoscope A long tubular telescope-like instrument passed through the abdominal wall to examine structures within the peritoneal cavity.

Specific treatment Treatment of underlying cause of disease.

Symptomatic treatment Treatment of symptoms rather than underlying cause of disease.

CASE 1-1

An eighteen-year-old college student suffers a four hour episode of mild abdominal pain and nausea that localizes in the **periumbilical** (near the belly button) region. She initially attributes this to "an upset stomach." As the pain continues to increase, the patient suffers severe nausea, cramping, and feels feverish. Her roommates take her to student health services. Because of the symptoms presented, the student is immediately transferred to the emergency room (ER) of a nearby hospital.

In the ER the pain continues to increase and localizes to the right lower quadrant (RLQ) of the abdominal region. On physical examination, the following is noted:

- A moderately elevated oral temperature (38.7 °C).

- An elevated number of white cells in the blood (23,000 per microliter; normal is about 8,000). Most of these cells are granulocytes.

- An area of local tenderness located on a line between the umbilicus and **iliac crest**, closer to the iliac crest.

- Right sided rectal tenderness.

Appendicitis is strongly suspected, and the patient is prepared for a CT scan of her abdomen. An axial CT scan through the upper pelvic region shows a dilated appendix containing a **appendicolith**, a calcified stone visible in the several sequential images (**FIGURE 1-15**).

The patient is prepared for laparoscopic surgery. An **edematous** (fluid-filled) red appendix is removed at surgery (**FIGURE 1-16**), which when opened contained several appendicoliths. The patient recovered uneventfully.

Discussion

The combination of patient symptoms and signs are sensitive indicators of appendicitis in young adults but lack specificity. The elevated temperature and increased numbers of white cells (particularly granulocytes) are strong indicators of a response to tissue injury, which is most likely the result of a bacterial infection. The localization of the pain to the specific region of the abdomen (sometimes called **McBurney's point**) and the right sided rectal tenderness suggest the infectious process may involve the appendix based on pelvic anatomy. However, a number of infectious diseases involving the intestine (as well as other illnesses) can present with similar signs and symptoms. The CT scan is a highly accurate test for appendicitis with a specificity approaching 95 percent. In young children; ultrasound is often used instead of CT to lower radiation exposure.

Etiology and Pathogenesis

Appendicitis is an inflammation of the appendix. The disease is most commonly related to blockage of the outlet of the appendix to the bowel (by stones representing calcified fecal material or sometimes by intestinal parasites). This results in bacterial overgrowth by gut microorganisms within the appendix and an inflammatory response. As you will learn in the presentation of inflammation, this response can lead to tissue injury and ultimately to rupture of the appendix (described more fully in the presentation on the gastrointestinal tract).

Questions

1. An elevated number of white cells is a sensitive indicator of systemic inflammation present in the above case. Why was a radiological study ordered prior to surgery?

2. Another patient comes to the ER complaining of pain on the center to left lower quadrant of her abdominal region. Is acute appendicitis ruled out? What are several additional potential diagnoses?

3. What are some of the potential advantages of the use of laparoscopic surgery (as opposed to "open" surgery) in this case? Consider the possibility that the diagnosis might have been uncertain.

Periumbilical Abdominal area near belly button.

Iliac crest Area of hip bone in abdomen.

Appendicolith A calcified stone in the appendix.

Edematous Filled with fluid.

McBurney's point Localization of pain to region of abdomen specific for appendicitis.

(continues)

CASE 1-1 (*Continued*)

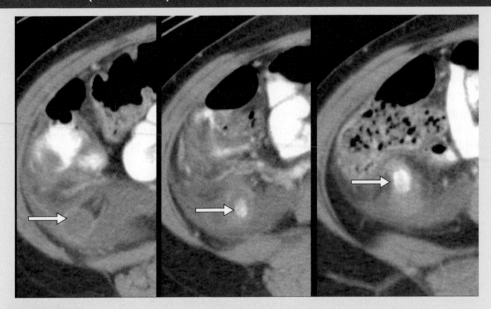

FIGURE 1-15 Sequential CT images from the upper pelvic region of a patient with appendicitis. The appendix is identified (*arrows*) and the appendicolith is visible in the last two images.

Image courtesy of Dr. David Warshauer, Department of Radiology, University of North Carolina at Chapel Hill.

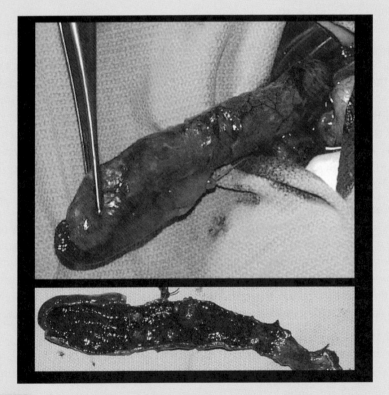

FIGURE 1-16 Inflamed appendix exposed during laparoscopic surgery (*upper* image). The removed appendix opened to reveal several appendicoliths (*lower* image).

Image courtesy of Dr. David Warshauer, Department of Radiology, University of North Carolina at Chapel Hill.

QUESTIONS FOR REVIEW

1. What are the major categories of disease?
2. What are the definitions of the following terms: *etiology, symptom of disease, sign of disease, diagnosis, prognosis,* and *pathogenesis*?
3. Describe the process of taking a patient history.
4. What principal factors does the physician evaluate in arriving at a diagnosis?
5. What is the difference between specific and symptomatic treatment?
6. What are the major categories of diagnostic tests and procedures that can help the practitioner make a diagnosis? Give some examples.
7. Compare and contrast the terms *sensitivity* and *specificity*.
8. How are cells and tissues used in diagnosis obtained?
9. What are the physical principles on which the following procedures are based: x-ray (plain film) examinations, CT scans, MRI, PET analysis, and ultrasound?

SUPPLEMENTARY READINGS

A large number of texts are written for undergraduate medical students and other health professionals and may serve as useful references for this material. The texts listed here are popular and frequently updated.

A note about online material: There are many accurate, reputable online sites for information on human disease. However, it is often difficult to decide which sources are reliable. Many students turn to Wikipedia as an initial online reference. This is a group sourced product always subject to change, so caution is urged. Many Wikipedia articles are first rate; however, information on controversial areas must be checked against other sources and the dates of provided references carefully examined.

Government sources such as the Center For Disease Control (www.cdc.gov), the MedlinePlus Medical Encyclopedia(www.nim.nih.gov), and major medical centers (for example, www.mayoclinic.org/diseases/) are often a good place to start. Other specific online resources are cited as appropriate.

Kumar, V., Abbas, A. K., and Aster, J. 2013. *Robbins Basic Pathology*. 9th ed. Philadelphia: Elsevier Saunders.

Rubin, E., and Reisner, H. M., ed. 2014. *Essentials of Rubin's Pathology*. 6th ed. Philadelphia: Wolters Kluwer Lippincott Williams & Wilkins.
  ► These two books are the shorter versions of the leading pathology texts used in medical education.

Bickley, L., and Szilagyi, P. G. 2013. *Bates' Guide to Physical Examination and History Taking*. 11th ed. Philadelphia: Wolters Kluwer, Lippincott Williams & Wilkins.
  ► A classic guide to the details of the physician–patient interaction.

Grobbee, D. E., and Hoes, A. W. 2015. *Clinical Epidemiology*. 2nd ed. Burlington, ME: Jones & Bartlett Learning.
  ► A serious and thorough text for the student with a mathematical bent interested in the details of clinical research.

Herring, W. 2012. *Learning Radiology: Recognizing the Basics*. 2nd ed. Philadelphia: Elsevier Saunders.
  ► An introductory text that does a good job of providing additional background on the diseases illustrated.

Laposata, M. 2014. *Laboratory Medicine*. 2nd ed. New York: McGraw Hill, Lange.
  ► A detailed description of the role of the clinical laboratory in diagnosing human disease.

Moini, J. 2012. *Anatomy and Physiology for Health Professionals*. Burlington (MA): Jones & Bartlett Learning.
  ► An easy to read and well-illustrated text on normal human anatomy and physiology.

American Society for Investigative Pathology. http://www.asip.org/

▶ This is the major research and teaching organization (although its major focus is not clinical). It is an excellent source for those interested in educational opportunities in the area.

Lab Tests OnLine. http://labtestsonline.org

▶ This is a public resource provided by laboratory professionals. It is an invaluable resource for those interested in any laboratory test. Its section on screening tests is of particular interest, presenting a nonbiased view of a very controversial area.

Geisel School of Medicine, Dartmouth Department of Anatomy. *Introduction to Radiology.* http://www .dartmouth.edu/~anatomy/Intro-to-radiology/

▶ This is an easy-to-follow, well-illustrated introduction to the area. Additional in-depth resources are available at the site.

Costello, J. A., Cecava, N. D., Tucker, J. E., and Bau, J. I. 2013. CT radiation dose: Current controversies and dose reduction strategy. *American Journal of Roentgenology (AJR)* 201:1283–90.

▶ Uses clinical examples to explore benefit, risk, and dose reduction strategies. Has an interesting review of models of cancer risk from CT.

Mansi, L., Ciarmiello, A., and Cuccurullo, V. 2012. PET/MRI and the revolution of the third eye. *European Journal of Nuclear Medicine and Molecular Imaging* 391:1519–24.

▶ An overview of combined PET/MRI imaging with particular emphasis on functional MRI; a field of rapidly growing importance.

Pyeritz, R. E. 2012. The family history: The first genetic test and still useful after all those years? *Genetics in Medicine* 14:3–9.

Vento, J. M. 2012. Family history: A guide for neurologists in the age of genomic medicine. *Seminars in Pediatric Neurology* 19:160–66.

▶ Two references that go together well. The first is a history of the role of the family history in patient evaluation up to the age of molecular genetics. The second (although the title sounds off-putting to the nonphysician) is an excellent introduction to the analysis of family history and pedigree analysis. Although the examples given involve neurological disease, it is a primer for genetic risk analysis, which has become an important component in clinical encounters.

Hoffman, R. M. 2011. Screening for prostate cancer. *New England Journal of Medicine* 365:2013–19.

▶ A case vignette is followed by a thorough discussion of the pluses and minuses of what is now a controversial screening procedure.

Horvath, A. R. 2013. From evidence to best practice in laboratory medicine. *Clinical Biochemist Reviews* 34:47–60.

▶ How does one implement a new diagnostic test? Describes how evidence-based medicine can be used to select clinically valid, clinically effective, and cost effective tests.

Woreta, T. A., and Alqahtani, S. A. 2014. Evaluation of abnormal liver tests. *Medical Clinics of North America* 98:1–16.

▶ Liver "function" tests are some of the most widely used assays in the clinical laboratory. What do they tell the physician and why? A guide to the appropriate use of laboratory information, in the diagnoses of disease.

Cells and Tissues: Their Structure and Function in Health and Disease

LEARNING OBJECTIVES

1. Make a sketch of the general structure of a typical cell.
2. Explain how cells are organized to form tissues. Diagram the fundamental structure of the four basic types of tissues: epithelium, connective, muscle, and nerve.
3. Explain how tissues are organized to form organs.
4. Write a general description of the three germ layers and their derivatives.
5. Illustrate how materials move in and out of cells. List five processes by which cells adapt to changing conditions.
6. Explain how cells adapt to changing conditions.
7. Compare and contrast cell injury, cell death/necrosis, and apoptosis.
8. Explain three ways in which an aging cell becomes increasingly vulnerable to injury.

Organization of Cells

The **cell** is the basic structural and functional unit of the body. Groups of similar cells arranged to perform a common function form **tissues.** Sets of tissues in turn are grouped together to form **organs,** and groups of organs functioning together form **organ systems.** Finally, the various organ systems are integrated to form a functioning organism. Communication between cells, tissues, and organs is carried out either by direct contact between cells (**juxtacrine** signaling) or by soluble mediators that act near groups of cells (**paracrine** signaling) or that act at a distance via the circulation (**endocrine** signaling). Cells have specialized **receptors** on their surface to recognize such signals and transmit the information into the cell, directing cellular functions. Dysfunction at any of these levels of organization or of communication between the levels of organization will cause disease.

The Cell

Although different functions of cells may be reflected in cell structure, all cells have certain features in common (**FIGURE 2-1**). Each cell consists of a nucleus surrounded by the cytoplasm. The nucleus contains the genetic information stored in the cell and much of the "switching mechanism" that controls the action of components of

Cell The basic structural and functional unit of the body.

Tissue A group of similar cells joined to perform a specific function.

Organs A group of different tissues organized to perform a specific function.

Organ systems A group of organs that function together as a unit, such as the various organs of the gastrointestinal tract.

Juxtacrine Cell to cell communication by direct contact.

Paracrine Cell to cell communication by soluble mediators acting near groups of cells.

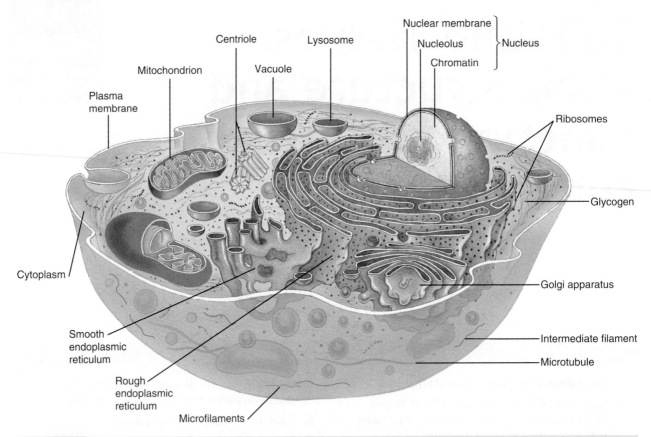

FIGURE 2-1 Structure of a typical cell. Note that the cell is divided into two compartments, the nuclear and cytoplasmic. The cytoplasm contains a variety of structures called organelles.

Endocrine Cell to cell communication by direct contact through soluble mediators acting across a distance between cells.

Receptor Cell surface signal receiver.

Organelle A small structure present in the cytoplasm of the cell, such as a mitochondrion.

Deoxyribonucleic acid (DNA) The nucleic acid present in the chromosomes of the nuclei of cells that carries genetic information.

Chromosome Cell structure organizing the molecules of DNA. Individual structural units of DNA which are best seen in dividing cells.

Chromatin Tightly wound DNA in the nucleus; formed in part from nucleosomes.

the genetic information. The expression of genes (See discussion of Chromosomes, Genes, and Cell Division) directs the metabolic functions of the cell and the structures in the cytoplasm, which carry out these directions. Within the cytoplasm are numerous small structures called **organelles**, which play an important part in the functions of the cell.

THE NUCLEUS

The nucleus contains two different types of nucleic acid combined with protein. **Deoxyribonucleic acid (DNA)** is contained in the **chromosomes**, which are long and thin in the nondividing cell. Although the chromosomes cannot be identified as distinct structures in a nondividing cell, they form the complex structure termed **chromatin**. Unwound, the DNA in the nucleus would stretch to a length of about 3 feet, but it must be compacted to fit into the nucleus, which has a diameter of only 0.0002 inches. The basis of this packaging is the **nucleosome**, a core consisting of nuclear proteins (**histones**) around which a segment of DNA is wound. Chromatin fibers in the nucleus are formed from nucleosomes, which are connected in a continuous strand by extended stretches of DNA (often described as "beads on a string"). However, these beads on a string are further packed together and folded into loops. The geometry of DNA compaction is of great importance in determining which segments of the DNA will function (**FIGURE 2-2**). Further compaction of these loops form the chromosomes which are visible through the microscope in a dividing cell (see discussion of cell division).

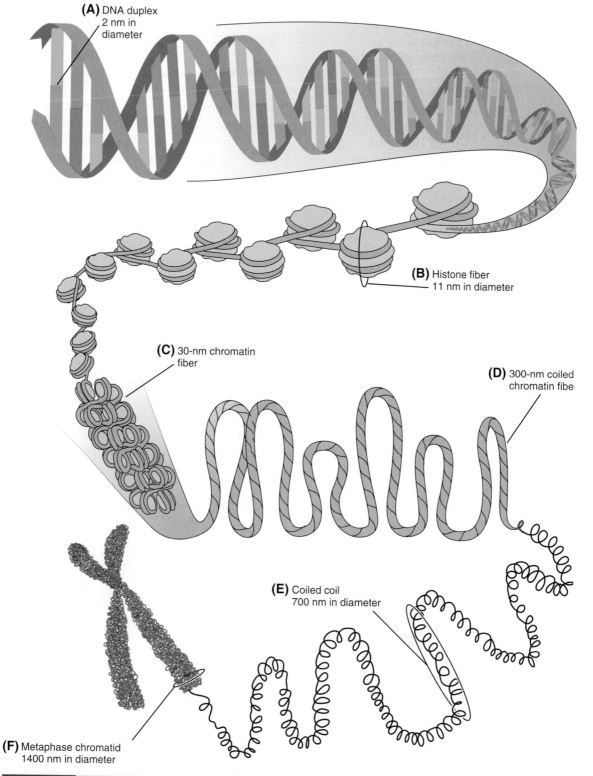

(A) DNA duplex 2 nm in diameter

(B) Histone fiber 11 nm in diameter

(C) 30-nm chromatin fiber

(D) 300-nm coiled chromatin fiber

(E) Coiled coil 700 nm in diameter

(F) Metaphase chromatid 1400 nm in diameter

FIGURE 2-2 Structure of chromatin. DNA **(A)** is packaged into nucleosomes **(B)** and further folded **(C, D, E)** to form chromosomes visible in a dividing cell **(F)**.

Ribonucleic acid (RNA) is contained in spherical intranuclear structures called **nucleoli** (singular, nucleolus). The nucleus is separated from the cytoplasm by a double-layered nuclear membrane. Small pores in the nuclear membrane permit the nucleus and cytoplasm to communicate.

Nucleosome Basis of packaging of DNA.

Histone Nuclear proteins forming the nucleosome.

Ribonucleic acid (RNA)
A type of nucleic acid contained in the nucleoli of cells. A component of messenger, transfer, and ribosomal RNA.

Nucleoli Structure containing RNA in the nucleus.

Alcoholic steatosis Condition of abnormal intracellular accumulation of lipid in the liver following ingestion of quantities of ethanol.

Mitochondria Rod-shaped structures in the cell capable of converting foods into energy to power the cell.

Adenosine triphosphate (ATP) A high-energy phosphate compound that liberates energy to power numerous cellular metabolic processes.

Endoplasmic reticulum A mass of hollow tubular channels within the cytoplasm of the cell, frequently bordered by ribosomes.

Rough endoplasmic reticulum (RER) Cell structure containing ribosomes and synthesizing protein.

Smooth endoplasmic reticulum (SER) Cell structure containing enzymes and synthesizing lipids.

Ribosome A small cytoplasmic organelle that serves as the site of protein synthesis. Ribosomes are usually attached to the endoplasmic reticulum but may be free in the cytoplasm.

THE CYTOPLASM

The gel-like cytoplasm contains many highly concentrated molecules including nutrients critical for cellular function. A cell membrane envelops the cytoplasm and acts selectively to allow some materials to pass into and out of the cell while it restricts the passage of others in either a passive or active process. (see presentation on Movement of Materials into and Out of Cells). The cytoplasm contains various organelles and may also contain products that accumulate within the cell, such as glycogen and fat. The most important organelles are the mitochondria, endoplasmic reticulum, Golgi apparatus, lysosomes, centrioles, and the tubules and filaments comprising the cytoskeleton of the cell. Inappropriate or excessive accumulation of products such as fats are an indicator of cellular dysfunction and disease. For example, excessive consumption of alcohol can lead to an abnormal intracellular accumulation of lipids, resulting in a "fatty liver" better termed **alcoholic steatosis** (see Case 2-1 and presentation of material on the liver). The cytoplasm, nucleus, and organelles are surrounded by membranes composed of lipid and protein molecules, which separate these structures from one another (see Figure 2-1).

MAJOR CELL ORGANELLES AND THEIR FUNCTIONS

TABLE 2-1 lists the major cell organelles.

    Mitochondria are membrane bound sausage-shaped structures that contain enzymes capable of converting food materials into energy by oxidizing them. The cell uses this energy to manufacture a high-energy compound called **adenosine triphosphate (ATP)**, the fuel that powers the chemical reactions in the cell.

    The **endoplasmic reticulum** is an interconnected network of tubular channels enclosed by membranes. This network communicates with both the nuclear membrane and the cell membrane. The **rough endoplasmic reticulum (RER)** has numerous small nucleoprotein particles called **ribosomes** attached to the external surfaces of its membranes. Its name derives from the knobby appearance that the attached ribosomes

TABLE 2-1	**Major Cell Organelles and Their Functions**
Organelle	**Function**
Mitochondria	Convert food materials into energy to make adenosine triphosphate (ATP) used to power the chemical reactions in the cell
Rough endoplasmic reticulum (RER)	Tubular ribosome-containing channels that synthesize protein to be secreted by cells
Smooth endoplasmic reticulum (SER)	Tubular channels containing enzymes that synthesize lipids and some other compounds within the cells
Golgi apparatus	Flat sacs located near nucleus attach carbohydrate molecules to the proteins synthesized by RER
Lysosomes	Spherical organelles in cytoplasm containing digestive enzymes that break down worn-out cell organelles and material brought into cell by phagocytosis
Centrioles	Short cylinders that form the mitotic spindle that separates chromosomes during cell division
Cytoskeleton	Protein tubules and filaments that form structural framework of cells and promote cell functions such as motility and phagocytosis

give the membranes, and its function is to synthesize protein that will be secreted by the cell. The attached ribosomes synthesize protein molecules that accumulate within the tubules of the RER and are eventually secreted. Digestive enzymes and antibody proteins, for example, are produced in this way. The second type of endoplasmic reticulum lacks ribosomes and is called the **smooth endoplasmic reticulum (SER)**. Its membranes contain enzymes that synthesize lipids and some other substances.

The **Golgi apparatus** consists of groups of flattened membrane-like sacs located near the nucleus. These sacs are connected with the tubules of the RER. The proteins produced by the ribosomes attached to the RER pass through the RER tubules into the Golgi apparatus. There the large carbohydrate molecules are synthesized and combined with the proteins, are formed into secretory granules, and eventually are discharged from the cell.

Lysosomes are cytoplasmic organelles made by the Golgi apparatus that are filled with digestive enzymes that function as the "digestive system" of the cell. Lysosomes break down material brought into the cell by phagocytosis; they also degrade worn-out intracellular components such as mitochondria and other organelles, making the breakdown products available to be recycled or excreted from the cells, a process called **autophagy**. When particulate material is ingested by **phagocytosis**, the particle becomes enclosed within a membrane-lined vacuole called a **phagocytic vacuole**. A lysosome then merges with the phagocytic vacuole, and their cell membranes fuse, allowing the digestive enzymes contained in the lysosome to flow into the phagocytic vacuole and digest the engulfed material. Digestion is accomplished entirely within the phagocytic vacuole, which prevents digestive enzymes from leaking into the cyto-plasm of the cell and causing injury to the cell (**FIGURE 2-3**). The same type of digestive

Golgi apparatus A group of membrane-lined sacs found in the cytoplasm of the cell near the nucleus; functions with the endoplasmic reticulum to synthesize and package secretory granules.

Lysosome A small cytoplasmic vacuole containing digestive enzymes.

Autophagy Process by which cellular organelles are degraded and recycled by the cells.

Phagocytosis Ingestion of particulate foreign material by cells.

Phagocytic vacuole Membrane-lined vacuole used to contain the foreign material.

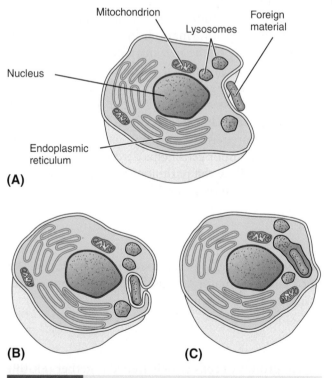

FIGURE 2-3 Digestion of engulfed material by lysosomes. **(A)** Extensions of cytoplasm from phagocytic cell begin to surround particulate material. **(B)** Cytoplasmic extensions engulf material and form phagocytic vacuole containing the engulfed material. **(C)** Lysosome and phagocytic vacuole merge, and enzymes from lysosome digest the engulfed material.

Peroxisome A cytoplasmic organelle containing various enzymes, including those that decompose potentially toxic compounds through the production of hydrogen peroxide.

Centrioles Short, cylindrical structures located adjacent to the nucleus that participate in the formation of spindle fibers during cell division.

Mitotic spindle Formed by the centriole during cell division.

Cytoskeleton Protein tubules and filaments that form the structural framework of cells.

Actin microfilament One type of cell framework filament.

Microtubule Largest type of cell framework filament.

Intermediate filaments Small, tough filaments of high tensile strength within the cell cytoplasm.

Keratin filament Type of filament in epithelial cells.

Vimentin filament Type of filament in connective and muscle cells.

Neurofilament Type of filament in nerve cells.

Lamin filament Type of filament involved in nuclear structure in all cells.

Anaplastic cell Type of tumor cell whose structure is so deranged as to make identification of origin difficult.

Parenchymal cell The functional cell of an organ or tissue.

Parenchyma The functional cells of an organ, as contrasted with the connective and supporting tissue that forms its framework.

process is involved when worn-out components are broken down within cells. In some diseases the lysosomal enzymes are unable to function properly and incompletely digested material accumulates within lysosomes, disrupting cell functions.

Closely related to lysosomes are smaller structures called **peroxisomes**, which contain enzymes that break down various potentially toxic intracellular molecules. The name of this organelle comes from hydrogen peroxide (H_2O_2), a toxic by-product of enzyme action. The hydrogen peroxide produced is used to oxidize the potentially toxic substances (such as ethanol) and is converted to water in the process. Excess hydrogen peroxide is promptly decomposed by enzymes in the peroxisome. Peroxisomes are also important in the synthesis of components of the myelin sheath of nerve cells.

Centrioles are short cylindrical structures located adjacent to the nucleus. In cell division, they move to opposite poles of the cell and form the **mitotic spindle**. The spindle fibers attach to the chromosomes and pull them apart in the course of cell division.

The cytoplasm also contains three types of filaments of structural proteins that form the framework (**cytoskeleton**) of the cell. **Actin** filaments or **microfilaments** (the smallest) are especially plentiful in contractile cells (such as muscle). **Microtubules** (the largest) are of particular importance in cell division and help organize the sorting of genetic information into daughter cells. **Intermediate filaments** are small tough filaments of high tensile strength that reinforce the interior of the cell, hold the organelles in proper position within the cell, and along with the other cytoskeletal structures are responsible for the characteristic shape of each specific type of cell. There are four classes of intermediate filaments. Three of the classes are cytoplasmic and can be identified in cells by specific histological techniques. Each of these classes is characteristic of a specific type of cell: **keratin filaments** in epithelial cells, **vimentin filaments** in connective and muscle cells, and **neurofilaments** in nerve cells. The fourth class (**lamin filaments**) is involved in the nuclear structure and is found in all cells.

Identification and characterization of intermediate filaments in cells often provide both diagnostic and prognostic information. In some diseases such as Alzheimer's disease, a degenerative disease of the nervous system (described in the discussion on the nervous system), the intermediate filaments exhibit characteristic abnormalities that help to establish the diagnosis of the disease. Identification of the type of intermediate filaments in cells is also useful in the diagnosis of tumors (described in neoplastic disease discussion). In cases in which the originating cell of a tumor is difficult to identify, the cells are termed **anaplastic cells**. Identifying the specific type of intermediate filament in the tumor cells helps determine the type of cell from which the tumor arose. This may allow the pathologist to make a more precise diagnosis and aid the clinician in selection of a suitable therapy.

Tissues

A tissue is a group of similar cells joined together to perform a specific function. Tissues are classified into four major groups: epithelium, connective and supporting tissues, muscle tissue, and nerve tissue.

EPITHELIUM

Epithelium consists of groups of cells closely joined together (**FIGURE 2-4**) that cover the exterior of the body and line the interior body surfaces that communicate with the outside, such as the gastrointestinal tract, urinary tract, and vagina. Epithelium forms glands such as the thyroid and pancreas and also makes up the functional cells (often called **parenchymal cells** or **parenchyma**) of organs that have excretory or secretory functions, such as the liver and the kidneys. The individual cells may be flat and

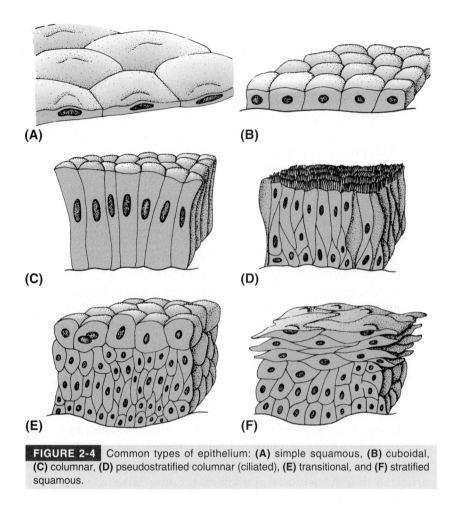

FIGURE 2-4 Common types of epithelium: **(A)** simple squamous, **(B)** cuboidal, **(C)** columnar, **(D)** pseudostratified columnar (ciliated), **(E)** transitional, and **(F)** stratified squamous.

platelike (**squamous cells**), cube-shaped (**cuboidal cells**), or tall and narrow (**columnar cells**). Many columnar epithelial cells have become specialized to absorb or secrete, and some contain hairlike processes called **cilia**. Epithelial cells may be arranged in a single layer (simple epithelium) or may be several layers thick (stratified epithelium).

The interiors of the heart, blood vessels, and lymphatic vessels are lined by a layer of simple squamous epithelium called **endothelium**. A similar appearing type of epithelium lining the pleural, pericardial, and peritoneal cavities is called **mesothelium**. Although these linings are classified as types of epithelium, they arise along with the connective tissues from the embryonic germ layer called the **mesoderm** and are therefore much more closely related to connective tissue than to other types of epithelium. Consequently, they are considered separately and are given distinct names. Tumors arising from endothelium or mesothelium have unique patterns of behavior and are considered apart from those arising from surface, glandular, or parenchymal epithelium. This subject is considered in the discussion on neoplastic disease.

The Structure of Epithelium

Epithelial cells are supported by a thin basement membrane. The cells are joined to each other, and the deeper layers of epithelium are firmly anchored to the basement membrane so that the epithelial cells remain relatively fixed in position. There are no blood vessels in epithelium. The cells are nourished by diffusion of material from capillaries located in the underlying connective tissue. Epithelia are characterized by both the shape and number of layers of cells of which they are comprised.

Squamous cells Flat, platelike cells.

Cuboidal cells Cube-shaped cells.

Columnar cells Tall, narrow cells.

Cilia Specialized hairlike processes on cells.

Endothelium The internal lining of blood vessels and interior of the heart.

Mesothelium A layer of flat, squamous epithelial cells that covers the surfaces of the pleural, pericardial, and peritoneal cavities.

Mesoderm The middle germ layer of the embryo, which gives rise to specific organs and tissues.

Simple Epithelium

Simple epithelia consist of a single layer of cells. The distribution of simple squamous epithelium composed of flat platelike cells is limited. It forms the lining of the pulmonary air sacs, the endothelial lining of the vascular system, and the mesothelial lining of the body cavities. Simple columnar epithelium lines most of the gastrointestinal tract. Pseudostratified columnar epithelium is a type of simple columnar epithelium in which the cells are so tightly packed together that their nuclei appear to lie at different levels. This gives an appearance of stratification. Pseudostratified epithelium is often ciliated. This type of epithelium lines most of the respiratory tract and is present in a few other areas.

Stratified Epithelium

Stratified epithelia contain multiple layers and often serve a protective function. Stratified squamous epithelium forms the external covering of the body and also lines the oral cavity, esophagus, and vagina. Stratified epithelium is named for the appearance of the most superficial cell layer. Consequently, this epithelium is designated "stratified squamous" based on the flat platelike appearance of the most superficial (exterior) layers of cells even though the deeper layers are composed of cuboidal cells (**FIGURE 2-5A**). The stratified squamous epithelium that forms the top layer of the skin undergoes a process called **keratinization**, in which the top layers of squamous cells accumulate a fibrous protein called **keratin**, lose their cellular structure, and are shed. This fibrous protein forms a dense layer that protects the underlying cells. The deeper layers adjacent to the basement membrane consist of dividing cells that replenish the epithelial cells shed from the surface as they move upward. Transitional epithelium, consisting of a layer of large superficial cells covering a deeper layer of cuboidal cells, is the characteristic lining of the bladder and other parts of the urinary tract. The superficial cells of transitional epithelium become flattened when the bladder is distended and resume their original shape when the bladder is empty.

Functions of Epithelium

Epithelium performs many different functions. All types of epithelium perform a protective function. Columnar epithelium, such as that lining the intestinal tract, is specialized to absorb and secrete. Other types of epithelium form glands that secrete mucus, sweat, lipid, enzymes, hormones, or other products (**FIGURE 2-5B**). Glands, such as the pancreas, that discharge their secretions through a duct onto an epithelial surface are called **exocrine glands**. **Endocrine glands**, such as the thyroid and adrenals, discharge their secretions directly into the bloodstream.

Keratinization
Accumulation of a fibrous protein called keratin inside cells.

Keratin An insoluble sulfur-containing protein that is the principal constituent of the hair and nails.

Exocrine glands
A gland that discharges its secretions through a duct onto a mucosal surface, in contrast to an endocrine gland that delivers its secretions directly into the bloodstream.

Endocrine glands
A gland that discharges its secretions directly into the bloodstream, in contrast to an exocrine gland that discharges its secretion through a duct onto a mucosal surface.

(A)

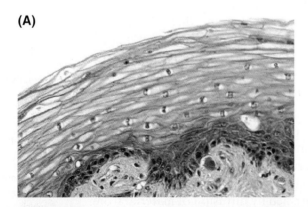

(B)

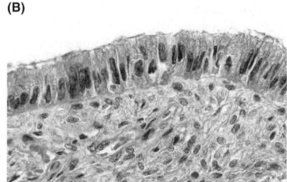

FIGURE 2-5 Two types of epithelial cells from the cervix. **(A)** Nonkeratinized stratified squamous epithelium from the exocervix serves a protective function. **(B)** Columnar epithelium from the endocervix secretes mucus.

Courtesy of Department of Pathology and Laboratory Medicine, University of North Carolina at Chapel Hill.

CONNECTIVE AND SUPPORTING TISSUES

Connective and supporting tissues consist of relatively small numbers of cells incorporated in a large amount of extracellular material called matrix in which are embedded various types of fibers. The proportions of cells, fibers, and matrix vary greatly in different types of connective tissue. Connective tissue fibers are of three types. Collagen fibers are long, flexible fibers composed of a protein called collagen. They are strong but do not stretch. Elastic fibers are composed of a protein called elastin. They are not as strong as collagen but stretch readily and return to their former shape when the stretching force is released. Reticulin fibers are very similar to collagen but are quite thin and delicate and help support organs with a high density of cells. The matrix in which the fibers are embedded (often termed ground substance) contains a large amount of water bound to complex long and unbranched polysaccharides termed glycosaminoglycans (GAGs). Some GAGs are bound to proteins to form extremely large molecules called proteoglycans or mucoproteins. The specific array of GAGs and connective tissue fibers define the specific properties of the connective tissue.

Connective and supporting tissues include various types of loose and dense fibrous tissue, elastic tissue, reticular tissue, adipose tissue, cartilage, and bone. Hematopoietic tissue (blood-forming tissue) and lymphatic tissue (lymphocyte-forming tissue) also are classified as types of connective tissue, primarily because, like other types of connective tissue, they originate from the mesoderm although they are often considered separately by pathologists (hematopathologists) who specialize in their study.

Fibrous connective tissue performs a variety of functions that connect and support the various parts of the body. Loose fibrous tissue, which is the most widely distributed, forms the tissue just beneath the skin (subcutaneous tissue, dermis) and also fills in around organs. Dense fibrous tissue forms ligaments and tendons, which reinforce joints and attach muscles to bone.

Elastic tissue forms membranes that are wrapped around the walls of blood vessels and are responsible for the characteristic distensibility of large arteries. Elastic membranes also form part of the walls of the trachea and bronchi.

Reticular tissue is a special type of connective tissue characterized by a fine meshwork of reticulin fibers that form the supporting framework of various organs such as the liver, spleen, and lymph nodes.

Adipose tissue is a variety of loose fibrous tissue containing large numbers of fat cells. Fat is a stored form of energy and also functions as padding and insulation.

Cartilage is a type of supporting tissue in which the cells are dispersed in a dense matrix. There are three types of cartilage. Hyaline cartilage is the most common. It is blue and translucent and contains only a few fine collagen fibers suspended in the abundant matrix. Hyaline cartilage covers the ends of bones where they form movable joints, forms the greater part of the laryngeal and tracheal cartilages, and connects the ribs to the sternum. Elastic cartilage contains yellow elastic fibers in the matrix and is found in only a few locations, such as the cartilaginous portions of the ears. The elastic fibers impart a flexibility to the cartilage that is lacking in other types of cartilage. Fibrocartilage contains many dense collagen bundles embedded in the matrix. It is found in areas where cartilage is subjected to marked weight-bearing stresses. It forms the disks between the vertebral bodies and some of the cartilages in the knee joints; it is also present in a few other locations.

Bone is a highly specialized, rigid supporting tissue in which the matrix containing the bone-forming cells is impregnated with calcium salts.

MUSCLE TISSUE

Muscle cells contain filaments of specialized intracellular contractile proteins called actin and myosin, arranged in parallel bundles. During contraction of a muscle fiber,

---

Matrix Material in which connective tissue cells are embedded.

Collagen fibers Fibers that are strong but do not stretch.

Collagen Main constituent of fibrous proteins in the human.

Elastic fibers Fibers made of elastin that stretch.

Elastin Component of elastic fibers.

Reticulin fibers Very thin fibers made of collagen.

Ground substance Matrix in which the fibers are embedded.

Glycosaminoglycans (GAGs) Long, unbranched polysaccharides making up the ground substance.

Proteoglycans/ mucoproteins Extremely large molecules in connective tissue.

Hematopoietic tissue Tissue that forms the blood.

Lymphatic tissue Tissue that forms the lymphatic system.

Hematopathologist Pathologist who specializes in the study of blood forming tissue.

Reticular tissue A special type of connective tissue characterized by fine reticulin fibers.

Adipose tissue Loose, fibrous tissue containing fat cells.

Cartilage A type of supporting tissue in which cells are dispersed in a dense matrix.

Hyaline cartilage Most common type of cartilage; contains only a few fine collagen fibers.

Elastic cartilage Contains elastic fibers.

Fibrocartilage Contains many dense collagen bundles.

Actin Contractile protein that cause muscles to shorten.

Myosin Contractile protein that cause muscles to lengthen.

Smooth muscle Muscle that functions automatically.

Striated muscle Muscle that moves the skeleton; under voluntary control.

Cardiac muscle Muscle found only in the heart; has features of both striated and smooth muscle.

Neuron A nerve cell, including the nerve cell body and its processes.

Glia cells/neuroglia Supporting cells of tissue of the nervous system.

Astrocyte A large stellate cell having highly branched processes. Forms the structural framework of the nervous system. One of the neuroglial cells.

Oligodendroglia/Schwann cells One type of neuroglia that surrounds nerve fibers within the central nervous system/peripheral nervous system.

Myelin Covering of nerve fibers to protect and speed the rate of signal transmission.

Microglia Phagocytic cells of the nervous system; comparable to macrophages in other tissues.

Organ Group of different tissues integrated for perform a specific function.

Stroma The tissue that forms the framework of an organ.

actin filaments slide inward on the myosin filaments, somewhat like pistons, causing the fiber to shorten. There are three types of muscle fibers. **Smooth muscle** is located primarily in the walls of hollow internal organs such as the gastrointestinal tract, biliary tract, and reproductive tract; in the walls of the blood vessels where the muscle regulates the caliber of the vessels to control blood flow to the tissues; and in the skin where they attach to hair follicles and control elevation of the hairs. Smooth muscle functions automatically and is not under conscious control. **Striated muscle** moves the skeleton and is under voluntary control. **Cardiac muscle** is found only in the heart. It resembles striated muscle but has some features common to both smooth and voluntary muscle.

NERVE TISSUE

Nerve tissue is composed of nerve cells called **neurons**, which transmit nerve impulses, and supporting cells called **glial cells or neuroglia**. Neuroglial cells are more numerous than neurons. They are of three different types. **Astrocytes** are long, star-shaped cells having numerous highly branched processes that interlace to form a meshwork. Astrocytes form the structural framework of the central nervous system in the way that the connective tissue fibers form the framework of internal organs. **Oligodendrocytes** (in the central nervous system; the brain and spinal cord) and **Schwann cells** (in the peripheral nervous system) are small cells with scanty cytoplasm that wrap around certain individual nerve cells in the nervous system and produce the **myelin** covering that protects the nerve and speeds up the rate of signal transmission. **Microglia** are phagocytic cells comparable to the macrophages found in other tissues.

Organs and Organ Systems

An **organ** is a group of different tissues that is integrated to perform a specific function. Generally, one tissue performs the primary function characteristic of the organ, and the other tissues perform a supporting function, such as providing the vascular and connective tissue framework for the organ. The functional cells of an organ are often called the parenchymal cells, and the total mass of functional tissue is called the parenchyma. The supporting framework of the organ is called the **stroma**. In the liver, for example, the parenchymal cells are formed by cords of epithelial cells that perform the many metabolic functions characteristic of the liver, such as the synthesis of protein and the excretion of bile. The cord cells are supported by a framework of connective tissue fibers. Numerous thin-walled blood vessels are interspersed between the cell cords, and the entire liver is surrounded by a capsule composed of dense fibrous tissue.

An organ system is a group of organs that is organized to perform complementary functions, such as the reproductive system, the respiratory system, and the digestive system. Finally, the various organ systems are integrated into a functioning individual.

The Germ Layers and Their Derivatives

The highly complex structure of the entire body evolves from a single cell, the fertilized ovum, by a complex process that includes periods of cell multiplication, differentiation, and organization to form organs and organ systems (prenatal development is considered in the discussion on prenatal development and diseases associated with pregnancy). As the fertilized ovum grows, its cells differentiate into two groups. The peripheral group of cells is called the **trophoblast**. This, along with maternally derived

TABLE 2-2 Derivatives of the Germ Layers		
Ectoderm	Mesoderm	Endoderm
Epidermis	Dermis	Lining of the digestive system
Hair, nails, sweat glands	All muscles of the body	Lining of the respiratory system
Brain and spinal cord	Cartilage	Urethra and urinary bladder
Cranial and spinal nerves	Bone	Gallbladder
Retina, lens, and cornea of eye	Blood	Liver and pancreas
Inner ear	All other connective tissue	Thyroid gland
Epithelium of nose, mouth, and anus	Blood vessels	Parathyroid gland
Enamel of teeth	Reproductive organs Kidneys	Thymus

tissue, forms the placenta and other structures that will support and nourish the embryo. The inner group of cells, the **inner cell mass**, are the cells that will give rise to the embryo, arranging themselves into three distinct layers called the **germ layers**. Each layer will form certain specialized tissues and organs (**TABLE 2-2**). The outer layer, called the **ectoderm**, forms the external covering of the body and the various organs that bring the individual into contact with the external environment: the nervous system, eyes, and ears. The inner layer, called the **endoderm**, forms the internal "lining": the epithelium of the pharynx, the respiratory tract, the gastrointestinal tract and the organs closely associated with it (the liver, biliary tract, and pancreas), and some parts of the urogenital tract. The **mesoderm** is the layer of cells sandwiched between the other two layers. These cells are the ancestors of the various supporting tissues (connective tissues, cartilage, and bone), muscle, the circulatory system (heart, blood, and blood vessels), and major portions of the urogenital system. Each normal cell in the body is part of a community of cells and is integrated with its neighbors so that it functions along with other cells to meet the body's needs.

Movement of Materials Into and Out of Cells

In order for the cell to function properly, oxygen and nutrients must enter the cell, and waste products must be eliminated. The proper balance of charged ions (such as Na^+, K^+, and Ca^{++}) must be maintained between the outside and inside of the cell. Materials entering and leaving the cell must cross the cell membrane, which limits the passage of some molecules and is freely permeable to others. Materials cross the cell membrane in three ways: diffusion and osmosis, active transport, and phagocytosis and **pinocytosis** (a process analogous to phagocytosis but in which fluid is engulfed).

DIFFUSION AND OSMOSIS

Diffusion is the movement of dissolved particles (solute) from a more concentrated to a more dilute solution. **Osmosis** is the movement of water molecules from a dilute solution to a more concentrated solution (**FIGURE 2-6**). Both are passive processes that do not require the cell to expend energy. If the membrane is freely permeable to both water and solute particles (Figure 2-6A, B), the solute particles diffuse from the higher solute concentration on the right side of the membrane into the lower solute concentration on the left side. At the same time, water molecules diffuse in the

Trophoblast Cell derived from the fertilized ovum that gives rise to the fetal membranes and contributes to the formation of the placenta.

Inner cell mass A group of cells derived from the fertilized ovum that are destined to form the embryo.

Germ layers The three layers of cells derived from the inner cell mass; each layer is destined to form specific organs and tissues in the embryo.

Ectoderm The outer germ layer in the embryo that gives rise to specific organs and tissues.

Endoderm The inner germ layer of the embryo that gives rise to specific organs and tissues.

Mesoderm The middle germ layer of the embryo that gives rise to specific organs and tissues.

Pinocytosis Process similar to phagocytosis but for the ingestion of water.

Osmosis The movement of water molecules from a dilute solution to a more concentrated one.

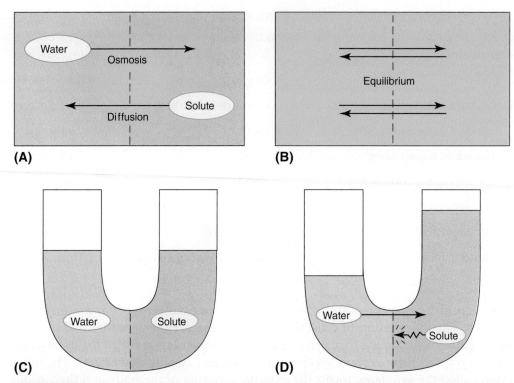

FIGURE 2-6 **(A)** Processes of osmosis and diffusion across a porous membrane (*dashed line*). **(B)** At equilibrium, the concentrations of water and solute molecules are equal on both sides of membrane. **(C)** The left compartment of U tube contains water; the right compartment contains solute impermeable to the membrane. **(D)** Water molecules diffuse freely across the membrane, but solute molecules are unable to diffuse. The volume of solute is increased by diffusion of water molecules into the solute. The volume of water in left limb of the U tube falls as water moves into the solute in the right limb of the U tube.

opposite direction, from the more dilute solution on the right side of the membrane into the more concentrated solution on the left side. At equilibrium, the concentrations of solute particles and water molecules are the same on both sides of the membrane. Solute and water molecules continue to move in both directions across the membrane after equilibrium is attained, but the net movement is equal in both directions, which does not change the equilibrium volume and concentration of the solutions on the two sides of the membrane.

The situation is quite different if the membrane is not permeable to the solute particles in the solution on one side of the membrane (Figure 2-6C, D). Water molecules move by osmosis from the left side of the membrane into the more concentrated solution on the right side (containing fewer water molecules). Because diffusion of solute is restricted by the membrane but movement of water molecules across the membrane is not, the volume of the solution on the right side of the membrane increases, and its solute concentration falls as the water molecules move by osmosis across the membrane. Eventually, the solutions on both sides of the membrane have the same concentration of solute but their volumes are quite different.

Osmotic Pressure, Osmolarity, and Tonicity

The "water-attracting" property of a solution, which can be measured, is called its **osmotic activity** or **osmotic pressure** and is related to the concentration of dissolved particles in the solution. The more concentrated the solution, the higher its osmotic pressure. The quantitative expression of the osmotic pressure of a solution is called **osmolarity**. Osmolarity reflects the number of dissolved particles in the solution, not the molecular weight or valence of the particles. For a substance such as glucose, which does not

Osmotic activity/ osmotic pressure "Water attracting" property of a solution.

Osmolarity A measure of the osmotic pressure exerted by a solution.

dissociate in solution, 1 mole (the molecular weight of the substance in grams) dissolved in water to a volume of 1 liter has an osmolarity of 1 osmole per liter (abbreviated Osm/L). However, 1 mole of a substance that dissociates into two univalent ions (such as sodium chloride) has an osmolarity of 2 Osm/L. Movement of water and solute between the extracellular fluid (interstitial fluid and fluid components of blood and lymph) and the intracellular fluid (fluid within the cells) is regulated by the cell membrane, which is permeable to water and some solutes but relatively impermeable to others. The osmolarity of extracellular fluids varies from about 280 to 295 mOsm/L (1 Osm = 1,000 mOsm) and the intracellular osmolarity is the same, as the two fluid compartments are in equilibrium. Most of the solutes in the extracellular fluid that contribute to its osmolarity are sodium (Na^+), chloride (Cl^-), and bicarbonate (HCO_3^-) ions. In contrast, the major intracellular ions are potassium (K^+) and phosphate (PO_4^{-3}). The sodium–potassium ion differences on the two sides of the cell membrane, which are essential for normal cell functions, are controlled by the cell. A special term for osmotic pressure, **oncotic pressure**, is used when the solute is a very large molecule such as the proteins found in the blood and other extracellular fluids. Such large proteins do not diffuse across cell membranes or exit from normal blood vessels. Blood proteins (in particular albumin) are responsible for maintaining the fluid content of the blood. If the level of blood protein drops (such as in liver disease because albumin is synthesized in the liver), the fluid retained in blood vessels diffuses into tissue. The result is **ascites**, the swelling of the abdominal area and legs by excess extracellular fluid.

The term **tonicity**, which is sometimes used to refer to the osmotic effects produced by a solution, is not quite the same as osmolarity because it is determined only by those solutes that cannot cross the membrane (most often the membrane of a cell). An **isotonic solution** is osmotically equivalent to the patient's own body fluids and can safely be administered intravenously to patients without causing changes in the volume of cells or fluid in the interstitium of tissue, the extracellular fluid (ECF). Generally, only isotonic solutions are used for intravenous administration. A **hypertonic solution** is more concentrated. Cells exposed to a hypertonic solution shrink because water moves by osmosis from the cells into the hypertonic fluid. In contrast, a **hypotonic solution** is a dilute solution, and cells exposed to a hypotonic solution swell as water moves by osmosis from the hypotonic fluid into the cells where the osmolarity is higher. If a hypotonic solution is administered intravenously, the flow of water into cells, such as red cells, might be so great that the cell membranes become damaged, causing hemoglobin to leak from the cells, a process termed **hemolysis**.

Normally, the osmotic pressures within the cell and in the ECF are kept equal; therefore, the shape and water content of the cells do not change. This cannot be accomplished by diffusion alone. For example, in the tubules of the kidney where urine is processed, the concentration of solute (particularly sodium ions, Na^+) is much higher than that within the epithelial cells that line the tubules of the kidney. Diffusion constantly acts to increase the Na^+ concentration within the cells. This tendency is counteracted by an active "pumping out" process requiring energy (in the form of ATP) produced by the mitochondria. If this pump fails (as happens in numerous disease states), Na^+ accumulates within the cells and water diffuses into the epithelial cells from the ECF (urine) in the tubule. If unchecked, the epithelial cells swell and ultimately die (a special type of cell death termed **oncosis**) resulting in kidney failure.

ACTIVE TRANSPORT

Active transport is the transfer of a substance across the cell membrane from a region of low concentration to one of higher concentration, counter to diffusion. The process requires the cell to expend energy because the substance must move against a

Oncotic pressure Osmotic pressure when solute is a very large molecule such as blood proteins.

Ascites Swelling of abdominal area and legs caused by excess extracellular fluid.

Tonicity Measure of ionic concentration determined only by solutes that cannot cross the membrane.

Isotonic solution A solution having essentially the same osmolarity as body fluids so that cells neither shrink nor swell when exposed to the solution.

Hypertonic solution A solution having a greater osmolarity than body fluids, which causes cells to shrink in such a solution because water moves by osmosis from the cells into the hypertonic solution.

Hypotonic solution A solution having a lower osmolarity than body fluids, causing cells in the solution to swell because water moves by osmosis from the hypotonic solution into the cells.

Hemolysis Hemoglobin leakage from red cells caused by damaged cell membranes.

Oncosis Cell death due to swelling of epithelial cells caused by failure of pumping out Na^+ ions. A type of necrosis.

Active transport Transfer of materials against a concentration gradient that is necessary to a maintain proper concentration of intracellular and extracellular ions.

concentration gradient. Many metabolic processes depend on active transport of ions or molecules. For example, for the cell to function normally, the intracellular potassium concentration must be higher than the concentration in the ECF, and the intracellular sodium concentration must be much lower. This is accomplished by a mechanism that actively transports potassium into the cell and simultaneously moves sodium out, the ATP-dependent pump mentioned previously. Active transport of ions is critical to many body processes including nerve and muscle function.

Adaptations of Cells to Changing Conditions

Cells respond to changing conditions in various ways. Common adaptive mechanisms are atrophy, hypertrophy and hyperplasia, metaplasia, dysplasia, and increased enzyme synthesis.

In many instances, the adaptation enables the cells to function more efficiently. Skin cells increase in number (undergo hyperplasia) to form a protective callus when subject to increased wear. This is an example of a **physiological adaptive change**. Sometimes, however, the adaptive change may be detrimental to the cell, a pathologic adaption. The hyperplasia of skin cells in a wart is the result of inappropriate (maladaptive) hyperplasia, which is the result of a viral infection, which may also occur in dysplasia. Atrophy, hyperplasia, hypertrophy, and metaplasia may be adaptive or maladaptive. Dysplasia is always maladaptive.

ATROPHY

Atrophy is a reduction in the size of cells (and hence organs) in response to diminished function, inadequate hormonal or neuronal stimulation, or reduced blood supply. The cell decreases in size to "get by" under the less favorable conditions. For example, skeletal muscles are reduced in size when an extremity is immobilized in a cast for long periods or if innervation is damaged. The breasts and genital organs shrink after menopause as a result of inadequate estrogen stimulation. A kidney becomes smaller if its blood supply becomes insufficient due to narrowing of the renal artery. Sometimes atrophy is part of a normal physiological process; for example, the reduction in size of the uterus after childbirth and of the breast when lactation ceases.

HYPERTROPHY AND HYPERPLASIA

If cells are required to do more work, they may increase either their size or their number to accomplish their task. **Hypertrophy** is an increase in the size of individual cells without an actual increase in their numbers. The large muscles of a weight lifter, for example, result from hypertrophy of individual muscle fibers. The number of fibers is not increased, but the size of individual muscle cells increases. Similarly, the heart of a person with high blood pressure often enlarges as a result of hypertrophy of the individual cardiac muscle fibers. This occurs because the heart must work harder to pump blood at a higher than normal pressure (**FIGURE 2-7**).

Hyperplasia is an increase in the size of a tissue or organ caused by an increase in the number of cells. Hyperplasia occurs in response to increased demand. For example, the glandular tissue of the breast becomes hyperplastic during pregnancy in preparation for lactation. Endocrine glands such as the thyroid may enlarge to increase their output of hormones. Hyperplasia in response to hormone balance may also be pathologic. An increase in the number of glandular and smooth muscle cells in the prostate results in benign prostatic hypertrophy, which often leads to difficulty in urination in elderly men.

Physiological adaptive change Cell or organ response to changing conditions.

Atrophy Reduction in size of cells or organs in response to diminished function.

Hypertrophy An enlargement or overgrowth of an organ caused by an increase in the size of its constituent cells.

Hyperplasia An increase in the number of cells.

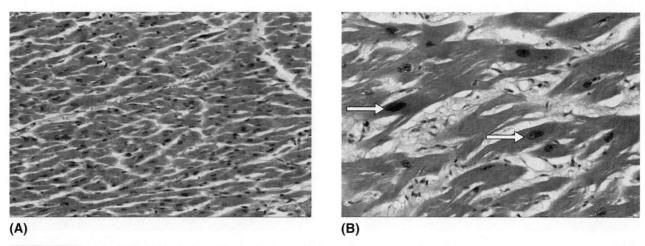

FIGURE 2-7 **(A)** Normal cardiac muscle. **(B)** Hypertrophic cardiac muscle from an individual with high blood pressure (both images at the same magnification). Note the greatly increased fiber size and very large nuclei (*arrows*). Although hypertrophic cardiac muscle cells do not divide, the DNA in the nuclei does, resulting in increased size.

Courtesy of Department of Pathology and Laboratory Medicine, University of North Carolina at Chapel Hill.

METAPLASIA

Metaplasia is a change from one type of cell to another type that is better able to tolerate some adverse environmental condition. For example, if the lining of the trachea is chronically irritated by the chemical agents in cigarette smoke, the normal ciliated columnar epithelial lining may assume the characteristic structure of a layer of squamous epithelium. The metaplastic epithelium is presumed to be more resistant to irritation and is better able to protect the tracheal wall. However, the metaplastic area is the locus at which common forms of lung cancer begin (**FIGURE 2-8**). The same is true of metaplasia that may occur in the esophagus (as a protection from acid reflux) or on the cervix (possibly as a protection from the acid environment of the vagina). In all cases, the metaplasia may initially be protective but ultimately often becomes the site of dysplasia.

> **Metaplasia** A change from one type of cell to a more resistant cell type.

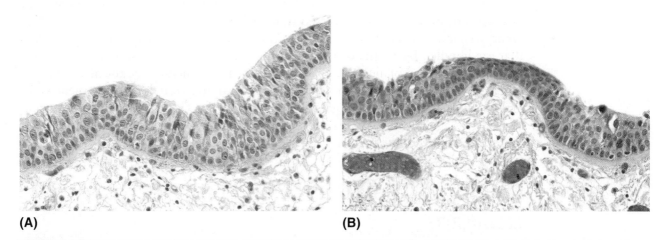

FIGURE 2-8 **(A)** An area of normal pseudostratified ciliated columnar epithelium from the trachea of a smoker (cilia not visible at magnification). **(B)** An area demonstrating metaplasia from the same tissue sample. The tissue appears as squamous epithelium (*center*).

Courtesy of Department of Pathology and Laboratory Medicine, University of North Carolina at Chapel Hill.

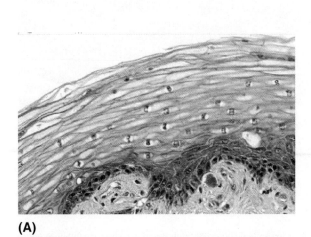

(A)

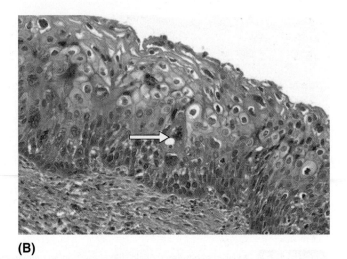

(B)

FIGURE 2-9 **(A)** Comparison of normal, squamous epithelium from exocervix with **(B)** dysplastic cervical epithelium. Note the variation in nuclear size, shape, and polarity. An abnormally dividing cell is also shown (*arrow*).
Courtesy of Department of Pathology and Laboratory Medicine, University of North Carolina at Chapel Hill.

DYSPLASIA

Dysplasia Abnormal maturation of cells.

Nuclear pleomorphism Irregular nuclear structures seen in groups of dysplastic cells.

Neoplasia A form of uncontrolled cell growth that may follow dysplasia and lead to formation of a tumor.

Dysplasia is a condition in which the development and maturation of cells are disturbed and abnormal. The individual cells vary in size and shape, and their relationship to one another is also abnormal. Nuclei differ from cell to cell and may show abnormal structure, termed **nuclear pleomorphism** (**FIGURE 2-9**). Dysplasia of epithelial cells may be associated with chronic irritation or inflammation. In some cases, dysplasia may progress to formation of a tumor; this is called **neoplasia**. The metaplastic epithelium of the uterine cervix is a common site of dysplasia, and cervical epithelial dysplasia sometimes progresses to cervical cancer. This subject is discussed in the female reproductive system.

INCREASED ENZYME SYNTHESIS

Increased synthesis of enzymes is another adaptive change that occurs in cells. Sometimes cells are called on to inactivate or detoxify drugs or chemicals by means of the enzymes present in the smooth endoplasmic reticulum (SER). If increased demands are placed on the cells, they respond by synthesizing more SER enzymes so that drugs or chemicals can be processed more efficiently. After the cells increase their ability to handle such chemicals or drugs, they can rapidly eliminate other substances that are handled by means of the same enzyme systems. A person accustomed to heavy consumption of alcohol, for example, is able to metabolize the alcohol more efficiently because of this adaptive change. Such an individual may also metabolize and eliminate other drugs at a greatly accelerated rate. Consequently, if a physician administers a medication that is metabolized by the same enzyme systems, the usual therapeutic doses of the medications may be ineffective.

Cell Injury, Cell Death, and Cell Necrosis

CELL INJURY

Injury to a cell may be reversible when the injurious agent is removed and normal cell function is restored. For example, cell swelling and fatty change (steatosis) are common morphologic abnormalities demonstrated by injured cells. If the injury

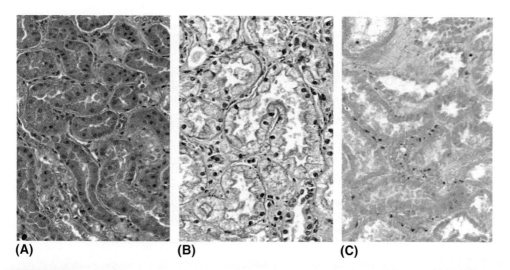

(A) (B) (C)

FIGURE 2-10 Comparison of **(A)** normal, **(B)** swollen (hydropic), and **(C)** necrotic renal tubular epithelial cells. The swollen cells retain normal appearing nuclei, are intact, and remain attached to the underlying basement membrane. The necrotic cells have lost their nuclei and are no longer intact. They show blebbing (formation of small blister) of the cytoplasmic membrane and appear to be detaching from the basement membrane.

Courtesy of Department of Pathology and Laboratory Medicine, University of North Carolina at Chapel Hill.

exceeds the ability of the cell to recover, the cell will die. It is not always easy for a pathologist to determine whether the cellular injury is irreversible. The most certain sign is nuclear damage or loss, but other changes (including the nature of staining) may provide a hint.

Cell Swelling

A normally functioning cell actively transports potassium into the cell and moves sodium out. This process requires the cell to expend energy. If the cell is injured and unable to function normally, the transport mechanism begins to fail. Sodium diffuses into the cell, and water moves into the cell along with the sodium, causing the cell to swell. If the swelling continues, fluid-filled vacuoles may accumulate within the cell, a process sometimes called **hydropic swelling**. The process is potentially reversible if energy production recommences (**FIGURE 2-10A, B**).

Fatty Change

If the enzyme systems that metabolize or export fat are impaired, leading to accumulation of fat droplets within the cytoplasm, fatty change (steatosis) results. This condition is a common manifestation of liver cell injury because liver cells are actively involved in fat metabolism (see Case 2-1).

CELL DEATH AND CELL NECROSIS

A cell dies if it has been irreparably damaged. This often occurs because of a failure in energy production by the cell. All cells ultimately depend on oxidative metabolism for energy production by the mitochondria. In the absence of an oxygen supply to the cell, such as occurs if blood circulation to the tissue is impaired (a process termed **infarction**), the cells in the tissue will die, a process termed **necrosis**. For example, impairment of coronary (heart) blood circulation leads to a myocardial infarct, a "heart attack." Tissues differ in how long they can survive in the absence of an oxygen supply: the brain, minutes; connective tissue, far longer. But ultimately all cells will

Hydropic swelling Cell swelling as a result of excessive water uptake by a cell. Associated with failure of active transport of ions.

Infarction Impaired blood supply to tissue.

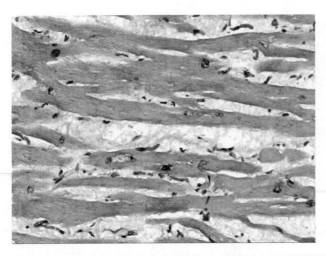

FIGURE 2-11 Cardiac muscle cells from a heart demonstrating chronic lack of oxygen (chronic ischemia). Many muscle fibers show either abnormal, fragmented, or absent nuclei. Compare with normal cardiac muscle cells in Figure 2-7A (same magnification).

Courtesy of Department of Pathology and Laboratory Medicine, University of North Carolina at Chapel Hill.

die without oxygen supplied by blood circulation. Lack of energy production also impairs the "ion pumps" necessary to prevent cellular swelling, resulting in a form of necrosis sometimes termed oncosis (Figure 2-10A, C).

Minutes to hours after the cell dies, various structural changes begin to take place within the nucleus and cytoplasm. Mitochondria undergo a series of shape changes and may have calcium deposited within them. Lysosomal enzymes are released and begin to digest the cell, and the cell membrane may bleb or rupture. The nucleus shrinks and either dissolves or breaks into fragments. With time, visible calcium deposition may occur within the dead tissue. These structural changes are microscopically detectable indicators of **necrosis**. All necrotic cells are dead, but a dead cell does not necessarily appear necrotic because the structural changes that characterize cell death as seen by the pathologist under the microscope take several hours to develop. With time, necrotic cells become easily recognizable on histologic examination because they appear quite different from normal cells in both their structural and their staining characteristics (**FIGURE 2-11**).

PROGRAMMED CELL DEATH: APOPTOSIS

Not all cell death results from cell injury. Cell death may result from a programmed, energy requiring active process that is part of normal organism function. This form of programmed cellular self-destruction is termed **apoptosis**. Contraintuitively, failure of cell death by apoptosis may result in disease because apoptosis is critical for normal development and function. During fetal development, certain body structures form and then disappear (such as webs between fingers and toes). Loss of this "unneeded tissue" is accomplished by apoptosis. The loss of uterine tissue during menstruation is accomplished by apoptosis as a result of changes in hormone balance. Death of virally infected cells may be a result of apoptosis induced in infected cells. Irremediable changes to DNA (mutations) result in the "turning on" of apoptosis within the mutated cell. If this fails, cancer may result. Certain lymphoid cells are programmed to die after a fixed number of divisions; if apoptosis fails, lymphoma (cancer of the lymphatic cells in lymph nodes) will result. Necrosis is "unwanted and unexpected" and is recognized as injury by our host defense systems, provoking a response that may, in itself, be destructive (think of the fever and malaise resulting from a viral or

Necrosis Unprogrammed cell death as a result of injury and the structural changes of cells that result. Often results in a host response.

Apoptosis Programmed cell death that does not provoke a host protective response.

bacterial infection). Apoptosis does not provoke a protective host response. Apoptotic cells neatly form small membrane bound fragments that are not recognized as injurious or foreign by our host defense systems.

Aging and the Cell

All organisms grow old and eventually die, and each species has a predetermined life span. Human life expectancy has increased over the years chiefly because early deaths from infectious diseases, accidents, and other conditions have been greatly reduced; however, the human life span appears constant. Just as humans as a whole have an ultimate life span, so do our cells. Normal cells of humans (and all higher organisms) undergo a fixed number of divisions before they die (called the **Hayflick limit** in honor of the scientist who first noted it). This is related to damage that occurs at the ends of our chromosomes (telomeres) each time they divide. In the absence of an enzyme system (telomerase transcriptase complex), the damage cannot be repaired. When the Hayflick limit is reached, the DNA damage results in the cell undergoing apoptosis. Only cells that serve to continually repopulate organs (stem cells) are immune to this limit. Many cancer cells activate telomerase and hence gain the ability to divide indefinitely. Somewhat surprisingly, the Hayflick limit differs greatly between species and does not correlate well with species life span.

The causes of aging are not well understood but reside within the cells themselves and are likely coded within our genetic material. A variety of mutations in single genes can result in **progerias**, diseases characterized by dramatic and premature aging in which a teenager appears to be elderly and suffers those diseases found in the aged.

The life span of an individual reflects the survival of the various populations of cells that together form the individual. Certain organ systems appear to be particularly susceptible to the effects of aging. Death and debility is often related to disease of the cardiovascular and nervous system. Aging changes in the brain appear to be caused by the wearing out and eventual death of neurons, which are not capable of cell division. The degenerative changes in the walls of arteries, called arteriosclerosis, are thought to be partially caused by a gradual failure of the endothelial cells lining the blood vessels as a result of deposition of lipids into the arterial walls. The common type of arthritis seen in older people involves aging-dependent change in the cartilage covering the ends of the bones. Organ systems containing constantly dividing epithelial cell populations (such as the gut) are particularly prone to cancer as one ages.

As a cell ages, many of its enzyme systems become less active, and the cell becomes less efficient in carrying out its functions. The cell becomes more susceptible to harmful chemical influences such as **reactive oxygen species (ROS)** which can damage and destroy the genetic material, cellular proteins, and the lipids that make up cell membranes. ROS may be the environmental agents or may be products of the cells own mitochondrial metabolism.

Another example of aging change in cells that affects the organism as a whole can be seen in our immune system. The cells of the immune system become less efficient as they age. Consequently, the aging individual becomes more susceptible to various infectious diseases, which can shorten the life span. The aging immune system also may becomes less able to eliminate abnormal cells that arise sporadically within the body, leading to the formation of malignant tumors that occur with increased frequency in the elderly.

In summary, cells have a finite life span. However, the less they are exposed to harmful environmental influences and the more efficient they are in repairing their own malfunctions, the greater their chances for survival to a "ripe old age."

Hayflick limit Fixed number of cell divisions possible for a normal cell.

Progerias Diseases characterized by dramatic and premature aging.

Reactive oxygen species (ROS) Harmful chemicals either environmental or self-produced that can damage cells.

CASE 2-1

A nineteen-year-old female high school senior has been involved in a serious single-driver automobile accident. She is brought into a surgical trauma unit suffering from massive internal bleeding. Attempts to stabilize her prior to surgery are unsuccessful. She suffers from severe hypotension (low blood pressure) and shock and expires. Blood alcohol testing demonstrates that she was legally intoxicated. This is considered to be a likely cause of her accident. The county medical examiner requests an autopsy.

Findings Pertinent to This Case

The decedent was noted to be moderately obese. The cause of internal bleeding was discovered to be multiple sites of injury to major vessels relating to the crush injury of her thorax (chest). The autopsy was otherwise remarkable for the finding of hepatomegaly (hypertrophy of the liver). The liver weighed 2,200 grams (normal about 1,400 grams in a young female) and was noted to be pale and fatty appearing. Histologic investigation of the liver disclosed macrovesicular steatosis, the presence of excess lipid within hepatocytes (cells of liver parenchyma) as large vesicles. Liver cells contained large clear vesicles that displaced the position of the nucleus on routine hematoxylin-eosin (H&E) stained material (tissue processing removes lipid). Frozen tissue sections processed to maintain lipid showed positive staining of the vesicles with a stain for lipids (**FIGURE 2-12**). No other abnormality of the liver was noted.

The decedent's parents were interviewed and stated that their daughter drank large amounts of beer and other alcoholic beverages. This usually occurred as binge drinking during weekends. They estimated that it was common for their daughter to consume five to six cans of beer per day on an average weekend. Neither parent felt this amount to be excessive and denied their daughter was an alcoholic.

Discussion

Steatosis or fatty liver disease (FLD) can occur in the obese as a result of a number of metabolic diseases of the liver or with the ingestion of potentially toxic agents such as some drugs or notably alcohol (ethanol). FLD results when the liver's ability to export fat is lower than the intake of exogenous and/or the production of endogenous lipids. Both decreased export and increased synthesis may occur in alcoholic FLD (AFLD). AFLD is almost always found in heavy drinkers, but even modest consumption of alcohol may result in the condition. Prolonged consumption of modest amounts of alcohol (about 50 grams per day, equivalent to about four twelve-ounce cans of beer) will result in AFLD in more than 40 percent of individuals. There is great individual variation in susceptibility to AFLD (and the more serious consequences of alcohol consumption). Females, the obese, and binge drinkers show much increased risk. Although AFLD is usually asymptomatic and is reversible with abstinence, continued alcohol consumption is likely to lead to serious and irreversible liver disease (cirrhosis see presentation on the liver).

Etiology and Pathogenesis

The etiologic agent is the toxic agent ethanol. Consumption of excess ethanol leads to derangement of liver metabolism and the deposition of lipid within the cells of the liver (alcoholic steatosis or AFLD). With continued consumption, this may progress to alcoholic hepatitis (inflammation of the liver) and alcoholic cirrhosis (scarring of the liver), resulting in hepatic failure and other systemic diseases.

Questions

1. Why are hepatocytes (liver parenchymal cells) particularly susceptible to deposition of lipid within the cells?

2. Why are frozen sections necessary to demonstrate steatosis in the liver?

3. What would have happened to the liver had the individual survived her accident and stopped drinking? What if she continued drinking?

CASE 2-1 (Continued)

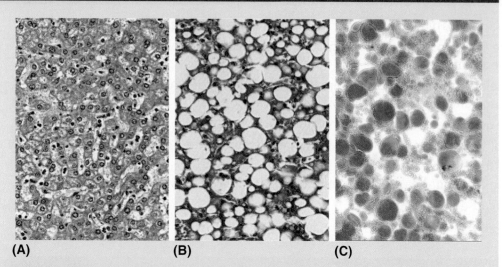

(A) **(B)** **(C)**

FIGURE 2-12 A section of liver from a patient with alcoholic fatty liver disease (AFLD alcoholic steatosis). **(A)** Normal liver, routine processing (stained with hematoxylin-eosin). **(B)** Liver from a patient with AFLD. Routine processing of tissue for staining with hematoxylin-eosin removes lipids leaving clear vesicles. **(C)** A section from the same liver processed to retain lipids (frozen section). The lipids have been stained with a special dye (oil red O).

Courtesy of Department of Pathology and Laboratory Medicine, University of North Carolina at Chapel Hill.

QUESTIONS FOR REVIEW

1. How does the nucleus direct the activities of the cell? What molecules are involved?

2. What are the functions of the following organelles: rough endoplasmic reticulum, ribosomes, lysosomes, and centrioles?

3. How is epithelium classified, and what are its functions? Why are mesothelium and endothelium considered separately from other types of epithelium?

4. What are the germ layers, and what are their functions?

5. What is the difference between atrophy and hypertrophy, between metaplasia and dysplasia, and between cell necrosis and apoptosis?

6. What morphologic abnormalities are manifested by an injured cell? Why do they develop?

7. What factors cause a cell to age?

SUPPLEMENTARY READINGS

Alberts, B., Bray, D., Hopkin, K., et al. 2014. *Essential Cell Biology*. 4th ed. New York: Garland Science, Taylor & Hall.

▶ An excellent and exhaustive primer on cell biology. For all its detail an extremely readable and well-illustrated text.

Chiras, D. D. 2012. *Human Biology*. 7th ed. Sudbury, MA: Jones & Bartlett Learning.

▶ A good overview of human physiology and cell biology. Has an interesting critical approach to current issues in the field.

Reisner, H. M. Ed. 2014. *Pathology: A Modern Case Approach*. New York: McGraw-Hill Professional Lange.

▶ The second chapter provides a detailed overview of cell injury, necrosis, and apoptosis. The text has many additional illustrated cases.

Fairbanks, K. D. 2012. *Alcoholic liver disease*. Cleveland Clinic. http://www.clevelandclinicmeded.com /medicalpubs/diseasemanagement/hepatology/alcoholic-liver-disease/

▶ Must reading for those who make light of excessive drinking. Covers the essentials of alcoholic liver disease and provides references on many additional aspects of alcohol toxicity.

Genes, DNA, Chromosomes, and Cell Division

1. Describe the inheritance pattern of genes and define dominant, recessive, codominant, and sex-linked inheritance.

2. Describe how chromosomes are studied. Explain how a karyotype is determined.

3. Describe the process used by the cells to synthesize a gene product using information contained in the DNA.

4. Describe how cells utilize the genetic code within DNA chains to convey genetic information to daughter cells during cell division.

5. Compare and contrast mitosis and meiosis.

6. Compare and contrast spermatogenesis and oogenesis. Explain the implications of abnormal chromosome separations in the course of meiosis in older women.

Introduction

Transmission of genetic information was initially studied through the analysis of the inheritance of detectable traits (**phenotypic traits**) from parent through successive generations of offspring using **patterns of inheritance**. These phenotypic traits are now understood as the expression of the **genotype** of the individual; that is, the genes that are the functional manifestation of the chemical code of the **DNA** organized in **chromosomes** in the nucleus of the cell. The human **genome** contains about 20,000 genes. The information encoded by those genes in the chromosomes defines the proteins critical to the structure, metabolism, and regulation of all aspects of cellular function. This information is transmitted to each newly formed cell during cell division, either to make two identical **daughter cells** (in the process of **mitosis**) or to form sperm or ovum (**meiosis**). All nongerminal cells of the body are **diploid** (have a 2N chromosome number, 46, arranged as 23 pairs), with one of each pair of chromosomes derived from each parent during fertilization of the ovum by a sperm. Members of a chromosome pair are called **homologous chromosomes**. During the formation of ova and sperm, a **reduction division** results in the formation of a **haploid** (N chromosome number, 23, with no chromosome pairs) that recombines traits from the maternal and paternal chromosome set of the individual. Fertilization restores the diploid chromosome number and produces a unique individual with a mixture of traits derived from the maternal and paternal genome. The genome of the fertilized egg (**zygote**) also contains the blueprint for the development of the new individual,

Phenotype Collection of inherited/phenotypic traits detectable in an individual.

Phenotypic traits Characteristics apparent in the individual.

Pattern of inheritance Inheritance of detectable traits across generations in a family.

Genotype DNA/ chromosome basis of inherited traits in an individual.

DNA Deoxyribonucleaic acid (DNA) is the molecule carrying the coding information for genes.

Chromosome Cell structure organizing the molecules of DNA Individual structural units of DNA which are best seen in dividing cells.

Genome The total of all the genes contained in a cell's chromosomes.

Daughter cell A cell resulting from division of a single cell (called the parent cell).

Mitosis The type of cell division of most cells in which chromosomes are duplicated in the daughter cells and are identical with those in the parent cell. The characteristic cell division found in all cells in the body except for the gametes.

Meiosis A special type of cell division occurring in *gametes* (ova and sperm) in which the number of chromosomes is reduced by one-half.

Diploid Cell containing 2N (pairs) of each chromosome.

Homologous chromosomes A matched pair of chromosomes, one derived from each parent.

Reduction division Process occurring in meiosis reducing the 2N pairs of chromosomes to 1N.

Haploid Cell containing 1N of each chromosome, a gamete.

Zygote Fertilized egg.

Autosomal chromosomes Chromosomes other than sex chromosomes. A human has 22 pairs of autosomes.

Sex chromosomes The X and Y chromosomes that determine genetic sex. A human has 1 pair of sex chromosomes.

the formation of the body plan that defines us as human. In the new individual, 22 of the chromosome pairs consist of **autosomal chromosomes** and one pair are the **sex chromosomes**, an XY pair determining a male, XX a female. The 23 pairs of chromosomes make up the **karyotype**.

Genes and Inheritance Patterns

The alternate forms of a gene found on the maternal and paternal chromosomes pair are called **alleles**. The chromosome site of a given gene is called a **locus**. Different alleles may produce easily detectable differences in the individual (such as eye color), more subtle differences (blood type, or the level of activity of a particular protein detectable only in the laboratory), or differences so subtle as to be undetectable in an individual. Deleterious alleles, the result of inherited alterations in the gene (**mutations**), can result in dysfunction and disease. The inherited differences between alleles at multiple loci (**polymorphisms**) are what define us as individuals and help define populations (which differ in the frequency of particular alleles for many genes). The much misused term "race" represents frequency differences in many polymorphic genes that define populations historically derived from different areas. Such differences are likely to be of evolutionary significance. Populations of African origin have alleles for a number of genes that result in higher levels of skin pigment, which protect against the deleterious effects of solar ultraviolet radiation. Scandinavian populations tend to have alleles resulting in lower levels of skin pigments, perhaps to capture scanty northern solar radiation important in the biosynthesis of vitamin D.

An individual is **homozygous** for a gene if both alleles are the same and **heterozygous** if the alleles are different. Alleles of different genes differ in how they are expressed. A **recessive gene** produces a detectable phenotype only in the homozygous state. An example is the ABO blood group. An individual will have blood type O only if he or she inherited the O allele for the ABO gene from each parent and is homozygous for this allele. A **dominant gene** expresses itself in either the heterozygous or the homozygous state. The A and B alleles of the ABO blood group are dominant. Individuals inheriting either one or two A or B alleles have blood types A and B, respectively. In some cases, there are detectable differences between homozygous or heterozygous expression of a dominant allele. Such **dosage effects** can result in higher levels of expression of a gene product when two doses of a dominant allele are present. Sometimes both alleles of a pair are expressed. Such alleles are called **codominant**. If one A and one B allele is present at the ABO gene locus, the individual has blood type AB, and his or her red cells will have both the A and B substance. Genes carried on sex chromosomes are called **sex-linked genes**; the effects they produce are called **sex-linked traits**. The small Y chromosome carries few genes other than those that direct male sex differentiation, but the much larger X chromosome carries many genes in addition to those concerned with sexual development. Most X-linked traits are recessive. The female carrier of a recessive X-linked trait is usually normal because the effect of the defective allele on one X chromosome is offset by the normal allele on the other X chromosome. The male, however, possesses only one X chromosome. Consequently, he can be neither heterozygous nor homozygous for X-linked genes and is called **hemizygous** for genes carried on the X chromosome. If the male receives an X chromosome containing a defective gene, the defective X-linked gene functions like a dominant gene when paired with the Y chromosome. Such is the case for the well-known disease hemophilia (resulting in excessive bleeding) because the genes responsible for the most common forms of this disease (hemophilia A and hemophilia B) are sex linked. Females who inherit an allele responsible for hemophilia are most often normal because the allele is recessive. They are, however, carriers of the disease. If their offspring inherits the maternal chromosome having the defective hemophilia allele and also the Y chromosome from the male parent, the result is a male child who is hemizygous for the defective allele and has the disease hemophilia. It is of interest to note that female hemophiliacs do occur (although rarely) for reasons to be discussed. The inheritance pattern of genes can be traced through a family tree or **pedigree** (**FIGURE 3-1**). The pattern of appearance of a trait or disease in a pedigree offers clues to the nature of the allele studied (i.e., dominant, recessive, or sex-linked). For example, in the case of dominant inheritance, the trait (disease) is expected to appear in one of the parents of the affected child. In the recessive case, neither parent will be affected (but both will be carriers). In the case of recessive gene transmission, parents are most often related and have the same recessive allele because they share a common ancestor. An example of this is a first-cousin

Karyotype Chromosomes from a single cell arranged in pairs in descending order according to size of the chromosomes and the positions of the centromeres used to visualize the chromosome composition of an individual.

Allele One of several related forms of a single gene.

Locus The position of a gene on a chromosome.

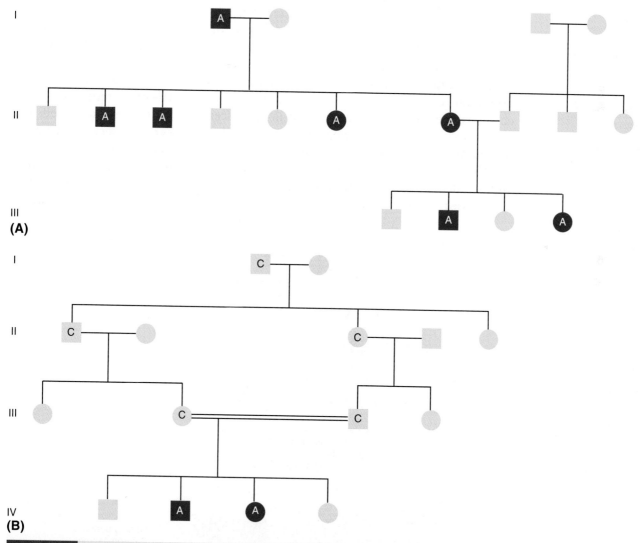

FIGURE 3-1 Examples of family trees (pedigrees) tracing dominant and recessive traits. Pedigrees use standard symbols. Males are shown by squares, females by circles. Matings are indicted by a horizontal line connecting male and female symbols. A double line indicates a mating between related individuals. Offspring of a mating are connected by vertical lines. Each generation of individuals is shown on a horizontal line that is given a Roman numeral. Affected individuals are shown by filled-in symbols (in this example containing an "A"). **(A)** Pedigree for a dominant trait. A parent of each affected individual is also affected. In the example given two nonrelated families intermarry. Only one family expresses the trait. **(B)** Pedigree for a recessive trait. The parents of affected individuals are most often not affected but are each carriers (heterozygous) for the trait. In the case of uncommon traits, the carrier parents are most often related by descent from a shared relative who carried the trait. This example shows a first-cousin marriage. Carriers of the trait are indicated by a "C" within the symbol. Sex-linked pedigrees are discussed in the case at the end of the chapter.

Courtesy of Department of Pathology and Laboratory Medicine, University of North Carolina at Chapel Hill.

Mutation Inherited or somatic alteration in a gene.

Polymorphism Collection of alleles for a single gene.

Homozygous Presence of the same alleles at a given gene loci on the chromosome pair.

Heterozygous Presence of two different alleles at given gene loci on the homologous pair of chromosomes.

Recessive gene A gene that expresses a trait only when present in the homozygous state.

Dominant gene A gene that expresses a trait in the heterozygous state.

Dosage effects Differing amounts of gene product in the heterozygous and homozygous states.

Codominant gene Products of both genes are expressed in the heterozygous state.

Sex-linked gene Gene present on the X or Y chromosome.

Sex-linked trait Product of gene present on X or Y chromosome.

Hemizygous A term applied to genes located on the X chromosome in the male.

Pedigree Formal pattern displaying the inheritance of traits or gene products through generations of a family.

Aneuploidy Condition of having extra or missing chromosomes.

Heterochromatin Small dense mass of condensed chromatin appearing in inactivated X chromosomes.

marriage. Sex-linked (recessive) traits appear only in males. Fathers are not affected (they donate their normal Y chromosome to their male offspring) but male uncles or grandfathers are likely to show the trait.

X CHROMOSOME INACTIVATION: THE LYON HYPOTHESIS

Having the proper number of chromosomes is critical to normal human development. Defects in the number of chromosomes, having extra or missing chromosomes (**aneuploidy**), is always associated with disease and often fatal prior to birth. In normal individuals, all autosomal chromosomes occur in pairs. This is not the case with sex chromosomes: females who are XX appear to have twice the X chromosomal DNA of XY males. Female cells, however, function as though they contained only genetic material equivalent to that of the single X chromosome of the male. The reason for this behavior is that almost all of one of the X chromosomes is inactivated and nonfunctional. In the female, the genetic activity of both X chromosomes is essential only during the first week of embryonic development. Thereafter, one of the X chromosomes in each of the developing cells is inactivated. With only rare exceptions, the inactivation occurs in a random manner (**FIGURE 3-2**). After the initial inactivation of an X chromosome has occurred, the same paternal- or maternal-derived X chromosome will also be inactivated in all descendants of the precursor cell. The inactivated X chromosome appears as a small, dense mass of condensed chromatin (**heterochromatin**) attached to the nuclear membrane of somatic cells.

The inactivated X chromosome can be identified in the cells of a normal female and is called a sex chromatin body, or **Barr body**, after the man who first described it. Because the inactivation occurs at random, females are a **mosaic** for genes that are

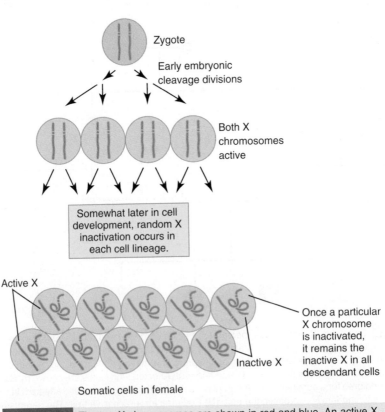

FIGURE 3-2 The two X chromosomes are shown in red and blue. An active X is depicted as a straight chromosome, an inactive X as a tangle. Each cell has just one active X. The particular X that remains active is a matter of chance, but it remains active in the progeny of that cell.

sex linked. If a female is heterozygous for a sex-linked gene (which has an "A" allele and a "B" allele), about half the cells in the women would be expected to express A and half B. The situation is actually more complex and is further described in the Case 3-1 and in later sections dealing with X-linked genetic diseases.

CHROMOSOME ANALYSIS

The chromosome composition (karyotype) of a human can be studied with great accuracy to determine the presence of abnormalities in chromosome number or structure. This is accomplished by using a drug to arrest dividing cells (usually from the blood) at a stage in which the chromosomes are condensed and have become separate and distinct. The complex structure of the chromosomes in such cells can be established by using special stains that allow microscopic visualization of the details of chromosome structure or by using a molecular biological technique that identifies specific regions of chromosomes using **fluorescent probes**, a technique termed "chromosome painting."

Artificially synthesized stretches of DNA that bind (hybridize) to specific chromosomes are linked to a series of fluorescent dyes in order to identify chromosomes by color. **FIGURE 3-3** illustrates the appearance of a cell arrested in mitosis with the chromosomes well separated. A normal dividing cell arrested in mitosis contains 46 chromosomes, each consisting of two chromatids joined at their centromeres. Each chromosome has its own unique structure and is classified according to size, the location of the centromere, the relative lengths of the chromatids that extend outward from the centromere (called the arms of the chromosome), and the pattern of light and dark bands along the chromosome. The separated chromosomes from a single cell are photographed and arranged in pairs in a standard pattern called a karyotype. **FIGURE 3-4** illustrates a karyotype produced using the technique of chromosome painting. Each pair of chromosomes is "painted" a specific color using a fluorescent probes.

Barr body The inactivated X chromosome attached to the nuclear membrane in the female. Sex chromatin body.

Genetic mosaic Condition of having different genes inactivated at random on the X chromosome.

Fluorescent probes Artificial pieces of DNA labeled with a dye.

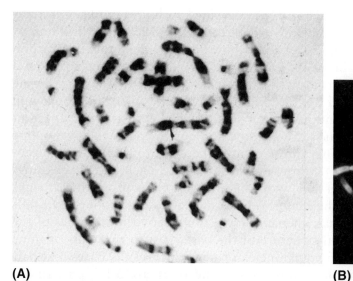
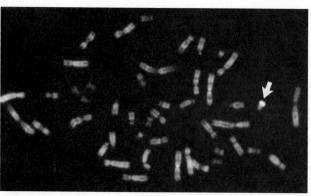

(A)   **(B)**

FIGURE 3-3 The appearance of chromosomes from a single cell arrested in mitosis, illustrating the banded pattern that facilitates the identification of individual chromosomes. The two chromatids composing each chromosome lie side by side. **(A)** Giemsa stain (photograph courtesy of Dr. Jorge Yunis). **(B)** Fluorescent stain showing intensely stained (*arrow*) Y chromosome (photograph courtesy of Patricia Crowley-Larsen).

Courtesy of Leonard V. Crowley, MD, Century College.

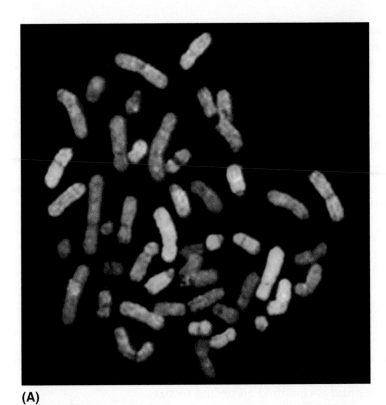

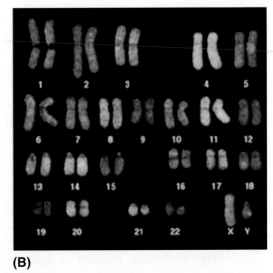

(A)

(B)

FIGURE 3-4 Result of human chromosome painting in which each pair of chromosomes is stained a different color by hybridizing with a specific fluorescent probe. **(A)** The appearance of stained chromosomes from a single cell arrested in mitosis. Each pair can be identified by both structure and color. **(B)** A karyotype in which the chromosomes have been grouped in pairs and arranged in a conventional order depending in part on size.

The Structure of DNA in the Chromosomes

Genetic code The information carried by DNA molecules in chromosomes. The DNA basis of the phenotype/genotype.

Nucleotide Basic structural unit of DNA consisting of a phosphate group linked to a five-carbon sugar, deoxyribose or ribose, which is linked to a nitrogen-containing compound called a base, either purine or pyrimidine.

The chromosomes are composed of DNA combined with protein. The information on the DNA is referred to as the **genetic code**. The basic structural unit of DNA, called a **nucleotide**, consists of a phosphate group linked to a five-carbon sugar, deoxyribose, which in turn is joined to a nitrogen-containing compound called a base (**FIGURE 3-5**). There are two different types of DNA bases: a purine base, which contains a fused double ring of carbon and nitrogen atoms, and a pyrimidine base, which contains only a single ring. There are four different bases in DNA: the purine bases are adenine and guanine, and the pyrimidine bases are thymine and cytosine. Consequently, there are four different nucleotides in DNA, each containing a different base (**FIGURE 3-6A, B**). The nucleotides are joined together in long chains, with the nitrogen bases projecting at right angles from the long axes of the chains. A DNA molecule consists of two strands of DNA held together by weak chemical attractions between the bases of the adjacent chains. The chemical structure of the bases is such that only adenine can pair with thymine and only guanine can pair with cytosine. Bases that pair in this way are called complementary bases, and there are 3 billion pairs of complementary bases (base pairs) in the human genome. However, less than 2 percent of the base pairs code for proteins. The DNA chains are twisted into a double spiral somewhat like a spiral staircase, with the sugar and phosphate groups forming the two railings and the complementary base pairs forming the steps (**FIGURE 3-6B, C**).

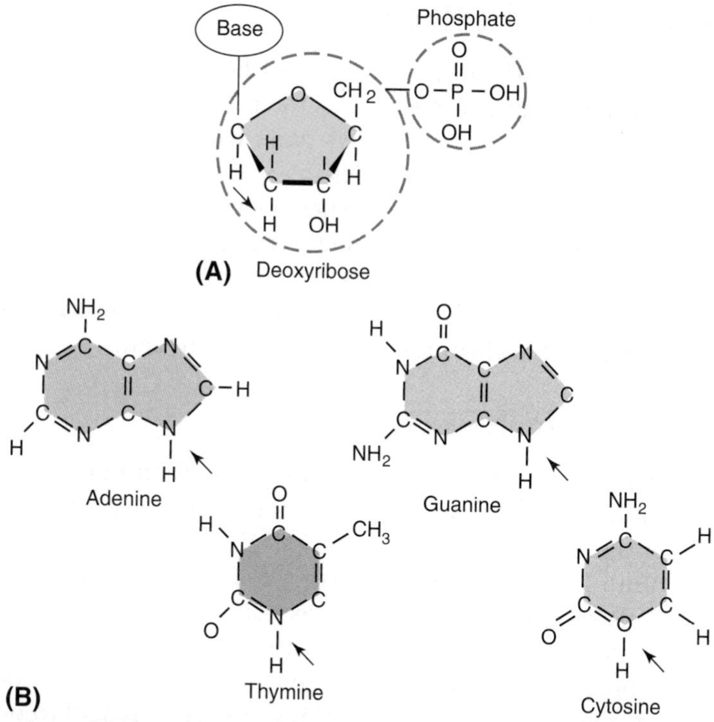

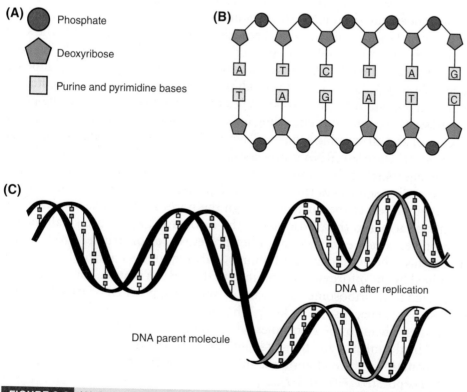

FIGURE 3-5 General structure of DNA nucleotide. **(A)** Deoxyribose is identical with ribose except for the absence of an oxygen atom (site of missing oxygen indicated by *arrow*). **(B)** Structure of the bases showing sites (*arrows*) at which bases are joined to deoxyribose.

FIGURE 3-6 **(A)** Components entering into the formation of DNA molecule. **(B)** Structure of double stranded DNA. **(C)** Duplication (replication) of DNA molecule.

Semiconservative replication Production of duplicating DNA strands using complementary strands as a guide.

Codon Triplet of bases coding for one piece of information or for one amino acid.

Degenerate code Condition in which each amino acid has many different codons.

Messenger RNA (mRNA) Molecule encoding information from DNA to the ribosomes. Similar to DNA but single-stranded and contains ribose rather than deoxyribose.

Transcription Process of copying information from DNA to mRNA.

Complementary The relationship between the base sequence of the two strands in a DNA molecule. During DNA replication, either strand can make an exact copy of the other. Complementary DNA strands bind to each other by base pairing.

Exon The part of a chromosomal DNA chain that codes for a specific protein or enzyme.

Intron A noncoding part of a chromosomal DNA chain.

Transfer RNA (tRNA) RNA molecule that "picks up" appropriate amino acid to build the gene product.

Translation Process of building a gene product using information from the mRNA.

Anticodon Code complementary to the codon on the mRNA, which allows the correct amino acid to be deposited by the tRNA.

DUPLICATION (REPLICATION) OF DNA

As a cell prepares to divide, the double strands of DNA duplicate themselves. The two chains separate, and each chain serves as the model for the synthesis of a new chain (Figure 3-6C). Because adenine always pairs with thymine and guanine with cytosine, the arrangement of the nucleotides in the original chains determines how the nucleotides will reassemble to form the new chains. The process of duplication (**semiconservative replication**) forms two double complementary strands, each containing one of the original strands plus a newly formed strand. In this way, each of the two daughter cells produced by cell division receives an exact duplicate of the genetic information possessed by the chromosomes of the parent cell.

TRANSLATION OF DNA INTO PROTEINS

The DNA in the nucleus directs the synthesis of enzymes and other proteins by the ribosomes located in the cytoplasm. The information is coded into the DNA as a series of three contiguous bases (a triplet) in a DNA strand. The triplet of bases defines a **codon**. With four bases there are sixty four possible unique codons. One codon is a "start" instruction, three codons are stop (termination) instructions, and the remaining sixty codons each specify one of the amino acids that form the building blocks for the proteins expressed by the gene. There are more codons than the twenty amino acids that are coded for in DNA, so the code is said to be **degenerate**; several different codons specify the same amino acid. The "instructions" are carried by **messenger RNA (mRNA)**, so named because it carries the message encoded in the DNA to the ribosomes in the cytoplasm. Messenger RNA is quite similar to DNA but consists of only a single rather than a double strand. It also differs by containing the five-carbon sugar ribose instead of deoxyribose and a base called uracil instead of thymine. During synthesis of mRNA, the DNA chains partially separate, and the DNA serves as the model on which the mRNA is assembled. Therefore, the information **transcribed** into the mRNA strand is an exact **complement** of the genetic information possessed by the nuclear DNA because the mRNA is composed of the sequence ribose bases that are complementary to the sequence of DNA bases being copied.

At this stage the mRNA is in a precursor form (termed pre-mRNA). Before the pre-mRNA leaves the nucleus, it is modified by a number of processing steps. Most genes do not contain continuous stretches of information coding for the protein to be expressed. The information coding for functional proteins (**exons**) is separated by stretches of an "intervening sequence" (**introns**) that does not code for the expressed gene product. The pre-mRNA is processed by removal of the RNA coding for introns and splicing together the exons to produce a mature mRNA molecule containing only the coding sequences that specify the protein to be constructed. The mature mRNA strand leaves the nucleus through the pores in the nuclear membrane and becomes attached to the ribosomes in the cytoplasm, which are small nucleoprotein particles where enzymes and other proteins are constructed from individual amino acids. The combination of amino acids required to assemble the protein is determined by the information contained in the mRNA strand. The amino acids are transported to the ribosomes by means of another type of RNA called **transfer RNA (tRNA)**, so named because it "picks up" the required amino acids from the cytoplasm and transfers them to the ribosomes where they are assembled in proper order, as specified by the mRNA and **translated** into protein. The tRNA contains an **anticodon** complementary to the codon on the mRNA, which ensures that the correct amino acid is incorporated (**FIGURE 3-7**).

In addition to mRNA, tRNA, and the RNAs that form part of the structure of ribosomes, there are several classes of regulatory RNAs that control how certain

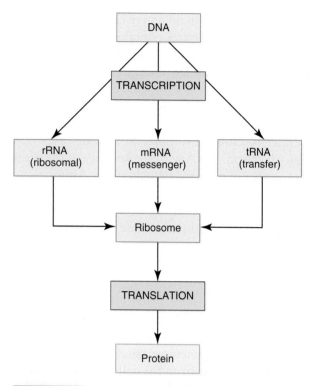

FIGURE 3-7 The central dogma of molecular genetics. DNA codes for RNA. RNA codes for protein. The DNA to RNA step is transcription. The RNA to protein step is translation and occurs on the ribosome.

genes are expressed. **MicroRNAs (miRNAs)**, so called because they are smaller than other RNA molecules, have the function of regulating the activity of groups of genes sharing certain common sequences. MiRNAs pair with the target mRNAs that have complementary sequences to "silence" them by blocking expression. About 500 different miRNA molecules have been described, each regulating the activity of a specific group of genes. In addition, there are sequences of DNA that regulate the expression of known genes and sequences whose function is currently unknown.

MicroRNA (miRNAs) Small RNA molecules that regulate the activity of sets of individual genes.

MITOCHONDRIAL GENES AND INHERITANCE

Chromosomes are not the only site where genes are located in the cell. Mitochondria (described in the chapter on cells and tissues), the site of oxidative metabolism and ATP generation in the cell, also have small amounts of DNA containing some of the genes required for synthesis of energy-generating mitochondrial proteins. The DNA in mitochondria is circular and has several similarities to the DNA found in bacteria. These similarities have led to the suggestion that mitochondria derived during evolution from trapped bacteria.

Although most of the genes involved in ATP synthesis are located on the chromosomes in the cell nuclei and are inherited like other genes, some of the ATP-generating components are coded as mitochondrial genes and are inherited differently from those on chromosomes. As mitochondria wear out, other mitochondria divide to replace them. Mutations occur frequently as the mitochondrial DNA duplicates (replicates). Because there are several mitochondrial DNA molecules in each mitochondrion and several hundred mitochondria in an active cell, a cell may contain a mixture of normal mitochondria and mitochondria containing mutated DNA. Mitochondrial DNA mutations do not affect cell function unless there are such a large number of mitochondrial DNA mutations that the energy-generating capability of the cells is impaired.

The human ovum contains a very large number of mitochondria, but sperm contain very few. Consequently, transmission of abnormal mitochondrial DNA is almost invariably from mother to child. A number of rare diseases result from inherited abnormalities of mitochondrial DNA with the severity of the disease manifestations related in part to the number of mutated mitochondria. Although mitochondrial DNA is not unique to an individual, mitochondrial DNA has proven useful in identifying the relationship of an individual to a family. Because there are multiple copies of the mitochondrial genome in cells, useful samples are often obtainable from decomposed or skeletal remains.

Cell Division

There are two types of cell division. Mitosis is characteristic of somatic cells. Meiosis is a specialized type of cell division that occurs during the development of the eggs (ova) and sperm, a process called **gametogenesis**. In mitosis, each of the two new cells (called the daughter cells) resulting from the cell division receives the same number of chromosomes that were present in the precursor cell (called the parent cell). In meiosis, the number of chromosomes is reduced so that the daughter cells receive only half of the chromosomes possessed by the parent cell.

MITOSIS

Mitosis is characteristic of somatic cells, but not all mature cells are able to divide. Some mature cells, such as cardiac muscle cells and nerve cells, do not divide. Others, such as connective tissue cells and liver cells, divide as needed to replace lost or damaged cells or to heal an injury. Yet others divide continually, such as those lining the digestive tract and those in the bone marrow that continually replace the circulating cells in the bloodstream. Regardless of the frequency of cell division, the rate of cell division is controlled closely to match the body's needs, and excess cells are not normally produced.

Many factors regulate cell growth and cell division. Often the stimulus that induces a cell to divide does not originate within the cell itself but comes from other cells. Various soluble growth-promoting substances called **growth factors** are secreted by neighboring cells and bind to receptors on the cell membrane of the target cell, which activates the receptors. The activated receptors in turn transmit biochemical signals to the "machinery" inside the cell, which induces the cell to divide. Genes within the cell also play an important role. Some promote cell growth by directing the production of the receptors on the cell surface to which the growth factors can attach. Other genes generate inhibitory signals that suppress cell growth and division. Depending on the signals, either the cell is induced to grow and divide or its growth is inhibited. These intracellular communications allow normal cells to divide often enough to accomplish their functions and to replenish cell losses from injury or normal aging but restrain excessive proliferation. Moreover, normal cells cannot continue to divide indefinitely. They are programmed to undergo a limited number of cell divisions, and then they die. Defects in the regulation of cell division can occur and result in the process of **neoplasia** (dysregulated cell growth), which ultimately may result in cancer.

Gametogenesis The development of mature eggs and sperm from precursor cells.

Growth factor A soluble growth promoting substance produced by cells that attaches to receptors on the cell membrane of other cells, which activates the receptors and initiates events leading to growth or division of the target cells.

Neoplasia Dysregulated cell growth possibly leading to the development of cancer.

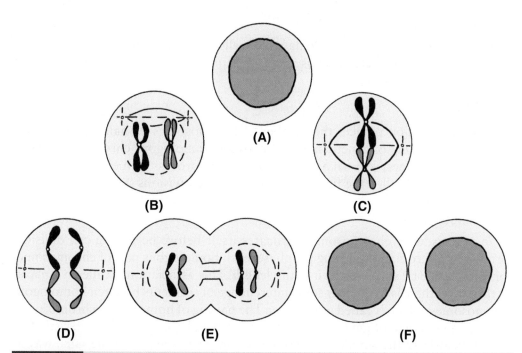

FIGURE 3-8 Stages of mitosis. The behavior of only one pair of homologous chromosomes is shown. **(A)** Prior to cell division. **(B)** Prophase. **(C)** Metaphase. **(D)** Anaphase. **(E)** Telophase. **(F)** Daughter cells resulting from mitosis, each identical to the parent cell.

Before a cell begins mitosis, its DNA chains are duplicated to form new chromosome material (the s phase prior to cell division). Each chromosome and its newly duplicated counterpart lie side by side. The two members of the pair are called **chromatids**. Mitosis is the process by which chromatids separate. (The use of the terms chromosomes and chromatids may at times be confusing. Each chromosome duplicates itself before beginning cell division. Because there are normally 46 chromosomes in each somatic cell, just prior to cell division there are actually the equivalent of 92 chromosomes in the cell [i.e., 46 × 2]. When the chromosomes condense in the course of cell division, each chromosome consists of two separate chromosomes still partially joined where the **spindle fibers** attach. The term chromatids is applied to the still-joined chromosomes at this stage. As soon as they separate, they are again called chromosomes.)

Mitosis is divided into four stages (**FIGURE 3-8**): prophase, metaphase, anaphase, and telophase.

Prophase

Each chromosome thickens and shortens. The **centrioles** migrate to opposite poles of the cell and form the mitotic spindle, which consists of small fibers radiating in all directions from the centrioles. Some of these spindle fibers attach to the chromatids. The nuclear membrane breaks down toward the end of prophase.

Metaphase

The chromosomes line up in the center of the cell. At this stage, the chromatids are partially separated but still remain joined at a constricted area called the **centromere**, which is the site where the spindle fibers are attached.

Anaphase

The chromatids constituting each chromosome separate to form individual chromosomes, which are pulled to opposite poles of the cell by the spindle fibers.

Chromatid One of two newly formed chromosomes held together by the centromere.

Spindle fibers The structure critical for proper alignment and separation of chromosomes during mitosis and meiosis.

Centromere/centriole The structure that joins each pair of chromatids formed by chromosome duplication.

Telophase

The nuclear membranes of the two daughter cells reform and the cytoplasm divides, forming two daughter cells. Each is an exact duplicate of the parent cell.

MEIOSIS

Meiotic cell division reduces the number of chromosomes by half and also leads to some intermixing of genetic material between homologous chromosomes via a **recombination** process known as **crossing over**. The process of meiosis entails two separate divisions called the first and second meiotic divisions (**FIGURE 3-9**).

First Meiotic Division

As in mitosis, each chromosome duplicates itself before beginning cell division, forming two chromatids. During prophase, each homologous pair of chromosomes come to lie side by side over their entire length. This association is called a **synapse**. At this stage, there is frequently some interchange of segments between homologous chromosomes, which is called a crossover. The pairing of homologous chromosomes and the interchange of genetic material during prophase is the characteristic feature of meiosis. In the female, the two X chromosomes synapse in the same way as autosomes, but in the male, the X and Y chromosomes synapse end to end and do not exchange segments. Rates of crossing over are greater in females than in males.

Recombination/ crossover Interchange of genetic material between homologous chromosomes during synapse and meiosis. Recombination between genes can be observed.

Synapse Pairing of homologous chromosomes in meiosis.

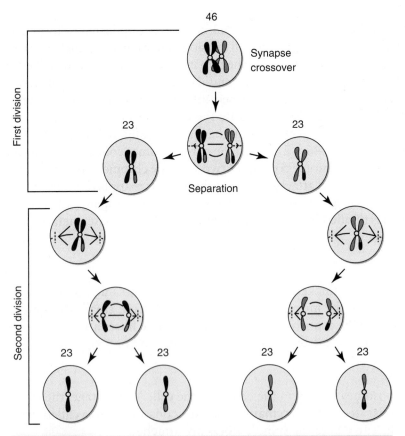

FIGURE 3-9 Stages of meiosis. The behavior of only one pair of homologous chromosomes is indicated. In the first meiotic division, each daughter cell receives only one member of each homologous pair, and the chromosomes are not exact duplicates of those in the parent cell. The second meiotic division is like a mitotic division, but each cell contains only 23 chromosomes.

In metaphase, the paired chromosomes become arranged in a plane within the middle of the cell. During anaphase, the homologous chromosomes separate and move to opposite poles of the cell. Each chromosome consists of two chromatids, but they do not separate at this stage. In telophase, two new daughter cells are formed. Each daughter cell contains only one member of each homologous pair of chromosomes; consequently, the chromosomes in each daughter cell are reduced by half. The chromosomes in the daughter cells are also different from those in the parent cell because of the interchange of genetic material during synapse.

Second Meiotic Division

The second meiotic division is similar to a mitotic division. The two chromatids composing each chromosome separate and two new daughter cells are formed, each containing half of the normal number of chromosomes.

Gametogenesis

The testes and ovaries, called **gonads**, contain precursor cells called germ cells, which are capable of developing into mature sperm or ova. The mature germ cells are called **gametes**, and the process by which they are formed is gametogenesis. The development of sperm (spermatogenesis) and of ova (oogenesis) is similar in many respects (**FIGURE 3-10**).

Gonad A general term referring to either the ovary or the testis.

Gametes Reproductive cells, eggs, and sperm, each containing 23 chromosomes, which unite during fertilization to form a zygote containing 46 chromosomes.

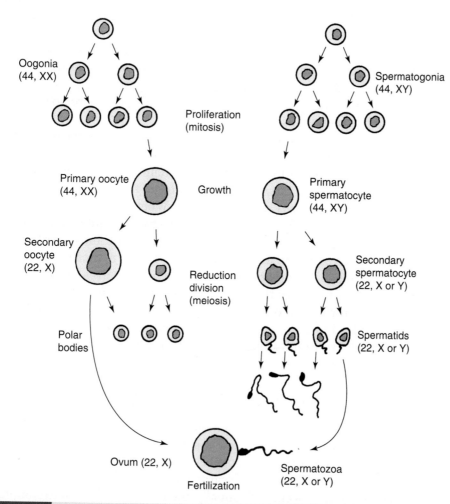

FIGURE 3-10 Sequence of events in gametogenesis. The numbers and letters in parentheses refer to the chromosomes in the cell. Numbers indicate autosomes; letters designate sex chromosomes.

SPERMATOGENESIS

The precursor cells in the testicular tubules are called **spermatogonia** (singular, spermatogonium). Each contains a full complement of 46 chromosomes. Spermatogonia divide by mitosis to form primary **spermatocytes**, which, like the precursor cells, contain 46 chromosomes. The primary spermatocytes then divide by meiosis. In the first meiotic division, each primary spermatocyte forms two secondary spermatocytes, each containing 23 chromosomes. Each secondary spermatocyte completes the second meiotic division and forms two **spermatids**, also containing 23 chromosomes, and the spermatids mature into sperm. The entire process of spermatogenesis takes about two months, and sperm are being produced continually after sexual maturity is reached.

OOGENESIS

The precursors of the ova are called **oogonia** (singular, oogonium). Each contains 46 chromosomes. Oogonia divide repeatedly in the fetal ovaries before birth, forming primary **oocytes**, which contain 46 chromosomes. The oocytes then become surrounded by a single layer of cells called **granulosa cells**, or follicular cells, forming structures called primary follicles. The primary oocytes in the follicles begin the prophase of the first meiotic division during fetal life but do not carry the division through to completion. A very large number of primary follicles are formed, but many of them degenerate during infancy and childhood. Up to 20 percent of oocytes show defects in chromosome complement (aneuploidy) and are likely to represent the degenerating population. However, about half a million of the primary follicles persist into adolescence, and the loss continues throughout the woman's reproductive years. During each reproductive cycle, several oocytes begin to mature; however, usually only one is ovulated, and the others degenerate. At menopause, only a few thousand oocytes remain, and the decline continues until, eventually, there are no oocytes left in the ovaries of a postmenopausal woman.

The ovaries with their contained primary follicles remain inactive until puberty. Then cyclic ovulation begins under the influence of the **pituitary gonadotrophic hormones**, follicle-stimulating hormone (FSH), and luteinizing hormone (LH). During each menstrual cycle, a number of primary follicles begin to grow, but normally only one follicle comes to full maturity and is ovulated. When the oocyte is discharged, it completes its first meiotic division and gives rise to two daughter cells, which are unequal in size. One daughter cell, which receives half of the chromosomes (one member of each homologous pair) and almost all of the cytoplasm, is called a secondary oocyte (23 chromosomes). The other daughter cell, which receives the remaining 23 chromosomes but almost none of the cytoplasm, is called the first **polar body** and is discarded. The newly formed secondary oocyte promptly begins its second meiotic division, which will lead to the formation of the mature ovum and a second polar body, each containing 23 chromosomes. The meiotic division is not completed, however, unless the ovum is fertilized.

COMPARISON OF SPERMATOGENESIS AND OOGENESIS

Spermatogenesis and oogenesis have two major differences. First, four spermatozoa are produced from each precursor cell in spermatogenesis, but only one ovum is formed from each precursor cell in oogenesis. The other three "daughter cells" derived from the meiotic divisions are discarded as polar bodies.

Second, spermatogenesis occurs continually and is carried through to completion in about two months. Consequently, seminal fluid always contains relatively "fresh" sperm. In contrast, the oocytes are not produced continually. All of the oocytes present

---

Spermatogonia Precursor cells of sperm.

Spermatocytes Precursor cells to sperm formed by mitotic division of spermatogonia.

Spermatids Germ cells in a late stage of sperm development just before complete maturation to form mature sperm. *Spermatogonia* and *spermatocytes* are terms for an earlier stage.

Oogonia Precursor cells of oocyte.

Oocyte Germ cells in a late stage of egg development.

Granulosa cells Cells lining the ovarian follicles.

Pituitary gonadotrophic hormones Hormones controlling cyclic ovulation.

Polar body Structure extruded during the meiosis of the oocyte. Contains discarded chromosomes and a small amount of cytoplasm.

in the ovary were formed before birth and have remained in a prolonged prophase of the first meiotic division from fetal life until they are ovulated. This may be why congenital abnormalities that result from abnormal separation of chromosomes in the course of gametogenesis are more frequent in older women. The ova released late in a woman's reproductive life have been held in prophase for as long as forty-five years before they finally resume meiosis at the time of ovulation. If the chromosomes do not separate normally in meiosis, an ovum may end up with either an excess or a deficiency of chromosomes. If the abnormal ovum is fertilized, a fetus that has an abnormal number of chromosomes may be conceived. This subject is considered in the discussion on congenital and hereditary diseases.

New Research on Genes

Starting with the Human Genome Project in 1990, tremendous strides have been made in our ability to determine the entire sequence of DNA in individuals. Currently, limited regions of the genome of individuals are sequenced using automated technology on a routine basis to obtain information for clinical diagnosis of disease and as an aid in selecting therapies. Major medical centers are beginning to routinely sequence multiple genes in individuals with a variety of cancers to determine genetic lesions involved in the causation and progress of the disease. This has led to the concept of personalized therapy in which specific drugs are matched to defects in genes responsible for particular diseases (so-called drugable genes). As previously noted, defects in growth factors and receptors may lead to unregulated cell growth and cancer. In many cases, the specific defect in the genome (mutation) responsible for unregulated growth may be determined by sequencing, and, in some cases, drugs have been tailored to inhibit the defect and slow down (although not cure) the disease. Differences in how individuals respond to drugs are often related to variation in specific genes in the genome. Technology exists to detect those differences and tailor drug therapy to prevent inappropriate dosing, which can result in dangerous drug reactions.

Although still somewhat costly and time consuming, the sequence of all expressed genes (the **exome**) or even the 3 billion base pairs of a single individual, can be determined. This has led to massive databases available for study and to the development of the study of **bioinformatics**. Bioinformatics as applied to studies of the human genome (**genomics** is a commonly used term for such) involves complex mathematical comparisons between data from the genome of many individuals to find base sequences that may be associated with the susceptibility to disease (or to resistance to particular diseases). Obviously, such information can be used for the prognosis, early therapy, or, potentially, the prevention of diseases in the human population.

> **Exome** The set of all expressed genes.
>
> **Bioinformatics** Massive databases used for the study of the human genome.
>
> **Genomics** Bioinformatic techniques applied to studies of human genome.

SINGLE NUCLEOTIDE POLYMORPHISMS

The sequence of base pairs in the human genome is about 99.9 percent identical between humans. (In comparison, we differ from our closest primate cousin by about 4 percent.) At the gross level, human genomes appear to be nearly identical. However, the remaining 0.1 percent of 3 billion base pairs means that average humans differ in about 3 million base pairs. In fact, as is familiar to all from popular media productions involving the science of forensics, no two individuals have exactly the same genome except identical twins. Determination of identity does not require complex sequencing of the genome because particular regions of DNA show great variation. Simple technology allows rapid typing of individual DNA samples (from body fluids or tissue such as hair) in a manner somewhat analogous to blood typing.

Single nucleotide polymorphisms (SNPs) Minor variations in the nucleotides contained in the individual genes of different individuals.

Genomewide association studies (GWAS) Process using tests of many SNPs to identify genes associated with particular diseases or traits.

Recombinant DNA technology/genetic engineering/gene splicing Methods for combining a gene from one organism, such as a gene specifying insulin synthesis, with genes from another organism, such as a bacterium.

Expression vector A set of DNA sequences necessary for the expression of a foreign gene in an organism. Often engineered to promote high levels of production of the gene product.

Monoclonal antibodies Antibodies of a unique specificity for use in treating human disease, produced in tissue culture.

Many of the minor variations in the nucleotides contained in the individual genes of different individuals may or may not have direct significance. These variations are called **single nucleotide polymorphisms (SNPs)**, usually pronounced "snips." Some SNPs may affect how the gene functions, such as how rapidly a cell enzyme inactivates a drug or environmental toxin or repairs damage to cell DNA. Genes in individuals within specific groups having risk factors for some disease or condition can be analyzed (constructing a "gene profile") to see if there is a correlation with particular SNPs. Although some SNPs lie within genes and may directly affect how a gene functions, many SNPs occur in the 98 percent of the genome that does not contain genes expressing a protein product. Such SNPs are important because their position within the genome is known and also because they easily can be typed without the need for direct DNA sequencing. This has allowed for the ever-increasing use of **genomewide association studies (GWAS)** to identify genes associated with particular diseases or traits. In such studies, the frequency of a very large number of SNPs spread across the entire genome is compared between a population with the particular condition or disease and a control population without the disease. Statistical studies are undertaken to see if the presence of particular SNPs correlates with the presence (or absence) of the disease in question. Because the position of the SNPs in the genome is known, an association suggests areas of the genome (or particular genes) that are associated with the condition. GWAS are particularly useful in studying complex chronic conditions such as heart disease and neuropsychiatric disorders that may be associated with differences in multiple genes found in different areas of the genome.

GENES AND RECOMBINANT DNA TECHNOLOGY (GENETIC ENGINEERING)

Overuse of terms such as **recombinant DNA technology** (because genes from two different sources are being recombined in a single unit), **genetic engineering** (because genes are being manipulated), or **gene splicing** (because genetic material is being reassembled in a given order) have made them both difficult to define and of limited utility. At its heart genetic engineering involves the techniques used to manipulate how and where individual genes and their products are expressed and to modify such genes to produce products of desired characteristics. The initial stages of the technology involved understanding how bacterial genes and their products could be manipulated. Currently gene products derived from viruses, bacteria, fungi and higher organisms can be manipulated to be expressed in essentially any host cell desired. When the product is to be used for human therapy (such as human growth factors, or proteins involved in coagulation used to treat deficiency diseases), the source of the gene coding for the product is most often human. This is inserted into an **expression vector**, a cassette of DNA sequences necessary for expression of the gene, which in turn is introduced into a mammalian cell grown in culture for expression. Both the gene and the expression vector are optimized to result in high levels of expression and increased stability of the desired product, which optimally will be secreted into the medium in which the mammalian cells are growing. An exception to the use of human genes is in the production of antibodies of a unique specificity (**monoclonal antibodies**) for use in treating human disease. Very often the gene may be derived from a mouse immunized to produce the desired antibody. A common example are antibodies to human inflammatory proteins used to treat diseases such as rheumatoid arthritis (which results in chronic joint inflammation). Because the use of animal proteins in a human may result in a serious immunological reaction, the mouse genes are altered to make them more "humanlike" before they are expressed.

It is also possible to introduce genes into living organisms or to control the expression of genes in an organism. Although news accounts of animals made to "glow" by the introduction fluorescent proteins trivialize this still difficult technique, the approach could be used to cure diseases associated with the deficiency of a protein related to a genetic mutation (so-called **gene therapy**). A prime example of this would be the introduction of the gene for a clotting factor into an individual with hemophilia. The area is complex and still lacks notable success. There are obvious problems with this approach;

1. One must identify and select the correct gene to insert into the cell.
2. One must choose the proper cell to receive the gene.
3. One must select an efficient means of getting the gene into the cell.
4. One must ensure that the newly inserted gene can function effectively long enough within the cell to make the therapy worthwhile and doesn't disrupt other important cell functions.

The gene may be expressed in a small segment of DNA that does not become a permanent part of the genome (and tends to be lost with time), or it may be integrated into the chromosome much as some viral DNAs to become part of the human genome. As can be imagined, insertion of DNA into the genome at random can have serious consequences by interrupting the synthesis of other genes. In summary, although many of the pieces of this technology are present, putting the pieces together for successful human therapy remains to be achieved.

Proposed gene therapy in humans targets somatic cells, not the germ cells that produce eggs and sperm. Gene therapy directed at germ cells is currently not considered to be feasible, ethical, or desirable. However, related technology has been used with great success to "knock out" genes in animals (most often mice and pigs) in such a way as to modify the animal's germ cells to produce animal strains that can be bred as models of particular human diseases. For example, there are strains of mice that exhibit "human hemophilia" and can be used as a model in studies of gene therapy.

An often ignored aspect of genetic engineering is the ability to chemically synthesize "artificial" segments of DNA or to modify segments of naturally occurring gene sequences to serve as diagnostic tools. The area is very complex but relies on the ability of DNA sequences to bind (hybridize) specifically to their complement. For example, if one wished to detect a pathogen in human samples (e.g., the TB bacteria), one would label a complementary sequence (a probe) for a common gene found in the bacterium that could detect the target organism's DNA. Thus one can label a relatively short segment of "manufactured" DNA with an indicator (such as a fluorescent dye or enzyme) and use the probe to detect a complementary DNA sequence in a sample by its ability to bind and "light up." This technique is often used in the microbiology laboratory to diagnose the presence of an infectious agent in a human sample. Manufactured small stretches of DNA that subtend an area of the genome can be used to artificially amplify the subtended area up to millions of times, greatly increasing the sensitivity of detection. The most common amplification technology uses the **polymerase chain reaction (PCR)**. Using such technology, the AIDS viral genes can be amplified to a level where even fifty copies of the viral genome can be detected in a single ml of patient blood.

The ability to use such technology raises difficult ethical questions, not only for the molecular biologist but for all of us who potentially might benefit. How much manipulation of human embryos is appropriate? Many would say yes to techniques aimed at curing genetic disease, but what about manipulating cosmetic factors such as attempting to increase muscle mass, height, or intelligence? Such questions most certainly will occur in the future.

Gene therapy
Introduction of genes into cells with the object of curing diseases associated with the deficiency of a protein related to a genetic mutation.

Polymerase chain reaction (PCR) Technology used to amplify stretches of DNA.

CASE 3-1

Hemophilia B results from a mutation of the F.IX B gene, causing a decrease in the ability of the F.IX protein to function in coagulation. At the age of eighteen months, a female child (individual II.2 in the pedigree in **FIGURE 3-11**) fell while playing with her fraternal twin sister and hit her knee on a table leg. She suffered a serious bleeding event in the injured knee joint that required hospital therapy. At that time, she was found to have a F.IX level 2 percent of normal and was diagnosed as being a female with hemophilia B. She required therapy with recombinant F.IX.

The family history indicated that her father (individual I.1 in the pedigree) also has the bleeding disease hemophilia B. Because his F.IX activity is less than 1 percent of normal levels, he requires therapy with human recombinant F.IX produced using genetic engineering technology in animal cells grown in tissue culture. If not treated, he suffers from spontaneous bleeding into his joints (**hemarthrosis**), which ultimately can result in severe joint damage. He is also at risk for life-threatening hemorrhages in his brain. His wife (individual I.2) has no bleeding tendencies and has normal levels of F.IX (about 100 percent of normal). She has no family history of bleeding diseases.

The parents have two offspring (II.1 and II.3) in addition to II.2. The older sibling (II.1) is a male with normal levels of F.IX. The younger siblings are female fraternal (not identical) twins. The sister (II.3) has not suffered from bleeding and has a F.IX level of 60 percent, which is sufficient to provide normal coagulation. (Bleeding is usually only noted when F.IX levels are below about 20 percent of normal.) As far as could be determined, the karyotype of all members of the family (including II.2) was normal.

Discussion

The normal level of F.IX in the male sibling is expected as he would have had to inherit his father's Y chromosome (to be male) and one of the mother's two normal X chromosomes. However, because hemophilia B is a recessive sex-linked disorder, all daughters of an affected father are obligate carriers (both individuals II.2 and II.3). They must inherit their father's single X chromosome, which carries the defective gene. Even as carriers, they would be expected to be normal (in terms of hemophilia B), having inherited one of their mother's normal X chromosomes as well as their father's mutated X chromosome. However, individual II.2 is not normal.

Female hemophiliacs do occur occasionally in families in which defects of the Factor IX gene are found. There are two general reasons this might occur.

1. Suppose the mother was actually not normal, but a carrier for hemophilia B. In such a case daughter II.2 would have received her father's affected X chromosome and had a 50 percent chance of inheriting her mother's single affected X chromosome. If she had, II.2 would be homozygous for a mutation in the F.IX gene and expected to be affected. In this case, this is unlikely because the mother's family did not demonstrate a history of bleeding disease and her normal level of F.IX strongly argues against her being an unknown carrier. However, females with homozygous hemophilia are known to occur (although very rarely).

2. A more likely reason for the low level of F.IX in II.2 is nonrandom X chromosome inactivation. As noted in this chapter, about half the cells in a female should have the paternally derived X chromosome inactivated and half the maternally derived chromosome. However, random inactivation does not always occur. A number of defects in the structure of the X chromosome (such as certain deletions and other chromosomal abnormalities) can result in the faulty chromosome being selectively inactivated. In such a case, if the structurally defective chromosome was from the mother (and hence normal in terms of the F.IX gene), the father's chromosome (carrying the hemophilia B gene) might be selectively expressed.

Hemarthrosis Arthritic condition caused by bleeding into the joint.

CASE 3-1 (Continued)

To determine whether nonrandom X inactivation did occur, the distribution of active maternal and paternal X chromosomes in the patient was examined using an X-linked SNP, which could differentiate the maternal and paternal X chromosomes of the patient. Ninety-seven percent of X chromosome product bearing the SNP in II.2 was from the paternal (affected) chromosome. In the unaffected twin sibling (II.3), the distribution was nearly random (about 40 percent was from the affected paternal chromosome).

Etiology and Pathogenesis

The most likely cause of female hemophilia in II.2 was extreme nonrandom X inactivation resulting in overrepresentation of the paternal X chromosome bearing a mutated Factor IX gene. However, this conclusion does not explain why this occurred in II.2 but not her sister, II.3. The great majority of female hemophiliacs result from unbalanced nonrandom X chromosome inactivation with no evidence of defects in the structure of the X chromosomes.

Questions

1. Suppose the mother in the family was a carrier of hemophilia B. How would this change the probability of disease in the offspring (and in future offspring)?

2. If the twins (II.2 and II.3) were identical, would this change your explanation for the occurrence of female hemophilia?

3. It is noted that recombinant human F.IX was used in therapy for affected individuals in the family. Why might recombinant human F.IX be preferable to F.IX isolated from pools of human blood?

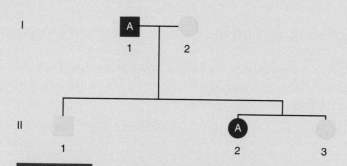

FIGURE 3-11 Case pedigree for sex-linked hemophilia B.

Courtesy of Department of Pathology and Laboratory Medicine, University of North Carolina at Chapel Hill.

QUESTIONS FOR REVIEW

1. What is meant by the following terms: *homologous chromosomes, autosomes, Barr body, gene, gametogenesis,* and *exome*?

2. Compare and contrast transcription and translation.

3. How does the process of mitosis compare with meiosis?

4. What are the differences between spermatogenesis and oogenesis?

5. What is a chromosome karyotype? How is it obtained? How is it used?

6. What pattern in a pedigree is typical of the inheritance of a recessive gene?

7. What is a SNP? How is it used?

SUPPLEMENTARY READINGS

Human Genome (Wikipedia). http://en.wikipedia.org/wiki/Human_genome

Introductory Genetics Online. Genetics Courses from the Hussman Institute for Human Genomics, Miller School of Medicine, University of Miami. http://hihg.med.miami.edu/educational-programs/online-genetics-courses

All about the Human Genome project (HGP) National Institute of Health. http://www.genome.gov/10001772

▶ These three references provide an excellent introductory online guide to human genetics. The third reference contains an extensive list of online resources of interest to both students and teachers.

Wirth, T., Parker, N., and Yla-Herttuala, S. 2013. History of gene therapy. *Gene* 525:162–69.

▶ An overview of gene therapy providing an introduction to the technology used and some current applications. There is a brief discussion of ethical issues.

Fan, N., and Lai, L. 2013. Genetically modified pig models for human diseases. *Journal of Genetics and Genomics* 40:67–73.

▶ Genetic modification of animals to produce models of human disease has been one of the most successful applications of genetic engineering to biomedical research. The recent extension of this technology from mice to pigs has yielded disease models in a species more comparable in size and metabolism to humans.

Walters, L. 2012. Genetics and bioethics: How our thinking has changed since 1969. *Theoretical Medicine and Bioethics* 33:83–95.

Robillard, J. M., Roskams_Edris, D., Kuzeljevic, B., et al. 2014. Prevailing public perceptions of the ethics of gene therapy. *Human Gene Therapy* 25:1–7.

▶ These two articles review how both professional bioethicists and the public view the ethics of gene therapy.

Altman, R. B. 2012. Translational bioinformatics: Linking the molecular world to the clinical world. *Clinical Pharmacology and Therapeutics* 91:994–1000.

▶ Describes how bioinformatics is used to translate basic biological discoveries into the clinic.

Visscher, P. M., Brown, M. A., McCarthy, M. I., et al. 2012. Five years of GWAS discovery. *American Journal of Human Genetics* 90:7–24.

▶ The use of genomewide association studies (GWAS) to detect genetic associations with disease has received much attention in the press. This is a balanced overview of the role of GWAS in biomedical research examining both its strengths and weaknesses.

Okumura, K., Fujimori, Y., Takagi, A., et al. 2008. Skewed X chromosome inactivation in fraternal female twins results in moderately severe and mild haemophilia B. *Haemohilia* 14:1088–93.

Peeters, S. B., Cotton, A. M., and Brown C. J. 2014. Variable escape from X-chromosome inactivation: Identifying factors that tip the scales toward expression. *Bioessays* 36:1–11.

▶ The first reference is the source on which the chapter case was modeled (in part) and contains additional details explaining how the pattern of X chromosome inactivation was determined in the family. The second reference provides additional information on the mechanism of X chromosome inactivation, which is far more interesting (and complex) than presented in the chapter.

Courtesy of Department of Pathology and Laboratory Medicine, University of North Carolina at Chapel Hill.

Congenital and Hereditary Diseases

LEARNING OBJECTIVES

1. Describe some of the more important malformations resulting from intrauterine injury.

2. List the common causes of congenital malformations and their approximate incidence.

3. Describe some of the common genetic abnormalities, and explain their methods of transmission.

4. Describe the role of chromosome deletions and translocations in congenital disease.

5. List the causes of Down syndrome, and describe its clinical manifestations. Explain why it is important to identify a carrier of a 14/21 chromosome translocation.

6. List four abnormalities of sex chromosomes, and describe their clinical manifestations.

7. Compare the methods of transmission and clinical manifestations of phenylketonuria and hemophilia.

8. Explain multifactorial inheritance. Give an example of a multifactorial defect, and describe the relevant factors.

9. Understand the various methods available to make a diagnosis of a congenital abnormality in the fetus.

Introduction

The term **congenital** disease refers to any abnormality that is present at birth (hereditary or not), even though it may not be detected prior to birth; this broad category encompasses all abnormalities caused by disturbed prenatal development, regardless of their nature. A congenital **malformation** is an intrinsic defect in development that may be genetic, environmental, or of mixed origin. Major malformations are of medical or social concern and require intervention. They are recognized in about 3 percent of all newborn infants. An additional 2 to 3 percent of developmental defects are not recognized at birth but become apparent as the infants grow older as is commonly the case with certain defects in cardiac development. Congenital defects are often incompatible with intrauterine development or extrauterine life. At least 50 percent and perhaps as high as 90 percent of recognized pregnancies that are lost are associated with chromosomal abnormalities in the conceptus. Studies of apparently normal preimplantation embryos suggest that half harbor chromosomal abnormalities and would likely be lost prior to recognition of pregnancy by the mother.

Congenital Present at birth.

Malformation Intrinsic defect in development.

Minor congenital malformations may be predominantly of cosmetic significance (such as partial fusion of several toes, extra nipples, or abnormal scalp hair whorls), and they occur in more than 10 percent of live births. A single example of a minor abnormality in an individual may be considered part of normal human variation rather than a malformation. However, the co-occurrence of multiple "minor" malformations in an individual is likely to indicate the presence of a congenital **syndrome**, a more serious defect characterized by a common set of abnormalities related to a single cause.

Although the majority of congenital abnormalities are intrinsic defects of development and hence termed malformations, extrinsic forces such as maternal uterine tumors or malformations and lack of amniotic fluid (oligohydramanios) can lead to **fetal deformation** due to compression or mispositioning during intrauterine development. An example would be a misshapen or asymmetric skull. Somewhat related to deformations are developmental **fetal disruptions**. This most commonly occurs when fibrous bands present in the amniotic fluid encircle and trap part of the developing fetus, leading to amputation of a developing limb.

The major factors known to induce congenital malformations include chromosomal abnormalities, abnormalities of individual genes, intrauterine injury to embryo or fetus, environmental factors, or a combination of environmental and genetic factors.

Intrauterine Injury

The embryo or fetus may be injured by drugs, radiation, or an infection that disrupts prenatal development and leads to congenital malformations. The effects of the injury to the developing embryo vary depending on the nature of the harmful agent and the stage of gestation. The embryonic period from the third to the eighth week after conception, when the organ systems are forming, is the time when the embryo is most vulnerable to the injurious effects of environmental agents.

HARMFUL DRUGS AND CHEMICALS

Many drugs are known to harm the developing embryo. The classic example is thalidomide, which was widely used in Europe in the 1960s to treat nausea and vomiting associated with pregnancy (morning sickness) but was never marketed in the United States. The drug produced a highly characteristic malformation called **phocomelia** in which the bones of the extremities were much reduced or absent, with the hands or feet arising from the trunk (**FIGURE 4-1**). Either upper or lower limbs or all four extremities were affected, depending on when the drug was taken during pregnancy. In addition to causing limb defects, the drug also caused malformations of the heart, gastrointestinal tract, eyes, and ears. The correlation between thalidomide and congenital malformations is species specific and was not detected in initial toxicity studies using rodents. The thalidomide tragedy clearly demonstrated to the medical profession the disastrous effects of a supposedly innocuous drug taken by a mother during a critical phase of embryonic development and resulted in more stringent testing procedures prior to approval of drugs for use in pregnancy.

Despite the hazard of thalidomide to the fetus, the drug has some properties that make it potentially useful for treating some diseases including leprosy and multiple myeloma, a form of lymphoid cell cancer. Because of the extreme hazard of the drug on fetal development, physicians prescribing the drug are required to take great precautions to be certain that the patient is not pregnant and will not become pregnant while taking the drug.

Syndrome Defect characterized by a common set of abnormalities related to a single cause.

Fetal deformation Misshapen fetus caused by compression or mispositioning during fetal development.

Fetal disruptions Congenital abnormality caused by physical disruption of the fetus.

Phocomelia Reduction of bones of the extremities.

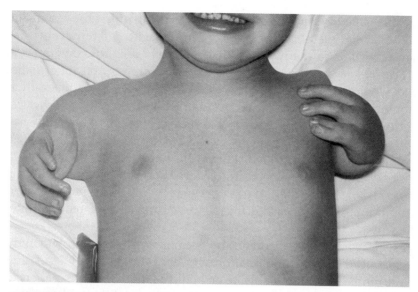

FIGURE 4-1 Characteristic limb deformities caused by thalidomide.
© Wellcome Images/Custom Medical Stock Photo.

Many other drugs, although less hazardous than thalidomide, also may cause congenital malformations. Currently, all drugs used in the United States are rated in five categories by the FDA according to the degree of possible risk to the fetus balanced against the drug's potential benefit to the patient (**TABLE 4-1**). Ratings range from "A" for drugs that are generally considered safe for use in pregnancy through "D" for drugs that may injure the fetus but are of enough benefit to the patient that their use may outweigh the risk to the fetus. "X"-rated drugs are contraindicated in pregnancy because the severe risk to the fetus outweighs any possible benefit to the patient.

Cigarettes and alcoholic beverages are not without risk. Cigarette smoking leads to retarded intrauterine growth with birth of smaller than normal infants and

TABLE 4-1 Five Categories of All Drugs Used in the United States Rated by the FDA According to Degree of Possible Risk to the Fetus

Category interpretation	
A	No risk to fetus demonstrated in well-controlled studies in humans.
B	No evidence of risk to fetus. Either animal studies show risk but human studies do not or there are no adequate human studies but animal studies do not indicate risk.
C	Risk to fetus cannot be ruled out. No human studies available to assess risk. Animal studies either are not available or indicate possible risk.
D	Positive evidence of risk to fetus; however, drug is needed to treat patients, and no safer alternative drug is available. Potential benefit to patients outweighs risk to fetus.
X	Absolutely contraindicated in pregnancy. Severe risk to fetus greatly outweighs any possible benefit to patients.

Sudden infant death syndrome (SIDS) Unexplained death of child under the age of one year.

Fetal alcohol syndrome Developmental abnormalities related to heavy alcohol consumption during pregnancy.

TORCH complex Mnemonic for organisms causing maternal infections injurious to the developing fetus.

premature births. **Sudden infant death syndrome (SIDS),** an otherwise unexplained death of a child under the age of one year, has been related to maternal smoking during pregnancy as well as to many other factors. Heavy alcohol consumption during pregnancy can result in a characteristic pattern of developmental abnormalities called **fetal alcohol syndrome.** Affected infants are both physically and mentally retarded, exhibit abnormal cranial and facial development, and may have other congenital malformations affecting the genital tract and cardiovascular system. Consequently, women with severe drinking problems should be cautioned not to become pregnant until their alcoholism is controlled. The level of alcohol consumption that puts a fetus at risk is controversial. Hence, it is generally considered unsafe for a pregnant woman to consume any alcohol during pregnancy (although most studies indicate that consumption of one or two drinks a week is not associated with measurable risk to the fetus).

Drugs such as heroin, methadone, and cocaine impair fetal growth and development and may lead to congenital malformation, as well as to addiction in both the fetus and the mother. The infant born to an addicted mother may experience narcotic withdrawal symptoms within a few days after delivery. Maternal cocaine use may also disturb blood flow through the placenta, leading to intrauterine fetal death, as described in the discussion on prenatal development and diseases associated with pregnancy.

Because of the established relation between drugs and congenital defects, physicians recommend that pregnant women refrain from indiscriminate use of drugs or other medications, especially during the early part of pregnancy when the embryo is especially vulnerable. This is particularly true of drugs of abuse whose contents are often unknown. Many new drugs and antibiotics are not recommended for use in pregnancy because the possible effects of the drugs on the developing embryo are not known.

RADIATION

Exposure of a pregnant woman to radiation may harm the fetus. Consequently, a risk to benefit analysis must be undertaken prior to x-ray examinations or diagnostic tests using radioactive materials during pregnancy. This is particularly true during the first fifteen weeks of fetal development. Although controversial, there may be a risk of an increased rate of development of childhood leukemia with a radiation dose equivalent to one or two abdominal CT studies. Fetuses with an age greater than fifteen weeks have a lower radiation sensitivity.

MATERNAL INFECTIONS

Some infections acquired by a pregnant woman may injure the developing fetus. The agents are commonly termed the **TORCH complex** T toxoplasmosis, infection with the parasite *Toxoplasma gondii*; **R** rubella (German measles); **C** cytomegalovirus (CMV); **H** herpes simplex virus; with **O** being other including HIV, parvovirus syphilis, and several other agents with potential to harm the fetus. Rubella virus, cytomegalovirus, toxoplasma, and occasionally the herpes virus all produce a similar type of infection in the fetus, so it may not be possible to determine clinically which agent caused the disease in either the fetus or the mother unless the infectious agent can be identified by histologic examination, culture, or serologic methods. For this reason, the maternal medical history including exposure and immunization history as well as physical findings in the newborn are critical in diagnosis of the specific agent. Of these, CMV transmission in utero is the most common, affecting up to 1.5 percent of pregnancies.

Rubella

Rubella is a mild illness that is usually acquired in childhood; 90 percent of women of childbearing age have already had the disease or have been immunized and are immune. If a susceptible woman acquires rubella during pregnancy, particularly between the twelfth and sixteenth weeks of gestation, up to 20 percent of children carried to term will show congenital defects including congenital cataracts, cardiac malformations, deafness, and neurologic disturbances. The virus may also cause a chronic progressive infection in the fetus. Because of near universal immunization, congenital rubella has almost been eliminated in the United States.

Cytomegalic Inclusion Disease

The name of the cytomegalovirus derives from its characteristic property of producing marked enlargement of the cells it infects. The infected cells also contain characteristic large, basophilic, intranuclear inclusions, causing the virus-infected cell to have a distinctly characteristic histologic appearance (**FIGURE 4-2**). Cytomegalovirus infection is very common and is usually asymptomatic. At least 60 percent of women of childbearing age have had a previous cytomegalovirus infection and have formed antibodies against the virus, but latent cytomegalovirus persists within the tissues of the infected woman and may become reactivated during pregnancy in immunocompromised individuals, leading to intermittent excretion of the virus in cervical and vaginal secretions throughout the pregnancy. The fetus may become infected either from a new maternal infection acquired during pregnancy or from reactivation of a prior maternal infection. A newly acquired maternal infection poses the greatest risk to the fetus with a 30 to 40 percent risk of transmission; however, only about

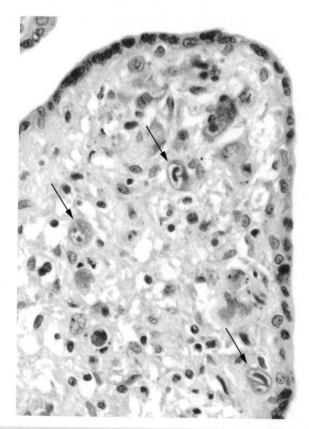

FIGURE 4-2 Cytomegalovirus. Three large cells with irregular nuclei (*arrows*) each have oddly shaped inclusions in a placental villus. The fetus died in utero of overwhelming cytomegalovirus infection involving lungs and brain.

Microcephaly Failure of the brain to develop normally.

10 percent of infected fetuses show symptoms. The virus may cause severe fetal damage, characterized by injury to the brain and eyes, leading to failure of the brain to develop normally (**microcephaly**), mental retardation, and blindness. Infection results in death of 30 percent of infants with severe disease. The cytomegalovirus may also cause a chronic systemic infection of the fetus similar to that caused by the rubella virus, and the virus can be identified in the tissues of the infected infant. Disease may also be contracted at the time of birth from genital secretions or breast milk. Asymptomatic neonates may develop hearing loss, retinal disease, and developmental delay within the first two years.

HIV

Vertical transmission of HIV from the infected mother to the child can occur before birth; however, infection usually occurs at the time of birth or soon thereafter by ingestion of infected breast milk. Intrauterine infection may result in growth retardation and facial abnormalities although this finding remains uncertain. Transmission from the mother is responsible for about 80 percent of all pediatric HIV disease. The risk of transmission by an infected mother depends on the level of HIV in the blood and the degree of contact between the neonate and maternal blood and genital secretions. Hence, appropriate drug therapy for the mother is critical. Cesarean delivery is suggested when the mother has a high viral load. The risk of perinatal transmission without treatment may be as high as 40 percent. Postpartum prophylactic drug therapy in the neonate much reduces the risk. Even when born to untreated mothers, transmission rates may be reduced to below 3 percent by optimal neonatal drug therapy. Maternal therapy is associated with a potential risk to the fetus, so careful consideration of risk versus benefit is important in counseling women of childbearing age who test positive for HIV. Essentially all states require "opt-out" testing for HIV for pregnant women.

Other Virus Diseases in Pregnancy

The herpes simplex virus, the same virus that causes fever blisters, may at times cause intrauterine and neonatal infections. Intrauterine infection is uncommon and results in skin and eye lesions and microcephaly; 90 percent of infections result from passage through an infected genital tract. Neonatal herpes (herpes neonatorum) may be localized to the eye, skin, or mucous membrane or result in severe disseminated disease involving the nervous system, liver, and lung with a very high mortality rate (**FIGURE 4-3**). For this reason, offspring of infected mothers may be treated prophylactically with antiviral therapy. Some other viruses may occasionally be transmitted to the fetus and cause disease in the fetus. Parvovirus B19 (responsible for "fifth disease," a mild rash-associated disease in children) may be responsible for more than 10 percent of intrauterine fetal death, fetal anemia, and in some cases hydrops fetalis, a condition discussed with diseases related to pregnancy. Recently characterized Zika virus infection appears to be similar to other congenital infections.

Toxoplasmosis

Toxoplasma gondii is a small, ovoid, intracellular parasite. described in the discussion on animal parasites. Adults acquired the infection by eating raw or partially cooked meat that is infected with the parasite or by contact with infected cats, which excrete an infectious form of the organism (oocysts) in their feces. As with cytomegalovirus infection, more than 50 percent of women of childbearing age have had a previous inapparent infection and have formed antibodies to the parasite. These women are immune, and the prior infection does not put the fetus at risk.

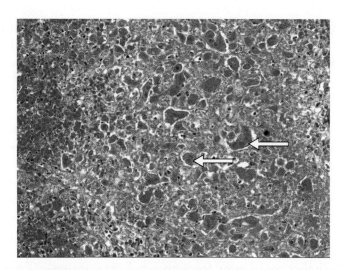

FIGURE 4-3 **Neonatal herpes.** Liver from a fatal case. Much of the liver is necrotic with no intact cells. Many cells have multiple nuclei with red inclusions (*arrows*) containing masses of herpes virus.

Courtesy of Department of Pathology and Laboratory Medicine, University of North Carolina at Chapel Hill.

A hazard to the fetus exists if a susceptible mother acquires the infection during pregnancy. In the fetus, the parasite causes severe injury to the brain and eyes, leadin to abnormal development of the brain (microcephaly); obstruction of the ventricles of the brain, causing hydrocephalus (discussion on the nervous system); and commonly visual disturbances or blindness. Many cases of fetal infection result in death. The infected fetus may be born with evidence of a systemic toxoplasma infection that is clinically quite similar to that caused by rubella and the cytomegalovirus. Primary infection during pregnancy is a major risk factor. Young women show low rates of immunity (less than 20 percent) and hence are of greatest risk. Although the risk of infection in such women is low (under 1 percent), pregnant woman should avoid eating incompletely cooked meat and should exercise caution in contact with cats and, in particular, cat litter boxes.

Genetic Disease

A **hereditary or genetic disease** results from a chromosome abnormality or a defective expression of a gene due to mutation within the gene or at a region important for normal gene function. Chromosomal abnormalities account for about 6 percent of genetic disease, and all known single gene defects (of which at least 6,000 have been described) account for an additional 7.5 percent. It is likely that 20 to 30 percent of birth defects are the result of multiple genes with complex patterns of inheritance or have both a genetic and an environmental component. Relatively common defects such as congenital heart disease, cleft lip and palate, and defects in the formation of the neural tube (brain and spine) fall into this category. Nongenetic, postconception factors such as chemical or physical agents, maternal illness and infection, and medicinal and recreational drugs (including excess alcohol consumption during pregnancy) account for an additional 5 to 10 percent of birth defects. About half of birth defects are of unknown cause although undoubtedly a proportion of these are related to unrecognized defects in chromosomal structure and mutations in genes.

> **Hereditary or genetic disease** Condition resulting from a chromosome abnormality or defective expression of a gene.

Chromosomal Abnormalities

Chromosomal abnormalities leading to congenital malformations may result from failure of homologous chromosomes in the germ cells to separate normally, from abnormal breaks and rearrangements of chromosomes in the germ cells as they are maturing, or at times from failure of chromosomes to separate normally in the fertilized ovum (zygote) as the cells divide by mitosis during early prenatal development.

Occasionally, homologous chromosomes in germ cells fail to separate from one another in either the first or the second meiotic division. This is called **nondisjunction** and leads to abnormalities in the distribution of chromosomes between germ cells (**FIGURE 4-4**). One of the two germ cells derived from the abnormal chromosome division has an extra chromosome, and the other cell lacks a chromosome. Nondisjunction may involve either the sex chromosomes or the autosomes. If it occurs during gametogenesis, one daughter cell will have 24 chromosomes and the other will have 22. If a gamete having an abnormal number of chromosomes fuses with a normal gamete during fertilization, the resulting zygote will either have an extra chromosome or be lacking one of the homologous pair of chromosomes; a condition termed **aneuploidy**. The presence of an extra chromosome in a cell is called a **trisomy** of the chromosome present in triplicate. Absence of a chromosome is called a **monosomy** of the missing chromosome. Complete monosomy for autosomal chromosomes is not viable; however, monosomy for the X chromosome (45, X) results in an individual with **Turner syndrome** (although only a small percentage of 45, X conceptuses survive to term). The most common autosomal chromosomal defect resulting in a viable birth is trisomy 21, resulting in Down syndrome. Such individuals may survive into the fifth decade, albeit with significant physical and developmental defects. Fetuses with trisomy for chromosome 13 (Patau syndrome) and chromosome 18 (Edward syndrome) may survive to birth; however, unlike individuals with Down, they generally die soon after birth.

CHROMOSOME DELETIONS AND TRANSLOCATIONS DURING GAMETOGENESIS

Sometimes a chromosome breaks in the course of meiosis, and the broken piece is lost from the cell. This is called a **chromosome deletion**. In some cases, the broken piece is

Nondisjunction Condition resulting from failure of homologous chromosomes to separate during meitosis.

Aneuploidy Condition denoting abnormal number of chromosomes.

Trisomy The presence of an extra chromosome within a cell; having three of a given chromosome instead of the usual pair.

Monosomy A condition of a cell in which one chromosome of a homologous pair is missing.

Turner syndrome A congenital syndrome usually caused by absence of one X chromosome in the female.

Chromosome deletion Loss of part of a chromosome during meiosis.

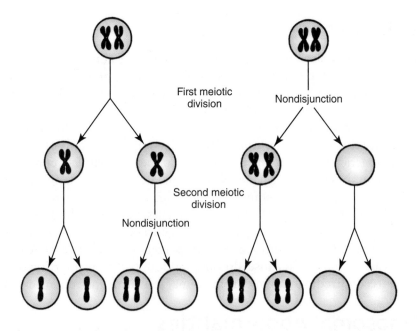

FIGURE 4-4 Effects of nondisjunction in meiosis, leading to formation of gametes with an extra or missing chromosome. Only the chromosome pair involved in nondisjunction is illustrated. Nondisjunction at second meiotic division (*left*). Nondisjunction at first meiotic division (*right*).

not lost but becomes attached to another nonhomologous chromosome with which it is carried along during meiosis. A misplaced chromosome or part of a chromosome attached to another chromosome is called a **translocation**. In a reciprocal translocation, pieces of chromosomes (containing different sets of genes) are reciprocally exchanged between two nonhomologous chromosomes. Such an accident may not disturb the function of the cell because there is no loss or gain of genetic material (although the expression of individual genes adjacent to break points may be affected). However, if the translocation occurs in a germ cell, an egg or sperm containing either a deficiency or an excess of chromosomal material may form during meiosis. If such a chromosomally abnormal gamete unites with a normal gamete during fertilization, the fertilized ovum (zygote) contains an abnormal amount of chromosomal material. As noted previously, most abnormal zygotes are spontaneously aborted, but some survive and give rise to defective fetuses. **FIGURE 4-5** demonstrates a case in which a chromosome 14/21 translocation may result in a case of inherited **Down syndrome** (**D**) or in a carrier for the disease (**C**). This is an uncommon cause of the disease (as we shall see) because most cases are not inherited.

The literature contains many descriptions of clinical abnormalities that are associated with extra chromosomes, chromosome translocation, or loss of entire chromosomes or portions of chromosomes (**TABLE 4-2**). Chromosomal abnormalities can be detected when abnormalities in chromosome size, configuration, or the band

Translocation A transfer of a piece of one chromosome to a nonhomologous chromosome.

Down syndrome Condition resulting from trisomy for chromosome 21.

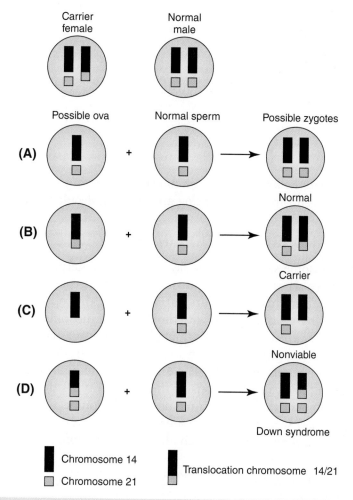

FIGURE 4-5 Possible ova produced by a female carrier of a 14/21 translocation chromosome and possible zygotes that could result from fertilization by normal sperm.

TABLE 4-2 Chromosome Abnormalities per 100,000 Recognized Human Pregnancies

Chromosome constitution	Number among spontaneously aborted fetuses	Number among live births
Normal	7,500	84,450
Trisomy	–	–
13	128	17
18	223	13
21	350	113
Other autosomes	3,176	0
Sex chromosomes	–	–
47,XYY	4	46
47,XXY	4	44
45,X	1,350	8
47,XXX	21	44
Translocations	–	–
Balanced (euploid)	14	164
Unbalanced (aneuploid)	225	52
Polyploid	–	–
Triploid	1,275	0
Tetraploid	450	0
Others (mosaics, etc.)	280	49
Total	15,000	85,000

pattern is detected in the karyotype. Even more subtle chromosomal defects may be characterized using chromosome painting and other molecular techniques.

CHROMOSOME NONDISJUNCTION IN THE ZYGOTE

Failures of chromosome separation are not restricted to germ cells. Sometimes the chromosomes fail to separate during mitosis in one of the cells of the zygote during prenatal development. When this occurs during mitosis, the cell lacking the chromosome is unable to survive, but the cell with the extra chromosome continues to divide along with the other chromosomally normal cells. As a result, the embryo eventually becomes composed of a population of normal cells and another population of cells having a chromosome trisomy (**FIGURE 4-6**). Such individuals are termed **chromosomal mosaics**. The relative proportions of the two cell types depend on how early in prenatal development the chromosome nondisjunction occurred and impacts on the severity of disease were seen. For example, Down syndrome mosaics are often more mildly affected than those in which all cells are trisomic.

Chromosomal mosaics Individual with both normal cells and cells having a chromosomal abnormality.

SEX CHROMOSOME ABNORMALITIES

When detailing the number of chromosomes in a cell, it is customary to indicate first the total number of chromosomes in the cell and then indicate the sex chromosomes. For example, a normal male is designated 46,XY, and a normal female is 46,XX.

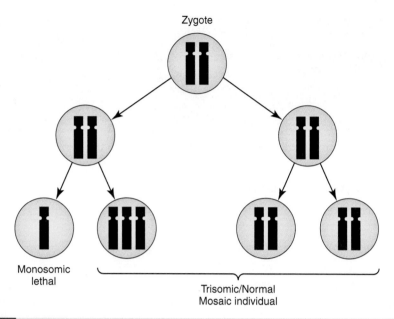

Zygote

Monosomic
lethal

Trisomic/Normal
Mosaic individual

FIGURE 4-6 Formation of two chromosome populations (chromosome mosaic) resulting from chromosome nondisjunction during mitosis in the zygote.

Unlike disorders of autosomal chromosome number (which most often result in fetal death or severe disease) defects in sex chromosome number are relatively mild and may be consistent with normal or near normal development into adulthood. Although most (but not all) genes on one X chromosome are inactivated in normal XX females and there are few active genes on the Y chromosome, both X- and Y-linked genes are critical for normal sexual development. If the Y chromosome is absent, the body configuration is female. Hence, it is not surprising that 45,X females (Turner syndrome) are female in body form (are **phenotypically** female) but do not show sexual maturation. Normal female sexual development requires two active copies of some X-linked genes (**pseudoautosomal genes**). The presence of one or more extra X chromosomes (**Triple X syndrome**) has very little effect on the female because the additional X chromosomes are inactivated. The Y chromosome directs male sexual differentiation, and its presence is almost invariably associated with a male body configuration regardless of the number of X chromosomes present. However, presence of one or more extra X chromosomes adversely affects masculine development. Thus, 47,XXY individuals (**Klinefelter syndrome**) are phenotypically male but do not sexually mature and invariably have very small gonads. An extra Y chromosome (47,XYY, **Double Y syndrome**) does not cause significant changes in the appearance of the affected individual because the Y chromosome carries little genetic material other than genes concerned with male sexual differentiation. The principal characteristics of these syndromes are summarized in **TABLE 4-3**.

In addition to conditions associated with abnormal numbers of sex chromosomes, the **fragile X syndrome**, although associated with a defect in an X-linked gene, can under some circumstances be detected as an abnormal karyotype.

Turner Syndrome

Turner syndrome results from either lack of or structural abnormalities in one of the X chromosomes that leads to loss of a portion of that chromosome. Sixty percent of patients have the 45,X karyotype; others have more subtle deletions in one of the X chromosomes. The reported frequency of about 1 in 2,500 female births represents

Phenotype Appearance of individual as opposed to genes present.

Pseudoautosomal genes Genes carried on the X chromosome not subject to random X inactivation.

Triple X syndrome Presence of one or more extra X chromosomes.

Klinefelter syndrome A congenital syndrome caused by an extra X chromosome in the male.

Double Y syndrome The presence of an extra Y chromosome in the male.

Fragile X syndrome Condition resulting from defects in a gene on the X chromosome associated with mental retardation.

TABLE 4-3 Syndromes Resulting from an Abnormal Complement of Sex Chromosomes

	Usual genotype	Approximate incidence	Unusual number of Barr bodies	Unusual number of Y fluorescent bodies	Fertility
Turner syndrome	45,X	1:2,500 females	0	0	Sterile
Triple X syndrome	47,XXX	1:850 females	2	0	Usually not impaired
Klinefelter syndrome	47,XXY	1:750 males	1	1	Usually sterile
XYY syndrome	47,XYY	1:850 males	0	2	Usually not impaired

only the 1 percent of Turner embryos that survive to be born alive. At least 75 percent (and possible nearly all) Turner patients are mosaic, and it has been suggested that at least some 46,XX cells must be present for viability. Severity of the syndrome is linked to the proportion of normal cells present. The most characteristic feature of Turner patients is short stature related to the absence of two copies of the X-linked *SHOX* gene (one of the pseudoautosomal genes that remain active on both X chromosomes of normal females). Characteristically, Turner patients, although showing normal ovarian development during fetal development, suffer what has been called "premature menopause" with loss of all oocytes by the age of two. Ovaries become completely atrophic and failure of puberty and amenorrhea (lack of menses) occurs without hormonal therapy. A variety of additional development defects include a webbed neck, kidney malformations, and defects in the cardiovascular system. Turner syndrome patients usually have normal intelligence; only subtle defects in nonverbal learning sometimes occur.

Triple X Syndrome

The presence of an extra X chromosome in the cells of the female is a relatively common abnormality with an incidence of about 1 in 1,000 female births. There are no specific abnormalities of body form. Sexual development and fertility are usually normal. Learning disabilities and delayed motor development sometimes occur.

Klinefelter Syndrome

Having an incidence of about 1 in 750 male births, Klinefelter syndrome (usual genotype 47,XXY) is one of the most common sex chromosome abnormalities. The external genital organs are male, but the testes are atrophic and puberty is either delayed or incomplete. Defects in the structure of the penis also occur. Usually no spermatozoa are produced, and the individual is sterile. The body configuration is somewhat feminine and "long-legged," and there may be moderate breast hypertrophy. Learning disabilities and delayed language development occur although mental retardation is uncommon.

XYY Syndrome

The sex chromosomal abnormality known as XYY syndrome has an incidence of about 1 in 1,000 male births. The individuals are usually taller than normal, but there are no specific abnormalities of body configuration or fertility. Delayed development of motor and language skills may occur along with behavioral and emotional difficulties, but intelligence is usually in the normal range. Autism disorders infrequently occur, and this may interfere with social interaction; however, individuals (contrary to early popular reports) are not aggressive.

Fragile X Syndrome

The condition called the fragile X syndrome is second only to Down syndrome as a major cause of mental retardation and is related to defects in the *FMR1* (for Fragile X Mental Retardation-1), or simply fragile X gene. The name derives from the fact that affected chromosomes show an inducible defect during karyotype studies, which cause a fragile, constricted area to form at the tip of the long arm of the X chromosome. The observed defect relates to expansion of a group of cytosine–guanine–guanine repeating sequences (**CGG repeats**) that occurs at the beginning of the *FMR1* gene (and are not translated into protein). Normal individuals have about 30 repeats, and affected individuals with **full mutations** have 200 to 4,000 repeats. The genetics of the disease is complex and does not follow simple Mendelian rules. Carrier individuals have 60 to 200 repeats, a condition termed a **premutation**, and are not affected. However, premutations are unstable and tend to grow from generation to generation as they are passed from father to grandchild through a female. The tendency for a mutation to become worse with each generation is termed **genetic anticipation**. The disease is expressed more frequently in males with full mutations than in females (for unknown reasons). About 1 in 1,600 males versus 1 in 8,000 females is affected. Affected females generally have a milder form of the disease. About half of females heterozygous for a chromosome with the full mutation express the disease.

The great excess of CGG repeats causes mental retardation because the large number of repeats blocks the function of the gene. As a result, no gene product is produced, interfering with the formation and function of synapses within the nervous system, which is the apparent cause of the mental retardation. Individuals with severe forms of the disease have markedly reduced IQs, a very long face with out-turned ears, and notably very large testicles (**macro-orchidism**). Although karyotype analysis was initially used to define the disease, modern techniques rely on molecular studies of the structure of the gene and, in particular, the number of CGG repeats.

CGG repeats Expansion of cytosine-guanine-guanine repeating sequences; defect responsible for fragile X syndrome.

Full mutation Large number of CGG repeats resulting in detectable disease.

Premutation Condition in carriers of fragile X; relatively few repeats.

Genetic anticipation Tendency for a mutation to become worse with each generation.

Macro-orchidism Large testicles.

AUTOSOMAL ABNORMALITIES

The presence of more than two copies of an autosome (trisomy) results in severe congenital abnormalities. Absence of an autosome (monosomy) results in the loss of so many genes that development is generally not possible and the embryo is aborted. Deletion of a small part of an autosome may be compatible with development, but it usually results in multiple severe congenital abnormalities in the infant. The most common autosomal trisomy seen in newborn infants is that of the small chromosome 21, which causes Down syndrome. Less frequent trisomy of a larger chromosome, such as chromosome 13 or chromosome 18, is associated with multiple severe congenital malformations. Trisomy of other large autosomes is almost invariably lethal.

Down Syndrome

Down syndrome, the most common chromosomal abnormality with an incidence of about 1 in 1,600 births (depending in large part on the age of the mother), is characterized by mental deficiency and a characteristic facial expression caused by the upward-slanting eyes and the prominent skin folds extending from the base of the nose to the inner aspects of the eyebrows (**FIGURE 4-7**). Other abnormalities of body form also are seen, including a protruding tongue and abnormal palmar creases. Congenital cardiac malformations occur frequently, as do major congenital defects in other organ systems. Acute lymphoblastic leukemia is a common occurrence, and early degenerative neurological changes similar to Alzheimer disease is seen by age forty. The reported incidence represents only the proportion of abnormal fetuses surviving to term. About 75 percent of trisomy 21 fetuses do not survive to be live-born, and 25 percent die in the first year of life.

Down syndrome may arise from nondisjunction during gametogenesis, translocation, or nondisjunction in the zygote. In about 95 percent of cases, Down syndrome results from nondisjunction of chromosome 21 during the first meiotic division of the oocytes in the female. Fertilization by a normal sperm produces a zygote containing 47 chromosomes, with chromosome 21 being present in triplicate. Down syndrome resulting from nondisjunction during oogenesis increases in frequency with advancing maternal age. The incidence is as high as 1 in 60 in the offspring of women over forty years of age, but even very young mothers can have Down offspring. Trisomy 21 occurs in 1 in 1,000 births in women between twenty-five and twenty-nine years of age.

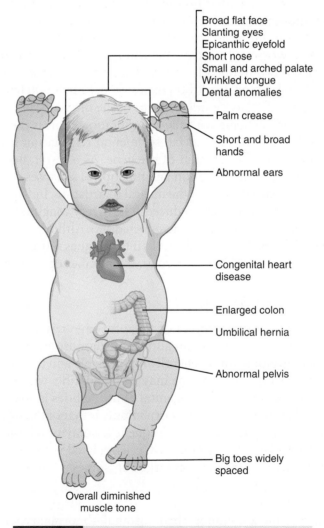

Broad flat face
Slanting eyes
Epicanthic eyefold
Short nose
Small and arched palate
Wrinkled tongue
Dental anomalies

Palm crease

Short and broad hands

Abnormal ears

Congenital heart disease

Enlarged colon

Umbilical hernia

Abnormal pelvis

Big toes widely spaced

Overall diminished muscle tone

FIGURE 4-7 Child with Down syndrome.

In a small number of persons with Down syndrome, the extra chromosome 21 is attached to another chromosome, usually chromosome 14. Although the total number of chromosomes is not increased in these individuals, one of the chromosomes is actually a composite chromosome resulting from the fusion of chromosome 21 with another chromosome; consequently, the affected person has extra genetic material derived from chromosome 21. The recognition of a translocation carrier is important because the carrier is capable of transmitting the abnormal chromosome to his or her children, resulting in translocation Down syndrome. However, the translocation chromosome is not always transmitted, as shown in Figure 4-5, which demonstrates the possible outcome of a pregnancy involving a female carrier of a 14/21 translocation chromosome.

In some individuals with Down syndrome, only some of the cells exhibit the characteristic trisomy 21 (i.e., they are mosaic for Down syndrome). Mosaic Down syndrome results from nondisjunction during mitosis of a normal cell to form a trisomy 21 cell and another cell lacking chromosome 21, which does not survive. Both the normal cells and the trisomy 21 cells continue to proliferate, and both cell populations are present in the developing embryo, as illustrated in Figure 4-6. Individuals with mosaic Down syndrome tend to suffer less disability than those in whom all of the cells contain an extra chromosome 21.

Because Down syndrome is frequent (particularly in the offspring of older mothers) and is associated with both mental and physical disabilities in the conceptus, prenatal screening for Down syndrome should be offered to all pregnant females. Such prenatal screening does not presuppose any particular choice by the parents who might choose to terminate the pregnancy or to carry the pregnancy to term. In the latter case, both the medical staff and parents are better able to cope with the difficulties associated with a Down neonate. Prenatal screening tests are complex and depend on biochemical markers in the mother's blood and imaging studies of the fetus. This combination results in a 85-percent detection rate and a 5-percent false positive rate. Sampling the fetal material (either obtained by amniotic fluid or chorionic villus sampling) provides more definitive information using either karyotypic or molecular testing of fetal cells and has a very low risk to the fetus. Recent advances (discussed in the section Prenatal Diagnosis of Congenital Abnormalities) allow fetal DNA to be sampled directly from the maternal circulation, obviating the need for invasive procedures. Tests using such technology have proven extremely accurate for Down syndrome, with 99 percent detection rates and nearly undetectable false positives.

Genetically Transmitted Diseases

Genetically determined diseases are the result of abnormalities of individual genes on the chromosome. Most hereditary diseases are transmitted on autosomes. A few are carried on sex chromosomes (TABLE 4-4). The chromosomes and the karyotype appear normal; however, using modern molecular techniques previously unrecognized, defects in chromosome or gene structure (e.g., small deletions or mutations) have been recognized in association with such diseases. Transmission of the abnormal gene is from parent to offspring, following the well-established patterns of inheritance described in the discussion on chromosomes, genes, and cell division.

Genes direct many functions within the cell. Some genes direct the synthesis of proteins. These may be proteins that form the structure of the cell (structural proteins) or enzymes that are necessary for cell function. Other genes function by regulating the activity of the genes that direct protein synthesis or are associated with the production of a variety of RNA species. Normally, genes in the germline are stable and

TABLE 4-4   Mode of Inheritance, Pathogenesis, and Major Manifestations of Some Common Genetic Diseases

Abnormality	Mode of inheritance	Defect	Manifestations
Phenylketonuria	Recessive	Phenylalanine hydroxylase deficiency	Mental retardation
Tay-Sachs disease	Recessive	Hexosaminidase A deficiency	Mental retardation, motor weakness, blindness
Cystic fibrosis of pancreas	Recessive	Dysfunction of mucous and sweat glands, thick mucus obstructs bronchioles, pancreatic ducts, and bile ducts	Chronic bronchopulmonary infections as a result of bronchial obstruction by mucus; pancreatic and liver dysfunction as a result of thick mucous obstruction of excretory ducts
Achondroplasia	Dominant	Disordered bone growth at ends of long bones (epiphyses)	Dwarfism with disproportionately short limbs
Congenital polycystic kidney disease	Dominant	Maldevelopment of nephrons and collecting tubules causes formation of multiple cysts in kidneys	Renal failure
Multiple neurofibromatosis	Dominant	Multiple tumors arise from peripheral nerves	Disfigurement and deformities caused by tumors; predisposition to malignant change in tumors
Sickle cell trait	Codominant	Red cells contain mixture of normal (A) and sickle (S) hemoglobin	None
Sickle cell anemia	Codominant	Red cells contain no normal hemoglobin	Severe anemia and obstruction of blood flow to organs by masses of sickled red cells
Hemophilia	X-linked recessive	Deficiency of protein required for normal coagulation of blood	Uncontrolled bleeding into joints and internal organs after minor injuries

are passed without change from parent to offspring. Occasionally, a gene undergoes a change called a **gene mutation**, which may occur spontaneously or as a result of exposure to chemicals or radiation. After a mutation has occurred in a germ cell, it can be transmitted from parent to offspring.

Sometimes, a gene mutation that induces only a minor change in the structure of a protein may cause a serious change in its properties. For example, **sickle hemoglobin** (hemoglobin S) differs from normal hemoglobin (hemoglobin A) only in a single amino acid, but it undergoes polymerization within the red blood cells when the oxygen content of the blood is reduced, leading to sickling and compromise to the circulation system.

If a mutation involves genes that control the synthesis of an enzyme, the enzyme may be defective and may lack normal functional activity. Metabolic processes regulated by the enzyme are disturbed, and the cell is unable to function normally.

The traditional diagnostic approach to genetic disease, based on the principles of classic genetics, is directed toward first identifying the abnormality in the patient; then identifying the gene product (most often a protein) that is responsible for the disease, such as an abnormal hemoglobin or an enzyme deficiency; and finally, attempting to identify the gene responsible for the abnormal gene product that caused the cell dysfunction. More recently, as a result of a better understanding of the sequence of DNA that constitutes the normal genome, there has been a shift toward molecular genetics approaches. Often the technique is to search for associations between the disease trait and other well-defined DNA markers that vary in populations (polymorphisms). Such polymorphisms occur throughout the entire human genome and serve as landmarks for such studies. For example, imagine that there is a polymorphism in a DNA sequence within or near a gene for a hemoglobin that has two detectable forms: A and B. If within families the presence of an unknown disease trait follows that of the marker (segregates with the marker) such that everyone in the family who has the disease also has marker A or B, it is likely that the gene for the unknown disease is located near (or perhaps contains) the marker. If we know where the marker is located in the genome (in this case hemoglobin), we then know that the gene for the new disease is near the gene for hemoglobin. The tendency for genes (or even noncoding segments of DNA) physically close in the genome to move together (i.e., to be inherited together) is termed **linkage**. Many complex statistical approaches are available for investigating these associations in many families and even in large groups of unrelated individuals (**genomewide association studies [GWAS]**). Having identified the location of the mutation, the human genetic map is searched to determine what genes are located at that position. One can than sequence such genes from individuals with the disease to determine how they differ from the normal gene, then determine the product of the gene, and finally evaluate how the abnormal gene and its gene product disrupt the functions of the cell. This approach has led to great advances in the prenatal diagnosis of many genetic diseases, as described later in the chapter.

AUTOSOMAL DOMINANT INHERITANCE

A dominant gene expresses itself in the heterozygous state. If either parent carries an abnormal dominant gene, either the abnormal gene or the corresponding normal allele may be passed to the offspring. Consequently, there is one chance in two that the offspring will receive the abnormal gene and will be affected with the hereditary disease. A common example of a genetic disease transmitted in this manner is **achondroplasia**, a type of dwarfism in which the limbs are disproportionately short (discussion on the musculoskeletal system). A second example is a type of autosomal dominant kidney disease (**adult polycystic kidney disease**), which is characterized by

Gene mutation Change in gene structure.

Sickle hemoglobin An abnormal hemoglobin that crystallizes under reduced oxygen tension.

Linkage Genes inherited together. Linked genes segregate together during meiosis.

Achondroplasia A type of dwarfism.

Adult polycystic kidney disease Autosomal dominant disease characterized by the formation of multiple cysts throughout both kidneys.

the formation of multiple cysts throughout both kidneys that progressively enlarge and eventually destroy renal function (discussion on the urinary system). A third genetic disease of this type is **multiple neurofibromatosis**, a condition characterized by the formation of multiple tumors that arise from peripheral nerves (discussion on the nervous system).

AUTOSOMAL RECESSIVE INHERITANCE

As noted in an earlier chapter a trait transmitted as an autosomal recessive is expressed only in the homozygous individual. Many diseases characterized by an enzyme deficiency within the cell are transmitted in this manner. The disease occurs only if both alleles are abnormal and no enzyme is produced. Therefore, for the offspring to be affected, both parents must carry the abnormal gene, and both must transmit the gene to the offspring. When the mutation is uncommon, it is likely that both parents are related and that the mutation is common by descent to both. (Hence, **inbreeding**, mating with individuals who are closely related genetically, raises concerns). When both parents carry an abnormal recessive gene, there is one chance in four that the mother will give birth to an abnormal infant who is homozygous for the defective gene. If only one parent transmits the recessive gene, the infant will be a carrier of the abnormal gene but will be normal because the normal allele will direct the synthesis of enough enzymes to keep the cell functioning normally. The many recognized types of genetically determined enzyme defects are sometimes called **inborn errors of metabolism**. Two of the more important ones are phenylketonuria and Tay-Sachs disease.

Phenylketonuria

Phenylalanine is an essential amino acid present in dietary protein. Much of it is converted in the body to tyrosine, which the body uses to make thyroid hormone, melanin, and other important compounds. A deficiency of the enzyme phenylalanine hydroxylase, which is required for normal metabolism of the amino acid phenylalanine, causes a disease called **phenylketonuria**. The enzyme deficiency causes no difficulty while the infant is still within the uterus being nourished by the mother. Soon after birth, however, the infant begins to drink milk. Because milk protein contains abundant phenylalanine, which the infant is unable to metabolize, this amino acid accumulates in the infant's blood and is excreted in the urine. The affected infant is able to convert some phenylalanine into phenylpyruvic acid (and other metabolites) by means of other metabolic pathways that do not require phenylalanine hydroxylase (**FIGURE 4-8**). Phenylpyruvic acid accumulates in the blood and is excreted in the urine along with phenylalanine. Permanent mental deficiency results from the disturbed phenylalanine metabolism, but it can be prevented by restricting the dietary intake of phenylalanine in the developing child. Phenylketonuria can be detected in the newborn infant by means of a screening laboratory test capable of detecting the elevated level of phenylalanine in the blood. Because this disease is a cause of preventable mental deficiency, a routine screening test to detect phenylketonuria (as well as many other inborn errors of metabolism) is required for all newborn infants.

Tay-Sachs Disease

Tay-Sachs disease occurs in the offspring of parents who carry the defective gene. The carrier rate is relatively high in some Jewish populations (those of Eastern European origin). In these groups, about 1 in 30 individuals carry the abnormal gene; however, other population groups also carry the gene at a high frequency (such as Cajuns and French Canadians).

Multiple neurofibromatosis Autosomal dominant disease characterized by formation of multiple tumors of nerve tissue.

Inbreeding Mating between closely related individuals.

Inborn errors of metabolism Genetically determined enzyme defects.

Phenylketonuria Autosomal recessive disease caused by the inability to convert phenylalanine to tyrosine.

Tay-Sachs disease Autosomal recessive disease caused by the absence of lysosomal enzyme hexosaminidase A.

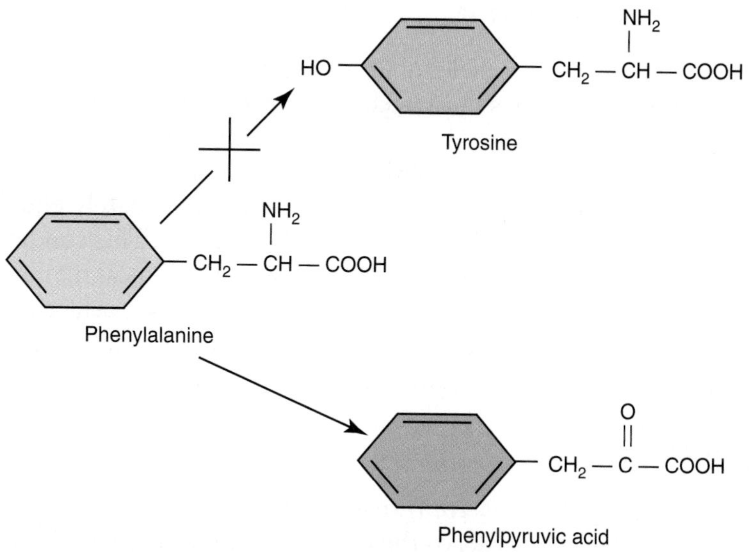

FIGURE 4-8 Metabolic defects in phenylketonuria. Infants with this disorder lack the enzyme phenylalanine hydroxylase, and their bodies are unable to hydroxylate phenylalanine to form tyrosine. Some phenylalanine is converted into phenylpyruvic acid (substitution of a keto group for the amino group in the molecule) by other metabolic pathways. Permanent mental deficiency results from disturbed phenylalanine metabolism and can be prevented by restricting dietary intake of phenylalanine.

The clinical manifestations result from absence of a lysosomal enzyme called hexosaminidase A. The enzyme deficiency causes a lipid called a ganglioside to accumulate within the lysosomes of nerve cells in the brain, spinal cord, autonomic nervous system, and the retina of the eye, causing cell dysfunction and, eventually, degeneration of the affected nerve cells. Clinically, the disease is characterized by progressive mental deterioration, neurologic dysfunction, and blindness. Onset of symptoms begins by about six months of age, and the disease is invariably fatal by the time the child is three or four years old.

Carriers of the abnormal gene can be detected by means of the low levels of hexosaminidase A in their serum and in their leukocytes. Tests for this enzyme can be used for screening. Tay-Sachs disease can be diagnosed prenatally by examining fetal cells obtained by amniocentesis.

Other Genetic Diseases

Two other relatively common and important diseases transmitted by autosomal recessive inheritance are cystic fibrosis of the pancreas and hemochromatosis. **Cystic fibrosis** is manifested by dysfunction of mucous and sweat glands related to a defective sodium ion transporter gene (cystic fibrosis transmembrane conductance regulator [*CFTR*]). The result of the defect is that mucous secretions in many organs of the body are abnormally viscid and tend to mechanically interfere with organ function. The most serious effect is recurrent infections of the lung that result in difficult to treat pneumonia and eventual loss of lung function. Plugging of the pancreas by thick secretions leads to loss of pancreatic secretions and defective digestion. Cystic fibrosis is the most common lethal autosomal recessive in white populations, with a gene frequency of about 1 in 30; but it is extremely rare in black populations. **Hemochromatosis** characterized by excessive absorption of iron, which accumulates within the body and disrupts the function of the liver, heart, and other organs, is discussed in the chapter on the hematopoietic and lymphatic systems

Cystic fibrosis Autosomal recessive disease caused by a defective sodium ion transporter gene.

Hemochromatosis An autosomal recessive genetic disease characterized by excessive iron absorption, leading to accumulation of excessive amounts of iron in the body, causing organ damage.

CODOMINANT INHERITANCE

In codominant inheritance, both alleles of a pair are fully expressed in the heterozygous state. This type of transmission is illustrated by the genes responsible for the synthesis of sickle (S) hemoglobin and other abnormal hemoglobins. These genes are abnormal alleles of the gene that directs the synthesis of normal hemoglobin. An individual heterozygous for the sickle hemoglobin gene will have approximately equal quantities of sickle hemoglobin and normal hemoglobin in the red cells. This condition is called **sickle cell trait** and usually causes no difficulties. Significant clinical manifestations are apparent, however, if the individual is homozygous for the sickle cell gene, resulting in no normal hemoglobin. This leads to a serious hereditary anemia called **sickle cell anemia**. This subject is considered in the hematopoietic and lymphatic systems discussion.

X-LINKED INHERITANCE

A number of hereditary diseases are transmitted on the X chromosome. The best-known example are the two forms of the disease hemophilia (hemophilia A and B), which are caused by deficiencies of proteins necessary for normal blood coagulation (F.VIII and F.IX, respectively).

Hemophilia is described in the discussion on abnormalities of blood coagulation and genetics.

MULTIFACTORIAL INHERITANCE

Many congenital defects do not result from single gene abnormalities and are not solely caused by environmental factors. Rather, they result from the combined effects of multiple genes interacting with environmental agents. This type of inheritance is called **multifactorial inheritance**.

Some of the common defects in which inheritance is multifactorial include cleft lip and palate, some congenital cardiac malformations, clubfoot, congenital dislocation of the hip, and certain congenital abnormalities of the nervous system called **anencephaly** and **spina bifida**, both congenital neural tube defects (NTDs).

NTDs may be related to environmental factors such as inadequate folic acid uptake, the use of the drug valproic acid, insulin dependent type 1 diabetes, and rarely from familial autosomal dominant or recessive inheritance. Most frequently, poorly defined multiple genetic and environmental factors play a role. Such multifactorial malformations have an incidence among newborn infants of from 1 in 500 to 1 in 2,000, depending on the malformation. The incidence is much higher, approximately 1 in 25, if one parent has the same type of congenital malformation or if other children born to the same parents have the malformation. This is likely because the genes that the parents are transmitting render their offspring more susceptible to disturbances in embryologic development, leading to specific types of congenital abnormalities. However, it is important to remember that sibs share environmental as well as genetic factors. The use of folic acid supplementation in wheat flour has markedly decreased the rate of NTDs. High-dose supplementation with folic acid in pregnant females who have had a previous NTD-associated pregnancy either abolishes (or much reduces) the risk in subsequent pregnancies, emphasizing the interaction of both environment and genetics.

Prenatal Diagnosis of Congenital Abnormalities

A wide variety of approaches is available to identify congenital abnormalities in the fetus. They include tests on maternal blood, examination of fetal cells obtained from amniotic fluid or the **chorionic villi** or ultrasound examination of the fetus and,

---

Sickle cell trait Condition in individuals heterozygous for the sickle hemoglobin gene.

Sickle cell anemia Condition in individuals homozygous for the sickle hemoglobin gene.

Multifactorial inheritance Inheritance of a trait or condition related to the combined effect of multiple genes rather than a single gene, as in Mendelian inheritance.

Anencephaly A congenital malformation: absence of brain, cranial vault, and scalp as a result of defective closure of the neural tube.

Spina bifida Incomplete closure of vertebral arches over the spinal cord, sometimes associated with protrusion of meninges and neural tissue through the defect (cystic spina bifida).

Chorionic villi examination Sampling of fetal derived placental cells.

most recently, analysis of fetal DNA obtained from the circulation of the mother. Currently, screening tests are offered to all pregnant women, not just to older women who are at higher risk for chromosomal abnormalities. Screening tests sometimes yield false-positive results, and positive screening test results must be confirmed by more definitive studies.

Tests on maternal blood to screen for possible fetal abnormalities measure the concentration of several substances normally present in the blood of pregnant women. Abnormal levels of such markers may indicate a fetal abnormality. One of the first maternal blood screening tests measured a protein called **alpha fetoprotein (AFP)**. The protein, produced by the fetus, diffuses into the amnionic fluid and then into the mother's blood. AFP is elevated when the fetus has a major central nervous system abnormality called an open neural tube defect (and NTD as mentioned above and described in the discussion on the nervous system). Because of its frequency and serious consequences, much effort has been placed on prenatal diagnosis of Down syndrome. A number of blood-based markers, including a lower than normal level of AFP and variation in the level of other circulating maternal proteins, combined with sonographic investigation of the neck region of the fetus allows for a 95-percent detection rate of Down syndrome with a 5-percent false-positive rate by the second trimester. (First trimester screening results in a lower detection rate of 85 percent.)

Fetal cells can be obtained from the amniotic fluid using a procedure called **amniocentesis** in which a needle is inserted through the mother's abdominal wall directly into the amnionic sac and a small amount of amniotic fluid is withdrawn, or by a procedure called chorionic villus sampling. Chorionic villi are frondlike structures of fetal origin that form part of the placenta and attach to the lining of the uterus (described in the discussion on prenatal development and diseases associated with pregnancy). The usual procedure involves passing a small catheter through the cervix to the site where the villi are attached to the uterus and suctioning out a small quantity of villi. Chorionic villus sampling has some advantages over amniocentesis because it can be performed at eight to ten weeks' gestation, whereas amniocentesis is usually performed between the fifteenth and twentieth week.

Both procedures are safe and show very little elevated risk of miscarriage (about 0.1 percent) when compared to spontaneous fetal loss and are strongly indicated in a number of situations (**TABLE 4-5**). Cytogenetic studies of fetal cells can detect chromosomal abnormalities. Genetic abnormalities also can be identified by biochemical tests performed on fetal cells or by analysis of DNA obtained from fetal cells. Thus, it possible to identify a large number of genetic diseases, including those listed in Table 4-2. The list of genetic diseases that can be identified prenatally continues to grow along with the rapid advances in the field of molecular genetics. Currently, such methods are being supplanted by direct measurement of cell free fetal DNA found in maternal blood during the first trimester. Such fetal DNA accounts for 10 percent of total DNA in maternal serum and is of placental origin. Although the separation

Alpha fetoprotein (AFP) Protein produced by fetal liver early in gestation. Level is elevated in amniotic fluid when fetus has a neural tube defect.

Amniocentesis Direct sampling of amniotic fluid.

TABLE 4-5 Main Indications for Amniocentesis or Chorionic Villus Sampling
1. Maternal blood tests (triple screen) indicating increased risk of fetal chromosome abnormality
2. Maternal age older than 35 years
3. Previous infant born with Down syndrome or other chromosomal abnormality
4. Known translocation chromosome carrier, or other chromosome abnormality in either parent
5. Risk of fetal genetic disease that can be detected by fetal cell biochemical or DNA analysis

of the fetal DNA "signal" from that of maternal DNA is complex, it allows the determination of Down syndrome (and other trisomies and potentially single gene mutations) with 99-percent accuracy and less than 0.1-percent false-positive rates. Such tests are available commercially at a cost of about $1,000.

By about sixteen weeks' gestation, ultrasound examination, described in the discussion on general concepts of disease: principles of diagnosis, can visualize the limbs and all of the major organs, including the brain and spinal cord, kidneys, bladder, and heart. The examination can detect major structural abnormalities of the nervous system called neural tube defects (anencephaly and spina bifida) and congenital hydrocephalus (discussion on the nervous system). Other structural abnormalities can be identified as well, including such defects as congenital obstruction of the urinary tract, failure of the kidneys to develop, or failure of the limbs to form normally.

If an abnormal fetus is identified by prenatal studies of the fetus, the parents are advised of the nature of the abnormality and its possible effects on the offspring. The parents must then reach a decision as to whether to terminate the pregnancy or allow it to continue to term.

Petechiae Small hemorrhages.

Seropositive Having antibodies to a pathogen.

CASE 4-1

The patient was an infant girl born after thirty-six weeks' gestation. A low birth weight for gestational age and small neonatal size with microcephaly were noted. The skin was covered with numerous small hemorrhages (**petechiae**) and appeared yellow (was jaundiced), indicating liver disease. The abdomen was markedly distended because of extreme enlargement of both the liver and the spleen (**FIGURE 4-9**). A CT scan of the head disclosed multiple defects, with enlargement of the fluid-filled spaces (ventricles) of the brain and abnormal deposits of calcium. The infant was moderately anemic, and the platelet count was reduced, which accounted for the widespread hemorrhages in the skin. Elevation of liver-specific enzymes in the infant's blood suggested serious liver disease. The infant was considered to be seriously ill as a result of a prenatal infection acquired from the mother. Diagnostic possibilities considered were congenital rubella, cytomegalic inclusion disease, systemic herpes virus infection, or toxoplasmosis. The infant died from widespread infection about five hours after examination before further diagnostic studies could be undertaken. The autopsy revealed the infection was caused by the cytomegalovirus. Pneumonia was detected, and characteristic cytomegalovirus inclusions were found in the lung. The diagnosis of congenital CMV infection was confirmed by additional laboratory tests (**FIGURE 4-10**).

Discussion

Cytomegalovirus infection (CMV) is the most common congenital infection, infecting between 0.6 and 1.0 percent of all births in the developing and developed world. CMV is a herpes virus that usually leads to asymptomatic disease in adults and children with normal immune systems. In developing countries, nearly 100 percent of people have been infected and have acquired antibodies to the virus (are **seropositive**) early in life. The number of seropositive people in developed countries reaches only about 50 percent in young adults. Although the risk of congenital CMV is greatest when the mother is first infected during pregnancy (and in particular during the first half), having antibodies to the virus does not rule out potential infection in utero. In a population in which more than 95 percent of pregnant women were seropositive, 1 percent of neonates were infected at birth and almost all were born of mothers who were seropositive prior to pregnancy.

Only 10 percent of CMV-infected neonates show signs of disease at birth, although this group is almost always born to mothers who have had their first CMV infection during

CASE 4-1 *(Continued)*

pregnancy. Such neonates are most frequently severely affected (as described in Case 4-1). The 90 percent of CMV-infected neonates who do not show disease at birth have a 10 to 20 percent risk of developing sequelae during childhood; most commonly hearing loss. Antiviral therapy may be considered in children with severe disease, but this is associated with significant side effects.

Etiology and Pathogenesis

The etiology is CMV infection in utero followed by multiorgan damage as a result of viral infection.

Questions

1. The physician attending the child considered a limited number of diseases to explain the symptoms observed. Why were these particular agents considered?

2. A definitive diagnosis was made at autopsy. How was this achieved?

3. Assume the child had survived. What other laboratory procedures could have been undertaken to establish a diagnosis of CMV?

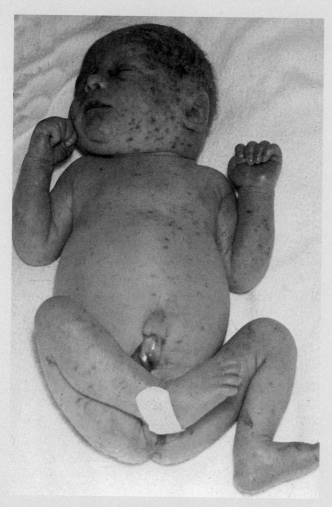

FIGURE 4-9 Severe systemic disease in newborn infant caused by an inapparent infection of the mother during pregnancy, as described in Case 4-1.

Courtesy of Leonard V. Crowley, MD, Century College.

(continues)

CASE 4-1 (Continued)

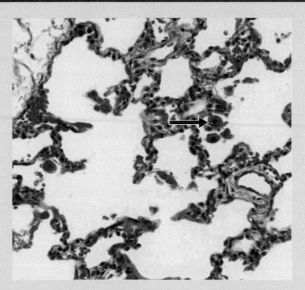

FIGURE 4-10 Characteristic CMV inclusions (*arrow*) in the lung of a newborn infant with congenital cytomegalovirus disease.

Courtesy of Department of Pathology and Laboratory Medicine, University of North Carolina at Chapel Hill.

QUESTIONS FOR REVIEW

1. What is the result of maternal infection? What can be the result of maternal alcohol use?

2. What are the consequences of chromosome nondisjunction? What is Down syndrome?

3. What are the karyotypes of an individual with Down syndrome? Klinefelter syndrome? Turner syndrome? What is fragile X syndrome?

4. What is the approximate incidence of congenital abnormalities? What are the major causes of congenital abnormalities?

5. What methods are available to sample fetal tissue?

SUPPLEMENTARY READINGS

Hartl, Daniel L. 2011. *Essential Genetics: A Genomic Perspective*, 5th ed. Sudbury, MA: Jones & Bartlett Learning.
▶ The study of congenital and hereditary disease is based on an understanding of modern genetics. An excellent general introduction to the area (with additional details of human disease) may be found here. Chapter 5 is of particular interest.

Viera, A. 2014. *Genes and disease.* Scitable by Nature Education. http://www.nature.com/scitable/topic/genes-and-disease-17
▶ There is a nearly limitless amount of reference material on congenital and hereditary disease available online. This article is good place to start and provides a gateway to additional information on topics covered in the chapter. The Explore This Subject list provides extensive additional resources on birth defects and specific diseases.

McKusick-Nathans Institute of Genetic Medicine. *OMIM.* http://www.ncbi.nlm.nih.gov/omim
▶ This is one of the most comprehensive and authoritative sources for genetic disease and genetic medicine. Although complex to use, it is a source that anyone interested in human genetics should consult.

An additional on-line source of authoritative information is the Center for Disease Control and Prevention (CDC). http://www.cdc.gov/ncbddd/birthdefects/index.html provides information on birth defects

The CDC Public Health Genomics Site http://www.cdc.gov/genomics/public/ provides information on specific genetic diseases including a list of current specific references.

Additional information relating to the CMV case may be found in the following review Schleiss, M. Pediatric Cytomegalovirus Infection Medscape Reference http://emedicine.medscape.com/article/963090-overview.

Inflammation and Repair

LEARNING OBJECTIVES

1. Compare/contrast innate and adaptive immunity.

2. Compare/contrast acute and chronic inflammation with special attention to the timeline of the response.

3. Name the chemical mediators of inflammation. Explain how they interact to intensify the inflammatory process. Include both cell and blood plasma derived mediators.

4. Describe the harmful effects of inflammation. Explain why it is sometimes necessary to suppress the inflammatory process.

5. Compare inflammation and infection. Name some of the terms used to describe infections.

Introduction: Host Defense

The body uses two approaches to respond to cell injury. Both are critical; defects in either rapidly result in disease. **Innate immunity** allows a quick response to a predetermined array of chemical signals that are associated with either invading **pathogens** (**Pathogen Associated Molecular Patterns [PAMPs]**) or injury to our cells (**Damage Associated Molecular Patterns [DAMPs]**). The innate immune response is limited to specific PAMPs and DAMPs, but these include the large array of pathogens and types of traumatic tissue injury that have occurred during human evolution. The injury related signals are detected by specific **receptor molecules (Pattern or Pathogen Recognition Receptors [PRRs])**. Similar PRRs occur throughout the animal kingdom, and related molecules are even found in insects. The second approach is termed **adaptive immunity**. This form of immunity can be relatively slow but has the ability to adapt itself to challenges never previously encountered by the organism. Even newly synthesized chemical toxins can be dealt with through adaptive immunity. Such challenges are remembered, and the adaptive response gets better with time to produce an even stronger, more specific response (**immune memory**). The PRR proteins for adaptive immunity are unique in having **variable regions** that adapt to fit the injurious substance. Such variable regions are found only in immunoglobulin protein molecules and on the PRRs found on T and B cells of the immune system. These adaptive immune responses are often simply termed "immune" and are the purview of the **immunologist** or **immunopathologist**. This is discussed in the chapter on immunology.

Innate immunity Quick response to predetermined array of chemical signals.

Pathogens Disease causing microorganisms.

Pathogen Associated Molecular Patterns (PAMPs) Microbial products that stimulate innate immunity.

Damage Associated Molecular Patterns (DAMPs) Molecules that can initiate and perpetuate immune response in the noninfectious inflammatory response.

Receptor molecules/ Pattern/Pathogen Recognition Receptors (PRRs) Receptors on cells recognizing molecular markers of disease causing microorganism.

Adaptive immunity
Immune response that can change based on intruding molecules.

Immune memory
Enhancement of immune response upon secondary encounter with antigen in adaptive immunity.

Variable region Region on the immunoglobulin molecule specific for a particular pathogen. Amino-terminal end of the immunoglobulin chain; part that recognizes antigen.

Immunologist Person who studies the immune response.

Immunopathologist Physician who studies the immune response associated with disease or who uses immunological-based testing tools.

Parasites Organism that lives in or on another organism deriving nutrients at the host's expense.

Acute inflammation Earliest phase of the inflammatory response.

Cellular component Circulating blood cell part of acute inflammation.

Neutrophils Polymorphonuclear neutrophils (PMNs) are actively phagocytic.

Phagocytic Engulf injurious agents into the cell.

Platelets Blood cells that adhere to collagen and mediate blood coagulation.

Mast cell A specialized connective tissue cell containing granules filled with histamine and other chemical mediators.

Chronic inflammation Cellular reaction leading to repair.

Although innate and adaptive immunity provide the "one-two punch" against tissue damage, they also often result in "bystander" injury to tissue or go awry and result in immune diseases.

The Inflammatory Reaction

The inflammatory reaction is part of the innate immune response to agents that cause cell injury. The agent may be physical (such as trauma, heat or cold), chemical (such as a caustic or irritating chemicals), microbiologic (such as a bacterium or virus), or multicellular **parasites**. The inflammatory reaction is characterized by predominantly local but also systemic effects (**FIGURE 5-1**).

The earliest phase of the inflammatory response, **acute inflammation**, occurs immediately after injury and lasts for twenty-four to forty-eight hours. Acute inflammation has both a vascular component (blood vessel related) and a **cellular component**, which relies on cells that circulate in the blood (**FIGURE 5-2**). The most important cells are **neutrophils** (polymorphonuclear neutrophils, PMNs), which are actively **phagocytic**. They engulf injurious agents (such as bacteria) and attempt to destroy them. **Platelets** adhere to collagen at the site of blood vessel injury and mediate the coagulation of blood to control hemorrhage related to tissue trauma. **Mast cells** found in the tissue (often in association with blood vessels) are important in the very early vascular phase of acute inflammation.

As acute inflammation winds down, **chronic inflammation** commences and continues, to some degree, until repair is complete, sometimes for weeks or months. Chronic inflammation, unlike acute inflammation, is predominantly a cellular reaction involving **macrophage-like cells (monocytes)** from the blood and tissue that produce a variety of **chemical mediators of inflammation**, clean up the debris produced early in acute inflammation, and also begin the healing process (**FIGURE 5-3**). **Lymphocytes**

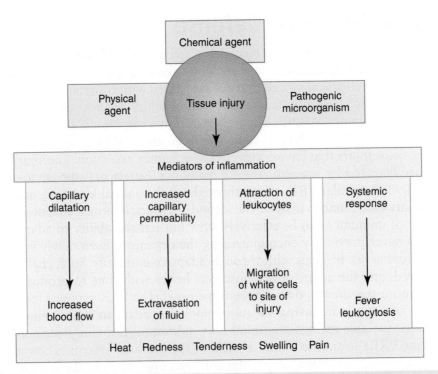

FIGURE 5-1 Local and systemic effects of tissue injury caused by various injurious agents.

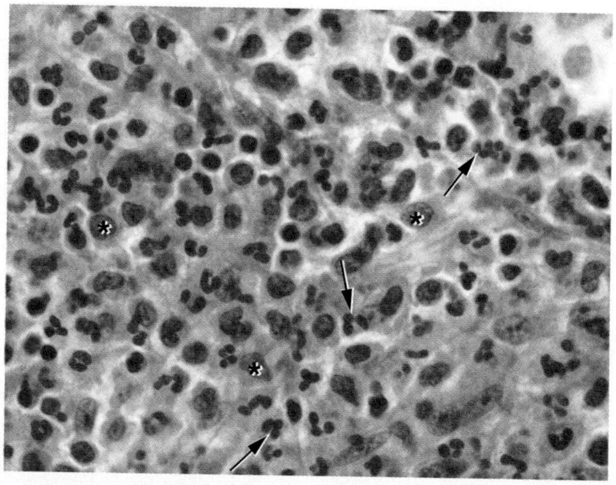

FIGURE 5-2　Acute inflammation is characterized by the presence of numerous neutrophils (polymorphonuclear leukocytes) (*arrows*). Several macrophages (*) are also present.

and related cells of the adaptive immune system are important in adaptive immunity and also play an important role in chronic inflammation.

The earliest part of acute inflammation is the vascular phase. The characteristic effects of the vascular phase of inflammation were clearly described by the Roman writer Celsus in the first century CE (but were also described in much older Egyptian medical texts). They are termed the **cardinal signs of inflammation**: the heat, swelling, redness, and pain observed at the site of injury. These signs can be observed after a relatively minor injury such as a scratch to the skin. All are the result of dilatation (expansion) of blood vessels and increased vascular permeability. The increased warmth and redness of the inflamed tissues are caused by dilatation of capillaries and increase of blood flow through the vessels (**hyperemia**). Swelling occurs because the **extravasation** (leakage) of plasma from the dilated and more permeable vessels causes the volume of fluid in the inflamed tissue to increase (**FIGURE 5-4**). The tenderness and pain are caused by irritation of sensory nerve endings at the site of the

Macrophage-like cells/monocytes　Type of white blood cell important in the immune response.

Chemical mediators of inflammation　Messenger molecule that acts on blood vessels, inflammatory cells, or other cells to contribute to an inflammatory response.

Lymphocytes　Cells important in adaptive immunity.

Cardinal signs of inflammation　Heat, swelling, redness, and pain observed at the site of injury.

Hyperemia　Increased blood flow through vessels.

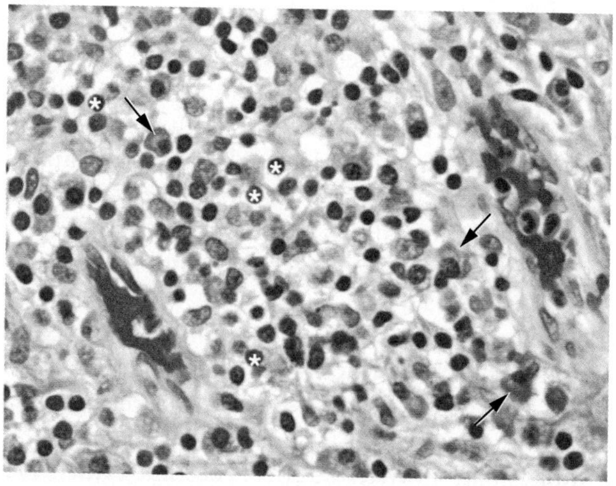

FIGURE 5-3　Chronic inflammation is characterized by an infiltrate composed of lymphocytes (*white* *), plasma cells (*black arrows*), and macrophages. Eosinophils (demonstrating red cytoplasm) are also present as are red cells in several capillaries.

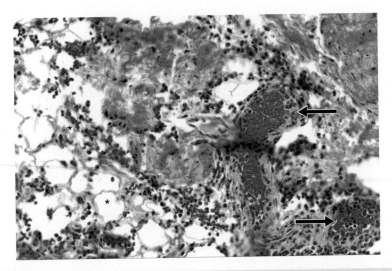

FIGURE 5-4 Photomicrograph of connective tissue removed during a surgical procedure illustrating neutrophils adherent to small blood vessel endothelium and migrating through wall to site of tissue injury. Several examples are shown at arrows. The open spaces in tissue (examples at *) represent exudation. Some hemorrhage of red cells into tissue is also present.

Courtesy of Department of Pathology and Laboratory Medicine, University of North Carolina at Chapel Hill.

Extravasation Leakage of plasma from dilated vessels.

Activated neutrophil Neutrophil stimulated by various substances resulting in degranulation.

Emigration Cells move through walls of blood vessels.

Chemotaxis Process of active movement of inflammatory cells to the site of the injury.

Exudate The fluid, leukocytes, and debris that accumulate as a result of an inflammation.

Serous Fluid-rich exudate.

Purulent Neutrophil-rich exudate, also called pus.

Fibrinous Fibrin-rich exudate.

Hemorrhagic Red-cell-rich inflammatory fluid.

Adhesions Bands of fibrous tissue that form subsequent to an inflammation and bind adjacent tissues together.

White cell count Count of number and type of white cells present in the blood. A test for inflammation.

inflammatory process, both as a result of the swelling and also as a result of specific chemical mediators of pain produced at the injured site.

Local and Systemic Effects

During inflammation a change in the permeability of venules and capillaries occurs as well as leakage of protein rich fluid into the tissue at sites of inflammation. PRRs on the neutrophil become activated (**activated neutrophil**) by recognition of the PAMPs and DAMPs, inciting the inflammatory response, and are primed to adhere to the endothelium of the small blood vessels, forcing their way through the walls (**emigration**) and migrating to the area of tissue damage (Figure 5-4). In doing so, the neutrophils (and likewise the macrophage-like monocytes of chronic inflammation) sense the molecules associated with either pathogens or tissue damage and actively move toward the site of injury in a process termed **chemotaxis**. The protein rich fluid in combination with neutrophils, which have either actively emigrated from vessels (as part of the cellular phase of acute inflammation) or are found in tissue as a result of damage to blood vessels, is called **exudate**. Although the proportions of protein and inflammatory cells vary in different exudates, along with its appearance, in general an exudate can be described as **serous** (fluid rich), **purulent** (neutrophil rich, pus), **fibrinous** (rich in the protein fibrin derived from fibrinogen in the blood), or **hemorrhagic** (rich in red cells). The terms are sometimes combined as in "fibrinopurulent" rich in fibrin and cells (**FIGURE 5-5**).

If a fibrinous exudate involves two surfaces in close proximity, such as adjacent loops of small intestine, the surfaces may stick together. In such cases, healing may result in fibrous scar tissue termed **adhesions** bridging the adjacent surfaces (**FIGURE 5-6**).

In more severe inflammation, systemic effects become evident. The individual feels ill, and the temperature is elevated. The bone marrow accelerates its production of neutrophils and monocytes, producing the elevated **white cell count** used to monitor for the presence of diseases associated with inflammation. The liver produces several

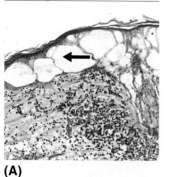 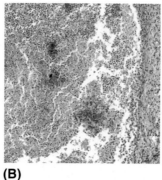 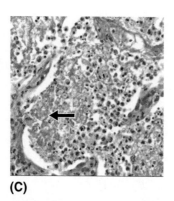

(A) **(B)** **(C)**

FIGURE 5-5 Examples of exudates: **(A)** Serous exudate; blister fluid in burned skin (*arrow*), **(B)** Purulent exudate; accumulation of neutrophils, many of which are necrotic in a liver abscess, **(C)** Fibrinopurulent; accumulation of neutrophils and fibrin (*arrow*) in the lung of a patient with bacterial pneumonia.

Courtesy of Department of Pathology and Laboratory Medicine, University of North Carolina at Chapel Hill.

proteins called **acute phase proteins** that are released into the bloodstream in response to tissue injury or inflammation, which help protect the body from the tissue injury caused by the inflammation. One of the best known of these proteins is **C reactive protein**, which is often measured to monitor the activity of diseases characterized by tissue inflammation. Another is **fibrinogen**, important in blood coagulation. The proteins concerned in the coagulation of the blood are considered in the discussion on abnormalities of blood coagulation. Increases in fibrinogen levels in the blood are responsible for an increased **erythrocyte sedimentation rate (ESR)**, a measure of how quickly red cells settle out of the blood placed in a tube. The ESR is a much used and very sensitive (but not very specific) test that detects inflammation in a patient.

The outcome of inflammation depends on how much tissue damage has resulted from the inflammation. If the inflammation is mild, it soon subsides, and the tissues return to normal. This process is called **resolution**. If the inflammatory process is more severe, tissue is destroyed to some extent and must be repaired. During healing, damaged cells are replaced, and the framework of the injured tissue is repaired as an ingrowth of cells produces connective tissue fibers and new blood vessels forming **granulation tissue**, an intermediate step in the repair process. Scar tissue is formed from

Acute phase proteins Proteins produced by the liver in response to inflammation.

C reactive protein An acute-phase protein.

Fibrinogen An acute-phase protein important in blood coagulation.

Erythrocyte sedimentation rate (ESR) A laboratory test to measure the speed red cells settle out of the blood; used to detect inflammation.

Resolution Regression of an inflammatory process without significant tissue destruction and with return of the tissues to normal.

Granulation tissue Normal part of the healing process.

FIGURE 5-6 Multiple fibrous adhesions (*arrows*) between loops of small intestine resulting from previous abdominal inflammation.

Courtesy of Leonard V. Crowley, MD, Century College.

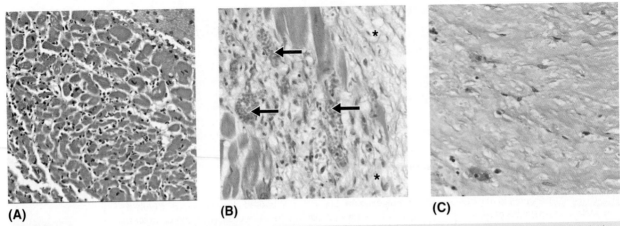

(A)　　**(B)**　　**(C)**

FIGURE 5-7　Injury and repair in a myocardial infarct (heart attack): **(A)** Acute inflammation; note the presence of neutrophils in the injured tissue (twenty-four hours post infarction), **(B)** Healing with the formation of granulation tissue; note the formation of new blood vessels (*arrow*) and new collagen deposition (*) (ten days post infarction), **(C)** Scar formation; note the dense fibrous (scar) tissue and lack of heart muscle cells see in (A).

Courtesy of Department of Pathology and Laboratory Medicine, University of North Carolina at Chapel Hill.

Myocardial infarct/ heart attack Necrosis of heart muscle as a result of interruption of its blood supply. May affect full thickness of muscle wall (transmural infarct) or only part of the wall (subendocardial infarct).

Mediators of inflammation Chemicals causing inflammatory response.

Histamine Chemical released by mast cells.

Vasodilator A substance that dilates blood vessels.

Serotonin A vasoconstrictor mediator of inflammation released from platelets.

Prostaglandin A series of derivatives of archidonic acid that have widespread physiologic effects.

Leukotriene A prostaglandin-like mediator of inflammation.

the granulation tissue in the area of damage. Sometimes, the scarring subsequent to a severe inflammation is so severe that function is seriously disturbed. Thus, even though scar tissue is a necessary patch to heal damage to an organ, the functional cells (parenchyma) of the organ may not be replaced if they cannot divide. For example, damage to the circulation supplying the heart causes a **myocardial infarct (heart attack)** characterized by the death of heart muscle cells. Release of DAMPs from the dying cells results in acute and then chronic inflammation, followed by the formation of granulation tissue, which will with time become a fibrous scar. However, the heart muscle cells cannot divide to repair the damage, so the individual is left with a "patched" area of the heart, a fibrous scar made of collagen that cannot contract. The heart, although repaired, can no longer function as effectively, and the patient may show signs of heart failure (**FIGURE 5-7**).

CHEMICAL MEDIATORS OF INFLAMMATION

The inflammatory reaction just described is a nonspecific, stereotyped response to tissue injury and is much the same no matter what caused the injury. The inflammatory response is not directly caused by the tissue injury but is caused by chemical agents called **mediators of inflammation** that are formed and released when damage to tissue is detected by PRRs. Some mediators are derived from cells, and others are formed from proteins in the blood plasma that accumulate in the injured area.

Cell-Derived Mediators

Mast cells, a major source of cell-derived mediators, are specialized cells that are widely distributed throughout the connective tissues of the body but often found proximate to blood vessels. Their cytoplasm is filled with preformed granules containing **histamine** and other chemicals. If tissue is injured, the mast cells discharge their granules, liberating the chemicals to initiate the inflammatory process. Histamine is a potent **vasodilator** and also greatly increases vascular permeability. Blood platelets also contain histamine and another mediator called **serotonin**, which are released when platelets adhere to collagen fragments at the site of blood vessel injury. Other important cell-derived mediators are a group called **prostaglandins** and a group of similar compounds called **leukotrienes**. These biologically active compounds are synthesized by cells from arachidonic acid present in cell membranes in response to stimuli that induce inflammation, and they function as mediators that intensify the inflammatory process. Many of the cells important in the inflammatory response including neutrophils; should be, macrophage-like cells and endothelial cells lining blood vessels synthesize specific types of prostaglandins and leukotrienes. Aspirin and other **nonsteroidal anti-inflammatory drugs (NSAIDs)** such as ibuprofen and naproxen function by inhibiting the production of prostaglandins. **Cytokines** are small proteins released by cells important in both adaptive and innate immunity that serve to modulate such reactions. They may act locally to affect nearby cells but also systemically. Cytokines may be pro-inflammatory or in some cases anti-inflammatory. **Interleukin-1 (IL-1)** and **tumor necrosis factor alpha (TNF-α)** are pro-inflammatory and act locally to help neutrophils adhere to and exit from blood vessels in injured areas. Acting systemically they are responsible for the fever and malaise associated with inflammation and the increased synthesis of acute-phase reactants previously mentioned.

Mediators from Blood Plasma

Blood plasma contains various protein substances that circulate as inactive compounds and leak from the permeable capillaries into the area of tissue damage where they become transformed (activated) by a complex process into chemical mediators. One important group of mediators formed in this way is called **bradykinins** (or simply kinins). The series of reactions that leads to the formation of bradykinins is triggered by one of the proteins concerned with blood coagulation, which is activated by tissue injury. Kinins are important in producing vasodilation, help recruit neutrophils to injured sites, and are responsible for much of the pain associated with inflammation.

Mediators of inflammation are also formed from another group of blood proteins called **complement**. Complement consists of at least fifty protein components, some of the best known of which are numbered as C_1 through C_9, The proteins interact in a regular sequence to yield a series of by-products, some of which function as mediators of inflammation. Complement (abbreviated as C′) participates in both the nonspecific and specific responses to cell injury. It is activated when an antigen combines with an antibody (specific response) but may also be activated in other ways that do not require an antigen–antibody interaction such as by pathogen components containing certain sugars (mannans). The various functions of the complement system are considered in connection with immunity, hypersensitivity, allergy, and autoimmune diseases.

FIGURE 5-8 illustrates how the various mediators interact. The release of mediators from any source not only initiates the inflammatory process but also induces release of more mediators from other sources, setting off a "chain reaction" that intensifies the inflammatory process.

Non-steroidal anti-inflammatory drugs (NSAIDs) Drug such as ibuprofen and naproxen that inhibit the production of prostaglandins.

Cytokine Small protein released by cells that modulate the production of mediators of inflammation.

Interleukin-1 (IL-1) Pro-inflammatory cytokine.

Tumor necrosis factor alpha (TNF α) Pro-inflammatory cytokine.

Bradykinin A chemical mediator of inflammation derived from components in the blood plasma.

Complement Group of proteins interact to produce by-products, some of which act as mediators of inflammation.

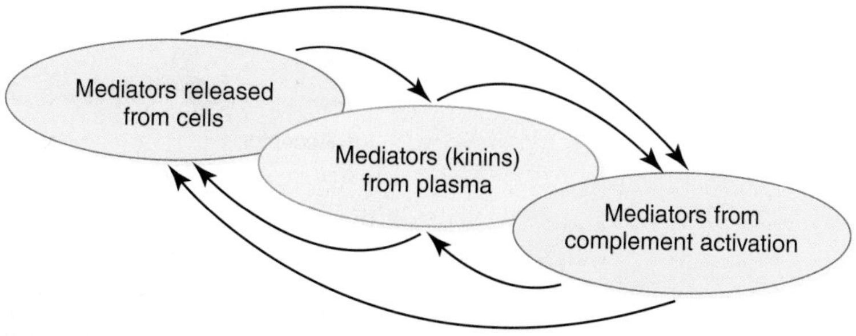

FIGURE 5-8 Interaction of mediators of inflammation. Activation of mediators from any source also leads to the formation of mediators from other sources, which intensifies the inflammatory reaction.

THE ROLE OF LYSOSOMAL ENZYMES IN THE INFLAMMATORY PROCESS

The cytoplasm of phagocytic neutrophils and monocytes that are attracted to the site of inflammation by chemical mediators contains organelles called **lysosomes**. Lysosomes contain potent enzymes that are capable of digesting the material brought into the cytoplasm of the cells by **phagocytosis**. During phagocytosis, bacteria or other foreign materials become enclosed within phagocytic vacuoles in the cell cytoplasm, and the lysosomes dissolve the material by discharging their enzymes into the vacuoles, as described in the discussion on cells and tissues (**FIGURE 5-9**). In addition to lysosomal-mediated destruction, potent **oxidizing agents** such as hydrogen peroxide and hypochlorous acid (laundry bleach) are synthesized by neutrophils and discharged into phagocytic vacuoles where they are important in destroying bacteria and fungi.

Much of the tissue injury in an area of inflammation is a result of the destructive effect of the lysosomal enzymes released from leukocytes. In the course of any inflammatory reaction, lysosomal enzymes are released from damaged neutrophils and monocytes. Some lysosomal enzymes and oxidizing agents also escape from intact leukocytes during phagocytosis. The tissue injury in turn generates more mediators, and this induces further inflammatory changes. Lack of oxidative killing of pathogens is associated with a serious inherited disease (**chronic granulomatous disease**) in which patients suffer from life-long and repeated infections by bacteria and fungi.

Lysosomes Cytoplasmic organelles containing digestive enzymes.

Phagocytosis Process by which cell engulfs foreign material.

Oxidizing agents Chemicals synthesized by neutrophils that help destroy bacteria and fungi.

Chronic granulomatous disease Disease caused by lack of oxidative killing of pathogens.

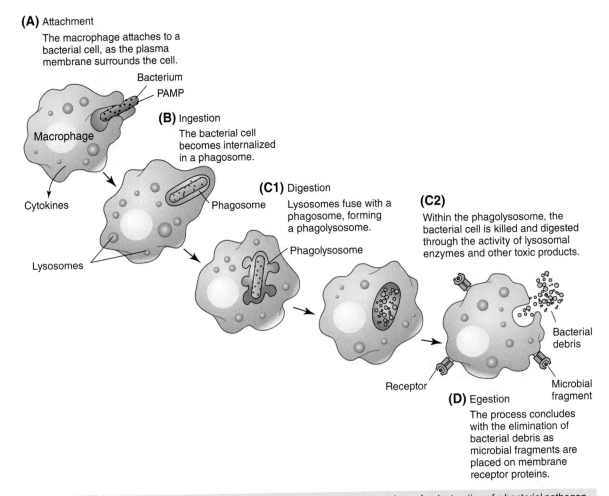

(A) Attachment
The macrophage attaches to a bacterial cell, as the plasma membrane surrounds the cell.

Bacterium
PAMP
Macrophage
Cytokines
Lysosomes

(B) Ingestion
The bacterial cell becomes internalized in a phagosome.

Phagosome

(C1) Digestion
Lysosomes fuse with a phagosome, forming a phagolysosome.

Phagolysosome

(C2)
Within the phagolysosome, the bacterial cell is killed and digested through the activity of lysosomal enzymes and other toxic products.

Receptor

Bacterial debris

Microbial fragment

(D) Egestion
The process concludes with the elimination of bacterial debris as microbial fragments are placed on membrane receptor proteins.

FIGURE 5-9 The mechanism of phagocytosis: The stages of phagocytosis are shown for destruction of a bacterial pathogen.

HARMFUL EFFECTS OF INFLAMMATION

The tissue injury that results from inflammation is due in part to the injurious agent and in part to the inflammatory reaction itself. In most cases, the inflammatory process is self-limited and subsides when the harmful agent has been eliminated. At times, however, an inflammatory process may persist and cause extensive, progressive tissue injury. If this occurs, the inflammatory process may need suppression by administering **adrenal corticosteroid hormones (steroids)** to reduce the tissue damage that would result if the inflammatory process were not restrained. Milder effects are treated with NSAIDs. (Suppression of the immune response is considered in the discussion on immunity, hypersensitivity, allergy, and autoimmune diseases.)

Role of Inflammation in Infection

FACTORS INFLUENCING THE OUTCOME OF AN INFECTION

The nonspecific inflammatory process plays a role in the body's ability to fight off an infection by bacteria or other microbiologic agents. Bacteria and other microbiologic agents vary in their ability to cause disease. The term **virulence** refers to the ease with which a pathogenic organism can overcome the defenses of the body. A highly virulent organism is one that is likely to produce progressive disease in the majority of susceptible individuals. In contrast, an organism of low virulence is capable only of producing disease in a highly susceptible individual under favorable circumstances.

The outcome of any infection depends on two factors: the virulence of the organism combined with the numbers ("dosage") of the invading organisms and the resistance of the infected individual (often called the **host**). These may be considered balanced against one another, as indicated diagrammatically in **FIGURE 5-10**. When large numbers of organisms of high virulence are introduced into the body, especially when host resistance is lowered, the balance is tipped in favor of the invader and progressive or fatal disease develops. When the virulence or dosage of the organism is low or the body's resistance is high, the balance is tipped in favor of the host. The **infection** is then overcome and healing occurs.

Role of Inflammatory Cells in Antimicrobial Defense

Neutrophils and macrophage-like cells (monocytes when in the blood) internalize and digest foreign material including pathogenic microorganisms by a process termed phagocytosis. There is some specialization as to which cells deal with particular types of pathogens. The acute inflammatory response characterized by the presence

> **Adrenal corticosteroid hormones/steroids** Chemicals that suppress the inflammatory process.
>
> **Virulence** The ability of an organism to cause disease.
>
> **Host** Individual infected with a disease-producing organism.
>
> **Infection** Inflammation caused by a disease-producing organism.

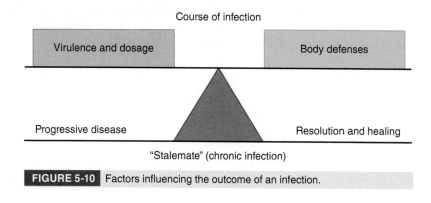

FIGURE 5-10 Factors influencing the outcome of an infection.

of neutrophils at the site of tissue injury is characteristic of bacterial disease. Viral and fungal disease most commonly presents as chronic inflammation without a preliminary acute inflammatory phase. Hence, the response to these pathogens is characterized by "mononuclear" cells including macrophage-like cells and lymphocytes. For this reason, a physician noting a higher than normal level of neutrophils in the blood suspects a bacterial etiology. An increase in mononuclear cells (usually lymphocytes) suggest a viral disease. However, there are many exceptions to this rule.

Both neutrophils and macrophages are attracted to the foreign material (undergo chemotaxis) when it is coated with plasma proteins collectively called **opsonins**, which are either derived from complement or are immunoglobulins produced as part of the adaptive host response. Microorganisms that have mechanisms to evade this process are more virulent. The role of inflammatory cells is crucial in degrading microbes but also contributes to further cell damage and inflammation as a result of release of lysosomal enzymes and oxidizing agents into tissue. The importance of these cells in antimicrobial defense is further emphasized by the frequency and severity of infections when these cells are decreased due to the neutropenia resulting from cancer chemotherapy or congenital diseases or when cells are incapable of killing the phagocytosed material.

TERMINOLOGY OF INFECTION

The term *infection* is used to denote an inflammatory process caused by disease-producing organisms. A number of different terms are used to refer to infections in various sites. Generally, the ending *-itis* is appended to the name of the tissue or organ to indicate an infection or inflammatory process. For example, the terms *appendicitis, hepatitis, colitis,* and *pneumonitis* refer to inflammation of the appendix, liver, colon, and lung, respectively. An acute spreading infection at any site is called **cellulitis**. Usually, this term is used to refer to an acute infection of the skin and deeper tissues. The term **abscess** is used when an infection is associated with breakdown of the tissues and the formation of a localized mass of pus (Figure 5-5B). If a localized infection spreads into the lymphatic channels draining the site of inflammation, the term **lymphangitis** is used. **Lymphadenitis** refers to infection in the regional lymph nodes draining the primary site of infection. The term **septicemia** is used to refer to an overwhelming infection in which pathogenic bacteria gain access to the bloodstream.

Chronic Infection

Sometimes, the organism and host are evenly matched. Neither can gain the advantage; the result is a stalemate. Clinically, this results in a chronic infection, characterized by a relatively quiet, smoldering inflammation that is usually associated with continued attempts at healing on the part of the host. The balance between the host and the invader is precarious. The infection may flare up at times when the pathogen obtains a temporary advantage, or it may become quiescent at other times when the defenses of the host gain the upper hand. Lymphocytes, plasma cells, and monocytes are the predominant cells in chronic inflammatory processes.

Opsonins Plasma proteins that attract neutrophils and macrophages to foreign material.

Cellulitis An acute spreading inflammation affecting the skin or deeper tissues.

Abscess A localized accumulation of pus in tissues.

Lymphangitis An inflammation of lymph vessels draining a site of infection.

Lymphadenitis An inflammation of lymph nodes draining a site of infection.

Septicemia An infection in which large numbers of pathogenic bacteria are present in the bloodstream.

CASE 5-1

Jane is an eighteen-year-old college freshman dressed in shorts who is playing a game of touch football on a grass field when she stumbles. She lands on a broken beer bottle and suffers a **laceration** on the **dorsal** surface of her thigh. Her friends suggest that she visit student health, but she has an examination in the afternoon. She washes the wound, places several large gauze pads on it. and wraps it to stop bleeding. She changes the pads every day, but five days after receiving the injury she notes some pus on the surface of the **eschar** and an **exophytic** growing mass of tissue (**FIGURE 5-11**). Alarmed, she visits the health service. The physician explains she has developed a minor infection in the wound. The mass is composed of granulation tissue, an excessive amount of what is a normal part of the healing process. However, because of the infection and large mass of granulation tissue, the physician **debrides** the wound. He explains that because she did not immediately seek medical attention and have the wound sutured she is likely to be left with a large scar.

Discussion

During wound healing, granulation tissue is the matrix in which new blood vessels form and in which fibroblasts proliferate to produce collagen, a process termed **fibrosis** (scar formation). Figure 5-11 (inset) shows an area rich in the formation of small capillaries oriented upward toward the wound surface. In addition, many mononuclear inflammatory cells and the elongated nuclei of fibroblasts are present. In cases where wound healing is delayed (as it was by infection in Case 5-1), cytokine production by inflammatory cells may promote the growth of excessive granulation tissue that can gape above the wound (sometimes termed **proud flesh**). With time, the granulation tissue will be replaced by a large scar. This form of healing of a large unsutured wound is termed **secondary union**. Sutured wounds oppose the injured surfaces, leaving little space for granulation tissue to form. Such healing by **primary union** leaves a small scar (**FIGURE 5-12**). Plastic and reconstructive surgeons go to great effort to carefully suture wounds to minimize scarring and to produce esthetically satisfactory results.

Etiology and Pathogenesis

The etiology is traumatic injury (laceration) resulting in superficial bacterial infection. The pathogenesis demonstrates healing of a wound by secondary union combined with excess production of granulation tissue.

Questions

1. Suppose Jane had immediately sough medical attention. What steps might the physician have taken in treating the wound?

2. Granulation tissue consists of mononuclear inflammatory cells, fibroblasts, and new capillaries. What role does each play in wound healing?

3. Careful examination of Figure 5-11 might disclose some neutrophils in the wound bed. Why do you think this is likely?

Laceration An irregular jagged wound.	
Dorsal Front surface.	
Eschar Scab.	
Exophytic Outward growing mass of tissue protruding from the wound.	
Debrides Removes dead, infected, and excess granulation tissue from the wound bed.	
Fibrosis Scar formation.	
Proud flesh Growth of excessive granulation tissue that can gape above the wound.	
Secondary union Form of healing of a large unsutured wound.	
Primary union Form of healing of a sutured wound.	

(continues)

CASE 5-1 *(Continued)*

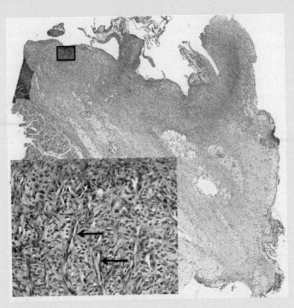

FIGURE 5-11 Debrided granulation tissue from wound. Inset (taken from boxed area) shows tissue at high power. Arrows indicate developing capillaries.

Courtesy of Department of Pathology and Laboratory Medicine, University of North Carolina at Chapel Hill.

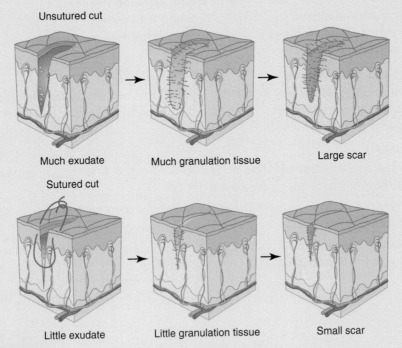

FIGURE 5-12 Repair of sutured and unsutured skin cut leading to secondary and primary union, respectively.

QUESTIONS FOR REVIEW

1. What is the inflammatory reaction? What are its clinical manifestations?
2. What factors influence the outcome of an infection?
3. What are mediators of inflammation? How do they function?
4. What is meant by the following terms: *chronic infection, pathogenic, complement?*
5. What is the relationship of innate and adaptive immunity?

SUPPLEMENTARY READINGS

Murphey, H. S., Chapter 2 "Inflammation," and Sephel, G. C., and Davidson, J. M., Chapter 3 "Regeneration and Fibrosis." 2014. In *Essentials of Rubin's Pathology*, edited by E. Rubin and H. M. Reisner. Baltimore and Philadelphia: Lippincott Williams & Wilkins.

▶ Detailed discussion of the aspects of inflammation and repair are of importance in undergraduate medical education. Hence, medical textbooks are the best source for concise and timely discussion of these complex areas. This text does a good job of presenting details in a concise manner.

IPLab (http://peir.path.uab.edu/wiki/IPLab)

▶ There are a number of web-based resources for the study of pathology. IPLab, an instructional resource for pathology education, is an excellent source for additional information and particular case studies with excellent illustrative material. "Lab 3: Inflammation and Repair" is of particular interest.

Greaves, N. S., et al. 2013. Current understanding of molecular and cellular mechanisms in fibroplasia and angiogenesis during acute wound healing. *Journal of Dermatological Science* 72:206–17.

▶ This article provides an up-to-date review of molecular and cellular aspects of wound healing.

Immunity, Hypersensitivity, Allergy, and Autoimmune Diseases

Courtesy of Department of Pathology and Laboratory Medicine, University of North Carolina at Chapel Hill

LEARNING OBJECTIVES

1. List the basic features of cell-mediated and humoral immunity. Explain the role of lymphocytes in the immune response.

2. List the five classes of antibodies, and explain how they differ from one another.

3. Describe the four types of hypersensitivity. Describe the pathogenesis of allergic manifestations and the role of IgE in allergy. Compare the methods of treatment.

4. Explain why it is sometimes necessary to suppress the immune response, and describe how this is accomplished.

5. Describe the causes and clinical manifestations of immunodeficiency disease.

6. Compare and contrast tolerance and autoimmune disease, including the clinical manifestations and the methods of treatment.

Introduction: The Body's Defense Mechanisms

Innate immunity, discussed in the presentation of the inflammatory response, is quick to respond but only to the predetermined array of molecular patterns associated with pathogens or those molecules characteristic of injured cells. The innate immune response is limited to specific challenges that have frequently occurred during human evolution.

Unlike us, many pathogens have the ability to quickly evolve to counter our host defenses. Even during the course of an infection, organisms may develop mechanisms to thwart our innate defenses mechanisms. In addition, the movement of populations and changes in the environment constantly exposes us to new challenges with which innate immunity may be unable to cope.

First found in lower vertebrates with jaws (cartilaginous fish such as sharks), **adaptive immunity**—comprised of **cell-mediated immunity** and **humoral immunity**—provides us with the ability to detect and adaptively respond essentially to any molecular structure foreign to us (even one never before encountered). The aspects of *adaptive recognition* and *response to foreign structures* and *immune memory* define adaptive immunity and differentiate it from innate immunity. Innate immunity can only adapt to new challenges with evolution, whereas adaptive immunity can cope with previously unrecognized agents nearly in "real time." Unfortunately, the adaptive immune system may err, recognizing the self as foreign and resulting in **autoimmune disease**.

Innate immunity
Preprogrammed immune response.

Adaptive immunity
Immune response with the ability to respond to almost any foreign molecule.

Cell-mediated immunity
Immunity associated with population of sensitized lymphocytes.

Humoral immunity
Immunity associated with formation of antibodies produced by plasma cells.

Autoimmune disease A disease associated with formation of cell-mediated or humoral immunity against the subject's own cells or tissue components.

INNATE VERSUS ADAPTIVE IMMUNITY

Innate immunity has a very rapid time of response and involves multiple classes of blood cells (e.g., mast cells, neutrophils, and macrophages) and a large number of chemical mediators, some produced by stimulated cells, others that circulate in the blood. Although low levels of cells, such as neutrophils, or a defect in one of the chemical mediators may result in disease, the many overlapping mechanisms of the innate immune system ensure that broad immunodeficiency to a wide array of opportunistic pathogens does not occur. The pattern recognition receptors (PRR) used by innate immunity are encoded into the genome and have fixed specificity. Several sets of these receptors are found on the surface of cells, within membrane bound vesicles, or free in the cytoplasm. All of the receptors of a given type are identical and invariant, and can cope with only a limited array of pathogen structures. Although the pathogen structures recognized by the PRR are often essential to pathogen infectivity; they are liable to mutation by the pathogen thus allowing the pathogen to circumvent the innate immune system. In summary, innate immunity is a rapidly acting first line of defense that often slows the infectious process but cannot eliminate it. Innate immunity primes the adaptive immune system, buying time for the adaptive system to respond as a second line and highly effective mechanism for host defense.

Adaptive Immunity

Adaptive immunity can be divided into two tightly interrelated systems: humoral immunity and cell-mediated (or cellular) immunity. Lack of either system will result in susceptibility to pathogens (albeit of a somewhat different nature) and can result in life-threatening disease. Humoral immunity absolutely requires an intact cellular immune system to function effectively.

Humoral immunity is associated with the production of antibodies, soluble proteins of the immunoglobulin class. Antibodies circulate in the blood and body fluids and function by binding to and eliminating foreign material. Humoral immunity is the body's major defense against many bacteria and bacterial toxin threats that are predominantly extracellular. Cell-mediated immunity is characterized by the formation of a population of lymphocytes (**T lymphocytes** or simply **T cells**) that can attack and destroy the foreign material. Cell-mediated immunity is the main defense against viruses, fungi, parasites, and some bacteria (particularly those that are intracellular). Cell-mediated immunity is also the major mechanism by which the body rejects transplanted organs and eliminates the abnormal cells that sometimes arise spontaneously in cell division (although humoral immunity can play a role in both processes under certain circumstances) (**TABLE 6-1**).

T lymphocyte/T cell
A type of lymphocyte associated with cell-mediated immunity.

TABLE 6-1 Comparison of Humoral and Cell-Mediated Immunity	
Humoral	**Cell-mediated**
Principal cellular agent is the B cell.	Principal cellular agent is the T cell.
B cell responds to bacteria, bacterial toxins, and some viruses.	T cell responds to cancer cells, virus-infected cells, single-cell fungi, parasites, and foreign cells in an organ transplant.
When activated, B cells form memory cells and plasma cells, which produce antibodies to these antigens.	When activated, T cells differentiate into memory cells, cytotoxic cells, suppressor cells, and helper cells; cytotoxic T cells attack the antigen directly.

Adaptive immunity is critical to host defense. However, the functioning of adaptive immunity can also lead to disease (**autoimmunity**) resulting from a failure of our immune systems to distinguish the self (the host) from foreign material. Autoimmune diseases tend to be chronic, debilitating, and difficult to control (short of making the patient immunodeficient to some degree). Certain damaging aspects of adaptive immunity are termed **hypersensitivity reactions,** implying excessive immunity. More often inappropriate immunity, such as occurs in allergic responses, is the cause. The plant products that result in "hay fever" allergies are foreign to us and recognized as such by our adaptive immune system. However, plant pollens are not of themselves harmful. The allergic individual produces a particular type (class) of **immunoglobulin (IgE)** that is ultimately responsible for the dripping nose and sneezing. However, IgE immunoglobulins are likely to be critical for host defense against parasites. So the allergic individual is not making too much immunoglobulin but rather is responding to something that is not a danger in a way that causes disease. Hypersensitivity reactions are classified in a manner depending on the nature of the damaging reaction and whether it is part of humoral immunity (as is allergy) or is related to cellular immunity. The reaction that a person exposed to tuberculosis has to a tuberculin test (in which a material derived from the bacteria tuberculin is injected into the skin) is a form of hypersensitivity mediated by cellular immunity. It is often referred to as **delayed hypersensitivity** because it may take a while to appear. (This is the reason a tuberculin skin test is read several days after testing.) The reaction tells us that our host defense system has recognized the tuberculosis bacteria and may be keeping it in check. But the reaction to tuberculin also results in some degree of tissue damage. To understand the two sides of the coin, the essential protective role of adaptive immunity and its potentially damaging role, one must understand how the complex system of adaptive immunity functions.

THE ROLE OF LYMPHOCYTES IN ADAPTIVE IMMUNITY

The key cells of the adaptive immune system are the lymphocyte (**FIGURE 6-1**), which responds to foreign antigens, and the macrophages and related cells that process the antigen and "present" it to the lymphocytes. Both functional lymphocytes and **antigen presenting cells (APC)** are necessary for response to a foreign substance, broadly termed an **antigen**. Antigens are circularly defined as any substance that can bind to an **antibody** (the immunoglobulin molecule that binds a particular antigen) or that can bind to the antigen recognition molecule on T lymphocytes responsible for cellular immunity (**T cell receptor**). Antigens must be foreign to the host and have certain other chemical characteristics. T cell receptors bind small peptides, whereas antibodies have a much broader range and bind larger proteins, carbohydrates, nucleic acids,

Autoimmunity Immunological activity against self antigen markers.

Hypersensitivity reaction A state of abnormal reactivity to a foreign material.

Immunoglobulin The class of proteins that includes antibodies.

IgE Immunoglobulin molecule with the E heavy chain type.

Delayed hypersensitivity A state of abnormal reactivity to a foreign material that takes time to develop.

Antigen presenting cell (APC) Cell that displays the foreign material.

Antigen Foreign substance.

Antibody Immunoglobulin molecule that can recognize a foreign substance.

T cell receptor Antigen recognition molecule.

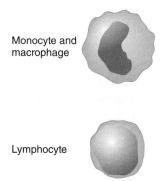

Monocyte and macrophage

Lymphocyte

FIGURE 6-1 Lymphocyte and macrophage (diagram).

Immunogen Antigen that can provoke an adaptive immune response as well as bind to antigen receptors.

B lymphocyte A lymphocyte that differentiates into plasma cells and is associated with humoral immunity.

Primary lymphoid organs Bone marrow and thymus.

Secondary lymphoid organs Lymph nodes, spleen bone marrow, and mucosal-associated lymphoid tissue.

Heavy chains (H chains) Longer of two types of chains making up an immunoglobulin molecule.

Light chains (L chains) Shorter of two types of chains making up an immunoglobulin molecule.

Heterodimer T cell receptor formed from an alpha and beta chain.

Somatic recombination Process during which gene segments are spliced together to form a mature antigen receptor molecule.

Variable region Amino-terminal end of the immunoglobulin chain; part that recognizes antigen.

and other substances. Some substances, such as small organic molecules, can bind to antibodies but cannot by themselves provoke an immune response. Antigens that can provoke an adaptive immune response as well as bind to antigen receptors are termed **immunogens**.

Development of Immune Competence

FORMATION OF ANTIGEN BINDING REGIONS IN T AND B CELLS

The precursor cells of the lymphocytes initially come from stem cells in the bone marrow, and they eventually develop into one of two groups of lymphocytes, depending on where (the fetal thymus or bone marrow) they undergo further development (i.e., develop immune competence). In the fetus, some of these precursor cells migrate from the marrow into the thymus where they undergo further maturation, developing into cells that are destined to form a specific type of lymphocyte called T (thymus-dependent) lymphocytes. Other lymphoid cells remain within the bone marrow, where they differentiate into cells destined to form a second specific type of bone marrow lymphocyte called **B lymphocytes**. This process does not require the presence of antigen. The bone marrow and thymus, where this early antigen independent process occurs, are termed **primary lymphoid organs**. The mature lymphocytes that can recognize specific antigens will repeatedly circulate through the body and home to **secondary lymphoid organs** (lymph nodes, spleen, bone marrow, and gut and mucosal-associated lymphoid tissue) where additional antigen dependent selection will improve the binding of receptor to antigen and amplify the number of cells that detect specific antigens during the process of host defense (**FIGURE 6-2**).

The programming process by which lymphocytes acquire immune competence involves a rearrangement of genes within the developing B and T lymphocytes. Both the B cell receptor, which is the immunoglobulin (Ig) or antibody molecule, and the T cell receptor are initially present in immature lymphocytes as sets of individual gene segments. Ig molecules are formed from two identical **heavy (H) chains** (of which there are several types) and either of two identical κ or λ **light (L) chains.** T cell receptors are formed from an α-chain and a β-chain (and are termed **heterodimers**). (Both the immunoglobulin molecule and the T cell receptor are discussed in detail later in this chapter.)

Maturation for either T or B cells occurs by a process termed **somatic recombination** during which particular gene segments are spliced together to form a mature antigen receptor chain (**FIGURE 6-3**). As an example, the immature H chain that will become part of the antibody molecule starts as a series of roughly 100 variable (V) chain gene segments, 25 diversity (D) segments, and 5 joining (J) segments that are present in tandem on the chromosome. During development, one of each type of segment is joined together more or less at random to form a mature Ig antigen binding region. Simple recombination would yield about 10,000 types of H chain antigen binding regions. The portion of the antigen receptor region assembled out of these pieces is termed the **variable region** and constitutes the amino-terminal end of the chain. The single constant region gene that is linked to the variable region defines the chain type (e.g., IgG, IgM). Many more types of variable regions are generated because the joining of the V, D, and J segments is not perfect, and different DNA sequences are generated at the junctions, greatly increasing the number of possible mature variable regions. Through a very similar process, variable regions are formed for Ig light chains and for the α-chain and β-chain of the T cell receptor, each chain type being assembled from its own set of gene segments. Considering all the possible types of variable regions for Ig molecules and for T cell receptors, it is easy to understand

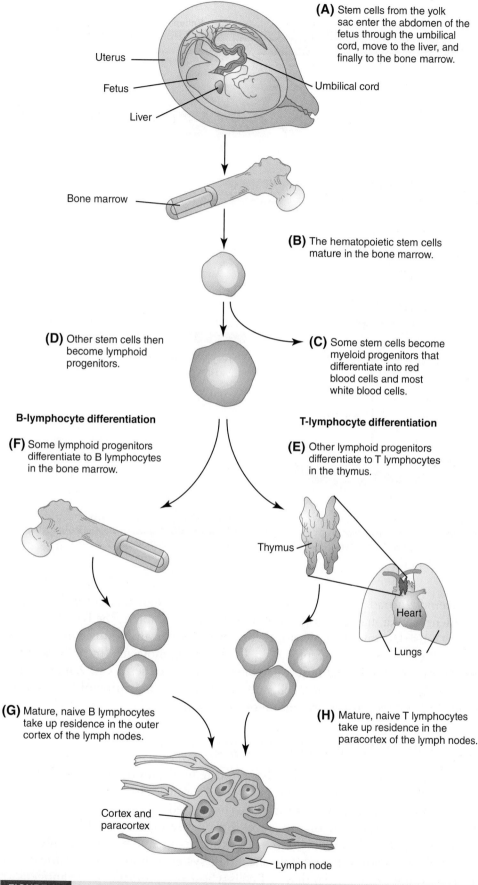

(A) Stem cells from the yolk sac enter the abdomen of the fetus through the umbilical cord, move to the liver, and finally to the bone marrow.

Uterus

Fetus

Liver

Umbilical cord

Bone marrow

(B) The hematopoietic stem cells mature in the bone marrow.

(D) Other stem cells then become lymphoid progenitors.

(C) Some stem cells become myeloid progenitors that differentiate into red blood cells and most white blood cells.

B-lymphocyte differentiation

T-lymphocyte differentiation

(F) Some lymphoid progenitors differentiate to B lymphocytes in the bone marrow.

(E) Other lymphoid progenitors differentiate to T lymphocytes in the thymus.

Thymus

Heart

Lungs

(G) Mature, naive B lymphocytes take up residence in the outer cortex of the lymph nodes.

(H) Mature, naive T lymphocytes take up residence in the paracortex of the lymph nodes.

Cortex and paracortex

Lymph node

FIGURE 6-2 Development of T and B lymphocytes.

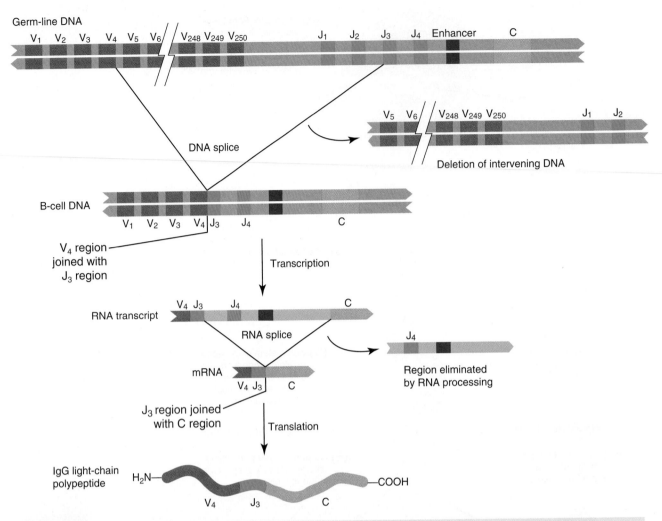

FIGURE 6-3 Formation of a gene for the light chain of an antibody molecule. One variable (V) region is joined with one randomly chosen J region by deletion of the intervening DNA. The remaining J regions are eliminated from the RNA transcript during RNA processing. A similar process occurs with Ig heavy chains (which also have a D region) and with the T cell receptor molecule.

the extremely broad range of antigens that can be recognized. Once the assembly of segments into a mature antigen binding region is complete, the lymphocytes can produce only that one type of antigen receptor—either an Ig molecule on the surface of a B cell or a T cell receptor on a T cell. The Ig molecule (initially having a μ type constant region linked to its variable region and either a κ or λ light chain) is expressed on the surface of the B cell, and a particular combination of α- and β-chain forming a T cell receptor is present on the T lymphocyte.

SELECTION OF ANTIGEN RECEPTORS

At this stage of antigen independent lymphocyte maturation, the T and B cells have a very large array of antigen receptors on their surface. The receptors were formed nearly at random, and each receptor type is expressed on a single cell. Now the host defense system must ensure that the receptors are useful; they must bind to "important" antigens while not binding to the host (the person) and producing autoimmune disease (i.e., that we develop **self-tolerance**). The system is both complex and remarkable. The example discussed is that of T cells whose receptors recognize antigens only when they are presented by (complexed with) those proteins that are important in

Self-tolerance Selection process to remove ability to recognize self.

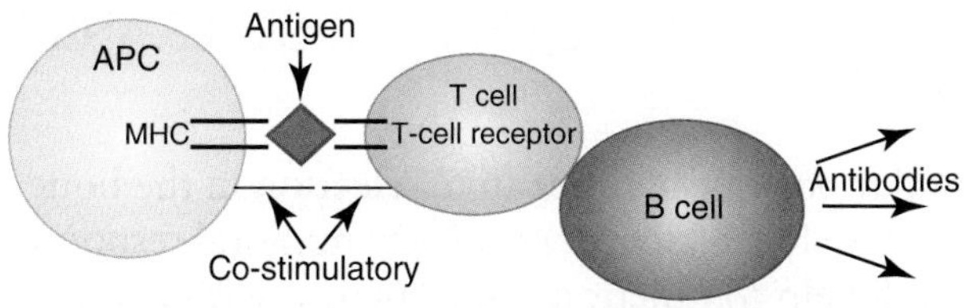

FIGURE 6-4 Antigen presentation. The antigen presenting cell (APC) cradles the antigen in the peptide arms of the MHC (HLA) molecule allowing engagement by the T cell receptor. If the MHC (HLA) is class II, it will engage a T helper cell; if it is class I, it will engage a cytotoxic T cell. T helper cells are necessary for antibody production by B cells.

self-recognition, which is called the **major histocompatibility complex (MHC)**. This process is called **MHC restriction** or **dual recognition** because the T cell receptor recognizes an antigen only in the presence of the MHC protein that initially presented the antigen. In humans the MHC is called the **HLA system**, which will be subsequently discussed. (It is the HLA system that prevents free transplantation of cells and organs between nonidentical individuals (**FIGURE 6-4**).

The process of antigen independent T lymphocyte maturation has two steps. First, immature T lymphocytes enter the thymus and are **positively selected**. An immature T cell in the thymus must bind to one of the person's HLA molecules in complex with a self antigen (a peptide) presented as a complex in the thymus. Like all cells in the body, thymic cells have HLA molecules as a surface component, but they also express a multitude of other small peptides found in our bodies. If binding does not occur, the lymphocyte self-destructs. The next step, **negative selection**, removes lymphocytes that have strong binding to self-peptides complexed with our HLA molecules. Such potentially autoreactive T cells also self-destruct, leaving a population of T cells that can react with a wide range of peptide antigens in complex with (restricted by) our own HLA molecules, but which cannot react with our own antigens to produce autoimmune disease. There is one further complication in the system, T cell types.

T CELL TYPES

T cells are divided into classes depending on the type of HLA molecule they recognize. HLA molecules are either class I or class II, a designation based on their structure and cells that express them. T cells that recognize class II molecules become CD4+ type T cells. T cells that recognize class I HLA molecules become CD8+ (Figure 6-4). The CD designation refers to immunologically detectable markers on the lymphocyte surface that help define the function of the cell. CD8+ T cells are often termed cytotoxic T cells because they function to lyse (dissolve) virally infected cells (and possibly also tumor cells). They recognize viral peptides in combination with HLA class I molecules. Because HLA class I molecules are present on essentially all cells, viruses affecting any cell type can be recognized and responded to. CD4+ T cells are referred to generically as T helper (Th) cells. Th cells have multiple functions and have been divided into a number of subtypes. Th1 cells mediate inflammation via the secretion of a number of pro-inflammatory cytokines, protect against intracellular pathogens (often by activating other cells such as macrophages), and play a role in the production of delayed hypersensitive reactions. Th2 helper T cells are important in providing help for humoral B cell mediated immunity and antibody production. CD4+ T helper cells recognize antigen only in combination with class II HLA antigens, which are found on specialized antigen presenting cells, such as macrophages. Hence, T helper cells require the presence of antigen presenting cells to recognize and respond to antigens.

Major histocompatibility complex (MHC) A group of genes on chromosome 6 that determine the antigens on the surface of cells.

MHC restriction/dual recognition Process needing presentation by MHC antigens to present antigen.

HLA system The genes of the histocompatibility complex and the antigens that they determine on the surface of cells.

Positive/negative selection Immature T lymphocytes must bind to self HLA molecules to remain positively selected; T lymphocytes with strong binding to self are removed (negative selection).

MATURATION OF OTHER CELL TYPES (B CELLS AND NATURAL KILLER CELLS)

B cells undergo similar positive and negative selection in the bone marrow, but they are not restricted by the MHC system. Most B cell humoral responses have an absolute requirement for T cell help to function. Thus, people with defective or diminished T helper cells (as is the case of people with active AIDS) have ineffective B cell-mediated immunity and cannot produce antibodies to many antigens.

A unique subset of lymphocytes characterized by their large size and multiple granules are **natural killer cells (NK cells)**, which make up about 10 percent of circulating lymphocytes and those in secondary lymphoid organs. NK cells are not part of either the cell-mediated or the humoral immune defense system but rather are part of the innate immune system; however, their functions are regulated by the adaptive immune system. Although NK cells show no antigen specificity, they play an important role in killing virally infected cells and cancer cells. Stimulated by the protein products of active macrophages and T cells, NK cells activate macrophages by releasing cytokines (notably interferon-γ, which has antiviral activity) and detect and lyse cells that do not express class I HLA antigens (such as cells that are virally infected or likely to form tumors). NK cells also recognize cells that have been coated by the product of humoral immunity (antibodies) and destroy them, a process called **antibody-dependent cellular cytotoxicity (ADCC)**.

ANTIGEN DEPENDENT LYMPOCYTE MATURATION

When the antigen independent programming process has been completed, many millions of different T and B cells have formed. About two-thirds of the circulating lymphocytes are T lymphocytes and one-third are B lymphocytes, all programmed to recognize and respond to a different antigen. Although a single lymphocyte can respond to only a single antigen, there is such an enormous population of lymphocytes that some T or B cell can respond to almost any antigen the individual may ever encounter. However, this circulating population of naive lymphocytes, never having seen their cognate antigen (i.e., the one to which they respond), is not yet ready to play an effective role in host defense.

Antigen Processing and Antigen Processing Cells

Entry of a foreign antigen into the body triggers a chain of events that involves interactions between T and B lymphocytes and antigen processing cells (APC). For T cells to recognize foreign antigens, the antigen must be "processed" within the APC, combined with MHC (HLA) molecules, and presented on the APC cell surface to the T cell antigen receptor. Macrophages, monocytes, that have left the bloodstream and taken up permanent residence in the tissues throughout the body, play a role in this process. However, the most important group of APC are widely distributed bone marrow derived antigen processing cells called dendritic cells, named from their long cytoplasmic processes that resemble the dendrites of a nerve cell. Initially, dendritic cells are present in all epithelial and subepithelial sites, including the skin (Langerhans cells), respiratory system, and gastrointestinal tract, where pathogens are likely to be first encountered. At epithelial sites, dendritic cells capture invading pathogens using a variety of cell surface receptors. Activation of innate immunity at such peripheral sites leads to the activation of dendritic cells, which then lose their ability to adhere to the epithelium and migrate into peripheral lymphoid organs (lymph nodes) that drain the epithelial sites. The activated dendritic cells process the captured antigen and move to areas in the lymph node rich in naïve T cells that

Natural killer cells (NK cells) Lymphocytes capable of destroying foreign or abnormal cells although they have not had any prior antigenic contact with the cells.

Antibody-dependent cellular cytotoxicity (ADCC) Recognition and destruction of cells coated with antibody.

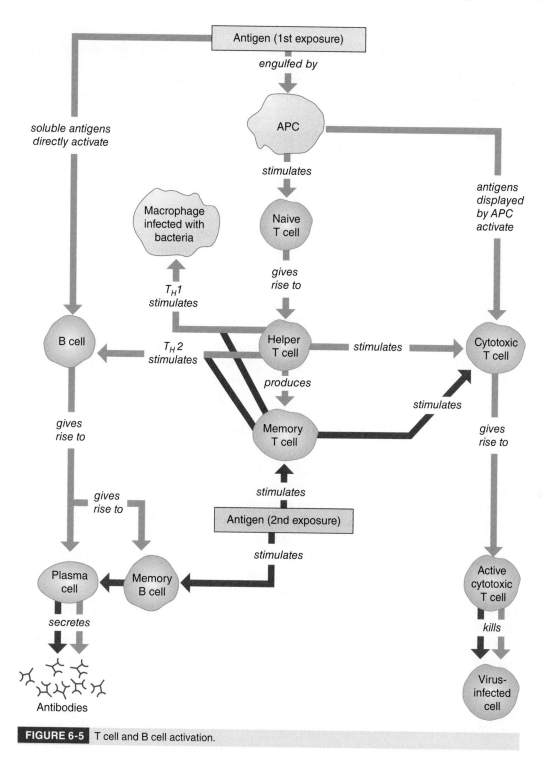

FIGURE 6-5 T cell and B cell activation.

continuously circulate through the nodes. Pathogens that reach the blood stream and circulate are captured by APC in the spleen and similarly presented to splenic T cells. Splenectomy (removal of the spleen) leaves people at particular risk for certain bacterial pathogens such as *Streptococcus pneumoniae*. Macrophages and B cells can also function as APC. B cell APC function is of particular importance in developing humoral immunity to protein antigens. **FIGURE 6-5** and **TABLE 6-2** present overviews of this complex process.

TABLE 6-2	Classification and Functions of Immune System Cells	
Cell function	**Cell type**	**Action of cell**
Antigen processing	Macrophages, B lymphocytes, dendritic cells	Process antigen and present to lymphocytes
Regulate immune response	Regulator T cells (CD4+)	Cytokines regulate immune system activity
Promote cytotoxic immune response	Cytotoxic T cells (CD8+)	Produce cytokines that destroy foreign or abnormal cells displaying antigen fragments combined with MHC Class I antigens
Promote delayed hypersensitivity response	Delayed hypersensitivity T cells (CD4+)	Respond to antigen-processing cells presenting foreign antigen fragments combined with MHC Class II antigens; produce cytokines that activate and stimulate macrophages, cytotoxic T cells, and NK cells
Destroy virus-infected cells and cancer cells	NK cells	Cytokine-mediated cell destruction; no previous contact with antigen required
Produce antibodies	Plasma cells	Antigen processed by B lymphocytes and presented to responding T cells stimulates B lymphocytes to mature into plasma cells and make antibodies

Antigen Dependent Lymphocyte Proliferation: T Cells

Initially, only a very small proportion (perhaps one in a million) naïve T cells would be expected to respond to a given antigen. Rapid activation and proliferation of the initially naïve T cell, which has recognized and interacted with its cognate antigen presented by the dendritic cell within the lymph node, is critical for the function of adaptive immunity. Stimulation and proliferation between APC and T cell requires not only recognition of the MHC bound antigen on the surface of the APC by the T cell receptor but also interaction of additional pairs of molecules on each cell. For example, the CD4 protein and CD8 protein on the respective T cell classes must interact with class II and class I MHC (HLA) molecules on the APC. Also, **costimulator molecules** (e.g., the CD28 molecule on the surface of the T cell and the B7-1 and B7-2 molecules on the APC) must interact for activation of the T cell to occur.

Once activated, T cells produce a host of specialized soluble proteins that influence the function of both themselves and other cells. Those secreted by lymphocytes are called **lymphokines. Cytokines,** a general term used to designate any chemical messengers that take part in any function of the immune system, have many specific names. Those that act by interfering with the multiplication of viruses within cells are called **interferons.** Those that send regulatory signals between cells of the immune system are called **interleukins.** For example, the cytokine IL-2 enhances the response of CD4+ T cells to itself (an **autocrine** response). IL-2 acts as a T cell growth factor and enhances the survival of T cells.

Once the antigen recognition process has been completed, antigen dependent T cells proliferate through the process of **clonal expansion** into a much increased population of antigen binding daughter progeny, all with an identical T cell receptor and identical specificity for the antigen. The degree of clonal expansion can be remarkable. It is estimated that CD8+ T cells reactive against viruses may expand 10,000 fold, CD4+ T cells may expand 100 to 1,000 fold. The expanded clone of T cells continues to differentiate into the various classes of **effector T cells,** which are active in host defense and circulate throughout the body. These classes of T cells are

---

Costimulator molecules Additional molecules on the surface of the T cell and APC needed for the immune response.

Lymphokine A soluble hormone-like substance liberated by lymphocytes.

Cytokine A general term for any protein secreted by cells that functions as an intercellular messenger and influences cells of the immune system. Cytokines are secreted by macrophages and monocytes (monokines), lymphocytes (lymphokines), and other cells.

Interferon A broad-spectrum antiviral agent manufactured by various cells in the body.

Interleukin A lymphokine that stimulates growth of lymphocytes.

Autocrine Cytokine that enhances the response of T cells to itself.

distinguished by their respective functions and the cytokine profiles they secrete. Pools of effector T cells are short-lived. Without the constant presence of their cognate antigen, their numbers rapidly decline. A small proportion of the clonal population of cells differentiate into **memory T cells**, which are long-lived and do not require the continued presence of cognate antigen to survive (in some cases as long as their host). The **primary response** to an antigen may lag by a week or more, during which time clonal expansion and effector generation occurs. The presence of memory cells (which are also produced in humoral B cell-mediated immunity) allows the host defense system to respond more rapidly to a subsequent challenge (termed a **secondary response** as opposed to the initial primary response).

Effector Functions of T Cell Subsets

Mature T cells also function as effector cells for host defense. During the differentiation and maturation of different T cells, different sets of genes become active (e.g., the cytokine gene of CD4+ helper T cells and genes for cytotoxic proteins in CD8+ cytotoxic T cells, which are active in the host defense against viruses).

For effector T cells (such as Th1, Th2, or cytotoxic cells) to function, they must leave the lymph node and migrate through the circulation to sites where they are needed. For example, the surface properties of the vascular endothelial cells (cells that line blood vessels) are modified during the inflammatory response to pathogens. This change in the blood vessel surface allows both the adherence of effector (but not naïve) T cells at the site of inflammation and the migration of the effector cells out of the blood vessel toward the site of inflammation (similar to the migration of neutrophils toward sites of inflammation during acute inflammation as discussed previously). Although the migration process is not antigen specific, those effector T cells that encounter their cognate antigen tend to stick at the site of the pathogen and play a role in its destruction.

In brief, the major role of effector Th1 cells is the activation of macrophages at the site of the pathogen, which allows the macrophage to kill microbes it has ingested. Activation of macrophages and the consequent release of pro-inflammatory tissue destructive molecules at the site of reaction may result in a local, delayed hypersensitivity reaction similar to the previously mentioned tuberculin skin test.

Th2 cells secrete cytokines (Il-4 and Il-5), which promote production of a class of immunoglobulin (IgE) and activate eosinophils, both of which are important in the host defense against parasites. Th2 cells also promote a type of macrophage activation that leads to the initiation of the healing process. The particular subclass of Th cell predominant in the host defense against an organism can be critical. The most often cited example is that of the disease leprosy, caused by the mycobacterium *M. leprae*. Certain individuals who develop leprosy cannot eliminate the bacteria and develop a destructive lepromatous disease associated with progressing destructive tissue lesions. These individuals are unable to mount a Th1 response (but may mount a Th2 response). Individuals who mount a Th1 response develop a generally less destructive form of the disease called tuberculoid leprosy.

Cytotoxic T cells (CTL) attack and destroy body cells infected with viruses or intracellular bacteria. The infected cells are marked for destruction by having some of the bacterial or viral antigen debris transported to the cell surface combined with MHC class I proteins. The CTL forms a tight association with the infected cells and synthesizes the protein perforin, which dissolves the membrane of the infected cell at the point of contact, as well as the protein granzyme B, which turns on the programmed cell death pathway (apoptosis) leading to the death of the infected cell (**FIGURE 6-6**). CTL can also attack cancer cells, which display antigens different from normal cell antigens combined with MHC class I proteins, and function in the rejection of transplanted organs, which also contain foreign antigens. The response

Clonal expansion Proliferation of a population from a single cell.

Effector T cell Cell active in host defense.

Memory T cells Long-lived cells that are primed to respond to an antigen.

Primary response Initial response to foreign substance.

Secondary response Rapid response, part of immune memory.

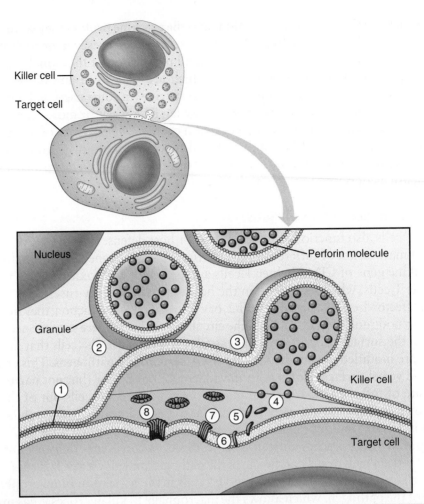

FIGURE 6-6 How cytotoxic T cells work. Cytotoxic T cells containing perforin-1 granules bind to their target and release perforin-1. Perforin-1 molecules form a pore in the target cell plasma membrane. Granzyme-B enters through the pore and induces the death of the target cell. (Illustration courtesy of Dana Burns.)

Reproduced from Cohn Z.A. and Yound J.D.-E. Sci Am 258 (January 1988) 38-44 Illustration courtesy of Dana Burns.

to foreign MHC (HLA) antigens is particularly strong because a high percentage of T cells in a nonimmune donor will recognize foreign MHC molecules. Remember that during negative selection only lymphocytes reacting strongly to self MHC and peptide are deleted. Lymphocytes reactive with foreign MHC molecules are not lost, and every cell on a transplant bears the foreign MHC.

Humoral Immunity

T CELL INDEPENDENT AND DEPENDENT HUMORAL RESPONSES

T cell-mediated immunity relies on close range interactions between the immune effector T cell and the target, resulting in the direct killing of pathogen infected (or cancerous) host cells by cytotoxic lymphocytes or the production of a multiplicity of cytokine-like proteins by antigen responding effector T helper cells. The cytokines stimulate additional cell populations (such as macrophages) to act at the site of infection. Such cytokine-mediated host defenses also amplify aspects of innate immunity such as the inflammatory response.

Humoral immunity is different. As the names implies, immunoglobulin molecules (antibodies), the product of antigen stimulated B cells, become widely disseminated through the vascular system and many mucosal sites specifically binding antigen. For this reason, humoral immunity is most effective against extracellular pathogens likely to come in contact with the antibody molecule. T cells respond only to small peptide antigens presented in the context of MHC (HLA) molecules. B cells can respond to a wide variety of polysaccharide, lipid nucleic acid and protein-based antigens in two general ways: **T cell independent** or **T cell dependent**. Antigens such as carbohydrates, nucleic acids, and lipids consist of chemically similar repeated components. These molecules contain multiple similar or identical **antigenic determinants (epitopes)**, each of which can react with the same antigen recognition molecule that activates B cells (e.g., Ig molecules expressed on the naïve B cell surface). The response by B cells to such polymeric antigens is T cell independent. T cell independent antigens elicit antibodies with limited properties for host defense, which are produced for a short time only and most often do not result in immune memory. These antibodies do not improve with time in their ability to bind (as do the antibodies to T cell dependent protein antigens). T cell independent antigens provoke a response critical in rapid host defense, but the response is limited.

Protein-based antigens are quite different. Proteins are made of chains of amino acids that differ along the length of the protein chain (thus determining the properties of the protein), and the majority of protein antigens do not consist of a large number of very similar or identical epitopes. Rather, protein antigens contain a series of different epitopes (about ten amino acids in length), each one binding to a different Ig molecule on a different B cell. These protein antigens are T cell dependent. They require T helper cell interaction (**T cell help**) to produce a B cell humoral response.

T cell dependent responses are quite different from those considered T cell independent, having several unique properties including being very long-lived. T cell dependent antigens result in B memory cells and effector cells (plasma cells that are "factories" for antibody production) that can persist throughout the life of the host. The antibodies produced against T cell dependent antigens can **class switch**, that is, change the nature of the antibody molecule's constant region. As discussed later the type of constant region defines the antibody class, each with different effector properties in host defense. Perhaps most surprising, the antibody produced by a single B cell can improve its ability to bind to antigen with time and with subsequent interactions with antigen. This process of **affinity maturation** of the antibody results from somatic mutations that occur at those DNA residues that code for the areas of the antibody variable region that closely interact with the antigen. As will be discussed, a process of positive selection for strong antibody binding B cells (among this now mutated population) repeatedly occurs within an area of the lymph node (the **germinal center**), resulting in a new population of B cells making ever better (stronger binding) antibodies.

ANTIGEN DEPENDENT LYMPHOCYTE PROLIFERATION: B CELLS

As was previously discussed, antigen independent maturation of immature B cells within the bone marrow results in a population of naïve B cells positively selected for their ability to synthesize an antibody molecule and negatively selected to eliminate self-reactive clones. The naïve B cell population carries IgM and IgD class immunoglobulin (antibody) molecules on the cell surface (B cell antigen receptors) that display the antibody specificity of the B cell. The constant region of the Ig molecule is attached to the B cell membrane, the variable region faces out into the environment. The naïve B cells circulate (much as do naïve T cells) but are activated when they encounter cognate antigen within a B cell rich area of the lymph node (the **follicle**). Cross-linking of the B cell surface Ig by binding to the cognate antigen results in initial activation of the B cell, turning it into an efficient antigen processing cell in a manner

T cell independent/T cell dependent Whether T cells are needed or not needed for a response from B cells.

Antigenic determinants/ epitopes Number of antigenic sites on a single molecule.

T cell help Requirement of a T cell to present antigen for a B cell humoral response.

Class switch A change in the immunoglobulin constant region using the same variable region.

Affinity maturation Improvement in ability to bind antigen by immunoglobulin resulting from somatic mutations.

Germinal center Site in lymph node where selection for strong binding B cells occurs.

Follicle B cell rich area of the lymph node.

analogous to dendritic or other APC. The activated B cell internalizes, processes, and presents the protein antigen as a series of peptides on its surface in combination with class II MHC (HLA) molecules. However, the activated B cell cannot proliferate and undergo further differentiation without T cell help.

The process of T cell help requires (remarkably) that a T helper cell *independently* be activated by the same antigen and express a T cell receptor molecule and specific costimulator molecules. This occurs in the T cell rich region of the lymph node at a site different from that where the B cell was activated. The activated T helper cell migrates toward the B cell rich lymphoid follicle while the activated B cells move to the edge of the follicles into an area called the parafollicular zone of the lymph node. After close contact, the T helper cell interacts with the B cell much as T helper cells interact with macrophages. The antigen class II MHC complex is presented to and binds with the T cell receptor; at the same time, additional costimulator molecules on the T helper cell and B cell interact, triggering B cell proliferation (clonal expansion) and antibody production. Secretion of cytokines by the T helper cell enhances the process. At this point, antibody production in the parafollicular region by B cells is both short-lived and weakly binding, requiring subsequent maturation of B cells within the follicle to produce a specialized structure termed the germinal center. Once the germinal center is produced, the processes of class switching and affinity maturation (mentioned above) results in production of mature plasma cells and B memory cells.

B CELL CLASS SWITCHING, AFFINITY MATURATION, AND PLASMA CELL PRODUCTION

The subsequent complex steps in the B cell maturation process are presented only in overview. A small number of the activated B cells from outside the follicle will migrate back into the B cell rich follicular region along with a proportion of the activated T helper cells, which become follicular T helper cells (T fH cells). In the presence of T fH cells, the clone of immune activated B cells rapidly divides and expands to form a germinal center within the follicle. In the germinal center, the clone of B cells (initially all expressing the same Ig variable region) undergo class switching. The cells express different constant regions, each with specialized effector functions (combined with the same variable antigen binding region). For example, the IgA immunoglobulin (having an α-chain constant region) form antibodies important in mucosal immunity in the oropharynx and vagina; IgE immunoglobulin (having an ε-chain constant region) is important in defense against parasitic worms and plays a role in allergic reactions. (The structure and types of the Ig molecules will be subsequently discussed). Antibodies with the same variable region can have different constant regions because switching occurs independently in different cells derived from the same clonally expanded population within the germinal center.

Affinity maturation refers to the positive selection of B cells within the germinal center having an increased affinity for (i.e., bind better to) antigen and the negative selection (and death) of B cells that bind less well. Somatic mutation of the variable region genes of B cells results in daughter cells (subclones derived from the original nonmutated cell) that may bind antigen better (or worse). The process of somatic mutation (hypermutation) is up to one million times as frequent in the variable region as in nonvariable region genes.

Survival of B cells within the germinal center depends on their ability to bind antigen. A specialized cell population (follicular dendritic cells, not related to the peripheral dendritic cells) binds small amounts of antigen within the germinal center. The mutated B cells compete for the limited amount of antigen, so those that bind best survive (and may undergo additional rounds of mutations); those that bind poorly lose out in the competition and do not survive. The result is the production of an increasingly more efficient population of antigen specific B cells. Some of the antibody secreting cells of the germinal center migrate through the vascular system into the bone marrow where they mature into long-lived plasma cells, the terminally differentiated cells that are the engines for antibody production. A small number of the germinal center B cells migrate to other tissue sites where they become memory B cells, which do not secrete antibody but can respond quickly when they detect cognate antigen (**FIGURE 6-7**).

(A)

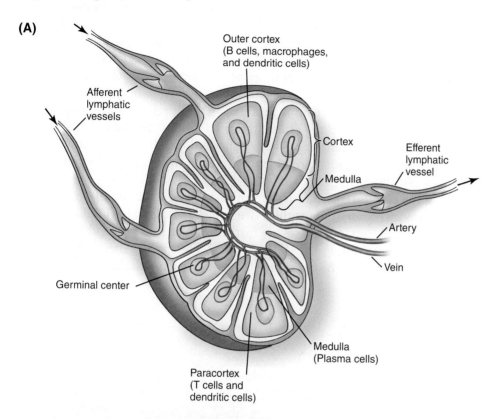

(B)

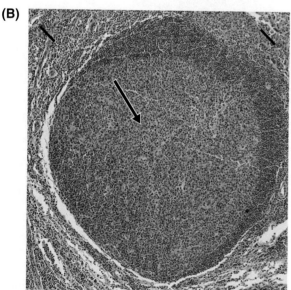

FIGURE 6-7 **(A)** Lymph node (diagram). **(B)** Germinal center: a high power photomicrograph of an active germinal center. The pale central region (*arrow*) contains both B and T cells and pale staining follicular dendritic cells and macrophages. The central region is surrounded by a mantle of darker staining transient B cells entering and exiting the central area. External to this (*line*) is the parafollicular zone rich in T helper cells.

Courtesy of Department of Pathology and Laboratory Medicine, University of North Carolina at Chapel Hill.

EFFECTOR MOLECULES OF HUMORAL IMMUNITY: IMMUNOGLOBULINS

The effector molecule of the humoral immune reaction is the immunoglobulin molecule (Ig) predominantly synthesized by plasma cells (terminally differentiated lymphocytes specialized to synthesize and secrete large amounts of protein). Although the term *antibody* should be used to refer to an Ig molecule known to react with a given antigen (be it a pathogen or some other defined molecule), in common usage antibody and immunoglobulin tend to be used interchangeably. Although the immunoglobulin classes differ somewhat from one another in chemical composition, molecular weight, and size of their constant regions, they all have the same basic structure: two identical pairs of polypeptide (protein) chains. One pair is called heavy chains. The second pair, light chains, is only half as long as the heavy chains. The variable regions (antigen binding regions) are unique to a given Ig molecule and make up the amino terminal half of the light chain and the amino terminal 20 or 25 percent of the heavy chain (depending on the chain type). The heavy chain variable regions are identical to each other as are the light chain variable regions (**FIGURE 6-8**).

The class of the immunoglobulin is determined by the structure of the constant region of the heavy chain. In humans there are five classes: IgA, IgM, IgG, IgD, and IgE. In addition, the IgA and IgG classes are further divided into two and four closely related subclasses (respectively, IgA_1, IgA_2, and IgG_{1-4}). The specific effector function of the antibody is determined by the constant region of the heavy chain (i.e., the Ig class

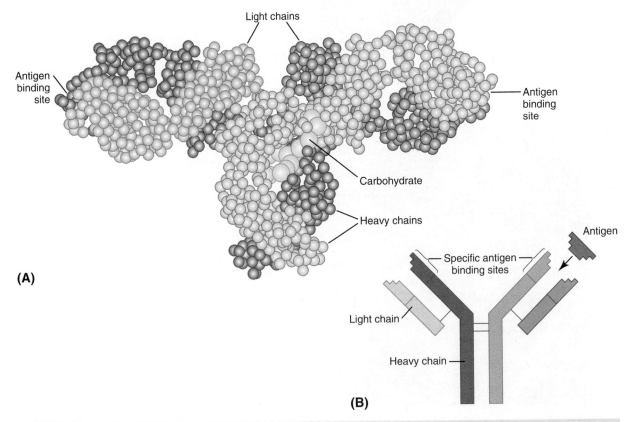

FIGURE 6-8 Antibody structure. **(A)** A three-dimensional model of an antibody showing the four chains. The molecule is T shaped before binding to antigen. As it binds, it becomes Y shaped. **(B)** A diagrammatic representation of the structure of an antibody molecule that shows the four protein chains, two large (heavy chains) and two small (light chains). Note that the antigen binds to the arms of the molecule.

and subclass); specificity of the antibody for a given antigen (such as a pathogenic virus or bacterial toxin) is conferred by the variable region. Humoral responses, even to very simple antigens, are almost always **polyclonal**; that is, they contain antibodies produced by a large number of individual clones of B cells. The antibodies in such a response may be of several classes due to class switching. The variable regions of the antibody show great diversity and, if separated by a charge using electrophoresis, appear as a blur of overlapping proteins. In special cases antibodies may be **monoclonal** (the product of only a single clone of B cells), for example, if there is a cancer of the plasma cells as in the disease multiple myeloma. Such tumors derive from a single plasma cell and have a uniform variable region. On electrophoresis they form a single sharp peak (**M spike**). Occasionally such monoclonal proteins can be shown to be "real antibodies" and bind to a known antigen. An important advance in biotechnology is the ability to produce monoclonal antibodies to desired antigens at will. The most common method (hybridoma production) fuses antibody producing cells with plasma cells (generally of animal origin). Such fused cells produce unlimited amounts of uniform monoclonal antibody of the desired specificity when grown in tissue culture devices. These monoclonal antibodies have important uses in therapy and will be described later.

All Ig molecules have the same basic four chain unit structure, but some immunoglobulins characteristically aggregate to form clusters of individual units. For example, IgM is usually a cluster of five individual units, and IgA is usually a pair of units.

An antibody molecule is not a rigid structure. The junction of its constant and variable parts is quite flexible (the hinge region). This feature allows the variable end of the Y shaped molecule to adapt to the configuration of the antigen. Treatment with enzymes breaks an immunoglobulin molecule into three fragments. The variable region yields two fragments called the F_{ab} fragments (antibody-combining fragments), each consists of a light chain and the associated part of the heavy chain. The other fragment is called the F_c fragment (constant fragment) and is in the constant region of the molecule (see Figure 6-8).

IgM is present in the blood as a cluster of five individual molecules (a pentamer) joined together in a star-shaped configuration with the antigen binding ends projecting outward and the opposite ends of the molecules directed toward the center of the cluster. It is the first antibody to be synthesized in a primary immune response because it does not require class switching. The pentamer of IgM forms a large antibody cluster that is efficient in combining with large particulate antigens such as fungi.

Monmeric IgM molecules and IgD molecules (neither of which is released from the cell) serve as the initial antigen receptors on naïve B cells. IgG, a much smaller antibody molecule, is the principal type of antibody molecule formed in response to the majority of infectious agents. IgA is produced by antibody-forming cells located in the respiratory, gastrointestinal, and genitourinary mucosa and is present in secretions from these areas. IgA apparently functions by combining with potentially harmful ingested or inhaled antigens. IgE is normally present in only small quantities in the blood of most people, but its concentration is greatly increased in allergic individuals. It binds specifically to mast cells via its F_c region where it plays a role in defense against parasites and also in provoking certain forms of allergy. **TABLE 6-3** summarizes the types and functions of the various immunoglobulins.

IMMUNOGLOBULIN EFFECTOR FUNCTIONS

Binding an antibody to a microbe or the toxic products of a microbe can block the ability of the microbe to infect cells or neutralize the damaging effect of the toxin.

Polyclonal antibodies Humoral response consisting of antibodies produced by a number of clones of B cells.

Monoclonal antibodies Product of a single clone of B cells.

TABLE 6-3	Types and Functions of Immunoglobulins	
Immunoglobulin	**Usual type of secretion**	**Properties and functions**
IgM	Pentamer	First Ig formed in response to foreign antigen (primary immune response). Present in bloodstream but not in tissues. Large pentamer antibody cluster very effective for combining with foreign antigen.
IgG	Monomer	Most prevalent Ig produced rapidly in large amounts (secondary immune response) to replace IgM. Found in blood and tissues. Crosses placenta to protect fetus until infant immune system can produce antibodies.
IgA	Dimer	Present in bloodstream, in secretions produced by mucous membranes (respiratory and GI tract), and in breast milk to provide maternal antibody protection to infant.
IgD	Monomer	Small amount in bloodstream and on surface of B lymphocytes. Undetermined functions.
IgE	Monomer	Present in bloodstream and attaches to mast cells and basophils, which causes allergic response when sensitizing antigen encountered. IgE evolved to protect against parasitic infections common in developing countries, but in developed countries causes allergy problems in susceptible (atopic) persons.

Once a pathogen is bound to the antibody via the variable region, the Fc (constant region) of the antibody is a signal to clear the pathogen from sites of infection; many cells that play a role in host defense have **Fc receptors** on their surface. A particular class of receptor (FcγR1 phagocytic receptor) is present on neutrophils and macrophages. Microbes coated with antibody (a process termed opsonization) are readily phagocytized by such cells via interaction with the Fc portion of the bound antibody, internalized, and destroyed. The Fc regions of IgG (and in particular of IgG$_1$ and IgG$_3$) are the most efficient at binding to the phagocytic receptor. Other types of Fc receptors are found on different cells important in host defense. The FcεR1 receptor found on mast cells (and the related basophils) specifically binds the Fc region of IgE molecules and plays a role in the defense against helminthes (parasitic worms) as well as allergic reactions. **FIGURE 6-9** summarizes the several roles of antibodies in host defense.

Fc receptor Cell surface receptor for the constant region of the immunoglobulin molecule.

The Role of Complement in Immune Responses

A number of systems of soluble proteins play a critical role in self-defense as discussed under inflammation. The complement system consists of a large number of interacting protein factors, which function in concert with humoral immunity to destroy or inactivate many bacterial pathogens, particularly organisms that have a capsule (such as *Streptococcus pneumonia*, *Haemophilus influenza*, and *Neisseria meningitides*). Individuals lacking critical components of complement have a much higher susceptibility to these pathogens and may suffer lethal infections. As described in the discussion on inflammation and repair, complement can be activated in several ways. The classical pathway, which is triggered by antigen—antibody interactions, is dependent on humoral immunity. Two other methods of complement activation, the alternative pathway and the lectin pathway, do not involve humoral immunity but

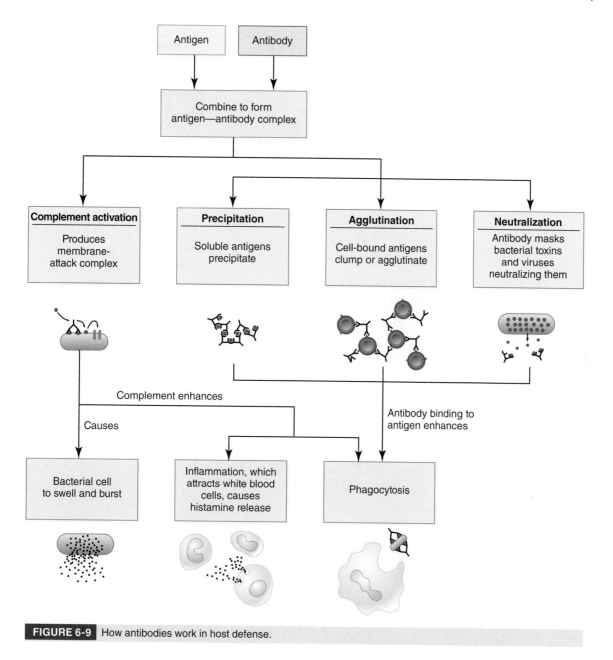

FIGURE 6-9 How antibodies work in host defense.

depend on the ability of complement proteins to recognize and bind to components of the surface of microbial pathogens. When complement is activated, the complement components interact to accomplish several important host defense functions. Some components function as mediators of inflammation. Other components coat the surface of invading bacteria, which makes them easier for macrophages and neutrophils to phagocytose. Finally, the interaction of the complement components generates a group of complement molecules called an **attack complex**, which destroys the target micro-organism or abnormal cell by "punching holes" in its cell membrane (**FIGURE 6-10**). IgM antibodies are most efficient in activating complement.

In addition to its role in host defense, complement plays an important role in clearing **immune complexes** from circulation. Immune complexes consist of antibody bound to its cognate antigen. Because there are at least two antigen binding sites on Ig molecules and antigens many have many antigenic sites on them, antibody bound to antigen can form "lattices" of variable size. These complexes may bind to parts of

Attack complex Group of complement molecules that destroys the target micro-organism or abnormal cell.

Immune complex Combination of antibody and antigen forming a lattice.

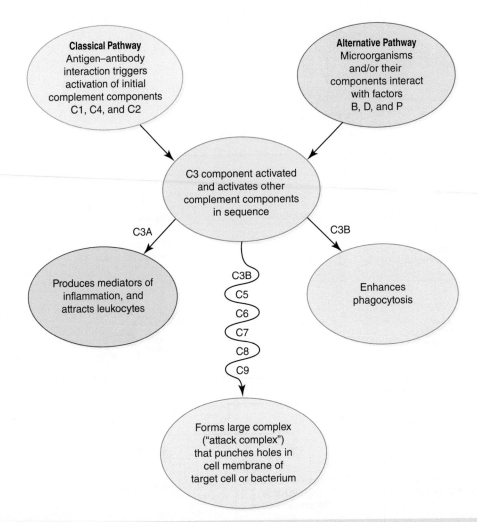

FIGURE 6-10 Components and pathways of complement activation that "complement" the body's immune defenses. Individual components named C1 through C9 and factors B, D, and P. Note that the lectin pathway (not shown) is similar in detail to the classical pathway substituting a carbohydrate binding protein (lectin) for the C1 Ig binding complex.

the vascular system and trigger hypersensitivity reactions (which will be subsequently discussed). Such complexes may also promote certain autoimmune diseases such as systemic lupus erythematosus (SLE). People with a genetic deficiency for certain complement components are highly susceptible to this disease.

HLA Types and Susceptibility to Disease

Although MHC proteins were originally considered of interest only with respect to organ transplantation, they have a much larger role in antigen presentation and are critical in the development of both cellular and humoral immunity as previously noted.

The surface proteins within the HLA system (the major MHC system in humans) fall into two major groups, designated MHC class I proteins and MHC class II proteins. The class I proteins are controlled by HLA-A, HLA-B, and HLA-C genes; class II proteins are controlled by HLA-D genes. More than 1,200 different allelic genes can occupy the gene loci within the HLA system.

The presence of certain HLA types predisposes individuals to specific diseases. The most striking example of such an association is between HLA-B27 and a particular type of arthritis of the spine and the sacroiliac joints, ankylosing spondylitis. HLA-B27 is present in about 5 percent of the random white population but is found in over 95 percent of people affected with this type of arthritis, indicating that a B27-positive individual is much more likely to develop this disease than is a person of a different HLA type. However, the presence of the B27 type indicates only a predisposition to the disease. It does not mean that any given individual will invariably be affected because no more than about 25 percent of B27-positive people ever develop this type of arthritis. In the case of ankylosing spondylitis (and a number of related forms of arthritic disease), gastrointestinal infection with certain microbial pathogens is a likely environmental trigger for the disease in B27-positive people. Predisposition to other diseases also has been associated with this HLA type.

Similar associations exist between certain class II HLA types and specific diseases, which are considered in other chapters. The diseases include type 1 diabetes, prone to develop in children and young adults (discussion on pancreas and diabetes mellitus), and rheumatoid arthritis (RA) (discussion on musculoskeletal system). These diseases tend to have an autoimmune component. The association of a particular class II HLA allele with an autoimmune disease relates to the ability of the MHC molecule specified by the gene to bind and present particular autoantigens. Certain types of RA are related to a specific form of postsynthetic protein modification that forms citrullinated peptides (i.e., containing the amino acid citrulline), which are derived from joint proteins. Such peptides bind to the particular class II MHC (HLA) alleles associated with severe rheumatoid arthritis. Smoking is also a risk factor for severe RA and results in the production of citrullinated peptides in the lung. Such peptides may be the immune trigger for RA and result in the production of humoral immunity to such modified peptides. Many (but not all) of the genes involved in propensity for a particular form of immune response (and in particular autoimmune response) are related to the MHC (HLA) system.

Hypersensitivity Reactions: Immune System—Related Tissue Injury

The immune system protects us from foreign substances that could harm us, but the immune response also may damage tissues. This undesirable effect is called hypersensitivity. As previously noted, hypersensitivity reactions often do not result from too much immunity but from inappropriately directed immunity (such as a response to poison ivy) or from "bystander" damage to normal tissue adjacent to a site of an immune reaction. The previously mentioned positive reaction to a tuberculin test is a clinically mild example. A far more serious example of bystander effect is the severe liver damage in hepatitis C infection mediated by immune T cells attempting to destroy hepatocytes chronically infected with virus.

Hypersensitivity reactions are classified based on how the immune system caused the injury using the Gell and Coombs system (named after the two immunologists who devised it) (TABLE 6-4). Four different types of hypersensitivity reactions, usually designated by roman numerals, are recognized. The first three types are related to antibodies formed in response to antigenic material, and the fourth type is a cell-mediated hypersensitivity reaction. Although most hypersensitive reactions involve more than one of the four defined types and some types of hypersensitivity reactions do not fit well into any of the categories, the system is still used by clinicians to describe hypersensitivity disease.

TABLE 6-4 Mechanisms of Immunologic Injury

Type	Mechanism	Examples
I: Immediate hypersensitivity	IgE antibodies fix to mast cells and basophils. Later contact with sensitizing antigen triggers mediator release and clinical manifestations.	Localized response: hay fever, food allergy, etc. Systemic response: bee sting or penicillin anaphylaxis, etc.
II: Cytotoxic hypersensitivity reactions	Antibody binds to cell or tissue antigen, and complement is activated, which damages cell, causes inflammation, and promotes destruction of antibody-coated cell by phagocytosis.	Autoimmune hemolytic anemia. Blood transfusion reactions. Rh hemolytic disease. Some types of glomerulonephritis
III: Immune complex disease	Circulating antigen-antibody complexes form, which activate complement and cause inflammatory reaction.	Some types of glomerulonephritis. Lupus erythematosus. Rheumatoid arthritis
IV: Delayed (cell-mediated) hypersensitivity	Sensitized (delayed hypersensitivity) T cells release lymphokines that attract macrophages and other inflammatory cells.	Tuberculosis. Fungus and parasitic infections. Contact dermatitis

TYPE I. IMMEDIATE HYPERSENSITIVITY REACTIONS: ALLERGY AND ANAPHYLAXIS

Type I hypersensitivity reactions follow contact with foreign antigens that induce formation of specific IgE antibodies in the sensitized person. IgE has the distinctive property of attaching to the surface of mast cells (and to similar cells circulating in the blood called basophils) via the Fc region. Cross linking of two or more IgE molecules by antigen binding to the variable region of the IgE molecule pointing away from the mast cell causes the mast cell to release preformed cytoplasmic granules filled with histamine, proteases, and cytokines, all of which serve as potent mediators of inflammation and attractants for other inflammatory cells such as eosinophils and neutrophils. Activation of mast cells by antigen binding to IgE also initiates the synthesis of other mediators in a time-dependent manner that promote T and B cell immunity and continue to attract eosinophils to the area. Type I hypersensitivity reactions (also called immediate hypersensitivity reactions) may be localized (allergic reactions including asthma) or may evoke a widespread systemic reaction called **anaphylaxis (FIGURE 6-11).**

Allergy

Individuals who develop localized IgE-mediated reactions are predisposed to form specific IgE antibodies (become allergic) to ragweed, other plant pollens, and various antigens that do not affect others, a process termed atopic allergy. Although there is a clear genetic component to atopic allergies, the exact mechanism remains unclear, and many genes appear to play a role. The sensitizing antigen is called an allergen,

Anaphylaxis A widespread systemic hypersensitive reaction.

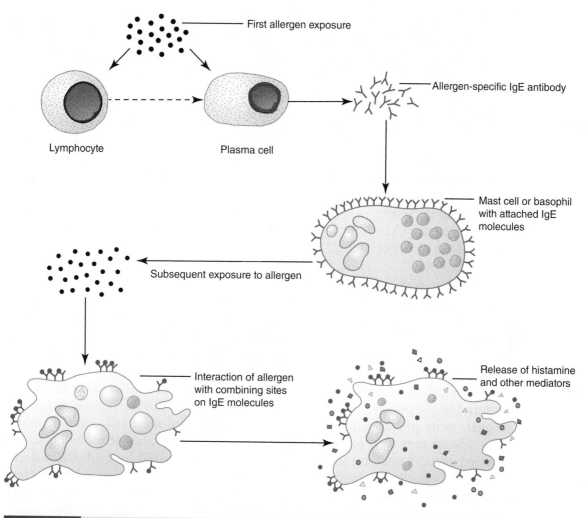

FIGURE 6-11 Pathogenesis of allergy. First exposure to allergen induces formation of specific IgE antibody in susceptible individual, which binds to mast cells and basophils by the nonantigen receptor end of the molecule. Subsequent exposure to the allergen leads to an antigen—antibody interaction, liberating histamine and other mediators from mast cells and basophils. These mediators induce allergic manifestations.

and the allergic manifestations are localized to the tissues that are exposed to the allergens, for example, swollen itchy eyes, stuffy nose, and sneezing in a ragweed-sensitive person.

Because histamine is one of the mediators released from the IgE-coated cells, antihistamine drugs (which block the effects of histamine) often relieve many of the allergic symptoms. A more specific method of treating an allergic individual consists of immunizing the person to the offending allergen by repeated subcutaneous injections of the antigen that induced the allergy, such as an extract of ragweed pollen in a ragweed-sensitive person. This method of treatment, called **desensitization**, induces the formation of IgG antibodies against the offending allergen. The IgG may act by combining with the allergen before it can affix to the cell-bound IgE, thus preventing the release of mediators although other mechanisms such as inducing unresponsiveness (generating tolerance) in T cells may play a role.

Desensitization Treatment for allergy that induces the formation of IgG antibodies.

Asthma

Asthma is defined by airway obstruction related to hyperresponsiveness of the smooth muscles of the bronchi. Although many pro-inflammatory triggers can result in asthma, type I (immediate) hypersensitivity involving an environmental inhaled allergen is most often the cause. Animal dander (especially from cats), house mites, bird feathers, and seasonal allergens such as tree and grass pollens also may trigger attacks in affected individuals. Asthma can have serious consequences and can even result in death if not appropriately treated using bronchodilators, steroid drugs, and other immunosuppressive agents. Although mediators produced by activated mast cells and eosinophils (which are prevalent in the respiratory tissue of asthmatics) result in an acute attack, the initial trigger is from sensitized Th2 cells that have an IgE type response to the inciting allergen. Individuals brought up in an environment containing numerous pathogens and allergens (such as farms) tend to be less likely to develop asthma, possibly because early exposure to environmental allergens results in a Th1 immune response, which does not stimulate IgE production and is protective. This concept has been termed the hygiene hypothesis. (A little dirt for children may, in fact, be a good thing!)

Anaphylaxis and Anaphylactoid Reactions

A severe generalized IgE-mediated hypersensitivity reaction, called anaphylaxis, may be life-threatening. The condition results from an initial exposure to a substance (allergen) that induces an extreme degree of sensitization in a susceptible person. Commonly implicated allergens include penicillin, bee stings, peanuts (a legume, not a true nut), tree nuts, latex products, some fruits that contain latex-like chemicals (Kiwi fruit, bananas, and others) as well as various other sensitizing agents. Once sensitization has occurred, a later exposure to the sensitizing antigen triggers widespread mediator release from IgE-coated mast cells and basophils. This release may lead to a fall in blood pressure with circulatory collapse and is often accompanied by severe respiratory distress caused by mediator-induced spasm of smooth muscle in the walls of the bronchioles, restricting airflow into and out of the lungs. Prompt treatment of this immunologic catastrophe with epinephrine and other appropriate agents is essential. A similar condition, called an **anaphylactoid reaction**, resembles an anaphylactic reaction but is not caused by IgE but by direct action on mast cells or by activating complement. Aspirin, other non-steroidal anti-inflammatory drugs, some antibiotics, and radiopaque iodine containing contrast material used for x-ray examinations may trigger an anaphylactoid reaction. An unusual form of anaphylactoid reaction (scombroid poisoning) occurs when bacteria acting on improperly stored dark meat fish convert the amino acid histidine in the fish flesh to histamine and related compounds (which are not degraded by cooking). The ingested histamine can produce a severe (and occasionally fatal) reaction. The treatment for anaphylactoid reactions is the same as for an anaphylactic reaction.

Anaphylactoid reaction Immune response resembling an anaphylactic reaction but by direct action on mast cells or by activating complement.

TYPE II. HYPERSENSITIVITY REACTIONS

Type II hypersensitivity reactions result from the deleterious effects of antibody (most often autoantibody) binding to a cell or neutralizing or blocking the physiological effect of an essential protein. The injurious effects may involve complement activation, opsonization of cells and neutrophil activation, or the direct effects of antibody binding. After IgG or IgM antibody react with a cell-associated antigen, complement is activated, and the products of complement activation directly or indirectly damage the target. The complement components interact to form an attack complex that directly damages the target cell membrane. Inflammatory cells such as neutrophils also are attracted and contribute to the tissue injury by releasing destructive enzymes; they may also destroy the antibody-coated target cells by phagocytosis. Examples of such type II reactions include transfusion reactions caused by administration of incompatible blood, hemolytic disease of newborn infants caused by Rh incompatibility in prenatal development, some types of chronic hemolytic anemia associated with autoantibodies directed against red blood cells in the hematopoietic and lymphatic systems, and a type of kidney disease caused by autoantibodies directed against basement membranes of glomerular capillaries in the urinary system.

In Graves disease autoantibodies to the TSH receptor on thyroid cells inappropriately stimulates the cells to make an excess of thyroid hormone resulting in hyperthyroidism. Autoantibodies directed to the acetylcholine receptors on motor endplates of muscle block the transmission of neuronal signals from the nerve, resulting in muscle fatigue and partial paralysis, a condition called myasthenia gravis. Patients may also develop antibodies against therapeutic proteins that inactivate them. Some individuals with severe hemophilia A totally lack the coagulation protein F.VIII. To prevent hemorrhage, these patients are treated with recombinant human F.VIII. Because the patients have had a total lack of the protein during development, the immune system may see the therapeutic F.VIII as foreign and produce antibodies (termed **inhibitors**) that render the protein useless.

TYPE III. TISSUE INJURY CAUSED BY IMMUNE COMPLEXES ("IMMUNE COMPLEX DISEASE")

In type III hypersensitivity, antigen bound to antibody forms immune complexes within the circulation that can be deposited in the tissues. Because antibodies have multiple binding sites for antigen (two on IgG, potentially 10 on IgM) and because most antigens have multiple sites (epitopes) to which antibody can bind, the interaction of antigen and antibody often form latticelike structures (immune complexes) that differ in size and chemical properties. The ability to bind to tissue (often within the vascular system) and the site of binding is determined by the properties of the immune complexes. The deposited antigen—antibody complexes activate complement, and the activated complement components, along with the inflammatory cells that they attract, damage the tissues. Often, the immunologic reaction within the tissues is quite severe and leads to thrombosis of blood vessels and considerable tissue necrosis.

An example of organ damage in the urinary system caused by immune complexes is a type of kidney disease called immune-complex glomerulonephritis, in which the complexes are trapped within the glomeruli as the blood flows through the kidneys. This leads to the accumulation of neutrophils within the glomerulus and destruction of the renal filtration mechanism, leading to renal failure. An example of this process is acute postinfectious glomerulonephritis, which sometimes occurs following infection by β-hemolytic strep infections in children ("strep throat"). The hypersensitivity reaction usually occurs ten days to two weeks after the infection starts. At this time, antibodies to and antigens derived from the bacteria are present in the circulation and bind to each other, forming complexes that deposit in glomerular capillary walls and activate complement at that site. The complement, along with neutrophils and macrophages attracted to the site, produce local inflammation and glomerular damage. The disease usually resolves spontaneously in several weeks although in rare cases the glomerular injury may be long-lasting. Another important diseases in which tissue injury is related to immune complexes is lupus erythematosus, considered in connection with autoimmune disease.

TYPE IV. DELAYED (CELL-MEDIATED) HYPERSENSITIVITY REACTIONS

In type IV hypersensitivity (delayed hypersensitivity reactions), T lymphocytes rather than antibodies are responsible for the tissue injury. Unlike immediate hypersensitivity reactions, a cell-mediated inflammatory reaction requires from twenty-four to forty-eight hours to develop, the delay being the time necessary for sensitized T cells to accumulate at the site and generate an inflammatory reaction. The most common examples of delayed hypersensitivity involve the reaction of immune T helper cells recognizing a soluble antigen in tissue. This results in the recruitment of macrophages and additional lymphocytes and local damage to tissue. The reaction is usually self-limited with a peak occurring one or two days followed by subsidence. The example of a TB skin test reaction has already been described. Contact dermatitis (inflammation of the skin), caused by exposure to plant derived oily resins from *Rhus* species (poison ivy, oak, and sumac), is another example with a characteristic delayed hypersensitive reaction. On first exposure, low molecular weight chemical in the resin binds to a skin-derived protein on the surface of a dendritic cell present in the skin. After about a week, a population of Th1 cells is generated that will react with the plant resin when the material subsequently contacts the skin. The results are well known to those who suffer from "poison ivy" and consist of intense itching and a red blistered rash that may last for several weeks. Corticosteroids (either locally applied or taken systemically) lessens the reaction.

Suppression of the Immune Response

Cell-mediated and humoral immune responses protect against potentially harmful micro-organisms and other foreign substances. However, we may want our immune system to accept a foreign protein as self such as is the case with organ transplants, or immune responses may be misdirected toward self, resulting in autoimmune disease. In such cases, a number of chemical agents (drugs) and biological agents can interfere with the immune response at several levels and can suppress the immune reaction.

CHEMICAL AGENTS (DRUGS)

Corticosteroids (derived from hormones produced by the adrenal cortex) discussed under the endocrine gland have a broad range of anti-inflammatory effects, the most important of which is in preventing activation of neutrophils and macrophages and preventing the production of cytokines and other chemical mediators important in inflammation. As is the case with many immunosuppressive agents, use of corticosteroids increases the risk of infection. Corticosteroids also interfere with wound healing and can lead to serious endocrine dysfunction. A number of cytotoxic drugs interfere with DNA synthesis and prevent the division of cells necessary for immune responses. Azathioprine causes a decrease in lymphocytes and NK cells. Because it suppresses the bone marrow, there is often a fall in granulocytic cells (such as neutrophils) and platelets as well. The DNA alkylating agent cyclophosphamide has little effect on inflammation but causes dose-dependent decreases in cytotoxic and helper T cells. It is widely used to treat serious autoimmune disease and in preparing patients for hematopoietic stem cell transplants (as discussed under hematopoietic and lymphoid systems). Calcineurin inhibitors, a more recently developed class of drugs, inhibit the production of the cytokine IL-2 and block the division of T helper cells. Cyclosporine and the closely related drug tacrolimus are both highly effective in prolonging graft survival and are essential for transplant procedures.

BIOLOGICAL AGENTS (MONOCLONAL ANTIBODIES)

The ability to produce essentially unlimited amounts of highly specific monoclonal antibodies (Mab) to desired cell surface antigens on cells important in the immune response allows such agents to be used to treat autoimmune and inflammatory diseases and to help prevent organ rejection. The list of agents is long and rapidly growing. Mab are available that inhibit activated T cells, T helper cells, B cells, and many pro-inflammatory proteins such as TNF-α.

A major problem in the past was that many Mabs were based on murine Ig molecules and could sometimes be recognized by humans as foreign and inactivated by our host defenses. Currently, humanized antibodies are being increasingly used. Such Mabs are 95 percent human in structure and are not recognized as foreign. As might be predicted, use of such potent immunosuppressive agents can be associated with susceptibility to bacterial and viral pathogens.

Pools of random human Ig given intravenously (IVIg) are often effective in treating autoimmune diseases. The exact mechanism is unknown but may involve blockading Fc receptors on cells, resulting in the more rapid destruction of endogenous antibody responsible for the disease. Eliminating a foreign antigen before the immune system can respond to the antigen is another effective way to suppress an immune response and is used routinely to prevent hemolytic disease of newborn infants caused by Rh incompatibility. Postdelivery administration of Rh immune globulin containing potent Rh antibodies to an Rh negative mother who has given birth to an Rh positive infant eliminates any antigenic Rh positive fetal cells that may have entered the mother's bloodstream during delivery. Because the antigenic fetal cells are rapidly removed from the mother's circulation, the mother does not form Rh antibody, preventing Rh hemolytic disease in subsequent pregnancies. This application is described in connection with prenatal development and diseases associated with pregnancy.

Immunodeficiency Disease

Primary immunodeficiency diseases are the result of intrinsic congenital defects that result in defects in the host immune response. Such defects may be global and result in a total lack of immune responses (severe combined immunodeficiency diseases [SCID]). The most severe form of SCID, reticular dysgenesis, is an extremely uncommon genetic disease characterized by early failure of bone marrow development, resulting in a total lack of granulocytes (such as neutrophils) and a near total lack of lymphocytes. The thymus and lymph nodes are absent or underdeveloped, and there is a lack of both innate and adaptive immunity. Severe recurrent infections in the neonatal period occur and result in death in the absence of hematopoietic stem cell transplantation. as discussed in post natal development.

Other rare genetic diseases resulting in SCID are X-linked SCID or RAG1/2. X-linked SCID, the most common, is caused by a lack of functioning receptors for a number of cytokines necessary for immune function. These receptors have a common polypeptide γ-chain that is defective in the disease. Another relatively common cause of SCID is RAG1/2. RAG enzymes are critical for the formation of both T cell receptors and Ig variable region synthesis, and affected individuals lack functioning antigen receptors. Congenital genetic defects also can result in isolated defects of either T cell or B cell development. Even in the presence of functional B cells, isolated T cell defects will result in very limited humoral immunity. SCID and isolated T cell deficiencies are generally treated by stem cell transplantation (as mentioned above).

Primary defects in humoral immunity are somewhat more common. Common variable immunodeficiency disease is a collection of disorders that is most often associated with low IgG and IgA. The disease varies in severity and is sometimes not detected until adulthood. X-linked agammaglobulineamia (Bruton disease) is associated with a failure of B cell maturation and a lack of plasma cells. Affected individuals have little or no circulating Ig of any class. Isolated B cell defects are effectively treated by aggressive replacement of Ig, which is necessary to prevent recurrent bacterial infections. These examples represent only a selection of the most commonly encountered of these rare, but devastating conditions.

Other congenital diseases include a degree of immunodeficiency as part of a broader syndrome. DiGeorge syndrome results in an abnormal or absent thymus, and defects in cellular immunity combined with cardiac and other abnormalities (such as very widely spaced eyes and defects in facial development). The disease results from a small deletion in chromosome 22. Although DiGeorge syndrome does result in immunodeficiency, it is best considered as a localized developmental defect.

Secondary defects in host defense, such as AIDS, are extensive and covered elsewhere. Malnutrition, leukemia and lymphoma therapeutic drugs, and other infectious agents all may result is some degree of immunodeficiency. Loss of proteins from the circulation, which occurs is some renal diseases (discussed with the urinary system), or extensive burns also may result in immunodeficiency states. A common surgical intervention (splenectomy) results in greatly increased susceptibility to *Streptococcus pneumoniae* and occasionally death if the lack of a spleen is not recognized. Immunization to pneumococcus is critical in such patients.

Tolerance and Its Failure: Autoimmune Disease

MECHANISMS OF TOLERANCE GENERATION

Central tolerance Part of the development of cellular and humoral immunity; cells reacting against self-antigen are removed during development.

The process of self-recognition (immunological tolerance) is central to the properly directed function of host defense. Failure results in self-reactivity and autoimmune disease. **Central tolerance** is discussed as part of the development of cellular and humoral immunity. Positive and negative selection of self-reactive T cells and B cells in the thymus and bone marrow is necessary for self-recognition. For this to function properly, the self-antigen must be expressed in those locations during immune development. This is not universally the case. Self-antigens from poorly vascularized tissue or structural proteins such as collagen or cartilage may not generate self-tolerance, and a low level of autoreactivity to these proteins (not associated with disease) is sometimes detected. Antibodies directed toward the proteolytic products of Ig breakdown are universally present in normal individuals and may play a physiological role in removing these products from the circulation. A more striking example is that of sperm antigens, which are not present in fetal development and are not presented to developing T cells in the thymus. Traumatic or surgical damage to the testes or spermatic ducts in an adult can expose sperm-related antigens to the immune system and result in immune reactivity toward host sperm. Sperm autoantibodies occasionally result in male sterility after such interventions.

The development of autoimmune disease in 3 percent of the population suggests that an ongoing process must occur and that failure results in self-recognition. Certain groups of individuals are more prone to developing autoimmunity. Women are up to eight times more susceptible to certain autoimmune conditions than men, which may be related to endocrine hormone production. (There are some exceptions to this. The above mentioned HLA B27-related disease ankylosing spondylitis presents far more commonly in men.) There is a clear genetic component to the development of autoimmune disease, and these diseases run in families. In some cases, the genes of the MHC (HLA) system are implicated, but in many cases the nature of the genetic factors responsible is unclear.

At some level, autoimmune disease is likely to be related to a failure in ongoing peripheral T and B cell tolerance, which appears to be an ongoing active process during life. **Anergy** is the continued nonresponsiveness of T cells to a host (or foreign antigen) that occurs when the antigen is presented to the T cell without necessary costimulatory signals (B7 cell receptor) from an antigen presenting cell. APC express B7 in limited locations, primarily lymph nodes, but not in tissue. A T cell encountering a self-antigen in tissue (outside the lymph node) will become anergic and be unable to respond to the self-antigen. During thymic development, a population of long-lived **regulatory T cells** develop that are specific for self-antigens. These cells block activation of autoreactive T cells, perhaps by producing inhibitory cytokines or possibly by capturing IL-2 necessary for T cell activation. An uncommon genetic disease that ablates the development of this regulatory cell population results in IPEX, which is an autoimmune disease directed toward multiple endocrine glands. Exposure of T cells to self-antigen may trigger apoptotic cell death although the mechanism remains unclear. Although different in detail, the mechanisms for peripheral B cell tolerance have a similar function.

FAILURE OF TOLERANCE: AUTOIMMUNE DISEASE

The reasons an individual forms an **autoantibody** to his or her own cells or tissue components are not well understood. Unfortunately, after an individual develops an autoimmune disease, it usually "doesn't go away." Although the affected person experiences periods when the disease is in remission or the manifestations are controlled by treatment, the disease persists and often progresses. Several mechanisms have been postulated to explain the pathogenesis of autoimmune diseases. As previously noted, many autoimmune diseases have a genetic component (which is often complex). Localized infections may provoke an autoimmune disease by allowing inflammatory antigen presenting cells to present necessary costimulatory signals normally not present at the tissue site. Experimentally it is possible to induce self-reactive antibodies in animals by presenting either a self-antigen or a closely related antigen along with potent inflammatory chemicals. Molecular mimicry can occur when a foreign antigen is sufficiently similar to a self-antigen (cross reactive to a self-antigen) that autoimmunity can occur. The group A streptococcal M protein is likely to result in the autoimmune reaction responsible for rheumatic fever. Cross reactive viral proteins may play a role in type 1 diabetes, which is clearly an autoimmune disease. (as discussed with valvular disease of the cardiovascular system and with diabetes and the pancreas). Certain drugs may induce autoimmune destruction of cells by altering their surface properties to promote immune recognition (**FIGURE 6-12**).

TABLE 6-5 summarizes the features of some of the more important diseases in which autoantibody formation appears to play a role. A presentation of lupus erythematosus follows; the other diseases are considered in greater detail in discussions of the appropriate organ systems.

LUPUS ERYTHEMATOSUS

Lupus erythematosus, one of the most common and serious autoimmune diseases, is seen most frequently in young women and is characterized by widespread damage to the vasculature in the skin, articular tissues, heart, serous membranes (pleura

Anergy Continued nonresponsiveness of T cells to a host or foreign antigen.

Regulatory T cells Cells specific for self-antigens that block the activation of autoreactive T cells.

Autoantibody An antibody formed against the host's own cells or tissue components.

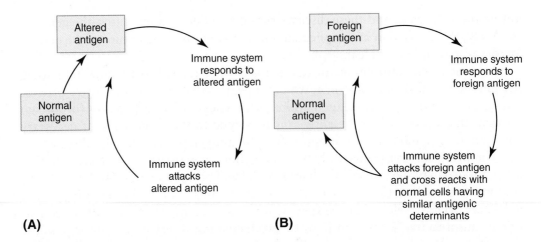

FIGURE 6-12 Two mechanisms postulated to induce autoimmunity. **(A)** Normal self-antigens altered, generating an immune response. **(B)** Immune response directed against foreign antigen cross reacts with similar antigenic determinants in normal self-antigens.

TABLE 6-5 Etiology and Clinical Manifestations of Common Autoimmune Diseases

	Probable pathogenesis	Major clinical manifestations
Rheumatic fever	Antistreptococcal antibodies cross-react with antigens in heart muscle, heart valves, and other tissues.	Inflammation of heart and joints
Glomerulonephritis	Some cases caused by antibodies formed against glomerular basement membrane; other cases caused by antigen-antibody complexes trapped in glomeruli.	Inflammation of renal glomeruli
Rheumatoid arthritis	Antibodies formed against serum gamma globulin.	Systemic disease with inflammation and degeneration of joints
Autoimmune blood diseases	Autoantibodies formed against platelets, white cells, or red cells; in some cases, antibody apparently is formed against altered cell antigens, and antibody reacts with both altered and normal cells.	Anemia, leukopenia, or thrombocytopenia, depending on nature of antibody
Lupus erythematosus, scleroderma, and related collagen diseases	Various autoantibodies cause widespread injury to tissues and organs.	Systemic disease with manifestations in several organs
Thyroiditis (Hashimoto thyroiditis)	Antithyroid antibody causes injury and inflammatory cell infiltration of thyroid gland.	Hypothyroidism

TABLE 6-5   Etiology and Clinical Manifestations of Common Autoimmune Diseases (*Continued*)

	Probable pathogenesis	Major clinical manifestations
Diffuse toxic goiter (Graves disease)	Autoantibody mimicking thyroid-stimulating hormone (TSH) causes increased output of thyroid hormone	Hyperthyroidism
Diabetes (Type 1)	Autoantibodies and activated T lymphocytes destroy pancreatic islet beta cells	Diabetes mellitus caused by insulin deficiency
Pernicious anemia	Autoantibodies destroy gastric mucosa cells	Macrocytic anemia and nervous system damage resulting from adequate absorption of vitamin B_{12}
Vasculitis (various types of blood vessel inflammation)	Autoantibody-mediated damage to small, medium, and large blood vessels	Blood vessel damage interferes with blood vessel function and blood supply to tissues
Various skin conditions and diseases causing loss of skin pigment or skin blisters	Some autoantibodies damage pigment-producing cells in skin; others attack intercellular connections between skin cells	Pigment cell loss causes areas of skin depigmentation (vitiligo); blisters result from loss of skin intercellular connections
Myasthenia gravis	Autoantibodies destroy acetylcholine receptors at muscle-nerve junctions	Muscle weakness resulting from inadequate transmission of impulses from nerves to muscles

and pericardium), and kidneys. The skin rash often has a characteristic appearance and is called a *malar rash* because it affects both cheeks (*mala* = cheek) joined by an extension across the bridge of the nose. The rash is also sometimes called a *butterfly rash* from its fancied resemblance to a butterfly with spread wings (**FIGURE 6-13**). The hemolytic anemia, leukopenia, and thrombocytopenia that are frequent hematologic manifestations of lupus are caused by autoantibodies. Patients may die of renal failure resulting from the severe renal glomerular injury.

Patients with lupus develop a variety of autoantibodies directed against nuclear components of the cell, including double-stranded DNA and a variety of nucleo-proteins and phospholipids. Circulating antigen—autoantibody complexes (immune complexes) containing these nuclear antigens form and are deposited in kidney glomeruli and blood vessels in many locations. The malar rash is related to immune complex deposition in the skin (**FIGURE 6-14**). Complement is activated, which generates an inflammatory reaction where the immune complexes are deposited. Renal

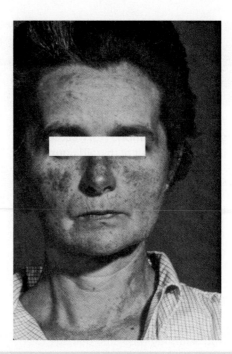

FIGURE 6-13 Characteristic butterfly rash in woman with lupus erythematosus.
Courtesy of Leonard V. Crowley, MD, Century College.

disease (lupus glomerulonephritis) is one of the most serious consequences of the disease (and can result in rapid renal failure), but neurological, vascular disease, inflammation of the linings of organs, and arthritis all occur likely as a result of the systemic deposition of immune complexes. These complexes interact with complement in promoting tissue damage. Decreases in the levels of complement components in the circulation of an SLE patient heralds disease exacerbation. Diagnosis of the disease depends on the detection of the particular types of autoantibodies most characteristically associated with SLE such as autoantibodies to double-stranded DNA and other nuclear components.

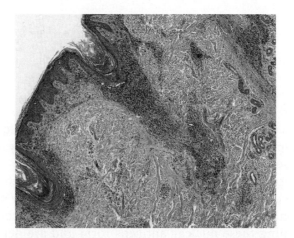

FIGURE 6-14 Vasculitis (vascular inflammation) in the skin of a patient with SLE. Blue inflammatory cell nuclei mark areas rich in dermal blood vessels.
Courtesy of Department of Pathology and Laboratory Medicine, University of North Carolina at Chapel Hill.

The pathogenesis of lupus is not well understood but appears to be related to a failure in cellular mechanisms that clear immune complexes (hence the strong association of SLE with genetic defects in early complement components important in binding to immune complexes). These complement components are likely to also play a role in clearing cellular debris and degraded DNA. Solar damage to the skin can provoke dermal disease in a patient with SLE, probably because of UV's ability to cause photodamage to cells (and specifically DNA). Variation in genes important in innate and adaptive immunity increase the risk of SLE, but no one gene has a strong effect. A combination of multiple genetic factors and intrinsic factors (including the presence of estrogen in females) plays a role in the pathogenesis of the disease. Many other diseases are also autoimmune in etiology (see Table 6-5).

CASE 6-1

George was sort of a hard luck guy. Now eighteen years old, he had a history of repeated sinus infections and his pediatrician previously had concerns about potential chronic bronchial infections caused by common bacteria. (The medical records mentioned *Haemophilus influenzae* and *Strep pneumoniae*.) His mother told him that when he was very young (about two years old) he had a series of "crouplike" episodes (inflammation of the larynx and trachea with "noisy" breathing) that seemed resistant to antibiotics. These were diagnosed as viral and became less frequent as George got older. Because George had repeated cases of bacterial respiratory infections through puberty, his pediatrician considered the possibility of immunodeficiency and evaluated him further at age thirteen. He had a mildly elevated neutrophil count along with a normal lymphocyte count with a normal ratio of B and T cells. His total immunoglobulin level was slightly low (on the lower borderline of normal). At that time, levels of individual immunoglobulin classes (IgG, IgA, and IgM) were not done. George mentioned that he was extremely sensitive to poison ivy, and, based on that, the pediatrician assumed that delayed hypersensitive reactions (dependent on T cell and macrophage function) were normal. The pediatrician considered the possibility that George had a mild deficiency in B cell function (humoral immunity). She prescribed a course of broad spectrum antibiotics, gave George an intramuscular injection of "gamma globulins" (a crude preparation of Ig prepared from pooled plasma), and asked George to return in two months for further evaluation and possible gamma globulin therapy. George felt much better over the next month with no further sinus or respiratory problems. He did not care for the gamma globulin injection and did not return for further evaluation. George did relatively well over the next four years. He had far fewer sinopulmonary infections but did develop an allergy to a variety of pollens that progressed to mild asthma, which was treated with occasional use of bronchodilators. At age seventeen George began to have mild gastrointestinal problems with bloating, cramping, and diarrhea. His girlfriend Shelly had given up gluten containing products and suggested George try it. George was a skeptic, but to his surprise a gluten free diet helped. It was clear that eating grain products made his gastrointestinal problem worse. George's pediatrician was doubtful but agreed to order testing when George showed her a food diary that linked his symptoms to gluten consumption. She ordered a TTG-IgA test (which is both highly specific and sensitive for the presence of celiac disease), and it was negative. The pediatrician diagnosed a mild food intolerance (but not celiac disease). George continued his low gluten diet, which made his gastrointestinal condition better (and pleased his girlfriend Shelly).

Now George's luck has become worse. While riding on his motor bike, he hit a wet patch on the road, skidded, and slid into a tree. His blood pressure was low when the emergency responders arrived, and George was rushed to the local hospital. His blood pressure

(continues)

CASE 6-1 (*Continued*)

remained low, and he was evaluated for internal bleeding as a result of splenic rupture. His surgeon ordered that blood be available for transfusion should it be needed. There was considerable bleeding during surgery, and transfusion was required postsurgery. Immediately on starting the transfusion, the nurse noted wheezing, hypotension, flushing, and signs of shock. An anaphylactic transfusion reaction was diagnosed, the transfusion was immediately stopped, and intravenous epinephrine and hydrocortisone was administered. George responded satisfactorily and recovered from surgery without further problems.

Discussion

Transfusion reactions can occur from a wide variety of causes (both immune and nonimmune mediated); however, such reactions are uncommon, occurring in about 0.24 percent of all transfusions in the United States. Anaphylactic transfusions are rare, with a reported incidence of 0.005 percent of all units transfused. Death from anaphylaxis related to transfusion is possible but has only been recorded once in the literature (as of 2015). Nevertheless, such reactions are of great concern to transfusion services and are investigated with care. Significant effort is expended to prevent this. So what was George's problem?

Samples of George's blood plasma were obtained after the reaction and tested for levels of immunoglobulin. He had normal levels of IgG (and associated IgG subclasses), somewhat high IgM, but less than 0.07 g/l IgA (none detectable at the limit of test sensitivity). Normal levels in an adult have a lower limit of about 0.7 g/l IgA. Based on this, George was diagnosed as having **selective IgA deficiency (SAD),** by far the most common primary immunodeficiency disease. These individuals have no detectable IgA in their blood and secretions. About 1 in 600 Caucasoids have the condition (which some consider an underestimate). The disease is relatively rare in Asian populations. Considering that IgA is the Ig isotype produced in the greatest amount (and second only to IgG in plasma level) and that it is believed to have a critical role in mucosal immunity to bacteria, it is surprising that 90 percent of individuals with SAD are asymptomatic. This figure may underestimate the morbidity associated with SAD because several careful recent studies in Scandinavia indicate a relatively higher mortality in SAD individuals as younger patients (within the first ten to fifteen years of diagnosis).

Individuals with SAD have a tenfold or greater prevalence of diseases with an autoimmune component such as celiac disease or type I diabetes and also have a greater prevalence for several others including SLE and rheumatoid arthritis. There is also a less certain indication that allergic disease and possibly certain cancers occur at a somewhat elevated rate. The mechanism for such a propensity for immune disease in SAD remains unknown.

Although SAD is often familial, the mechanism of inheritance remains uncertain. It is likely in some cases to be linked to the HLA locus, and a number of other genes have been implicated, but this remains controversial. The B cell defect seems to reside in a stem cell population: (inadvertent) transplantation of hematopoietic stem cells from a SAD donor into a previously normal donor resulted in an IgA defect in the recipient, whereas transplantation of normal stem cells into a SAD recipient cured the disease.

George had no IgA (presumably this was a congenital condition), so he has no self-tolerance to IgA. SAD patients are considered to be at risk of anaphylaxis following exposure to IgA containing materials. George's early exposure to pooled Ig (gamma globulin) probably resulted in the formation of IgE antibodies to human IgA present in the blood transfusion. The demonstration of such antibodies in SAD patients following anaphylaxis is often unsuccessful, possibly due to a technical issue as IgE antibodies can be difficult to detect. (In any case, George was not tested posttransfusion.) Although there is controversy over how likely anaphylaxis is in SAD patients following transfusion, transfusion services

CASE 6-1 (*Continued*)

make a great effort to prevent the exposure of such patients to IgA. For example, red cells to be transfused into SAD patients are repeatedly washed to remove plasma IgA. Some blood transfusion services prepare low IgA IG preparations for use in therapy.

George demonstrates the characteristic set of diseases expected in a SAD patient. In particular, celiac disease would not be unlikely. Why was George's test for the disease negative? The best test for celiac disease depends on finding IgA autoantibodies to a protein termed TTG. Because George has no IgA, his test was negative. Other tests that detect IgG autoantibodies might have been positive (but these tests are considered less reliable than those detecting IgA antibodies). George now wears a med-alert bracelet to warn of his sensitivity to plasma therapy and remains on a gluten free diet.

Etiology and Pathogenesis

Primary immunodeficiency; isolated IgA deficiency, and consequent impaired immunity to sinorespiratory infections. Increased susceptibility to autoimmune disease with celiac disease probable.

Questions

1. Suppose SAD had been diagnosed at age thirteen. What difference (if any) would this have made in George's medical history?

2. How would George's medical condition differed if he had X-linked (Bruton) agammaglobulinemia?

3. It is expected that an initial (primary) immunization is necessary prior to the occurrence of anaphylaxis. In many cases of transfusion-related anaphylaxis, no primary exposure to antigen can be demonstrated. What are some potential explanations for this finding?

4. George objected (with good reason) to intramuscular gamma globulin injections, which can be quite painful. What alternative form of medication is currently in common use to treat humoral immunodeficiency?

5. Why might autoimmune diseases such as celiac disease be more common in individuals with SAD?

QUESTIONS FOR REVIEW

1. What is meant by the following terms: *acquired immunity, cell-mediated immunity, humoral immunity,* and *hypersensitivity*?

2. What is the role of the lymphocyte in acquired immunity? What is the role of the macrophage?

3. How does the physician manipulate the body's immune reaction to allow transplantation?

4. What is meant by the following terms: *B lymphocyte, T lymphocyte,* and *lymphokine*?

5. What are immunoglobulins? What is their basic structure? How do they function?

6. What is meant by the following terms: *anaphylaxis, allergy,* and *immune deficiency*?

7. How can tolerance be induced?

8. What is an autoantibody? What are some of the postulated mechanisms that result in autoantibody formation? What is the effect of autoantibody directed against the patient's own blood cells?

9. What are antigen—antibody complexes? How do they cause tissue injury?

10. How can the immune response be suppressed? Why is this sometimes necessary?

SUPPLEMENTARY READINGS

Loeffler, A. G., and Hart, M. N. *Introduction to Human Disease*. 6th ed. Burlington, MA: Jones & Bartlett Learning.

Abbas, A. K., Lichtman, A. H., and Pillai, S. 2014. *Basic Immunology*. 4th ed. Philadelphia, PA: Elsevier Saunders.

Chapel, H. et al. 2014. *Essentials of Clinical Immunology*. 6th ed. Oxford, UK: Wiley Blackwell.

▶ The area of immunology is so complex that specialized texts are a sensible place to start a search for additional information on the subjects covered in this chapter. In the first reference, Chapter 17 is a useful introduction to the basics of immunology and immune disease, which is an excellent starting place. The second entry is a short version of a much used immunology text with excellent diagrams that will step you through some of the complexities not dealt with in the chapter. The third entry is a medically oriented text that concentrates on immunologic disease (not basic immune function). It is an excellent reference work.

Kasamatsu, J. 2013. Evolution of innate and adaptive immune systems in jawless vertebrates. *Microbiology Immunology* 57:1–12.

▶ One of the more mysterious areas in host defense is the evolution of adaptive immunity. Where did it come from? This article covers a more primitive system of host immunity that may, or may not, be an ancestor to that of higher vertebrates. It makes for fascinating reading.

Leavy, O. 2015. B Cells: Mediators of central tolerance. *Nature Reviews Immunology* 15:404.

▶ Central B cell tolerance is not as well understood as the mechanisms for T cell central tolerance. An overview of some recent work.

Aas-Hanssen, K., Thompson, K. M., Bogen, B., and Munthe, L. A. 2015. Systemic lupus erythematosus: Molecular mimicry between anti-ds DNA CDR3 idiotype, microbial and self peptides—As antigens for Th cells. *Frontiers in Immunology* 6:382

Niewold, T. B. 2015. Advances in lupus genetics. *Current Opinion in Rheumatology* 5:440–47.

▶ The first entry is a somewhat technical exploration of a possible role for molecular mimicry in the pathogenesis of SLE. The second entry explains the role of DNA polymorphisms in SLE susceptibility.

Hwang, J. K., Alt, F. W., and Yeap, L. S. 2015. Related mechanisms of antibody somatic hypermutation and class switch recombination. *Microbiology Spectrum* 3:325-348

▶ A review of mechanisms only briefly discussed in the chapter that are at the heart of the generation of antigen receptor diversity.

Yel, M. 2010. Selective IgA deficiency. *Journal of Clinical Immunology* 30:10–16.

Wang, N., and Hammarström, L. 2012. IgA deficiency: What is new? *Current Opinion in Allergy and Clinical Immunology* 12:602–8.

Immune Deficiency Foundation. 2013. *Selective IgA deficiency*. http://primaryimmune.org/about-primary-immunodeficiencies/specific-disease-types/selective-iga-deficiency/
► Three sources for the Case. The third entry is a great go-to source for information on all forms of immunodeficiency.

Neoplastic Disease

LEARNING OBJECTIVES

1. Compare the general characteristics of benign and malignant tumors. Explain how tumors are named.
2. Describe the stepwise process of the development of malignancy.
3. Differentiate between infiltrating and in situ carcinoma.
4. Understand the role of activated oncogenes and disturbance in suppressor gene function on the pathogenesis of tumors.
5. Understand how susceptibility to cancer can be inherited.
6. Explain the mechanisms of the body's immunologic defenses against tumors.
7. Summarize the principal modalities of tumor treatment including physiology, advantages, disadvantages, and common side effects of each technique.
8. Explain the role of the Pap smear in early diagnosis of neoplasm.
9. Compare the incidence and survival rates for various types of malignant tumors. Explain the mechanisms of late recurrence. Describe the role of adjuvant therapy in preventing late recurrence.

Introduction

All cells in the body are subject to control mechanisms that regulate their growth rate. Some cell populations continually divide. These **labile cell populations** such as those found in the gut are constantly renewed. Other populations are **stabile** and show little division but can be rapidly renewed from a specialized cell population when needed. Hepatocytes in the liver are a good example. Yet other cell populations are **permanent** and have no (or perhaps extremely limited) ability to divide as is the case with cardiac myocytes. In all cases, the process of cell division, maturation, and, in many cases, cell death is under physiological control. In contrast, a neoplasm (*neo* = new + *plasm* = growth) is an inappropriate growth of cells not subject to the control mechanisms that normally regulate cell growth and differentiation. Neoplasms often do not resemble the tissue from which they are derived, and their growth is not controlled by the same mechanisms that control growth in the tissue of origin. Neoplasms are **clonal** in origin; that is, they derive from a single cell and perpetuate the genetic alteration that occurred within the cell. The alteration is most often somatic, occurs in a nongerminal cell of the body, and is not inherited. However,

Labile cell populations Cells that divides continually.

Stabile Population of cells that show little cell division.

Permanent Population of cells have no ability to divide.

Clonal Derived from a single cell.

TABLE 7-1 Comparison of Benign and Malignant Tumors		
	Benign tumor	**Malignant tumor**
Growth rate	Slow	Rapid
Character of growth	Expansion	Infiltration
Tumor spread	Remains localized	Metastasis by bloodstream and lymphatics
Cell differentiation	Well differentiated	Poorly differentiated

sometimes the genetic changes associated with the development of cancer represent inherited mutations.

CLASSIFICATION AND NOMENCLATURE

The terms neoplasm and **tumor** are often used interchangeably but should not be. *Tumor* is derived from the Latin word for swelling. Although it is true that in common usage tumors are most often neoplasms (i.e., masses of cells), many (perhaps most) neoplasms do not start as tumors but as localized areas of dysregulated growth (**dysplasia**) that are not readily apparent. Such lesions are (as we shall see) often found in flat areas of epithelium that may or may not project above the normal tissue but differ in visual appearance from the surrounding tissue. A good example is melanoma, a neoplasm of epithelial pigment cells. Melanomas start out as flat, pigmented lesions and certainly would not be called tumors, at least not initially. With time, many neoplasms begin to grow and displace normal cells and warrant being described as tumors. Neoplasms may be defined as either **benign** or **malignant**; these terms have a specialized medical definition (**TABLE 7-1**). Benign neoplasms do not spread to sites distant from their origin (they do not **metastasize**), but a benign neoplasm can certainly cause local injury and in some cases be lethal. A neoplasm of the meninges of the brain may be classified as benign in the sense that it will remain localized to that tissue layer within the brain. However, if it cannot be completely removed, it may grow large enough to become lethal by occupying space within the skull. Malignant tumors can metastasize (i.e., travel to distant sites), usually by cells migrating through the lymph or bloodstream to sites where they can establish themselves and divide. The terms *cancer* or *tumor* are used to refer to malignant neoplasms. The distinction between benign and malignant neoplasms is not always absolute and can, at times, depend on the specifics of a given case. Depending on their location, tumors can be **solid** (and often embedded in, but discrete from, host tissue), **invasive** within (and not discrete from) host tissue, or derived from a blood cell or blood cell precursor and found in the circulation (**leukemia**) or in the lymph nodes or spleen (**lymphoma**).

COMPARISON OF BENIGN AND MALIGNANT TUMORS

Generally, a benign tumor grows slowly and remains localized. Although it pushes surrounding normal tissue aside, it does not infiltrate surrounding tissues (is said to be **well-circumscribed**), nor does it spread by blood and lymphatic channels to distant sites. A benign tumor often can be completely removed surgically without difficulty (**FIGURE 7-1, FIGURE 7-2,** and **FIGURE 7-3**). Histologically, the cells in a benign tumor typically appear mature and closely resemble the normal cells from which the tumor was derived. **Grade** refers to how closely the neoplasm resembles the cell of origin. Benign tumors are generally low grade because they closely resemble the cell of origin.

Tumor A benign or malignant overgrowth of tissues that serves no normal function which is no longer under homeostatic control.

Dysplasia Localized areas of dysregulated growth.

Benign Neoplasms that do not spread to sites distant from their origin.

Malignant Neoplasms that spread to sites distant from their origin.

Metastasize The spread of cancer cells from the primary site of origin to a distant site within the body.

Solid Tumor type that is embedded in host tissue.

Invasive Tumor type that infiltrates host tissue.

Leukemia A neoplastic proliferation of leukocytes.

Lymphoma A neoplasm of lymphoid cells limited to lymph nodes and sometimes spleen.

Well-circumscribed Tumor with a clear border.

Grade Term describing how closely the neoplasm resembles host tissue.

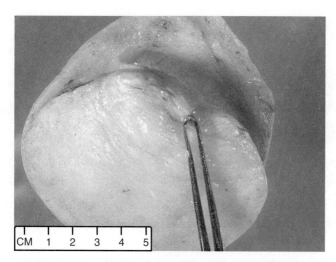

FIGURE 7-1 Well-circumscribed benign tumor. The capsule of the tumor is held by a clamp. Surrounding normal tissues have retracted, indicating an absence of infiltration.

Courtesy of Leonard V. Crowley, MD, Century College.

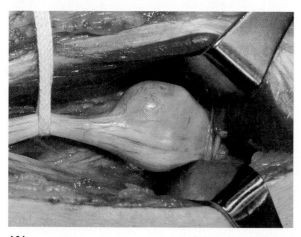

(A)

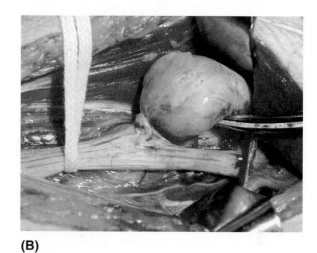

(B)

FIGURE 7-2 **(A)** Benign tumor (neuroma) arising from the sciatic nerve. **(B)** Tumor dissected from surrounding nerve. The cleavage plane is easily established, indicating that the tumor is sharply circumscribed and does not infiltrate the adjacent nerve.

Courtesy of Leonard V. Crowley, MD, Century College.

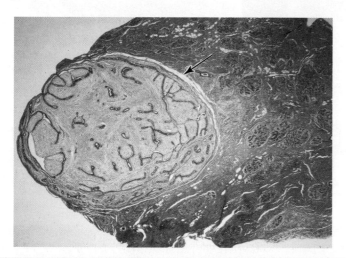

FIGURE 7-3 Low-magnification photomicrograph of benign breast tumor (fibroadenoma). Note the sharp demarcation between the tumor and surrounding breast tissue (*arrow*).

Courtesy of Leonard V. Crowley, MD, Century College.

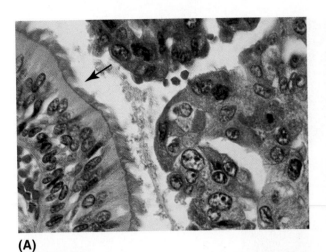

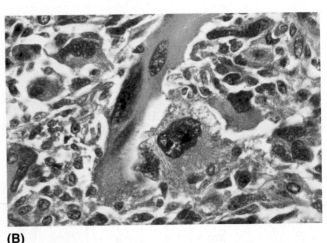

(A)   **(B)**

FIGURE 7-4 Cellular abnormalities in malignant tumors. **(A)** Biopsy of a bronchus from a patient with lung carcinoma, comparing normal respiratory epithelium (*arrow*) with clusters of neoplastic cells from a lung carcinoma. Cancer cells grow in a haphazard pattern and exhibit great variation in size and structure. **(B)** Malignant tumor of smooth muscle (leiomyosarcoma), illustrating large, bizarre, elongated tumor cells showing little resemblance to normal smooth muscle cells from which the tumor arose.

Courtesy of Leonard V. Crowley, MD, Century College.

Primary site Tissue of origin for neoplasm.

Secondary site Site of tumor following metastic growth.

In contrast to benign tumors, a malignant neoplasm is composed of less well-differentiated cells and is high grade (**FIGURE 7-4**), grows more rapidly, and infiltrates the surrounding tissues rather than growing by expansion (**FIGURE 7-5**). Frequently, the infiltrating strands of tumor find their way into the vascular and lymphatic channels. Tumor cells from the **primary site** may establish **secondary sites** of metastatic tumor growth not connected with the original tumor (**FIGURE 7-6** and **FIGURE 7-7**). If a malignant tumor is not eradicated promptly, it may eventually become widely disseminated throughout the body and may either directly or indirectly be responsible for the patient's death. For example, a primary tumor of the colon may metastasize via the blood to the liver. Multiple secondary metastatic tumors in the liver will grow, occupy space, lead to hepatocyte injury, and, ultimately, liver failure and death. This may occur even if the primary colonic tumor is removed.

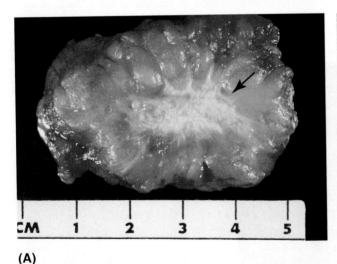

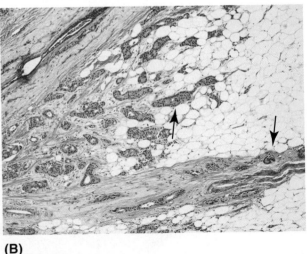

(A)   **(B)**

FIGURE 7-5 Breast carcinoma. **(A)** Breast biopsy illustrating breast carcinoma (*arrow*) infiltrating adjacent fatty tissue of the breast. There is no distinct demarcation between tumor and normal tissue. **(B)** Low-magnification photograph illustrating the margin of infiltrating breast carcinoma. Small clusters of tumor cells (*arrows*) infiltrate adipose tissues of breast (original × magnification ×20).

Courtesy of Leonard V. Crowley, MD, Century College.

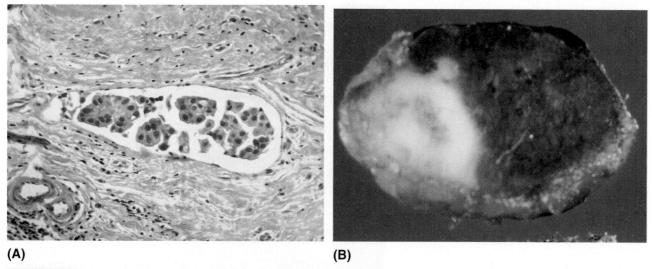

(A)

(B)

FIGURE 7-6 Lymphatic spread of carcinoma. **(A)** Cluster of tumor cells in lymphatic vessel (original magnification ×400). **(B)** Deposit of metastatic carcinoma (white mass within node) that has spread via lymphatic channels into a small regional lymph node.

Courtesy of Leonard V. Crowley, MD, Century College.

The primary factor used to classify any tumor, be it benign or malignant, is the cell or tissue of origin. Therefore, understanding the tissue classifications, including their structure and function in health and disease, is helpful in understanding the names of tumors. Although tumor nomenclature is not completely uniform, sometimes being based on historical names or jargon, certain generalizations are possible.

Benign Tumors

A tumor that projects from an epithelial surface is usually called a **polyp** or **papilloma** (**FIGURE 7-8**). Papillomas are wartlike benign growths often caused by the human papillomavirus (HPV). The term *polyp* is most often used to refer to epithelial lesions that project from the surface of an organ into the lumen (examples being colonic and uterine polyps). Polyps are generally benign when discovered but can become (or sometimes are) malignant. Benign neoplasms are named by adding the suffix *-oma*

> **Polyp/papilloma** Wart-like benign tumor often associated with viral infection.

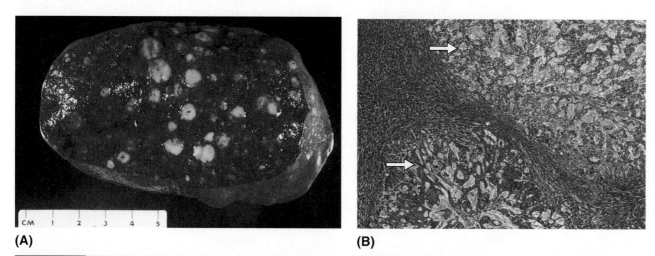

(A)

(B)

FIGURE 7-7 **(A)** Multiple nodules of metastatic carcinoma in spleen. **(B)** Multiple nodules of metastatic adenocarcinoma in the liver (*arrows*). Liver cells show damage from expanding nodules (pressure atrophy) (*).

(A) Courtesy of Leonard V. Crowley, MD, Century College; (B) Courtesy of Department of Pathology and Laboratory Medicine, University of North Carolina at Chapel Hill.

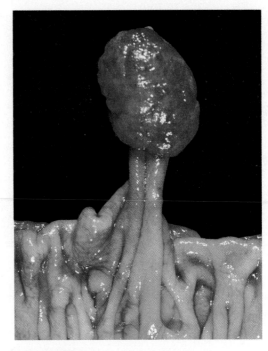

FIGURE 7-8 Benign polyp of colon.

Courtesy of Leonard V. Crowley, MD, Century College.

to the prefix that designates the cell of origin, as shown in **TABLE 7-2**. For example, a benign tumor arising from glandular epithelium is called an adenoma. A benign tumor of blood vessels is an angioma, one arising from cartilage is designated a chondroma, and from bone an osteoma.

MALIGNANT TUMORS

Carcinoma A malignant tumor derived from epithelial cells.

There are many types of malignant tumors (cancers), but most can be classified based on their tissue of origin into three groups: (1) **carcinomas** (from epithelium),

TABLE 7-2	Common Prefixes Used to Name Tumors
Prefix	**Meaning**
Adeno-	Gland
Angio-	Vessels (type not specified)
Chondro-	Cartilage
Fibro-	Fibrous tissue
Hemangio-	Blood vessels
Lymphangio-	Lymph vessels
Lipo-	Fat
Myo-	Muscle
Neuro-	Nerve
Osteo-	Bone

(2) **sarcomas** (from connective tissue), or (3) leukemias/lymphomas (from blood cells or their precursors).

A carcinoma is any malignant tumor arising from surface, glandular, or parenchymal (organ) epithelium. (The term is not applied, however, to malignant tumors of endothelium or mesothelium, which behave more like malignant connective tissue tumors.) A carcinoma is classified further by designating the type of epithelium from which it arose and whether it is of glandular or epithelial origin. For example, a malignant tumor arising from the urothelium of the urinary bladder is called a urothelial carcinoma of the bladder. A carcinoma arising from the glandular epithelium of the pancreas is termed an adenocarcinoma of the pancreas (*aden* = gland), and a tumor arising from the squamous epithelium of the esophagus is called a squamous cell carcinoma of the esophagus.

Sarcoma is a general term referring to a malignant tumor arising from connective tissue. The exact type of sarcoma is specified by prefixing the term designating the cell of origin. For example, a malignant tumor of cartilage is designated as a chondrosarcoma. Fibrosarcoma, liposarcoma, myosarcoma, osteosarcoma, and angiosarcoma indicate, respectively, malignant tumors of fibroblasts, fat cells, muscle cells, bone-forming cells, and blood vessels.

The term *leukemia* is applied to any neoplasm of blood-forming tissues found in the bone marrow or circulating in the blood. Neoplasms arising from the precursors of white blood cells usually do not form solid tumors. Instead, the abnormal cells proliferate within the bone marrow, where they overgrow and crowd out the normal blood-forming cells. The neoplastic cells also "spill over" into the bloodstream, where large numbers of abnormal cells can circulate in the peripheral blood. In some cases, these neoplastic cells may populate lymph nodes and spleen rather than circulate. Then the term *lymphoma* is used.

There are some inconsistencies and exceptions to the general principles of nomenclature. As mentioned previously, melanomas are malignant tumors derived from melanocytes. Benign neoplasms of these cells are called *benign nevi*. Seminomas are malignant testicular tumors. **Teratomas** are germ cell–derived tumors of multiple tissue types and may be either benign or malignant. Pediatric malignant neoplasms are sometimes denoted with the suffix "blastoma"; some examples being retinoblastoma and nephroblastoma (commonly called Wilms tumor). These cancers are derived from primitive (immature) retinal and renal cells, respectively. Do not be unduly concerned about the exceptions; overall, the general principles of naming tumors are followed.

TABLE 7-3 summarizes the general principles used to name malignant tumors.

DEVELOPMENT OF MALIGNANT NEOPLASMS

Studies of the development of epithelial neoplasia of the cervix, colon, lung, and breast indicate the development of cancer is a stepwise process that involves an ongoing series of genetic changes. (This is not necessarily true in the development of leukemia and lymphoma, however.) This concept is important from a clinical point of view because the progress of neoplasia from an initial event to the development of a cancer that can widely metastasize may take years. This slow progression gives the **oncologist** (a physician who specializes in the treatment of cancer) a wide window of time to diagnose and treat the disease before it becomes life-threatening. Colonoscopy (to diagnose potential adenocarcinoma of the colon by physically examining the lower digestive tract) need be done only every seven to ten years in older people because it takes time for the benign polyp detected by the test to become malignant, spread through the colon, and metastasize.

Sarcoma A malignant tumor arising from connective and supporting tissues.

Teratoma A tumor of mixed cell components.

Oncologist Physician specializing in treatment of cancer.

TABLE 7-3 Names of Malignant Neoplasms	
Cell or tissue of origin	Name
Epithelium	
Site not specified	Carcinoma
Squamous epithelium	Squamous cell carcinoma
Basal cells of epithelium	Basal cell carcinoma (unique to skin)
Colonic mucosa	Adenocarcinoma of colon
Breast glands	Adenocarcinoma of breast
Bronchial epithelium of lung	Bronchogenic carcinoma
Prostatic glands	Adenocarcinoma of prostate
Bladder mucosa	Urothelial carcinoma
Endometrium	Adenocarcinoma of endometrium
Cervix	Squamous cell carcinoma of cervix
Stomach mucosa	Adenocarcinoma of stomach
Pancreatic ducts	Adenocarcinoma of pancreas
Connective tissue and muscle	
Site not specified	Sarcoma
Lymphoid tissue	Lymphoma
Bone marrow	Leukemia
Plasma cells in bone marrow	Multiple myeloma
Cartilage	Chondrosarcoma
Bone	Osteosarcoma
Fibrous tissue	Fibrosarcoma
Smooth muscle	Leiomyosarcoma
Other	
Site not specified	Malignant neoplasm
Glial cells	Glioma
Melanocytes	Malignant melanoma
Germ cells	Teratoma

Transition zone Area of cervix where the columnar music producing epithelial cells meet the squamous epithelial cells.

Many neoplasms arising from surface epithelium remain localized within the epithelium for many years before evidence of spread into the deeper tissues or to distant sites occurs. This has been well documented for squamous cell carcinoma of the cervix (**FIGURE 7-9** and **FIGURE 7-10**). Most often cervical cancer begins in an area of the cervix (the **transition zone**) where the columnar, mucin producing epithelial cells of the cervical canal leading to the uterus meet the squamous epithelial cells that line the face of the cervix. During sexual maturation, the transition zone

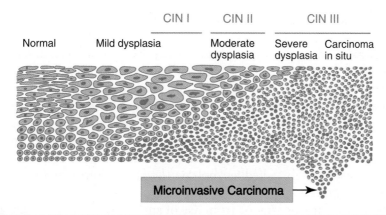

CIN I   CIN II   CIN III

Normal   Mild dysplasia   Moderate dysplasia   Severe dysplasia   Carcinoma in situ

Microinvasive Carcinoma →

FIGURE 7-9 Cervical intraepithelial neoplasia (CIN). Drawing illustrates progressive changes in cervical epithelium with time, leading to carcinoma in situ.

Courtesy of Department of Pathology and Laboratory Medicine, University of North Carolina at Chapel Hill.

moves further onto the face of the cervix, exposing the secretory cells to the acidic environment of the vagina. Perhaps as a response to injury, the columnar secretory cells undergo **metaplasia** (conversion of one differentiated tissue type to another) and become squamous cells. This area of metaplasia is susceptible to the initiation of the process of neoplasia. The process begins with the development of cervical dysplasia, a combination of abnormal cytological appearance and abnormal tissue architecture (and, at least in some cases, somatic genetic alterations) in the mucosa that defines early **cervical intraepithelial neoplasia (CIN)**. In a strict sense, the area of dysplasia is **precancerous** until the neoplastic cells traverse the basement membrane into the body of the cervix. The pathologist defines increasing degrees of dysplasia (CIN I to CIN III) as the neoplasia subtends more of the thickness of the epithelial layer. When dysplastic cells occupy the full thickness of the epithelium, the lesion is termed CIN III or **carcinoma in situ** (in-site carcinoma). An abnormal Pap test indicates the detection of dysplastic epithelial cells scraped from the surface mucosa of the cervix; if detected early in the course of cervical neoplasia, this is easily treated. However, once the neoplastic cells have traversed the basement membrane, metastasis to distant sites becomes possible and the disease is no longer CIN but cervical cancer. Although most clearly demonstrated in the cervix, the gradual progression of metaplasia to dysplasia (early "precancer") to carcinoma in situ, followed in time by invasion and metastasis (cancer or malignant neoplasia), has also been described in the breast, bronchus and lung, urinary tract and skin. The slow progression of histological changes is accompanied by the neoplastic cells gaining additional mutations,

Metaplasia Conversion of one differentiated tissue type to another.

Cervical intraepithelial neoplasia (CIN) Precancerous condition characterized by cervical dysplasia in mucosa of cervix.

Precancerous Area of dysplasia in early stages of cancer development.

Carcinoma in situ Neoplasm occupying full thickness of the epithelium.

Normal   CIN I   CIN II   CIN III
Carcinoma *in situ*

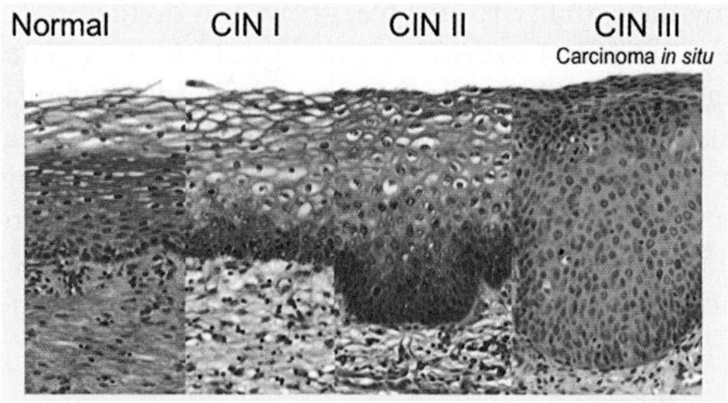

FIGURE 7-10 Cervical intraepithelial neoplasia (CIN). Cervical biopsies from four patients illustrating progressive stages of CIN.

Courtesy of Department of Pathology and Laboratory Medicine, University of North Carolina at Chapel Hill.

which are responsible for an increasing degree of malignancy as has been best studied in the colon.

Although a determination of dysplasia is made by a pathologist based on changes seen at the cell or tissue level, certain precancerous neoplasms can be visually recognized. Because these lesions have a likelihood of eventually developing into cancer, it is important to recognize them. Prolonged exposure to sunlight, for example, not only causes premature aging of the skin but also causes small, crusted, scaly patches to develop on sun-exposed skin called **actinic keratoses** ("actinic" refers to sun rays). Untreated, many keratoses eventually develop into skin cancers. Precancerous, thick, white patches descriptively called **leukoplakia** (*leuko* = white + *plakia* = patch) may develop in the mucous membranes of the mouth as a result of exposure to tobacco tars from pipe or cigar smoking or from use of smokeless tobacco (snuff and chewing tobacco) and may give rise to squamous cell cancers of the oral cavity (see the discussion on the gastrointestinal tract). Somewhat similar precancerous changes may take place in the epithelium of the vulva (discussion on the female reproductive system) and may develop into vulvar cancer. These neoplastic precancerous conditions should always be treated appropriately to prevent malignant change, which occurs in many, but not all, cases.

GROWTH OF NEOPLASMS

The great majority of neoplasms are monoclonal and derive from a single cell "gone bad" that perpetuates the genetic change responsible for its uncontrolled growth. Some neoplasias appear to be initiated in a particular population of cells present in many organs that serve as a continuing source of differentiated cells to replace populations that are damaged or have died. Such **stem cells** constitute a self-renewing pool of cells that normally give rise to mature differentiated progeny. Stem cells may undergo a mutational event to give rise to cancer stem cells (CSC), which in turn may serve as a source of malignancies. These CSC populations have a low rate of division and are resistant to anticancer drugs, which require dividing cells, and hence are difficult to eradicate. The CSC is a subpopulaton within the cancer that provides a continuing source of malignant cells.

Although a neoplasm starts from a single cell, the population of cells within a tumor shows great diversity (**tumor heterogeneity**). As the tumor grows, additional mutations occur; the mutated cells are selected for rapid growth, survival, ability to escape immune killing, and resistance to therapeutic drugs. The acquisition of mutations that support additional mutations (e.g., by preventing DNA repair or interfering with apoptosis in response to DNA damage) occurs as neoplasia become increasingly malignant. The cells in a malignancy undergo a "selection of the fittest," which is defined by their ability to survive, grow, and divide.

Although there are many exceptions, malignant lesions generally grow more rapidly than benign lesions. However, the apparent sudden expansion of tumors is a result of exponential growth. It may take thirty cell doublings for a tumor to be just detectable (about 1 gram and 10^9 cells), but only ten more doublings would result in 10^{12} cells having a weight of 1 kg, and perhaps only a month more to grow to a lethal cell number and mass. Of course, this assumes that all cancer cells grow and divide, which does not necessarily occur because tumors may outgrow their blood supply.

Necrosis in Tumors

Tumors derive their blood supply from the tissues they invade but may outgrow that blood supply. Malignant tumors frequently induce new blood vessels to proliferate in

---

Actinic keratosis A precancerous warty proliferation of squamous epithelial cells in sun-damaged skin of older persons.

Leukoplakia A white patch of hyperplastic and usually atypical squamous epithelium on the oral mucosa or genital tract mucosa.

Stem cells A self-renewing pool of cells that normally give rise to mature differentiated progeny.

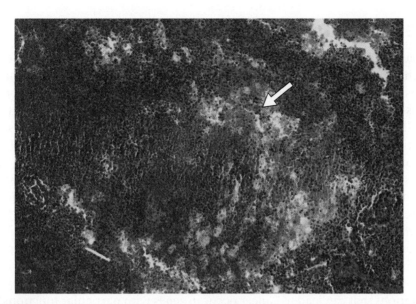

FIGURE 7-11 Central area of necrosis in a rapidly growing small cell carcinoma of the lung (*arrow*).
Courtesy of Department of Pathology and Laboratory Medicine, University of North Carolina at Chapel Hill.

the adjacent normal tissues to supply the demands of the growing tumor. When the blood supply is no longer sufficient, the parts of the tumor with the poorest blood supply undergo necrosis (**FIGURE 7-11**). If the tumor is growing within an organ such as the lung or kidney surrounded by normal tissue, the blood supply is best at the junction of the tumor and adjacent normal tissue, and poorest in the center of the tumor, which often degenerates. In contrast, if the malignant tumor is growing outward from an epithelial surface, such as the colon, the best blood supply is at the base of the tumor. The poorest blood supply is at the surface, which frequently becomes necrotic and sloughs, leaving a shallow crater covered with degenerated tissue and inflammatory exudate (**FIGURE 7-12**). Exposed small blood vessels in the ulcerated base of the tumor may bleed, eventually leading to anemia from chronic blood loss into the stool. This is the basis for the use of stool blood tests to detect colon cancer. Sometimes the ulcerated tumor may be the source of a severe hemorrhage.

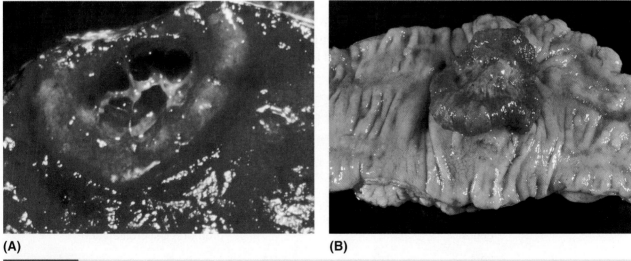

(A)   **(B)**

FIGURE 7-12 **(A)** Carcinoma of lung with central necrosis. **(B)** Carcinoma of colon exhibiting superficial ulceration.
Courtesy of Leonard V. Crowley, MD, Century College.

Genetic Change in Neoplastic Disease

The basic process common to all neoplasms is an alteration (mutation) of the genes on the chromosomes of a cell so that the cell no longer responds to normal control mechanisms and proceeds to proliferate without regard for the needs of the body. This change is then perpetuated in the offspring (clonal products) of that cell. In the body, many billions of cells are dividing all the time. They are also continually subjected to radiation, various chemical carcinogens (cancer-producing substances), viruses, and agents that are the products of cellular metabolism that can alter the structure of genes. Although robust error correction systems are built into our genome, these systems are not perfect and uncorrected mutations can accumulate in our DNA. The increase in rate of many types of cancer with age probably reflect both the accumulation of errors and a gradual failure of the error correction systems. Although mutations can be in the germline (cells that will become ova or sperm), resulting in an inherited disposition to cancer, the somatic mutations occurring in dividing cell populations are far more common and are responsible for most cases of cancer.

Mutations that can lead to cancer occur in genes with particular functions such as controlling cell growth, programmed cell death, or DNA repair. Mutations in genes that (1) control cell growth can result in cells that no longer respond to physiological inhibitors of growth. The cells may be able to undergo unlimited divisions without undergoing cellular senescence as discussed in cells and tissue. They may gain the ability to stimulate the formation of new blood vessels (promote sustained **angiogenesis**) and hence not outgrow local blood supplies. Mutations in genes (2) required for **apoptosis** or its suppression (see also presentation on cells and tissue) can allow cells to continue to grow indefinitely, even in the presence of DNA damage that would normally activate apoptotic pathways and result in cell death. Mutations in genes (3) required for the repair of DNA and for genome stability allow the neoplastic cell to accumulate additional mutations and further promote malignancy. In addition, secondary mutations may result in cells able to invade and metastasize by altering their surface properties and their ability to adhere to neighboring cells or allowing them to secrete enzymes that break down normal cell and tissue barriers. Genes in which derangements are associated with **carcinogenesis** are classified into three large groups proto-oncogenes, tumor suppressor genes, and DNA repair genes (**TABLE 7-4**).

PROTO-ONCOGENES

Human chromosomes contain a number of normal "growth genes" that promote some aspect of cell growth, differentiation, or mitotic activity. **Proto-oncogenes** are closely related to genes carried by viruses that cause tumors in experimental animals

Angiogenesis The formation of new blood vessels.

Apoptosis Programmed cell death that occurs after a cell has lived its normal life span.

Carcinogenesis Development of cancer.

Proto-oncogenes A gene promoting cell growth, differentiation or mitotic activity associated with neoplasia.

TABLE 7-4	Gene Mutations That Disrupt Cell Function	
Gene	**Normal function**	**Malfunction**
Proto-oncogenes	Promotes normal cell growth	Point mutation, amplification, or translocation forms an oncogene, resulting in unrestrained cell growth
Tumor suppressor genes	Inhibit cell proliferation	Both genes inactivated in same cell promotes cell proliferation
DNA repair genes	Correct errors in DNA duplication	Gene inactivation increases mutation rate

and are named from the tumor viruses they resemble. A proto-oncogene is a gene that regulates some normal growth function in a cell, but a proto-oncogene can be converted into an **oncogene** (*onkos* = tumor), an abnormally functioning gene that stimulates excessive cell growth leading to unrestrained cell proliferation. An oncogene is a gene that is important in causing cancer.

Conversion of a proto-oncogene into an oncogene (activation of an oncogene) may occur with a change in a single nucleotide in the DNA of the gene (a point mutation), or chromosomal changes may generate multiple copies of the same gene, a process called **gene amplification**, which greatly increases the activity of the gene. Translocation of a proto-oncogene to another chromosomal location may form an oncogene because of the way in which genes are related on individual chromosomes. For example, the translocation may bring the proto-oncogene to a new location on another chromosome where it is freed from the inhibitory genes that formerly controlled its activities. Alternatively, the translocation may bring the proto-oncogene to a new location on another chromosome adjacent to another gene that stimulates its functions. Mutations that create oncogenes mutations are dominant **gain of function** mutations; so called because the oncogene now has an altered function that interferes with normal control of cell growth and replication.

A straightforward example is the oncogene c-Sis (named for the simian sarcoma virus). In normal (non-neoplastic) cells, the proto-oncogene for c-Sis codes for a growth factor (beta PDGF, a platelet-derived growth factor) under physiological control that is synthesized only when needed to support the generation of new blood vessels during tissue repair. The oncogen c-Sis can mutate so that beta PGDF is produced constantly. This mutation results in inappropriate clonal cell growth, and each "daughter" cell also constantly produces excess growth factor. This **autocrine** (self-acting) loop is found in many cancers (particularly glioblastomas, malignant tumors of the glial cells of the brain) and is responsible in part for the uncontrolled growth and tumor formation.

The best-known chromosomal abnormality resulting in gene activation, called Philadelphia chromosome (named after the city where it was discovered), can be demonstrated in the white cells of patients with chronic granulocytic leukemia (described in the discussion on leukemia). The abnormality is a reciprocal translocation of broken end pieces between chromosomes 9 and 22. In this translocation, a proto-oncogene (*abl*) on chromosome 9 is moved to a position on chromosome 22. There it becomes fused with another gene (*bcr*) to form a composite gene (*bcr/abl*) that directs the synthesis of an uncontrolled, extremely active **tyrosine kinase** enzyme that produces multiple effects concerned with cell growth and cell division. It is the excessive unregulated activity of this enzyme that stimulates the unrestrained proliferation of white blood cells characteristic of chronic granulocytic leukemia (**FIGURE 7-13**). The same type of translocation also occurs in some patients with acute lymphocytic leukemia, but the composite gene *bcr/abl* resulting from the translocation is slightly different, which leads to a different and more aggressive type of disease.

TUMOR SUPPRESSOR GENES

Tumor suppressor genes are groups of different genes that suppress cell proliferation. Loss of suppressor gene function by mutation or another event disrupts cell functions and can lead to unrestrained cell growth. Tumor suppressor genes often function by preventing cells from undergoing DNA replication and completing mitosis in an uncontrolled manner. In the absence of a functioning tumor suppressor gene, the cell may repeatedly divide without restraint and form a malignant tumor. Tumor suppressor genes exist as paired alleles at corresponding gene loci on homologous

Oncogene An abnormally functioning gene that causes unrestrained cell growth leading to formation of a tumor. Results from mutation or translocation of a proto-oncogene.

Gene amplification Generation of multiple copies of a gene, increasing gene activity.

Autocrine Self acting loop in cancer responsible for uncontrolled growth.

Tyrosine kinase Enzyme that produces multiple effects concerned with cell growth and cell division by phosphorylation of tyrosine residues in a protein.

Tumor suppressor gene Gene that normally functions to suppress abnormal cell growth.

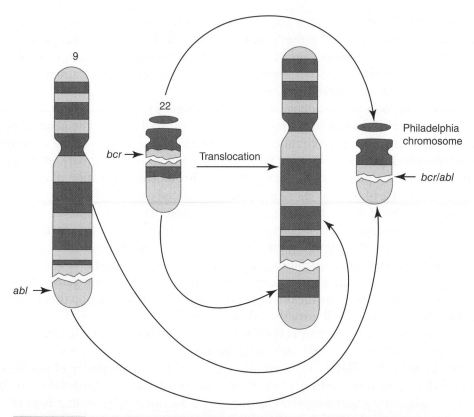

FIGURE 7-13 Reciprocal translocation between broken pieces of chromosomes 9 and 22, forming the Philadelphia chromosome containing the composite gene that disrupts normal cell functions.

chromosomes, so both alleles must cease to function before the cell malfunctions. Hence, tumor suppressor genes are recessive. However, a carrier (heterozygote) for a mutation at this locus has a greatly increased risk of developing cancer because a somatic mutation in a single cell may inactivate the one functioning copy of the tumor suppressor gene. This results in **loss of heterozygosity (LOH)** of the tumor suppressor gene, leading to potential tumor formation. Tumor suppressor genes may also inhibit "pro-growth" metabolic pathways, be part of DNA repair mechanisms, or help maintain stability of the genome. Loss of function of specific tumor suppressor genes has been correlated with specific tumors, and the suppressor genes are often named from the tumors with which they have been associated.

The classic example is retinoblastoma, an uncommon childhood tumor illustrated in **FIGURE 7-14**. This tumor is also a typical example of how tumor suppressor genes control cell function and how loss of control can cause a tumor. Retinoblastoma is a malignant tumor of primitive retinal cells occurring in infants and children that is caused by loss of function of a tumor suppressor gene called *RB*. Normal *RB* genes exist as alleles, one on each of the homologous pair of chromosome 13, so both *RB* genes must be nonfunctional in a retinal cell before a tumor arises. About 40 percent of retinoblastomas are hereditary; the rest occur sporadically, without any hereditary predisposition. The hereditary form of retinoblastoma is probable if a child inherits a defective, nonfunctional *RB* gene from a parent. The affected child has only a single functioning *RB* gene in all body cells, including those in the retina, but the single functioning *RB* gene is sufficient to maintain control of cell functions. However, if a chance mutation occurs in the remaining single functional *RB* gene within a retinal cell, loss of heterozygosity occurs, and all *RB* gene function in the affected cell is lost. The affected cell then proliferates to form a clone of unregulated cells, eventually becoming a malignant retinal tumor. Hereditary retinoblastomas may occur in

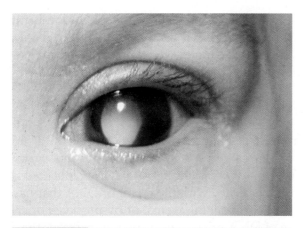

FIGURE 7-14 Retinoblastoma of an eye that appears as a pale mass of tissue seen through the dilated pupil.

Courtesy of Leonard V. Crowley, MD, Century College.

both eyes because retinal cells in both eyes are equally vulnerable to similar random *RB* gene mutations in other single functioning *RB* genes. In the sporadic form of retinoblastoma, both *RB* genes in the same retinal cell must undergo mutation to deregulate cell function and give rise to a retinoblastoma, so tumors in both eyes are unlikely. **FIGURE 7-15** summarizes the pathogenesis of this tumor. The hereditary

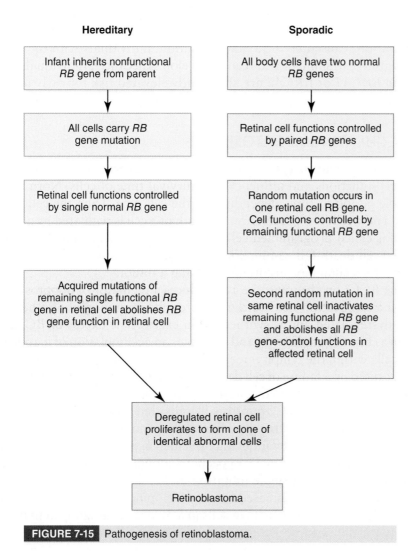

Hereditary

Infant inherits nonfunctional *RB* gene from parent

↓

All cells carry *RB* gene mutation

↓

Retinal cell functions controlled by single normal *RB* gene

↓

Acquired mutations of remaining single functional *RB* gene in retinal cell abolishes *RB* gene function in retinal cell

Sporadic

All body cells have two normal *RB* genes

↓

Retinal cell functions controlled by paired *RB* genes

↓

Random mutation occurs in one retinal cell RB gene. Cell functions controlled by remaining functional *RB* gene

↓

Second random mutation in same retinal cell inactivates remaining functional *RB* gene and abolishes all *RB* gene-control functions in affected retinal cell

Deregulated retinal cell proliferates to form clone of identical abnormal cells

↓

Retinoblastoma

FIGURE 7-15 Pathogenesis of retinoblastoma.

form of retinoblastoma is transmitted as a Mendelian dominant trait because the transmission of a single defective *RB* gene from parent to child places the child at very high risk of developing this tumor, even though the second *RB* gene must become nonfunctional in a retinal cell before the neoplasm actually arises.

DNA REPAIR GENES

DNA repair gene Gene that normally functions to repair DNA.

DNA repair genes are part of the cell's "quality control" and repair system. These genes regulate the processes that monitor and repair any errors in DNA duplication that may occur when the cell's chromosomes are replicated in the course of cell division; they are also concerned with the repair of DNA that has been damaged by radiation, chemicals, environmental agents, or by-products of cellular metabolism. Consequently, failure of DNA repair gene function increases the likelihood of DNA mutations within the affected cell being maintained and passed on to daughter cells. A high rate of uncorrected mutations within cells predisposes the individual to tumors because some mutations may affect cell functions that promote unrestrained cell growth.

Like tumor suppressor genes, DNA repair genes also exist in pairs in homologous chromosomes, and both must become nonfunctional before the repair functions regulated by the genes are compromised. People with an inherited mutation of a DNA repair gene are at increased risk of some tumors; if a spontaneous mutation of the other gene occurs, the affected cell will accumulate mutations. Mutations in DNA repair genes may be related to increased risk for particular types of cancer. *Xeroderma pigmentosum* results from an inability of skin cells to repair a particular class of mutations caused by ultraviolet radiation. Individuals with the disease are extremely sensitive to sunlight and readily develop skin cancer. Individuals inheriting mutations in *BRCA1* or *BRCA2* are at a greatly elevated risk for early onset breast and ovarian cancer.

GENES REGULATING APOPTOSIS

Another group of genes plays a more limited but nevertheless important role in regulating cell functions and influences the survival time of cells. Normal cells live for a variable period of time, depending on the cell type. Then the cell dies and is replaced by a new cell. The predetermined death of a cell is regulated by genes within the cell and is called programmed cell death, or apoptosis. If the genes regulating programmed cell death fail to function properly, the cells don't die as they should and continue to accumulate, eventually forming a tumor.

The gene *BCL2* on chromosome 18 produces a regulator of apoptosis. If *BCL2* undergoes a translocation next to the gene for the immunoglobulin heavy chain, it becomes dysregulated and is synthesized in excess. The excess of *BCL2* inhibits apoptosis in a class of lymphocytes and promotes an accumulation of inappropriately long-lived cells within the lymph node. This results in a lymphoid tumor (follicular lymphoma) caused by a failure of cell death rather than by excess proliferation of cells.

The most commonly mutated gene in human cancers, *TP53*, is a tumor suppressor that is critical in inducing apoptosis in cells that have undergone irreparable DNA damage. Referred to as "the guardian of the genome," *TP53* provides the final protection against neoplasia by inducing "suicide" in cells that have mutations that cannot be repaired. Mutations in *TP53* occur in about half of all cancers. Individuals who are heterozygous for a single mutation in *TP53* have Li-Fraumeni syndrome and have a twenty-five-fold increased risk of developing cancer as a result of somatic mutation and loss of heterozygosity in cells in a manner analogous to that seen with mutations in *RB*. Because loss of *TP53* function allows rapid additional accumulation of mutations in neoplastic cells, it is often associated with the occurrence of high-grade disseminated cancer. Because many anticancer drugs work by inducing apoptosis in cancer cells, tumors with inactivation of *p53* function may become resistant to the drug's anticancer activity.

MULTISTEP PROGRESSION OF GENETIC CHANGES LEADING TO CANCER

In most cases, cancers do not result from mutation of a single gene. Rather, they are the result of multiple genetic "insults" to the genome characterized by activation of oncogenes along with loss of function of one or more tumor suppressor genes. The transition, for example, from a benign polyp of the colon to an invasive colon cancer requires activation of an oncogene (*ras*) and inactivation of three distinct tumor suppressor genes (*APC*, *DCC*, and *p53*) (**FIGURE 7-16**).

Once a cell has been deregulated and has formed a tumor, additional random genetic changes may take place in the tumor cells, which now have a very unstable genome. Often individual genes may undergo additional mutations, or they may reduplicate themselves by gene amplification, forming multiple copies of a single gene. Chromosomes may fragment; pieces of chromosomes may be lost from the cells or be translocated to other chromosomes. Some of these mutations in the unstable tumor cell genome may produce new mutant cells that exhibit more aggressive growth than the original tumor cells, and the new mutant may eventually outgrow the other cells in the tumor. Clinically, this event may be manifested by more rapid growth and aggressive behavior of the tumor, and as noted, often the tumor may become less

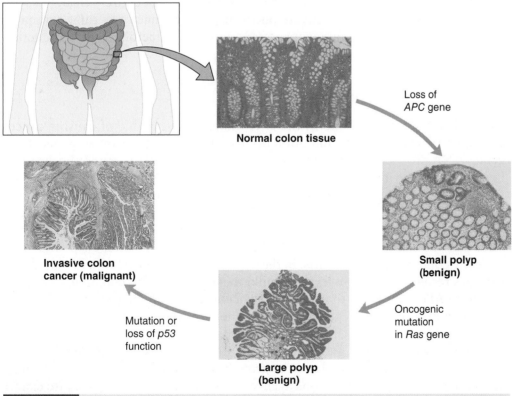

FIGURE 7-16 Somatic mutations and cell morphology in the progression of colon cancer. (Loss of *DCC* is not shown.)

Photographs courtesy of Dr. Kathleen R. Cho, University of Michigan Medical School.

responsive to the anticancer drugs that formerly could control it. Leukemias present an exception to the pattern of stepwise accumulation of mutations associated with malignancy because a single chromosomal translocation and associated oncogene activation can result in the production of aggressive disease.

VIRUSES

Many types of tumors in animals are caused by viruses and can be readily transmitted by appropriate methods to animals of the same or a different species. In some instances, a single type of virus is capable of producing many different types of tumors in various species of animals. Some of the cancers in humans also appear to be caused by viruses. Some unusual types of leukemia and lymphoma are caused by a virus called the human T cell leukemia–lymphoma virus (HTLV-1), which is related to the virus that causes the acquired immune deficiency syndrome (AIDS). The HTLV-1 genome contains a gene called *tax* that has an oncogene-like action in T lymphocytes. Some strains of the human papilloma virus (HPV) that cause genital condylomas (discussion on the female reproductive system) are responsible for cervical carcinoma and are also responsible for some squamous cell carcinomas of the mouth, throat, and larynx (oropharyngeal carcinomas). Oncogenic strains of HPV integrate into the host cell genome and secrete proteins that inactivate the tumor suppressor genes *Rb* and *Tp53*. Chronic viral hepatitis (discussion on the liver and the biliary system) predisposes to primary carcinoma of the liver. Kaposi's sarcoma, which occurs predominantly in AIDS patients, is caused by a herpes virus, designated human herpesvirus 8 (HHV-8). Some types of nasophyngeal carcinoma and some types of lymphoma appear to be related to infection with Epstein-Barr virus, the same herpesvirus that causes infectious mononucleosis. The mechanism by which herpesviruses result in cancer is complex and not entirely clear, but viral genes may function both to activate oncogenes and to inactivate tumor suppressors. In addition, host immunosuppressant acts as a cofactor for the production of cancer.

CHEMICAL CARCINOGENS

Many chemical agents found in the environment are capable of causing cancer through a two-step process. **Initiation** occurs when a highly reactive chemical targeting DNA produces a nonlethal mutation in the genome that cannot be repaired. In many cases, the mutation occurs at random in the DNA and will result in cancer only, if by chance, the mutation occurs within a critical gene. However, some chemical agents have a degree of specificity in their action. For example, the carcinogen aflatoxin B_1 is produced by a mold that infects improperly stored grains and nuts. The toxin is either directly ingested by humans or enters the food chain and inadvertently contaminates foodstuffs. In the southern United States, contaminated feed for cows results in aflatoxin levels in milk; the toxin may also contaminate peanut products. Aflatoxin tends to mutate a particular codon in the gene for *TP53* that ultimately may result in hepatocellular carcinoma (liver cancer). This cancer is far more common in areas of Africa and Asia where ingestion of contaminated products is common. Contact with an initiating carcinogen alone is not sufficient to cause cancer; a **promotor** that stimulates the growth of initiated cells must also be present. Promotors may be exogenous agents that do not, in themselves, cause cancer but do encourage cell division, such as certain drugs and hormone preparations. Endogenous promoters include persistent inflammation and excess production of estrogen-like hormones.

Promotor Substance needed to stimulate growth of cells after contact with carcinogen.

FAILURE OF IMMUNOLOGIC DEFENSES

A neoplasm may produce proteins and cell surface components (glycolipids and glycoproteins) that are either not present or altered from those found in a normal cell. Such cell products are sometimes recognized as abnormal by the immune system, which attempts to destroy the cell by various cell-mediated mechanisms. These new or altered products may be produced by mutated genes directly involved in carcinogenesis or may be overexpressed or inappropriately expressed products of cellular genes, which result from changes in cellular metabolism induced by neoplasia. For example, some tumors produce **oncofetal antigens**, which are proteins normally synthesized at high levels only during fetal development but also occur in high amounts in some cancers.

> **Oncofetal antigens** Proteins normally synthesized only during fetal development and associated with neoplasia.

The role played by the immune system in surveillance and destruction of neoplastic cells is still unclear. The immune system must be imperfect in destroying potential cancer causing cells because immunocompetent people do get cancer. Severely immunocompromised individuals are at much increased risk for some, but not all, cancers. The majority of the high-risk cancers are mature B cell neoplasms (lymphomas), often associated with an Epstein-Barr virus infection.

The limited role of the immune system in the suppression of cancer may be related, in part, to the ability of cancer cells to evade immune killing. Cancer cells may mutate and no longer express antigens necessary for immune killing and may lose expression of HLA molecules necessary for recognition by immune cells. Cancer cells may secrete immunosuppressive agents or turn on cellular pathways that inhibit immune activation. Cancer cells may exploit immune checkpoints, physiological regulators of the immune response, to prevent immune destruction. A major goal in developing new cancer therapies is to learn how to better use the immune system to destroy cancer cells and to circumvent the mechanisms used by these cells to prevent immune-mediated killing.

Heredity and Tumors

Although well-defined hereditary (germline) mutations are responsible for a small proportion of all cancers, individuals bearing these mutations are at greatly increased risk. A person whose parent or sibling has been afflicted with a breast, colon, or lung carcinoma has about a three times greater risk of developing a similar tumor than do other people. The predisposition is apparently the result of a multifactorial inheritance pattern in which the individual at risk has inherited sets of genes that influence some hormonal- or enzyme-regulated biochemical process within the body that slightly increases the susceptibility to a specific cancer. The increased risk may be caused by genetic differences in various biochemical or physiologic activities that influence cell functions, such as differences in circulating hormone levels that could influence cell growth rates, variations in the rate at which the cell can metabolize and inactivate cancer-causing chemicals, variations in the ability to repair DNA that has been damaged by injurious agents, or variations in the efficiency of the immune system in eliminating abnormal cells as they arise.

Heredity does play an important role in some tumors. The best known of these are autosomal dominant mutations of tumor suppressor genes. Hereditary gene mutations are responsible for a small percentage of breast carcinomas, and the affected individuals are at increased risk of ovarian carcinoma as well. Two different genes are involved. Some hereditary breast and ovarian carcinomas can be traced to an inherited mutation of a tumor suppressor gene designated *BRCA1* (breast carcinoma 1), which has been localized to chromosome 17. Other cases are related to a mutation of a second tumor suppressor gene designated *BRCA2* (breast carcinoma 2), which is located on chromosome 13. The pathogenesis of hereditary breast and ovarian carcinoma related to either a *BRCA1* or *BRCA2* mutation is comparable to that of hereditary retinoblastoma caused by an inherited mutant *RB* gene (see Figure 7-15). *BRCA* mutations are considered to be inherited as dominant traits because the inheritance of a single *BRCA* mutant gene from either parent is responsible for the increased susceptibility to both breast and ovarian carcinomas.

A condition called multiple polyposis of the colon, also a dominant trait, is characterized by the formation of multiple polyps throughout the colon, and usually one or more of them eventually becomes malignant. Another condition transmitted as an autosomal dominant trait is multiple neurofibromatosis (discussion on the nervous system). Many of the nerves throughout the body give rise to benign tumors called neurofibromas, and often one of these tumors eventually undergoes malignant change. Another hereditary tumor syndrome, also an autosomal dominant transmission, is multiple endocrine adenomatosis, which is characterized by the formation of adenomas arising in several different endocrine glands, as the name indicates.

There are many other examples of tumors related to hereditary gene mutations, but it is important to remember that they make up only a small fraction of the benign and malignant tumors afflicting humans.

Diagnosis of Tumors

EARLY RECOGNITION OF NEOPLASMS

The American Cancer Society publicizes a number of signs and symptoms that should arouse suspicion of cancer (**TABLE 7-5**). In general, any abnormality of form or function may be an early symptom of a neoplasm and should be investigated by a physician. For example, a lump in the breast, an ulcer on the lip, or a change in the character of a wart or mole may be considered an abnormality of form. Vaginal bleeding in a postmenopausal woman or a change in bowel habits manifested by constipation or diarrhea is an abnormality of function. Early diagnosis of specific cancers is furthered by routine screening tests such as mammograms and routine fecal stool blood tests and colonoscopy in selected groups at increased risk, most often persons above a particular age.

A complete medical history and physical examination by the physician are the next steps in evaluating suspected abnormalities. The physical examination may include special studies such as an examination of the rectum and colon by means of a special instrument, a vaginal examination and Pap smear in women, or examination of the esophagus and stomach with special devices, and various types of x-ray studies.

TABLE 7-5 American Cancer Society Warning Signals
1. Change in bowel or bladder habits
2. A sore that does not heal
3. Unusual bleeding or discharge
4. A thickening or lump in the breast or elsewhere
5. Indigestion or difficulty in swallowing
6. An obvious change in wart or mole
7. A nagging cough or hoarseness

If a tumor is discovered, exact diagnosis requires biopsy or complete excision of the suspected tumor. Histologic examination of the tissue by the pathologist provides an exact diagnosis and serves as a guide to further treatment. If the tumor is benign, simple excision is curative. If the tumor is malignant, a more extensive operation or additional types of treatment may be required.

CYTOLOGIC DIAGNOSIS OF NEOPLASMS

Tumors shed abnormal cells from their surfaces, and these cells can be recognized in the body fluids and secretions that come into contact with the tumor. Often the abnormal cells can be recognized when the neoplasm is only microscopic in size and is still confined to the surface epithelium. These observations have been applied to the cytologic diagnosis of tumors. The method is named after the physician who played a large part in developing and applying cytologic methods, Dr. George Papanicolaou. The microscopic slides of the material prepared for cytologic examination are called Papanicolaou smears, or simply **Pap smears** (**FIGURE 7-17**). This subject is considered further in the discussion on the female reproductive system.

Cytologic methods can also be applied to the diagnosis of neoplasms in other locations by examining sputum, urine, breast secretions, and fluids obtained from the pleural or peritoneal cavities.

Pap smear A study of cells from various sources, commonly used as a screening test for cancer.

FINE NEEDLE ASPIATION

Cells for cytologic and histopathologic study can also be examined by aspirating material from organs or tissues by means of a fine needle attached to a syringe and preparing slides from the aspirated material (fine needle aspiration [FNA]). This technique can be used to evaluate nodules in the thyroid or breast, and often the nature of the nodule can be determined by the appearance of the aspirated cells, avoiding the need for a biopsy. However, many fine needle aspirations require a follow-up biopsy to better determine whether a neoplasm is benign or shows signs of malignancy. Suspected tumors in the lung, liver, pancreas, kidney, and other internal

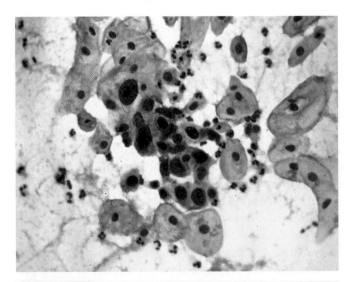

FIGURE 7-17 Photomicrograph of Pap smear, illustrating a cluster of abnormal cells from in situ carcinoma of the cervix. Cells appear much different from adjacent normal squamous epithelial cells.

Courtesy of Leonard V. Crowley, MD, Century College.

organs can be examined by fine needle aspiration. When attempting aspiration from internal organs, the precise location of the suspected tumor must be determined by means of a CT scan or other x-ray examination or by ultrasound. The needle is then inserted into the suspected tumor under x-ray guidance. In general, the diagnostic accuracy of fine needle aspiration is not as good as a biopsy but may be adequate for diagnosis, avoiding a more extensive biopsy procedure. Because FNAs are less traumatic to the patient, safer, and often provide results rapidly and at less expense, these procedures are widely used in the initial diagnosis of suspicious lesions.

Frozen-Section Diagnosis of Neoplasms

Many times, it is important that a surgeon learn immediately whether a tumor discovered in the course of an operation is benign or malignant because the extent of surgery performed may depend on the nature of the neoplasm. The surgeon must also find out during the operation whether a tumor has been excised completely and whether it has spread to lymph nodes or distant sites. A pathologist can provide the surgeon with a rapid **intraoperative** histologic diagnosis and other information by means of a special technique called a **frozen section**. In this method, a portion of the tumor or other tissue to be examined histologically is frozen solid at a subzero temperature. A thin section of the frozen tissue is cut by means of a special instrument called a cryotome, and slides are prepared and stained. The slides can then be examined by the pathologist, and a rapid histologic diagnosis can be made. The entire procedure takes only a few minutes as compared to routine histologic diagnosis which can take several days.

TUMOR-ASSOCIATED ANTIGEN TESTS

As discussed earlier in this chapter, some cancers secrete substances called **tumor-associated antigens**. These are either absent from normal mature tissues or present only in trace amounts. Many tumor-associated antigens are carbohydrate–protein complexes (glycoproteins) that are secreted as a coating on the surface of the cancer cells. Some of the glycoprotein gains access to the circulation, where it can be detected by means of specialized laboratory tests performed on the blood of patients with cancer.

A well-known tumor-associated oncofetal antigen is **carcinoembryonic antigen (CEA)**, so named because it resembles a glycoprotein antigen secreted by the cells lining the fetal intestinal tract. CEA is produced by most but not all malignant tumors of the gastrointestinal tract and pancreas and by many cancers of the breast and lung as well as other cancers. Moreover, elevation of CEA levels is not specific for any one type of cancer. CEA is usually not elevated in the blood of people with small, early cancers, and it occurs at low levels in diseases other than cancer. For these reasons, it is not a useful screening test. However, CEA levels are related to tumor size and may be very high in people with large tumors or tumors that have metastasized. The level of CEA falls after the tumor has been removed and often rises again if the tumor recurs or metastasizes (**FIGURE 7-18**). If CEA falls after removal of the tumor and later becomes elevated, this usually means the tumor has recurred and additional treatment is needed.

Other products secreted by tumor cells that can be used to monitor tumor growth are discussed in the discussion on the male reproductive system. They include **alpha fetoprotein (AFP)**, a protein produced by fetal tissues but not normally produced by adult cells, and **human chorionic gonadotropin (HCG)**, the hormone normally produced by the placenta in pregnancy, which are often elevated in patients with testicular carcinoma and in females with certain gynecologic tumors. Alpha fetoprotein is

Intraoperative During surgery.

Frozen section A method of rapid diagnosis of tumors used by the pathologist; tissue is frozen solid, cut into thin sections, stained, and examined microscopically.

Tumor-associated antigen An antigen associated with growing tumor cells that serves as an indicator of tumor growth in the body.

Carcinoembryonic antigen (CEA) A tumor-associated antigen that resembles the antigen secreted by the cells of the fetal gastrointestinal tract.

Alpha fetoprotein (AFP) Protein produced by fetal liver early in gestation. Sometimes produced by tumor cells. Level is elevated in amnionic fluid when fetus has a neural tube defect.

Human chorionic gonadotropin (HCG) A hormone made by the placenta in pregnancy that acts in a way similar to pituitary gonadotropins. Same hormone is made by neoplastic cells in some types of malignant testicular tumors.

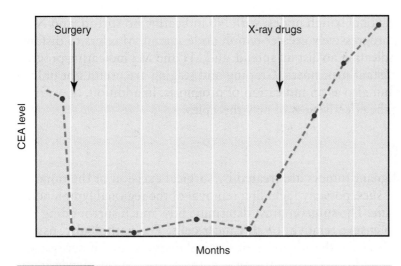

FIGURE 7-18 The use of CEA to monitor response to therapy. An elevated CEA level falls after resection of colon cancer and then rises when tumor recurs, indicating the need for additional treatment.

frequently elevated in patients with primary carcinoma of the liver. Prostatic-specific antigen (PSA), produced by prostatic epithelial cells, often is elevated in the bloodstream of men with prostatic carcinoma. The PSA test is used to detect early prostate carcinoma before symptoms develop and to monitor the response to treatment. Many other tumor-associated substances have been described, which are used to monitor patients with various types of lung, breast, and ovarian carcinoma.

Treatment of Tumors

Benign tumors may be completely cured by surgical excision. Malignant tumors are much more difficult to treat. Four major forms of treatment directed against malignant tumors are surgery, radiotherapy, hormone treatment, and chemotherapy.

The method of treatment depends on the type of tumor and its extent, and sometimes several methods are combined. In many cases, treatment eradicates the cancer, and the patient is cured. In less favorable cases, cure is no longer possible but the growth of the cancer is arrested and life is prolonged. Before a course of treatment is selected, further information obtained by grading and staging the tumor is needed.

GRADING AND STAGING MALIGNANT TUMORS

After a biopsy has established the diagnosis of a malignant tumor, selection of the appropriate treatment is based on the characteristics of the tumor cells and the extent of the tumor. Grading the tumor is used to predict the behavior of the tumor from the biopsy material based on the differentiation of the tumor cells, their growth rate based on the number of mitoses, and any characteristics of the tumor cells that would influence the type of treatment selected, such as the response of the tumor cells to estrogen in the case of a breast carcinoma (as described in the discussion on the breast). Staging the tumor determines whether the tumor is still localized or has spread to regional lymph nodes or distant sites, which is useful additional information to guide selection of the best treatment. The various characteristics of a tumor identified by grading and staging often are expressed in a classification called the TNM system. The *T* refers to the size of the primary tumor with T0 indicating an in situ lesion, and T1 through T4 indicating increasing size. *N* refers to the spread of tumor to regional lymph nodes, with N0 indicating no spread, and N1 through N3 indicating progressively greater lymph node spread. *M* refers to distant metastasis, with M0 indicating no distant spread, and M1 and M2 indicating progressively more extensive distant metastases. Grading and staging are useful not only for selecting treatment but also as an indication of prognosis. In addition, they are important in evaluating the effectiveness of new therapies.

SURGERY

Many malignant tumors are treated by surgical excision of the tumor and the surrounding tissues, possibly including removal of the regional lymph nodes that drain the tumor site. The surgeon must determine how much surrounding tissue must be removed to ensure removal of all cancer cells. The pathologist, using frozen sections, will check for the adequacy of **surgical margins**, and, if necessary, the surgeon may remove additional tissue from the surgical area. Surgical excision is successful if the tumor has not already spread to distant sites. Unfortunately, many cancers have metastasized when first detected and may no longer be curable by surgery alone. Other methods of treatment must be used frequently in combination with surgery.

RADIOTHERAPY

Malignant lymphomas and some other tumors are quite radiosensitive and can be destroyed by radiotherapy alone or in combination with surgical excision. In some cases, antibodies can be used to deliver radiotherapy to the tumor cells. For example, radiation may be administered preoperatively to reduce the size of a tumor, thereby facilitating its surgical resection. In other instances, radiotherapy is given after a malignant tumor has been resected (cut out) to destroy any cancer cells that may have been left behind. Radiotherapy is also used to control the growth of widespread tumors and to treat deposits of metastatic tumor that cause pain and disability. The treatment relieves symptoms and makes the patient more comfortable, even though the cancer is not curable. Radiotherapy may be delivered from an external source (x-rays being a common example) or by implanting radioactive "seeds" or pellets at the site of the tumor, a technique used in treating prostate cancer.

HORMONE THERAPY

Some malignant tumors require hormones for their growth and are called hormone responsive; these tumors regress temporarily if deprived of the required hormone. For example, many prostate tumors require testosterone and are inhibited by removal of the testes (eliminating the source of testosterone) or by administration of drugs that suppresses testosterone secretion. Many breast carcinomas in postmenopausal women are estrogen responsive and can be controlled by drugs that block estrogen so that the tumor cells are no longer stimulated by estrogen.

Adrenal cortical hormones (corticosteroids) also inhibit the growth of many malignant tumors. Corticosteroids inhibit protein synthesis, thereby suppressing the growth and division of the tumor cells. Tumors of the lymphatic tissues are especially susceptible to the effects of corticosteroids.

ANTICANCER DRUGS

Chemotherapy of cancer is an extraordinarily complex and rapidly changing area. At a basic level, the chemotherapeutic agent most useful in cancer therapy interferes with some metabolic pathway in a cancer cell without causing unacceptable damage in normal cells. Broadly speaking, such drugs are selectively **cytotoxic** (causing cell death) to cancer cells as opposed to other cells in the body. **Antimetabolites** are drugs that interfere with some well-defined metabolic target within the cell, and the cause of their cytotoxicity is usually well known. Surprisingly, the reason a particular antimetabolite is specific for cancer cells is often unclear because the target metabolic pathway is present in both normal and cancer cells. A goal of those designing chemotherapeutics is to produce agents that have near absolute specificity for a the mutated protein involved in cancer production. If a drug specific for the mutated product responsible for malignant transformation of a cell can be found, that drug would be specific for treating the cancer, with no side effects (or much reduced side effects) on normal cells. Such agents are now available for some cancers and are used in the clinic.

The various drugs differ in their mechanisms of action. Some inhibit the synthesis of either DNA or RNA. Others alter the structure of DNA or disturb its function. Still others inhibit protein synthesis or prevent the mitotic spindle from forming so the cell cannot divide. Frequently, several different anticancer drugs are administered simultaneously, each drug blocking a different phase in the cell's metabolic processes. Another group of anticancer drugs act by suppressing the proliferation of the blood vessels that nourish the tumor, thereby inhibiting tumor growth by interfering with its blood supply.

Most anticancer drugs work best against fast-growing tumors that contain large numbers of actively growing and dividing cells. They are usually less effective against slowly growing tumors because only relatively small numbers of the tumor cells are in the stages of cell growth or division susceptible to the injurious effects of the drugs. However, even within a rapidly growing tumor, many cells have a very low rate of division. Although rate of cell division may play a role in the selectivity of anticancer drugs, this cannot be the only answer.

One important group of anticancer drugs is **alkylating agents**. These drugs interact with both strands of the paired DNA chains in the nucleus and bind them together so they cannot separate. This reaction is called cross linking of the DNA chains. It disrupts the function of DNA because the chains must separate for duplication of the DNA chains and for synthesis of RNA. Alkylating agents also disturb cell function by altering the structure of the DNA chains. In contrast to most anticancer drugs, these agents are effective against nondividing ("resting") cells as well as actively growing cells. Similarly, some drugs chemically alter one of the DNA bases (often guanine) within the DNA strands. These changes are not removed by the DNA repair process and can lead to apoptotic cell death. For this reason, inactivation of the tumor suppressor *Tp53* interfering with the death of mutated cells can lead to resistance to such agents.

Although they have some degree of selectivity for cancer cells, most anticancer drugs are quite toxic to normal cells as well. Therefore, they must be administered very carefully to ensure maximum damage to tumor cells without irreparable injury to normal cells. Lymphoid tissue is quite susceptible to the destructive effects of these potent drugs; consequently, one unavoidable side effect of anticancer drugs is impairment of cell-mediated and humoral immunity.

Recently, several less toxic and more cell-specific anticancer drugs have been developed that function by blocking the action of specific cell components that stimulate the tumor cells. Some of these drugs suppress tumor growth by blocking growth factor receptors on the surface of the tumor cells so that growth factors produced by normal cells cannot attach to the receptors and stimulate the tumor cells. For example, antibodies directed against HER2, which is overexpressed on the surface

Cytotoxic Causing cell death.

Antimetabolite A substance that competes with or replaces another substance (metabolite) required for cell.

Alkylating agent An anticancer drug that disrupts cell function by binding DNA chains together so they cannot separate.

of some breast cancer cells, is an effective therapy for HER2 positive breast cancer. Other drugs inhibit the functions of important intracellular proteins, such as the tyrosine kinases that act as oncoproteins (active oncogene products) in some cancers.

No matter how effective the drug, cancer cells ultimately develop resistance to chemotherapeutic drugs. This is related to the large number of cancer cells and their ability to mutate. If, by chance, a single cell in a tumor mutates and develops resistance to a drug, the cell and all its progeny will be at a growth advantage and ultimately lead to resistance. One way around this is to use multidrug therapies; it is unlikely that a single cancer cell will simultaneously become resistant to several agents. Another is to design additional drugs capable of acting against the mutant cells.

Early detection of localized cancers certainly can result in cures, but this is unlikely in most cases of widespread cancer. Although life span can be prolonged, ultimately the cancer becomes resistant and leads to death.

ADJUVANT CHEMOTHERAPY

Sometimes surgical resection of a cancer appears to be successful, but metastases appear several years later and eventually prove fatal. The operation fails to eradicate the tumor because small, unrecognized metastases have already spread throughout the body. Even though the main tumor has been removed, the minute metastases continue to grow until eventually they form many large, bulky deposits of metastatic tumor that kill the patient.

To forestall the development of late metastases, a current trend is to administer a course of anticancer drugs either immediately before or after surgical resection of some tumors. This is called **adjuvant chemotherapy** (*adjuvare* = to assist). The drugs destroy any small, undetected foci of metastatic tumor before they become large enough to produce clinical manifestations. In many cases, adjuvant chemotherapy combined with surgery appears to achieve better results than surgery alone (as discussed in the section on breast cancer). Anticancer drugs are quite toxic, and the potential benefits of adjuvant chemotherapy must be weighed against the harmful effects of the drugs on normal tissues.

IMMUNOTHERAPY

The immune system has evolved a number of ways to deal with abnormal cells that can proliferate and form tumors and to deal with established tumors. Cytotoxic T cells recognize antigens on tumor cells that are displayed along with the cells' own MHC class I proteins and can damage the tumor cells by secreting destructive lymphokines. Natural killer lymphocytes can attack and destroy tumor cells without prior antigenic stimulation, and some killer lymphocytes specialize in attacking antibody-coated tumor cells. Activated macrophages can destroy tumor cells by phagocytosis and by secreting tumor necrosis factor along with other cytokines that stimulate lymphocytes to attack tumor cells. Antibodies formed against tumor cell antigens can attach to tumor cells and activate complement; products of complement activation attract lymphocytes and macrophages and form destructive attack complexes that damage the cell membranes of the tumor cells.

Despite this array of immunologic defenses, many tumors circumvent or overwhelm the body's immune defenses, which then become ineffective and no longer retard the growth of the tumor. Treatment of tumors by stimulating the body's

Adjuvant chemotherapy Anticancer chemotherapy administered before or after surgical resection of a tumor in an attempt to destroy any small, undetected foci of metastatic tumor before they become clinically detectable.

immune defenses is called **immunotherapy.** Nonspecific immunotherapy is directed toward bolstering the patient's own immune defenses to help the patient deal more effectively with the tumor. Specific immunotherapy directs the immune system against the specific antigens present in the patient's own tumor.

Nonspecific Immunotherapy

Recent approaches for immunotherapy administer various cytokines that either stimulate cells of the immune system or act against the tumor cells. The two cytokines that have been used with greatest success against tumors are **interferon alpha** and **interleukin-2.**

In general, interferon consists of a group of carbohydrate-containing, "broad-spectrum" antiviral protein substances produced by cells in response to viral infection. Interferon also regulates the functions of the immune system and regulates cell growth, inhibiting the growth of rapidly dividing cells. Interferon has proved useful in treating some types of leukemia, multiple myeloma (a leukemia-like disease), malignant melanoma, and kidney cancer. Interferon is much less toxic than many anticancer drugs, and treatment by subcutaneous injection several times per week is usually well tolerated although flulike symptoms and disorders in the production of red cells and platelets are common.

Interleukin-2, a lymphokine produced by T cells, stimulates natural killer cells and cytotoxic T cells that can destroy tumor cells, but it has no direct effects against the tumor cells. Interleukin-2 administered in multiple courses has produced beneficial effects in the treatment of metastatic melanoma and renal cell carcinoma. High doses of interleukin-2 produce a variety of serious toxic effects that limit its use.

Specific Immunotherapy

Specific immunotherapy targets the patient's own tumor cells for attack. Four different approaches appear promising: (1) administration of cytotoxic T lymphocytes directed against the tumor, which are called tumor-infiltrating lymphocytes; (2) administration of tumor vaccines; (3) administration of antitumor antibodies; and (4) "blockading" (inhibiting) immune checkpoints, which inhibit the role of the immune system in destroying tumor cells.

Adoptive T-cell transfer therapy uses cytotoxic T cells isolated from within a patient's tumor. The cells are grown in the laboratory using a variety of cytokines, including interleukin-2. The expanded cytotoic T cells are then reinfused into the patient. The cells may also be genetically modified before reinfusion to allow them to specifically attach to a cell surface component of the tumor. Although initially used to treat malignant melanoma, the technique shows promise for use in treating a number of tumors.

Tumor vaccines prepared from the patient's own tumor also have been used to immunize the patient against the tumor in an effort to reduce the likelihood that the tumor will recur or metastasize after it has been resected. Tumor cells are obtained from the resected tumor, grown in the laboratory, and then killed so they cannot proliferate in the patient but can still generate an immune response. They are then used to prepare a vaccine that will stimulate an immune response to the resected tumor. Tumor vaccines have been used as an additional treatment after resection of a malignant melanoma or a colon carcinoma when the patient is considered at high risk of recurrence.

Immunotherapy
Treatment given to retard growth of a disseminated malignant tumor by stimulating the body's own immune defenses.

Interferon alpha A broad-spectrum antiviral agent manufactured by various cells in the body.

Interleukin-2 (IL-2) A lymphokine that stimulates growth of lymphocytes.

For *tumor antibody therapy*, antibodies are prepared against tumor cell antigens, and then linked to an antitumor drug or toxin that can kill tumor cells. The antibodies with attached drug or toxin are then infused back into the patient to seek out and destroy the tumor cells without damaging normal cells.

Immune checkpoint blockades prevent tumors from shutting down the immune response by inappropriately activating physiological pathways that regulate and control the immune response. Blockading immunosuppressive receptors with monoclonal antibodies "reactivates" the patient's immune system and has had impressive success in treating tumors with vaccines directed against specific tumor antigens.

Although the results of immunotherapy have been mixed to date, the combination of immune checkpoint blockade with additional modes of therapy is promising. There have been some notable successes, as in the use of interferon therapy for one type of leukemia called hairy cell leukemia, or in cases involving specific types of widespread tumors when no other methods of treatment are available to control the tumor. No single method works against all types of tumors. Unfortunately, most patients treated with immunotherapy have advanced diseases, and often the body's immune defenses are incapable of dealing with such large amounts of tumor even when stimulated by immunotherapy.

Survival Rates in Neoplastic Disease

Malignant neoplasms are a leading cause of disability and death. Cancer is second only to heart disease as a cause of death in the United States, accounting for about 25 percent of all deaths in this country. Although prostate carcinoma is the most common malignant tumor in men, and breast carcinoma is the most frequent in women, lung cancer is responsible for the greatest number of cancer deaths in both sexes. Carcinoma of the intestine is quite common in both sexes. The survival rate for patients with malignant tumors depends on whether the disease has been diagnosed and treated early, before it has spread. The chances for survival are significantly reduced if the tumor has metastasized to regional lymph nodes or to distant sites.

The curability of the various types of cancer can be assessed in terms of five-year survival rates, which range from more than 98 percent for patients with thyroid cancer to a discouraging 7 percent for those with pancreatic carcinoma (**TABLE 7-6**). Attempts are being made to improve survival rates by means of earlier diagnosis and more effective therapy. Unfortunately, five-year survival does not necessarily indicate that the patient is cured. Some types of malignant tumors may recur and prove fatal many years after initial treatment. Breast carcinoma and malignant melanomas are two tumors prone to late recurrence. For all stages of breast carcinoma combined, the overall five-year survival rate is approximately 89 percent. The ten-year rate is 83 percent, and the fifteen-year survival rate is 78 percent due to late recurrences and metastases. In cases of late disease, the existing metastatic deposits may have been held in check by the body's immune defense mechanisms, which have now failed. The five-year survival rate is highly dependent on the stage of disease. Localized breast cancer has a five-year survival rate of 99 percent, but the rate falls to 25 percent for individuals with metastatic disease.

TABLE 7-6   Five-Year Relative Survival Rates* (%) by Stage at Diagnosis, US, 2004–2010

	All stages	Local	Regional	Distant
Breast (female)	89	99	85	25
Colon & rectum	65	90	71	13
Esophagus	18	40	21	4
Kidney[†]	72	92	65	12
Larynx	60	75	43	35
Liver[‡]	17	30	11	3
Lung & bronchus	17	54	27	4
Melanoma of the skin	91	98	63	16
Oral cavity & pharynx	63	83	61	37
Ovary	45	92	72	27
Pancreas	7	26	10	2
Prostate	99	>99	>99	28
Stomach	28	64	29	4
Testis	95	99	96	73
Thyroid	98	>99	98	55
Uninary bladder[§]	77	69	34	6
Uterine cervix	68	91	57	16
Uterine corpus	82	95	68	18

*Rates are adjusted for normal life expectancy and are based on cases diagnosed in the SEER 18 areas from 2004–2010, all followed through 2011. [†]Includes renal pelvis. [‡]Includes intrahepatic bile duct. [§]Rate for in situ cases is 96%.

Local: an invasive malignant cancer confined entirely to the organ of origin. **Regional:** a malignant cancer that 1) has extended beyond the limits of the organ of origin directly into surrounding organs or tissues; 2) involves regional lymph nodes; or 3) has both regional extension and involvement of regional lymph nodes. **Distant:** amalignant cancer that has spread to parts of the body remote from the primary tumor either by direct extension or by discontinuous metastasis to distant organs, tissues, or via the lymphatic system to distance lymph nodes.

Cases diagnosed 1975–2011. Survival for all ages based on stage. Average survival for both sexes used when neoplasm occurs in both sexes. Data from Howlander, N., Noone, A. M., and Krapo, M. Eds. *SEER Cancer Statistics Review 1975–2011.*

Data from Howlander N, Noone AM, Krapo M, et al. SEER Cancer statistics Review, 1975–2011.

CASE 7-1

John is a seventy-year-old who has not been seen by his primary care physician for several years. He has noticed increasing fatigue and weight loss of about 10 pounds in the last two months. He is concerned that he may have seen signs of rectal bleeding in the past year (but attributed them to hemorrhoids). The physician orders a stool blood test, which is positive and detects iron deficiency anemia. John also has a moderate elevation in blood CEA levels. The physician notes that John has not had any of the recommended screening procedures for the detection of colorectal cancer such as colonoscopy or flexible sigmoidoscopy and is

(continues)

CASE 7-1 *(Continued)*

concerned about the possibility of such. John is unaware of any history of colorectal cancer in his large number of relatives. The patient is scheduled for colonoscopy, to which he objects, but the physician notes that other diagnostic procedures such as a double contrast barium enema or CT-based colonography also require preliminary bowel preparation and are likely to require subsequent colonoscopy either for definitive diagnosis or therapy. John undergoes successful colonoscopy during which several small polyps are found in the descending colon and removed. However, the endoscopist is unable to fully examine the colon because the lumen of the colon is stenosed (constricted) in the ascending portion, preventing further passage of the scope. The stenosed area appears to be associated with a large tumor that cannot be removed using the endoscope. The endoscopist tattoos the area with ink to note the area of concern and refers the patient for surgery. The surgeon notes a suspicious lesion of the right (ascending colon) and performs a right hemicolectomy, removing the lesion and the right colon, reattaching the small intestine to the transverse colon to preserve bowel function. During surgery, the surgeon also removes adjacent lymph nodes for analysis. The surgical specimen and nodes are sent to pathology for evaluation (**FIGURE 7-19**). Microscopic analysis indicates the lesion to be an adenocarcinoma that has infiltrated through almost the entire colon (**FIGURE 7-20**). No tumor is detected in lymph nodes. John is given a course of adjuvant chemotherapy with a cytotoxic agent. The patient remains healthy. His CEA level fell to normal and has shown no elevation in the five years since surgery.

Discussion

John is lucky. The only potential cure for colon cancer is surgical removal of the lesion. TMN analysis of his lesion would be T3; cancer has grown through the muscular layers but has not penetrated beyond the outer layer, or serosa, of the colon. N0 (no cancer in adjacent nodes), and M0 (no distant spread). T3N0 disease has almost an 80 percent five-year relapse-free survival rate. Adjuvant chemotherapy is not always used with John's stage of disease but is likely to improve relapse-free survival. However, there is a moral to this case. It is extremely likely that John would never have had colon cancer had he followed routine cancer screening guidelines. Colon cancer peaks in both sexes at about age sixty-five. Hence, screening for polyps in the colon and rectum should start at age fifty (in the absence of other risk factors such as a strong family history or a defined hereditary disease). Because most colon cancer starts as a detectable precancerous lesion, removal of these lesions (colon and rectal adenomatous polyps) via endoscopy prevents colon cancer from occurring. Even removal of lesions showing marked dysplasia or localized cancer is likely to be curative.

Because colon cancer progresses slowly, screening tests need not be undertaken frequently if no suspicious lesions are found. Colonoscopy at ten-year intervals allows examination of the entire colon and cecum and is considered to be the most sensitive screening test. It also allows for therapeutic removal of lesions. Alternatively, flexible proctosigmoidoscopy every five years is recommended. This procedure (unlike colonoscopy) generally does not require anesthesia and is often done by a trained physician rather than a gastroenterologist. It is less costly than colonoscopy and requires less patient preparation (generally two disposable enemas as opposed to the thorough bowel cleaning needed for colonoscopy). However, proctosigmoidoscopy (as the name implies) can examine only the descending colon. Detection of multiple polyps in this region suggests the presence of additional undetected polyps in the transverse or ascending colon, necessitating colonoscopy. Several other techniques are available for use in special cases (CT-based colonography, double contrast barium enema, and, recently, examination of the colon by orally ingested camera-containing capsules). None of these techniques allow for removal of lesions, and suspicious findings require follow-up colonoscopy. Annual fecal blood testing and tests that detect DNA mutations in the stool that derive from colonic cells may also be of value.

CASE 7-1 *(Continued)*

Etiology and Pathogenesis

Colonic adenocarcinoma T3N0 treated by surgery and adjuvant chemotherapy with no signs of recurrence five years postoperation.

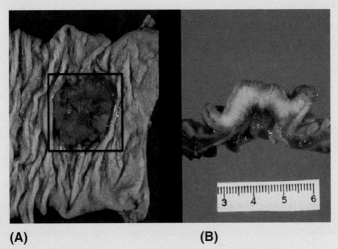

(A)   **(B)**

FIGURE 7-19 **(A)** Opened loop of the colon removed at colectomy showing lesion (*boxed*). **(B)** Cross section of lesion seen on edge. White-tan tumor infiltrates into the bowel wall.

Courtesy of Department of Pathology and Laboratory Medicine, University of North Carolina at Chapel Hill.

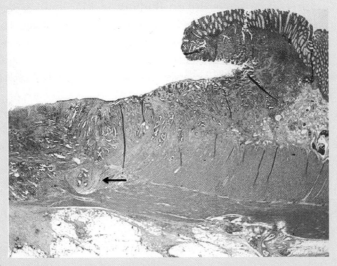

FIGURE 7-20 Microscopic examination of lesion in Figure 7-19 showing adenocarcinoma infiltrating into the muscular wall (muscularis) (*arrow*).

Courtesy of Department of Pathology and Laboratory Medicine, University of North Carolina at Chapel Hill.

Questions

1. There is dispute over the cost effectiveness of colonoscopy versus proctosigmoidoscopy. What factors should be taken into account in establishing the procedure that should be recommended?

2. Stool-based DNA testing has been licensed for use in the detection of colon cancer. What potential advantages and disadvantages does such a test have?

3. There is some controversy about the use of adjuvant chemotherapy in this patient's disease. What factors might argue for and against its use?

QUESTIONS FOR REVIEW

1. What are the major differences between a benign and a malignant tumor?

2. How are tumors named? What are the common prefixes used in naming tumors?

3. What are proto-oncogenes, tumor suppressor genes, DNA repair genes, and genes regulating apoptosis? What is their role in the development of neoplasms?

4. What is the role of viruses in causing cancer?

5. How does the body defend itself against abnormal cells that arise spontaneously in the course of cell division? What is the consequence of failure of these defense mechanisms?

6. What is a lymphoma? What is the difference between a nevus and a melanoma? What is a teratoma?

7. What is the significance of a Pap smear containing atypical cells?

8. What is a frozen section? How is it used in the diagnosis of tumors?

SUPPLEMENTARY READINGS

Rubin, E., and Reisner, H. M. 2014. *Essentials of Rubin's Pathology*. 6th ed. Baltimore, MD: Wolters Kluwer/ Lippincott Williams & Wilkins.

Weinberg, R. A. 2014. *The Biology of Cancer*. 2nd ed. New York, NY: Garland Science/Taylor and Francis Group.

Hartl, D. L. 2011. *Essential Genetics. A Genomics Perspective*. 5th ed. Burlington, MA: Jones & Bartlett Learning.

▶ The area of neoplastic disease is so broad and intensely studied that the interested individual would be wise to read an overview prior to undertaking detailed reading. The first entry presents an up-to-date pathologist's view of cancer and its diagnosis in Chapter 5, Neoplasia. The second entry provides a detailed text on all aspects of neoplastc disease; strong on experimental concepts. The third entry contains a very readable overview of cancer genetics and cell cycle control in Chapter 13, Molecular Genetics of the Cell Cycle and Cancer.

Bordon, Y. 2015. Checkpoint parley. *Nature Reviews Cancer/Research Highlight 15*:3.

Gubin, M. M., Zhang, X., Schuster, H., et al. 2014. Checkpoint blockade cancer immunotherapy targets tumour-specific mutant antigens. *Nature 515*(7528):577–81.

Leavy, O. In press. A triple blow for cancer. *Natures Review Cancer*.

Bachireddy, P., Burkhardt, U. E., Rajasage, M., and Wu, C. J. 2015. Haematological malignancies: At the forefront of immunotherapeutic innovation. *Nature Reviews Cancer 15*:201–15.

▶ One of the most exciting and recent advances in cancer immunotherapy is the concept of checkpoint blockade. The approach has resulted in a major advance in concepts of cancer therapy (and some striking clinical results). The first article provides a brief overview to introduce the area. The other three present additional details of current experimental and clinical applications.

Wang, H., Zhang, X., Teng, L., and Legerski, R. J. In press. DNA damage checkpoint recovery and cancer development. *Experimental Cell Research*.

▶ A recent overview of the mechanism by which DNA damage (and its control) results in cancer development.

Franco, S. S., Raveh-Amit, H., Kobolak, J., et al. 2015. The crossroads between cancer stem cells and aging. *BMC Cancer 15*(suppl 1):51.

Takaheshi, R., Miyazaki, H., and Ochiya, T. 2014. The role of microRNAs in the regulation of cancer stem cells. *Frontiers in Genetics* vol. 4: article 29.

▶ The concept of cancer stem cells has been briefly addressed in the text and remains controversial. In addition the role of microRNA in neoplastic disease is gaining increasing attention. These articles cover current concepts of both areas and how they may intersect.

Kalia, M. 2015. Biomarkers for personalized oncology: Recent advances and future challenges. *Metabolism Clinical and Experimental 64*:516–21.

▶ Cancer biomarkers have proven of very limited utility in current practice. However, the recognition of specific molecular defects not only may serve as a biomarker for cancer but also as an important therapeutic target.

Alderton, G. K. 2015. Metastasis: Spreading the seed. *Nature Reviews Cancer 15*:255.

▶ The molecular changes associated with tumor metastasis are still poorly defined but could be important therapeutic targets. This article provides a recent overview of work in this area.

Uspeert, J. E. G., Medema, J. P., and Dekker, E. 2015. Colorectal neoplasia pathways: State of the art. *Gastrointestinal Endoscopy Clinics of North America 25*:169–82.

▶ The title says it all. A thorough overview that presents a molecular overview of the case in this chapter.

Pathogenic Microorganisms

1. Explain how bacteria are classified. List and describe the major groups of pathogenic bacteria.

2. Describe the mechanism by which antibiotics inhibit the growth and metabolism of bacteria.

3. Explain the adverse effects of antibiotics.

4. Explain the mode of action of virus infections, and describe how the body's response to viral infection leads to recovery.

5. List the common infections caused by chlamydiae, mycoplasmas, and rickettsiae.

6. Discuss the spectrum of infections caused by fungi. Explain the factors that predispose people to systemic infections. Describe the methods used to treat fungus infections.

Introduction

Of the wide spectrum of microorganisms found in nature, only a relatively small proportion cause disease in humans. These pathogenic microorganisms are classified into several large groups: bacteria, viruses, chlamydiae, rickettsiae/ehrlichiae, mycoplasmas, and fungi. In addition, humans serve as host to a number of animal parasites capable of causing illness or disability. A small number of microbiologic agents are extremely **virulent**. Such virulence is often associated with specific genes; **virulence factors** may be part of the bacterial chromosome or be inherited as a plasmid, most often a small circular DNA element in the bacterial cytoplasm that can replicate and be transmitted independently of the bacterial chromosome. Others are of very low virulence and are capable of causing disease only when the body's normal defenses have been weakened by a debilitating illness.

Virulence/virulent Ability to cause disease.

Virulence factors Elements of microbe that cause disease.

Gram stain Staining process used to identify bacteria.

Bacteria

CLASSIFICATION OF BACTERIA

Bacteria are classified on the basis of four major characteristics: shape, **Gram stain** reaction, antigenic structure, and biochemical and cultural characteristics. A bacterium

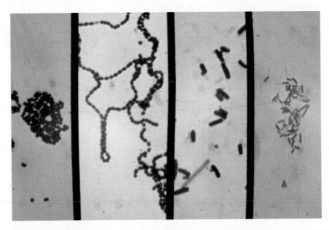

FIGURE 8-1 Appearance of bacteria as seen in Gram stains. From left to right: gram-positive cocci in clusters (staphylococci), gram-positive cocci in chains (streptococci), gram-positive bacilli, gram-negative bacilli (original magnification ×1,000).

Courtesy of Leonard V. Crowley, MD, Century College.

Coccus Spherical bacteria.

Bacillus Rod-shaped bacteria.

Porins Unique proteins on bacteria outer membrane contributing to resistance to antimicrobial agents.

Flagellum/flagella A whiplike process that propels an organism or sperm.

Aerobic organisms Microbes that grow best in the presence of oxygen.

Anaerobic organisms Microbes that grow best in the absence of oxygen.

Spores A highly resistant spherical structure produced by some bacteria to assure survival under adverse conditions.

may be spherical (**coccus**) or rod shaped (**bacillus**), or have a spiral or corkscrew shape. Cocci may grow in clusters (staphylococci), in pairs (diplococci), or in chains (streptococci). Gram staining is an identification technique using two different dyes. A dried, fixed suspension of bacteria, prepared on a microscope slide, is stained first with a purple dye (hematoxylin) and then with an iodine solution. Next, the slide is decolorized with alcohol or another solvent and is then stained with a red dye (eosin). Bacteria that resist decolorization and retain the purple stain are called gram-positive, whereas those that have been decolorized and accept the red counterstain are termed gram-negative (**FIGURE 8-1**). The Gram stain reaction is based on differences in the structure of the bacterial cell wall between the two classes of bacteria, which affect certain significant biochemical properties of the bacteria such as susceptibility to host defense mechanisms and particular antibiotics (**FIGURE 8-2**).

Each type of bacterium contains a large number of antigens associated with the cell body, the capsule of the bacterium, and the **flagella** (in the case of motile organisms). The antigenic structure can be determined by special methods, defining a system of antigens unique for each group of bacteria.

Some bacteria are quite fastidious and can be grown only on enriched media under carefully controlled conditions of temperature and acidity (pH). Other bacteria are hardy and capable of growing on relatively simple culture media under a wide variety of conditions. Many bacteria grow best in the presence of oxygen (**aerobic organisms**). Some bacteria are able to grow only in the absence of oxygen or under extremely low oxygen tension. These are called **anaerobic bacteria** (without oxygen). Others grow equally well under either aerobic or anaerobic conditions.

Many bacteria have special structural characteristics. Some bacteria have flagella: hairlike processes covering their surface. Flagella give a bacterium its motility; organisms that lack flagella are nonmotile. Some bacteria form **spores**, spherical structures found within the bacterial cell that can survive under conditions (e.g., elevated temperature and desiccation) that would kill an actively growing bacterium. Spores may be considered as a dormant, extremely resistant bacterial modification that forms under adverse conditions. Spores can germinate and give rise to actively growing bacteria under favorable conditions.

Most bacteria have distinct biochemical characteristics. Some types of bacteria are capable of fermenting carbohydrates and can promote many different biochemical reactions under suitable cultural conditions. Each type of bacterium has its own

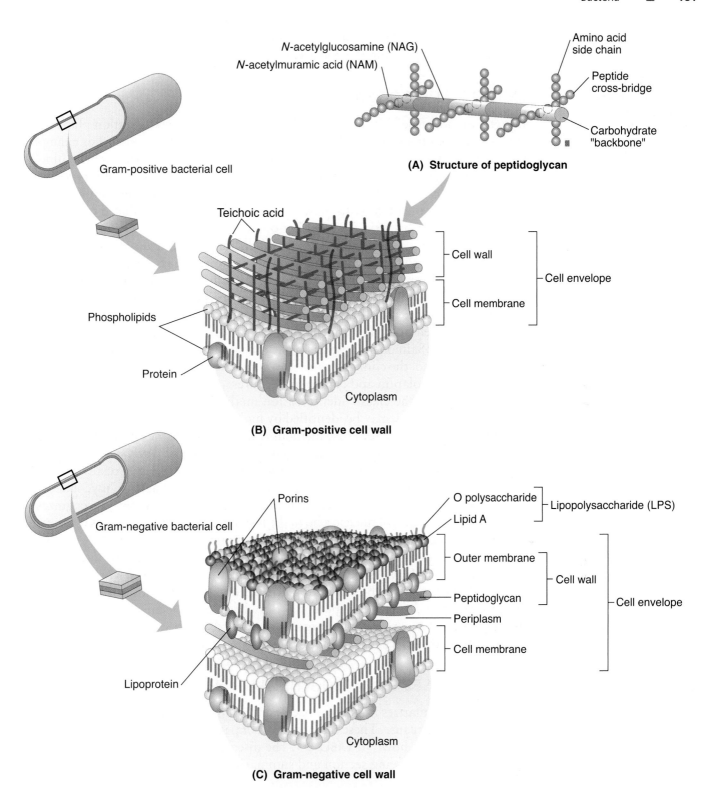

N-acetylglucosamine (NAG)
N-acetylmuramic acid (NAM)

Amino acid side chain
Peptide cross-bridge
Carbohydrate "backbone"

(A) Structure of peptidoglycan

Gram-positive bacterial cell

Teichoic acid

Cell wall
Cell membrane
Cell envelope

Phospholipids

Protein

Cytoplasm

(B) Gram-positive cell wall

Porins

O polysaccharide
Lipid A
Lipopolysaccharide (LPS)

Gram-negative bacterial cell

Outer membrane
Cell wall
Peptidoglycan
Periplasm
Cell envelope
Cell membrane

Lipoprotein

Cytoplasm

(C) Gram-negative cell wall

FIGURE 8-2 A comparison of cell walls of Gram-positive and Gram-negative bacterial cells. **(A)** The structure of peptidoglycan of the cell wall is shown as units of NAG and NAM joined laterally and vertically by amino acids. **(B)** The cell wall of a gram-positive bacteria is composed of multiple peptidoglycan layers combined with teichoic acid (a bacterial polysaccharide). **(C)** In the gram-negative cell wall, the peptidoglycan layer is much thinner and lacks teichoic acid. In addition, the cell wall has both an outer and inner cell membrane. Gram-negative bacteria are also unique in having lipid A (a lipopolysaccharide important in bacterial virulence) and unique proteins called porins in the outer membrane that contribute to the resistance of this class of bacteria to certain antimicrobial agents.

Media Special food for bacteria.

Genetic probes Preparations of nucleic acid devised to identify specific sequences in bacteria.

Blood agar plates Bacteria media incorporating red blood cells.

Hemolysis Destruction of blood cells around bacterial colonies.

"biochemical profile," which aids in its identification. This biochemical profile can be determined by growing the bacteria on different **media**.

IDENTIFICATION OF BACTERIA

Bacteria are identified by algorithms that use microscopic visualization plus different test methods to determine the previously discussed characteristics. For example, an organism has been isolated from the blood of a patient with a febrile illness. The organism is a gram-negative bacillus that is not fastidious and not anaerobic. The organism is motile but does not form spores. At this point, the number of possible organisms consistent with these characteristics has been reduced to relatively few gram-negative bacteria. The number of possibilities is narrowed still further by testing with various biochemical tests that indicate the bacterium does not ferment lactose but is able to ferment glucose and certain other sugars. These and other biochemical and immunological tests support the conclusion that the organism is a type of pathogenic bacterium called Salmonella, which is found in the gastrointestinal tract and is capable of causing a typhoid-like febrile illness. The bacterial antigens present on the cell body and flagella of the bacteria can be identified to determine the exact type of Salmonella responsible for the patient's illness. Once the organism has been identified, the clinician can select appropriate antibiotics and, if necessary, institute proper isolation and control procedures.

In addition to the classic identification methods of culture and visualization, microorganisms today may be identified by molecular methods that detect the presence of specific nucleic acid. These methods can demonstrate the organisms in patient specimens as well as identify isolated organisms. This is particularly useful for microorganisms such as mycobacteria that are difficult to culture. Commercially available **genetic probes** can detect specific nucleic acid sequences in bacteria, mycobacteria, and fungi. Methods used are direct hybridization, in which the probe recognizes a complementary strand of nucleic acid in the test material, or various types of amplification assays (making additional copies of the test nucleic acid) such as PCR, followed by a detection method. Molecular-based quantitative assays are also available for pathogens such as HIV. These tests can determine the level of HIV RNA in patients with HIV infection, which is used to guide the highly active antiretroviral therapy used to treat the disease. One potential drawback of molecular methods are that they detect dead as well as living organisms. Hence, this test may be inappropriate for measuring the effects of antibiotic therapy on bacteria.

MAJOR CLASSES OF PATHOGENIC BACTERIA

This section summarizes important bacteria that infect humans along with the principal diseases they cause. These major groups of pathogenic bacteria and their Gram stain reactions are shown in **TABLE 8-1**. The diseases caused by these organisms are described in the following section and summarized in **TABLE 8-2**.

Staphylococci

Staphylococci, normal inhabitants of the skin and nasal cavity, are generally not pathogenic. Some staphylococci are pathogens and may be extremely virulent. Pathogens usually can be distinguished from nonpathogenic staphylococci by the appearance of their colonies on media containing blood (**blood agar plates**). Pathogenic staphylococci produce zones of complete **hemolysis** around the growing colonies (**FIGURE 8-3**) in contrast to nonpathogenic staphylococci, which do not hemolyze red cells.

TABLE 8-1   Important Pathogenic Bacteria

Type	Gram-stain reaction	
	Gram-positive	Gram-negative
Cocci	Staphylococci	Gonococci
	Streptococci	Meningococci
	Pneumococci	
Bacilli	*Corynebacteria*	*Haemophilus*
	Listeria	*Gardnerella*
	Bacilli	*Francisella*
	Clostridia	*Yersinia*
		Brucella
		Legionella
		Salmonella
		Shigella
		Campylobacter
		Cholera bacillus
		Colon bacillus (*Escherichia coli*) and related organisms
Spiral organisms	*Treponema pallidum*	
	Borrelia burgdorferi	
Acid-fast organisms	Tubercle bacillus	
	Leprosy bacillus	

Pathogenic staphylococci are a common cause of boils, other skin infections, and postoperative wound infections. Occasionally, staphylococci cause serious pulmonary infections and other types of systemic infections. Staphylococci infections are difficult to manage in hospitals where patients have had recent surgical operations or have various chronic diseases associated with impairment of the body's normal defenses against bacterial infection. Some strains of staphylococci are highly resistant to antibiotics, and infections caused by antibiotic-resistant staphylococci are extremely difficult to treat.

Streptococci

Streptococci are classified on the basis of their serologic group designated by a capital letter, and on the type of hemolysis the organism produces when grown on a solid medium containing blood. Generally, both the letter group and the type of hemolysis are specified when describing a streptococcus.

The serologic classification, called the Lancefield system, divides the streptococci into twenty major groups based on differences in the carbohydrate antigens present in their cell walls. These groups are designated A through H and K through V, with most of the streptococci of medical importance in groups A, B, and D. The classification based on hemolysis describes the organisms as producing either

TABLE 8-2 Summary of Major Bacterial Pathogens and the Diseases They Cause

Cocci	Disease
Staphylococcus aureus	Various localized and systemic infections.
Beta hemolytic streptococcus, Group A	Pharyngitis, systemic infections, skin and muscle necrosis. Hypersensitivity response to organism causes rheumatic fever, nephritis.
Beta hemolytic streptococcus, Group B	Urinary tract and wound infections, systemic infection. Newborn infection acquired from vaginal organisms in mother.
Streptococci, other groups	Wound and urinary tract infections.
Streptococcus pneumoniae (Pneumococcus)	Middle ear and sinus infections. Systemic infection. Lobar pneumonia. Meningitis.
Neisseria gonorrhoeae (Gonococcus)	Genital tract infections. Bacteremia causing endocarditis, osteomyelitis, septic arthritis.
Neisseria meningiditis (Meningococcus)	Meningococcal meningitis.
Aerobic gram-positive rods	
Corynebacterium diphtheriae	Diphtheria. Clinical manifestations caused by toxin production.
Listeria monocytogenes	Systemic infection. Pregnant women may infect fetus. Persons with impaired immune system are very susceptible.
Aerobic spore-forming rods	
Bacillus anthracis	Primarily a disease of animals. People infected from contact with wool or animal products. Localized and systemic infection. Potential germ warfare agent.
Anaerobic spore-forming rods	
Clostridium perfringens	Gas gangrene. Muscle necrosis and hemolytic anemia caused by toxin. Gas formation in infected tissues.
Clostridium tetani	Tetanus (lockjaw) caused by toxin-induced spasm of voluntary muscles.
Clostridium botulinum	Botulism. Neuroparalytic toxin produced in improperly processed or canned foods.
Clostridium difficile	Antibiotic-associated colitis. Loss of normal intestinal flora caused by antibiotics allows overgrowth of *Clostridia*. Toxin produced by *Clostridia* damage bowel mucosa.
Gram-negative rods	
Haemophilus influenzae	Pulmonary infections. Meningitis in susceptible children.
Yersinia pestis	Plague. Disease of wild rodents transmitted to humans by fleas. Causes systemic infection. Can spread person-to-person if infection spreads to lungs (pneumonic plague).
Brucella species	Brucellosis. Febrile illness from contact with infected animals or consumption of raw milk from infected animals.
Francisella species	Tularemia. Febrile illness acquired from flesh of infected animals, usually wild rabbits, or transmitted to humans by bite of infected ticks or deer flies.

TABLE 8-2   Summary of Major Bacterial Pathogens and the Diseases They Cause   (*Continued*)

Cocci	Disease
Legionella pneumophila	Legionnaires' disease. Organisms live in water and cause pulmonary infection in persons who inhale aerosolized droplets from showers, air conditioners, or other water sources. No person-to-person spread.
Salmonella species	Gastroenteritis and systemic infections. Infection acquired from contaminated food or water sources.
Shigella species	Dysentery with frequent watery stools. Spread by person-to-person contact, or by contaminated food and water.
Campylobacter species	Gastroenteritis. May cause systemic infection. Infects many animals. Humans infected from contaminated water, undercooked meat or poultry, or contact with infected animals.
Escherichia coli	Gastroenteritis, urinary tract and systemic infections. Some strains (0157:H7) produce toxins that cause hemolytic anemia and kidney damage.
Spiral organisms	
Treponema pallidum	Syphilis. Considered in the discussion on communicable diseases.
Borrelia burgdorferi	Lyme disease, transmitted from rodents to humans by ticks. Causes febrile illness and arthritis with lesion at site of tick bite.
Acid-fast bacteria	
Mycobacterium tuberculosis	Pulmonary tuberculosis. Considered in the discussion on the respiratory system.
Mycobacterium avium complex	A normally nonpathogenic organism that may cause an opportunistic infection in AIDS patients.

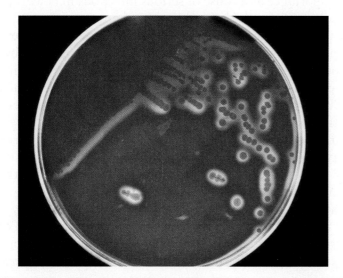

FIGURE 8-3 Bacteriologic culture plate (blood agar) containing colonies of hemolytic staphylococci. Enzymes produced by the bacteria break down (hemolyze) the blood cells in the culture medium, which causes the clear zones surrounding the colonies.

Courtesy of Leonard V. Crowley, MD, Century College.

alpha hemolysis, beta hemolysis, or no hemolysis on blood agar plates. Usually, both the Lancefield group and the type of hemolysis are specified when describing a streptococcus.

Alpha hemolytic streptococci (or simply alpha streptococci) produce green discoloration of the blood immediately around the colony and are often called *Streptococcus viridans* because of this growth characteristic (*viridans* = green). These organisms are normal inhabitants of the mouth and throat and usually are not pathogenic. They cannot be classified in the Lancefield system because they lack the carbohydrate antigen possessed by other streptococci.

Beta hemolytic streptococci (or simply beta streptococci) produce a narrow zone of complete hemolysis around the growing colony. One of the most important beta streptococci is in Lancefield group A and is called a group A beta streptococcus. Many group A beta streptococci are extremely pathogenic, causing streptococcal sore throat, scarlet fever, serious skin infections, and infections of the uterus after childbirth. Some produce a toxin that causes a toxic shock syndrome similar to that caused by toxin-producing staphylococci. One particularly virulent toxin-producing group A beta streptococcal strain causes a rapidly progressive, destructive infection of the subcutaneous tissues and the fibrous tissue (fascia) covering the adjacent muscles. This condition, called **necrotizing fasciitis**, may be complicated by necrosis (**gangrene**) of the overlying skin and by necrosis of the muscles in the infected area (streptococcal myositis).

In addition to causing infections in various tissues, some strains of group A beta streptococci are capable of inducing a state of hypersensitivity in susceptible individuals, leading to development of **rheumatic fever** or a type of kidney disease called **glomerulonephritis**. These diseases are considered in greater detail in the sections on the circulatory system (discussion on the cardiovascular system) and kidneys (discussion on the urinary system). Fortunately, group A beta streptococci still remain quite sensitive to penicillin and other antibiotics.

Beta streptococci in other Lancefield groups are also of medical importance. Group B beta streptococci may cause urinary tract and wound infections, but they are of greatest importance as a cause of serious infections in newborn infants. They often inhabit (colonize) the rectum and vagina of pregnant women, and the infant may become infected during labor and delivery. Because of the potential hazard of a life-threatening infection in an infant born to a mother colonized by group B beta streptococci, routine rectal and vaginal cultures to detect the organism are recommended for all pregnant women late in pregnancy. Those women who are colonized are treated with intravenous antibiotics during labor to reduce the risk of a serious group B beta streptococcal infection in the infant.

Group D streptococci and streptococci of other Lancefield groups may also cause various types of infections, but it is the group A beta streptococcus that is responsible for almost all of the late immunologic complications: rheumatic fever and glomerulonephritis.

Closely related to group D streptococci but classified separately are organisms that inhabit the intestinal tract called enterococci (*enteron* = bowel). These organisms are often very resistant to multiple antibiotics. Consequently, a wound or urinary tract infection caused by an enterococcus may be very difficult to treat.

Pneumococci

Pneumococci (*Streptococcus pneumoniae*) are gram-positive cocci and are classified with the streptococci. They grow in pairs and short chains and have certain biochemical characteristics setting them apart from other streptococci. Pneumococci are a common cause of bacterial pneumonia.

Necrotizing fasciitis Destruction of subcutaneous tissues in beta streptococcal infection.

Gangrene Tissue death caused by bacterial infection or lack of blood circulation.

Rheumatic fever Inflammatory disease that occurs following a *Streptococcus pyogenes* infection that can involve the heart, joints, skin, and brain.

Glomerulonephritis An inflammation of the glomeruli caused by either antigen-antibody complexes trapped in the glomeruli or by antiglomerular basement membrane antibodies.

Gram-Negative Cocci

Most gram-negative cocci are nonpathogenic members of the genus *Neisseria* and are normal inhabitants of the upper respiratory passages. This group has two pathogenic members. The meningococcus (*Neisseria meningitidis*) causes a type of meningitis (inflammation of the membranes surrounding the brain and spinal cord) that frequently occurs in epidemics. The gonococcus (*Neisseria gonorrhoeae*) causes gonorrhea. This disease is transmitted by sexual contact and is discussed in greater detail in the discussion on communicable diseases.

Gram-Positive Bacilli

There are several important groups of gram-positive rod-shaped bacteria that can be subdivided on the basis of their oxygen requirements and on their ability to form spores. The two important groups of non–spore-forming aerobic bacteria are *Corynebacteria* and *Listeria*. The two important groups of spore-forming organisms are *Bacilli*, which are aerobic microorganisms, and *Clostridia*, which are anaerobic organisms.

Aerobic Non–Spore-Forming Gram-Positive Organisms. *Corynebacteria* are a large group of microorganisms. Most are nonpathogenic inhabitants of the skin and other squamous epithelium-lined body surfaces (mucous membranes). However, one member of this group (*Corynebacterium diphtheriae*) causes diphtheria. The organism causes an acute ulcerative inflammation of the throat and produces a potent toxin that can injure heart muscle and nerve tissue.

One important member of the *Listeria* group of microorganisms, called *Listeria monocytogenes*, can cause a very serious infection. The organism is widely distributed in nature: in the soil, on plants, and in the intestinal tract of people and animals. The organism may contaminate dairy products, raw vegetables, and other food products such as soft cheeses, hot dogs, and delicatessen foods. People become infected by eating *Listeria*-contaminated foods, and those at greatest risk for serious infections are infants and older people, pregnant women, and people whose immune system is impaired. *Listeria* infection is a very serious systemic illness that may be complicated by spread of the organism to the brain and meninges, causing a meningitis or brain abscess. In pregnant women, the organism may also spread through the placenta to infect the unborn infant, leading to intrauterine fetal death or life-threatening infection of the infant.

Aerobic Spore-Forming Gram-Positive Organisms. Spore-forming aerobes are called *Bacilli*. Only one member of this group is highly pathogenic. This organism is *Bacillus anthracis*, which causes anthrax.

Anthrax is primarily a disease of animals that is rare in the United States, but is a more common animal infection in some other countries. Anthrax spores are highly resistant, can survive for many years in the soil, and can contaminate the hair, wool, or other tissues of animals from countries where anthrax is prevalent. If anthrax spores enter the body of a susceptible animal or person, the spores can germinate to form very large numbers of rapidly growing bacteria, which causes the disease anthrax.

Inhalation of anthrax spores from spore-contaminated wool, yarn, or other animal products causes a severe life-threatening pulmonary and systemic infection with extremely high mortality. The spores germinate within the pulmonary alveoli, actively proliferate, and produce lethal toxins that cause extensive tissue destruction. Other spores are ingested by macrophages and transported to regional lymph nodes, where they continue to germinate and produce toxins. A vaccine to immunize against anthrax has been available for many years, and it is recommended for people at high risk of exposure to anthrax, such as veterinarians and employees of textile mills that process imported wool or similar animal products. The U.S. military establishment has been quite concerned that anthrax spores may be used as a germ warfare agent because inhalation of spores is potentially lethal.

Concerns about the use of anthrax spores as a bioterrorism germ warfare agent became a reality in 2001 when a letter containing anthrax spores was mailed to a U.S. senator, processed at a postal facility in Washington, D.C., and opened in a senate office building. The spores contaminated the postal facility and senate office building, caused acute inhalation anthrax in five postal workers who worked in the facility where the letter was processed, and also exposed a number of people who worked in the office building.

People who may have been exposed to anthrax spores require a prolonged course of antibiotics to prevent development of pulmonary anthrax. Antibiotics effective against the germinated form of the anthrax bacillus are not effective against the spore form of the organism, and many spores do not germinate as soon as they are inhaled. Some are ingested by macrophages and transported to the regional lymph nodes, where they may continue to germinate for as long as two months after the initial exposure. The long course of antibiotics is required to destroy the antibiotic-sensitive vegetative bacteria as they germinate at various times from antibiotic-resistant spores.

Anaerobic Spore-Forming Gram-Positive Organisms. Anaerobic spore-forming bacilli are called *Clostridia*. These are normal inhabitants of the intestinal tract of animals and humans and are also found in the soil. Members of this group produce potent toxins and cause several important diseases. Some *Clostridia* cause gas gangrene. Some cause tetanus (lockjaw). Some cause botulism, and others cause an intestinal infection.

Gas gangrene, caused by *Clostridium perfringens* and related organisms, develops in dirty, spore-contaminated wounds. These anaerobic organisms germinate and proliferate in dead or devitalized tissues, especially in wounds where considerable necrosis of tissue has taken place. The *Clostridia* produce large amounts of gas by fermenting the necrotic tissues, and they also release powerful toxins that destroy tissues and cause widespread systemic effects.

Another clostridial species, *Clostridium tetani*, produces a potent toxin that causes spasm of voluntary muscles. The common term "lockjaw" comes from the marked rigidity of the jaw muscles that is a common feature of the disease. Tetanus may be fatal because of respiratory failure resulting from spasm of the muscles concerned with respiration.

Clostridium botulinum produces a potent neuroparalytic toxin. **Botulism** can generally be traced to eating improperly processed or canned foods in which the organism has grown and produced toxin. Botulism is a poisoning caused by the ingestion of toxin in food rather than a bacterial infection. Although botulism was more common when home canning was prevalent, outbreaks of botulism have also been traced to contamination of home cured ham, some meats, and even raw carrot juice left unrefrigerated for several days. Infantile botulism can occur when infants consume contaminated honey or corn syrup and toxin is absorbed from bacteria proliferating in the intestine. For this reason, even commercially produced honey should not be fed to infants.

Clostridium difficile is the organism responsible for the intestinal infection called *antibiotic-associated colitis* that sometimes follows use of broad-spectrum antibiotics and is considered in the discussion on the gastrointestinal tract.

Gram-Negative Bacteria

There are many gram-negative organisms of clinical importance. Several different groups cause important diseases in humans. These are named *Haemophilus*,

Botulism Food poisoning caused by ingestion of a neurotoxin produced by an anaerobic spore-forming bacillus *Clostridium botulinum* growing in improperly canned or preserved food.

Francisella, Yersinia, Brucella, and *Legionella.* Members of the genus *Haemophilus* are normal inhabitants of the respiratory tract. One member of this group, *Haemophilus influenzae,* sometimes causes meningitis in infants and young children. Occasionally, it produces respiratory infections in patients with chronic lung disease. Another closely related organism was previously classified as *Haemophilus* but has been renamed *Gardnerella.* In conjunction with other bacteria, this organism causes a common vaginal infection called *nonspecific vaginitis* (discussion on the female reproductive system). One member of the genus *Yersinia* is responsible for bubonic plague. A member of the genus *Francisella* produces a somewhat similar illness called *tularemia.* Members of the genus *Brucella* cause disease in cattle, goats, and hogs that can be transmitted to people from contact with meat or other tissues from infected animals, or from drinking unpasteurized milk from infected cows or goats. In humans, the disease is a febrile illness without any specific features and responds to appropriate antibiotics. *Legionella* causes a serious respiratory illness called *Legionnaires disease.*

Other gram-negative organisms of medical importance include a number of closely related organisms that live in the gastrointestinal tract of people and animals. Other members of this group are free-living organisms, widely distributed in nature. Important pathogenic members of the group include Salmonella, Shigella, Campylobacter, and the cholera bacillus (*Vibrio cholerae*). These organisms cause various types of febrile illness and gastroenteritis. The organisms are excreted from the gastrointestinal tract in the feces of infected patients and are transmitted by contaminated food or water.

An organism closely related to *Campylobacter* but now designated *Helicobacter* is of medical importance because it appears to cause chronic inflammation of the stomach lining (chronic gastritis) and stomach ulcers. This organism is considered in connection with the gastrointestinal tract (discussion on the gastrointestinal tract).

Other members of this large group are of only limited pathogenicity but sometimes produce disease when they are outside of their normal habitat in the gastrointestinal tract. These organisms may cause wound infections, urinary tract infections, and pulmonary infections in susceptible individuals. The best-known enteric bacterium is the colon bacillus (*Escherichia coli*), which is the predominant organism found within the intestinal tract of humans and animals. Some strains of the colon bacillus can produce various toxins that can cause intestinal symptoms ranging from a cholera-like diarrhea to a dysentery-like acute inflammation of the intestinal tract. One well-known pathogenic strain is designated *E. coli 0157:H7,* the numbers referring to the antigens contained in the bacterial cell and its flagellae. This organism's toxin causes an acute inflammation of the colon characterized by bloody diarrhea and abdominal pain. Sometimes there is also an associated destruction of the patient's red blood cells, with marked anemia and impaired renal function with renal failure, called the hemolytic uremic syndrome. This pathogenic organism is present in the intestinal tract of infected cattle, and people usually become infected by consuming contaminated, incompletely cooked beef or by drinking raw milk. Recent outbreaks were caused by consumption of improperly cooked hamburgers prepared from beef contaminated with the organism and by consumption of leafy vegetables contaminated in the field. In 2011, almost 4,000 Europeans were infected by a closely related *E. coli* organism, resulting in more than fifty deaths. The organism *E. coli 0104:H4* contaminated fenugreek seed derived beansprouts.

Spiral Organisms

The spiral organisms can cause a wide variety of illnesses. The best-known member of this group is *Treponema pallidum,* which causes syphilis—one of the sexually transmitted diseases. These diseases are considered in the discussion on communicable diseases. Another spiral organism in this group is *Borrelia burgdorferi*, which causes **Lyme disease**. Named after a town in Connecticut where the disease was first recognized, it is now widespread in North America, Europe, and Australia. Transmission to humans is by the bite of an infected tick (*Ixodes dammini* and other *Ixodes* species). Most infections occur in the summer when exposure to ticks is frequent. Untreated Lyme disease typically progresses through three stages. In the first stage, a roughly circular, localized skin rash appears at the site of the tick bite and is frequently associated with flulike symptoms of fever, chills, and headaches, along with muscular and joint aches and pain. The rash and other manifestations eventually subside, but weeks or months later many patients develop various neurologic, cardiac, and joint manifestations, which characterize the second stage of the disease. The third stage, which eventually develops in some untreated patients, is characterized by chronic arthritis and various neurologic problems. Diagnosis is usually made by means of various serologic tests, and the disease is usually treated with a tetracycline antibiotic.

> **Lyme disease**
> A tick-borne systemic infection caused by a spiral organism, *Borrelia burgdorferi*, characterized by neurologic, joint, and cardiac manifestations.

Acid-Fast Bacteria

Acid-fast bacteria have a waxy capsule that is stained with difficulty by means of certain red dyes. After the organism has been stained, the stain-impregnated capsule resists decolorization with various acid solvents. This property, attributable to the capsule, is the reason for the term *acid-fast*, used to refer to this type of organism. Acid-fast bacteria cause a special type of chronic inflammatory reaction, called a chronic granulomatous inflammation, rather than the polymorphonuclear inflammatory reaction usually seen with bacterial infections.

The best-known acid-fast bacterium is the tubercle bacillus (*Mycobacterium tuberculosis*) responsible for tuberculosis. Mycobacteria, other than the tubercle bacillus, may at times cause a tuberculosis-like disease affecting lungs, lymph nodes, or skin, and some may cause severe systemic infections in immunocompromised individuals. (Disseminated infection caused by *Mycobacterium avium* complex in people with the acquired immune deficiency syndrome is described in the discussion on communicable diseases.) Another acid-fast bacterium (*Mycobacterium leprae*) causes leprosy.

ANTIBIOTIC TREATMENT OF BACTERIAL INFECTIONS

The discovery of antibiotic compounds and their widespread use to treat various types of infections has been one of the great advances in medicine. Antibiotics are substances that destroy bacteria or inhibit their growth. They are useful clinically because of their ability to injure bacterial cells without producing significant injury to the patient.

The bacterial cell is a complex structure containing genetic material, a protein-synthesizing mechanism, numerous enzyme systems concerned with intracellular metabolic functions, a semipermeable cell membrane, and a rigid cell wall. The bacterial genetic material is arranged as a circular DNA molecule that is attached to the cell membrane. Some bacteria also contain smaller circular DNA molecules, called plasmids, that contain genes coding for various properties useful to bacteria but often harmful to the people infected by the bacteria. Such properties include resistance to antibiotics, toxin production, and formation of soluble factors that inhibit growth of normal bacterial flora, so the plasmid-bearing bacterium has a growth advantage over the bacterial flora with which it must compete. Antimicrobial substances act by interfering with the structure or function of the bacterial cell in one or more ways (**FIGURE 8-4**).

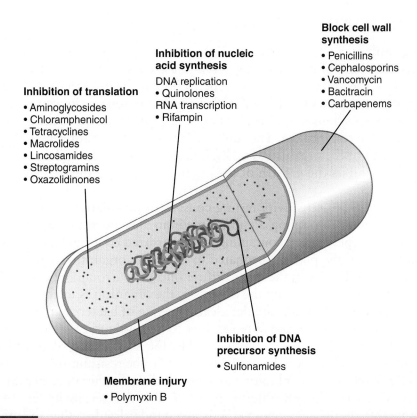

Inhibition of translation

- Aminoglycosides
- Chloramphenicol
- Tetracyclines
- Macrolides
- Lincosamides
- Streptogramins
- Oxazolidinones

Inhibition of nucleic acid synthesis

DNA replication
- Quinolones
RNA transcription
- Rifampin

Block cell wall synthesis

- Penicillins
- Cephalosporins
- Vancomycin
- Bacitracin
- Carbapenems

Inhibition of DNA precursor synthesis
- Sulfonamides

Membrane injury
- Polymyxin B

FIGURE 8-4 The targets for antibacterial agents. There are five major targets for antibacterial agents: the cell wall, cell membrane, ribosomes (protein synthesis), nucleic acid synthesis (RNA and DNA synthesis), and metabolic reactions vital to the bacteria.

Inhibition of Cell-Wall Synthesis

The bacterial cell has a high internal osmotic pressure, and the rigid outer cell wall maintains the shape of the bacterium. In some respects, the function of the cell wall can be compared with a corset or girdle supporting the enclosed cell. Penicillin and several other antibiotics act by inhibiting the synthesis of the bacterial cell wall so that the cell body is exposed. Because of the high osmotic pressure inside the bacterium, the relatively unsupported cell swells and eventually ruptures.

Inhibition of Cell-Membrane Function

The cell membrane is a semipermeable membrane surrounding the bacterial protoplasm. It controls the internal composition of the cell by regulating the diffusion of materials into and out of the cell. Some antibiotics act by inhibiting various functions of the cell membrane. Loss of the selective permeability of the cell membrane leads to cell injury and death.

Inhibition of Metabolic Functions

Some antibiotics interfere with nucleic acid or protein synthesis by bacteria so that the organisms are unable to carry out essential metabolic functions.

Inhibition of Nucleic Acid and Protein Synthesis

A large number of antibiotic agents inhibit bacterial protein synthesis by binding to either the 30s or 50s subunits of the bacterial ribosome and interfering with their activity. One of the most commonly used class of antibiotics (the fluroquinolines) block DNA synthesis in both gram-positive and gram-negative organisms.

ANTIBIOTIC SENSITIVITY TESTS

In selecting antibiotics to treat a bacterial infection, the practitioner is aided by laboratory tests called antibiotic sensitivity tests. These tests measure, under standardized conditions, the ability of the antibiotic to inhibit the growth of the organism isolated from the patient. One method, called a tube dilution sensitivity test, consists of preparing various dilutions of antibiotics in test tubes and inoculating the tubes with the organism to be tested. The tubes are then incubated for a period of time to permit growth of the organism. Finally, determination of the highest dilution of antibiotic that inhibits the growth of the organism indicates the sensitivity of the organism to the drug.

Another method of sensitivity testing consists of inoculating the organism on a bacteriologic plate containing a culture medium. Several filter paper disks are then placed on the plate, each containing a standardized concentration of a different antibiotic. Next, the plate is incubated to allow the organism to grow. During incubation, the antibiotics in the disks diffuse into the surrounding culture. If the antibiotic is capable of inhibiting the organism, the organism is unable to grow in the area around the disk, and a circular clear zone free of bacterial growth appears (**FIGURE 8-5**). The organism is said to be sensitive to the antibiotic. On the other hand, if the growth of the organism is not influenced by the antibiotic, growth will not be inhibited around the disk, and the organism is said to be resistant to the antibiotic. The diameter of the zones of inhibition around the disks further indicates the sensitivity of the organism. The tube dilution and disk diffusion sensitivity test methods yield comparable results. The two methods are standardized so that the diameter of the zone of inhibition obtained by the disk diffusion method correlates with the antibiotic concentration required to inhibit the organism, as measured by the tube dilution method.

A bacteriology laboratory report that the organism is sensitive to a given antibiotic means that the organism probably can be inhibited by giving the patient the

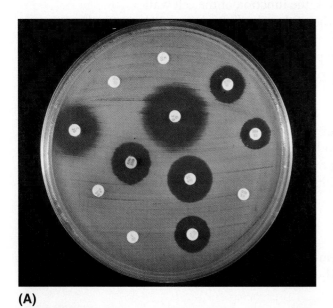

(A)

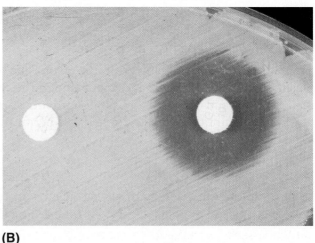

(B)

FIGURE 8-5 **(A)** Sensitivity test, illustrating antibiotic-impregnated filter paper disks on surface of culture plate. The clear zone around disk indicates that the antibiotic in the disk has inhibited bacterial growth. **(B)** Closer view of two disks on plate. The antibiotic contained in the disk (*left*) fails to inhibit growth of organism, which is *resistant* to antibiotic. The clear zone around the antibiotic (*right*) indicates that the antibiotic in the disk inhibits the growth of the organism, which is *sensitive* to the antibiotic.

Courtesy of Leonard V. Crowley, MD, Century College.

usual therapeutic dose of that drug. A report that the organism is resistant to an antibiotic indicates that a therapeutic dose of antibiotic is unlikely to inhibit the growth of the organism.

It should be emphasized, however, that the sensitivity of an organism to an antibiotic is only one factor influencing a patient's response to an infection. Other factors include the patient's own resistance and the antibiotic's ability to diffuse in sufficient quantities into the site of the infection.

ADVERSE EFFECTS OF ANTIBIOTICS

Toxicity

Antibiotics are useful because they are much more toxic to bacteria than they are to the patient. Antibiotics vary in their effects on people, but all are toxic to some degree. Some injure the kidneys; others injure nerve tissue or the blood-forming tissues. Penicillin and other antibiotics that act by interfering with bacterial cell-wall synthesis are relatively nontoxic, probably because the body cells have no structure comparable to the bacterial cell wall. Some antibiotics that interfere with bacterial metabolic functions can sometimes produce similar derangements in the patient's own metabolic functions. For example, tetracycline is a relatively nontoxic antibiotic, excreted chiefly by the kidneys. If renal function is impaired, very high blood levels of antibiotic may develop after administration of the usual therapeutic doses of the drug; this may cause severe and often fatal impairment of the patient's own cellular metabolic functions.

Hypersensitivity

Some antibiotics induce a marked hypersensitivity that can lead to a fatal reaction if the drug is later administered to a sensitized patient. Penicillin is capable of inducing extremely severe anaphylactic reactions, although the antibiotic itself has a very low toxicity.

Alteration of Normal Bacterial Flora

The normal bacterial flora in the oral cavity, the colon, and other locations may be altered by antibiotics. If the normal bacteria are destroyed, there may be overgrowth of resistant bacteria and fungi previously controlled by the normal flora. These resistant organisms may cause infections in susceptible patients.

Development of Resistant Strains of Bacteria

Some bacteria that are initially sensitive to antibiotics eventually become resistant. There are two ways in which an organism becomes resistant. It may undergo a spontaneous mutation that conveys resistance, or it may acquire a plasmid that contains resistance genes from another bacterium.

Spontaneous mutations do not occur frequently in cell division, but many bacteria divide so rapidly that spontaneous mutations can present a problem if the rapidly dividing bacteria are not quickly eliminated by the antibiotic. After a mutation that conveys antibiotic resistance occurs, the mutant organism has an advantage over its antibiotic-sensitive counterpart because it can flourish in the presence of the antibiotic while the antibiotic-sensitive organisms are eliminated.

Plasmid-acquired resistance can be a major problem because the transferred plasmid may convey resistance to multiple antibiotics, and plasmid transfers can take place between bacteria of different types. In this process, a bacterium with antibiotic-resistant genes carried on one of its plasmids (the donor) extends a thin cytoplasmic tube to contact another bacterium (the recipient), "reels in" the bacterium that it has contacted, and passes a copy of its plasmid to the recipient bacterium. Now both bacteria possess antibiotic-resistance plasmids, which they in turn can pass to other bacteria.

There are a number of mechanisms by which resistant bacteria can circumvent an antibiotic's effect. Such mechanisms include (1) developing enzymes to destroy the antibiotic, (2) either changing their cell-wall structure so that the antibiotic is unable to get into the cell or developing mechanisms to expel the antibiotic as soon as it enters the cell and before it can disturb bacterial functions, or (3) changing their intracellular "metabolic machinery" so that the antibiotic is no longer able to disturb bacterial functions.

A few examples serve to illustrate the ingenuous adaptations of bacteria that thwart our efforts to eliminate them. A bacterium that is penicillin sensitive may develop an enzyme, penicillinase, that inactivates the antibiotic and allows the bacterium to survive in the presence of the drug. An antibiotic that acts against an enzyme required for a bacterial function, such as constructing a cell wall, may be rendered ineffective if the bacterium slightly alters the structure of its enzyme so that the antibiotic can no longer bind to the enzyme and inactivate it. An antibiotic that attaches to bacterial ribosomes, preventing protein synthesis, may be rendered ineffective if the bacterium slightly changes the structure of the ribosome so that the antibiotic can no longer act against it.

Widespread use of an antibiotic predisposes to the development of resistant strains. This may complicate the treatment of patients who become infected with antibiotic-resistant organisms. Staphylococci, in particular, have raised this problem because many strains isolated from hospital patients have been found to be highly resistant to a large number of antibiotics. Treatment of gonorrhea also has been complicated by the development of a high degree of penicillin resistance in many strains of gonococci; consequently, prolonged courses of therapy and much larger doses of antibiotic are required to eradicate the infections. Even the pneumococcus is no longer uniformly sensitive to penicillin, as it was in the past. Some strains are resistant to penicillin and other drugs normally used against them. Resistant strains of tubercle bacilli also have developed, hindering treatment of tuberculosis with antituberculosis drugs. On the other hand, some bacteria still remain quite sensitive to antibiotics. For example, group A beta streptococci remain sensitive to penicillin, despite widespread use of penicillin to treat streptococcal infections. *Treponema pallidum*, the organism responsible for syphilis, also has remained quite sensitive to penicillin, even though the drug has been used to treat syphilis for many years.

There is current concern over the use of antibiotic additives in livestock production. The use of antibiotics in raising meat animals increases weight at slaughter and prevents disease in herds. However, such antibiotics lead to the generation of bacteria with antibiotic resistance that may either directly infect humans or serve as a source of resistance bearing plasmids, which may be transferred to human pathogens.

Chlamydiae

Inclusion bodies
Spherical structures in the nucleus or cytoplasm of virus-infected cells or intracytoplasmic clusters of organisms such as Chlamydiae within a cell.

The chlamydiae are very small, gram-negative, nonmotile bacteria once thought to be large viruses. They are deficient in certain enzymes and can live only as parasites inside of the cells of the individual that they infect. They are taken into the cells of the host by phagocytosis, where they divide to form large intracytoplasmic clusters of organisms called **inclusion bodies**. These resemble inclusion bodies formed in some viral diseases. Their growth can be inhibited by various antibiotics that inhibit protein synthesis.

Chlamydiae cause several different types of diseases. The most common chlamydial disease affects the genital tract and is transmitted by sexual contact. In the male, it causes an inflammation of the urethra called *nongonococcal urethritis*. In the female, it causes an inflammation of the uterine cervix that may spread to the fallopian tubes and ovaries as well. If a mother has a chlamydial infection of the cervix, infected secretions may get into her infant's eyes during childbirth and cause an inflammation called *inclusion conjunctivitis*. The name is based on the fact that characteristic inclusions can be demonstrated in the infected cells of the infant's conjunctiva. Other chlamydiae cause pulmonary infections. One species causes a disease of birds called psitticosis that is transmissible to humans and is manifested clinically as a type of pneumonia. Another species of chlamydiae causes an uncommon sexually transmissible disease called lymphogranuloma venereum. This disease is characterized by marked enlargement and inflammation of the lymph nodes in the groin and around the rectum. (See the presentation of communicable and sexually transmitted disease.)

Rickettsiae and Ehrlichiae

Rickettsiae are very small intracellular bacteria that can only multiply within the cells of an infected person. Many small animals and dogs are infected. The rickettsiae are transmitted to humans by insect bites (often from ticks), and they multiply in the endothelial cells of small blood vessels, which become swollen and necrotic, leading to thrombosis, rupture, and necrosis. Clinically, a rickettsial infection usually causes a febrile illness, often associated with a skin rash. Typhus and Rocky Mountain spotted fever are the most common rickettsial diseases. These organisms are sensitive to some antibiotics. Similar organisms transmitted by ticks infect white blood cells rather than endothelial cells and are called Ehrlichiae (named after an early immunologist, Paul Ehrlich). There are several species. Some infect neutrophils and others infect monocytes. The infected white cells contain small, compact clusters of organisms called morulae (singular, morula), which can be identified in blood smears. Ehrlichiosis is a febrile illness similar to infections caused by rickettsiae and may be associated with a skin rash. Ehrlichiosis can be treated successfully with antibiotic therapy.

Mycoplasmas

The mycoplasmas are very small bacteria that are very fragile because they lack a cell wall. One member of this group causes a type of pneumonia called primary atypical pneumonia (or sometimes "walking pneumonia"). Mycoplasmas respond to several antibiotics.

Viruses

Viruses are the smallest infectious agents. A typical virus consists of a molecule of nucleic acid (either DNA or RNA), its genome, enclosed within a protein shell called a **capsid**. The capsid is made of subunits called **capsomeres**, which are arranged in a precise geometric fashion around the genome. Many viruses are also covered by an outer lipid envelope acquired from the cytoplasm of the host cell when the virus buds from the cell that it has infected. Projections from the surface of the virus allow the virus to attach to the cell that it will infect. Viruses vary greatly in size. The smallest are only slightly larger than protein molecules, whereas the largest viruses approach the size of a bacterium.

Capsid The protein covering the central nucleic acid core of a virus.

Capsomere One of the subunits that make up the protein shell (capsid) of a virus.

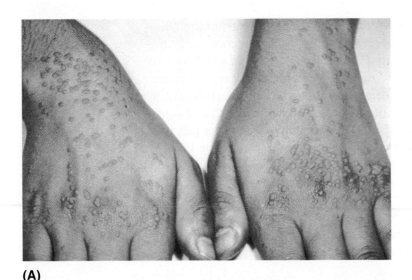

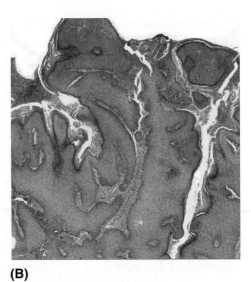

(A) (B)

FIGURE 8-6 **(A)** Multiple dermal warts on skin of hands. **(B)** Photomicrograph of a dermal wart at low power demonstrating extreme hyperplasia of the epidermis and the multiple clefts that give warts their characteristic appearance.

(A) Courtesy of Leonard V. Crowley, MD, Century College; (B) Courtesy of Department of Pathology and Laboratory Medicine, University of North Carolina at Chapel Hill.

Latent A viral infection producing no symptoms.

Papilloma Otherwise known as a wart, produced after human papilloma virus infection.

The nucleic acid of the virus genome may be arranged in either a single or a double strand, and the complexity of the viral genome varies. Some viruses have as many as 400 genes within their nucleic acid structure, whereas others have as few as 8. Viruses have few metabolic enzymes and therefore must rely on the cells of the infected person to carry out their activities. When a virus invades the cell, the viral genome directs the metabolic processes of the cell to synthesize more virus particles. In many respects, the virus may be likened to a criminal who takes over a business, forcing it to function for the criminal's benefit rather than for the benefit of the owner. Viral infection of a cell may be **latent** and produce no symptoms at the time of infection only to reactivate and cause disease in the future. Viruses may cause either acute cell necrosis or a slow progressive injury. In addition, viral infection may cause cell hyperplasia and may ultimately lead to a malignant neoplastic disease. For example, warts (**papillomas**) are a benign neoplasm commonly found on the hands and feet that are caused by strains of the human papilloma virus (**FIGURE 8-6**). Other strains of the papilloma virus are associated with venereal warts and cervical and penile cancer.

CLASSIFICATION OF VIRUSES

An older classification of viruses was based on the major clinical features of the viral infection, and viruses were classified on the basis of the portion of the body or organ system in which the viral infection produced the most prominent clinical manifestations. A more modern classification categorizes viruses on the basis of their nucleic acid structure, size, structural configuration, and biologic characteristics. In this classification, several large groups of viruses are recognized, and a large number of viruses are identified in each group. **TABLE 8-3** presents a simplified classification of viruses and the diseases they cause.

HEMORRHAGIC FEVERS

Hemorrhagic fevers include Ebola and Marburg fevers, the former now a major public health problem in West Africa. Ebola is caused by infection with one of the four infectious strains of ebola virus. In earlier outbreaks, approximately 80 percent of

TABLE 8-3   Common Viruses Infecting Humans

	Virus	Disease
DNA viruses	Adenoviruses	Respiratory infections
	Hepatitis B virus	Hepatitis B
	Herpes viruses	
	Herpes simplex type 1	Cold sores
	Herpes simplex type 2	Genital herpes
	Epstein-Barr virus	Infectious mononucleosis
	Varicella-zoster virus	Chickenpox, herpes zoster (shingles)
	Cytomegalovirus	Mononucleosis-like illness, hepatitis
	Herpesvirus 8	Kaposi's sarcoma
	Papilloma virus	Warts, condylomas (benign tumors)
RNA viruses	Arboviruses	Encephalitis
	Noroviruses	Gastroenteritis
	Coronavirus	Respiratory infections
		Severe acute respiratory syndrome (SARS)
	Hantavirus (bunyavirus)	Acute respiratory illness
	Hepatitis viruses	
	Hepatitis A virus (picornavirus)	Hepatitis
	Hepatitis C virus (flavivirus)	Hepatitis
	Hepatitis D virus (coated with HbsAg)	Hepatitis
	Hepatitis E virus (calicivirus)	Hepatitis
	Myxoviruses	
	Influenza viruses	Influenza
	Parainfluenza viruses	Respiratory infections, croup
	Respiratory syncytial viruses	Respiratory infections
	Measles virus	Measles
	Mumps virus	Mumps
	Picornaviruses	
	Coxsackie viruses	Pharyngitis, myocarditis, pericarditis
	Echoviruses	Respiratory infections, gastroenteritis
	Hepatitis A virus	Hepatitis A
	Polioviruses	Poliomyelitis
	Rhinoviruses	Respiratory infections
	Rabies virus (rhabdovirus)	Rabies
	Retroviruses	
	HIV	AIDS
	HTLV 1	Adult T-cell leukemia
	Rubella virus (togavirus)	German measles

infected people died. Uninfected people can be exposed to the virus by direct contact with the blood or secretions of symptomatic infected people or through contact with contaminated objects. The Ebola virus damages endothelial cells, causing massive internal bleeding and hemorrhage. The infected individual often suffers from severe fluid loss or bleeds to death before an immune response can be mounted. Although still uncertain, bats appear to be the animal host of the virus, particularly the Marburg virus. Infected primates used as a food source may also contribute to epidemics. Poor and overcrowded neighborhoods in urban centers have led to outbreaks of epidemic proportion and the collapse of public health and medical facilities in the worst affected countries. Marburg fever was first identified in green monkeys imported into Germany from Africa. Recent outbreaks have been traced to exposure to fruit bats. Symptoms are similar to those for Ebola, but the disease is generally milder, with a lower fatality rate.

MODE OF ACTION

A distinction is sometimes made between a viral infection and a viral disease. A condition in which a virus infects a cell without causing any evidence of cell injury is considered a latent viral infection. Many viruses are capable of coexisting with normal cells in lymphoid tissue and the gastrointestinal tract, and probably in other sites, without causing cellular injury. Such viruses are able to live for long periods within the cells of the infected host while they continually discharge virus particles. Other viruses are more virulent and regularly produce cell injury, manifested by necrosis and degeneration of the infected cell. This is called a cytopathogenic effect. Some viruses induce cell hyperplasia and proliferation rather than cell necrosis (Figure 8-6B). Many viruses induce various combinations of cell damage and cell hyperplasia.

Under certain circumstances, a latent asymptomatic viral infection may become activated, leading to actual disease. The herpes virus, which infects both the oral cavity and the genital tract, may persist in the tissues of the host for many years. The virus periodically becomes activated and causes crops of painful vesicles that may recur during an intercurrent febrile illness when the patient's immunologic defenses have been disrupted by a neoplasm or by various other diseases, or sometimes for no apparent reason (**FIGURE 8-7**).

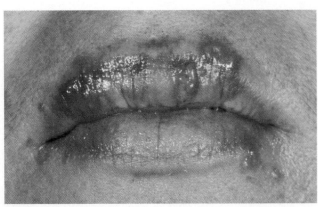

(A)

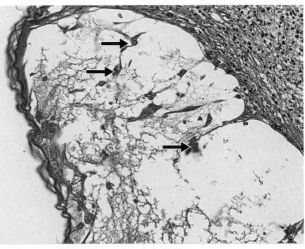

(B)

FIGURE 8-7   Herpes virus infection. **(A)** Recurrent oral herpes is most often caused by herpes virus type 1. **(B)** Section of a small herpes blister. Virus infected cells demonstrating intranuclear viral inclusions (*arrows*) have become necrotic, leading to separation of epidermal tissue and blister formation.

(A) Courtesy of Leonard V. Crowley, MD, Century College; (B) Courtesy of Department of Pathology and Laboratory Medicine, University of North Carolina at Chapel Hill.

Another member of the herpes group of viruses is the varicella-zoster virus, named from its two different manifestations. The initial contact with the virus causes chickenpox (varicella), which is an extremely contagious disease characterized by an itchy skin rash that usually soon subsides, almost always without any serious complications. A person who has had chickenpox develops an immunity and cannot contract chickenpox again. However, the virus is not eradicated by the immune system and remains dormant within sensory nerve ganglia. Sometimes the virus becomes active again within a sensory ganglion many years later and then travels in the nerve associated with the ganglion to the skin, where it causes a characteristic bandlike vesicular skin rash in the segment of skin supplied by the sensory nerve. The recurrent infection is **herpes zoster**, which is often called **shingles**, from a Latin word, *cingulum*, which means a belt or girdle. The term refers to the beltlike band of skin vesicles along the course of a spinal nerve that partially girdles the trunk, as illustrated in **FIGURE 8-8**.

Herpes zoster is a late complication of the varicella-zoster virus (VZV) infection and is often complicated by chronic pain in the distribution of the previously affected nerve, which is called post–herpes-zoster neuralgia. Chickenpox had been a very common disease before the introduction of a live virus varicella-zoster vaccine in 1996. More than 95 percent of people living in the United States had developed chickenpox by the time they were twenty years old, and they were at risk for later reactivation of the virus followed by development of herpes zoster. However, they had also developed a cell-mediated immune response resulting from chickenpox, which tended to suppress reactivation of the latent virus. The cell-mediated immunity of previously infected adults declines as they age, which increased the risk that the latent virus might become activated to cause herpes zoster and its associated complications. A high dose form of the live virus varicella-zoster vaccine helps to prevent herpes

Herpes zoster A skin rash caused by reactivation of the varicella-zoster virus that caused chickenpox.

Shingles Another name for herpes zoster.

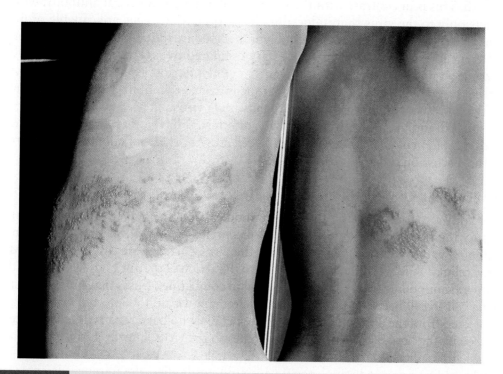

FIGURE 8-8 One type of herpes virus infection (called shingles or herpes zoster) characterized by clusters of vesicles that occur in a segment of skin (dermatome) supplied by a sensory nerve. The subject was photographed beside a mirror to illustrate the bandlike distribution of the rash in the segment of skin supplied by a spinal nerve.

Courtesy of Leonard V. Crowley, MD, Century College.

zoster and is recommended for older adults to help boost their immunity against VZV. The vaccine is over 60 percent effective, but it is not effective once herpes zoster has developed. To treat patients with herpes zoster, a number of medications similar to acyclovir (used to treat oral and genital herpes) are helpful to shorten the duration and severity of herpes zoster and may also reduce the pain often associated with the skin rash.

Inclusion Bodies in Viral Disease

Tissues infected with virus frequently contain spherical, densely staining structures called inclusion bodies (Figure 8-7B) that are also illustrated in the presentation of congenital and genetic diseases. They are present within the nucleus or the cytoplasm, or in both locations. Inclusion bodies consist of masses of virus or products of virus multiplication. The presence of inclusion bodies may be of considerable diagnostic aid in recognizing viral infection and determining the type of viral disease present.

BODILY DEFENSES AGAINST VIRAL INFECTIONS

The body responds to a viral infection by forming a protein substance called **interferon** and by activating **humoral immunity** and **cell-mediated defense mechanisms**.

Formation of Interferon

Interferon A broad-spectrum antiviral agent manufactured by various cells in the body.

Interferon is a general term for a group of carbohydrate-containing proteins produced by cells in response to viral infection and was named from its ability to "interfere" with viral multiplication. Interferon functions as a nonspecific, broad-spectrum antiviral agent. It inhibits not only the virus that induced its formation but other viruses as well. This is in contrast with the behavior of a specific antiviral antibody, which reacts only to the virus that induced its formation. Many cells are capable of producing interferon, but monocytes and lymphocytes are the primary sources. Several different interferons are produced, each designated by a Greek letter. Interferons provide a rapid "first-line" defense against a viral infection. By slowing viral growth during the early phase of the infection, time is gained to mobilize humoral and cell-mediated responses directed against the invading virus.

Humoral immunity Immunity associated with formation of antibodies produced by plasma cells.

In addition to their antiviral activity, interferons have other actions concerned with regulation of the immune system and cell growth. These functions are considered in the discussion on neoplastic disease.

Humoral and Cell-Mediated Immunity in Viral Infections

Cell-mediated defense mechanism The defense against foreign antigens provided by a population of T lymphocytes that can attach and destroy the foreign antigens.

The body also forms specific antiviral antibodies capable of inactivating viruses and destroying virus particles in the presence of complement. Antiviral antibodies cannot combine with the virus, however, unless the virus particles are discharged into the extracellular fluid where they are exposed to the action of the antibody. Consequently, antiviral antibodies are relatively inefficient in combating viruses that spread directly from cell to cell because the virus particles remain within the infected cells and are protected from the antibody. For example, people who have recurrent fever blisters caused by the herpes virus possess antibodies to the virus, but the antibody is often unable to eradicate the intracellular virus particles.

In addition to producing specific antiviral antibodies, the immune defenses of the host are directed against the virus-infected cells. This occurs because viruses that invade cells often induce the formation of new antigens on the surface of the infected cells. These antigens are recognized as foreign by the host's immune defenses and induce both humoral and cell-mediated immune reactions directed against the virus-infected cells. Antibodies are formed that affix to the infected cells and destroy them in the presence of complement. Sensitized lymphocytes release lymphokines, which damage the cells, and they also produce interferon, which inhibits the multiplication of viruses. Chemical mediators that induce an acute inflammatory reaction also are liberated (see discussion on inflammation and repair). In many viral infections, much of the tissue injury is caused not by proliferation of the virus within the cells of the host but by the inflammation and tissue destruction caused by the body's attempts to rid itself of the virus-infected cells.

TREATMENT WITH ANTIVIRAL AGENTS

Because viruses are simple structures lacking a cell wall, a cell membrane, and the complex "metabolic machinery" of bacteria, they are not susceptible to the disruptive actions of antibiotics. Some chemotherapeutic agents that are active against viruses have been developed, however. Some antiviral agents active against DNA viruses either block synthesis of DNA or induce the formation of an abnormal, nonfunctional DNA, thereby preventing virus multiplication. Another agent active against RNA viruses causes the formation of an abnormal messenger RNA that disrupts viral multiplication. Unfortunately, many compounds that block viral multiplication by such mechanisms also have a similar adverse effect on the host cells and may be as toxic to the host as to the virus. For this reason, antiviral agents have had limited application in the treatment of most viral disease. They are, however, the mainstay in the treatment of HIV. Because the reverse transcriptase enzyme is found only in virally infected cells, many anti-HIV drugs use the reverse transcriptase as a target. The drug acyclovir is effective against some infections caused by the herpes group of viruses. The drug is activated within the virus-infected cells by a viral enzyme to yield the active antiviral compound that selectively inhibits synthesis of viral DNA within the cells in which the virus is replicating.

Fungi

Fungi are plantlike organisms without chlorophyll and are subdivided into two large groups: yeasts and molds. Yeasts are small ovoid or spherical cells that reproduce by budding. Molds, when grown on suitable media at room temperature, form large colonies composed of multiple branching filamentous structures called **hyphae** (singular, hypha). The matted mass of hyphae, which is called a **mycelium**, is responsible for the characteristic appearance of the colony (**FIGURE 8-9**). Some pathogenic fungi exhibit two different growth phases, forming typical mycelial colonies on laboratory culture media but forming small yeastlike structures in the tissues of the infected individual.

> **Hyphae** Filamentous branching structures formed by fungi.

> **Mycelium** Matted mass of hyphae forming a fluffy colony characteristic of fungi.

Some fungi live on the skin and only occasionally cause minor discomfort. Others are found in small numbers in the oral cavity, gastrointestinal tract, and vagina, where they live in harmony with the normal bacterial flora. Most fungi have a limited ability to cause disease. Under special circumstances, however, fungi may produce serious localized or systemic infections in susceptible individuals. Two major factors predispose to systemic fungal infections: disturbance in the normal bacterial flora and impaired immunologic defenses.

After intensive therapy with broad-spectrum antibiotics, the normal bacterial flora of the oral cavity, colon, vagina, and other areas may be altered or completely eradicated, disturbing the normal balance between the bacterial flora and fungi. Normally, the predominance of the bacterial flora holds the fungi in check. When the bacteria are eliminated, the fungi may proliferate and cause disease.

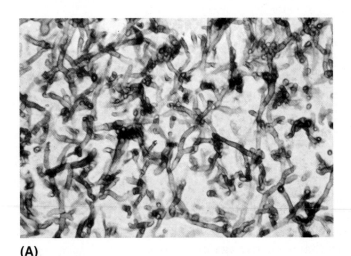

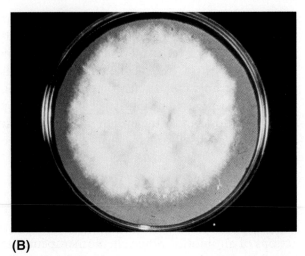

(A) **(B)**

FIGURE 8-9 **(A)** A low magnification photomicrograph illustrating a cluster of fungal hyphae. **(B)** Appearance of fungus colony growing on a laboratory culture medium.

Courtesy of Leonard V. Crowley, MD, Century College.

Patients with various types of chronic debilitating diseases may be susceptible to fungal infections. Infections of this type are also encountered in patients whose immunologic defense mechanisms have been depressed by various drugs and chemicals or by radiation therapy. Patients with certain types of cancer, particularly those treated with cytotoxic drugs, may also develop systemic fungal infections.

SUPERFICIAL FUNGAL INFECTIONS

The common superficial fungal infections of the skin are caused by a group of fungi called **dermatophytes**. They cause itchy, scaling skin lesions on the scalp and on other parts of the body. Some have been given such picturesque, popular names as "athlete's foot" and "jock itch." A common superficial fungal infection of the mucous membranes is caused by a yeastlike fungus called *Candida albicans*. This organism is a common cause of superficial infections of the tongue, mouth, and esophagus (termed **thrush**) in the newborn and in immunosuppressed individuals (**FIGURE 8-10**). Vulvovaginal infections, producing symptoms of itching and vaginal discharge, are common in pregnant women and those taking broad-spectrum antibiotics. A number of antifungal drugs are available that can be applied locally to treat infections caused by dermatophytes and *Candida*.

HIGHLY PATHOGENIC FUNGI

Although most fungi are at best only potential pathogens of low virulence, several are highly infectious and frequently produce disease in humans. They can be identified by biopsy or by culture of infected tissues.

Various species of the fungus *aspergillus* (most often *Aspergillus fumigatus*), a common fungus found in decaying plant material in the soil, can cause both pulmonary disease from inhaled spores and serious, potentially fatal systemic disease in immunocompromised individuals. In the lung, the fungus is responsible for allergic bronchopulmonary aspergillosis, a condition that complicates (and may contribute to) allergic asthma. Individuals with pulmonary cavities (as may occur in those who have had tuberculosis) may develop aspergillomas, fungal balls that reside in such spaces but generally do not invade lung tissue. Invasive aspergillosis most often

Dermatophyte A fungus that causes a superficial infection of the skin.

Thrush Superficial infection of mouth caused by *Candida albicans*.

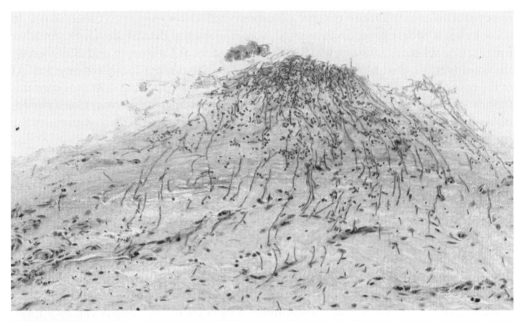

FIGURE 8-10 Esophageal candidiasis in an immunocompromised patient. Both hyphae and yeast forms (small spheres) of the organism are present in this eroded area of the mucosa.

Courtesy of Department of Pathology and Laboratory Medicine, University of North Carolina at Chapel Hill.

occurs in severely immunocompromised patients with very low numbers of circulating neutrophils (**FIGURE 8-11**). In such cases, the fungi may invade blood vessels and spread widely.

The fungus *Histoplasma capsulatum*, which is found in many parts of the United States, causes the disease **histoplasmosis**. This organism is found in the soil. People become infected by inhaling dust containing spores of the fungus. In most cases, the fungus produces an acute, self-limited respiratory infection. Less commonly,

Histoplasmosis
An infection caused by the fungus *Histoplasma capsulatum*.

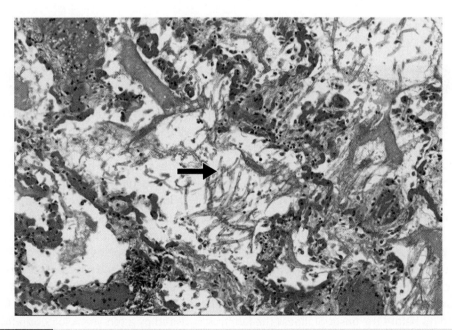

FIGURE 8-11 Invasive aspergillosis in the lung of an immunocompromised patient. Fungal hyphae (*arrow*) are visible in the alveolar spaces.

Courtesy of Department of Pathology and Laboratory Medicine, University of North Carolina at Chapel Hill.

the organism causes a more chronic pulmonary infection similar to tuberculosis. In some cases, a progressive, disseminated, sometimes fatal disease develops. Another fungus, *Coccidioides immitis*, which is found in parts of California and elsewhere in the southwestern part of the United States, causes the disease **coccidioidomycosis**. As in the case of histoplasmosis, humans become infected by inhaling dust that contains fungus spores. The symptoms are similar to those of histoplasmosis. Coccidioidomycosis is usually manifested as an acute pulmonary infection, but sometimes the fungus causes chronic or severe progressive systemic disease.

OTHER FUNGI OF MEDICAL IMPORTANCE

Two other pathogenic fungi of medical importance are *Blastomyces dermatitidis*, which causes the disease **blastomycosis**, and *Cryptococcus neoformans*, which causes *cryptococcosis*. Infections caused by these organisms are less common than either histoplasmosis or coccidioidomycosis. Both organisms are found in the soil, and infection is caused by inhalation of dust containing the organisms.

Clinically, blastomycosis is similar to histoplasmosis and coccidioidomycosis. Most infections are acute and self-limited. Occasionally, the fungus causes a more chronic pulmonary infection or a widespread systemic disease.

Cryptococcus neoformans is a yeastlike organism that has a large mucoid capsule. The organism initially causes a pulmonary infection but then may be transported in the bloodstream to the meninges of the brain, where it causes a chronic meningitis. The organisms can be identified in smears and cultures of spinal fluid.

TREATMENT OF SYSTEMIC FUNGAL INFECTIONS

Acute pulmonary infections caused by fungi frequently subside spontaneously and do not require treatment. Chronic or progressive systemic fungal infections are treated with various systemic antifungal antibiotics; local superficial infections are treated topically.

Coccidioidomycosis A disease caused by the pathogenic fungus *Coccidioides immitis*.

Blastomycosis A systemic fungus infection caused by the fungus *Blastomyces dermatitidis*.

CASE 8-1

A six-year-old male child attending a small private preschool is noted to have a high fever (103° F). He has malaise (is tired) and has lost his appetite (anorexia). His mother notes that his eyes appear red (conjunctivitis), and he has a cough and runny nose (coryza). When the child complains of pain on eating, spots are noted on the mucosa of his mouth opposite his molars (Koplik spots). Soon after, an itching rash appears initially behind his ears that within a day spreads to cover much of his body. The child complains of itching. The rash is "dusky" red and macropapular (has large red areas not raised above the skin that have small raised bumps also termed morbilliform, which look similar to measles) (**FIGURE 8-12A**). The child's pediatrician diagnoses measles (rubeola). The child appears to recover over the next five days. However, on day six he develops a crouplike cough and earache that by day seven progresses to respiratory distress diagnosed as measles pneumonia (**FIGURE 8-12B**). Aggressive respiratory support is provided, but the child dies. The clinical history notes that ten days before the onset of illness the family was visited by a ten-year-old cousin from Central Africa. On questioning, the relatives' parents state that their child had also suffered from a "measleslike" illness but had recovered.

CASE 8-1 (*Continued*)

Discussion

Measles is an extremely contagious viral disease spread by droplets. The virus initially infects tracheal and bronchial epithelia but spreads via lymphatics systemically. The **viremia** produces a notable general immunosuppression that can outlast the acute disease for weeks. The immunosuppression may lead to progressive fatal disease in patients who have preexisting compromise of their immune system. Although measles is considered a benign disease by many, this is not the case. In developing countries, particularly in areas with childhood malnourishment, measles is a major cause of childhood death. Most of these deaths have

Viremia Presence of large numbers of viral particles.

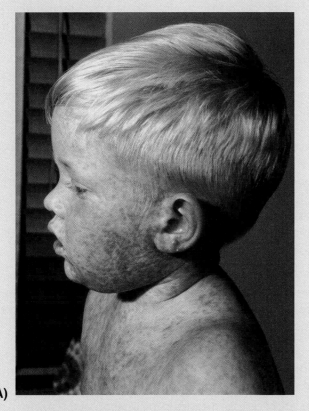

(A)

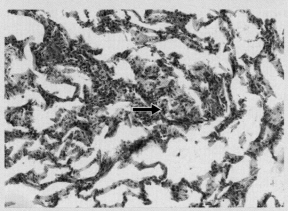

(B)

FIGURE 8-12 **(A)** Macular (morbilliform) rash of measles. **(B)** Measles pneumonia. Note the large number of mononuclear cells in the alveolar walls characteristic of viral disease (interstitial pneumonia). Measles pneumonia is characterized by groups of large multinucleated cells (giant cells) that are virally infected (*arrow*).

(B) Courtesy of Department of Pathology and Laboratory Medicine, University of North Carolina at Chapel Hill.

(*continues*)

CASE 8-1 (Continued)

occurred in Africa and Southeast Asia in areas with poor vaccination programs. It is also a major cause of blindness. In the United States, measles mortality is rare (about 0.1 percent of cases) and generally occurs in children who are immunosuppressed for other extant conditions. In this case, the medical history indicated the child was under therapy for childhood allergic asthma using inhaled corticosteroids, and the child's parents had refused measles vaccination. The asthma therapy may have produced sufficient immunosuppression to account for the progressive viral pneumonia. Other complications of measles are not uncommon and occur in about 30 percent of cases. These complications include ear infection and subsequent hearing loss, diarrheas, and, as noted, pneumonia, which can occur in 5 to 10 percent of cases. Viral encephalitis is an uncommon complication, and, more rarely, a fatal neurodegenerative disease (subacute sclerosing panencephalitis SSPE) may occur five to ten years following measles infection.

Vaccination against measles early in childhood is an extremely effective method of disease prevention. However, the unfounded rumors and inaccurate information that have linked measles vaccination to childhood autism and other diseases have led to a decline in vaccination rates and a resurgence of measles in the United States. Since 2013, there has been a marked increase in reported cases of measles resulting in localized outbreaks in more than twenty states. In the first eight months of 2014, 600 cases of measles were reported, compared to fewer than 100 in 2012. Nearly all of the cases started with importation of disease into the United States by an unvaccinated individual. It is important to realize that in the case of effective vaccination programs, the small number of unvaccinated individuals are protected by herd or community immunity. The unvaccinated remain at high risk of disease by imported infections.

Etiology and Pathogenesis

The etiologic agent is the RNA measles virus, a paramyxovirus closely related to that causing canine distemper. The virus causes systemic infection and immunosuppression, leading to a significant incidence of secondary infections and complications.

Questions

1. A mother asks you why it is necessary to immunize her child against measles as it is a very mild disease. How would you answer her?

2. Over 95 percent of cases of measles in the United States result from disease imported from outside the country. Why is this?

3. The term "herd or community immunity" is used in the case discussion. What does the term mean?

QUESTIONS FOR REVIEW

1. By what standards are bacteria classified? Name the classifications.

2. What is the Gram stain test procedure? What important diseases are caused by the following bacteria: staphylococci, beta streptococci, pneumococci, gonococci, and acid-fast bacteria?

3. What is meant by the following terms: *granulomatous inflammation, gram-positive organism,* and *Legionella?*

4. How do antibiotics inhibit the growth of bacteria? How does penicillin kill bacteria?

5. How do bacteria become resistant to an antibiotic?

6. What are some of the potential harmful effects of antibiotics?

7. What is meant by the following terms: *sensitivity test, resistant organism,* and *cell membrane?*

8. How does a viral infection affect a susceptible cell?

9. What is a latent (asymptomatic) viral infection? Give an example.

10. What is meant by the following terms: *inclusion body, chlamydiae,* and *mycoplasma?*

11. What factors render a patient susceptible to an infection by a fungus of low pathogenicity?

12. What are the names of the two highly pathogenic fungi? What type of disease do they produce?

13. A young woman receives a course of antibiotics and soon afterward develops a vaginal infection caused by a fungus. Why?

SUPPLEMENTARY READINGS

Shors, T. 2011. *Understanding Viruses*. 2nd ed. Burlington, MA: Jones & Bartlett Learning.
▶ This book contains additional information on all aspects of virology, including HIV and Ebola.

Pommerville, J. C. 2014. *Fundamentals of Microbiology*. 10th ed. Burlington, MA: Jones & Bartlett Learning.
▶ Additional information on all aspects of microbiology, including Ebola, can be found in Chapter 16.

Alby, K., and Gilligan, P. H. 2013. Identification of pathogens by classical clinical tests. In *The Prokaryotes*. 4th ed., Vol. 5: *Human Microbiology*, edited by E. Rosenberg, E. F. DeLong, S. Lory, E. Stackebrandt, and F. Thompson. Devon, UK: Springer-Verlag Berlin Heidelberg.
▶ Detailed information on identification of organisms using microscopic examination and culture methods is included in this article on pages 1–45.

Omer, S. B., Salmon, D. A., Orenstein, W. A., et al. 2009. Vaccine refusal, mandatory immunization, and the risks of vaccine-preventable diseases. *New England Journal of Medicine 360*:1981–88.
▶ The success of an immunization program depends on high rates of acceptance and coverage. Rates of refusal of immunization are increasing, and clustering of refusals leads to outbreaks of vaccine-preventable diseases. Children with exemptions from school immunization requirements, which is a measure of vaccine refusal, are at increased risk for measles and pertussis. In turn, they can infect others who are too young to be vaccinated, cannot be vaccinated for medical reasons, or were vaccinated but did not achieve a sufficient immunologic response. Clinicians can play a crucial role in promoting vaccination by respectfully listening to parents' concerns and discussing the risks and benefits of immunization.

Chen, S. P. 2015. *Measles*. Medscape. http://emedicine.medscape.com/article/966220-overview
▶ The details used to construct the case and additional detailed information on the disease can be found here.

Centers for Disease Control. *Ebola (Ebola Virus Disease)*. http://www.cdc.gov/vhf/ebola/index.html
▶ The ongoing Ebola outbreak in Central West Africa has led to a large number of publications detailing the epidemiology and clinical details of the disease as well as the molecular biology of the virus. An excellent starting place for detailed information can be found here.

Parasitic Disease

1. List the common types of parasites and their associated human infections.

2. Describe a typical parasite life cycle.

3. Compare and contrast parasitic disease in humans and animals.

4. Explain how these infections are acquired.

5. Describe their clinical manifestations, and explain their clinical and economic significance.

The Parasite and Its Host

Animal parasites are organisms adapted to living within or on the body of another animal, called the **host**, and are no longer capable of free-living existence. Many animal parasites have a complex life cycle. An immature form of a parasite may spend part of its cycle within the body of an animal or fish (the **intermediate host**) before the mature parasite eventually takes up residence within the body of the final host (the **definitive host**). Because many animal parasites live in the intestinal tract and discharge eggs in the feces, transmission is favored by conditions of poor sanitation and by relatively high temperature and humidity, which enhance survival of the parasite in its infective stage. Therefore, parasitic infections are common in tropical climates but are much less frequent in cold or temperate climates. Specific drugs are available to treat almost all parasitic infections effectively. Insect **vectors** may transmit the parasite from the intermediate or definitive host to humans who may serve as an **opportunistic (accidental) host**.

Animal parasites are classified into three large groups: **protozoa**, which are simple, one-celled organisms; **metazoa**, which are more complex, multicellular structures; and **arthropods**, which are small insects. Parasitic diseases, particularly those involving helminths (worms), may be accompanied by eosinophilia (high circulating eosinophil count). These white cells in the blood may play a role in the host defense against such parasitic agents.

Host Individual infected with a disease-producing organism.

Intermediate host Place of residence of an immature form of a parasite.

Definitive host Residence of mature form of a parasite.

Vectors Transmission agent of parasite; may be insects or other animals.

Opportunistic host Accidental host of parasite; often humans.

Protozoa Simple one-celled animal parasites, such as the plasmodium causing malaria.

Metazoa Complex multicelled animal parasites, such as worms and flukes.

Arthropod Invertebrate animal with jointed limbs and segmented body, such as insect and spider. Important arthropods that parasitize humans include the crab louse and the organism causing scabies.

Parasitic diseases are often thought of as being limited to populations in less developed countries, but the Centers for Disease Control (CDC) notes that these diseases can infect anyone regardless of socioeconomic status. There is no doubt that parasitic diseases are a major health burden in developing nations, malaria being a prime example, and minorities, immigrants, and people living under disadvantaged conditions are at the highest risk. Parasitic diseases affect a significant number of individuals with what may be a severe disease and, in some cases, one that can be easily prevented and treated. Five so-called neglected parasitic diseases have been singled out by the CDC to improve awareness among physicians and the public in the United States: Chagas disease, neurocysticercosis, toxocariasis, toxoplasmosis, and trichomoniasis. These diseases are discussed in the appropriate sections along with other parasitic diseases of importance.

Infections Caused by Protozoa and Related Organisms

Some of the more important protozoal infections in humans include malaria, caused by various species of *Plasmodium*; amebic dysentery, caused by a pathogenic, ameba *Entamoeba histolytica*; Chagas disease (American trypanosomiasis caused by *Trypanosoma cruzi*), a systemic disease causing serious damage to the heart; Leishmaniasis, caused by various species of the protozoan *Leishmania*, resulting in ulcerating skin lesions and a multisystem visceral disease termed kala azar; trichomonad infections of the genital tract, caused by the parasite *Trichomonas vaginalis*; Giardiasis, caused by *Giardia lamblia*, which infects the small intestine; Toxoplasmosis, caused by *Toxoplasma gondii*, which may infect the fetus and cause congenital malformations; and Cryptosporidiosis, caused by a parasite called *Cryptosporidium parvum*, which parasitizes the intestinal tract and can cause severe diarrhea (**TABLE 9-1**).

This list is not exhaustive. Other protozoal diseases may have serious consequences in animal husbandry and occasionally infect humans who serve as an opportunistic host when exposed to infected animals and insect vectors. An example is babesiosis, which is most often asymptomatic or produces only mild disease in humans. The organism can cause a malaria-like disease, destroying erythrocytes in asplenic or immunocompromised people. The primary host of the protozoan parasite (*Babesia* species) are rodents (most often deer mice in the United States). Deer ticks serve as a vector, and increased deer populations result in increased risk although the disease is seen in very limited regions including Cape Cod and the coastal area and islands of New England and Long Island.

MALARIA

Malaria is caused by several species of the protozoan parasite *Plasmodium*, which has a complicated life cycle. The parasite is transmitted to humans by the bite of the Anopheles mosquito, which breeds in swampy lowland areas. The name malaria dates to the time when in Italy the disease was thought to be caused by breathing night air near lowland marshes and swampy areas (*malo* = bad + *aria* = air). After the parasite and its mosquito vector were recognized, the marshy areas were known to be mosquito breeding grounds, with the mosquitoes most active in the evenings.

The initial source of the parasite is a blood meal taken by an anopheles mosquito from an infected person. The sexual stage of the parasite (gametocytes) reproduces within the insect host, producing the infectious stage of the parasite (sporocytes). Following delivery by a mosquito bite, the parasites begin their development within

TABLE 9-1   Some of the More Common Protozoal Diseases in Humans

Disease	Organism	Transmission	Site of infection	Manifestations
Trichomoniasis	*Trichomonas-vaginalis*	Sexual	• Vagina	• Itching, discharge
Giardiasis	*Giardia lamblia*	Fecal–oral	• Intestines	• Diarrhea • Abdominal pain • Nausea • Dehydration • Constipation • Gas production
Amebiasis	*Entamoebahis-tolytica*	Fecal–oral	• Intestines • Liver	• Diarrhea • Dysentery • Liver abscesses
Malaria	*Plasmodium sp.*	Mosquito bite	• Red blood cells	• Paroxysm (alternating coldness, rigor, and fever) • Symptoms referable to all organ-systems, including joint pain, respiratory distress, convulsions
Trypanosomiasis (Chagas disease)	*Trypanosoma-cruzi*	Bite and feces of "kissing bug"	• Heart • Esophagus	• Cardiomyopathy • Dilation of esophagus
Toxoplasmosis	*Toxoplasma gondii*	Fecal–oral Contaminated meat	• Brain	• Congenital: stunted CNS development • Immune compromised: mental status changes, seizures, encephalitis
Leishmaniasis	*Leishmania sp.*	Sandfly	• Skin • Mucous membranes • Visceral organs	• Skin ulcers • Nasopharyngeal ulcers • Lymphadenopathy • Hepatosplenomegaly • Can infect all tissues of the body, including bone marrow, kidneys, testes
Cryptosporidiosis	*Cryptosporid-ium parvum*	Fecal–oral	• Small intestine	• Diarrhea

the liver and after several weeks invade the red blood cells of the host. There they multiply, feeding on the hemoglobin, which becomes degraded to a product called malarial pigment. Soon, the rapidly multiplying parasites destroy the invaded red cells, releasing masses of new parasites along with red cell debris and malarial pigment into the circulation. This event is associated with an elevated temperature and a shaking chill ("chills and fever"). The newly liberated parasites in turn attack other red cells, continuing the cycles of invasion–multiplication–red cell destruction. The

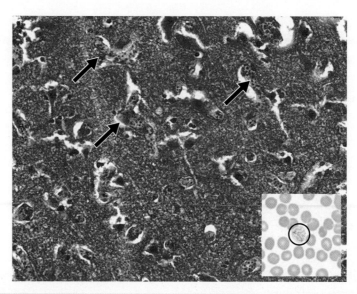

FIGURE 9-1 Cerebral malaria. Malarial parasites are plugging many of the small blood vessels (*arrows*). Inset: Malarial parasites in a red cell smear (*circled*).

Courtesy of Department of Pathology and Laboratory Medicine, University of North Carolina at Chapel Hill.

time required for each species of parasite to complete its cycle is constant, so the episodes of chills and fever tend to occur at regular intervals every forty-eight or seventy-two hours, depending on the species. In addition to suffering repeated, periodic chills and fever, infected individuals frequently become anemic because of the excessive red cell destruction. Often their spleens and livers enlarge when phagocytic cells in the spleen proliferate and become filled with debris and malarial pigment. In one type of malaria, clumps of parasitized red cells may plug small blood vessels in the brain (cerebral malaria), heart, or other vital organs. This serious complication impedes blood flow to the affected organs and may be fatal. Diagnosis of malaria is established by demonstrating the parasite in properly prepared and stained slides made from the blood of the infected patient (**FIGURE 9-1**).

Malaria is a major health problem in many parts of the world and is widespread in many less developed countries, including parts of Africa, Asia, Central America, and South America. More than 200 million people are affected at any given time, and 1 to 3 million people die of the disease each year. Few infectious diseases have had such a profound effect on the social and economic development of countries. Malaria is no longer a major public health problem in the United States, Canada, and Europe. Most of the 2,000 cases of malaria diagnosed in the United States are contracted by people who have traveled to or have immigrated from areas where malaria occurs frequently. Various antimalarial drugs are available to prevent infection when traveling in an endemic area and to treat an established infection. Unfortunately, parasites are becoming resistant to many of the commonly used antimalarial drugs, which makes treatment more difficult.

AMEBIASIS

Trophozoite Active, motile vegetative phase of a parasite

Amebiasis is an infection of the intestinal tract by a pathogenic ameba, *Entamoeba histolytica*. The life cycle of the parasite includes an active, motile, vegetative phase (called a **trophozoite**) and a relatively resistant cystic phase. Humans become infected by ingesting cysts of the parasite in contaminated food and water. The motile phase of the parasite develops from the cyst and invades the mucosa of the colon, producing mucosal ulcers and causing symptoms of inflammation of the colon. Occasionally,

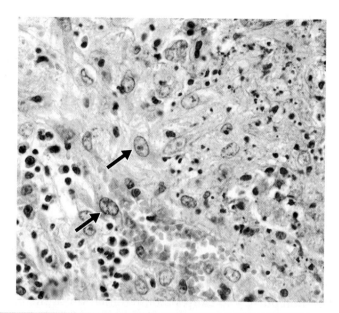

FIGURE 9-2 Amebic liver abscess. Several examples of trophozoites are highlighted (*arrows*).
Courtesy of Department of Pathology and Laboratory Medicine, University of North Carolina at Chapel Hill.

the amebas are carried to the liver in the portal circulation and may cause amebic hepatitis or amebic liver abscess (**FIGURE 9-2**).

CHAGAS DISEASE (AMERICAN TRYPANOSOMIASIS)

Chagas disease is caused by the protozoan *Trypanosoma cruzi*, which produces an endemic infection in both wild and domestic animals. The disease is transmitted to humans by a vector (triatomine insects or "kissing bugs"). The parasite and insect vector are present in animal populations in the Southwest of the United States, but the disease is most common in South and Central America where infection is associated with poor living conditions that allow insects entry into dwellings. The overwhelming majority of people with Chagas disease in the United States were infected in Mexico where the prevalence of the disease is about 1 percent. Overall about 10 million individuals in the United States are estimated to suffer from chronic Chagas disease. The organisms spread systemically after entry and parasitize muscle, most frequently the heart, resulting in severe acute myocarditis and necrosis of affected tissue. The disease may cause a chronic infected state with progressive heart failure and disease of the gastrointestinal tract. Chagas disease may also be transferred by blood products. Active insect eradication programs and screening of blood products has reduced disease frequency in many South American countries. Effective antiparasitic drug therapy is available.

LEISHMANIASIS

Leishmaniasis occurs as a variety of syndromes in different geographic areas depending on the particular species of the causative leishmanian protozoan responsible. The disease is endemic in a variety of animal populations and is transmitted to humans by the bite of phlebotomus sandflies. The disease is found in a cutaneous form, which produces ulcerating skin lesions (oriental or tropical sores) that often heal spontaneously. The disease is found in the Middle East, Asia, tropical and North Africa, and Central and South America. Rare cases have occurred in Texas and Oklahoma, but 75 percent of those diagnosed among civilians in the USA were acquired in tourist destinations such as Costa Rica. The action in Iraq and Afghanistan led to at least

2,000 cases in military personnel. The mucocutaneous form of the disease (found predominantly in Central and South America) produces progressive and disfiguring ulcers where the mucous membrane and skin meet (e.g., in the nasal septum and mouth) and requires antiprotozoan therapy. Visceral leishmaniasis (kala azar) is a systemic form of the disease with massive enlargement of the spleen and liver. The name comes from the Hindi for "black fever" because of a characteristic darkening of the skin in severely affected individuals. This form of the disease occurs predominantly in the Indian subcontinent and Brazil. Without treatment, kala azar leads to severe wasting and death. Although uncommon in the United States, there are an estimated 1 million cases of cutaneous and 0.3 million cases of visceral disease per year worldwide.

TRICHOMIAD GENITAL TRACT INFECTIONS

The trichomonads are small motile parasites. One species, *Trichomonas vaginalis*, sometimes causes an acute inflammation of the vagina characterized by itching, burning, and a profuse, frothy vaginal discharge. The infection can be transmitted to the male by sexual intercourse and causes an inflammation of the urethra. *T. vaginalis* infection is one of the most common sexually transmitted diseases (STDs). Infection increases the risk of HIV transmission and is associated with problems in pregnancy, including low birth weight and intrauterine infection (**FIGURE 9-3**).

GIARDIASIS

Giardia intestinalis is a small, pear-shaped parasite that inhabits the duodenum and upper jejunum and is the most commonly detected intestinal parasite in the United States. Giardiasis manifests with crampy abdominal pain, distention, and severe watery diarrhea and occurs in both animals and humans. Beavers are the source of contamination commonly found in much raw water from natural sources such as lakes or ponds. Since parasites are present in the stools of infected individuals, the disease is usually transmitted from humans by means of contaminated food and water. Giardiasis is relatively common in St. Petersburg, Russia, where many American tourists have been infected. Several epidemics caused by contaminated water supplies have occurred, most frequently in the western mountain regions of the United States.

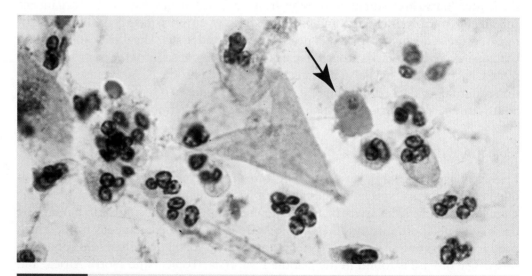

FIGURE 9-3 Vaginal secretions from women with trichomonad infection, illustrating a parasite (*arrow*) and many neutrophils.

Courtesy of Leonard V. Crowley, MD, Century College.

TOXOPLASMOSIS

Toxoplasma gondii is a small intracellular parasite that infects a large number of birds and animals as well as humans. Many cats are infected with the parasite and excrete an infectious form of the organism in their stools. The parasite is frequently present in the flesh of cattle and many other animals. People acquire toxoplasma infections by ingesting raw or partially cooked meat that is infected with the parasite or by contact with infected cats whose feces may contain an infectious form of the parasite called an **oocyst**. Usually the infection does not cause symptoms in healthy adults. About 50 percent of the adult population has had a previous inapparent infection and is immune. The importance of toxoplasmosis is related to its effect on the fetus. If a susceptible (nonimmune) woman acquires a toxoplasma infection during pregnancy, the parasite may be transmitted to the fetus. Infection of the fetus causes severe injury to fetal tissues and often leads to congenital malformations that are described in the discussion on congenital and hereditary disease.

Toxoplasmosis, like other parasitic diseases, is of increased risk to the immunocompromised. In these people, toxoplasmosis most commonly causes a disease of the brain, toxoplasmosis encephalitis (**FIGURE 9-4**). The disease may result either from a first exposure to the parasite or from reactivation of an infection acquired many years previously.

CRYPTOSPORIDIOSIS

Cryptosporidium parvum, *Cryptosporidium hominis*, and several other species found commonly in animals are protozoal parasites related to toxoplasma and are an important cause of severe diarrhea in both immunocompetent and immunocompromised people. Crptosporidosis became well-known when nearly half a million people in Milwaukee, Wisconsin, developed the disease in 1993. Many large outbreaks have occurred subsequently in the United States and in England and other European countries. The organism infects cattle, other farm animals, and people, who excrete large numbers of the infectious forms of the parasites called oocysts in their feces. Fecal material from farm animals can contaminate surface water flowing into rivers and lakes, and oocysts have been identified in 65 to 85 percent of surface water

Toxoplasma gondii
A small intracellular parasite of birds, animals, and humans. Causes the disease toxoplasmosis.

Oocyst Infectious form of a parasite.

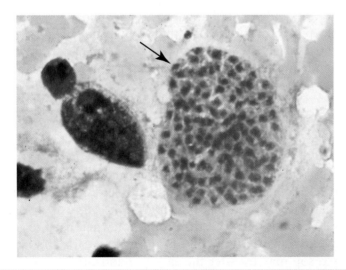

FIGURE 9-4 Cerebral toxoplasmosis demonstrated by brain biopsy. The cyst (*arrow*) is composed of a large cluster of organisms.

Courtesy of Leonard V. Crowley, MD, Century College.

samples tested throughout the United States. The infectious oocyst has a thick wall and is quite small, only about half the size of a red blood cell. It is highly resistant to chlorination of water supplies and must be removed from municipal water supplies by filtration. People can become infected by ingesting oocysts in unfiltered municipal water supplies, from oocyst-contaminated water in swimming pools, or by person-to-person fecal–oral transmission in the same way that other intestinal infections are transmitted. The infection is easily transmitted person to person in households and in child day care facilities.

When oocysts are ingested, the cyst wall disintegrates in the intestinal tract, releasing the infectious parasite, which multiplies and infects the intestinal epithelial cells. Only a few oocysts are enough to cause an infection, and people with diarrhea excrete large numbers of oocysts in their stool. People with normal immune defenses experience an acute self-limited diarrhea, but people with AIDS and other immunocompromised people develop a severe chronic life-threatening diarrheal disease. Antiparasitic therapy is of limited utility but appears to shorten the duration of the disease.

Metazoal Infections

The three large groups of metazoal helminthic (wormlike) parasites are roundworms (nematodes), tapeworms (cestodes), and flukes or flatworms (trematodes). Some of the more common examples are summarized in **TABLE 9-2**.

ROUNDWORMS

A number of nematodes are intestinal parasites in humans. For the most part, parasitization does not lead to clinical symptoms until the parasite load becomes very large. Intestinal nematodes are of greatest concern in tropical areas and regions of poor sanitation where shed eggs are passed in the feces from person to person, most often infecting children. The overall health burden of such infestation is high; it results in growth retardation and malnutrition with associated developmental problems. Fortunately, drug therapy is safe, effective, and inexpensive. However, hundreds of millions of people remain infected, particularly in developing countries, along with millions of individuals in the United States, particularly in the Southeast. The most important roundworms that parasitize the human intestine are the roundworm *Ascaris*, the pinworm *Enterobius*, the whipworm *Trichuris*, the threadworm *Strongyloides*, and a variety of hookworms. The tissue nematode *Trichinella spiralis*, although uncommon in the United States, is also discussed.

Ascaris

The *Ascaris lumbricoides* is the most commonly encountered parasitic worm, infecting an estimated 1 billion people worldwide. The roundworm is about the size of a large earthworm, lives in the intestinal tract, and discharges eggs in the feces. Direct person-to-person transmission of *Ascaris* eggs does not occur because the eggs expelled in feces are immature, and a maturation period of about a week is required before the eggs become infectious. Maturation of the immature eggs usually occurs in the soil when fecal material is defecated on the ground or when used to fertilize the soil. The mature eggs can survive in the soil for up to two years, and later contact with egg-contaminated soil may transfer the eggs to hands, then to food or beverages, and finally into the intestinal tract.

When mature *Ascaris* eggs are ingested, the larval worms are released from the eggs within the intestinal tract, and burrow through the intestine, where they

TABLE 9-2 Some Common Diseases Caused by Helminths

Organism	Disease	Route of infection	Infected organ(s)	Disease manifestations
Schistosoma sp.	Schistosomiasis (Bilharzia)	Infected water, across the skin	• Skin • Liver • Bladder • Intestine • Kidney • CNS	• Chronic disease • Anemia, malnutrition • Destruction of liver: portal hypertension • Cystitis and ureteritis, progressing to bladder cancer
Enterobius vermicularis	Pinworm	Fecal–oral	• Intestine	• Anal itching
Trichinella spiralis	Trichinosis	Undercooked meat (pork)	• Muscle • Heart	• Muscle pain
Taenia solium	Cysticercosis	Undercooked meat (pork)	• Brain	• Encysted larvae in braincause seizures, headaches
Echinococcus-granulosus	Echinococcosis	Food contaminated by dog feces	• Liver	• Hydatid cysts
Ascaris lumbricoides	Ascariasis	Fecal–oral	• Lung • Intestine	• Pneumonitis • Intestinal obstruction
Trichuris trichiura (whipworm)	Trichuriasis	Fecal–oral	• Intestine	• Abdominal pain • Anemia • Appendicitis • Rectal prolapse
Wuchereria bancrofti (and others)	Filariasis	Mosquito bites	• Lymphatic system	• Lymphatic obstruction, lymphedema, elephantiasis

enter the circulatory system of the liver and then the lungs where they may produce pneumonia-like symptoms. They are then coughed up, and eventually are swallowed, finding their way again into the small intestine where they grow to maturity. At times, mature worms may enter and block the bile or pancreatic ducts or plug the appendix. Rarely, a large mass of worms may completely block the lumen of the small intestine. Mature worms may also be coughed up (**FIGURE 9-5**). The mature worm has a limited life span, so persistent infections are the result of reexposure. An *Ascaris* infection is identified by detecting worm eggs in the fecal material of an infected person or by identifying an adult worm.

Dogs and cats may be infected with a similar type of roundworm that occasionally causes disease in humans. Infection by the animal worm is most common in children who are in close contact with an infected animal. The children transfer the eggs to their mouths by contaminated hands, toys, or other objects.

Whipworms (Trichuriasis)

Trichuriasis, caused by parasitization by *Trichuris trichiura*, is extremely prevalent in warm moist regions, and nearly a billion people may be infected worldwide. The

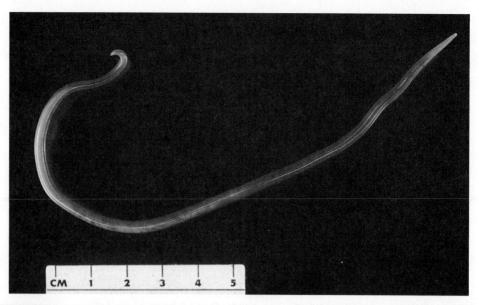

FIGURE 9-5 Large *Ascaris* that migrated into the back of patient's throat and was coughed up.
Courtesy of Leonard V. Crowley, MD, Century College.

disease is common in the Southeast of the United States, infecting several million. As has been seen with other nematodes, whipworm is transferred from fecally contaminated soil by ingestion of eggs. The eggs hatch in the intestine, and adult forms reside in the cecum and ascending colon. The worms burrow into the colonic mucosa, and if infection is heavy, they may cause colitis (although light infections are asymptomatic). Eggs shed by the female worm pass into the feces.

Pinworms

> **Pinworm** A small parasitic worm infecting humans. Lives in lower bowel and causes perianal pruritus.

The small roundworm *Enterobius vermicularis*, called simply the **pinworm** because of its small size, generally measures less than 1 cm in length. Pinworm infections are very common, second only to *Ascaris* infections in frequency, and often infect children, who may harbor a large number of worms in their intestinal tract. Often the infection spreads from the child to the rest of the family members. The infection is acquired from ingesting worm eggs that are transferred to the hands from contaminated bedclothes or other objects. The worms hatch in the duodenum and then travel to the ileocecal region, where they take up residence. Female egg-laden worms migrate out of the colon through the anus, often at night while the child is asleep, and deposit their eggs on the perianal skin. The main symptoms of pinworm infection are intense anal and perianal itching caused by irritation resulting from the migration of the worm although the incidence of appendicitis may be increased. Intravaginal infections can occur in females. Pinworm eggs are usually not found in fecal material. The diagnosis of a pinworm infection is made by identifying the eggs deposited by migrating worms on the perianal skin.

Hookworms

Hookworm disease is caused by *Necator americanus* (American hookworm) and several species of *Ancyclostoma*. Infection was once common in the American Southeast but is now nearly eradicated. In the United States, the disease is most commonly found in immigrant populations or in returning travelers. However, parasitic infection is extremely common in many subtropical and tropical areas. It has been estimated that 30 percent of the population of sub-Saharan Africa is infected. Unlike may other parasitic nematodes, hookworm infection occurs by direct contact with larvae in soil contaminated with human feces. Initially the larvae are inactive, but over time they mature into a stage that can rapidly penetrate undamaged skin, usually the hands and feet, where they often provoke extreme itching (ground itch). The larva migrate through the bloodstream into the lungs where they enter the alveoli, move up the respiratory tract and are swallowed, eventually arriving in the small intestine. During their peregrination they may cause pulmonary symptoms, sore throat, and cough. The worms mature and develop a specialized attachment organ (the **buccal plate**) and use this to attach themselves to the mucosa of the small intestine. They cause local bleeding by damaging vessels and secreting digestive enzymes and an anticoagulant substance. Sexually mature worms produce eggs that pass into the stool. Intestinal blood loss is the major clinical effect, which may lead to iron deficiency anemia, malnutrition, and potentially low levels of blood proteins because of worm ingestion in severe cases.

Buccal plate Specialized attachment organ of hookworms.

Strongyloidiasis

Strongyloidiasis (threadworm) infection by the nematode *Strongyloides stercoralis* has similarities to hookworm in mode of infection via intact skin. In the United States, the disease is most commonly found in immigrant populations. Most cases are asymptomatic; however, immunosuppressed individuals may suffer from hyperinfection syndrome where dissemination of parasites can occur and result in a critical illness requiring immediate therapy.

Trichinella

Another small roundworm, *Trichinella spiralis*, causes a severe parasitic infection called trichinellosis (formerly trichinosis). The organism parasitizes not only humans but also a wide variety of animals. Larval forms of the *Trichinella* are encapsulated as small cystic structures within the muscles of the infected human or animal host. People formerly became infected by eating improperly cooked pork from *Trichinella*-infected animals, but the disease has been eradicated from commercial meat products. Hence, the disease is very uncommon in the United States today, and is related to ingestion of undercooked wild game (bear meat being a common source). After the infected meat has been ingested, the larvae are released from their cysts and develop into mature parasitic worms in the small intestine. The worms then burrow into the intestinal mucosa and produce larvae, which gain access to the circulation and are carried throughout the body. They are filtered out in various tissues, where they incite an intense inflammatory reaction. The parasites that lodge in the muscles of the infected individual become encapsulated, forming small cysts within the muscle (**FIGURE 9-6**). These cysts are the infectious form of the parasite. The phase of larval migration is associated with severe systemic symptoms, and there may also be symptoms referable to disturbed function of organs that have been heavily infiltrated by the parasites. The disease is usually self-limited and ranges from mild to severe depending on parasite load. Initial symptoms (within days of ingestion) relate to gastrointestinal distress. With time, muscle pain and, less commonly, heart problems may occur.

TAPEWORMS

Tapeworms, long, ribbonlike worms that sometimes grow to a length of several feet, can inhabit the intestinal tract. In general, tapeworms cause no great inconvenience to the individual carrying them except for depriving the host of the food that nourishes the worm. Three species of tapeworms are recognized: the pork tapeworm,

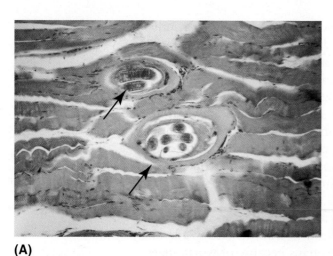

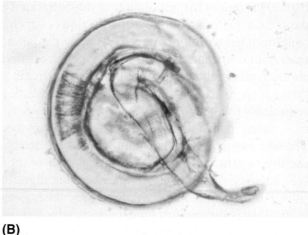

(A)   **(B)**

FIGURE 9-6 Trichinellosis. **(A)** Biopsy of skeletal muscle showing encysted larvae surrounded by fibrous capsules. Each cyst measures about 1 mm in diameter (original magnification × 100). **(B)** Higher magnification view of unstained coiled larva with the capsule removed (original magnification × 400).

Courtesy of Leonard V. Crowley, MD, Century College.

the beef tapeworm, and the fish tapeworm. Humans become infected by eating the flesh of an infected animal that contains the larval form of the parasite. Accidental ingestion of pork tapeworm (*Taenia solium*) ova can result in neurocysticercosis, a common parasitic disease of the nervous system in developing countries that is a common cause of acquired epilepsy. Infection can result from a human carrier or from contaminated food products. In the United States, the disease is found in immigrant populations, particularly among Hispanics in the Southwest, and appears to be increasing in frequency. Treatment of the disease is complex and depends on the stage of the infecting organism; it may require surgical removal of cysts from brain spaces and symptomatic therapy to reduce neurological consequences.

FLUKES

Flukes are thick, fleshy, short worms provided with suckers for attachment to the host; they have a complex life cycle involving one or more intermediate hosts. Flukes are classified according to the area of the body in which the development of the adult flukes is completed and the eggs are deposited. Some species of flukes live in the intestinal tract; others live in the liver; and one species lives in the lung. Some flukes, called Schistosomes or blood flukes, live in the portal venous system and its tributaries or in the veins draining the bladder, where the eggs cause severe inflammation and damage to the bladder and ureters, which is a major risk factor for development of bladder cancer (**FIGURE 9-7**). Fluke infections are an important cause of illness and disability in some Asiatic countries, but human fluke infections are not seen in the United States or Canada.

Although human fluke infections do not occur in North America, some animal schistosomes can infect humans but are more a nuisance than a cause of serious illness. Birds and mammals, infected with their own specific species of schistosomes, excrete them in their droppings into lakes and other bodies of water, where they develop into the infectious form of the parasite. People who swim in bird or animal schistosome-contaminated lakes may be "attacked" by the parasites, which can penetrate the skin of the swimmers. The parasites cause discrete areas of acute pruritic inflammation at the site where they entered the skin. They cannot cause a systemic

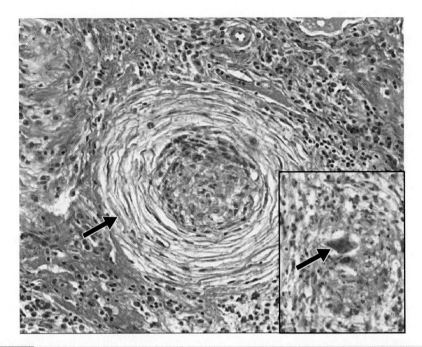

FIGURE 9-7 Schistosomal granuloma in tissue (*arrow*). Inset: Small granuloma surrounding schistosome egg (*arrow*).

Courtesy of Department of Pathology and Laboratory Medicine, University of North Carolina at Chapel Hill.

infection, however, because humans are not the normal host for the parasite, and the parasites are destroyed in the skin by the body's immune defenses. The condition is called *schistosome dermatitis* but is more commonly referred to as "swimmers itch." Many lakes in North America and some saltwater beaches are contaminated by bird or animal schistosomes.

Arthropods

Two common parasitic skin infestations caused by arthropods—scabies and lice—are transmitted by close physical contact and often are spread by sexual contact. Both infestations respond promptly to treatment with antiparasitic medications applied to the skin.

SCABIES

Scabies is caused by a small parasite called *Sarcoptes scabiei*, which burrows in the superficial layers of the skin, where it lays eggs that hatch in a few days. The infestation causes intense itching. The tracks made by the parasites as they burrow in the skin appear as fine, wavy, dark lines in the skin measuring from 1 mm to 1 cm in length. Common sites of involvement are the base of the fingers, the wrists, the armpits, the skin around the nipples, and the skin around the belt line.

CRAB LOUSE INFESTATION

The most common and best-known infectious louse is the **crab louse** (*Phthirus pubis*), which lives in the anal and genital hairs. The organism also causes intense itching. The louse lays eggs that become attached to the hair shafts. Diagnosis is established by identifying either the parasite or the eggs.

Crab louse A parasite of the pubic area; causes intense itching.

CASE 9-1

The patient is an eighteen-year-old female who initially noted a swollen warm area on her left cheek accompanied by a low grade fever, headache, muscle aches, and other nonspecific symptoms. Two days later she was alarmed when her right eye became pruritic, swollen, and painful. The condition progressed, and the patient consulted with an ophthalmologist who believed the condition to be either an allergic reaction or a bacterial infection of the conjunctiva and eyelid. Antibiotics were prescribed. The patient did not respond to the therapy and three days later sought attention at a local emergency room for increasing fever and headaches, lack of energy, and shortness of breath with no additional symptoms. In the ER the attending physician inquired about recent travel. The patient noted that she had returned about two weeks before from an eco-tour to Costa Rica. She had slept in a modern facility under insect netting in Puerto Viejo Limon but had gone on a several day raft trip up the Pacure River. During this trip she slept on an open platform covered with an insecticide-treated net. She noted that the net appeared old and had several torn areas. She did not apply insect repellent (as she had been instructed) because what was available was "not organic." She was referred to the infectious disease department for additional workup. Initial blood cultures and eye swabs showed only normal skin bacteria. Liver function tests noted a borderline abnormality. However, both electrocardiogram and transthoracic ultrasound disclosed a number of abnormalities suggestive of mild myocarditis. Analysis of her peripheral blood smear showed *Trypanosoma cruzi* organisms. The results were confirmed by the Center for Disease Control using PCR analysis. The patient was treated for four months with antiparasitic agents. The patient became negative by PCR analysis following three months of therapy.

Discussion

The case (based on one from the author's affiliated hospital with many modifications, see references) demonstrates a typical presentation of acute Chagas disease in a returning traveler from Central America. Chagas disease (American trypanosomiasis) is caused by parasitization by the protozoa *T. cruzi*. It is a zoonotic infection with a multiplicity of both wild and domesticated mammalian hosts. The disease vector is triatomine insects (kissing bugs), which transmit the disease between animal hosts and humans. Triatomines are obligate, nocturnal, blood feeding insects that defecate after feeding. Infection occurs when infected feces are deposited on mucosal surfaces or at the site of the bite. Triatomine insects tend to infest thatch roofs, adobe and brick homes, and substandard dwellings. Oral transmission of fecally contaminated food, congenital infections, and transmission via infected blood products (now much reduced by blood screening) can also occur. In this case, the initial swelling was likely to be the site of an insect bite (a chagoma), which may show local parasite infection or may be the result of an immune reaction to the bite. Such swellings are of minor medical concern. Unilateral eye swelling is a typical sign/symptom of disease and infection of the conjunctiva by the organism. Of more concern is systemic infection by the organism, which can produce acute myocarditis and infection of the brain and its coverings. Treatment is critical as the disease may become chronic and lead to severe cardiac and gastrointestinal disease that are difficult or impossible to treat.

Chagas disease is prevalent in South and Central America where it may produce more disability than malaria. Aggressive insect eradication programs for dwellings and donor blood screening programs have reduced disease frequency; however, deforestation has led to increased movement of insects to more heavily inhabited areas. Only a handful of autochthonous (indigenous) cases of insect vectored Chagas disease have been reported in the United States. This is quite surprising as both the insect vector and infected sylvatic (not domesticated, "wild") mammalian animal hosts, which are the disease reservoirs, are common in the southern United States. In the Southeast raccoons, opossums, and

CASE 9-1 (Continued)

armadillos serve as infected hosts; in the Southwest, woodrats and many other small mammals are infected. In addition, infected domestic dogs have been found in the South. Sylvatic animal dens are often colonized by the vector triatomine insects. Hence, the lack of "native" U.S. disease is likely related to the quality of housing and rarity of vector insect infestation. It is of interest that several of the "native U.S. cases" demonstrated triatomine insects in the dwelling.

Etiology and Pathogenesis

Travel-related infection by *Trypanosoma cruzi* producing acute Chagas disease characterized by cutaneous and ocular symptoms and mild myocarditis.

Questions

1. An essential part of taking a patient's history is to question recent travel outside of the United States. Why is this information of particular relevance in cases of suspected parasitic disease?

2. Parasitic infestation is often considered to be insignificant in the United States. Cite examples of protozoal parasitic disease that have caused significant public health problems in the United States.

3. Several roundworm (nematode) parasites still frequently occur in the United States, particularly in children. What simple precautions can be taken to prevent infestation?

QUESTIONS FOR REVIEW

1. What are some of the more important protozoal infections?
2. How is malaria transmitted?
3. What is trichinellosis? How is it transmitted?
4. What are the more important worm infestations? What are their manifestations?
5. What parasitic diseases are acquired from unclean water sources?
6. How do people become infected with pinworms? How do they acquire an *Ascaris* infection?
7. What is the source of most parasitic disease in the United States?

SUPPLEMENTARY READINGS

Centers for Disease Control and Prevention. *Parasites*. www.cdc.gov/parasites/

▶ A large number of texts discuss the study of parasitic disease (parasitology) in great detail. However, the CDC is an authoritative source that is readily available, up to the minute, and should always be consulted first.

Centers for Disease Control and Prevention. *Yellow Book* and *Travelers' Health*. www.cdc.gov/travel/

▶ This site has definitive information on travel-related health and provides links to the definitive "Yellow Book" with information on disease risks country by country.

Bern, C., Kjos, S., Yabsley, M. J., and Montgomery, S. P. 2011. *Trypanosoma cruzi* and Chagas' disease in the United States. *Clinical Microbiology Reviews 24*:655–81.

Carter, Y. L., Juliano, J. J., Montgomery, S. P., and Qvarnstorm, Y. 2012. Case report: Acute Chagas disease in a returning traveler. *American Journal of Tropical Medicine and Hygiene 87*:1038–40.

▶ Two useful references to *Trypanosoma cruzi* and Chagas disease with particular reference to the United States. (Note: The case is in part based on the second reference.)

Dorny, P., Praet, N., Deckers, N., and Gabriel, S. 2009. Emerging food-borne parasites. *Veterinary Parasitology 163*:196–206.

Ito, A., and Budke, C. M. 2014. Culinary delights and travel? A review of zoonotic cestodiases and metacestodiases. *Travel Medicine and Infectious Disease 12*(6):582–91.

▶ Two references for those interested in exotic foods and the parasites therein.

Omura, S., and Crump, A. 2014. Ivermectin: Panacea for resource poor communities?, *Trends in Parasitology 30*:445–55.

▶ A new pharmalogical approach to parasitic (and other) diseases.

Hartley, M. A., et al. 2014. The immunological, environmental and phylogenetic perpetrators of metastatic leishmaniasis, *Trends in Parasitology 30*:412–22.

▶ An article of particular interest in its treatment of antiparasite host defense.

Alonso, P. L., et al. 2011. A research agenda to underpin malaria eradication. *PLOS Medicine 8*:e1000406.

▶ An excellent series of articles on the current status of attempts to eradicate malaria. The supplement referenced contains a number of short review articles. Malaria is an increasing worldwide problem and is becoming harder to control because the organisms are becoming resistant to antimalarial drugs. About 1,000 new cases are reported annually in the United States, usually acquired outside the country by travelers, military personnel, and immigrants from malaria-endemic countries, but a small number of cases are acquired in the United States.

Communicable Disease Control and Sexually Transmitted Disease

LEARNING OBJECTIVES

1. Explain how communicable diseases are transmitted and controlled.

2. List the common sexually transmitted diseases. Describe their major clinical manifestations, complications, and methods of treatment.

3. Describe the symptoms of herpes infection in men and women. Explain the effects on sexual partners. Describe how herpes may affect a fetus or newborn infant of an infected mother.

4. Understand the pathogenesis of human immunodeficiency virus infections, the groups affected, and the effects of the virus on the immune system. List the major clinical manifestations of the infection, the significance of a positive test for antibody to the virus, and methods of preventing spread of the infection.

Methods of Transmission and Control

An infectious disease that is readily transmitted from person to person is considered a **communicable disease.** Such a disease is said to be **endemic** (*en* = within + *demos* = population) if small numbers of cases are continually present in the population without the need for the disease being imported. It reaches **epidemic** proportions (*epi* = upon + *demos* = population) when relatively large numbers of people are affected. Sometimes an endemic disease may flare up and assume epidemic proportions.

METHODS OF TRANSMISSION

A communicable disease may be transmitted from person to person by either direct or indirect methods. Direct transmission is either by direct physical contact, by contact with a contaminated inanimate object (**fomite**), or by means of droplet spread, such as by coughing or sneezing. Indirect transmission of an infectious agent is accomplished by some intermediary mechanism, such as transmission in contaminated water or by means of insects. A few communicable diseases are primarily diseases of animals and are transmitted to humans only incidentally (**FIGURE 10-1**).

For a communicable disease to perpetuate itself, there must be a continuous transmission of the infectious agent from person to person by either direct or indirect methods. Therefore, to eradicate or control the disease, the chain of transmission must be broken at some point.

Communicable disease
A disease transmitted from person to person.

Endemic disease
A communicable disease in which small numbers of cases are continually present in a population.

Epidemic disease
A communicable disease affecting concurrently large numbers of people in a population.

Fomite Contaminated inanimate object that can transmit disease.

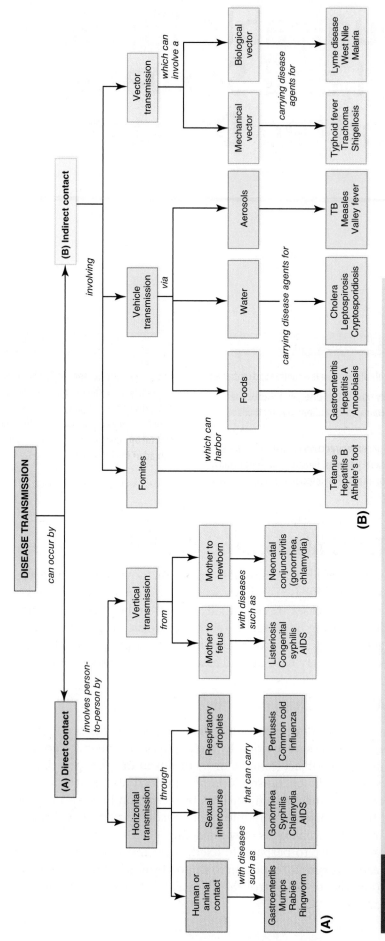

FIGURE 10-1 Transmission of microorganisms and viruses. **(A)** Transmission by direct contact. **(B)** Transmission by indirect contact.

METHODS OF CONTROL

This section deals with some of the methods that can be applied to control communicable diseases. In practice, multiple methods of control are applied whenever possible.

Immunization

If a large proportion of the population can be immunized against a communicable disease, the disease will eventually die out because there will be very few susceptible people in the population. This assumes there are no animal or other reservoirs that maintain the disease. Smallpox is an example of a disease that has no nonhuman reservoir and has been eliminated worldwide because of widespread immunization. Poliomyelitis is another disease that has been virtually eradicated in the United States as a result of widespread immunization of people at risk. Immunization can be used to protect susceptible people entering a foreign country where a communicable disease is endemic. The immunized person will no longer be susceptible to the disease, even though the disease is widespread in the native population.

Immunization may be either active or passive. **Active immunization** is accomplished by exposing the person to either killed or a noninfectious form of the pathogen to provoke an immune response, which will prevent (or moderate) the disease if the person is exposed to the pathogen. Active immunization is generally parenteral (subcutaneous or intramuscular and occasionally by oral or intranasal routes). Highly purified fragments of pathogens (sometimes produced using recombinant genetic technology) are often combined with substances termed **adjuvants** or are incorporated into other nonpathogenic microorganisms to enhance the immune response. **Passive immunization** relies on the transfer of the protein products of the immune system (immunoglobulins) from an immunized animal or human into the person to be protected. Passive immunization is relatively short-lived as the host does not produce protective immunoglobulins of its own. Passive immunization has been used in the past to prevent disease prior to its occurrence or to counteract the effect of toxins produced by an organism (such as in the case of tetanus or botulism). During the recent outbreak of Ebola viral disease, blood plasma containing immunoglobulins reactive with the virus from individuals who had survived the disease was used to treat acutely ill patients with some apparent success. Passive immunization is accomplished by parenteral routes: intramuscularly (using purified immunoglobulins) or intravenously (using specially treated purified immunoglobulins or in some cases whole blood plasma). Passive immunization using immunoglobulins from animals has the risk of provoking allergic reactions in the treated individual.

Active immunization Exposing a person to a non-infectious pathogen to provoke an immune response.

Adjuvant Substance that enhances an immune response.

Passive immunization Transfer of immunoglobulin from an immunized animal or person to the person to be protected.

Identification, Isolation, and Treatment of Infected People

The point at which an infected person becomes capable of transmitting the disease agent is critical. If a person is capable of transmitting disease prior to becoming symptomatic, identification of infected people is problematic (or impossible). For example, the Ebola virus outbreak led to calls for isolation of those capable of transmitting the disease. Transmission of Ebola (and many other viral diseases) depends on a sufficient level of virus to be present in body fluids or secretions. (Ebola is not spread by droplets as is influenza and other respiratory viruses but rather by direct contact with viremic body fluids.) The first sign of Ebola infection is fever; however, fever is a nonspecific indicator of many diseases likely to be present in a population. Gastrointestinal symptoms are next in the progression of Ebola pathogenesis, and it is clear that at this point transmission by contact with body fluids is possible. Current evidence suggests that individuals suffering the febrile prodrome of Ebola may not have detectable levels of virus in their blood. So at what point should individuals potentially exposed to Ebola be isolated? The question is of great concern to public health experts, epidemiologists, and the public at large. There is, however, no question that sick people should be identified and treated promptly to shorten the time during which they can infect others. Isolation of infected people prevents contact with susceptible people and stops the spread of the disease. Identification, isolation, and treatment are the primary methods used to control diseases when effective methods of immunization are not available. These measures are sometimes difficult to accomplish because some diseases produce relatively few symptoms in the infected individual until late in the course of the disease. For example, the person infected with tuberculosis or a sexually transmitted disease may spread the disease to others, but his or her own disease may not be recognized and treated because the person does not feel ill and does not seek medical treatment.

Control of Means of Indirect Transmission

Various control measures can be instituted, depending on the manner by which the infectious agent is transmitted. When the transmission is by means of contaminated food or water, methods of control include chlorination (or similar treatments) of water supplies and establishment of effective sewage treatment facilities, control of food handlers, and standards for monitoring the manufacture and distribution of commercially prepared foods. When a disease is transmitted by insects, either between people or between infected animals and people, it is necessary to eradicate or control the insects that transmit the disease. When a disease is spread from animals to people, control of the animal source of infection also is required.

Requirements for Effective Control

Application of effective control measures requires knowing the cause of the disease and its method of transmission. If this information is not available, control measures are often ineffective. For example, bubonic plague, the "black death" of the Middle Ages, decimated entire populations because the people understood neither the cause of the disease nor how it was transmitted and therefore were unable to protect themselves from its ravages. Although the forty-day quarantine enforced on trading vessels ensured that infection of sailors and traders would be obvious, the time period was insufficient to ensure the death of fleas present in trade goods (textiles, for example). We now know that plague is primarily a disease of rats and other rodents, that it is caused by a bacterium, and that it is transmitted to people by rat flea bites. In some cases, the plague bacillus causes a pulmonary infection in people. When this occurs, direct transmission from person to person can be through droplet spread, causing an extremely contagious and highly fatal pulmonary infection called *pneumonic plague*. In some parts of the Southwest and West United States, plague infection still persists in some rodent populations, but plague is no longer a serious problem if recognized because the disease can be largely prevented in people by controlling the infected animal population and by instituting measures that prevent close contact between potentially infected rodents and people. Transmission from person to person is prevented by prompt isolation and treatment of infected individuals using antibiotics.

Types of Communicable Disease

There are many types of communicable disease caused by microorganisms, virus, or parasites. For most, transmission is limited to a few people, and the disease is easily contained. Specific details on transmission and symptoms for these diseases are presented in discussions concerning the specific microorganisms or in discussions of the body organs affected. One exception to limited transmission are the sexually transmitted diseases, which remain a major public health problem and are discussed in this chapter. Because transmission of these diseases occurs during intimate (and most often private) interactions between individuals and because prevention of transmission requires modification of such interactions (such as the use of condoms during sexual contact), the sexually transmitted diseases are worthy of special consideration.

Sexually Transmitted Diseases Other Than HIV

Sexually transmitted diseases are communicable diseases that spread primarily by sexual contact and have reached near epidemic proportions. They can be transmitted by sexual relations between heterosexual or homosexual partners (more generally termed "men who have sex with men" [MSM] in the behavioral and epidemiological literature) both by genital-genital or genital-oral and anal contact. The four major sexually transmitted diseases are syphilis, gonorrhea, genital herpes infection, and genital chlamydial infections (**TABLE 10-1**). Although often not so classified, cervical

TABLE 10-1 Comparison of Four Major Sexually Transmitted Diseases

	Syphilis	**Gonorrhea**	**Herpes**	**Chlamydia**
Organism	*Treponema pallidum*	Gonococcus (*Neisseria gonorrhoeae*)	Herpes virus	*Chlamydia trachomatis*
Major clinical manifestations	Primary: chancre Secondary: systemic infection with skin rash and enlarged lymph nodes Tertiary: late destructive lesions in internal organs	Urethritis Cervicitis Pharyngitis Infection of rectal mucosa (proctitis)	Superficial vesicles and ulcers on external genitalia and in genital tract Regional lymph nodes often enlarged and tender	Cervicitis Urethritis
Tests used to establish diagnosis	Demonstration of treponemas in chancre Serologic tests	Culture of organisms from sites of infection Nonculture tests also available	Demonstration of intranuclear inclusions in infected cells Virus cultures Serologic tests in some cases	Detection of chlamydial antigens in cervical/urethral secretions Fluorescence microscopy Cultures Nonculture tests also available
Major complications	Damage to cardiovascular system and nervous system in tertiary syphilis may be fatal	Disseminated bloodstream infection Tubal infection with impaired fertility Spread of infection to prostate and epididymides	Spread from infected mother to infant	Tubal infection with impaired fertility Epididymitis
Treatment	Antibiotics	Antibiotics	Antiviral drug shortens infection but not curative	Antibiotics

cancer also may be considered as a sexually transmitted disease caused by human papilloma virus (HPV) infection. In a class by itself because of its devastating consequences and high mortality is the **acquired immune deficiency syndrome (AIDS)**, which is transmitted by either homosexual or heterosexual contacts and by blood and secretions from infected people.

Other common but less serious sexually transmitted diseases are anal and genital warts (condylomas) caused by HPV, nonspecific vaginitis caused by pathogenic microorganisms such as *Gardnerella* in conjunction with anaerobic vaginal bacteria, and trichomonal vaginitis caused by the protozoan parasite *Trichomonas vaginalis*. Other diseases including scabies and crabs, animal parasites, hepatitis B, and some gastrointestinal tract infections are also sometimes transmitted sexually.

SYPHILIS

Syphilis, caused by the spirochete *Treponema pallidum*, is a very serious sexually transmitted disease because it may cause severe damage in almost any organ of the body. If the disease is not treated, it progresses through three stages called primary, secondary, and tertiary syphilis. Each stage has its own characteristic clinical manifestations (**FIGURE 10-2**). Although often thought of as an uncommon disease well under control in the population, this is not the case. In the last eight years, the number of syphilis cases has doubled to almost 17,000 cases per year. Currently syphilis is primarily a disease of males (>90 percent) and much of the increase is among the MSM population. This serves as a reminder that to be effective, safe sex practices must be observed by all regardless of preferred sexual behavior.

Primary Syphilis

Contact with an infected partner enables the treponemes to penetrate the mucous membranes of the genital tract, oral cavity, or rectal mucosa, or to be introduced through a break in the skin. The organisms multiply rapidly and spread throughout the body. After an incubation period of up to several weeks, a small ulcer called a **chancre** develops at the site of inoculation. It is easily seen if it is on the penis or vulva, but it may be undetected if it is within the vagina, oral cavity, or rectum (**FIGURE 10-2A**).

The chancre, which is swarming with treponemes and is highly infectious, persists for about four to six weeks and eventually heals even if the disease is untreated. Even though the chancre has healed, however, the treponemes are widely disseminated through the body and continue to multiply.

Secondary Syphilis

The secondary stage of syphilis begins several weeks to months after the chancre has healed. The infected individual develops manifestations of a systemic infection characterized by elevated temperature, enlargement of lymph nodes, a skin rash, and shallow ulcers on the mucous membranes of the oral cavity and genital tract (mucous patches) (**FIGURE 10-2B**). This stage of the disease also is extremely infectious because the skin and mucous membrane lesions contain large numbers of treponemes. The secondary stage persists for several weeks and, like the chancre, eventually subsides even if no treatment is administered. Some subjects experience one or more recurrences of secondary syphilis, but each recurrence subsides spontaneously.

Tertiary Syphilis

After the second stage subsides, the infected individual appears well for a variable period of time, but the organisms are still active and may cause irreparable damage to the cardiovascular and nervous systems and to other organs as well. Gumma

Acquired immune deficiency syndrome (AIDS) An infection caused by the human immunodeficiency virus. The virus attacks and destroys helper T lymphocytes, which compromises cell-mediated immunity, leading to increased susceptibility to infection and some tumors.

Treponema pallidum The spiral organism causing syphilis.

Chancre Small ulcer at site of syphilis inoculation.

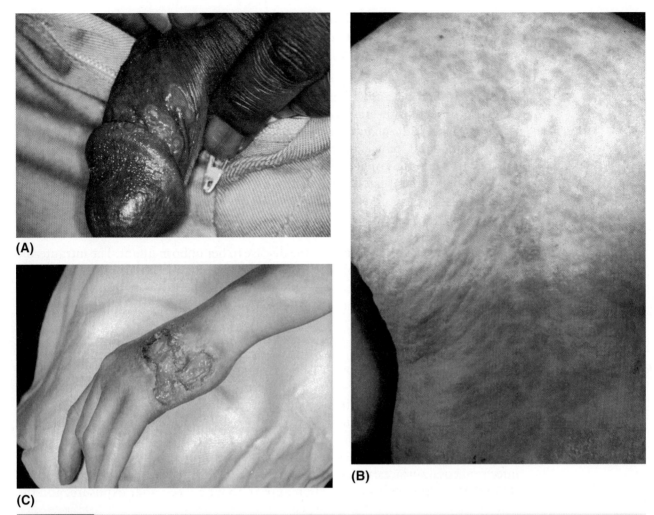

(A)

(B)

(C)

FIGURE 10-2 The stages of syphilis. **(A)** The chancre of primary syphilis as it occurs on the penis. The chancre has raised margins and is usually painless (Courtesy of M. Rein VD/CDC). **(B)** A skin rash is characteristic of secondary syphilis (Courtesy of Dr. Gavin Hart/CDC). **(C)** The gumma that forms in tertiary syphilis is a granular diffuse lesion compared with the primary chancre (Courtesy of Susan Lindsley/CDC).

(A) Courtesy of M. Rein VD/CDC; (B) Courtesy of Dr. Gavin Hart/CDC; (C) Courtesy of Susan Lindsley/CDC.

(granulomatous lesions often found in the skin or bones) are characteristic of this stage of the disease (**FIGURE 10-2C**). Chronic inflammation and scarring of the aortic valve lead to valve malfunction and heart failure. Often, the aortic wall just above the aortic valve also is damaged by the treponemes. This weakens the aortic wall, causing it to balloon out and eventually rupture. Degeneration of fiber tracts in the spinal cord caused by syphilis impairs sensation and disturbs walking. Damage to the brain and spinal cord by the treponemes (neurosyphilis) causes mental deterioration and eventual paralysis. The late manifestations of the disease, which can appear as long as twenty years after the initial infection, are called tertiary syphilis. This stage is not generally communicable because the organisms are relatively few and are confined to the internal organs.

Diagnosis and Treatment

Two different types of laboratory tests are used to diagnose syphilis:

1. Demonstration of treponemes by means of microscopic examination, in fluid squeezed from the ulcerated surface of the chancre. Specialized techniques and equipment are required.

2. Blood tests, called serologic tests for syphilis, that detect the various antibodies produced in response to a treponemal infection. The serologic tests become positive soon after the chancre appears and remain positive for many years.

Both types of tests are widely used; each has specific applications and limitations. Microscopic examination of material from a suspected chancre establishes the diagnosis of syphilis several weeks before a blood test will show positive results. On the other hand, if the chancre is in an inaccessible location and escapes detection, a positive blood test may be the only indication of syphilis in an individual who does not exhibit symptoms of active infection.

Syphilis can be treated successfully by penicillin and some other antibiotics. Treatment stops the progression of the disease and prevents serious late complications.

Congenital Syphilis

A syphilitic mother often transmits the disease to her unborn infant. The intrauterine infection may cause death of the fetus, or the infant may be born with congenital syphilis. An infected mother should be treated as soon as the maternal infection is identified without regard to the stage of her pregnancy.

GONORRHEA

Neisseria gonorrhoeae
Organism causing gonorrhea.

Gonorrhea, caused by the gonococcus *Neisseria gonorrhoeae*, is one of the most common communicable diseases and is the second most frequently reported disease to the CDC. The rate of infection dropped markedly during the last decades of the twentieth century, reaching a low point in 2009. However, since that time, the rate of gonorrhea infection has begun to climb, and just under 350,000 cases were reported in 2012. This figure is probably an underestimate. The organism primarily infects mucosal surfaces: the linings of the urethra, genital tract, pharynx, and rectum (**FIGURE 10-3**). Symptoms of infection appear about a week after exposure, and the clinical manifestations differ in the two sexes.

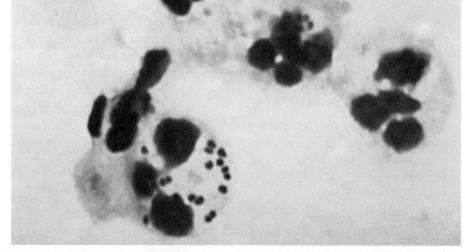

FIGURE 10-3 Gram stain of pus from the urethra, illustrating many gram-negative intracellular diplococci characteristic of gonorrhea (original magnification ×1,000).

Courtesy of Leonard V. Crowley, MD, Century College.

Gonorrhea in the Female

In the female, the gonococci infect chiefly the mucosa, uterine cervix and the urethral mucosa, and cause inflammation of the fallopian tubes (salpingitis). Therefore, it is a common cause of pelvic inflammatory disease (ascending infection of the female genital tract). The gonococcal infection may also spread into Bartholin glands, which are located adjacent to the vaginal orifice. The cervical infection usually causes profuse vaginal discharge; the urethral involvement is manifested by pain and burning on urination. Some women, however, have few or no symptoms of infection but are nevertheless capable of transmitting the disease to their sexual partners.

The gonococcal infection may also spread upward from the cervix through the uterus into the Fallopian tubes, where, as previously noted, it causes an acute salpingitis (*salpinx* = tube). Sometimes, the tubal infection is followed by the formation of an abscess within the fallopian tube or an abscess involving both the tube and the adjacent ovary. Gonococcal salpingitis is manifested by abdominal pain and tenderness together with elevated temperature and leukocytosis. Scarring following the tubal infection may delay transport of the fertilized ovum through the Fallopian tube, causing the pregnancy to develop in the tube instead of the uterus, a condition called an ectopic pregnancy (described in the discussion on prenatal development and diseases associated with pregnancy). Complete obstruction of both tubes by scar tissue blocks the transport of a fertilized ovum through the tubes and leads to sterility.

Gonorrhea in the Male

In the male, gonococci cause an acute inflammation of the mucosa of the anterior part of the urethra. The infection is usually manifested by a purulent urethral discharge and considerable pain on urination, and if untreated, urethral strictures. Occasionally the infected male may have relatively few symptoms although he is still capable of infecting others. However, gonorrhea is less likely to be asymptomatic in men than in women.

From the anterior urethra, the infection often spreads by direct extension into the posterior urethra, prostate, seminal vesicles, vasa deferentia, and epididymides. An infection in both epididymides and vasa deferentia may lead to sterility because the scarring after the infection may obstruct the duct system and thus block transport of sperm into the seminal fluid. More information is presented in the discussion of the male reproductive system.

Extragenital Gonorrhea

Recently, the incidence of gonococcal infection in extragenital sites has increased. Gonoccocal infection of the rectal mucosa causes anorectal pain and tenderness associated with purulent bloody mucoid discharge from the rectum. Rectal infection results from contamination of the rectal mucosa either by infected vaginal secretions or from anal intercourse. Gonococcal infection of the pharynx and tonsils results from oral–genital sex. The infection may be asymptomatic but often causes a sore throat. Neonatal gonorrhea, a result of infection during birth, is most often expressed as conjunctivitis. It is still a major cause of blindness in areas with poor neonatal care, but it is prevented by ocular antibiotic instillation in the United States.

Disseminated Gonococcal Infection

In a small proportion of infected patients, the organism gains access to the bloodstream and spreads throughout the body. This serious complication is characterized by elevated temperature, joint pain, multiple small abscesses in the skin, and sometimes infections of the joints, tendons, heart valves, and covering of the brain (meninges).

Diagnosis and Treatment

Diagnosis of gonorrhea is established by culturing gonococci from suspected sites of infection: urethra, cervix, rectum, and pharynx. Gonococci may also be cultured from the bloodstream in disseminated gonococcal infection. DNA-based tests are also available.

Recently, strains of gonococci resistant to the most commonly used antibiotics in therapy (ceftriaxone and azithromycin) have been isolated in several different parts of the world. Such resistance raises great concern, and consequently selecting an appropriate antibiotic to treat a gonococcal infection is more difficult than in the past.

HERPES

The herpes simplex virus is one of several herpes viruses that infect people. There are two forms of the herpes simplex virus, designated type 1 and 2 (HSV-1 and HSV-2). HSV-1 usually infects the oral mucous membrane, where it causes the familiar fever blisters. Most individuals are infected in childhood, and most adults have antibodies to the virus, indicating a previous infection. HSV-2 usually infects the genital tract, and most infections occur after puberty. However, the two types are not restricted in their distribution. Either HSV-1 or HSV-2 may infect either site. Genital herpes is responsible for about 250,000 initial doctors visits per year although infection is asymptomatic in about 80 percent of cases. Serological evidence of infection is common to both forms of the virus.

Genital herpes virus infection has increased significantly in recent years. The clinical course of genital disease caused by either HSV-1 or HSV-2 is indistinguishable although HSV-2 tends to reoccur more frequently. About 80 percent of genital lesions are associated with HSV-2. In some sexually active populations, up to 80 percent of people may show evidence of having been infected although many may have had no symptoms.

The lesions caused by the viral infection usually appear within a week after sexual exposure. They consist of clusters of very small, painful blisters (vesicles) that soon rupture, forming painful shallow ulcers that often coalesce. This may be accompanied by fever, headache, and other systemic symptoms. The lesions contain large quantities of virus and are infectious to sexual contacts. Usually the lymph nodes draining the infected areas are swollen and tender. In men, the vesicles usually appear on the glans or shaft of the penis (**FIGURE 10-4**). In women, the lesions may be quite extensive (**FIGURE 10-5**). They may be on the vulva, in the vagina, or on the cervix. Vulvar lesions are quite painful, but those deep in the vagina or on the cervix may cause little discomfort because these regions are relatively insensitive. The ulcers heal slowly in a few weeks. However, the virus persists in the tissues of the infected person and may flare up periodically, causing recurrent infections. Some patients have repeated flare-ups for several years after the initial infection.

Active herpetic ulcers shed large amounts of virus, and sexual partners of patients with active lesions are readily infected. Unfortunately, patients without active lesions also may excrete small amounts of virus periodically and infect their sexual partners even though they have no lesions or symptoms of infection.

Diagnosis and Treatment

Herpes can usually be suspected from the clinical appearance of the lesions and can be confirmed by smears obtained from the lesions, which reveal the characteristic intranuclear inclusions in infected cells (**FIGURE 10-6**).

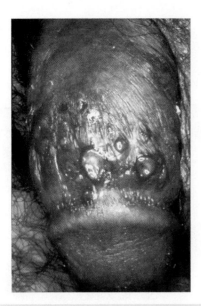

FIGURE 10-4 Several small superficial herpetic ulcers on shaft of penis behind glans.

Antiviral drugs are available that shorten the course and reduce the severity of an acute infection, but antiviral drugs do not eradicate the virus or prevent transmission. Depending on the severity of the infection, they can be administered intravenously or orally or applied as an ointment to the lesions. Patients with frequent and disabling recurrent infections sometimes benefit from long-term oral treatment, which seems to reduce the frequency and severity of recurrences.

Herpes Infection and Pregnancy

A pregnant woman with a genital herpes infection may infect her infant. If the mother has active herpetic lesions in her genital tract, the infant may acquire the virus when

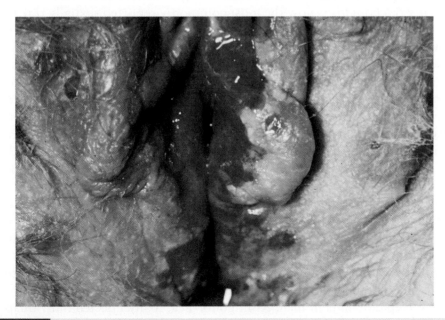

FIGURE 10-5 Multiple confluent ulcers of vulva as a result of herpes.

Courtesy of Leonard V. Crowley, MD, Century College.

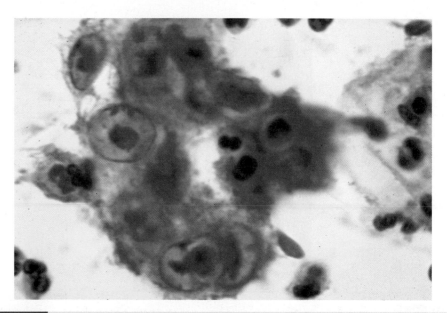

FIGURE 10-6 Vaginal smear illustrating clusters of herpes-infected epithelial cells containing intranuclear inclusions (original magnification ×1,000).
Courtesy of Leonard V. Crowley, MD, Century College.

passing through the genital tract during delivery. Consequently, a mother with an active infection is usually delivered by cesarean section to prevent infection of the newborn infant, which is likely if the infant is delivered vaginally. Neonatal herpetic infections may infect the CNS and many other visceral organs and, if untreated, have a high risk of mortality.

GENITAL CHLAMYDIAL INFECTIONS

Genital tract infection caused by the small obligate intracellular bacterial parasite *Chlamydia trachomatis* is now the most commonly reported sexually transmitted disease, with well over 3 million cases reported each year in the United States. The overall prevalence is about 2 percent, but in selected age and ethnic groups the prevalence may be over 10 percent. The incidence is more than two times that of gonorrhea. Part of this increase reflects the availability of new diagnostic tests that enable the physician to recognize chlamydial infections in patients who have few symptoms and whose cases probably would previously have gone undetected. Many chlamydial infections are asymptomatic, and detection is the result of routine screening. The risk of male–female transmission in unprotected sex is about 25 percent, and rates of transmission from infected mother to newborn are 50 percent or greater.

Chlamydia causes much the same type of inflammation and clinical symptoms as gonorrhea. In women, the initial infection is usually in the uterine cervix and is associated with moderate vaginal discharge. Men often develop acute inflammation of the urethra associated with frequency and burning on urination, which is called *nongonococcal urethritis*. Like gonorrhea, the chlamydial infection may spread to the Fallopian tubes in women, followed by scarring and impaired fertility, and may cause acute epididymitis in men. As in gonorrhea, many infected individuals may have no symptoms of infection but are still able to infect their sexual partners and may develop complications related to the spread of the infection to other parts of the genital tract.

Diagnosis and Treatment

Highly sensitive specific tests are available that can detect chlamydial antigens in cervical secretions and secretions from the male urethra, and the tests can also be performed on urine. Nucleic acid amplification tests, similar to the tests used to identify gonococci, can also be used to diagnose a chlamydial infection by identifying characteristic groups of chlamydial nucleic acids. Currently azithromycin and doxycycline are preferred for therapy and are 95 percent effective. Both the patient and the partner should be treated.

Human Immunodeficiency Virus Infections and AIDS

AIDS is the end-stage and most serious manifestation of an infection caused by a virus called the human immunodeficiency virus, or simply HIV. AIDS (the clinical end-stage of HIV infection) is a devastating disease that cripples the body's immune system by attacking and destroying helper T lymphocytes, making the affected individuals susceptible to a large number of both common and unusual infections and malignant tumors. Two viruses cause AIDS, designated HIV-1 and HIV-2, each of which has multiple closely related groups. HIV-1 is the virus that causes AIDS in most parts of the world; HIV-2 infections are seen mainly in West Africa and increasingly in India but are uncommon in the United States. HIV-1 and HIV-2 cause a very similar disease although HIV-2 may be slightly less virulent and is resistant to certain therapeutic agents.

HIV TRANSMISSION

Although HIV infection often is predominantly a sexually transmitted disease, HIV may also be transmitted congenitally, parenterally (most commonly via blood contaminated needles used by drug abusers), and, in the past, by contaminated blood products. In the United States, sexual transmission (occurring predominantly in the MSM population in Europe and the Americas) accounts for 65 percent of diagnoses, heterosexual contact is responsible for 25 percent of cases, and the balance is associated with intravenous drug abuse. There are also ethnic differences in the prevalence of HIV infections and AIDS. There is a disproportionately large number of AIDS cases in minority groups. African Americans and Hispanics comprise about 30 percent of the U.S. population, but they account for about 69 percent of all AIDS cases.

It should be noted, however, that in much of the world HIV is transmitted predominantly by heterosexual sex. Sub-Saharan Africa accounts for about 70 percent of HIV mediated disease with a predominantly heterosexual mode of transmission (much of which is related to multiple sexual partners and via professional sex workers). Infection by HIV does not occur by nonsexual transient exposure to infected individuals. Infection requires the transfer of blood, seminal fluid, cervical and vaginal secretions, or breast milk, which generally contain large amounts of virus and hence are infectious, whereas urine, stool, saliva, tears, and perspiration usually contain little if any virus and are not considered a risk. Even accidental needle sticks by health care workers have a low probability of infection (around 1 percent, which can be prevented by drug prophylaxis). The probability of HIV transmission per single act of heterosexual sex is estimated by some to be quite low (male to female transmission 0.002, female to male transmission 0.001). However, the risk is much increased as plasma HIV levels increase and in the presence of a variety of genital infections in the individual without HIV. Condom use and male circumcision decrease the risk of male–female transmission significantly. Receptive anal intercourse bears a much increased risk of 0.14 per act, which is presumably related to anatomical differences between the vagina and rectum.

HIV mediated disease in humans is relatively recent. HIV-1 is closely related to viruses found in chimpanzee populations in the southern Cameroons. Retrospective genetic studies suggest that cross-species transmission to humans (likely from the blood of contaminated "bushmeat") occurred early in the twentieth century. The virus was established in the human population of Kinshasa, Democratic Republic of Congo, by the 1950s. The disease spread across Africa via trade and railroad routes and entered the United States most likely via Haiti. The first cases of the disease that we now call AIDS were identified clinically in 1981 in a small group of homosexual men with an opportunistic lung infection caused by *Pneumocystis jiroveci*, an unusual fungal pathogen. The virus was identified in 1983, and a blood test to detect HIV infection became available in 1985. Recent molecular genetic studies on historical samples have identified the virus in patient material as early as 1959. Although durable cures have still not been achieved, we can slow the multiplication of the virus and arrest the progression of the disease that it causes.

HIV LIFE CYCLE

Retrovirus Class of RNA viruses including HIV.

Reverse transcriptase Enzyme included within the genome of the HIV virus necessary for viral replication.

Capsid Protein coat of the HIV virus.

HIV integrase Viral enzyme allowing the viral genes to direct the synthesis and assembly of more virus.

HIV protease Enzyme that cuts and assembles the virus protein.

HIV is an RNA virus that belongs to a class of viruses called **retroviruses**. The viral RNA and an enzyme called **reverse transcriptase** are enclosed within a protein coat (**capsid**), forming the core of the virus. The core is surrounded by an envelope, composed of a double layer of lipid molecules, acquired from the cell membrane of the infected cell when the virus is budded out.

The target of the HIV is the CD4 protein present on the cell membranes of helper T lymphocytes, as well as on monocytes, macrophages, and similar macrophage-like cells in the skin, lymph nodes, and within the central nervous system. The CD4 protein functions as a receptor and attachment point for the virus in combination with another cell surface receptor (CCR5). When the virus binds to the cell, the virus envelope fuses with the cell membrane, allowing the virus to enter the cell. Once inside the cell, the virus makes a DNA copy of its own RNA genetic material by means of its reverse transcriptase enzyme. The viral reverse transcriptase has a very high error rate, and HIV-1 has a very high mutation rate, leading to rapid formation of viruses selected for resistance to therapeutic drugs. The viral DNA copy is then inserted into the genetic material of the infected cell, a process assisted by another viral enzyme called **HIV integrase**, allowing the viral genes to direct the synthesis and assembly of more virus. The final stages of virus production requires a viral enzyme called **HIV protease**, which cuts and assembles the virus protein into small segments that surround the viral RNA, forming the infectious virus particles that bud from the infected cells. As the virus particles bud from the cells, they become coated by part of the cell membranes of the infected cells. The newly formed virus particles attack other susceptible cells within the lymphoid tissue throughout the body, where the virus replicates (proliferates) and releases more virus particles to infect still more susceptible cells. Helper T lymphocytes, which are the primary targets for the virus, are damaged and many are killed. Monocytes, however, which are also attacked, are quite resistant and survive, but the virus continues to replicate within the monocytes, releasing virus particles that infect other cells. In addition, the monocytes function as vehicles to transport the virus throughout the body and into the nervous system to infect the brain (**FIGURE 10-7**).

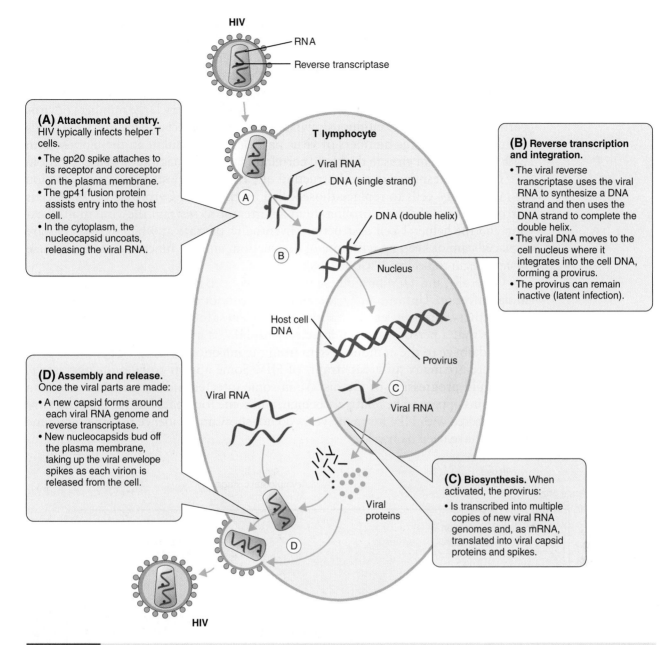

HIV
— RNA
— Reverse transcriptase

(A) Attachment and entry. HIV typically infects helper T cells.
- The gp20 spike attaches to its receptor and coreceptor on the plasma membrane.
- The gp41 fusion protein assists entry into the host cell.
- In the cytoplasm, the nucleocapsid uncoats, releasing the viral RNA.

T lymphocyte

Viral RNA
DNA (single strand)
DNA (double helix)
Nucleus

(B) Reverse transcription and integration.
- The viral reverse transcriptase uses the viral RNA to synthesize a DNA strand and then uses the DNA strand to complete the double helix.
- The viral DNA moves to the cell nucleus where it integrates into the cell DNA, forming a provirus.
- The provirus can remain inactive (latent infection).

Host cell DNA

Provirus

(D) Assembly and release. Once the viral parts are made:
- A new capsid forms around each viral RNA genome and reverse transcriptase.
- New nucleocapsids bud off the plasma membrane, taking up the viral envelope spikes as each virion is released from the cell.

Viral RNA

Viral RNA

Viral proteins

(C) Biosynthesis. When activated, the provirus:
- Is transcribed into multiple copies of new viral RNA genomes and, as mRNA, translated into viral capsid proteins and spikes.

HIV

FIGURE 10-7 Replication cycle of the human immunodeficiency virus (HIV). Replication is dependent on the reverse transcriptase enzyme.

Mother-to-Infant Transmission

Infected maternal blood or cervical–vaginal secretions are the source of infection of newborn infants born to infected mothers, so the likelihood of fetal infection depends to some extent on how much virus is present in the mother's blood and body fluids. Consequently, all infected pregnant women should receive highly active antiviral therapy to suppress HIV multiplication. With effective antiviral therapy, the amount of virus in the maternal blood can be reduced to an extremely low level, which greatly reduces the risk of fetal HIV infection.

MANIFESTATIONS OF HIV INFECTION

During the early stages of the infection, large amounts of virus can be detected in the blood and body fluids of the infected person, including large numbers of virus-infected lymphocytes in lymph nodes and other lymphoid tissue. During this phase, many infected individuals develop a mild febrile illness. The body responds to the infection by forming anti-HIV antibodies and by generating cytotoxic T lymphocytes. The amount of virus in the blood and body fluids declines as the acute phase of the infection subsides, but, unfortunately, the body's defenses are not able to eliminate the virus, and the infection enters a more chronic phase. Very large numbers of virus particles are produced continuously, which continue to infect and destroy CD4+ cells (helper T cells). Large numbers of virus particles also circulate in the bloodstream with the amount of virus in the blood correlating with the magnitude of the infection.

The body responds to the destruction of CD4+ cells by stepping up production of more CD4+ cells to replace those killed by the virus. Cytotoxic (CD8) T cells directed against the virus proliferate in an attempt to restrain the viral multiplication and the helper T cell destruction. Eventually, the rate at which CD4+ cells are replaced cannot keep up with rate of destruction, and the functions of the immune system begin to decline (**FIGURE 10-8**).

Generally, anti-HIV antibodies appear from one to as long as six months after the initial infection. Unfortunately, the antibodies cannot eradicate the virus or reduce its infectivity. Nevertheless, a confirmed positive test for virus antibodies is useful to indicate that a person has been infected with HIV, is infectious to others, and is at risk of damage to the immune system from the infection.

There are many different strains of HIV. Some appear to be quite aggressive, with rapid progression of the disease in some infected individuals. In contrast, a few strains appear to be relatively benign, and some fortunate individuals who have been infected with HIV for many years do not show any evidence that their immune systems have been damaged.

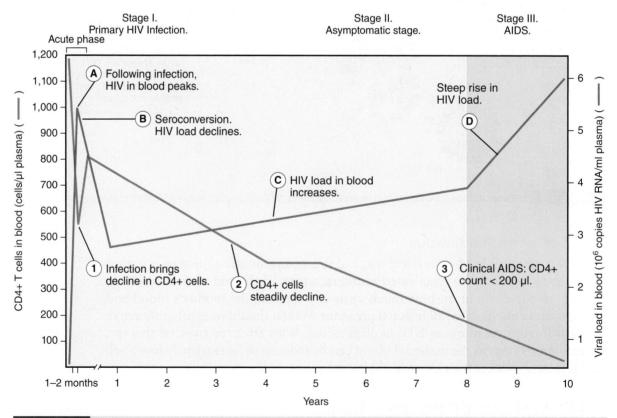

FIGURE 10-8 HIV infection and AIDS. Once infected with HIV, an immune response brings about an abrupt drop in the blood HIV population, which rises as the immune system fails (A–D). Without antiretroviral therapy, the T cell count slowly drops (1–3) until clinical AIDS occurs.

TABLE 10-2 Sequence of Events in HIV Infections and Their Significance	
Event	**Significance**
HIV invades CD4+ cells and becomes part of cell DNA	Individual is infected for life
Virus proliferates in infected cells and sheds virus particles	Virus present in blood and body fluids
Body forms anti-HIV antibody	Antibody is a marker of infection but is not protective
Progressive destruction of helper T cells	Compromised cell-mediated immunity
Immune defenses collapse	Opportunistic infections Neoplasms

TABLE 10-2 summarizes the sequence of events in HIV infection and their significance.

MEASUREMENT OF VIRAL RNA AND CD4 LYMPHOCYTES AS AN INDEX OF DISEASE PROGRESSION

Although HIV replicates in lymph nodes, not in the blood, the amount of viral RNA in the blood reflects the extent of viral replication in the lymphoid tissue throughout the body and can vary from over a million virus particles per milliliter of blood plasma in a patient with an acute infection to extremely low levels in a patient being treated successfully with agents effective against the virus. Currently, measurement of the level of viral RNA using PCR-based techniques is the key to determining disease progression and the efficacy of therapy.

A determination of the number of helper T lymphocytes in the blood allows one to estimate the extent of damage to the immune system. Normally, there are from about 800 to 1,200 helper T (CD4+) lymphocytes per microliter of blood, but this number declines progressively as the disease advances. When this number falls to about 500 cells per microliter of blood, the patient becomes at risk of opportunistic infections, and by the time the helper T lymphocyte count falls below 200 per microliter, the infected person is at very high risk of major complications from the disease.

COMPLICATIONS OF AIDS

The impaired cell-mediated immunity leads to two very serious problems: a greatly increased susceptibility to infection and a predisposition to various malignant tumors.

Infections

Many of the viruses, fungi, parasites, and other pathogens that attack AIDS patients do not usually cause disease in healthy people. (Infections of this type are often called **opportunistic infections.**) Formerly, one of the most common AIDS-related opportunistic infections was pneumonia, caused by the fungal parasite *Pneumocystis jiroveci*. However, recent advances in therapy have reduced the risk of this pathogen. Another relatively common and serious systemic infection is caused by a normally nonpathogenic acid-fast bacterium called *Mycobacterium avium* complex. Other serious infections are the parasitic infections toxoplasmosis and cryptosporidiosis, described in the discussion on animal parasites.

AIDS patients are also at risk for acquiring widespread, rapidly progressive tuberculosis or histoplasmosis, infections that normally are held in check in people with

Opportunistic infection
An infection in an immunocompromised person caused by an organism that is normally nonpathogenic or of limited pathogenicity.

TABLE 10-3	Common Infections in HIV Patients
Viruses	Herpes, cytomegalovirus, Epstein-Barr virus (infectious mononucleosis)
Fungi	Histoplasmosis, coccidioidomycosis, aspergillosis, *Candida* infections, *Pneumocystis jiroveci* pneumonia
Protozoa	Amebiasis, cryptosporidiosis, toxoplasmosis
Mycobacteria	Tuberculosis, *Mycobacterium avium-intracellulare* infections

normal immune systems. Many of the symptoms exhibited by patients with AIDS such as fever, cough, shortness of breath, weight loss, and enlarged lymph nodes are the result of severe opportunistic infections. **TABLE 10-3** lists some of the more common, severe, and often life-threatening infections in AIDS patients.

Malignant Tumors

The malignant tumors common in AIDS patients also are related to failure of the immune system, which helps to protect people from neoplastic disease such as tumors as well as infections. The most common malignant tumor in AIDS patients, which is rare in other people, is Kaposi sarcoma, which is caused by a herpes virus designated human herpes virus 8. This tumor, which is composed of immature connective tissue cells (fibroblasts) and blood capillaries intermixed with inflammatory and phagocytic cells, forms hemorrhagic nodules in the skin, mouth, lymph nodes, and internal organs (**FIGURE 10-9**). Malignant tumors of B lymphocytes also are common, as are cancers of the mouth, rectum, and uterine cervix.

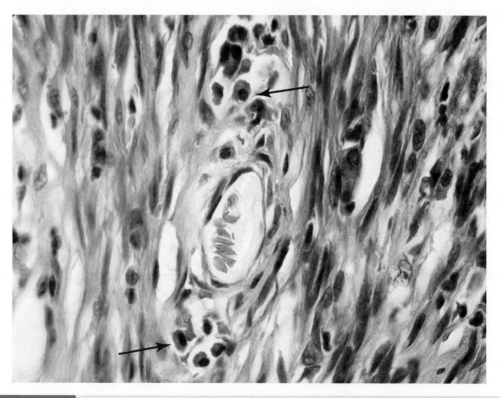

FIGURE 10-9 Kaposi sarcoma, illustrating proliferating spindle-shaped connective tissue cells (fibroblasts) surrounding a small blood vessel in the center of the field. Plasma cells (*arrows*) are intermixed with connective tissue cells (original magnification ×400).

Courtesy of Leonard V. Crowley, MD, Century College.

VACCINES AND PREVENTION OF HIV INFECTION

Infections and tumors in AIDS patients can be treated, but treatment of the underlying viral infection has been hampered by lack of a drug that can totally eliminate, rather than reduce, the virus load. Much effort is being directed toward finding ways to control or eradicate the virus and toward developing a vaccine to immunize against the virus. There are a number of potential drug targets within the viral life cycle. Currently HART (Highly Active Retroviral Therapy) uses a combination of drugs directed against several different viral targets. Molecular analysis of the particular strain of HIV-1 infecting the patient is used to search for mutations associated with drug resistance to select the best drug regimen on a patient-by-patient basis when possible. In areas where medical care is limited, the best combination of drugs based on efficacy, cost, and availability is chosen. Many drugs are available that can impede viral replication and slow the progression of the disease, and recently some that can reduce the probability of infection in selected noninfected individuals, but ultimately the most effective way to control the disease is to prevent further spread of the infection. On a personal level, this requires avoiding unprotected sex, be it genital–genital or genital–anal and avoiding the use of injected drugs and shared needles. The ready availability of condoms and needle-exchange programs has helped to lessen the spread. On a societal basis, programs to eradicate venereal disease, encourage male circumcision, and educate professional sex workers about risky behavior have lessened HIV transmission in many areas of the world.

TREATMENT OF HIV INFECTION

Current antiviral treatment has greatly improved the outcome of an HIV infection, which now can often be controlled for many years by appropriate treatment. Unfortunately, although the proliferation of the virus and associated damage to the immune system can often be suppressed, current antiviral drugs cannot completely eliminate the virus, which persists indefinitely in the tissues of the infected host. Current drug therapy has changed HIV infection from a relatively rapidly progressing fatal disease to a more slowly progressive chronic disease that can be controlled but cannot be cured.

When to Treat

Starting treatment requires balancing the advantages of suppressing viral multiplication against the cost, side effects, and inconvenience of treatment. Intensive treatment of HIV (HART) involves multiple drugs that must be taken on a precise schedule for life to arrest the progression of the disease. Side effects related to the drugs are relatively frequent and may be severe, and drug resistance often occurs, especially if the multiple drugs are not taken as prescribed. However, effective antiviral therapy inhibits viral multiplication, reduces the amount of virus in the circulation, and helps the immune system to recover.

Increasing evidence indicates immune system damage begins in the early asymptomatic phase of HIV infection. The risks associated with antiretroviral therapy (HART) have decreased. Current guidelines suggest beginning HART when the CD4 count is between 500 and 350 cells/μl. Many suggest considering therapy even in patients without symptoms who have higher CD4 counts. The goal is to achieve plasma HIV-1 RNA below the detection level of the most sensitive HIV test available. Delay in therapy is associated with treatment failure. Couples who are serodiscordant (where one partner may not yet be infected), people with hepatitis B, women who are pregnant or breastfeeding, and children under age five are candidates for immediate therapy. Such use of HART has nearly eliminated mother-to-child transmission and has reduced the risk of transmission of HIV to an uninfected partner.

Many drugs are now available to treat HIV infections, and more are being developed. The anti-HIV drugs are classified into six groups based on the phase of the viral life cycle inhibited by the drugs: (1) **non-nucleoside reverse transcriptase inhibitors**, (2) **nucleoside reverse transcriptase inhibitors** (nucleoside analogs), (3) **protease inhibitors**, (4) HIV fusion/entry inhibitors, (5) HIV integrase inhibitors, and (6) entry inhibitors (CCR5 co-receptor antagonists). A number of specific drug regimes are suggested for those starting therapy.

How the Drugs Act

Each class of drug attacks a different phase in the HIV life cycle, and they are generally given in combination. Such combinations usually are very effective inhibitors of viral replication, maintaining the function of the immune system and helping restore an immune system that has already been damaged by the virus. Infected individuals must be willing to continue lifelong treatment with various combinations of potent antiviral drugs to inhibit virus proliferation. In addition, other drugs are available that interfere with specific phases of virus proliferation.

Non-nucleoside reverse transcriptase inhibitors bind directly to reverse transcriptase and block DNA polymerase, which is required to convert viral RNA to DNA so it can be incorporated in the nucleus of the infected cell. Nucleoside reverse transcriptase inhibitors (nucleoside analogs) interrupt the formation of viral DNA from RNA by substituting a nucleoside analog (a "look-alike" compound) that resembles one of the normal nucleosides used by the virus to construct DNA. The virus cannot distinguish the analog from the "normal" nucleoside that it resembles. When the virus tries to incorporate the "look-alike" compound into the viral DNA, the viral DNA synthesis is interrupted and unable to continue.

Protease inhibitors block the enzyme that cuts the viral protein into short segments and assembles the protein segments around viral RNA to form the infectious virus particle. Inhibition of the protease enzyme leads to release of disorganized and noninfectious virus particles. **HIV entry inhibitors** and **fusion inhibitors** block the binding entry and fusion of HIV with the target cell. **Integrase inhibitors** block the enzyme responsible for inserting the HIV viral DNA into the genome of the host cell. This class of drugs has particular utility for people who have become resistant to other classes of agents. **CCR5 co-receptor antagonists** prevent the CCR5 receptor on CD4 T cells from interacting with the HIV protein gp120, a necessary step for fusion of the HIV viral envelope with the cell membrane. It is of interest that this class of drugs grew out of the finding that some professional sex workers were relatively resistant to HIV infection. It was found that a natural mutation of the CCR5 receptor was responsible for the resistance, suggesting that CCR5 was a reasonable target for anti-HIV agents.

Although much remains to be done, HART therapy has been responsible for a 29-percent decrease in AIDS-related deaths in the last ten years. There has been a fortyfold increase in antiretroviral drug therapy, with more than 10 million people having access to such therapy in low- and middle-income countries. In the United States, the annual HIV death rate has rapidly declined from a peak in 1994–1995 of 17 deaths per 100,000 to 7 deaths per 100,000 by 1997, due in part to antiretroviral therapy and better treatment of opportunistic infections. Since then, there has been a continuous slow decline in the death rate. However, HIV infection is still a leading cause of death in the twenty-five to forty-four year age range, particularly among African Americans.

Non-nucleoside reverse transcriptase inhibitors Drugs used to treat HIV infections that bind to reverse transcriptase, blocking DNA polymerase that converts RNA to DNA.

Nucleoside reverse transcriptase inhibitors Nucleoside analogs ("look-alike" compounds) that resemble the normal nucleosides a virus uses to construct DNA. Synthesis is disrupted when the analog substitutes for the required nucleoside.

Protease inhibitors Drugs used to treat HIV infection that block the enzyme that cuts the viral protein into segments and assembles them around the viral RNA to form the infectious virus particle. As a result, the virus particle is improperly constructed and is not infectious.

HIV entry inhibitors/fusion inhibitors Drugs that block the binding entry and fusion of HIV with the target cell.

Integrase inhibitors Drugs that block the enzyme responsible for inserting the HIV viral DNA into the cell DNA.

CCR5 co-receptor antagonists Drugs that prevent the CCR5 receptor on CD4 T cells from interacting with an HIV protein.

CASE 10-1

The patient, an eighteen-year-old female, is seen at the emergency room of a local hospital complaining of severe abdominal pain, vaginal bleeding, and delay in her expected menstrual period. She notes that she had unprotected vaginal intercourse about seven weeks prior and is concerned about a sexually transmitted disease. She experienced coitarche (initial sexual intercourse) at age fifteen and has been sexually active since that time with a variety of partners. She states that usually barrier protection was used by the male (condoms) but they did sometimes "forget." She notes that she has been seen in a venereal disease clinic several times in the past and was diagnosed with both gonorrhea and chlamydia infections for which she received antibiotic therapy "several times." A rapid pregnancy test is ordered, which is positive. Transvaginal ultrasound detects signs of an ectopic pregnancy (the fetuses is implanted in a site other than the uterus) located in the fallopian tube (oviduct), a so-called tubal pregnancy. She suffers a decrease in blood pressure with hemorrhage (hemorrhagic shock) and is rushed to surgery. At surgery blood is found in the abdominal cavity (hemoperitoneum) and an 8 cm left mass was found that encompassed both the left fallopian tube and ovary. The mass contained a nonviable fetus judged to be of eight weeks gestational age (**FIGURE 10-10**). Both the left ovary and fallopian tube were removed (salpingo-oophorectomy). The contralateral fallopian tube and ovary showed numerous adhesions that distorted their anatomy and were considered to be consistent with long-standing pelvic inflammatory disease. Recovery was complicated by ongoing infections, but she eventually recovered.

Discussion

Ectopic pregnancies have been observed since before 1000 CE. Because the developing fetus is detectable as a mass during examination in only about 50 percent of cases, the use of very sensitive assays for human chorionic gonadotrophin (hCG) to determine pregnancy combined with transvaginal ultrasound makes location of the conceptus possible very early in pregnancy. This has allowed for much improved medical management. In cases where no fetal heartbeat is detected and the fetus is small, it is possible to chemically terminate the ectopic pregnancy without the need for (often laparoscopic) surgery. However, extrauterine pregnancy accounts for about 9 percent of maternal deaths currently and a ten times greater risk than delivery in the third trimester. Hemorrhage and infection (as in the case) are the major risks, and medical or surgical intervention is necessary, even in the case of more advanced fetuses.

Currently ectopic pregnancies account for about 2 percent of all recognized conceptions. There is evidence that the frequency is increasing, and this is due, in part, to an increasing incidence of pelvic inflammatory disease (PID) related to untreated or recurrent infections with *Chlamydia trachomatis* and *Neisseria gonorrhea*. Any factor that causes anatomic obstruction or other abnormalities in tubal structure that delay or prevent passage of the embryo increase the risk of ectopic pregnancy.

PID is a preventable but increasingly diagnosed condition that affects more than 1 million women (about 8 percent of all of reproductive age). It is clearly most frequent in adolescents (about 1 in 5 cases occurring before the age of nineteen). Multiple sexual partners and early coitarche are also risk factors. Infection related to either of the above mentioned organisms can, if not properly treated, result in acute followed by chronic inflammation of the salpinx (fallopian tube, salpingitis), which, as was noted in the case, can lead to scarring distortion and adhesions of and within the tube affecting passage of the embryo (**FIGURE 10-11**).

Etiology and Pathogenesis

Ectopic pregnancy (tubal pregnancy) most likely resulting from tubal scarring and adhesions as a result of pelvic inflammatory disease subsequent to Neisserial and chlamydial infection.

(continues)

CASE 10-1   *(Continued)*

Questions

1. What actions could the patient have taken prior to being seen in the emergency room to have prevented the tubal pregnancy?

2. Many venereal disease clinics monitor patients as they take prescribed drugs. Do you think this is a reasonable approach and why?

3. There is increasing concern about antibiotic resistance developing in several of the pathogens responsible for venereal disease. Why is the problem increasing?

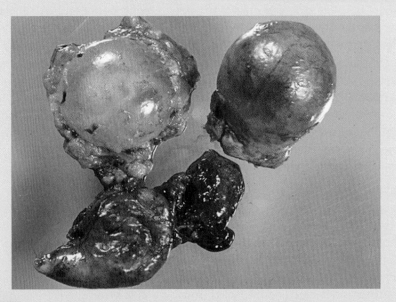

FIGURE 10-10 An ectopic (tubal pregnancy) removed during surgery. The nonviable fetus is visible within the membranous sack.

Image courtesy of Wesley C. Fowler, Jr., M.D. Professor of Obstetrics and Gynecology, Division of Gynecologic Oncology, The University of North Carolina School of Medicine.

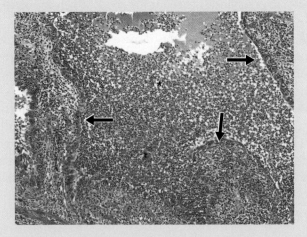

FIGURE 10-11 Fallopian tube (salpinx or oviduct) demonstrating acute inflammation as a result of Neisserial infection. The lumen of the tube (*) is filled with pus. The fingers (fimbrae) (*arrows*) line the tube and are covered with cilia that guide the embryo toward the uterus. After infection, scarring leads to adhesions between the fimbrae.

Courtesy of Department of Pathology and Laboratory Medicine, University of North Carolina at Chapel Hill.

QUESTIONS FOR REVIEW

1. How are communicable diseases transmitted? How are they controlled?
2. What is meant by the following terms: *epidemic disease, endemic disease, immunization,* and *sexually transmitted disease?*
3. How is syphilis transmitted? What are its clinical manifestations?
4. How is gonorrhea transmitted? What are its clinical manifestations? What is nongonococcal urethritis?
5. What are the manifestations of herpes infection of the genital tract?
6. What are the manifestations of chlamydial infection of the genital tract? How are chlamydial infections diagnosed and treated?
7. What is AIDS? What is its cause? What are its clinical manifestations? How can the spread of the infection be prevented or minimized?
8. What is the significance of a positive test for HIV antibody?

SUPPLEMENTARY READINGS

Pommerville, J. C. 2014. *Fundamentals of Microbiology.* 10th ed. Burlington MA: Jones & Bartlett Learning.

Shors T. 2013. *Understanding Viruses.* 2nd ed. Burlington MA: Jones & Bartlett Learning.
▶   Those interested in the study of infectious disease should start by consulting texts in the area of microbiology and virology. Although somewhat advanced, both of these texts are easy to read and up to date.

Centers for Disease Control. *Sexually Transmitted Diseases.* www.cdc.gov/std
▶   A first place to look for accurate and up to the minute information on any aspect of infectious disease is the United States Centers for Disease Control. This is a gateway to information on essentially all aspects of sexually transmitted disease.

Centers for Disease Control. www.cdc.gov/hiv
▶   This site provides accurate information on all aspects of HIV.

Centers for Disease Control. www.cdc.gov/hiv/library/slideSets/index.html
▶   At this site you will find slide sets in PowerPoint and other formats for use in both teaching and learning.

Avert. www.avert.org
▶   Many online sites have information on HIV, some reputable, some less so. This organization has multiple resources, many of which are aimed at prevention and at a younger audience.

Bennett, N. J. 2015. *HIV disease treatment & management.* emedicine.medscape.com/article/211316-treatment
▶   Consult this site for a summary of current practice in HIV disease treatment and management.

Faria, N. R., et al. 2014. The early spread and epidemic ignition of HIV-1 in human populations. *Science 346*:6205.

Hughes, J. P., et al. 2012. Determinants of per-coital act HIV-1 infectivity among HIV-1-serodiscordant couples. *Journal of Infectious Disease 205*:358.

Maartens, G., Celum, C., and Lewin, S. R. 2014. HIV infection: Epidemiology, pathogenesis, treatment and prevention. *Lancet 384*:258.
▶   The original scientific literature on HIV is endless. These three references review areas of research that have been of recent interest. The first article, although very technical in its details, presents a fascinating picture of how the AIDS epidemic developed and spread based on modern genetic technology. Although the title of the second article sounds specific (and perhaps off-putting), the discussion within the paper is an excellent introduction to risk factors involved in heterosexual HIV-1 transmission. A 2012 editorial in the same journal (*Journal of Infectious Disease 205*:351) provides an overview and skeptical comments. The third article is highly recommended for those looking for a recent review of HIV infection aimed at the health professional that is readable by the nonspecialist.

Gray-Swain, R. M., and Peipert, J. F. 2006. Pelvic inflammatory disease in adolescents. *Current Opinion in Obstetrics and Gynecology 18*:503.

Rolle, C. J., et al. 2006. Unilateral twin ectopic pregnancy in a patient with a history of multiple sexually transmitted infections. *Infectious Diseases in Obstetrics and Gynecology 2006*:1.

Marion, L. L., and Meeks, G. R. 2012. Ectopic Pregnancy: History, Incidence, Epidemiology, and Risk Factors, Clinical Obstetrics and Gynecology 55:376.

> ▶ The case presented in this chapter is based on information contained in the following three references. The third has a very interesting historical introduction.

The Cardiovascular System

1. Explain the basic anatomy and physiology of the heart and relate information to the common types of heart disease.

2. Explain how the heart beat is generated.

3. Describe the common causes of congenital heart disease and valvular heart disease. Explain the effects of these diseases. Describe the methods of treating congenital and acquired valvular heart disease.

4. Describe the pathogenesis of primary myocardial disease.

5. Describe the development and treatment of cardiac arrhythmias.

6. Describe the pathogenesis of myocardial ischemia. Describe the clinical manifestations of coronary heart disease. Explain the methods of treatment and their rationales.

7. List the major complications of myocardial infarction and describe their clinical manifestations.

8. Explain the general principles applied to the diagnosis and treatment of coronary heart disease and myocardial infarction.

9. Compare and contrast myocardial ischemia and myocardial infarct.

Cardiac Structure and Function

The heart is a muscular pump that propels blood through the lungs and to the peripheral tissues via the vasculature. Heart disease is caused by a disturbance in the function of the cardiac pump as a result of an intrinsic defect of pump function, a defect of the vasculature, or a combination of both. A working knowledge of the normal structure and function of the heart is essential to an understanding of the various types of heart disease.

The heart is a cone-shaped muscular pump that weighs about 350 g and is enclosed within a fibrous sac called the **pericardium** located in the **mediastinum**, the middle compartment of the thorax. The pericardium is lined by a layer of mesothelial cells that is continuous with a similar layer of mesothelial cells covering the external surface of the heart. The heart is composed of three layers: the **epicardium**, consisting of a layer of mesothelial cells overlying a small amount of loose fibrous and adipose tissue; the **myocardium**, a thick layer of muscle that forms the bulk of the heart; and the **endocardium**, a thin layer of endothelial cells that lines the chambers and covers the surfaces of the heart valves. The heart is divided into four chambers by partitions

Pericardium Fibrous sac enclosing the heart.

Mediastinum Middle compartment of the thorax.

Epicardium/myocardium/endocardium Three layers of the heart moving from outside in.

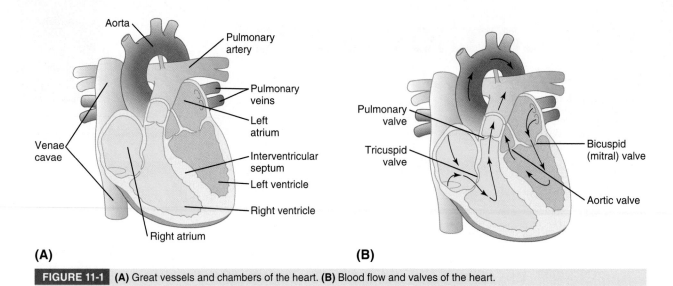

(A)   **(B)**

FIGURE 11-1 **(A)** Great vessels and chambers of the heart. **(B)** Blood flow and valves of the heart.

Atrium/atria Upper chambers of the heart.

Ventricles Lower chambers of the heart.

Fibrous framework Layer of dense fibrous tissue located between the atria and the ventricles.

Atrioventricular (AV) valve The flaplike heart valve located between the atrium and the ventricle.

(septae). The two upper chambers are separated by the interatrial septum into the right and left **atria**. The right atrium receives venous blood returning to the heart; the left atrium receives oxygenated arterial blood returning to the heart from the pulmonary circulation. The two lower chambers are separated by the interventricular septum into the right and left **ventricles**. The right ventricle pumps venous blood through the pulmonary artery to the lungs, where it is oxygenated and returned to the left atrium, and the left ventricle pumps oxygen-rich blood throughout the body, which is then collected into veins and returned to the right atrium. The right and left cardiac chambers work together, but no direct communications normally exist between the chambers on the right and left sides of the heart, so it is convenient clinically to consider each half as an independent structure. The "right heart" circulates blood into the pulmonary artery and through the lungs (the pulmonary circulation), and the "left heart" pumps blood into the aorta for distribution to the various organs and tissues in the body (the systemic circulation) (**FIGURE 11-1**). As will be discussed later, failure of the left side of the heart will, with time, lead to right-side failure as blood "backs up" through the pulmonary circulation and overloads the right side of the heart.

The atrial and ventricular muscles are arranged in bundles that encircle the heart and attach to a layer of dense fibrous tissue called the **fibrous framework**, which is located between the atria and ventricles and extends into the upper part of the interventricular septum surrounding the openings of the cardiac valves. The fibrous framework separates the atrial muscle fibers from those in the ventricles so that the atrial and ventricular muscles can function independently. Contraction of cardiac muscle reduces the size of the atria or ventricles, raising the pressure of the blood within the compressed chambers, and squeezing blood out of the chambers. The fibrous framework also provides a firm support to which the heart valves can attach, and contains a small opening to allow the atrioventricular bundle (bundle of His), part of the impulse conducting system, to carry impulses to the ventricles.

CARDIAC VALVES

The flow of blood into and out of the cardiac chambers is controlled by a system of four valves that normally permits flow in only one direction. The **atrioventricular (AV) valves** are flaplike valves surrounding the orifices between atria and ventricles.

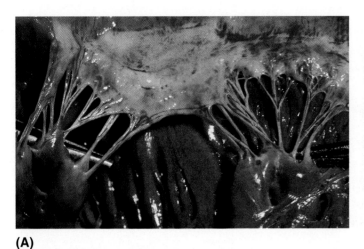

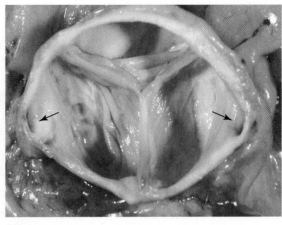

(A)

(B)

FIGURE 11-2 **(A)** Normal mitral valve, illustrating thin chordae extending from valve leaflets to papillary muscles. **(B)** Aortic valve viewed from above, illustrating a cup-shaped configuration of valve leaflets. Note the openings of coronary arteries (*arrows*) arising from the base of the aorta adjacent to aortic valve leaflets.

Courtesy of Leonard V. Crowley, MD, Century College.

The **tricuspid valve** separates the right atrium and ventricle; the **mitral valve** (so named because of it resemblance to a bishop's mitre) separates the left atrium and ventricle. The free margins of the valves are connected to the papillary muscles of the ventricular walls by narrow, stringlike bands of fibrous tissue called the **chordae tendineae** (**FIGURE 11-2A**). These bands prevent the valves from prolapsing (falling back) into the atria during **ventricular systole** (the period of ventricular contraction). The **semilunar valves** surrounding the orifices of the aorta (the **aortic valve**) and pulmonary artery (the **pulmonary valve**) are positioned so that the free margins of the valves face upward. This structural arrangement defines cuplike pockets between the free margins of the valves and the roots of the blood vessels to which the valves are attached (**FIGURE 11-2B**).

When the heart relaxes in **diastole** (ventricular relaxation), the chordae produce tension on the valves and pull the atrioventricular valves apart. When the ventricles contract in systole, the chordae are no longer under tension, and the force of the blood flow pushes the valves together so that no blood flows "backward" from the ventricles into the atria. During ventricular contraction, the semilunar valves are forced apart by the increased intraventricular pressure of blood, allowing it to leave the ventricles. When ventricular contraction ceases, the weight of the column of ejected blood forces the valves back into position, preventing reflux of blood into the ventricles during diastole. The atrioventricular and semilunar valves function reciprocally. Ventricular contraction relaxes tension on the chordae, causing the atrioventricular valves to close at the same time that the increased intraventricular pressure of blood opens the semilunar valves. Closure of the semilunar valves in diastole is also associated with opening of the atrioventricular valves. **FIGURE 11-3** illustrates the reciprocal action of the two sets of valves, which is responsible for the unidirectional flow required for normal cardiac function.

BLOOD SUPPLY TO THE HEART

The Left and Right Coronary Arteries

The heart is supplied by two large coronary arteries that arise from the aortic sinuses at the root of the aorta (**FIGURE 11-4**). The left coronary artery is a short vessel that

Tricuspid valve AV valve separating the right atrium and ventricle.

Mitral valve AV valve separating the left atrium and ventricle.

Chordae tendineae Bands of fibrous tissue connecting the margins of the valves to papillary muscles.

Ventricular systole Period of ventricular contraction.

Semilunar valve The cup-shaped valve located between the ventricles and the aorta or pulmonary artery.

Aortic valve Semilunar valve surrounding the orifices of the aorta.

Pulmonary valve Semilunar valve surrounding the orifices of the pulmonary artery.

Diastole Ventricular relaxation.

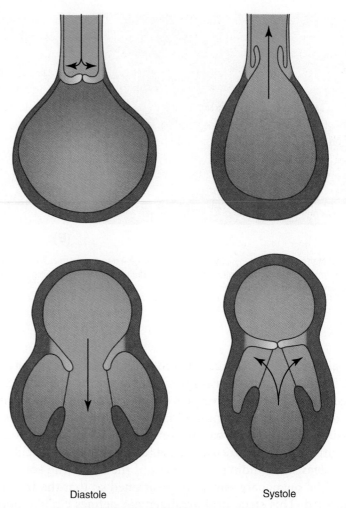

Diastole   Systole

FIGURE 11-3 Reciprocal action of atrioventricular and semilunar valves, resulting in unidirectional blood flow.

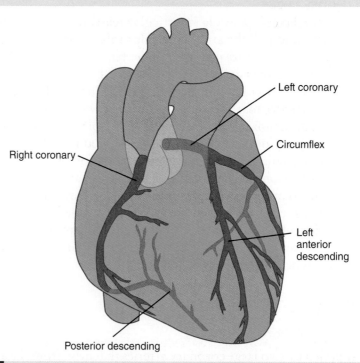

Left coronary

Circumflex

Right coronary

Left anterior descending

Posterior descending

FIGURE 11-4 Distribution of coronary arteries.

soon divides into two major branches. The left anterior descending artery supplies the front of the heart and the anterior part of the interventricular septum. The circumflex artery swings to the left (*circum* = around + *flex* = bend) to supply the left side of the heart. The right coronary artery swings to the right, supplying the right side of the heart, and then descends to supply the back of the heart and the posterior part of the interventricular septum. Each coronary artery has many branches that supply the heart muscle. The terminal branches of the coronary arteries frequently communicate with each other by means of connections called **anastomoses**. Because of these connections, obstruction of one of the arteries does not necessarily completely interrupt the blood flow to the tissues supplied by the blocked vessel. There may be enough blood flow through anastomoses with other arteries to supply the heart muscle. This is called a **collateral circulation**.

CONDUCTION SYSTEM OF THE HEART

The impulses that cause the heart to beat are initiated and propagated by groups of specialized muscle cells that depolarize spontaneously, which is called the conduction system of the heart (**FIGURE 11-5**). Impulses normally are generated in the sinoatrial (SA) node, which is located in the right atrium near the opening of the superior vena cava. Small bundles of fibers called internodal tracts connect the SA node to the atrioventricular (AV) node, which is located posteriorly in the lower part of the atrial septum. The atrioventricular bundle (bundle of His) is the continuation of the AV node, which transmits the impulse to the ventricles by passing through a small opening in the fibrous framework of the heart, the fibrous tissue that separates the atrial muscle from the ventricular muscle. After entering the ventricles, the AV bundle divides into right and left bundle branches in the upper part of the interventricular

Anastomosis
A communication between two blood vessels or other tubular structures. Also refers to a surgical connection of two hollow tubular structures, such as the divided ends of the intestine or a blood vessel (surgical anastomosis).

Collateral circulation
An accessory circulation capable of delivering blood to a tissue when the main circulation is blocked, as by a thrombus or embolus.

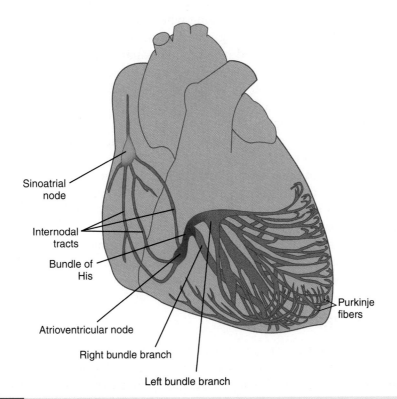

Sinoatrial node

Internodal tracts

Bundle of His

Atrioventricular node

Right bundle branch

Left bundle branch

Purkinje fibers

FIGURE 11-5 Diagram of the cardiac conduction system. The cardiac impulse originates in the SA node and is conducted to the ventricles via the internodal tracts, the AV node, the bundle of His, and the right and left bundle branches, which terminate in the network of Purkinje fibers.

septum, then descends in the septum and extends into the ventricles, where they terminate as Purkinje fibers that activate the heart muscle. The depolarization rate is also influenced by the autonomic nervous system. Sympathetic nervous system impulses increase the rate, and parasympathetic impulses slow it. The normal rhythm established by the cardiac conduction system is often called a normal sinus rhythm to emphasize that the normal cardiac rhythm is controlled by the sinoatrial node (which is often called simply the sinus node).

Although any part of the conduction system can depolarize spontaneously and generate an impulse, the SA node normally functions as the cardiac pacemaker because it depolarizes about 60 to 70 times per minute, which in turn depolarizes the other parts of the conduction system that depolarize at a slower rate. However, if impulse transmission from the SA node is interrupted by damage to the conduction system, the AV node, which discharges at about 50 times per minute, can take over, and if this system fails, then the bundle or bundle branches can initiate impulses but at a still slower rate of about 30 to 40 times per minute.

THE CARDIAC CYCLE

The sequence of events that occurs during a single contraction and relaxation of the cardiac chambers is called a cardiac cycle. During diastole, both the atria and ventricles are relaxed, the chambers are dilated, and the pressure of the blood within the chambers is very low. In a normal person at rest, each ventricle in diastole contains about 120 ml of blood, and much of the blood that fills the ventricles flows passively into the ventricles through the open atrioventricular valves. Late in diastole, atrial contraction expels an additional 30 ml of blood into the ventricles. If the heart rate is normal, the additional blood pumped into the ventricles by atrial contractions is not essential for reasonably normal cardiac function, but this extra amount makes a greater contribution to ventricular filling when the heart beats rapidly.

The ventricles contract following completion of atrial systole, ejecting blood into the aorta at high pressure and into the pulmonary artery at much lower pressure. Both ventricles contract at the same time, and each ventricle ejects the same volume of blood. Only about 70 ml is ejected from each ventricle during a systolic contraction, which is called the stroke volume, and is about 60 percent of the blood contained within the ventricles. The percentage of the ventricular volume ejected during systole is called the **ejection fraction**, a measurement that is often used when evaluating patients with heart failure.

Cardiac output is the output of blood from a single ventricle in one minute and is the product of the stroke volume (normally about 70 ml) multiplied by the heart rate (about 72 beats per minute), which equals about 5,000 ml per minute. This is approximately the total blood volume of the average adult. During vigorous activity, the normal heart of a healthy young person can double the stroke volume and greatly increase the heart rate, increasing cardiac output from four to seven times the resting cardiac output.

Ejection fraction
Percentage of the ventricular volume ejected during systole.

BLOOD PRESSURE

The flow of blood in the arteries is a result of the force of ventricular contraction. The pressure within the arteries varies rhythmically with the beating of the heart. The highest pressure is reached during ventricular contraction as blood is ejected into the aorta and its branches (systolic pressure). The pressure is lowest when the ventricles are relaxed (diastolic pressure); the recoil of the stretched arteries provides the force to propel the blood between contractions. The peripheral

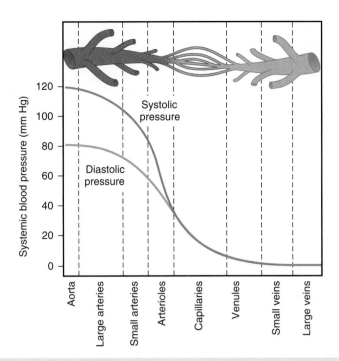

FIGURE 11-6 Changes in blood pressure as distance from the left ventricle increases.

Data from Shier, D.N., Butler, J.L., and Lewis, R. Hole's Essentials of Human Anatomy & Physiology, Tenth Edition. McGraw Hill Higher Education, 2009.

arterioles regulate the rate of blood flow into the capillaries by varying the degree of arteriolar constriction. Because of the resistance offered by the muscular arteries and arterioles, the blood pressure during cardiac diastole does not fall to zero but declines slowly as blood leaves the large arteries through the arterioles into the capillaries (**FIGURE 11-6**).

The elasticity of the large arteries also influences the systolic pressure. Some of the pressure rise caused by the blood ejected from the ventricle is absorbed by the stretch of the arteries, so the systolic pressure does not rise as high as it would if the arteries were more rigid and unable to stretch normally. In summary, blood pressure depends on cardiac output and the resistance of the peripheral vascular system. The systolic blood pressure is a measure of the force of ventricular contraction as blood is ejected into the large arteries and the resistance of the arterial system (sometimes called the tone of the system). The diastolic pressure is a measure of the rate of "run off" of blood into the capillaries, which is governed by the peripheral resistance caused by the small arterioles throughout the body. The mean (average) pressure of blood in the large arteries is approximately midway between systolic and diastolic pressure. Both cardiac output and vascular resistance are regulated by multiple physiologic systems to accommodate the body's need as discussed in the section on hypertension in the circulatory system.

Tools to Examine Cardiovascular Function

THE ELECTROCARDIOGRAM

The **electrocardiogram (ECG)** is a measure of the electrical activity of the heart as measured on the surface of the body by means of electrodes attached to the legs, arms, and chest. Voltage differences are recorded as a series of upward (positive) and downward (negative) deflections that form a characteristic pattern of deflections named in order: P, Q, R, S, and T. The P wave reflects the initial wave of depolarization associated with

Electrocardiogram (ECG)
A technique for measuring the serial changes in the electrical activity of the heart during the various phases of the cardiac cycle. (Often called ECG or EKG.)

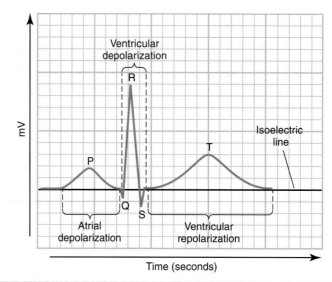

FIGURE 11-7   Characteristic features of a normal electrocardiogram.

atrial systole. The Q, R, and S waves, called collectively as the QRS complex, reflect the depolarization of the ventricles, which is followed by ventricular systole. The T wave represents repolarization of the ventricles during diastole. The time interval from the beginning of the P wave to the beginning of the QRS complex, which is called the PR interval, reflects the time required for the depolarization wave to pass through the AV bundle from the atria to the ventricles (**FIGURE 11-7**).

Usually, the positive and negative deflections are recorded on calibrated graph paper, each horizontal line representing a standard voltage difference and each vertical line representing a standard time interval. However, the ECG tracing also can be displayed on a fluorescent screen, which occurs when continuously monitoring a patient in a coronary care unit.

The ECG is a valuable diagnostic aid that can identify characteristic disturbances in the heart rate or rhythm (such as fibrillation discussed below) and abnormalities in the conduction of impulses through the heart. The ECG can also identify heart muscle injury, as occurs following a heart attack, and can determine the extent of the damage to the heart muscle (**FIGURE 11-8**).

ECHOCARDIOGRAPHY

Ultrasound examinations described in the discussion on general concepts of disease, principles of diagnosis, have many applications in medicine. An ultrasound examination of the cardiovascular system is usually called an **echocardiogram**. The procedure can identify valve and chamber abnormalities, and the dimensions of a narrowed valve orifice can be calculated from the rate of flow through the valve. The use of Doppler ultrasound allows the direction and velocity of blood flow to be determined, and abnormal blood flow patterns between chambers can be detected.

If a cardiac valve abnormality is suspected because a faint heart murmur was heard during a routine physical examination and the echocardiogram is normal, the echocardiogram can be used to determine whether this is a functional murmur resulting from turbulent blood flow within a normal heart. A normal echocardiogram can exclude a valve abnormality, an abnormal communication between adjacent atria or between adjacent ventricles, or an abnormal communication between the major blood vessels leaving the heart.

Echocardiogram
A record obtained from an ultrasound examination of the heart and related blood vessels; used to assist in the diagnosis of cardiovascular disease.

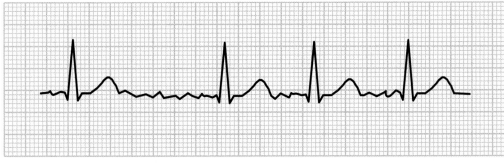

(A)

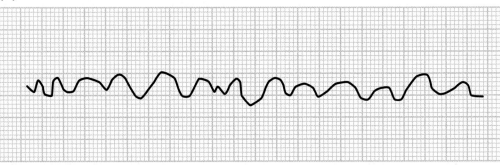

(B)

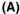 **FIGURE 11-8** **(A)** Atrial fibrillation illustrating absence of distinct P waves together with irregular ventricular rate, usually 140 to 160 beats per minute. **(B)** Ventricular fibrillation illustrating extremely abnormal chaotic cardiac rhythm without any evidence of synchronized electrical impulses.

Garcia, T. B., and Holtz, N. E. 2003. *Introduction to 12-Lead ECG*. Boston: Jones and Bartlett Publishers.

Heart Disease: An Introduction

Heart disease can result from congenital (and sometimes inherited) defects in the structure of the heart or in the contractile apparatus of cardiac myocytes. Infectious agents may damage heart valves and myocytes. Atherosclerotic disease of the coronary arteries will lead to compromised blood supply to the heart, termed coronary ischemia. If severe, such ischemia will result in cardiac myocyte necrosis, an event that defines a myocardial infarct (heart attack) with sequelae that may result in sudden cardiac death or some degree of chronic heart disease and failure. Systemic hypertension (excessive systemic blood pressure) will cause the heart to compensate by undergoing left ventricular hypertrophy. Ultimately the heart may not be able to compensate for the extra workload and fails.

Congenital Heart Disease

CARDIAC DEVELOPMENT AND PRENATAL BLOOD FLOW

The heart undergoes a complex developmental sequence. It is formed from a tube that undergoes segmental dilatations and constrictions along with considerable growth and change in configuration. Eventually the individual chambers, valves, and large arteries develop, culminating in the final structural characteristics of a normal fully developed heart.

As the heart is developing, the blood flow through the fetal heart differs from its final postdelivery flow pattern. Much of the blood flow in the pulmonary artery

Ductus arteriosus A fetal artery connecting the pulmonary artery with the aorta that permits pressure determined blood flow from pulmonary artery into the aorta, bypassing blood flow to the nonfunctional fetal lungs.

Foramen ovale An opening in the atrial septum covered by a one-way flap valve regulated by pressure differences between the atria, permitting blood flow from right to left atrium but not in the opposite direction, thereby bypassing blood flow from right cardiac chambers to the nonfunctional fetal lungs.

is diverted away from the lungs, which are nonfunctional in the fetus, and used instead to supply other fetal tissues. One bypass, called the **ductus arteriosus**, is a large communication connecting the pulmonary artery with the aorta that shunts much of the blood pumped into the pulmonary artery directly into the aorta. As soon as the infant is born and begins to breathe air, the lungs expand and the ductus arteriosus constricts, blocking blood flow. Consequently, pulmonary artery blood can then flow only into the newly expanded lungs; the nonfunctional ductus eventually becomes converted into a fibrous cord called the ligamentum arteriosum. The other bypass is an opening in the atrial septum called the **foramen ovale**, which maintains blood flow between the two atria as the atrial septum is developing. Blood (in part derived from maternal circulation via the umbilical vein and hence oxygen-rich) flow across the foramen ovale is controlled by a flap of atrial tissue on the left atrial side of the septum that covers (overlaps) the opening in the foramen ovale. In this position, the flap functions as a one-way valve that allows blood to flow from the right atrium into the left atrium but does not allow flow in the opposite direction (**FIGURE 11-9**). The right-to-left flow is determined by pressure differences between the two chambers. In the fetus, the blood pressure is higher in the right atrium than in the left atrium because only a relatively small volume of blood flows through the lungs and is returned to the left atrium. Most is directed into the aorta through the ductus arteriosus. After birth, the left atrial pressure rises when the lungs expand, allowing a large volume of blood to flow through the lungs and into the left atrium.

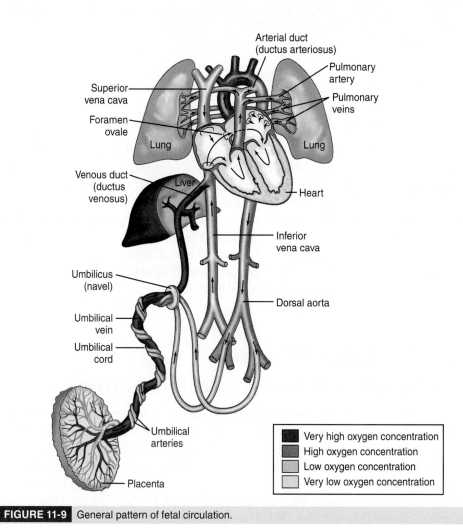

FIGURE 11-9 General pattern of fetal circulation.

The higher left atrial pressure presses the flap valve against the left atrial surface of the septum, closing the communication between the atria. Usually, the tissue flap fuses with the atrial septum to form a solid partition between the two atria. Sometimes, the fusion is incomplete but no flow of blood from right to left atria is possible as long as the left atrial pressure exceeds the pressure in the right atrium, which holds the flap against the atrial septum.

PATHOGENESIS AND MANIFESTATIONS OF CONGENITAL HEART DISEASE

Sometimes the heart fails to develop normally. Partitions between cardiac chambers may be defective, the cardiac valves may be malformed, or the large vessels entering and leaving the heart may not communicate normally with the appropriate atrium or ventricle. Some viral infections, such as rubella (German measles) or other maternal illnesses during the early phases of fetal development, may cause improper development of the heart as well as other organs. Some drugs or medications taken by the mother may disrupt normal fetal development. Some chromosomal abnormalities, such as Down syndrome, also are frequently associated with abnormal cardiac development. Genetic factors may account for some cardiac abnormalities, but often the reason for a congenital abnormality cannot be determined.

The effect of a structural abnormality depends on the nature of the defect and its effect on the circulation of blood. Most people with congenital heart abnormalities have a heart murmur caused by turbulent flow of blood within the heart, related to the cardiac malformation. Many congenital heart abnormalities result from abnormal communications between the systemic and pulmonary circulations that permit blood to be shunted between the adjacent chambers. The amount of blood shunted and the direction of the shunt depend on the size of the opening between the chambers, and the blood pressure difference between the chambers determines the direction of flow.

Most shunts are left-to-right shunts from left cardiac chambers (systemic circulation) into right cardiac chambers (pulmonary circulation). A left-to-right shunt mixes oxygenated blood from the left cardiac chambers with deoxygenated blood in the right chambers, but the admixture does not affect the oxygen content of the blood delivered to the tissues by the left ventricle. The amount of blood shunted depends on the size of the septal defect. A small defect shunts very little blood and has no significant effect on cardiovascular function. However, a large septal defect can shunt a large volume of blood, which puts an additional burden on the right ventricle, which is overfilled by the shunted blood. The larger volume of blood pumped into the lungs raises the pulmonary blood pressure, which eventually damages the lungs by causing thickening and narrowing of the pulmonary blood vessels. As the pulmonary vascular damage progresses and the pulmonary artery pressure continues to rise, the right ventricle has to work even harder to overcome the increasing resistance to blood flow through the lungs. The higher right ventricular pressure also causes the right atrial pressure to rise, reducing the pressure differences between the left and right atria. Consequently, the amount of blood shunted from the left to the right atrium also falls. Little or no blood shunting occurs when left and right atrial pressures equalize, and if right atrial pressure exceeds left atrial pressure, blood shunts between the atria in the opposite direction resulting in deoxygenated blood entering the circulation (a right-to-left shunt). This is termed **Eisenmenger syndrome** and has serious consequences.

Right-to-left shunts mix poorly oxygenated blood from the right cardiac chambers with normally oxygenated blood contained in the left cardiac chambers, which reduces the oxygen content of the blood pumped by the left ventricle to supply the

Eisenmenger syndrome Blood shunts between the atria in the opposite direction of normal.

body. The affected person's activities usually are severely restricted because of the low oxygen content of the arterial blood. The skin and mucous membranes acquire a blue color called **cyanosis**, which is caused by the low oxygen saturation of arterial blood, and congenital cardiovascular abnormalities associated with cyanosis are grouped together under the general term cyanotic congenital heart disease.

COMMON CARDIOVASCULAR ABNORMALITIES

The more common and important cardiovascular abnormalities fall into four major groups: failure of the normal fetal bypass channels to close; defects in the formation of the atrial and ventral septae; abnormalities that obstruct blood flow through the heart, pulmonary artery, or aorta; and malformations of the aorta and pulmonary artery or abnormal connection of the arteries to the appropriate ventricles.

Patent Ductus Arteriosus

Normally the ductus closes spontaneously soon after birth in full-term infants, in part due to falling levels of prostaglandins. A large patent ductus shunts blood from the aorta into the pulmonary artery and causes the same clinical manifestations and complications as an intracardiac left-to-right shunt. This is treated by the use of prostaglandin synthesis inhibitors (such as indomethacin) or, if necessary, surgical closure of the ductus.

Atrial and Ventricular Septal Defects

Usually, an atrial septal defect results from defective development of the partitions that divide the atria with the defect located in the middle of the septum at the site usually occupied by the foramen ovale. Small defects in children often close spontaneously and are often asymptomatic as discussed above. Larger defects should be closed, which usually can be accomplished using a device inserted into the heart through a peripheral vein. Sometimes an open surgical procedure is required to place a patch over the defect.

A common type of atrial septal defect is a patent foramen ovale. The foramen ovale normally becomes nonfunctional after birth, caused by the rapid postdelivery changes in atrial pressures. The left atrial pressure rises when pulmonary blood flow increases after the ductus arteriosus closes. The higher left atrial pressure pushes the flap valve of the foramen ovale against the atrial septum, where it usually fuses with the septum. In newborn infants, the foramen ovale may remain patent and functional if the infant has a congenital cardiac abnormality that is associated with a high right atrial pressure, which forces right-to-left blood flow through the foramen ovale. In about 25 percent of adults, the flap valve does not fuse completely, but the foramen ovale remains nonfunctional as long as the left atrial pressure remains higher than the right atrial pressure.

Ventricular septal defects are also very common (**FIGURE 11-10**). Many are less than 3 mm in diameter and often close spontaneously, but larger defects require surgical closure. Generally, all large septal defects need to be closed because of the harmful effects of a large defect.

Pulmonary or Aortic Valve Stenosis Caused by Semilunar Valve Maldevelopment

Abnormal development of the semilunar valve leaflets narrows the valve opening, which can vary from 2 to 10 ml diameter. The degree of obstruction depends on the diameter of the orifice (**FIGURE 11-11**). Pulmonary stenosis obstructs outflow from the right ventricle, and aortic stenosis impedes outflow from the left ventricle. Treatment consists of dilating the valve opening by inserting a balloonlike device into the narrow opening.

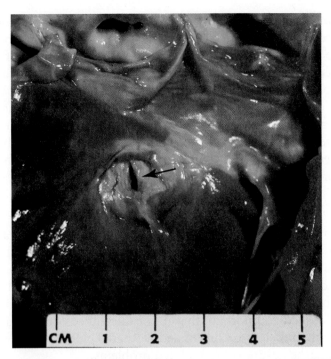

FIGURE 11-10 Small ventricular septal defect (*arrow*).

Courtesy of Leonard V. Crowley, MD, Century College.

Coarctation of the Aorta

Coarctation is a Latin word meaning "narrowing" that describes a localized narrowing of the proximal aorta restricting blood flow into the distal aorta. Usually, the constriction is located distal to the origin of the large arteries arising from the arch of the aorta. The blood pressure in the aorta and its branches proximal to the

Coarctation Localized narrowing of the proximal aorta.

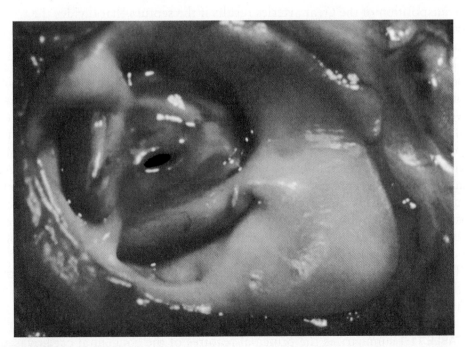

FIGURE 11-11 Congenital pulmonary stenosis. The valve orifice is reduced to a narrow slit, obstructing outflow from the right ventricle.

Courtesy of Leonard V. Crowley, MD, Century College.

coarctation is much higher than normal because the heart has to pump blood at a much higher pressure to deliver blood through the narrowed segment of aorta, possibly leading to left ventricular disease. The pressure and volume of blood flowing into the aorta distal to the coarctation are both lower than normal, and a collateral circulation develops to bypass the obstruction. An individual with a coarctation may appear normal except for high blood pressure identified when measuring pressure in the brachial arteries, but lower-than-normal blood pressure in the arteries of the lower extremities. Usually, the narrowed segment of aorta is relatively short and can be treated by resecting the constricting segment and reconnecting the aorta so that its caliber is normal throughout its entire length.

The Tetralogy of Fallot and Transposition of the Great Arteries

Both of these conditions result from abnormal division of a single channel called the truncus arteriosus, which extends from the developing ventricles and will be divided by a partition to form the aorta and the pulmonary artery. The partition takes a spiral course as it divides the truncus arteriosus, which is why the aorta and the pulmonary artery spiral around each other as they attach to their respective ventricles. The two abnormalities caused by abnormal division of the truncus arteriosus are relatively common, and both cause intermixing of deoxygenated blood with oxygenated blood, which leads to marked cyanosis and related problems.

The tetralogy of Fallot results if the septum that divides the truncus is misplaced and divides unequally. This results in the four abnormalities that comprise the tetralogy: a ventricular septal defect, pulmonary stenosis, an enlarged aorta that overrides the septal defect, and right ventricular hypertrophy that develops as a consequence of the pulmonary stenosis. In this condition, poorly oxygenated blood in the right ventricle flows through the septal defect to mix with blood from the left ventricle flowing into the aorta, which overrides the septal defect. Treatment consists of enlarging the opening of the narrowed pulmonary artery and closing the septal defect.

Transposition of the great arteries results if the septum that divides the truncus arteriosus does not follow its normal spiral course when it divides the truncus into the aorta and pulmonary artery. Consequently, the aorta and pulmonary artery develop parallel to each other. The aorta becomes located to the right of the pulmonary artery instead of behind and to the left of the pulmonary artery. The aorta becomes connected to the right ventricle and the pulmonary artery attaches to the left ventricle, which severely disrupts blood flow in both the pulmonary and systemic circulations. Consequently, the body is supplied by poorly oxygenated blood that is continuously circulated in the systemic circulation and the flow of oxygenated blood remains confined to the pulmonary circuit, where it serves no useful purpose. After birth, the condition is not compatible with life unless there is a communication that permits some intermixing of blood between the pulmonary and systemic circulations such as a patent foramen ovale, atrial septal defect, or ventricular septal defect (**FIGURE 11-12**). Generally, such communications do not provide enough oxygenated blood to supply the infant's needs.

The current treatment of this condition is called the arterial switch operation in which the aorta is connected to the left ventricle, and the pulmonary artery is attached to the right ventricle. It is also necessary to reposition the coronary arteries so they are connected properly to the artery supplying blood to the left ventricle.

TABLE 11-1 summarizes the principal features of the congenital cardiovascular malformations described in this section, which are also illustrated in **FIGURE 11-13**.

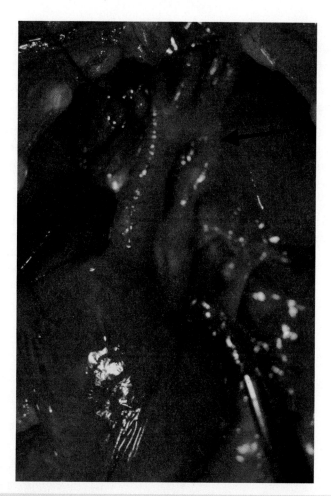

FIGURE 11-12 Transposition of the great arteries showing the parallel course of the aorta and pulmonary artery. Aorta is located to the right of the pulmonary artery (*left*) and is connected to the right ventricle, and the pulmonary artery is attached to the left ventricle. Some intermixing of blood between the aortic and pulmonary circulations is achieved by the large patent ductus arteriosus *(arrow)*, and also by the foramen ovale, which is not demonstrated in the photograph.

Courtesy of Leonard V. Crowley, MD, Century College.

TABLE 11-1   Features of Common Congenital Cardiovascular Abnormalities

Abnormality	Physiologic disturbance	Complications	Treatment
Patent ductus arteriosus	Aorta to pulmonary artery shunt	Pulmonary hypertension	Ligate or excise ductus
Patent foramen ovale	Right-to-left atrial shunt	Usually nonfunctional as long as left atrial pressure exceeds right atrial pressure	Usually no treatment required
Atrial, ventricular, and combined septal defects	Left-to-right shunt	Pulmonary hypertension damages lungs. Right ventricular hypertrophy	Close defect
Pulmonary stenosis	Obstructed outflow from right ventricle	Right ventricular hypertrophy	Dilate narrowed valve opening
Aortic stenosis	Obstructed outflow from left ventricle	Left ventricular hypertrophy	Dilate narrowed valve opening

(continues)

TABLE 11-1 Features of Common Congenital Cardiovascular Abnormalities (*Continued*)

Abnormality	Physiologic disturbance	Complications	Treatment
Aortic coarctation	Obstructed flow into aorta distal to coarctation	Hypertension in arteries supplying head and upper limbs	Excise coarctation and reconnect aorta
Tetralogy of Fallot	Right-to-left shunt. Ventricular septal defect straddled by enlarged aorta. Pulmonary stenosis. Right ventricular hypertrophy	Cyanosis. Polycythemia. Clubbing of fingers and toes	Enlarge pulmonary artery opening. Close septal defect
Transposition of great arteries	Aorta attached to right ventricle and pulmonary artery attached to left ventricle	Only communication between systemic and pulmonary circulations is through ductus arteriosus and foramen ovale	Reattach aorta and pulmonary artery to proper ventricles. Reposition coronary arteries

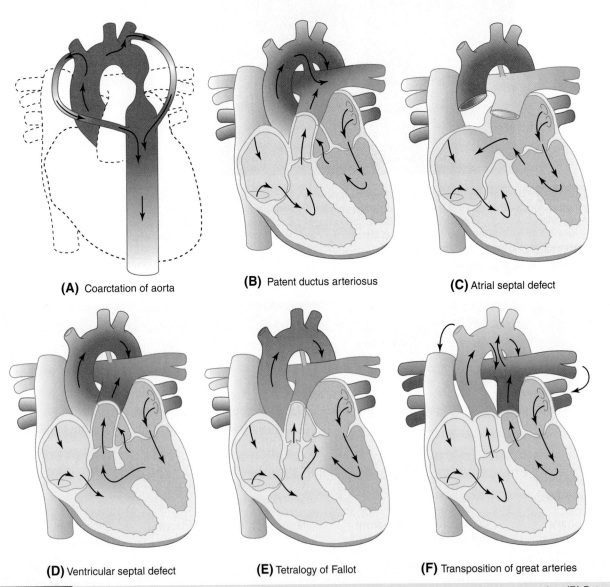

(A) Coarctation of aorta **(B)** Patent ductus arteriosus **(C)** Atrial septal defect

(D) Ventricular septal defect **(E)** Tetralogy of Fallot **(F)** Transposition of great arteries

FIGURE 11-13 Blood flow patterns in six common congenital abnormalities described in this section. **(A)** Aortic coarctation. **(B)** Patent ductus arteriosus. **(C)** Atrial septal defect. **(D)** Ventricular septal defect. **(E)** Tetralogy of Fallot. **(F)** Transposition of the great arteries.

Primary Myocardial Disease

In a small number of patients, heart disease results not from valvular or coronary disease or hypertension but from primary disease of the heart muscle itself. There are two major types of primary myocardial disease. One type results from inflammation of the heart muscle and is called myocarditis. The other type, in which there is no evidence of inflammation, is designated by the noncommittal term cardiomyopathy (*cardio* = heart + *myo* = muscle + *pathy* = disease).

MYOCARDITIS

Myocarditis is characterized by an active inflammation in the heart muscle associated with injury and necrosis of individual muscle fibers. In the United States, most cases are caused by viruses; coxsackievirus, adenovirus, and echovirus are the most common (**FIGURE 11-14**). Rarely myocarditis may be caused by parasites, such as *Trichinella* or the agent of Chagas disease (discussion on animal parasites) that lodge in the myocardium and cause an inflammation. Occasionally, other pathogens such as *Histoplasma* are responsible, especially in immunocompromised patients. Some cases are the result of a hypersensitivity reaction such as the myocarditis occurring in acute rheumatic fever (see below) and some drug reactions.

The onset of myocarditis is usually abrupt and may lead to acute heart failure. Fortunately, in most cases, the inflammation subsides completely and the patient recovers without any permanent heart damage. There is no specific treatment other than treating the underlying condition that caused the myocarditis and decreasing cardiac work by bed rest and limited activity until the inflammation subsides.

CARDIOMYOPATHY

The general term cardiomyopathy encompasses several different conditions of which dilated cardiomyopathy (DCM) and hypertrophic cardiomyopathy (HCM) are most

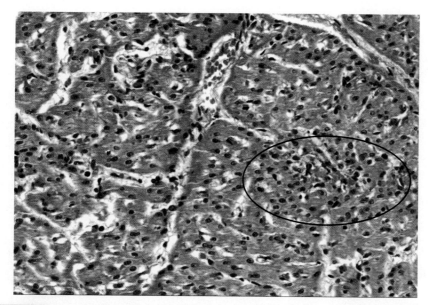

FIGURE 11-14 Photomicrograph of acute viral myocarditis in a child. There is infiltration of the heart by mononuclear inflammatory cells in response to the viral infection. The highlighted area shows a locus of inflammatory cells and destruction of cardiac myocytes.

Courtesy of Department of Pathology and Laboratory Medicine, University of North Carolina at Chapel Hill.

important. One third of DCM cases are hereditary and most are transmitted as dominant traits. More than fifty genes are associated with the disease. HCM is also often caused by dominant mutations, about 80 percent of the time of two genes (beta myosin heavy chain and myosin binding protein C). The responsible gene mutations often can be identified by genetic tests. Dilated cardiomyopathy is characterized by enlargement of the heart and dilatation of its chambers. The pumping action of the ventricles is greatly impaired, which leads to chronic heart failure.

Hypertrophic cardiomyopathy is characterized by disarray of muscle fibers that intersect at odd angles with no apparent organized pattern and marked hypertrophy of heart muscle to such an extent that the thick-walled chambers become greatly reduced in size and do not dilate readily in diastole. Frequently, the muscle of the septum is hypertrophied to a greater extent than the rest of the myocardium and hinders outflow of the blood from the ventricle into the aorta. At times, the thick septum may actually impinge on the anterior mitral valve leaflet, intermittently completely blocking the outflow of blood from the left ventricle (HCM with outflow tract obstruction) (FIGURE 11-15).

Patients with HCM that show outflow tract obstruction frequently exhibit manifestations related to inadequate cardiac output, such as episodes of excessive fatigue and lightheadedness related to exertion. The characteristic myocardial hypertrophy with greatly thickened septa can be identified by echocardiography (see discussion on general concepts of disease, principles of diagnosis). Treatment consists of administering drugs that slow the heart, allowing more time for ventricular filling, and that reduce the force of ventricular contraction, which tends to reduce the degree of obstruction caused by the hypertrophied septum. Commonly used drugs are those that block the sympathetic nerve impulses that normally increase heart rate and the force of contraction (beta blockers) and those that decrease myocardial contractility by impeding the flow of calcium into myocardial cells (called calcium channel blocking agents). People who do not respond to medical treatment may require surgical resection of part of the thickened septum.

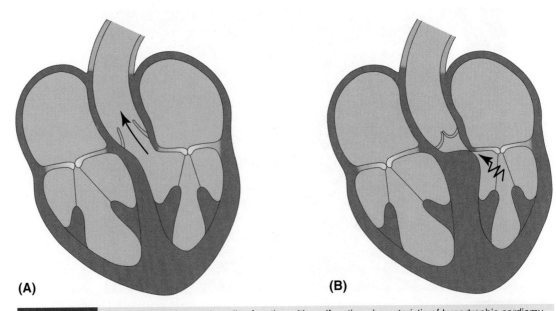

(A) **(B)**

FIGURE 11-15 A comparison of normal cardiac function with malfunction characteristic of hypertrophic cardiomyopathy. **(A)** Normal heart, illustrating unobstructed flow of blood from left ventricle into aorta during ventricular systole. **(B)** Hypertrophic cardiomyopathy, illustrating obstruction to outflow of blood from left ventricle by hypertrophied septum, which impinges on anterior leaflet of mitral valve.

Valvular Heart Disease

Rheumatic valvular heart disease has markedly declined, along with rheumatic fever, but other conditions that cause valve malfunction have assumed greater importance. These include various degenerative conditions of the aortic valve and an abnormality of the mitral valve that causes it to prolapse into the atrium during ventricular systole.

RHEUMATIC FEVER AND RHEUMATIC HEART DISEASE

Rheumatic fever is a complication of infection by the group A beta hemolytic strep-tococcus, the organism responsible for streptococcal sore throat and scarlet fever. Clinically, the affected individual has an acute arthritis affecting multiple joints (which is why the disease is called "rheumatic" fever) and evidence of inflammation of the heart.

Rheumatic fever is not a bacterial infection but a type of hypersensitivity reaction induced by various antigens present in the streptococcus. This reaction develops several weeks after the initial streptococcal infection. Apparently, some individuals form antibodies against antigens present in the streptococcus, and the antistreptococcal antibody cross-reacts with similar antigens in the individual's own tissues. The antigen–antibody reaction injures connective tissue and is responsible for the febrile illness. Fortunately, rheumatic fever develops in only a small proportion of people with group A beta streptococcal infections.

Patients with acute rheumatic fever rarely die as a result of severe inflammation of the heart and consequent acute heart failure; generally the fever and signs of inflammation eventually subside although healing is often associated with some degree of scarring. In the joints and in many other tissues, scarring causes no difficulties, but scarring of heart valves may produce deformities that impair function.

Rheumatic heart disease is caused by scarring of the heart valves subsequent to the healing of a rheumatic inflammation. This complication is relatively common and primarily affects the valves of the left side of the heart, the mitral and aortic valves (**FIGURE 11-16**). If the valve does not close properly, blood refluxes back through it (called **regurgitation**). Frequently, the damaged valve also does not open properly, and the valve orifice is narrowed. This is called a valve **stenosis**. Valve lesions impair cardiac function. When valvular stenosis is present, the heart must exert more effort than normal to force blood through the narrowed orifice. In regurgitation, a portion of the ventricular output is not expelled normally and leaks through the incompetent valve. This is a serious disadvantage because the heart must repump the volume of regurgitated blood to deliver the same amount of blood to the peripheral tissues.

When a person is seriously disabled by a rheumatic valvular deformity, it is possible to excise the abnormal, scarred heart valve surgically and replace it with an artificial valve (discussed later in this chapter).

NONRHEUMATIC AORTIC STENOSIS

Nonrheumatic aortic stenosis can be caused by aortic stenosis secondary to a bicuspid aortic valve or by the aging of the valve. In about 2 percent of people, the aortic valve has two rather than the usual three cusps. This abnormality is called a congenital bicuspid aortic valve. The valve functions satisfactorily for a time but is subjected to unusual stress during opening and closing because of its bicuspid configuration. As a result, the valve gradually becomes thickened and may eventually become calcified after many years, leading to marked rigidity of the valve when a person

Rheumatic fever A disease caused by hypersensitivity to antigens of the beta streptococcus, characterized by fever, joint pains, and inflammation of heart valves and muscle.

Regurgitation Backward flow of blood because valve does not close properly.

Stenosis Narrowing of a valve orifice.

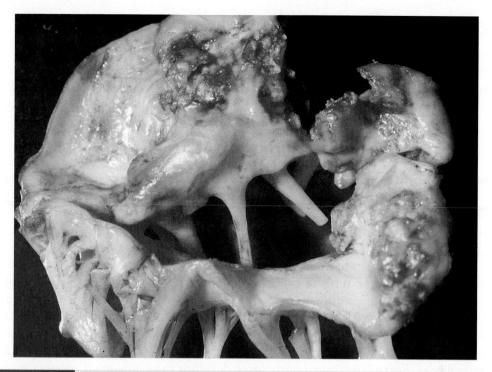

FIGURE 11-16 A poorly functioning scarred and calcified mitral valve resulting from valve damage caused by prior rheumatic fever. The valve was excised and replaced by an artificial heart valve.
Courtesy of Leonard V. Crowley, MD, Century College.

reaches middle age (**FIGURE 11-17**). This condition is called aortic stenosis secondary to bicuspid aortic valve.

Fibrosis and calcification of the valve leaflets of a normal three cusp aortic valve may also occur in older people when sometimes the valve becomes so rigid that it is unable to open properly. This entity is called calcific aortic stenosis (**FIGURE 11-18**).

Mild degrees of aortic stenosis may not greatly compromise cardiac function, but severe aortic stenosis places a great strain on the left ventricle, which must expel blood through the greatly narrowed and rigid valve orifice. This leads to marked left ventricular hypertrophy and eventual heart failure. Treatment of severe aortic stenosis consists of surgically replacing the stenotic valve with an artificial heart valve.

Aortic stenosis usually is considered to be caused by degenerative changes in valve leaflet connective tissue, which are similar to those seen in atherosclerotic disease discussed with diseases of blood circulation. As our population ages, aortic stenosis is becoming one of the most common types of valvular heart disease.

MITRAL VALVE PROLAPSE

Although mitral valve prolapse is a common condition, only a very small percentage of people ever develops any problems related to the prolapse. In this condition, one or both mitral leaflets is enlarged and prolapse into the left atrium during ventricular systole. Sometimes, the prolapsing free margins of the valve leaflets do not fit together tightly, which allows some blood to leak across the closed mitral valve into the atrium, called mitral regurgitation. The amount of blood that leaks into the left atrium through the prolapsing valve depends on how tightly the free margins of the prolapsing valve leaflets come together during ventricular systole (**FIGURE 11-19**).

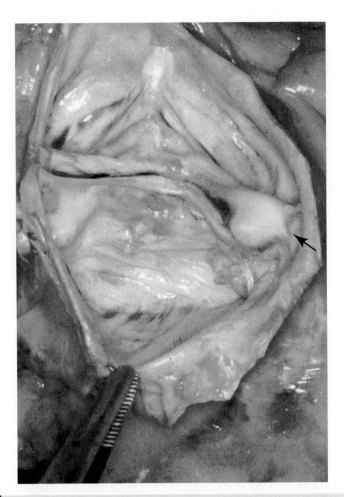

FIGURE 11-17 A congenital bicuspid aortic valve viewed from above. Beginning scarring is seen at the right margin of the valve (*arrow*).

Courtesy of Leonard V. Crowley, MD, Century College.

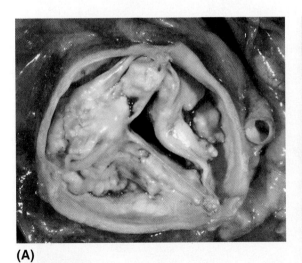

(A)

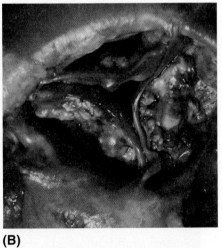

(B)

FIGURE 11-18 An aortic valve viewed from above, illustrating marked thickening and nodularity of valve leaflets. **(A)** Partial fusion of valve cusps (*left*). A normal coronary artery is seen in a cross section at right of aortic valve. **(B)** Severe calcific aortic stenosis. Extensive calcium deposits within cusps severely limit valve mobility.

Courtesy of Leonard V. Crowley, MD, Century College.

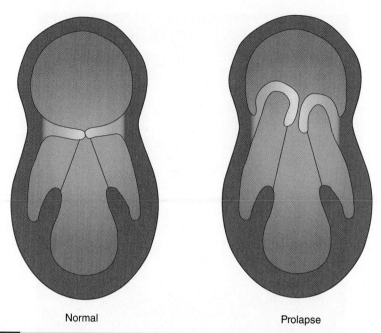

Normal   Prolapse

FIGURE 11-19 Normal mitral valve leaflets (*left*) compared with prolapsing mitral leaflets associated with mild mitral insufficiency (*right*).

In some cases, the prolapse appears to be caused by degenerative changes in the connective tissue of the valve leaflets, which permits the affected valve leaflets to gradually stretch as a result of the degeneration of the valve connective tissue. Eventually, one or both leaflets may become enlarged. When this occurs, the stretched prolapsing mitral valve, held at its margin by the chordae, somewhat resembles an open parachute (**FIGURE 11-20**); a significant amount of blood may reflux into the left

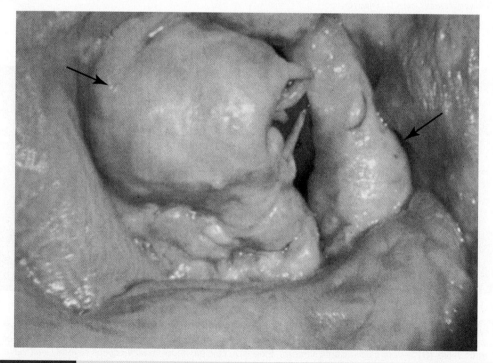

FIGURE 11-20 The interior of the left atrium viewed from above, illustrating prolapsing mitral valve leaflets ballooning into the left atrium (*arrows*). Prolapse was complicated by a rupture of mitral valve chorda tendinea.

Courtesy of Leonard V. Crowley, MD, Century College.

atrium. The prolapsing valve may also produce excessive strain on the chordae and papillary muscles, which may provoke bouts of ventricular arrhythmia. Sometimes the excessive stress causes one of the chordae to rupture. Mitral regurgitation may be related to any defect in the structure of the valve (e.g., caused by rheumatic disease or by certain tumors or drugs that increase the circulating level of serotonin) and, if severe, can be associated with acute and chronic disease. Surgical valvular repair or replacement may become necessary.

PROSTHETIC (ARTIFICIAL) HEART VALVES

A heart valve that has been so badly damaged by disease that it no longer can function adequately can be replaced by an artificial valve, which is usually called a prosthetic heart valve (*prosthesis* = replacement). The two major types are mechanical valves and bioprosthetic valves manufactured from porcine valves or bovine pericardial tissue. Because no prosthetic valve can function as well as a normal heart valve, each type has advantages and disadvantages. Mechanical valves, which are very durable, are composed of metal components. The valves are classified into three categories according to how they function: a caged-ball valve, tilting circular disk valve, or a two leaflet (bi-leaflet) valve (**FIGURE 11-21**). The valves come in various sizes. The

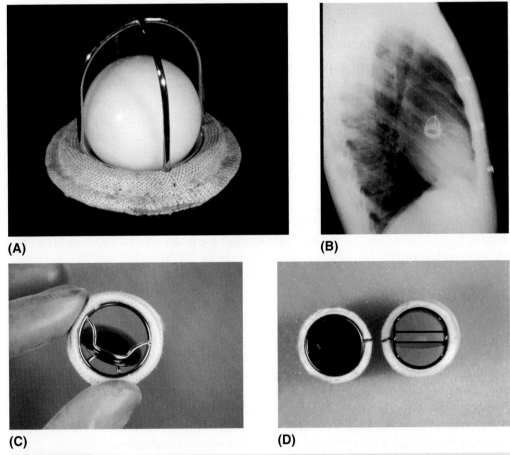

(A) **(B)** **(C)** **(D)**

FIGURE 11-21 **(A)** Caged-ball valve. **(B)** Lateral chest x-ray showing the caged-ball valve positioned to replace the aortic valve. The base of the valve is positioned in the aortic valve opening with the cage extending into the base of the aorta. The ball is not radio-opaque and is not seen in the x-ray film. **(C)** Tilting disk valve viewed from superior surface with the disc in open valve position to allow flow from atrium to ventricle during diastole, as when replacing a mitral valve. **(D)** Two views of two leaflet valves viewed from undersurface with leaflets closed (*left*) and opened (*right*).

Courtesy of Leonard V. Crowley, MD, Century College.

periphery of all valves has a rim of synthetic flexible material for attachment of sutures to hold the valve in proper position when anchoring it within the heart after the patient's own dysfunctional valve has been removed. In all prosthetic valves, as in the normal heart, the opening and closing of the valve is governed by blood pressure differences on opposite sides of the valve.

Although mechanical valves are more durable than bioprosthetic valves, they have one disadvantage. Blood clots can form on the metal parts of the prosthesis unless the patient takes an anticoagulant continuously to prevent formation of thrombi, which would disrupt the function of the prosthesis and could lead to embolic disease if pieces of blood clot break off from the prosthesis, blocking major systemic arteries. Bioprosthetic valves, which more closely resemble normal valves, are composed of specially treated animal tissues. Although the patient does not have to take anticoagulants, these valves are not as durable as mechanical valves and tend to wear out in ten to fifteen years, requiring replacement. Consequently, their use is usually limited to older individuals, such as elderly people with severe calcific aortic stenosis. About twice as many individuals with bioprosthetic valves rather than mechanical valves will require replacement within fifteen years (12 percent versus 7 percent of patients).

A person with a valve prosthesis has an increased risk of developing infective endocarditis, described in the following section. Infection of a prosthetic heart valve is a very serious complication because the infection is often at the site where the valve is attached to the myocardial tissues surrounding the valve opening.

Methods of Valve Replacement

The standard method for replacing a poorly functioning heart valve, such as a narrowed calcified aortic stenosis in an elderly patient (illustrated by the valve in Figure 11-18), requires an extensive surgical procedure. The sternum must be divided and separated to reach the heart, followed by a cardiopulmonary bypass procedure assisted by a heart lung machine to divert blood from the heart while the calcified valve is removed and usually replaced by a tissue valve, such as a pig valve. Many elderly patients with other health problems in addition to aortic stenosis may be too ill for such an extensive procedure. Consequently, other less invasive procedures to replace heart valves are being developed, such as passing the replacement valve retrograde into the heart through the femoral artery. Advances in valve design and development of newer ways to place the valves in the heart should improve the safety of valve replacement.

INFECTIVE ENDOCARDITIS

Infective endocarditis is an infection of a heart valve, usually caused by bacteria but occasionally by other pathogens. In most cases, the infection is in the mitral and aortic valves in the left side of the heart. It is customary to classify infective endocarditis as either subacute or acute infective endocarditis. The subacute form is caused by organisms of low virulence, may be a complication of any type of valvular heart disease, and is associated with relatively mild symptoms of infection. Acute infective endocarditis, caused by highly virulent organisms that infect previously normal heart valves, is associated with symptoms of a severe systemic infection.

Subacute Infective Endocarditis

An abnormal or damaged valve is susceptible to infection because small deposits of aggregated platelets and fibrin may accumulate on the roughened surface of the valve, serving as a site for implantation of bacteria. In normal people, transient bacteremia

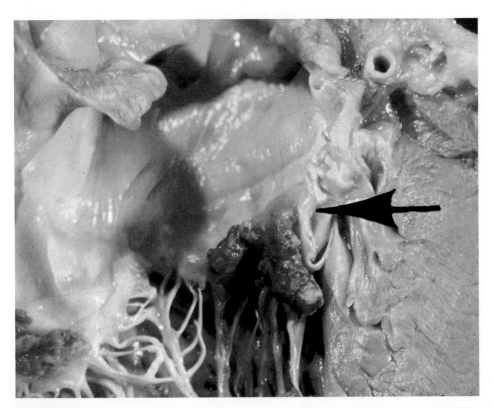

FIGURE 11-22 Bacterial endocarditis illustrating vegetations on mitral valve leaflet (*arrow*). Normal coronary artery is seen in cross section (*upper right*).

Courtesy of Leonard V. Crowley, MD, Century College.

causes no problems because the organisms are normally destroyed by the body's defenses. However, an individual with a damaged valve runs the risk that bacteria may become implanted on the valve and cause an inflammation (**FIGURE 11-22**). Frequently, thrombi form at the site of the valve infection, and bits of thrombus may be dislodged and carried as emboli to other parts of the body, producing infarcts in various organs.

Antibiotic Prophylaxis to Prevent Endocarditis

Infective (bacterial) endocarditis is relatively uncommon, but it is a very serious disease. Individuals with damaged heart valves or other cardiac abnormalities are at increased risk. Some surgical procedures and many dental procedures, such as cleaning and removal of dental plaque, tooth extractions, and root canal treatment, may cause a shower of bacteria to be discharged into the bloodstream, becoming a potential risk to patients with damaged or abnormal heart valves. The American Heart Association provides guidelines regarding who should receive antibiotic prophylaxis, the types of surgical procedures requiring antibiotic prophylaxis, the recommended antibiotics to use, and the recommended dosage and duration of antibiotic treatment. At present, prophylactic antibiotics are only recommended for dental patients who are at high risk of endocarditis such as those with heart valve damage, an artificial heart valve, or who have had surgically treated congenital heart disease.

Acute Infective Endocarditis

Acute infective endocarditis results when highly pathogenic organisms spread into the bloodstream from an infection elsewhere in the body and infect a previously normal

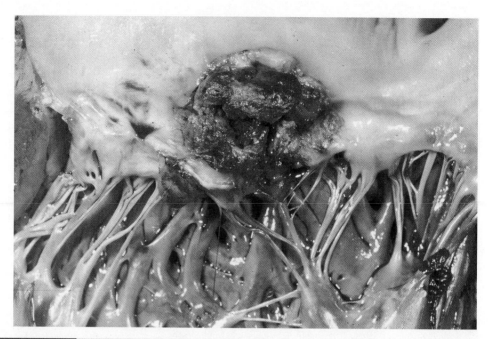

FIGURE 11-23 Severe bacterial endocarditis caused by staphylococcal infection of normal mitral valve. Infection has caused extensive destruction and perforation of valve leaflet.

Courtesy of Leonard V. Crowley, MD, Century College.

heart valve. Virulent staphylococci are a common cause of acute endocarditis and may cause considerable destruction of the affected valve (**FIGURE 11-23**).

Another group at high risk are intravenous drug abusers; in this group, the infection is usually in the tricuspid valve rather than the valves on the left side of the heart. Infection results from using unsterile materials to dissolve and inject the drug and from the normal skin flora.

Cardiac Arrhythmias

The orderly depolarization and repolarization of the conduction system that directs the contraction and relaxation of the atria and ventricles does not always function perfectly, leading to disturbances in the heart rate or rhythm, called cardiac **arrhythmias**. Such problems include atrial or ventricular fibrillation or heart block.

Arrhythmia An irregularity of the heartbeat.

ATRIAL FIBRILLATION

One of the more common abnormal cardiac rhythms is called atrial fibrillation (AF), in which the atria contract in an irregular pattern and at a very rapid rate. The condition often occurs in older people, especially those with cardiovascular disease or chronic pulmonary disease, but may also occur in people whose thyroid glands produce an excess of thyroid hormone (hyperthyroidism) and in a few other conditions. Occasionally, AF occurs in apparently normal healthy individuals for no apparent reason.

AF starts as an abnormal focus of electrical activity in the atrium, which abruptly evolves into multiple areas of depolarization throughout the atria that stimulate atrial muscle fibers continuously in a haphazard, disorganized manner at a very rapid rate of up to 400 impulses per minute. The intense disorderly stimulation of multiple groups of atrial muscle fibers causes the atrial muscle to quiver ineffectively instead of contracting normally. This allows blood to "pool" in the atria, which may result in thrombus (clot) formation. The abnormal electrical impulses are also relayed to the AV node, which is overwhelmed and unable to respond to such a large number of stimuli. Only a relatively small number of impulses are able to travel through the AV node and AV bundle (bundle of His) to reach the ventricles, which beat irregularly at about 140 to 160 times per minute (Figure 11-8A). At such a fast ventricular contraction rate, the duration of diastole is very short. The duration of diastole also varies from beat to beat because the rate at which impulses can be delivered to the ventricles from the quivering atria is not uniform. As a result, the time available for ventricular filling in diastole also varies from beat to beat, which causes the volume of blood filling the ventricles and ejected during each ventricular contraction (stroke volume) to vary. Some of the ventricular contractions occur before the ventricles are adequately filled with blood, and the volume of blood ejected may be insufficient, resulting in **hypotension** (abnormally low blood pressure) and **pulmonary congestion** (pooling of blood in the lungs). The diagnosis of atrial fibrillation is made by examination of the ECG, which reveals a lack of P waves (an indication that the atria are not contracting normally) along with some variability in the QRS complexes related to the variable ventricular stroke volumes (Figure 11-8A).

Hypotension Abnormally low blood pressure.

Pulmonary congestion Pooling of blood in the lungs.

TREATMENT OF ATRIAL FIBRILLATION

The first treatment step is to administer drugs that help regulate AV node function. This can be accomplished by giving medications that impede transmission of impulses through the AV node and bundle so fewer impulses reach the ventricles (beta blockers, calcium channel antagonists, and sometimes digitalis [digoxin], which decrease heart contractility).

When the heart rate has been slowed, the next step is to restore a normal heart rhythm by terminating the fibrillation. This can be accomplished either by an electrical cardioversion, which involves the application of an electrical shock by paddles applied to the patient's chest to terminate the arrhythmia, or by pharmacologic therapy, which uses drugs that terminate the arrhythmia by interfering with some phase in the abnormal impulse formation to "break up" the arrhythmia. Endoscopic techniques that ablate areas of the heart around the AV node may also be attempted if these therapies fail. Once the normal rhythm is restored, the patient may need to continue taking some medication to maintain the normal rhythm.

VENTRICULAR FIBRILLATION

In contrast to atrial fibrillation, ventricular fibrillation is incompatible with life because the ventricles are unable to contract normally and the circulation ceases (Figure 11-8B). Ventricular fibrillation sometimes occurs following a heart attack. If recognized promptly, it is often possible to stop the fibrillation by delivering an electric shock to the heart by means of electrodes applied to the chest. The procedure usually causes the ventricles to resume normal contractions.

HEART BLOCK

Heart block is a delay or complete interruption of impulse transmission from the atria to the ventricles. Usually, the condition results from arteriosclerosis of the coronary arteries in which parts of the conduction system fail to receive an adequate blood supply. In the mildest form, heart block is manifested only as a delay in the conduction of impulses from the atria to the ventricles. In a more marked degree of block (incomplete heart block), not all the SA node impulses are conducted through the damaged AV bundle. Every second, third, or fourth impulse may fail to reach the ventricle. In the most severe form (complete heart block), conduction of impulses through the AV bundle is completely interrupted. Impulses originating in the SA node cause the atria to contract normally, but the impulses are not transmitted normally to the ventricles. When this occurs, the conduction system distal to the block "takes over" as the source of impulses to activate the ventricles, but the impulses are generated at a much slower rate of 30 to 40 per minute. The extremely low ventricular rate may not provide sufficient blood flow to the brain, resulting in periodic episodes of dizziness or loss of consciousness. Complete heart block is treated by implanting an artificial pacemaker that consists of a small electrode inserted into the heart through a vein and positioned in the ventricle. The electrode is connected to a small device containing a battery that is implanted beneath the skin of the chest. The device can be programmed to generate impulses that stimulate ventricular contractions at a predetermined rate. Many different types of pacemakers are available, each having specific applications.

Myocardial Ischemia and Its Complications: A "Heart Attack"

> **Coronary thrombosis** Thrombus formation on the surface of a plaque blocking the coronary artery.

Several mechanisms may trigger a heart attack in a patient with coronary artery disease. Sudden blockage of a coronary artery may occur by a thrombus formation on the surface of an atheromatous plaque (atheroma), a process termed **coronary thrombosis**. This is most often related to some change in atheroma such as hemorrhage into the plaque (further narrowing the vessel's lumen), plaque rupture, or sudden damage to the plaque surface exposing the contents of the plaque to the blood (**FIGURE 11-24A**). Platelets accumulate at the site of the altered atheroma, followed by activation of the blood coagulation mechanism and formation of a thrombus at the site of plaque rupture (**FIGURE 11-24B**). Vigorous activities, such as running, snow shoveling, or tennis that abruptly increase cardiac output, raising myocardial oxygen consumption, can precipitate a myocardial infarct when the atherosclerotic

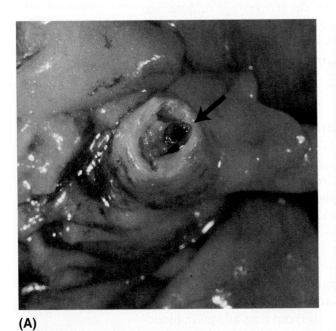

(A)

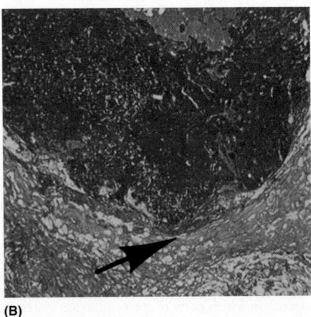

(B)

FIGURE 11-24 **(A)** Marked atherosclerosis of coronary artery with thrombus blocking artery (*arrow*). **(B)** Photomicrograph illustrating thrombosis of coronary artery at the site of a ruptured unstable atheromatous plaque. Note absence of fibrous tissue (*arrow*) covering the inner surface of the plaque.

Courtesy of Leonard V. Crowley, MD, Century College.

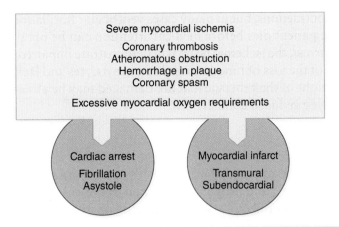

FIGURE 11-25   Causes and effects of severe myocardial ischemia, as described in the text.

coronary arteries are incapable of delivering an adequate blood supply to the heart muscle. Severe **myocardial ischemia** (inadequate blood flow reaching the heart muscle) then develops. Severe and prolonged myocardial ischemia may precipitate an acute episode called a "heart attack" (see **FIGURE 11-25** and **FIGURE 11-26**). This event may be manifested as either cessation of normal cardiac contractions, called a **cardiac arrest**, or damage and necrosis of heart muscle, which is termed a **myocardial infarction.**

CARDIAC ARREST

Myocardial ischemia may lead to disturbances of cardiac rhythm called cardiac arrhythmias. Damage to the conduction pathways of the heart, accumulation of toxic metabolites, and stimulation by the autonomic system all can play a role. A cardiac arrest occurs when an arrhythmia induced by prolonged or severe myocardial ischemia disrupts the pumping of the ventricles by causing ventricular fibrillation, a severe arrhythmia that is the most common cause of cardiac arrest and sudden death in patients with coronary heart disease as described previously in the discussion of cardiac arrhythmia. The application of an electric shock may cause the ventricles to

Myocardial ischemia Inadequate blood flow through the coronary arteries to the heart muscle.

Cardiac arrest Complete cessation of cardiac activity.

Myocardial infarction Necrosis of heart muscle as a result of interruption of its blood supply. May affect full thickness of muscle wall (transmural infarct) or only part of the wall (subendocardial infarct).

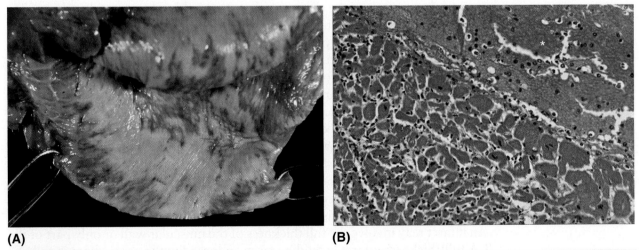

(A)   **(B)**

FIGURE 11-26   **(A)** Longitudinal section through infracted heart muscle, illustrating the pale zone of necrotic muscle that has been infiltrated by inflammatory cells. **(B)** Photomicrograph of a thirty-six-hour-old myocardial infarct demonstrating necrotic myocytes and infiltrating inflammatory cells. Upper right of image (*star*) is an area of hemorrhage into the heart tissue.

(A) Courtesy of Leonard V. Crowley, MD, Century College; (B) Courtesy of Department of Pathology and Laboratory Medicine, University of North Carolina at Chapel Hill.

resume normal contractions, but in many cases ventricular fibrillation occurs without warning, and the patient dies before medical attention can be obtained. Even in the absence of total arrest, the ischemic heart will demonstrate impaired ventricular contraction because of the loss of functioning cardiac myocytes and lack of synchronous contraction. Portions of the ventricle that are damaged may be **akinetic** or **hypokinetic** (lacking or showing reduced contraction).

ACUTE CORONARY SYNDROME

The manifestations of a myocardial infarct results from partial to complete obstruction of a coronary artery, and prognosis is related to the amount of muscle damage, which often can be minimized by prompt treatment to restore blood flow to the damaged heart muscle.

Compromised coronary function because of coronary thrombosis results in a pattern of injury of increasing severity. All patients with suspected inadequate blood flow to the heart muscle (myocardial ischemia) may be classified into three categories of progressively increasing severity based on the clinical manifestations, enzyme tests, and ECG findings. These categories include stable angina, unstable angina and **acute coronary syndromes (ACS)**.

Partial chronic blockage of the coronary vasculature results in **stable angina**. This results in temporary chest pain during stress and exertion that is relieved by rest or vasodilating drugs (such as nitroglycerin) and is not considered part of ACS as it is chronic in nature. The onset of the acute coronary syndrome occurs when there is a sudden increase in angina of prolonged duration that is resistant to therapy. This is now termed **unstable angina** and is associated with an acute worsening in the nature of coronary thrombosis. The anginal chest pain is a direct result of hypoperfusion of the heart muscle analogous to the cramping muscle pain that may result from overexertion. The patient requires treatment with antiangina drugs, but also anticoagulant and antiplatelet drugs, to prevent aggregation of platelets that may initiate a coronary thrombosis. Without treatment, unstable angina is likely to progress to non-ST elevation myocardial infarction (NSTEMI), which is related to the nature of ECG changes seen. A myocardial infarction is defined as necrosis of heart muscle resulting from ischemia. Non-ST elevation MI can be seen as a "mild-MI," but one in which death of cardiac myoctyes can be detected by observing the release of the contents of these cells into the serum (as discussed in blood tests to identify cardiac muscle necrosis in the following section). The ECG may show minor abnormalities but does not reveal the ST-segment elevation of a large infarct.

ST Elevation MI (STEMI) are a result of more severe cardiac necrosis related to total obstruction of the coronary artery and are often associated with shock and collapse. The extensive myocardial injury causes a characteristic elevation of the ST segment in the ECG and is also associated with marked elevation of cardiac muscle enzymes. An ST elevation myocardial infarction is a medical emergency and should be treated by an angioplasty or thrombolytic drugs to unblock the artery as soon as possible. The faster the blood flow can be restored through the blocked artery, the less severe the heart muscle damage and the better the prognosis. Acute coronary syndromes are diagnosed on a continuum related to the severity of cardiac ischemia and degree of myocyte necrosis (**TABLE 11-2**).

An infarct may involve the full thickness of the muscular wall or only part of the wall. A full-thickness infarct extending from endocardium to epicardium is called a transmural infarct (*trans* = across + *muris* = wall) and is usually the result of thrombosis of a major coronary artery. If only part of the wall undergoes necrosis, the term subendocardial infarct is used.

Akinetic/hypokinetic Lacking or showing reduced contraction.

Acute coronary syndromes (ACS) A classification of patients with coronary artery disease complaining of chest pain into one of three separate groups (unstable angina, non-ST elevation myocardial infarction, and ST elevation myocardial infarction) based on ECG and cardiac enzyme tests, used to assess prognosis and guide treatment.

Stable angina Temporary chest pain during stress or exertion caused by partial chronic blockage of the coronary vasculature.

Unstable angina Angina of prolonged duration resistant to therapy.

TABLE 11-2 Acute Coronary Syndrome (ACS) Classification of Coronary Heart Disease

Condition	ECG	Enzymes	Evaluation and treatment
Unstable angina	ST depression during angina returns to normal when angina subsides	Not elevated.	Treat angina. May progress to minor myocardial damage. Consider adding antiplatelet and anticoagulant drugs. Minimize cardiovascular risk factors.
Non ST-segment elevation myocardial infarction	ST-segment depression	Troponin elevated. Creatine kinase not elevated, if test is performed.	Minor myocardial damage caused by atheromatous debris from ruptured coronary plaque blocking distal branches of artery, or artery partially blocked by thrombus. Treat with anticoagulant and antiplatelet drugs to keep artery open. Consider angioplasty (percutaneous coronary intervention) if anticoagulant-antiplatelet treatment is not successful.
ST-segment elevation myocardial infarction	ST-segment elevation	Troponin elevated. Creatine kinase also elevated if test is performed.	Artery completely blocked. Identify site of block by arteriogram and open blocked coronary artery preferably by angioplasty (percutaneous coronary intervention) as quickly as possible to salvage as much cardiac muscle as possible. If facilities not available for angioplasty, attempt to dissolve clot by thrombolytic drugs.

The physician usually can assess the amount of heart muscle damage by correlating the changes in the ECG (**FIGURE 11-27**) with cardiac enzyme test results and the patient's clinical condition. The information helps to guide proper treatment and provides an indication of the patient's prognosis.

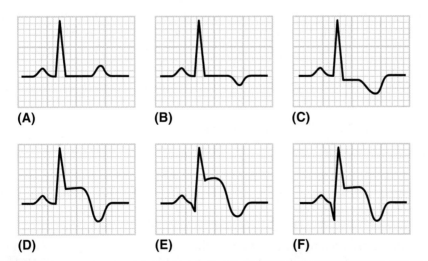

(A)   (B)   (C)

(D)   (E)   (F)

FIGURE 11-27 ECG ischemia and infarction patterns. **(A)** Normal ECG for comparison. **(B)** Mild ischemia demonstrated by inverted T wave. **(C)** Moderate ischemia demonstrated by slight ST-segment depression and inverted T wave. **(D)** and **(E)** ST-segment elevation myocardial infarction. **(F)** ST-segment myocardial infarction with prominent Q wave indicating more severe myocardial damage.

Slightly modified from Garcia, T. B., and Holtz, N. E. 2003. *Introduction to 12-Lead ECG.* Boston: Jones and Bartlett Publishers.

DIAGNOSIS OF MYOCARDIAL INFARCTION

Diagnosis of myocardial infarction rests on evaluation and interpretation of the medical history, physical examination, and laboratory data. The clinical history may at times be inconclusive because severe angina may be quite similar to the pain of a myocardial infarction. Conversely, many patients who develop subendocardial myocardial infarcts may have minimal symptoms. Physical examination will usually not be abnormal unless the patient exhibits evidence of shock, heart failure, or a heart murmur as a result of papillary muscle dysfunction. Consequently, the physician must rely on specialized diagnostic studies to demonstrate infarction of heart muscle. The most helpful diagnostic aids are the electrocardiogram (discussed previously) and determination of blood levels of various enzymes that leak from damaged heart muscle.

Blood Tests to Identify Cardiac Muscle Necrosis

Heart muscle is rich in proteins and enzymes that regulate the metabolic activities of cardiac muscle cells. When heart muscle is damaged, some of these components leak from the injured cells into the bloodstream, where they can be detected by laboratory tests on the blood of the affected patient. The most important proteins used as diagnostic tests of muscle necrosis are called cardiac troponin T (cTnT) and troponin I (cTnI), which are not detectable in the blood of normal people. Cardiac muscle damage causes the proteins to leak from the damaged cardiac muscle fibers.

Elevated troponin blood levels appear within three hours after muscle necrosis, with the highest levels attained within twenty-four hours, and the elevations persist for as long as ten to fourteen days. In general, the larger the infarct, the higher the troponin elevation and the longer it takes for the levels to return to normal. The pattern of rapid troponin rise and subsequent fall over the succeeding days is characteristic of myocardial necrosis. Troponin tests are so sensitive that even very small areas of muscle necrosis are sufficient to produce a positive test. Consequently, the troponin tests have become the preferred blood tests for evaluating patients with a suspected myocardial infarct because the tests can detect a very small area of heart muscle damage as well as a large myocardial infarct.

Another diagnostic test for heart muscle damage is measurement of the creatine phosphokinase (CK) enzyme present in heart muscle called CK-MB. The test is less sensitive than troponin tests but usually becomes positive when a large amount of heart muscle has been damaged. Muscle and other tissues have low levels of CK-MB and hence the test is not as specific nor as sensitive as the use of troponins.

TREATMENT OF ACUTE CORONARY SYNDROME (UNSTABLE ANGINA AND MYOCARDIAL INFARCTS)

Initial treatment may use drugs that decrease the heart's demand for oxygen. These include the previously mentioned nitroglycerin and also beta blocking agents (to reduce sympathetic nervous system stimulation of the heart) and calcium channel antagonists, which decrease heart rate and contractility. Antiplatelet agents and anticoagulant drugs are used to prevent further thrombosis. This conservative drug-based therapy may be sufficient for dealing with unstable angina or NSTEMI. However STEMI or progressing NSTEMI requires therapy to reestablish blood flow to the myocardium and limit cardiac damage. Two different methods can be used to reestablish blood flow through a thrombosed coronary artery; each has advantages and limitations. One method is fibrinolytic (clot dissolving) treatment, which attempts to dissolve the clot, and the second is a procedure called percutaneous coronary intervention (often abbreviated PCI), which is another name for an angioplasty procedure that is used to open the artery and place a short expandable metal mesh tube called a stent at the site of the occlusion to hold the artery open. The angioplasty procedure is more effective than thrombolytic therapy but requires a medical center staffed by personnel experienced with PCI procedures.

Fibrinolytic Treatment

Fibrinolytic therapy offers the advantage of ready availability. Various fibrinolytic drugs are available for intravenous administration based on recombinant human tissue plasminogen activator. The drugs act by binding to the fibrin within the clot in the coronary artery, where they convert plasminogen into plasmin, which is the fibrinolytic agent that dissolves the clot. (The coagulation and fibrinolytic mechanisms are described in the discussion on abnormalities of blood coagulation.)

Any physician can perform the procedure in a hospital or emergency room setting, which is an advantage when there are no personnel available who are skilled in performing angioplasty procedures, and the additional time required to transfer the patient to a coronary care facility would delay attempting to open the artery and would lead to further myocardial necrosis. Rapid use of this therapy (within thirty minutes of admission if possible) is critical for success. The benefit of thrombolytic therapy decreases progressively as the time interval between coronary thrombosis and clot lysis lengthens. After about six hours, administration of a thrombolytic drug is of little benefit because by this time the heart muscle has progressed from ischemia to complete infarction, and it can no longer be salvaged by restoring blood flow through the occluded vessel. The disadvantages are that up to 30 percent of patients are not suitable for fibrinolytic therapy because bleeding may be a serious side effect of therapy. Postsurgical or other patients for which bleeding might be expected or have serious consequences are not candidates for fibrinolytic therapy. The procedure is less effective than percutaneous coronary intervention.

Percutaneous Coronary Intervention (PCI)

The term percutaneous coronary intervention (PCI) is used frequently to describe a coronary angioplasty (*angio* = vessel + *plasty* = molding), which is used to open a blocked coronary artery, and is the preferred method of treatment if the procedures can be performed by an experienced physician within twelve hours after onset of symptoms and within ninety minutes after the patient reaches the hospital or coronary care unit where PCI is to be performed. The procedure is quite similar to the angioplasty procedure used to dilate stenotic coronary arteries described in detail under diseases of blood circulation. Generally, blood flow through the artery can be restored in about 90 percent of the patients, as compared with dissolving the clot with thrombolytic drugs, which has only a 70 to 80 percent success rate. Unfortunately, although good flow is restored through the blocked artery, the PCI procedure may dislodge small bits of thrombus and atherosclerotic plaque debris from the arterial wall when the artery is opened, which is carried downstream to block small arterioles and capillaries. Coronary care units in many hospitals can evaluate a suspected myocardial infarction patient and proceed with a PCI if necessary in as little as one hour. Success of the PCI procedure depends on how long the artery had been obstructed *before* the patient reached the coronary care unit. Many patients delay seeking treatment for several hours after onset of symptoms, which reduces the chance of a successful outcome in patients with an ST elevation myocardial infarction.

SUBSEQUENT TREATMENT AND PROGNOSIS OF MYOCARDIAL INFARCTION

After as much myocardium as possible has been salvaged by restoring flow through the occluded artery, further treatment of myocardial infarction consists of initial bed rest, gradually progressing to limited activity, and then to full activity. Sometimes, the injured heart is quite irritable and prone to abnormal rhythms. Therefore, various drugs are often given to decrease the irritability of the heart muscle. Development of heart block may require insertion of a cardiac pacemaker. The patient who has sustained a myocardial infarction may develop intracardiac thrombi if the endocardium is injured or may develop thrombi in leg veins as a result of reduced activity. Therefore, some physicians also administer anticoagulant drugs to reduce the coagulability of the blood and thereby decrease the likelihood of thromboses and emboli. If the patient shows evidence of heart failure, various drugs are administered to sustain the failing heart.

Patients recovering from a myocardial infarct are at increased risk of sudden death from a fatal arrhythmia or a subsequent second infarct, and the risk is greatest within the first six months after the infarct. Many physicians treat postinfarct patients for at least two years with drugs that reduce myocardial irritability (called beta blockers) because this seems to reduce the incidence of these postinfarct complications and improves survival. Ingesting a small amount of aspirin daily also is beneficial. As mentioned earlier, aspirin inhibits platelet function, making them less likely to adhere to roughened atheromatous plaques and initiate thrombosis in the coronary artery. Some physicians also recommend insertion of a cardioverter-defibrillator in postinfarct patients considered at high risk of a cardiac arrest or fatal arrhythmia. The device continually monitors the patient's heart rhythm. If ventricular fibrillation or other life-threatening arrhythmia is detected, the device automatically administers an electric shock to terminate the arrhythmia.

LOCATION OF MYOCARDIAL INFARCTS

Myocardial infarcts involve the muscle of the left ventricle and septum almost exclusively. Only rarely are the walls of the atria or right ventricle involved. This is because the left ventricle is much more vulnerable to interruption of its blood supply than are other parts of the heart. The left ventricular wall is much thicker than the walls of the other chambers, and works much harder because it must pump blood at high pressure into the systemic circulation. Consequently, it requires a very rich blood supply. In contrast, the other chambers have much thinner walls, pump blood under much lower pressures, need a less abundant blood supply, and can usually "get by" by means of collateral blood flow if a major coronary artery is blocked.

The size and location of myocardial infarcts are determined by both the location of the obstructions in the coronary arteries and the amount of collateral blood flow. Generally, an obstruction of the left anterior descending artery leads to an infarct of the anterior wall and often of the adjacent anterior part of the interventricular septum as well. If the circumflex artery is blocked, it is usually the lateral wall that is damaged. Occlusion of the right coronary artery generally causes an infarction of the back wall of the left ventricle and adjacent posterior part of the interventricular septum. A block of the main left coronary artery, which fortunately is quite uncommon, causes an extensive infarction of both the anterior and the lateral walls of the left ventricle and is frequently fatal.

MAJOR COMPLICATIONS OF MYOCARDIAL INFARCTS

Patients who sustain a myocardial infarct are subject to a number of complications. These include the previously discussed arrhythmias, cardiac rupture, intracardiac thrombus formation, and chronic heart failure. The latter is often called congestive failure because of the association with pulmonary congestion-related increased intrapulmonary pressure caused by left ventricular failure. Complications are not inevitable, and prompt restoration of blood flow through the blocked artery can reduce the damage sustained by the heart muscle and improve the patient's prognosis. On the other hand, the ventricle may be so badly damaged that it is unable to maintain normal cardiac function, and the heart fails. Heart failure may develop abruptly (acute heart failure) or more slowly (chronic heart failure), as described in a subsequent section, and may be difficult to treat.

Intracardial Thrombi

If the infarct extends to involve the endocardium, thrombi may form on the interior of the ventricular wall and cover the damaged endocardial surface, particularly in areas that are akinetic. These are called mural thrombi. Bits of the thrombus may break loose and be carried as emboli into the systemic circulation, causing infarctions in the brain, kidneys, spleen, or other organs. Some physicians attempt to forestall this complication by administering anticoagulants when a patient has sustained a severe infarction.

Cardiac Rupture

If a patient sustains a transmural infarct, a perforation may occur through the necrotic muscle (**FIGURE 11-28**). This permits blood to leak through the rupture into the pericardial sac, and as the blood accumulates, it compresses the heart so the ventricles cannot fill in diastole, a condition called **cardiac tamponade**. Eventually, the circulation ceases because the heart is no longer able to pump blood.

Cardiac tamponade Result of blood leaking through ruptured heart muscle compressing the heart.

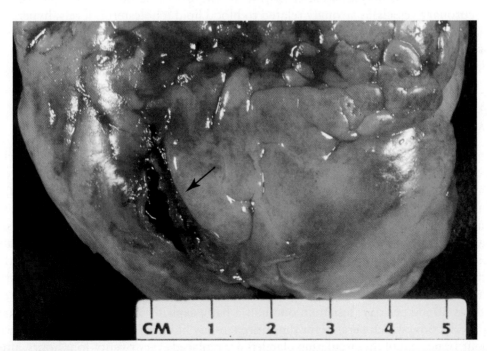

FIGURE 11-28 Rupture of heart (*arrow*) through large transmural myocardial infarct.

Courtesy of Leonard V. Crowley, MD, Century College.

SURVIVAL AFTER MYOCARDIAL INFARCTION

The survival rate of patients who have had a myocardial infarct depends on many factors, the more important being the size of the infarct, which is related to how rapidly the blood flow to the damaged muscle can be restored; the patient's age; the development of complications; and the presence of other diseases that would adversely affect the patient's survival.

Current thirty-day in-hospital survival rates are about 95 percent for all myocardial infarcts and about 85 percent for more severe cases. However, an additional 15 percent of severe cases die prior to hospital admission. Long-term survival rates are highly dependent on variables such as patient age. Overall five-year survival rates are about 80 percent. Major causes of death after myocardial infarction are fatal arrhythmia, heart failure, and cardiac rupture. Coronary care units staffed by specially trained personnel have reduced the mortality from cardiac arrhythmias, which are prone to occur in the first several days after myocardial infarction, but these facilities have not had any significant effect on the rates of death from heart failure or cardiac rupture.

Survival data also do not include patients with small infarcts that may not be detected clinically. Many small myocardial infarcts cause relatively mild symptoms and heal without complications. The patients may ascribe the chest discomfort associated with the infarction to indigestion or other causes and never seek medical attention. Some studies indicate that as many as 25 percent of all patients with myocardial infarcts have very few symptoms and do not consult a physician.

Risk Factors for Coronary Artery Disease

Coronary artery disease is the overriding risk factor for the acute coronary syndrome and concomitant occurrence of myocardial infarction. The risk of coronary artery disease (and specifically atherosclerosis, the formation of atheromatous plaques within the coronary vessels) is strongly related to blood lipid (cholesterol) levels, hypertension, diabetes, and smoking. Such risk factors are discussed in relation to atherosclerosis under diseases of blood circulation. There are ways to reduce this risk, such as taking low dose aspirin, refraining from cocaine use, and following a diet low in lipids.

TAKING ASPIRIN TO REDUCE THE RISK OF CARDIOVASCULAR DISEASE

Aspirin is now widely used in clinical medicine to reduce the risk of heart attacks and strokes. Aspirin works by interfering with platelet function (see discussion on abnormalities of blood coagulation). Aspirin permanently inactivates (acetylates) a platelet enzyme needed to produce a chemical compound called thromboxane A_2 that is released by platelets when they adhere to a roughened surface, which causes platelets to clump together and start the clotting process (discussed in abnormalities of blood coagulation). Blocking platelet function by taking aspirin reduces the likelihood that platelets will adhere to the roughened surface of an atherosclerotic plaque in a coronary or cerebral artery and cause a blood clot to plug the artery. As little as 30 mg per day (less than one-half a baby aspirin) inactivates thromboxane A_2 production, which persists for the entire ten-day life span of the platelets. Because about 10 percent of the circulating platelets are replaced every twenty-four hours, after about ten days almost no functionally normal platelets are present in the circulation.

Although taking aspirin to inactivate platelet function reduces the risk of cardiovascular disease as well as strokes caused by blood clots in cerebral blood vessels, aspirin use to reduce the risk of heart attacks slightly increases the risk of bleeding in the brain if the person does have a stroke.

COCAINE-INDUCED ARRHYTHMIAS AND MYOCARDIAL INFARCTS

Cocaine has very powerful effects on the cardiovascular system, and as the recreational use of cocaine has increased in recent years, so have the number of cocaine-related cardiac deaths.

The drug prolongs and intensifies the effects of sympathetic nerve impulses that regulate the heart and blood vessels. As a result, the heart beats faster and more forcefully, thereby increasing myocardial oxygen requirements. The heart muscle becomes more irritable, which predisposes to arrhythmias, and the peripheral arterioles constrict, which raises the blood pressure. Cocaine also constricts the coronary arteries and may induce coronary artery spasm, which leads to severe myocardial ischemia and may be followed by a myocardial infarction. Cocaine-related fatal arrhythmias and myocardial infarcts may occur in people with normal coronary arteries, and cocaine users who already have some degree of coronary atherosclerosis are at even greater risk.

Heart Failure

Heart failure exists whenever the heart is no longer able to pump adequate amounts of blood to the tissues. It may result from any type of heart disease. Rapid failing of the heart, when a large portion of muscle undergoes infarction, is called acute heart failure. In most cases, however, cardiac failure develops slowly and insidiously; this is called chronic heart failure. When the heart begins to fail, the pumping capability of both ventricles slowly declines, but initially not necessarily to the same extent. A disproportionate decline of left ventricular output causes the lungs to become engorged with blood, which is called left heart failure. The term right heart failure may be used when the right ventricle cannot "keep up" with the volume of venous blood being returned to the heart. The increased venous pressure in the distended veins causes the body tissues to accumulate fluid that usually is detected most easily in the feet and legs. When one compresses the swollen (edematous) skin with a fingertip, the indentation persists for a few minutes until the fluid refills the depression, which is called pitting edema. Because the most prominent feature in chronic heart failure is congestion of the tissues and at times the lungs as a result of engorgement by blood, the physician often uses the term congestive heart failure when referring to chronic heart failure and its attendant clinical manifestations. Although the term indicates that the heart is failing, it does not necessarily indicate a severe life-threatening condition. Although chronic heart failure is a slowly progressing condition, many patients respond well to effective treatment and can live comfortably in reasonably good health for many years.

PATHOPHYSIOLOGY AND TREATMENT

Heart failure is often categorized as being associated with either left or right ventricular failure (although left-sided failure will ultimately also effect the right side of the heart). The most common symptom of left ventricular failure is exertional dyspnea (shortness of breath on exertion). It may result from "back up" of venous blood in the lungs (exacerbated when the patient is in a prone position such as during sleep) and hence poor oxygenation or from insufficient cardiac output to muscles involved in respiration. Reduced cardiac output may also result in fatigue,

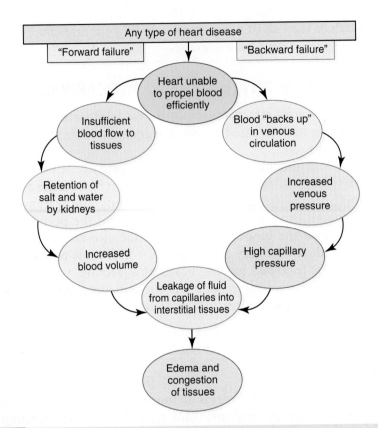

FIGURE 11-29 Mechanisms in the pathogenesis of congestive heart failure.

altered mental status, and decreased kidney function. Right-sided failure results in increased systemic venous pressure with abdominal discomfort. The high venous pressure and high capillary pressure cause excessive transudation of fluid from the capillaries, leading to edema of the tissues. In backward failure, the inadequate output of blood is considered to cause "back up" of blood within the veins draining back to the heart, leading to increased venous pressure, congestion of the viscera (leading to abdominal pain), and edema. **FIGURE 11-29** illustrates the interrelation of the various factors concerned in the development of cardiac failure. Treatment consists of diuretic drugs, which promote excretion of excess salt and water by the kidneys, thereby lowering blood volume. In addition, digitalis preparations are sometimes administered. They act to increase the efficiency of ventricular contractions. Other medications called ACE inhibitors are also frequently used. These drugs block an enzyme called angiotensin converting enzyme (ACE), which is part of a renal regulatory mechanism called the renin–angiotensin—aldosterone system (see discussion on the urinary system) that promotes retention of salt and water by the kidneys and raises blood pressure. Both of these effects are undesirable in heart failure patients, and blocking this mechanism by an ACE inhibitor has been shown to improve survival of patients in congestive heart failure.

ACUTE PULMONARY EDEMA

Acute pulmonary edema is a manifestation of acute heart failure and is a very serious life-threatening condition that requires immediate treatment. It is caused by a temporary disproportion in the output of blood from the ventricles. If the output of blood from the left ventricle is temporarily reduced more than the output from the right ventricle, the "right heart" will pump blood into the lungs faster than the "left heart" can deliver the blood to the peripheral tissues. This rapidly engorges the lungs with blood, raises the pulmonary capillary pressure, and produces transudation of fluid into the pulmonary alveoli. The patient becomes extremely short of breath because fluid accumulates within the alveoli, and oxygenation of the blood circulating through the lungs is impaired. The edema fluid becomes mixed with inspired air, forming a frothy mixture that "overflows" into the bronchi and trachea, filling the patient's upper respiratory passages. Treatment consists of supplementary oxygen to get more oxygen to the edematous pulmonary alveoli, intravenous diuretics and other medications to improve cardiac function by reducing the circulating blood volume, morphine to relieve anxiety, and measures directed toward correcting the underlying condition that precipitated the acute heart failure.

TYPES OF HEART FAILURE

The efficiency of ventricular function in heart failure patients can be measured, which allows the physician to determine whether the heart failure results primarily from inadequate ejection of blood from the ventricles in systole (heart failure with reduced ejection fraction, **systolic heart failure**) or from inadequate filling of the ventricles in diastole (heart failure with preserved ejection fraction, **diastolic heart failure**). Most patients with heart failure demonstrate systolic failure; the failing ventricles are distended with blood but are unable to expel a normal volume of blood during systole. Consequently, the left ventricular ejection fraction is significantly reduced and may fall from a normal value of about 60 percent to as low as 20 percent.

In contrast, the main problem in some heart failure patients is not with the impaired ejection of blood in systole but with inadequate filling of the ventricles during diastole. In this condition (diastolic heart failure), the volume of blood contained in the ventricles during diastole is lower than it should be, and the pressure of the blood within the chambers is elevated. This condition may occur in individuals with marked hypertension in whom the thick hypertrophied left ventricular wall cannot relax enough in diastole to allow the left ventricular chamber to expand normally. Consequently, less blood can flow into the ventricle, and the pressure of the blood within the ventricle is elevated. Some other less common conditions in which the ventricles are unable to relax normally in diastole may also reduce ventricular filling and raise intraventricular pressure. In all of these conditions, the left ventricle is underfilled in diastole (low end diastolic volume), and the stroke volume is also low because there is a smaller volume of blood available in the chamber to be ejected. However, the ejection fraction is normal because both end diastolic volume and stroke volume are reduced proportionately. Nevertheless, the cardiac output is inadequate to supply the body's needs. The clinical manifestations and methods of treatment of both systolic and diastolic heart failure are similar, although diuretics are the preferred treatment for patients with diastolic heart failure.

Systolic heart failure Heart failure caused by inadequate ejection of blood from the ventricles during systole, in contrast to diastolic heart failure in which filling of the ventricles in diastole is inadequate.

Diastolic heart failure Heart failure caused by inadequate filling of the ventricles during diastole, in contrast to systolic heart failure in which ejection of blood from the ventricles during systole is inadequate.

NATRIURETIC PEPTIDES IN HEART FAILURE

In heart failure patients, the unfavorable physiologic effects of the renin–angiotensin–aldosterone system resulting from reduced renal perfusion are counteracted to some extent by peptide hormones called natriuretic peptides that are released from cardiac muscle fibers when the fibers are stretched as a result of overdistension and increased pressure within the cardiac chambers, as occurs in patients with chronic heart failure. As the name indicates (*natrium* = sodium + *uresis* = urination), the peptides promote urinary loss of salt and water and also reduce blood volume and pressure, effects that oppose those caused by activation of the renin–angiotensin–aldosterone system.

The peptides are called atrial natriuretic peptide (ANP) released from the atria and B-type natriuretic peptide (BNP) released from the ventricles. Because ventricular pressures are higher than atrial pressures, the ventricular muscle cells are subjected to greater stretching forces. Consequently, BNP is of greater physiologic significance than is ANP.

A blood test to measure the level of BNP in a seriously ill patient who is very short of breath may help the physician determine whether the patient's marked dyspnea (shortness of breath) is caused by heart failure or by some other condition, such as lung disease. In heart failure, BNP is very high because the ventricular muscle fibers of the failing heart are overstretched. If BNP is not significantly elevated, the diagnosis of heart failure is unlikely, and other conditions must be considered to explain the patient's symptoms. BNP has been prepared for clinical use by recombinant technology and is sometimes used to treat patients in acute heart failure who are very short of breath. The intravenously administered BNP preparation promotes fluid loss and improves the patient's dyspnea.

CASE 11-1

John Strelow is a fifteen-year-old male child with no prior history of serious illness. He is a freshman at Brementown High School (ninth grade) and is interested in participating in the school's highly competitive athletics program. He wishes to join the school's freshmen football team. As a requirement for participation, he goes for a preparticipation health screening at his local pediatrician. The physician does a cardiac examination looking for heart murmurs and checks John's blood pressure in a sitting position, all of which are normal. He asks John if he has ever experienced chest pain, shortness of breath, or palpitations. John answers in the negative. Finally, the pediatrician asks John about heart disease or unexplained early death in his family. John replies that his father died in a farm accident having been crushed in a combine at age forty and that he has no other known paternal relatives. John's mother has been diagnosed with mild hypertension and elevated blood lipids but is otherwise healthy. John has a younger sister (age twelve) who has only minor medical problems. The pediatrician approves John's participation (warning him about adequate fluid intake and the danger of excessive exercise during periods of high heat and humidity).

John begins a preparticipation workout session at the school on a hot, humid September day and tells the coach he feels a bit dizzy and that his vision temporarily "grayed out." The coach instructs him to rest in the shade for a few minutes. Feeling better, John continues his workout telling the coach he feels fine. On returning home, John mentions the episode to his mother who is concerned. John has not told the coach (or his mother) that he felt short of breath for the entire workout. John participates in several additional training sessions and has several more episodes of shortness of breath coming close to fainting twice. He hides this from the trainer and coach, wanting to participate in the first freshmen team game against Muenster High. During the game, John collapses suddenly. Paramedical aid is on hand, but John cannot be resuscitated. He is pronounced dead on arrival at Saint Ann Regional Hospital.

His autopsy, requested by the county medical examiner, shows cardiac abnormalities. There is asymmetric thickening of the left ventricle with excess septal wall hypertrophy. The ventricular chamber is small, and there is a suggestion that vascular outflow from the left ventricle might have been impeded. A tissue sample from the left ventricle is examined and disorganization of the cardiac myocytes is noted. The medical examiner records the case as sudden cardiac death related to presumptive hypertrophic cardiomyopathy resulting in cardiac arrhythmia.

CASE 11-1 (Continued)

Discussion

Sudden cardiac death (SCD) in preadolescent and adolescent children is a tragic event and comes to general attention when those deaths are involved in school athletic programs. Because of understandable publicity, these deaths appear common when, in fact, they are unusual. A U.S. Registry of Sudden Death in Athletes has collected data for over thirty years. There are about 75 cardiovascular deaths per year in young athletes, compared to about 115 deaths among young athletes from all causes. The overall incidence of cardiac death in young athletes is estimated to be between 0.5 and 0.7 deaths per 100,000 person years. Deaths from motor vehicle accidents are 2,500 times more common in the same age group. It should be noted that estimates of SCD in school athletes have been criticized because they are difficult to interpret based on the large number of variables in these studies. Some believe the true figures to be twice as high (1 death per 100,000) or perhaps even higher. However, for U.S. high school students, the incidence of sudden cardiac death among athletes as compared to nonathletes was over 3.5 times higher. Clearly participatory high school athletics does present an elevated risk for SCD, but the overall risk is very small when compared to the more common causes of death among the young (notably trauma by accident, homicide, or suicide).

What is responsible for the increased risk of SCD in young athletes? In the above noted registry, hypertrophic cardiomyopathy (HCM), defined as increased asymmetric left ventricular wall thickness in the absence of other causes, was the most common cause of SCD in athletes, being responsible for 35 percent of deaths. Other studies report the incidence of proven and possible HCM in cases of SCD ranging from 11 percent (in NCAA athletes) to 7 percent (in the U.S. military) to 37 percent (in athletes in the United Kingdom). Myocarditis, often cited as a cause of SCD in young athletes, was less common (6 percent of deaths in the U.S. Registry).

The variation in frequency of HCM in SCD is likely related to differences in diagnostic criteria and, more important, to the fact that at least 60 percent of HCM cases are genetic in origin with mutations in three genes being responsible for over 80 percent of cases. The disease is most often dominant, and familial clusters of affected individuals may have a strong effect on observed frequencies. The disease is common with a prevalence of 1 in 500 and, although many cases are asymptomatic, 10 percent of patients ultimately develop heart failure. Stress accentuates symptoms in HCM patients, and in some cases the risk for SCD may be as high as 4 to 5 percent per year. Although certain high-risk HCM mutations have been defined, the correlation between mutations and presence and severity of cardiac disease is poor. Hence, there is considerable controversy about the utility of genetic analysis (although it may be useful in some families).

Considering the relatively high frequency of HCM in at least some populations and the publicity and trauma attendant with SCD in a young athlete, proposals have been made to increase screening criteria. Currently a fourteen-element preparticipation screen is suggested by the American Heart Association for competitive athletics (TABLE 11-3). Some, but not all, of these elements were utilized in this case. Major problems are standardization between screenings and qualifications for the person doing the screening. Even with effective screening, not all cases of HCM will be detected. Also, youth might be expected to be less than forthcoming in reporting symptoms. Screening using 12-lead ECG, which is effective in detecting ventricular hypertrophy, has been suggested as a mandatory component to screening. However, the test is costly, controversial in terms of specificity and sensitivity, and is technically challenging. Mandatory screening with 12-lead ECG is *not* recommended for young athletes and nonathletes by the American Heart Association or the American College of Cardiology because there is no evidence of benefit. Serious ethical concerns exist regarding the provision of specialized screening solely to athletes when in aggregate there are far more cases of HCM in the nonathlete population.

(continues)

CASE 11-1 (Continued)

When HCM is suspected, highly effective specialized, noninvasive diagnostic procedures are available (two-dimensional echocardiography and cardiac MRI investigations). Today these procedures are far too costly and too technically demanding for use in screening normal populations. Finally, a diagnosis of HCM need not prevent a person from engaging in a program of physical activity of a stress level appropriate to the specifics of their particular case.

Etiology and Pathogenesis

Sudden cardiac death likely from cardiac arrhythmia as a result of hypertrophic cardiomyopathy.

Questions

1. The case notes that there are far more cases in aggregate of HCM in nonathletes than in athletes. Why is this? Given that fact, would you support mandatory screening for high school athletes?

2. There are racial and sex-based differences in SCD frequency in athletes (not discussed in this case). What could be some of the factors responsible for these differences?

3. Based on the content in this chapter, suggest a plausible pathophysiological explanation for SCD in HCM.

4. Based on the case description, how thorough was the preparticipation screening given to John?

5. Under what circumstances might genetic screening for mutations be useful in evaluating the risk of HCM?

TABLE 11-3 American Heart Association Recommendations for Preparticipation Cardiovascular Screening for Competitive Athletes

Medical history

Chest pain/discomfort/tightness/pressure related to exertion

Unexplained syncope/near-syncope

Excessive and unexplained dyspnea/fatigue or palpitations associated with exercise

Prior recognition of a heart murmur

Elevated systemic blood pressure

Prior restriction from participation in sports

Prior testing for the heart ordered by a physician

Family history

Premature sudden death before fifty years of age attributable to hear disease in at least one relative

Disability from heart disease in close relative less than fifty years old

Close relative with hypertrophic or dilated cardiomyopathy, long-QT syndrome or other ion channelopathies, Marfan syndrome, clinically significant arrhythmias or genetic cardiac condition

Physical examination

Heart murmur

Femoral pulses to exclude aortic coarction

Physical stigmata of Marfan syndrome

Brachial artery blood pressure (sitting)

Modified from Marion et al. Assessment of the 12-lead electrocardiogram as a Screening Test for Detection of Cardiovascular Disease in Healthy General Populations of Young People (12–25 years of Age) J Am College of Cardiology 64 2014.

QUESTIONS FOR REVIEW

1. How do the heart valves function to provide unidirectional blood flow? What factors determine the level of the systolic and diastolic blood pressure?

2. What are the major causes of heart disease? What is the difference between rheumatic fever and rheumatic heart disease?

3. What is infective endocarditis? How does it arise? How is it prevented?

4. What is coronary heart disease? What are its manifestations? What is the difference between angina pectoris and myocardial infarction?

5. What is the effect of high blood pressure on the heart and the blood vessels?

6. What are the major complications of a large myocardial infarction?

SUPPLEMENTARY READINGS

Lilly, L. S. 2011. *Pathophysiology of Heart Disease: A Collaborative Project of Medical Students and Faculty*. 5th ed. Philadelphia, PA: Lippincott Williams & Wilkins.

▶ This book provides an in-depth overview of the topics covered in this chapter. The interested reader is urged to consult this resource for additional information on the cardiovascular system and, in particular, current clinical and therapeutic approaches to heart disease. The area of heart disease is so broad (and so detailed) that no set of readings can fully do it justice. This text presents a readable and somewhat technical overview aimed at medical and advanced undergraduate students. It is an excellent single source for additional background for this chapter and for the chapter on diseases of blood circulation. It is particularly strong on therapy.

American Heart Association. http://www.heart.org/HEARTORG/

American Heart Association. http://www.heart.org/HEARTORG/HealthcareResearch/Healthcare-Research_UCM_001093_SubHomePage.jsp

▶ The American Heart Association website is an essential resource for any area of cardiovascular disease. The first entry is for the introductory page, and the second entry provides a portal for scientific information. AHA statements and guidelines (which can be accessed from this page) are authoritative and carefully reviewed by all health care professionals. In-depth overviews of the topics covered in the chapter can be found at these websites. The interested reader is urged to consult them for additional information on the cardiovascular system and, in particular, current clinical and therapeutic approaches to heart disease.

American College of Cardiology. www.acc.org

Amsterdam, E. A., et al. 2014. AHA/ACC guideline for the management of patients with non-ST elevation acute coronary syndromes. *Journal of the American College of Cardiology 64e*:139–228. http://content.onlinejacc.org/article.aspx?articleid=1910086

▶ The American College of Cardiology website has a wealth of material, and much of it is updated immediately. It also acts as a gateway to scientific publications of extremely high quality, and many are publicly available. The second selection describes current therapeutic approaches to NSTEMI and has an excellent illustrated overview of the pathogenesis of the condition.

Zhelev, Z., et al. 2015. Diagnostic accuracy of single baseline measurement of Elecsys Troponin T high-sensitivity assay for diagnosis of acute myocardial infarction in emergency department: Systemic review and meta-analysis. *BMJ* 2015:*350*:h15. http://dx.doi.org/10.1136/bmj.h15

Daniels, L. B. 2014. Making sense of high-sensitivity troponin assays and their role in clinical care. *Current Cardiology Reports 16*:471.

▶ High-sensitivity troponin testing is becoming the standard for the rapid diagnosis of acute myocardial infarction. These two articles present an overview of the use of the assay, its sensitivity, and potential pitfalls.

Cowans, J. R., and Ware, S. M. 2015. Genetics and genetic testing in congenital heart disease. *Clinics in Perinatology 42*:373–93.

Bruno, C. J., and Havranek, T. 2015. Screening for critical congenital heart disease in newborns. *Advances in Pediatrics 62*:211–26.

▶ The first article has an excellent discussion of cardiac development and the genetics of congenital heart defects. The second article reviews the epidemiology and current screening procedures for congenital heart disease in the newborn. This is an excellent introduction to imaging and other diagnostic modalities used in early diagnosis.

Pollack, A., et al. 2015. Viral myocarditis—Diagnosis, treatment options, and current controversies. *Nature Reviews Cardiology 12*:670–80.

▶ Often diagnosed as a cause of sudden cardiac death, many areas surrounding this diagnosis are controversial. Although the review focuses on viral etiologies, it also reviews other causes of myocarditis.

Maron, B. J., Winkel, B. G., and Tfelt-Hansen, J. 2015. Perspectives on cardiovascular screening. *JAMA 313*:31–32.

Maron, B. J., et al. 2014. Assessment of the 12-lead electrocardiogram as a screening test for detection of cardiovascular disease in healthy general populations of young people: A scientific statement from the American Heart Association and the American College of Cardiology. *Journal of the American College of Cardiology 64*:1479–1514.

Maron, B. J., Friedman, R. A., and Caplan, A. 2015. Ethics of participation cardiovascular screening for athletes. *Nature Reviews Cardiology 12*:375–78.

Harmon, K. G., et al. 2014. Incidence of sudden cardiac death in athletes: A state-of-the art review. *Heart 100*:1227–34.

Maron, B. J., and Maron, M. S. 2015. The 20 advances that have defined contemporary hypertrophic cardiomyopathy. *Trends in Cardiovascular Medicine 25*:54–64.

▶ This set of five readings presents an overview of current thought on aspects of sudden coronary death in young athletes and the utility of additional preparticipation tests. The articles should be read with care by anyone involved in participatory athletics in an academic setting. These readings (and several others) were used in case preparation. The fifth selection takes a particularly interesting approach to reviewing hypertrophic cardiomyopathy.

Diseases of Blood Circulation

Courtesy of Vincent Moylin Department of Pathology and Laboratory Medicine, University of North Carolina at Chapel Hill

Blood Vessels

The heart pumps blood into a system of conduction and distribution vessels that differ in both their structure and function. It is convenient to consider them as four separate groups: the elastic arteries, the muscular arteries, the arterioles, and the capillaries. The large elastic arteries conduct the blood to various locations throughout the body. They distend as blood is ejected from the heart during systole and recoil during diastole to maintain flow between contractions and reduce pulsations in pressure. The muscular arteries distribute the blood from the large elastic arteries into individual organs. They are smaller vessels with muscular walls that regulate flow and reduce blood pressure from the large arteries into the capillaries. They also help to maintain systemic blood pressure by controlling resistance to flow. The arterioles are the smallest component of the arterial system and lack an elastic layer. Smooth muscle cells in their walls regulate blood flow into capillaries by contraction and expansion as necessary to regulate capillary flow as necessary. The capillaries are thin endothelium-lined channels that deliver nutrients to cells in the interstitial space and remove waste products. Veins return blood to the heart under low pressure and usually travel with the arteries (**FIGURE 12-1**).

A separate system of channels carrying fluid called lymph is part of the lymphatic system. Its functions and relation to the circulatory system are considered in the discussion on circulatory disturbances.

FACTORS REGULATING FLUID FLOW BETWEEN CAPILLARIES AND INTERSTITIAL TISSUE

The flow of fluid through the interstitial space between arteries and veins depends on capillary hydrostatic pressure, capillary permeability, osmotic pressure of blood proteins, and the presence of open lymphatic channels. The capillary hydrostatic pressure filters fluid from the blood through the capillary endothelium. The capillary permeability determines the ease with which the fluid can pass through the capillary endothelium and whether larger proteins can leak into the tissue. The osmotic pressure exerted by the proteins in the blood plasma (called colloid osmotic pressure) attracts fluid from the interstitial space back into the vascular compartment. Osmotic pressure, which was considered in the discussion on cells and tissues, may be defined as the property causing fluid to migrate in the direction of a higher concentration of molecules. The osmotic pressure of the plasma depends primarily on the concentration of the plasma proteins (termed the **plasma oncotic pressure**). Because normal capillaries are impermeable to protein, the protein tends to draw water from the interstitial fluid into the capillaries and to hold it there. However, changes in capillary permeability (as occur in inflammation) may allow proteins to leak into tissue, reducing the plasma oncotic pressure. Open lymphatic channels collect some of the fluid forced out of the capillaries by the hydrostatic pressure of the blood and return the fluid to the circulation. **FIGURE 12-2** illustrates the mechanism by which fluid flow is regulated through interstitial tissues.

> **Plasma oncotic pressure** Concentration of the plasma proteins in blood.

FLOW OF FLUID INTO AND OUT OF CAPILLARIES

The pressure of the blood at the arterial end of the capillary is higher than the colloid osmotic pressure, which causes fluid to be filtered through the endothelium of the capillaries into the interstitial space. The capillary endothelium acts as a semipermeable membrane and limits the rate at which fluid is filtered from the blood. At the venous end of the capillary, the hydrostatic pressure is lower than the

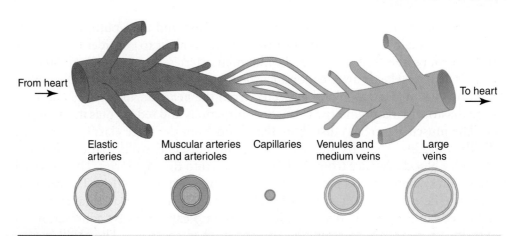

FIGURE 12-1 The composition and diameter of blood vessel walls varies with the type of blood vessel.

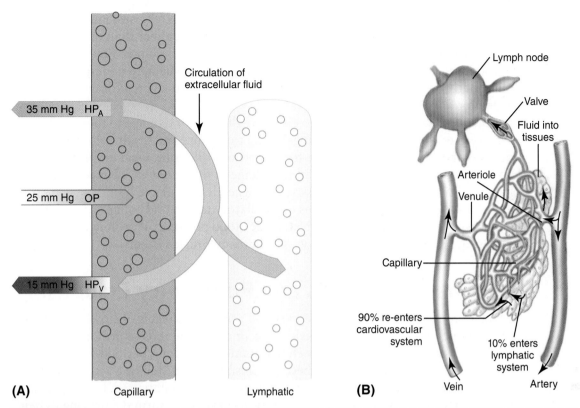

FIGURE 12-2 **(A)** Factors regulating the flow of fluid through the interstitial tissues. HP$_A$, hydrostatic pressure at the arterial end of the capillary. HP$_V$, hydrostatic pressure at the venous end of the capillary. OP, osmotic pressure. Pressures are indicated in millimeters of mercury (mm Hg). Fluid is forced from the arterial end of the capillary because the hydrostatic pressure exceeds the osmotic pressure. At the venous end of the capillary, the hydrostatic pressure is lower than the osmotic pressure and fluid returns. Lymphatic channels also collect some of the fluid forced from the capillaries by the hydrostatic pressure. **(B)** Excess tissue fluid is picked up by lymphatics that drain into larger vessels. Lymph nodes are interspersed along the vessels and act to filter the lymph.

colloid osmotic (oncotic) pressure, and fluid tends to diffuse back into the capillaries. In this way, the fluid containing dissolved nutrients is carried from the blood into the interstitial tissues to nourish the cells, and waste products are returned to the circulation for excretion.

Circulatory Disturbances: Introduction

Disturbances to the circulatory system can result from a variety of causes. Heading the list are disturbances to the flow of blood resulting from either complete or partial blockage of vessels. Normally, blood does not clot within the vascular system. Under unusual circumstances, however, **thrombosis**, or intravascular clotting, may occur. In the venous system this is the result of slowing or stasis of the blood flow, damage to the walls of the blood vessel, or an increase in the coagulability of the blood. These three factors leading to venous thrombosis are termed *Virchow's Triad* after the famous nineteenth-century pathologist who first defined them. Intravascular thrombi can also form within arteries and occasionally within the heart itself. Most commonly, arterial thrombi are related to the process of **atherosclerosis**, the formation of lipid-rich plaques in large and medium arteries. A clot in the vascular system may become detached and may be carried in the circulation. Such a clot is termed an **embolus** (embolus = plug or stopper); the process is termed *embolization*. Depending on where the blood clot was formed initially, the embolus may be carried

Thrombosis The formation of blood clots (thrombi) within the vascular system.

Atherosclerosis Formation of lipid-rich plaques in large and medium arteries.

Embolism A condition in which a plug composed of a detached clot, mass of bacteria, or other foreign material (embolus) occludes a blood vessel.

into either the pulmonary circulation or, less commonly, the systemic arterial circulation. Eventually, it is arrested in a vessel of smaller caliber than the diameter of the clot. When the embolus plugs the vessel, it blocks the blood flow to the tissue beyond (distal to) the obstruction, and the damaged tissue may undergo necrosis if the collateral blood supply is inadequate. The area of tissue breakdown is called an **infarct**, or an infarction.

Blood vessels may also undergo excessive dilation or damage to their walls leading to either **aneurysms** (outpouchings) likely to rupture and result in hemorrhage or demonstrate **varicosities** (excessive tortuosity and dilation). Changes in the permeability properties of vessels can lead to leakage of fluid content into tissue resulting in a condition termed **edema**. **Shock** results when low systemic blood pressure from any of a variety of causes progresses to circulatory failure and collapse. On the other hand, **hypertension** (excessively high systemic blood pressure), if prolonged, will result in damage to the heart and blood vessels in many organ systems.

Venous Thrombosis and Pulmonary Embolism

Formation of blood clots within leg veins is primarily a result of slowing, or stasis, of the blood in the veins. This is likely to occur during periods of prolonged bed rest or after a cramped position has been maintained for a long period of time such as prolonged airplane travel. Under these circumstances, the "milking action" of the leg musculature, which normally promotes venous return, is impaired, leading to stasis of the blood. Varicose veins or any condition preventing normal emptying of veins predisposes an individual to thrombosis by causing venous stasis.

Postoperative thrombosis in leg veins is a common problem. The surgical patient is susceptible to venous thrombosis because of the combined effects of venous stasis resulting from inactivity and increased blood coagulability resulting from an increased concentration of coagulation factors. (Blood coagulation factors usually increase as a result of tissue injury or necrosis from any cause.)

A venous thrombosis may partially block venous return in the leg, making the leg swell. However, the major complication of venous thrombosis is related to detachment of the clot from the wall of the vein. Since the thrombus often is not firmly attached to the vein wall, it may break loose, forming an embolus that is carried rapidly up the inferior vena cava into the right side of the heart. From there, it is ejected into the pulmonary artery, where it may become lodged in either the main pulmonary artery or one of its branches. The clinical manifestations of a pulmonary embolism depend on the size of the embolus and where it lodges in the pulmonary artery and may result in only mild pulmonary damage and pain or, in the case of occlusion of the main pulmonary artery, sudden death.

Venous thrombosis is treated by elevation of the leg, heat, and most important, by anticoagulant drugs. The anticoagulation stops the progression of the intravascular clotting process while the body's normal protective mechanisms remove the clot. The clot is dissolved by activation of the fibrinolytic mechanism and by ingrowth of connective tissue from the vein wall at the site where the clot adheres to the vein wall (discussed under abnormalities of blood coagulation). Damage to the vein wall and its valves after thrombophlebitis may disturb venous return and predispose the individual to later development of varicose veins.

LARGE PULMONARY EMBOLI

A large pulmonary embolus (PE) that completely blocks the main pulmonary artery or its two major branches obstructs the flow of blood through the lungs (**FIGURE 12-3**).

Infarct Necrosis of tissue caused by interruption of its blood supply.

Aneurysms Outpouching of walls of blood vessels.

Varicosities Excessive tortuosity and dilation of blood vessels.

Edema Accumulation of an excess of fluid in the interstitial tissues.

Shock A general term for any condition leading to such a marked fall of blood pressure that body tissues do not receive an adequate amount of oxygen, most often caused by acute blood loss or severe infection (sepsis).

Hypertension Excessively high systemic blood pressure.

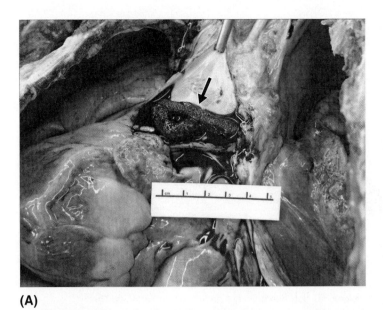
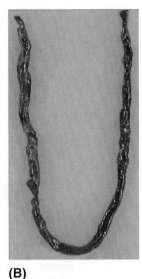

(A)   **(B)**

FIGURE 12-3   Massive pulmonary embolism. **(A)** Main pulmonary artery occluded by an embolus (*arrow*). The embolus resulted in sudden death of the patient. **(B)** Extracted embolus from case illustrated in figure.
Courtesy of Vincent Moylin Department of Pathology and Laboratory Medicine, University of North Carolina at Chapel Hill.

The right side of the heart becomes overdistended with blood because blood cannot be expelled into the lungs. The pulmonary artery leading to (proximal to) the obstructing embolus also becomes overdistended with blood, and the pressure in the pulmonary artery rises. Because less blood flows through the lungs into the left side of the heart, the left ventricle is unable to pump an adequate volume of blood to the brain and other vital organs. The systemic blood pressure falls, and the patient may go into shock and die. Blood still flows into the lungs from the bronchial arteries, which arise from the descending aorta and interconnect with the pulmonary arteries by means of collateral channels. This flow may lessen the degree of infarction but also allows blood to flow into the damaged tissue, leading to pulmonary hemorrhage in the damaged area (**FIGURE 12-4**).

Clinically, the patient becomes very short of breath, and the skin and mucous membranes assume a bluish coloration (cyanosis) because of inadequate oxygenation of the blood. If the massive embolism is not immediately fatal, some blood may be able to flow around the embolus and circulate through the lungs because the caliber of the pulmonary artery is increased by overdistention, and the high arterial pressure forces blood around the site of obstruction. In favorable circumstances, the embolus is eventually dissolved by the body's normal clot-dissolving mechanisms, and blood flow through the pulmonary artery is restored. In unfavorable cases, however, thrombus material builds up on the surface of the obstructing embolus and enlarges it. The sluggishly flowing blood in the branches of the pulmonary artery distal to the obstructing embolus may also become thrombosed. These events further impair pulmonary blood flow and may ultimately cause death several days after the initial embolization.

SMALL PULMONARY EMBOLI

If emboli are small, they may pass through the main pulmonary arteries and become impacted in the peripheral branches, usually in the arteries supplying the lower lobes of the lungs. Smaller emboli impede the flow of blood through the lungs and

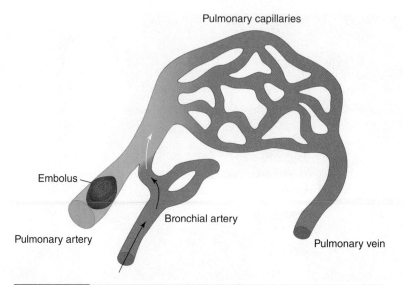

Pulmonary capillaries

Embolus

Bronchial artery

Pulmonary artery

Pulmonary vein

FIGURE 12-4   Anastomoses between bronchial and pulmonary arteries. The presence of an alternative pathway for blood flow often prevents infarction of the lung when the pulmonary artery is blocked by an embolus.

raise pulmonary artery pressure, but they have a less devastating effect than large emboli. Frequently, the segment of lung supplied by the obstructed pulmonary artery undergoes necrosis, resulting in a pulmonary infarct. The alveolar septa break down, and blood flows from the ruptured capillaries into the pulmonary alveoli, which become distended with blood. The typical infarct is a wedge-shaped hemorrhagic area that extends to the pleural surface (**FIGURE 12-5**). Infarction does not always follow a pulmonary embolism because anastomoses between the bronchial artery and pulmonary artery distal to the obstruction provide an alternative pathway for

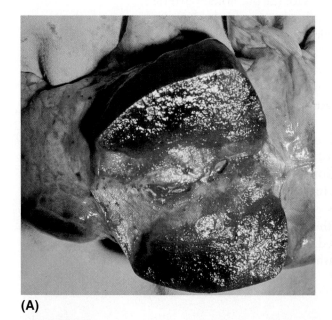

(A)

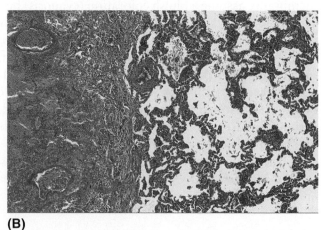

(B)

FIGURE 12-5   **(A)** Cut surface of a pulmonary infarct, illustrating the hemorrhage in the infarcted lung segment and the sharp demarcation between infarct and adjacent normal lung tissue. **(B)** Photomicrograph of a several days' old pulmonary infarct. Infarcted hemorrhagic area (*left third*) is shown as well as the adjacent lung tissue (*right*), which is spared.

(A) Courtesy of Leonard V. Crowley, MD, Century College; (B) Courtesy of Department of Pathology and Laboratory Medicine, University of North Carolina at Chapel Hill.

blood flow. If the pulmonary venous pressure is elevated, however, as occurs in heart failure or when the lungs are poorly expanded, an adequate collateral circulation often does not develop and the lung becomes infarcted.

The clinical manifestations of smaller pulmonary emboli are quite variable and are frequently minimal if the lung does not become infarcted. Common symptoms of pulmonary infarction are difficulty breathing (dyspnea), pleuritic chest pain, cough, and expectoration of bloody sputum. The chest pain occurs because the pleura overlying the infarct become inflamed and rub against the overlying parietal pleura as the lung expands and contracts during respiration. The cough is caused by irritation of the bronchi in the injured area. The bloody sputum appears because blood escapes from the infarcted segment of the lung into the bronchi and is subsequently coughed up.

DIAGNOSIS OF PULMONARY EMBOLISM

Unexplained dyspnea, cough, or pleuritic chest pain in a predisposed patient may be the only manifestations of a pulmonary embolism. These symptoms should alert the physician to undertake further diagnostic studies, particularly with evidence of venous thrombosis in the leg (a deep-vein thrombosis or DVT). Often, a blood test is helpful to confirm the physician's clinical impression of a possible pulmonary embolism. The test (called the *d-dimer test*) measures a by-product formed when fibrin within a blood clot is being broken down (fibrinolysis) by the body's normal clot-dissolving process, which would be activated in response to an intravascular thrombus or embolus. If the d-dimer concentration is not elevated, the possibility of a pulmonary embolism is less likely. On the other hand, although an elevated d-dimer concentration would support the physician's clinical evaluation, further studies are required.

Tools for Diagnosis

Some of the more useful studies are chest x-ray, ventilation perfusion lung scans, and pulmonary angiography using either a standard radiologic method or a computed tomography (CT) procedure. If the embolus has caused pulmonary infarction, a routine chest x-ray will often demonstrate the infarct, which appears as a wedge-shaped area of increased density in the lung. Because emboli cannot be visualized on x-ray films, the lung will appear normal if it is not infarcted.

A commonly used procedure to detect a pulmonary embolus is a **ventilation/perfusion scan**, or (**V/Q scan**). The test has two parts. First a radioactive gas or aerosol preparation is inhaled (the ventilation phase). The distribution of tracer is detected using a gamma ray camera to determine the area of the lung that is ventilated. In the subsequent perfusion phase, a solution of specially prepared albumin labeled with a radioisotope is injected into a peripheral vein. The injected material flows through the lung and is filtered out in the pulmonary capillaries. The radioactivity in the lungs, which is related to pulmonary blood flow, is likewise recorded. An area of the lung that shows a ventilation–perfusion mismatch (i.e., an area of the lung ventilated but not perfused by blood) is highly indicative of a pulmonary embolism. The V/Q study does not demonstrate the embolus; it only indicates that a part of the lung having the ability to be ventilated has a reduced blood supply, which is highly indicative of a PE (**FIGURE 12-6**). Consequently, the lung scan will be abnormal even when the lung is not infarcted, but the routine chest x-ray appears normal.

The definitive diagnostic method to identify a pulmonary embolism is a **pulmonary angiogram**, which directly visualizes the pulmonary artery and its branches. A catheter is inserted into a vein in the arm and advanced up the vein through the superior vena cava into the right side of the heart and out the pulmonary artery.

Ventilation/perfusion scan (V/Q scan) Procedure used to detect a pulmonary embolus.

Pulmonary angiogram Test that directly visualizes the pulmonary artery and its branches.

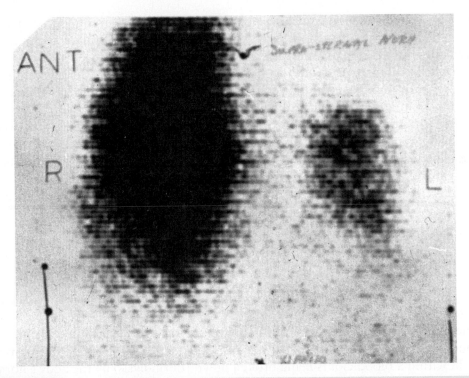

FIGURE 12-6 Lung scan illustrating impaired blood flow to left lung (*right*), representing decreased radio-activity. Radioactivity of the opposite lung is normal (uniform dark appearance), indicating normal pulmonary blood flow. This represents the perfusion phase of a V/Q scan.

Courtesy of Leonard V. Crowley, MD, Century College.

A radiopaque material is then injected, and the flow of the material through the pulmonary arteries is visualized by means of serial x-ray films or, optimally, using a specialized computed tomography technique that allows three-dimensional reconstruction of the pulmonary vasculature. If the pulmonary artery or one of its branches is completely obstructed by an embolus, no contrast material flows into the blocked vessel (**FIGURE 12-7**). If the embolus does not completely obstruct the artery, some contrast medium flows around the embolus, which appears as a filling defect in the column of contrast material within the partially occluded vessel.

TREATMENT OF PULMONARY EMBOLISM

Treatment of patients with pulmonary embolism includes general supportive care and administration of anticoagulants. Heparin, which has an immediate effect, is generally used initially, followed by administration of coumadin-type anticoagulants, which act by depressing hepatic synthesis of coagulation factors. The purpose of anticoagulant therapy is twofold: to prevent recurrent pulmonary emboli by preventing the formation of more thrombi in leg and pelvic veins and to prevent thrombus formation in branches of the pulmonary artery distal to the embolism. If adequate therapy is given, further thromboembolism is prevented, and the embolus will slowly dissolve. Less commonly, if the patient has sustained a massive embolus and is in critical condition because blood flow through a main pulmonary artery is blocked, an attempt may be made to dissolve the embolus rapidly by administering clot-dissolving (thrombolytic) drugs. These are the same drugs given to a heart attack patient to dissolve a thrombus blocking a coronary artery (discussion on the cardiovascular system).

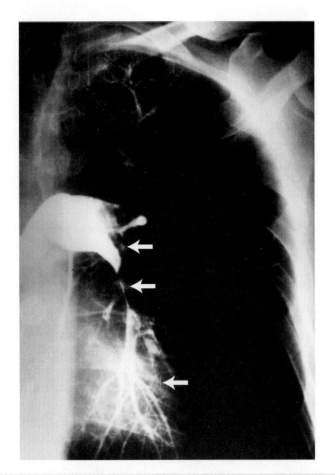

FIGURE 12-7 An angiogram used to identify pulmonary embolism illustrated by view of the left lung and pulmonary artery. A catheter has been inserted into the pulmonary artery, and radiopaque contrast material has been injected. Flow of contrast material is almost completely blocked (*upper arrow*) by a large pulmonary embolus obstructing the left main pulmonary artery. Only a thin trickle of contrast material flows around the embolus (*middle arrow*) to fill the pulmonary artery branches supplying part of the lower lobe (*lower arrow*).

Courtesy of Leonard V. Crowley, MD, Century College.

If the patient continues to have pulmonary emboli despite adequate anticoagulant therapy, a filter may be placed in the inferior vena cava percutaneously (through a skin incision). Such filters trap emboli and prevent them from reaching the lung. The filter may be removed at a later date if necessary.

Embolism as a result of Foreign Material

Most emboli are caused by blood clots, but other materials occasionally gain access to the circulation. Fat, air, and foreign particles within the vascular system may sometimes cause serious difficulties.

FAT EMBOLISM

After a severe bone fracture, fatty bone marrow and surrounding adipose tissue may be disrupted. The emulsified fat globules may be sucked into the veins and carried into the lungs, leading to widespread obstruction of the pulmonary capillaries. Some of the fat may be carried through the pulmonary capillaries and may reach the systemic circulation, eventually blocking small blood vessels in the brain and other organs (**FIGURE 12-8**).

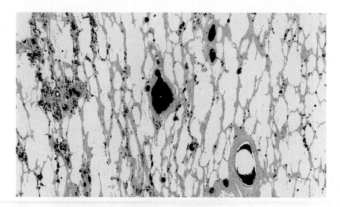

FIGURE 12-8 Multiple fat emboli in cerebral vessels of a patient who suffered severe lower limb trauma. Intravascular fat emboli are stained black using a fat-specific stain.

Courtesy of Department of Pathology and Laboratory Medicine, University of North Carolina at Chapel Hill.

AMNIONIC FLUID EMBOLISM

This condition is an uncommon but devastating complication of pregnancy that usually occurs during labor when the pressure of uterine contractions forces a large volume of amnionic fluid through a tear in fetal membranes into a torn uterine vein at the site of a cervical or uterine laceration. The amnionic fluid, which contains desquamated fetal epithelial cells and hair, fatty material (vernix), debris from the fetal respiratory and gastrointestinal tract, and thromboplastic material, is carried in the maternal venous circulation to the lungs, where it plugs the pulmonary capillaries. Manifestations are severe dyspnea, shock, and often an acute disseminated intravascular coagulation syndrome induced by the thromboplastic material in the amnionic fluid.

AIR EMBOLISM

Sometimes a large amount of air is sucked into the venous circulation after a chest wound with injury to the lung. Air may also be accidentally injected into the circulation in attempts at abortion by people without medical training. The air is carried to the heart and accumulates in the right heart chambers, preventing filling of the heart by returning venous blood. As a result, the heart is unable to pump blood, and the individual dies rapidly of circulatory failure.

EMBOLISM OF PARTICULATE FOREIGN MATERIAL

Various types of particulate material may be injected into veins by drug abusers, who crush and dissolve tablets intended for oral use and inject the material intravenously or who "cut" drugs with substances such as talc. The material is usually trapped within the small pulmonary blood vessels, producing symptoms of severe respiratory distress caused by obstruction of the pulmonary capillaries by the foreign material, or may, with time, result in pulmonary fibrosis (lung scarring).

Varicose Veins

Dilated tortuous veins are called varices or varicose veins. (*Varix* is a Latin word meaning dilated vessel; the plural term is varices.) Varicosities occur most often in leg veins but may occur in other veins as well. Venous thromboses also occur most commonly in leg veins, but sometimes clots form within veins elsewhere in the body. Inflammation of a vein is called **phlebitis** (*phleb* = vein + *itis* = inflammation). If there is an associated thrombosis of the affected vein, the term thrombophlebitis is used (**FIGURE 12-9A**).

Veins, both deep veins and superficial veins, return blood from the lower limbs with the deep veins carrying most of the venous return. These veins accompany the major arteries and drain into the iliac veins, which in turn empty into the inferior vena cava. The superficial veins form a network of intercommunicating channels that travel just beneath the skin in the subcutaneous tissue and eventually drain into the deep veins and constitute the saphenous system. Both the superficial and deep veins contain cup-shaped valves that are interposed along the course of the veins. The arrangement of the valves is such that blood can flow upward in the veins but cannot flow in the reverse direction. The superficial and deep venous systems are also interconnected by short communicating branches that contain valves arranged so that blood normally flows only from superficial to deep veins and not in the reverse direction.

Blood is propelled upward within the deep veins by contraction of the leg and thigh muscles, which intermittently compress the veins and force the blood upward within the veins against gravity with the valves preventing retrograde flow. In contrast, the superficial veins are relatively unsupported, and venous return is much less efficient (**FIGURE 12-9B**).

Varicose veins result if the saphenous veins become dilated and their valves become incompetent. As a result, the blood tends to stagnate in the veins instead

Phlebitis Inflammation of a vein.

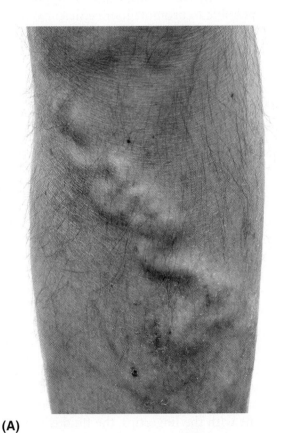

(A)

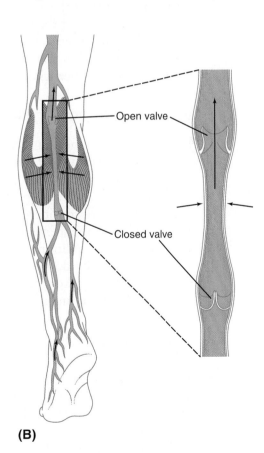

Open valve

Closed valve

(B)

FIGURE 12-9 **(A)** Varicose veins result from a restriction of venous blood flow to the heart. **(B)** Valves in veins. The slight hydrostatic pressure in the veins and the contraction of skeletal muscles propel the blood along the veins back toward the heart. The one-way valves stop the blood from flowing backward.

of flowing back normally to the heart, causing the veins to become elongated and tortuous. The condition is common, affecting 15 percent of people and tends to run in families, suggesting that the basic cause is a congenital weakness of the vein wall or its valves, which predisposes them to the varicosities. Varicose veins increase with age and are more common in women, particularly those who have been pregnant. Continued upright posture and obesity are also risk factors.

Varicose veins of the saphenous system also may develop if the deeper veins become blocked or if their valves become damaged by previous thrombophlebitis. As a result of damage to the deep veins, more of the venous return is shifted to the unsupported superficial veins, which are unable to cope with the increased flow and become varicose.

COMPLICATIONS OF VARICOSE VEINS

Complications result from stasis of blood in the veins leading to poor nutrition of the tissues caused by chronic venous engorgement. The skin of the distal leg and ankle becomes thin and atrophic and quite susceptible to infection. Skin ulcers may develop and heal poorly. The dilated veins are easily injured and may rupture, leading to extravasation of blood and chronic discoloration of the skin. Stasis of blood in the veins also predisposes individuals to repeated bouts of thrombophlebitis.

TREATMENT OF VARICOSE VEINS

Varicosities of the saphenous veins are treated by elastic stockings to support the veins and elevation of the legs whenever possible to promote more efficient venous return. Sometimes surgical removal of the varicose veins may be required. This is usually performed in conjunction with ligation of the communicating veins that interconnect the superficial and deep venous systems.

VARICOSE VEINS IN OTHER LOCATIONS

Hemorrhoids Dilated veins around the rectum.

Hydrothorax Accumulation of fluid in the pleural cavity.

Ascites Fluid accumulating in body cavities due to low albumin.

Dilated veins around the rectum are called **hemorrhoids** and are described in the discussion on disorders of the gastrointestinal tract. Varicose veins of the esophagus often occur in patients with a disease called cirrhosis of the liver. Esophageal varices may rupture and cause profuse life-threatening hemorrhage. Their pathogenesis and treatment are considered in the discussion on the liver and the biliary system. Varicose veins of the spermatic cord appear as a mass of vessels in the scrotum above the testicle. The condition is called a varicocele (*varix* = vein + *cele* = swelling). The varicosities usually do not cause symptoms but at times may cause mild scrotal discomfort. Rarely they may impair fertility in some men. Usually no treatment is required (discussed under the male reproductive system).

Edema

The term *edema* refers to accumulation of fluid in the interstitial tissues. Edema is most conspicuous in the skin and subcutaneous tissues of the dependent (lower) parts of the body and is usually noted first in the legs and ankles. When the edematous tissue is compressed by indenting the tissue with the fingertips, the fluid is pushed aside, leaving a pit or indentation that gradually refills with fluid. This characteristic is responsible for the common term pitting edema. Fluid may also accumulate in the pleural cavity (**hydrothorax**) or in the peritoneal cavity (**ascites**).

Edema may result from any condition in which the circulation of extracellular fluid between the capillaries and the interstitial tissues becomes disturbed.

PATHOGENESIS AND CLASSIFICATION OF EDEMA

Increased Capillary Permeability

Normally, the endothelium of the capillaries limits the amount of fluid filtered from the blood. If the capillaries are excessively permeable, filtration of fluid into the interstitial space is greater than normal. Increased capillary permeability is responsible for the swelling of the tissues associated with an acute inflammation such as a boil or a severe sunburn. Some systemic diseases also cause a generalized increase in capillary permeability, which leads to widespread edema of the subcutaneous tissues (**FIGURE 12-10**).

Low Plasma Proteins

If the concentration of plasma proteins is decreased, the colloid osmotic (oncotic) pressure is reduced correspondingly. Consequently, less fluid is attracted back into the capillaries, and the fluid accumulates in the tissues. A low concentration of plasma proteins may result from excessive loss of plasma proteins in the urine, as occurs in patients with some types of kidney disease, or from inadequate synthesis of plasma proteins as a result of malnutrition or starvation. Hypoproteinemia, caused by inadequate protein intake, may be encountered in patients with chronic debilitating diseases who are unable to eat an adequate amount of food and in patients with intestinal diseases in whom assimilation of food is impaired.

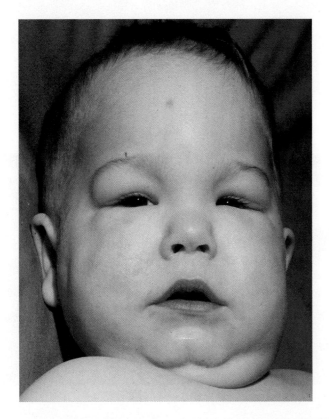

FIGURE 12-10 Edema as a result of increased capillary permeability. Note the swelling of the eyelids and face.

Courtesy of Leonard V. Crowley, MD, Century College.

Increased Hydrostatic Pressure

Increased pressure in the veins draining the capillaries is reflected as a higher than normal pressure at the venous end of the capillaries. As a result, more fluid is filtered from the capillaries, causing it to accumulate in the tissues. A localized increase in venous pressure may be encountered if the veins draining a part of the body become compressed, twisted, or obstructed by a blood clot that fills the lumen. More commonly, the increased venous pressure is a manifestation of heart failure, and the pressure is elevated in all the systemic veins (**FIGURE 12-11**).

Lymphatic Obstruction

Sometimes, lymphatic channels draining a part of the body become obstructed because of disease. The obstruction blocks a pathway by which fluid is returned from the interstitial space into the circulation and leads to edema in the region that is normally drained by the obstructed lymphatic vessels.

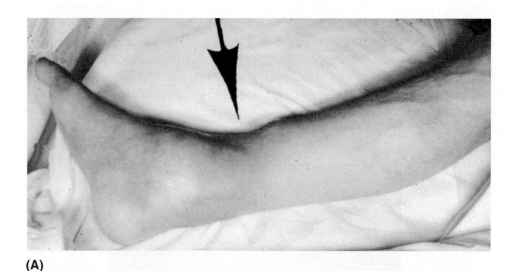

(A)

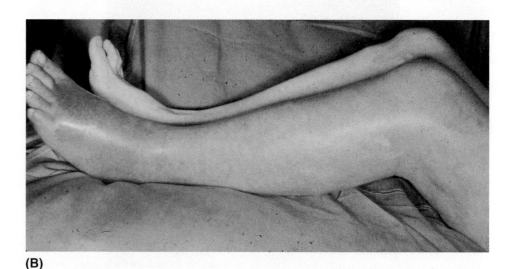

(B)

FIGURE 12-11 **(A)** Marked pitting edema of leg (*arrow*) as a result of chronic heart failure. **(B)** Localized edema of left leg caused by venous obstruction. Right leg appears normal.

Courtesy of Leonard V. Crowley, MD, Century College.

Shock

Shock is a general term to describe any condition in which the blood pressure is too low to provide adequate blood flow to the body cells and organs; it is a serious, potentially life-threatening condition. Shock results from a disproportion between the volume of blood in the circulatory system and the capacity of the vascular system that carries the blood. Blood pressure falls if the volume of blood filling the circulatory system falls or if marked dilation of blood vessels expands the capacity of the vascular system to such an extent that the existing blood volume is insufficient to fill the vessels adequately.

CLASSIFICATION

Shock can be classified in four categories based on its cause: hypovolemic, cardiogenic, septic, or anaphylactic shock. Hypovolemic shock is caused by low blood volume, leading to a corresponding drop in blood pressure. Most cases result from a large hemorrhage that significantly reduces the circulating blood volume, but any excessive depletion of body fluids such as fluid losses from a severe burn, from severe diarrhea, or from excessive fluid loss in urine resulting from diuretics can also reduce blood volume as fluid shifts from the vascular compartment into the depleted extravascular body fluids. Cardiogenic shock is caused by inadequate or impaired cardiac pumping function, which reduces cardiac output. Cardiogenic shock usually is a complication of a myocardial infarction, but the pumping function of the heart can also be impaired if the heart is compressed by accumulation of blood or fluid within the pericardial sac, which prevents filling of the heart in diastole, or by other conditions that cause acute heart failure. Septic shock results from the release of inflammatory mediators in response to infection (often by gram-negative organisms that release endotoxin, a potent inflammatory mediator). These mediators can increase capillary permeability, resulting in the decrease of plasma oncotic pressure and fluid loss. The infection also can result in endothelial cell injury and vasodilation as a result of endothelial cell stimulation.

Anaphylactic shock (described in the discussion on immunity, hypersensitivity, allergy, and autoimmune diseases) also results from excessive vasodilation caused by the widespread release of mediators of inflammation from mast cells and basophils, which is often followed by circulatory collapse.

PROGNOSIS AND TREATMENT

The outcome of shock depends on its cause and how quickly it is recognized and treated. Treatment consists of administering drugs that raise blood pressure by constricting blood vessels, restoring blood volume by intravenous fluids or blood if the shock is caused by a severe hemorrhage, and treating the underlying condition that leads to the shock. Unfortunately, septic shock or cardiogenic shock in an elderly patient with other medical problems has a very poor prognosis.

Thrombosis at Nonvenous Sites

ARTERIAL THROMBOSIS

Blood flow in arteries is rapid, and intravascular pressure is high; so stasis of blood is not a factor in arterial thrombosis. The main cause of arterial thrombosis is injury to the wall of the vessel, usually secondary to atherosclerosis. The effects of arterial thrombus formation depend on the location and size of the artery that has become obstructed. Blockage of a coronary artery frequently causes infarction of the heart muscle and consequent "heart attack." If a major artery supplying the leg is occluded, the extremity undergoes necrosis, usually called **gangrene.** (This differs from gas gangrene, which is caused by a species of *Clostridium*.) Occlusion of an artery to the brain leads to infarction of a portion of the brain, commonly called a "stroke."

Gangrene Tissue death caused by bacterial infection or lack of blood circulation.

INTRACARDIAC THROMBOSIS

Occasionally, blood clots may form within the heart itself. Thrombi may form within the atrial appendages when heart function is abnormal, as in heart failure, or when the atria are not contracting normally. Thrombi may also form on the surfaces of heart valves that have been damaged as a result of disease. Occasionally, thrombi may form on the internal lining of the ventricle adjacent to an area where the heart muscle is infarcted. Such thrombi, which adhere to the endocardium (inner layer of heart), are termed mural thrombi (*mural* is Latin for "wall") (**FIGURE 12-12**). Intracardiac thrombi may become dislodged and may be carried into the systemic circulation, resulting in infarction of the spleen, kidneys, brain, or other organs. The symptoms produced depend on the size and location of the infarction.

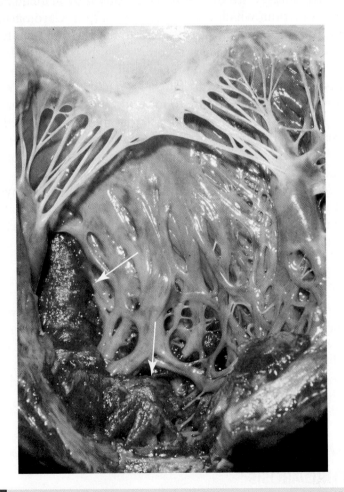

FIGURE 12-12 Interior of heart chamber (left ventricle), illustrating a mural thrombus adherent to the wall (endocardium) adjacent to a myocardial infarct (*arrows*). A normal heart valve (the mitral valve) and its components are seen at the top of the photo.

Courtesy of Leonard V. Crowley, MD, Century College.

THROMBOSIS IN PATIENTS WITH CANCER

Many patients with advanced cancer are predisposed to both venous and arterial thromboses. This tendency results from the release of thromboplastic materials into the circulation from the tumor. The same basic mechanism induces hemorrhage in patients with a disseminated intravascular coagulation syndrome (discussed in abnormalities of blood coagulation).

Atherosclerosis

THE RESPONSE TO INJURY HYPOTHESIS

Atherosclerosis is a chronic and progressive degenerative disease of large- to medium-sized elastic and muscular arteries such as the thoracic and abdominal aorta, the femoral and popliteal arteries, the internal carotids, various cerebral arteries, and the coronary arteries. The disease is believed to be triggered by endothelial injury and is associated with the gradual accumulation of cells, connective tissue, and lipid (mostly free cholesterol and cholesterol esterified to long-chain fatty acids) within the intima of the vessel wall. The normal artery consists of several layers. The non-thrombogenic single layer of endothelial cells (the endothelium) lining the lumen overlays the tunica intima, which is predominantly collagenous in nature and contains few fibroblasts or smooth muscle cells. Under this is the tunica media, composed of multiple concentric layers of smooth muscle cells that are rich in elastin in an elastic artery. The outer surface of the artery is the tunica adventitia, composed of connective tissue (**FIGURE 12-13**).

During the process of atherosclerosis, inflammatory and immune cells accumulate in the intima as do smooth muscle cells, which migrate from the media in response to cytokines liberated by inflammatory and immune cells. Damage to the endothelial cells due in part to blood flow, lipid products, inflammatory mediators, and possibly

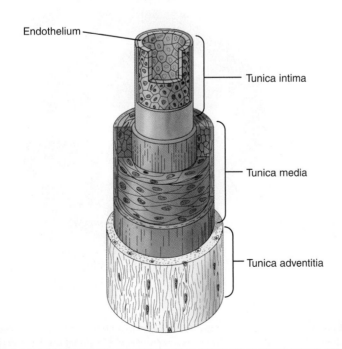

FIGURE 12-13 General structure of the blood vessel. The artery shown here consists of three major layers: tunica intima, tunica media, and tunica adventitia.

pathogens and their products interferes with the endothelial permeability barrier, allowing lipids to penetrate into the intima from the blood. In addition (and critical to the process), damaged endothelial cells express cell surface molecules that facilitate adherence of blood monocytes/macrophages to the damaged endothelium and migration of these inflammatory cells into the arterial wall. These macrophages carry lipids (as a component of low-density lipoprotein) from the blood into the intima where they accumulate as **foamy macrophages**. The macrophages release cytokines and growth factors, which stimulate smooth muscle cell, connective tissue, and additional inflammatory cell accumulation. The inflammatory cells and damaged endothelium promote oxidation of the deposited lipid carried by lipoproteins, and these oxidized lipids are a further source of tissue damage and inflammation. With time the hallmark lesion of atherosclerosis, the raised **atheroma** (*athere* = porridge), forms in the intima. The atheroma is a plaque with a necrotic core rich in lipid (and in particular cholesterol, which often deposits as crystals). The core is covered by a fibrous cap tissue containing immune and inflammatory cells (often foamy macrophages), smooth muscle cells, and other connective tissue. This lesion is termed a fibrofatty plaque (**FIGURE 12-14**). The gradual growth of the atheroma (likely over decades) leads it to encroach into the lumen of the artery where it compromises blood flow. The artery can initially remodel to enlarge the lumen, but this is a limited process that will ultimately result in arterial **stenosis** (narrowing) and reduced oxygenation to adjacent tissue. As the atheroma enlarges, the surface of the vessel over the atheroma becomes increasingly damaged and fibrotic (termed *complicated plaque*). Turbulent hemodynamic flow over the stenosed area will result in endothelial damage and possibly ulceration and plaque rupture, releasing thrombotic lipids and calcified damaged cellular debris into the circulation.

Hemorrhage into the plaque may occur suddenly, increasing the size and totally blocking blood flow. The damaged endothelium over the atheroma becomes

Foamy macrophages Macrophages carrying lipids.

Atheroma Formation of plaque with a necrotic core rich in lipids.

Stenosis Narrowing of a valve orifice.

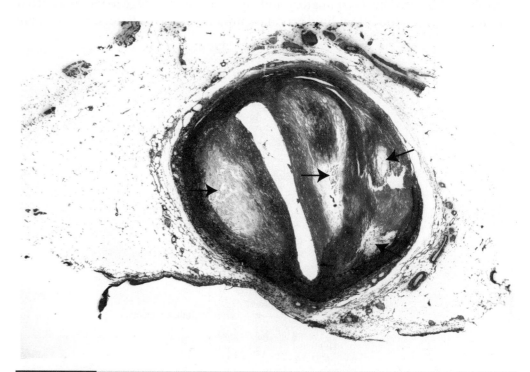

FIGURE 12-14 Low-magnification photomicrograph of coronary artery in cross section illustrating several atheromatous plaques (*arrows*) surrounded by dense fibrous tissue. Atheromatous deposits reduce lumen of artery to a narrow slit (original magnification ×40).

Courtesy of Leonard V. Crowley, MD, Century College.

increasingly prothrombotic as the endothelium is lost and the fibrous cap is exposed, leading to platelet adhesion and the formation of an adherent thrombus blocking arterial flow. The thrombus may detach and travel in the vessel to a distant site where it lodges as an embolus (**FIGURE 12-15**).

The ultimate effects of atherosclerosis depend on where it occurs. In coronary arteries, it results in cardiac ischemia. If atherosclerotic plaques narrow the coronary arteries by 50 to 75 percent, the arteries may still be able to supply enough blood to the heart muscle if the individual is not very active and no excessive demands are placed on the heart (**FIGURE 12-16**). However, the blood supply may become inadequate under exertion when the heart requires more blood to satisfy the increased demands. If the reduction in blood flow is sudden and sufficiently severe, a myocardial infarct (heart attack) will occur. In cerebral vessels, a **thrombotic stroke** leading to brain ischemia will result in damage and death of neural tissue. Death or compromise of function is a likely result.

The damaged aortic wall may balloon outward as an abdominal aortic aneurysm (often called an AAA, or "triple A") that can rupture with catastrophic results. Atherosclerosis of the arteries supplying the legs results in **vascular claudication** with severe cramping leg pain, impaired mobility, and potentially gangrene of the lower limb. Atherosclerosis of the renal arteries can lead to loss of kidney function; in the mesenteric vessels atherosclerosis can result in lethal necrosis of the gut.

NATURAL HISTORY OF ATHEROSCLEROSIS

A myocardial infarct is often a sudden and unexpected event occurring in individuals sixty years of age or older. However, the process of atherosclerosis that precipitated this event began far earlier in the person's life, perhaps as early as the first decade. The first signs of atherosclerosis are precursor lesions detectable in children in their

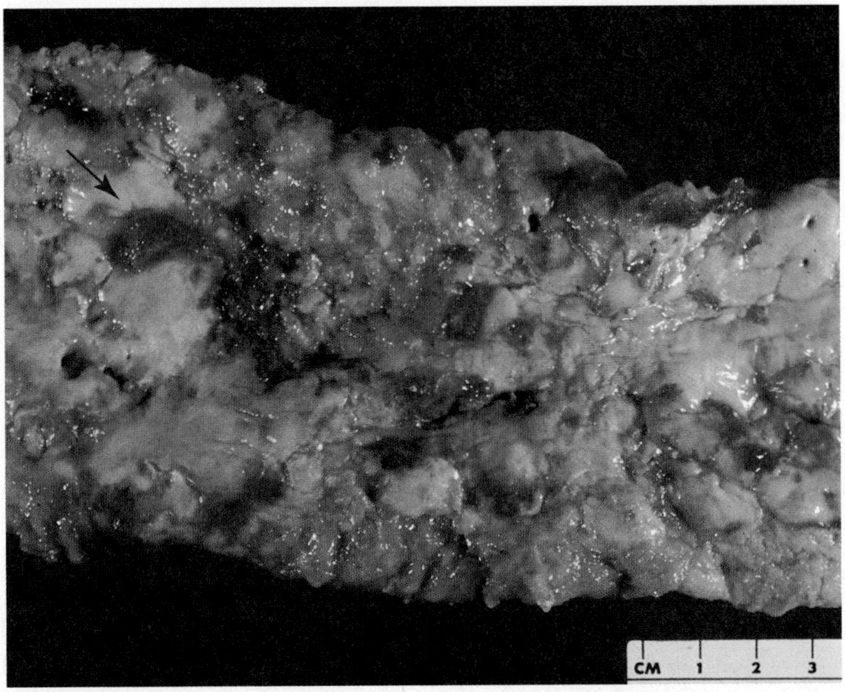

Thrombotic stroke
Reduction in blood flow in brain due to thrombus.

Vascular claudication
Severe cramping leg pain due to atherosclerosis of arteries in leg.

FIGURE 12-15 Advanced atherosclerosis of aorta. Many plaques are ulcerated and are covered by thrombus material (*arrow*).

Courtesy of Leonard V. Crowley, MD, Century College.

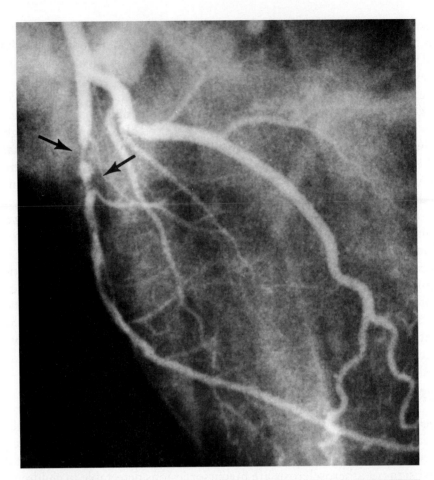

FIGURE 12-16 A coronary angiogram illustrating several areas of coronary artery narrowing (*arrows*). The individual demonstrated exertional chest pain (angina pectoris) on exercise.

Courtesy of Leonard V. Crowley, MD, Century College.

Fatty streak lesions Early sign of atherosclerosis as elongated flat accumulations of foam cells.

first and second decade. These **fatty streak lesions** are accumulations of lipid-rich foam cells within the intima. The lesions are often elongated (hence the term "streak") and parallel to the direction of blood flow. The lesions are mostly flat, so blood flow is not disturbed. Fatty streaks first appear in the thoracic aorta, but the distribution of these lesions does not mirror the location of atheromas in adults (which are not frequent in this location). Somewhat later in life, fatty streaks begin to appear in coronary vessels in locations where fibrofatty atheromas become common with age, suggesting the fatty streaks are a precursor lesion of atherosclerosis. With time fibro-fatty atheromas develop, a process that may take decades (**FIGURE 12-17**). This occurs at sites where endothelial injury occurs, a process in which blood flow dynamics plays a role. Initially the atheroma may be stabile, but as it begins to grow in size, it becomes clinically significant and causes luminal stenosis and reduced blood flow.

Reduced blood flow may result in some degree of cardiac ischemia when the heart is stressed by exercise or in some other way (Figure 12-16). This results in a cramping chest pain (cardiac angina) that can be relieved using vasodilators to increase the luminal diameter of the vessels (discussed in cardiovascular system, coronary vascular disease). As the process continues, changes to the plaque destabilize it and render it prothrombotic. Eventually (possibly in the late sixth or seventh decade) an acute change to a complicated lesion results in clinically evident (and possibly catastrophic) disease. Hence, atherosclerosis is a chronic,

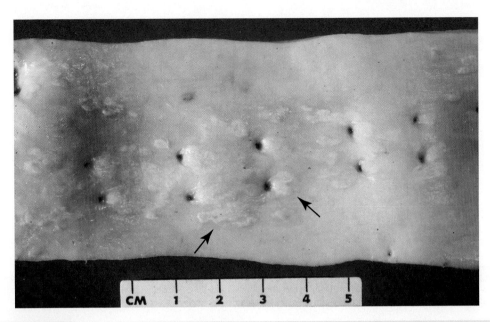

FIGURE 12-17 Interior of aorta, illustrating early atheromatous plaque (*arrows*) formation. Circular openings are orifices of intercostal arteries. Compare this to Figure 12-15, which demonstrates advanced atherosclerosis of the aorta.

Courtesy of Leonard V. Crowley, MD, Century College.

multidecade process. Prevention of atherosclerosis requires modification of risk factors and recognition that some risk factors may not be changed and require positive therapeutic intervention.

Risk Factors for Atherosclerotic Disease: Introduction

A number of modifiable factors are known to increase the risk of developing atherosclerotic vascular disease and its associated complications. Of the four major risk factors (elevated blood lipids, high blood pressure, cigarette smoking, and diabetes), the most important is elevated blood lipids (**hyperlipidemia**), and specifically **hypercholesterolemia**, which *even in the absence of other risk factors can promote atheroma development*. Most serum cholesterol is associated with **low-density lipoprotein (LDL)**, the plasma protein molecule that carries cholesterol to the tissue where it is metabolized. LDL cholesterol is often termed "bad lipid" and is strongly associated with increased risk. **High-density lipoprotein (HDL)** carries cholesterol from the periphery (and from atheromas) to the liver for excretion as bile and is often called "good lipid" as higher levels of HDL reduce risk to some degree (**FIGURE 12-18**).

The remaining major modifiable risk factors include high blood pressure, cigarette smoking, and diabetes. If one risk factor is present, the likelihood of coronary heart disease and heart attacks is twice that of an individual lacking risk factors. If two risk factors are present, the risk increases fourfold, and if three factors are present, the risk of heart attack is seven times that for an individual with none.

Other modifiable factors play a less important (or more poorly defined) role. Obesity and physical inactivity increase the risk of atherosclerotic disease, probably because such factors interact to promote high blood lipids, elevated blood pressure and the risk of metabolic syndrome and subsequent type II diabetes, which is discussed in diabetes mellitus and the pancreas sections. Elevated levels of blood

Hyperlipidemia Elevated blood lipids.

Hypercholesterolemia Elevated blood cholesterol.

Low-density lipoprotein (LDL) Plasma protein molecule carrying cholesterol to the tissue.

High-density lipoprotein (HDL) Plasma protein molecule carrying cholesterol away from the tissue.

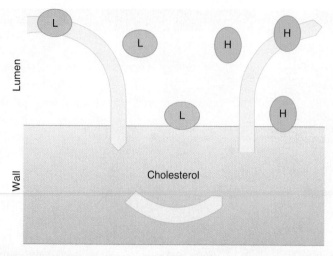

FIGURE 12-18 Role of lipoproteins in transport of cholesterol. Low-density lipoprotein (L) promotes atherosclerosis by transporting cholesterol into the arterial wall. High-density lipoprotein (H) protects against atherosclerosis by transporting cholesterol to the liver for excretion.

Homocysteine/ homocysteinemia Sulfur containing amino acid/ excessive levels of homocysteine.

C-reactive protein Acute phase reactant associated with inflammation.

homocysteine (homocysteinemia) are a major risk factor (which can in part be genetic). It is uncertain whether dietary therapy using B vitamins and folic acid reduce the incidence of cardiovascular disease. Likewise, an elevated level of the acute phase reactant **C-reactive protein**, associated with inflammation, is an independent risk factor for atherosclerosis; it is uncertain whether modification by drug therapy is effective in reducing this risk. A number of genetic diseases, including familial hypercholesterolemia and homocystinuria, an uncommon autosomal recessive condition related to defects in the metabolism of the amino acid methionine associated with grossly elevated plasma homocysteine, are associated with increased risk for atherosclerosis. Drug therapy using lipid lowering agents is highly effective for the former. Other major risk factors, such as age and male sex, obviously cannot be modified.

BLOOD LIPIDS

It is abundantly clear that elevated levels of serum cholesterol are associated with atherosclerosis and cardiovascular disease. Clinical risk is best measured by the level of low-density lipoprotein (LDL) because this protein carries with about 80 percent of serum cholesterol and is associated with tissue deposition of the lipid. Cholesterol is found in nutrients of animal origin (eggs, meats, and dairy products). Currently, it is unclear whether dietary cholesterol intake is associated with cardiovascular disease. Although prudence suggests some caution in excessive consumption, butter and eggs have lost much of their evil repute. Saturated fats (fats solid at room temperature and whose carbon atoms cannot accept additional hydrogen atoms having no double bonds between them) do raise LDL cholesterol levels, but there is still much controversy regarding whether this elevation increases the incidence of cardiovascular disease. Nevertheless, the American Heart Association recommends limiting saturated fat consumption to 5 to 6 percent of caloric intake. Examples of foods with saturated fats include tropical oils (such as coconut or palm kernel oil), beef fat, lard and cream, and many other meat and dairy products. Labels of prepared foods indicate the amount of saturated fat they contain. Not subject to controversy is both the ability of trans fats to raise LDL cholesterol and for reduction in consumption to reduce cardiovascular risk. Trans fats are solid fats chemically synthesized from unsaturated fats to improve shelf life and baking characteristics. Recognizing the risks, several governments have either banned or soon will ban trans fats from all food products (the "no trans fat" label is already common in the United States).

Triglycerides are the lipids used for storage of excess calories in fat cells for future use as an energy source (unlike cholesterol, which is used in cell membrane and hormone synthesis). High levels of triglycerides indicate excess caloric intake over energy needs and are associated with cardiovascular disease (and also obesity, metabolic syndrome, and type II diabetes). Triglyceride levels are best reduced by losing weight, cutting back on calories, and lifestyle modifications.

Several dietary lipids may *improve* lipid profiles by increasing HDL ("good" cholesterol) and lowering triglycerides. Monounsaturated fats (such as found in olive oil, avocados, almonds, and dark chocolate) do not raise LDL while raising HDL. Omega-6 polyunsaturated fatty acids (omega-6 PUFA found in seeds and nuts) and omega-3 polyunsaturated fatty acids (omega-3 PUFA found in fish oils) both have claimed benefits in terms of lipid metabolism (such as decreasing LDL cholesterol and triglycerides and increasing HDL cholesterol). The omega 3 and 6 indicate the position of an unsaturated double bond in the long carbon chain. Such claims are complicated by the finding that omega-6 PUFA might promote the synthesis of certain mediators of inflammation and that omega-3 supplementation in high-risk individuals has not demonstrated a reduction in cardiovascular disease. Although the American Heart Association currently suggests including 6 to 10 percent of calories as omega-6 PUFA from foods as part of a healthy diet, use of both omega-6 and omega-3 PUFA dietary supplements is not recommended for healthy individuals.

Therapeutic Approaches to Hyperlipidemia

The decision to actively lower blood lipid levels, and in particular cholesterol levels, is clinically based on the overall risk of cardiovascular disease. Individuals with known cardiovascular disease (including deposits in coronary arteries and also in other areas of the vasculature) or with genetic diseases that elevate cholesterol levels clearly benefit from drug-based therapy using a class of agents termed **statins** (although other generally less effective agents are available). Even individuals *without* known cardiovascular disease are likely to show reduced risk of developing disease (or exacerbation of undiagnosed early disease). Clinicians use risk calculation estimators (one is available online from the American Heart Association) to estimate the risk of a myocardial infarct in the next decade and base suggested intervention on the degree of future risk. Lifestyle modification—including weight loss, exercise, and diet modification—is often suggested in an initial attempt to improve cholesterol levels in individuals without current disease. These interventions provide an overall health benefit, but they have little if any effect on overall mortality from cardiovascular disease. Serum cholesterol levels depend on genetic factors, and once body mass is elevated, those levels respond poorly to dietary modification. For these reasons, the use of drug therapy with statins to lower serum cholesterol levels is clearly of benefit. Statins are a class of agents that inhibit the enzyme HMG-CoA reductase, which is critical to the synthesis of cholesterol by the liver. Potential side effects of statin use include muscle pain and (rarely) serious damage to muscles; drug cost is a potential problem for some. The decision of when to treat otherwise healthy individuals and how aggressively to attempt to lower cholesterol levels is complex and still not fully settled. Clearly individuals with very low serum cholesterol levels (below 70 mg/dl) would not demonstrate sufficient future risk to warrant therapy, but individuals with higher levels (and other risk factors such as low HDL) would likely benefit from reduced risk. Recent guidelines from the American College of Cardiology and the American Heart Association increase the suggested use of aggressive statin therapy in individuals without cardiovascular disease who have levels of 190 mg/dl LDL

Triglycerides Lipids used to store excess calories in fat cells.

Statins Drug agents effective against development of atherosclerosis.

cholesterol or greater (or at even lower levels given other indicators of increased future risk). More aggressive drug use is also suggested for individuals between the ages of forty and seventy-five.

There is no controversy regarding the benefit of aggressive attempts to lower serum cholesterol in individuals either with known cardiovascular disease or with very high risk of such (such as young individuals who have familial hypercholesterolemia, a relatively common autosomal dominant disease resulting in much increased levels of LDL cholesterol in childhood).

C-REACTIVE PROTEIN

C-reactive protein (CRP) is one of several proteins produced by the liver and released into the bloodstream in response to tissue injury or inflammation. The protein is one of the body's nonspecific defenses against infection and provides some protection against the harmful effects of inflammation by neutralizing various products produced by the cells that accumulate at the site of the inflammation. Measurement of CRP has been used for many years to monitor the activity of diseases associated with inflammation such as rheumatic fever and rheumatoid arthritis.

Recently, very sensitive tests have been developed that can detect slight CRP elevations in people who do not appear to have evidence of an inflammatory or infectious disease. Studies have demonstrated that an elevated CRP level in an otherwise normal person predicts an increased long-term risk of cardiovascular disease, probably because the elevated CRP is detecting the accumulation of macrophages, lymphocytes, lipids, and products of tissue injury within unstable plaques in coronary arteries. The increase in relative risk associated with CRP elevation is similar to (and slightly higher than) the relative risk attributable to hypertension and hyperlipidemia. The CRP test is recommended as an additional screening test to detect people at risk of coronary artery disease, who then can be offered treatment to reduce their risk factors.

HOMOCYSTEINE

Homocysteine is a sulfur-containing amino acid formed enzymatically from methionine, an essential amino acid abundant in animal protein. Homocysteine is then metabolized by other biochemical pathways in which vitamin B_6, vitamin B_{12}, and folic acid are required. Blood concentrations of homocysteine are higher in men than in premenopausal women but increase in women after the menopause. Renal function also influences homocysteine blood levels, which are elevated in people with kidney disease.

Abnormal homocysteine metabolism is characteristic of a rare hereditary disease called homocystinuria. The disease results from a gene mutation leading to an enzyme defect that impairs the normal metabolism of homocysteine. Affected individuals have an extremely high concentration of homocysteine in their blood and excrete the amino acid in their urine. Those affected show evidence of marked vascular disease, which has its onset at a very young age. These manifestations include atherosclerosis of coronary arteries and other major arteries, strokes, and blood clots in arteries and veins.

Clinical studies have demonstrated that many people with cardiovascular disease, strokes, and peripheral vascular disease have elevated homocysteine blood levels, and a high homocysteine blood level is a risk factor for atherosclerosis, comparable to the increased risk associated with hypercholesterolemia, smoking, and hypertension. In most people in whom renal function is normal, the elevated homocysteine level may be related to a deficiency of B vitamins and folic acid; however, it is unclear whether dietary supplementation reduces the risk of cardiovascular disease in individuals who do not have hereditary homocytinuria.

Hypertension and Hypertensive Cardiovascular Disease

PRIMARY HYPERTENSION

Hypertension is a critical and modifiable risk factor for cardiovascular disease, and attempts have been made to define a normal "ideal" blood pressure and set guidelines for therapy to reduce risk should this pressure be exceeded. Traditionally, normal blood pressure is considered to be below 120/80 (systolic/diastolic). A pressure consistently higher than 140/90 is called hypertension, whereas in-between values are considered to be "prehypertensive" and indicate a potential problem. The higher the pressure, the greater are its harmful effects. Normal blood pressures are defined on the basis of population studies and vary depending on age and sex among normal individuals. Rather than defining "normal," current guidelines set "blood pressure goals" above which antihypertensive therapy should be considered. Threshold values for an otherwise normal individual under age sixty are 140/90. For those over age sixty, threshold values are 150/90. Individuals of any age with diabetes or chronic renal disease have a goal of 140/90.

Ninety-five percent of cases of hypertension (so-called **essential hypertension**) have no easily identifiable cause but rather are multifactorial with genetics, salt intake, and vascular tone all playing a role. In the case of vascular tone, increased sympathetic activity can result in excessive vasoconstriction of the small arterioles throughout the body, which raises the diastolic pressure. Because of the high peripheral resistance, the heart needs to pump more forcefully to overcome the resistance created by the constricted arterioles and supply adequate blood to the tissues, which leads to a compensatory rise in systolic blood pressure. Therefore, both systolic and diastolic pressure rise when the primary problem is excessive arteriolar vasoconstriction.

Essential hypertension
High blood pressure with no identifiable cause.

Cardiac Effects

The heart responds to the increased workload resulting from the high peripheral resistance by becoming enlarged, particularly in the left ventricle, which serves as the pump for systemic circulation. Although the enlarged heart may be able to function effectively for many years, the cardiac pump is being forced to work beyond its "rated capacity." Eventually, the heart can no longer maintain adequate blood flow, and the patient develops symptoms of cardiac failure.

Vascular Effects

Because the blood vessels are not designed to carry blood at such a high pressure, the vessels wear out prematurely. Hypertension accelerates the development of atherosclerosis in the larger arteries and is a major risk factor for cardiovascular disease. The arterioles also are injured; they thicken and undergo degenerative changes, and their lumens become narrowed. This process is termed *arteriolosclerosis*. Sometimes the walls of the small arterioles become completely necrotic due to the effects of the sustained high blood pressure. Weakened arterioles may rupture, leading to hemorrhage. The brain is particularly vulnerable, and cerebral hemorrhage (hemorrhagic stroke) is a relatively common complication of severe hypertension.

Renal Effects

The narrowing of the renal arterioles decreases the blood supply to the kidneys, which, in turn, leads to injury and degenerative changes in the glomeruli and renal tubules. Severe hypertension may cause severe derangement of renal function and eventually leads to renal failure (**FIGURE 12-19**).

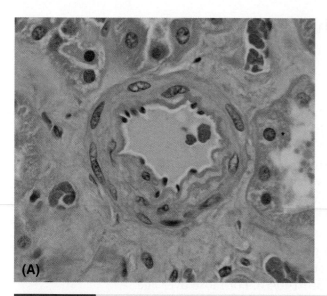
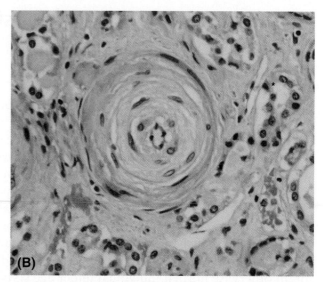

FIGURE 12-19 **(A)** Renal arteriole of normal size. Its wall is composed of a few concentric layers of smooth muscle cells. **(B)** Renal arteriole from a patient with long-standing hypertension. The wall is greatly thickened and contains many concentric layers of smooth muscle cells and a marked reduction in the size of the lumen. (The asterisk in both images marks a renal tubular cell for use in comparing the photos.)

SECONDARY HYPERTENSION

In 5 percent of patients, hypertension results from a known disease or condition such as chronic kidney disease (see discussion on the urinary system), endocrine gland dysfunction such as a pituitary or an adrenal tumor, or a hyperactive thyroid gland (see discussion on the endocrine glands). The high blood pressure associated with these conditions is called secondary hypertension because the cause of the hypertension is known. In many cases, successful treatment of the underlying condition cures the hypertension.

TREATMENT OF HYPERTENSION

Although the reason for hypertension cannot be determined in most instances, blood pressure can be reduced to more normal levels, thereby lowering the risk of complications of high blood pressure. This is accomplished by administering various drugs that lower the blood pressure using a variety of mechanisms. Commonly used drugs include thiazide-type diuretics that increase the ability of the kidney to remove salt and water from the circulation, thus lessening the "load" the heart must pump against. Calcium channel blockers inhibit the contraction of arteriolar smooth muscle cells, lowering peripheral resistance. ACE inhibitors reduce the production of angiotensin II, which is a potent vasoconstrictor. Several other classes of antihypertensive drugs also can be useful in particular clinical circumstances.

Hypertension and the Aorta: Aneurysms

An aneurysm is a dilatation of the wall of an artery, or an outpouching of a portion of the wall. Most aneurysms are acquired as a result of atherosclerosis, which causes weakening of the vessel wall. One type of aneurysm involving the cerebral arteries is the result of a congenital abnormality of the vessel wall and is considered in conjunction with the nervous system (see discussion on the nervous system).

ARTERIOSCLEROTIC ANEURYSM

A small artery that undergoes arteriosclerotic change becomes narrowed and may eventually become thrombosed. A large artery, such as the aorta, has a diameter so large that complete obstruction is uncommon. However, atheromatous deposits tend to damage the wall of the aorta, reducing its elasticity and weakening the wall. The aortic wall tends to balloon out under the stress of the high pressure within the vessel, forming an aortic aneurysm. Aortic aneurysms usually develop in the distal part of the abdominal aorta, where the pressure is highest and the atheromatous change is most severe (**FIGURE 12-20** and **FIGURE 12-21**). Usually, the interior of the aneurysm becomes covered with a layer of thrombus material, and the wall often becomes partially calcified. Aneurysms also occur in the thoracic aorta, usually in association with a history of tobacco use and hypertension.

Atherosclerosis is the major cause of aortic aneurysms, but there appears to be some genetic predisposition as well because 15 to 20 percent of patients with an aneurysm also have another affected family member. An aortic aneurysm usually enlarges slowly and does not produce symptoms initially. Because a small aneurysm is difficult to detect by physical examination, current guidelines recommend a routine ultrasound screening examination to identify an asymptomatic aneurysm in any adult

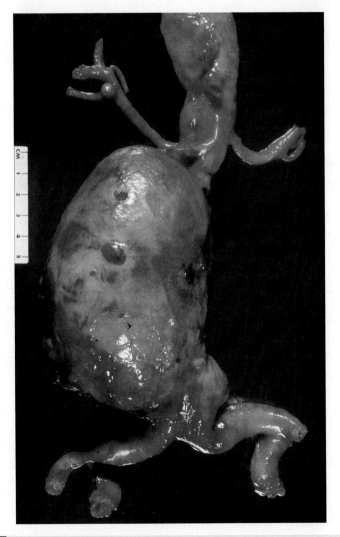

FIGURE 12-20 Large arteriosclerotic aneurysm extending from renal arteries (*above*) to iliac arteries (*below*).

Courtesy of Leonard V. Crowley, MD, Century College.

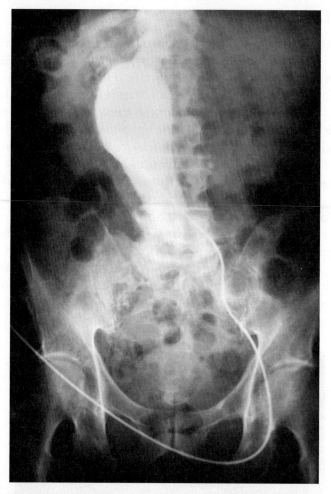

FIGURE 12-21 Aortic aneurysm demonstrated on x-ray by injection of contrast material into aorta.
Courtesy of Leonard V. Crowley, MD, Century College.

older than age sixty-five who has risk factors that predispose to atherosclerosis or who has a family history of an aortic aneurysm.

Aortic aneurysms are dangerous because they may rupture, leading to massive and often fatal hemorrhage. The normal cross-section diameter of the abdominal aorta is about 2 cm. An aneurysm exceeding about 5 cm in diameter may rupture and should be repaired. In general, the larger the aneurysm, the greater the likelihood of rupture (**FIGURE 12-22**).

The standard open surgical aneurysm repair procedure consists of opening the aneurysm and sewing a nylon or Dacron graft into the aorta above and below the aneurysmal segment so that the blood flowing through the aorta flows through the graft rather than through the aneurysm. It is not necessary to excise the aneurysm that has been bypassed by the graft, and usually the walls of the aneurysm are wrapped around the graft. This procedure is a well-established, reliable, and highly successful method of treatment, but it is a major surgical procedure and poses significant risks to older patients who may have coronary artery disease and other medical problems.

DISSECTING ANEURYSM OF THE AORTA

The thick middle layer of the aorta is called the media. It is composed of multiple layers of elastic tissue and muscle bonded together by fibrous connective tissue.

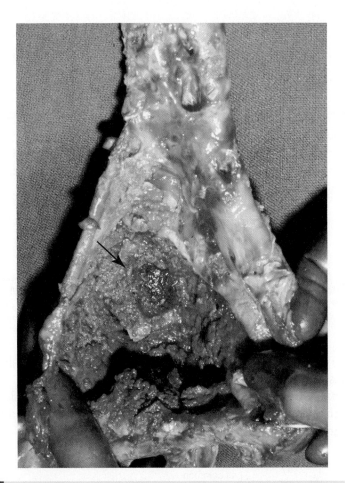

FIGURE 12-22 Interior of atherosclerotic aneurysm, illustrating marked degenerative change in wall. Extremely thin area in wall (*arrow*) predisposes to rupture.

Courtesy of Leonard V. Crowley, MD, Century College.

Degenerative changes sometimes occur in the media, causing the layers to lose their cohesiveness and separate (**FIGURE 12-23**). Then the pulsatile force of the blood flowing through the aorta may cause the inner half of the aortic wall to pull away from the outer half in the region where the media has degenerated, and sometimes the inner lining (intima) tears as the media separates. This complication is especially likely to occur in individuals with high blood pressure.

After an intimal tear has developed, blood is forced into the aortic wall. The area of medial degeneration forms a cleavage plane that permits the blood to dissect within the media for a variable distance. This event, a dissecting aneurysm of the aorta, is associated with severe chest and back pain. The term *dissecting* refers to the splitting (dissection) of the media by the blood, and the somewhat misleading term *aneurysm* was applied because the affected part of the aorta appears wider than normal. The widening results from the hemorrhage within the aortic wall, but the lumen of the aorta is not dilated.

The intimal tear that starts the dissection is usually either in the ascending aorta just above the aortic valve or in the descending aorta just beyond the origin of the large arteries that arise from the aortic arch (**FIGURE 12-24**). If the tear is in the ascending aorta, the blood often dissects proximally as well as distally within the aortic wall, extending into the base of the aorta where the aortic valve attaches and the coronary arteries arise leading to compromise of cardiac function. A dissection in the ascending aorta is often fatal because the blood frequently ruptures through

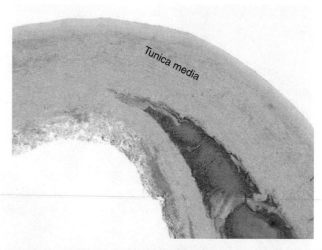

FIGURE 12-23 Characteristic degenerative changes in the media of the aortic wall (called cystic medial necrosis) has led to a loss of cohesion between the inner and outer layers of the aortic wall and allowed blood (bright red wedge) to dissect down the tunica media of the aorta.

Courtesy Dr. Daniel Yandow, Department of Radiology University of Wisconsin School of Medicine.

the outer wall of the aorta at the base of the heart, leading to extensive hemorrhage into the mediastinum or pericardial sac.

If the intimal tear is in the descending aorta, the blood dissects distally and may extend the entire length of the aorta, leading to impairment of blood flow to the kidneys, the intestines, or other vital organs.

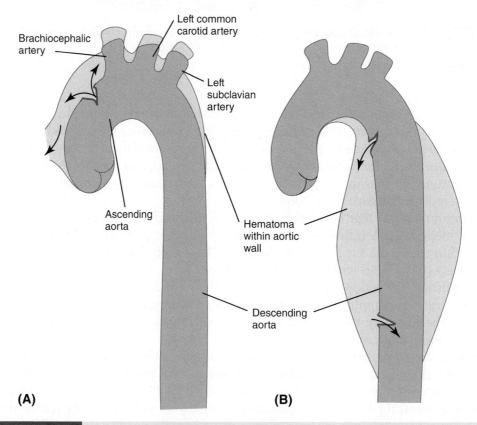

FIGURE 12-24 Sites of aortic dissection. **(A)** Tear in ascending aorta causes both proximal and distal dissection. **(B)** Tear in descending aorta may cause extensive distal dissection and may rupture back into lumen of aorta.

DIAGNOSIS OF CORONARY ARTERY DISEASE

Physicians can now evaluate the extent of coronary artery disease as well as the exact sites where the main coronary arteries are obstructed. This is accomplished by passing a catheter into the aorta and injecting a radiopaque dye directly into the orifices of the coronary arteries. The filling of the coronary arteries can be observed, along with the location and degree of arterial obstruction (Figure 12-16). This procedure is called a coronary angiogram (see discussion on general concepts of disease, principles of diagnosis). Echocardiograms of the heart using ultrasound are also useful in detecting coronary artery disease. Stress tests use exercise or drugs to stimulate the heart whose function is measured using either ECG or in some cases a radiotracer injected into the circulation to measure whether areas of the heart have diminished blood flow (nuclear stress test).

TREATMENT OF CORONARY ARTERY DISEASE

Medical Treatment

Medical treatment of coronary heart disease consists of administering drugs that reduce myocardial oxygen consumption and improve coronary circulation (antianginal drugs). If the patient exhibits cardiac irregularities, drugs that reduce myocardial irritability also are prescribed (antiarrhythmial drugs). Factors that potentiate coronary artery disease also are controlled or eliminated whenever possible: eliminate smoking, add hypertension control, improve diet, reduce weight, and increase exercise.

Surgical Treatment

Several surgical approaches, called myocardial revascularization procedures, have been devised to improve blood supply to the heart muscle. Surgery is often recommended for patients who do not respond satisfactorily to medical treatment. The usual surgical method is to bypass the obstructions in the coronary arteries by means of segments of saphenous vein obtained from the patient's legs. The proximal ends of the grafts are sutured to small openings made in the aorta above the normal openings of the coronary arteries, and the distal ends are sutured into the coronary arteries beyond the areas of narrowing (**FIGURE 12-25**). Myocardial revascularization operations are generally reserved for patients with severe sclerosis of all three major coronary arteries, and usually grafts are used to bypass all three arteries. The operation alleviates or greatly improves symptoms of angina and may also improve survival in some groups of patients. Unfortunately, the high arterial pressure carried by the vein grafts sometimes causes the grafts to undergo progressive intimal thickening, which may lead to complete occlusion of the grafts. Many of the grafts eventually also develop the same type of atherosclerosis that occurred in the coronary arteries.

The internal thoracic arteries, which are more often called by their older name of internal mammary arteries, also can be used to bypass obstructed coronary arteries. The internal mammary arteries are paired arteries that arise from the aorta and descend along the undersurface of the thoracic cavity just lateral to the sternum. They can be dissected from their normal location and connected to the coronary arteries, thereby delivering blood directly from the aorta to the coronary arteries beyond the narrowed or blocked areas. Because the arteries are able to carry blood under much higher pressure than veins, artery grafts are less likely to become narrowed or obstructed. In some patients, both vein grafts and internal mammary arteries are used to restore adequate blood flow to the myocardium.

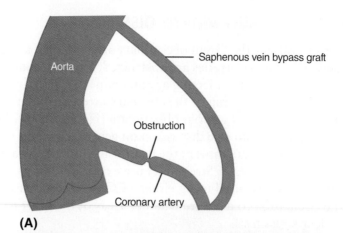

(A)

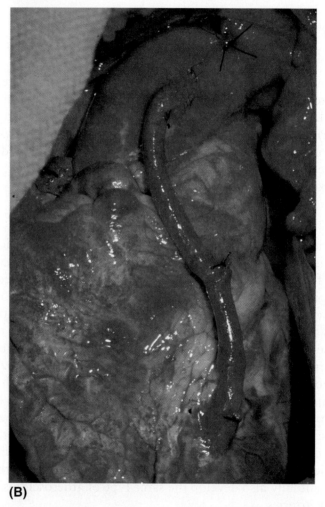

(B)

FIGURE 12-25 **(A)** Principle of surgical treatment of coronary heart disease by means of saphenous vein grafts that bypass obstructions in coronary arteries. **(B)** Vein graft extending from aorta above the origin of the coronary arteries to the anterior interventricular (descending) coronary artery distal to the site of arterial narrowing.

Courtesy of Leonard V. Crowley, MD, Century College.

Coronary Angioplasty

Many patients with less extensive coronary artery disease can be treated successfully by dilating narrowed areas in the coronary arteries instead of bypassing them, thereby avoiding major surgery. The procedure is called coronary angioplasty

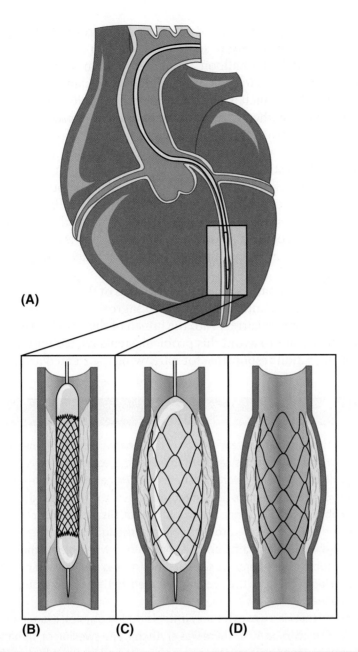

(A)

(B)   **(C)**   **(D)**

FIGURE 12-26 Principle of coronary angioplasty. **(A)** An overview illustrating the positioning of the guide catheter at the site of narrowing in the coronary artery. **(B)** A balloon catheter covered by unexpanded stent advanced through guide catheter and positioned within narrowed segment of artery. **(C)** Balloon inflated, relieving arterial obstruction by smashing plaque and simultaneously expanding the stent. **(D)** Balloon catheter withdrawn, leaving an expanded stent that forms a rigid support to maintain the caliber of the dilated artery.

(*angio* = vessel + *plasty* = molding) and is illustrated in **FIGURE 12-26**. By means of a technique similar to that used to perform a coronary arteriogram (see discussion on general concepts of disease, principles of diagnosis), a guiding catheter is introduced through the skin and into a large artery in the arm or leg, threaded under fluoroscopic control into the narrowed coronary artery, and positioned at the site of narrowing. Then the balloon catheter is threaded through the guide catheter until the balloon lies within the narrowed area. After the balloon is properly positioned, it is inflated briefly under high pressure, which smashes the plaque and pushes it into the arterial wall, enlarging the lumen of the artery and improving blood flow to the myocardium.

Successful dilatation of a narrowed coronary artery restores normal blood flow through the artery. Unfortunately, in some successfully treated patients, the stenosis recurs within six months after balloon angioplasty and may require redilatation. In an attempt to solve the problem of restenosis, most physicians now perform balloon angioplasty using a **stent,** which is often a short, expandable metal mesh tube that is placed over the balloon catheter with the metal mesh collapsed. The stent expands as the balloon is inflated to enlarge the lumen of the artery and functions as a rigid support to help keep the vessel open (Figure 12-26D). This procedure is usually supplemented by administration of drugs that prevent accumulation of platelets at the site where the stent was placed. The arterial wall responds to the metal stent by proliferation of connective tissue and smooth muscle cells that grow through the meshes in the stent and cover its inner surface, followed by gradual ingrowth of endothelial cells to provide a smooth interior lining for the stent. Consequently, platelets are less likely to adhere at the site of the stent placement and cause thrombosis of the stented vessel.

Although use of stents has been helpful, restenosis of the dilated artery still occurs in about 25 percent of patients, resulting from ingrowth of tissue extending from the inner layers of the stented artery into the lumen of the vessel between the meshes of the stent. In an attempt to avoid this problem, stents coated with drugs that suppress the cell proliferation responsible for narrowing the stented artery can be used.

> **Stent** Short tube often made of expandable metal mesh used to hold the blood vessel open.

CASE 12-1

Haruto, known as "Hari," is the four-year-old son of the Tonagas, a second generation Japanese American family. Hari has been fussy and irritable over the last several days. His parents felt he had a "spring cold" and initially were not concerned. He had a low grade fever during the day (38.5°C) that did not respond to acetaminophen. Over the next four days Hari became increasingly irritable. He vomited once and would not eat. His parents noticed that his hands and feet appeared red and seemed to be swollen. Although Hari usually ran around the house, walking now seemed painful and he complained when his mother asked him to play. His mother took his temperature several times during the day and noted that Hari's fever varied, peaking at 39.5°C in the evening. Alarmed, Hari's parents brought him to their pediatrician, Dr. Janet.

Dr. Janet noted that Hari was extremely irritable during physical examination. His temperature was confirmed to be 40°C. There was erythema and swelling of his hands and feet and movement of his limbs caused Hari to complain. He had cracks in his lips (fissures), his tongue was red and swollen (described as a "strawberry tongue"), and he had a "measlelike" rash on his back and groin. Dr. Janet noted that both of Hari's conjunctiva were red, and the superficial bulbar vessels were prominent (bulbar conjunctival injection). Hari had a single enlarged cervical lymph node on his right side. Dr. Janet was quite concerned about Hari's illness. She considered a number of infectious etiologies including adenovirus or measles infection and number of bacterial etiologies such as group A beta-hemolytic-streptococcal infection. However, Hari's symptoms (and to some extent his Asiatic background) suggested Kawasaki disease, an idiopathic condition for which there are no specific diagnostic test. Because 25 percent of untreated Kawasaki disease patients develop coronary artery disease, which is often serious and may ultimately result in death, Dr. Janet had Hari admitted to a pediatric referral center experienced in acute care. On admission Dr. Janet's initial impression of possible Kawasaki disease was confirmed. Hari was immediately treated with a single high dose of intravenous immunoglobulin (IVIG) given over a twelve-hour period. An initial blood sample showed a very high level of C-reactive protein

CASE 12-1 (*Continued*)

(a nonspecific marker of inflammation elevated in Kawaski disease). High-dose aspirin was also started, and echocardiography was performed. Hari's temperature and level of C-reactive protein were carefully monitored over the next days. C-reactive protein levels fell over three days post-IVIG therapy, and Hari was afebrile by day four. Low-dose aspirin therapy was continued for an additional ten days. Echocardiographic finding initially and two weeks after therapy showed abnormal width of the left anterior descending coronary artery (termed a z-score), raising concern over the possibility of coronary artery aneurysm formation (which can be associated with serious consequences such as chronic vascular disease and sudden cardiac death). A repeat echocardiogram at seven weeks posttherapy was considered normal, and Hari was scheduled for a repeat echocardiogram at six months.

Discussion

Kawasaki disease (first described by Tomisaku Kawasaki in the 1970s) is a potentially fatal disease, predominantly of young children. The frequency of the disease varies greatly with geographic area and ethnic background and is most frequent in Japan, Korea, and Taiwan. The current frequency in Japan is 260 cases per 100,00 children under age five (the ages at which the disease is most common) and the frequency appears to be increasing. The frequency of the disease is ten to twenty times lower in the United States and Europe (about 18 cases per 100,000 children under age five in the United States) with a stabile incidence. Individuals of Asiatic (predominantly Japanese) origin show a higher rate of disease incidence even when living in relatively low-incidence areas, and evidence suggests that susceptibility is familial. However, no one genetic factor is associated with the disease (although variation in several genes associated with immune response does confer increased risk of disease and serious clinical outcomes). Although Kawasaki disease is much more frequent in certain populations, the disease is not limited to these groups and occurs in all ethnicities.

There is strong evidence to suggest that the etiology of the disease depends on an infectious agent, but no agent has been definitively identified. The disease frequency shows seasonal variation, has occurred in widespread epidemics in Japan as well as smaller localized disease clusters, and is associated with the formation of IgA antibodies, which react with cytoplasmic inclusions found in patients and are believed to be an otherwise unknown RNA virus. Unfortunately, there is no good animal model for the disease.

The pathophysiology of the disease in relation to vascular effects is complex. Kawasaki disease results in an inflammation of the arteries (arteritis), most significantly in but not limited to the coronary arteries. The arteritis has an acute neutrophilic phase, resulting in a self-limited necrotizing pathology occurring during the first two weeks of the disease. The acute phase results in necrosis of the endothelium and media, occasionally extending to the adventitia, which can form large saccular aneurysms that thrombose and may rupture. Later in the disease, a more generalized chronic vasculitis occurs that is most prominent in the coronary arteries. This chronic phase is mediated by lymphocytic cells and eosinophils and affects the adventitia progressing inward. During this more chronic phase, a proliferation of medial "myofibroblasts" occurs (which is distinct from atherosclerotic disease). The proliferation may result in obstruction of vessels. The chronic phase may persist indefinitely and ultimately result in death from coronary vascular disease months or even years after Kawaski disease is first diagnosed.

Kawaski disease is currently believed to be an exaggerated response to an undefined infectious agent (or agents) in genetically susceptible individuals, which results in both acute and potentially chronic vasculitis and vascular abnormalities of greatest consequence in the coronary vessels.

(*continues*)

CASE 12-1 (Continued)

Although Kawaski disease results in marked increases in nonspecific indicators of inflammation, diagnosis is based on clinical signs and symptoms. The currently accepted clinical diagnostic criteria for the disease are detailed in the Supplementary Readings. Therapy with IVIG has an excellent response rate in the disease. The mode of action of the therapy is still not understood but is likely to rely on the generalized anti-inflammatory effects of IVIG and possibly the presence of specific antibody in the IVIG reactive with the putative infectious agent. Whatever the mechanism, rapid IVIG therapy prevents the appearance of the abnormalities in the coronary vasculature likely to result in serious cardiac disease. The effect of aspirin therapy is controversial but is likely to act as an anti-inflammatory (in high doses) and prevent platelet-mediated thrombosis in lower doses. More intensive treatment with immunosuppressive agents is needed for the approximately 20 percent of patients who are resistant to combined IVIG and aspirin therapy.

Etiology and Pathogenesis

Kawasaki disease with transient arteritis of the coronary arteries.

Questions

1. Given the signs and symptoms noted in the case, should the pediatrician have had an equally strong index of suspicion for Kawaski disease in a non-Asiatic patient?

2. What are other infectious diseases a pediatrician might consider in a similar case?

3. Why is C-reactive protein used as an index of disease severity in Kawaski patients?

4. Are C-reactive protein levels a useful initial screen for Kawaski disease in patients?

5. What might be the short- and long-term consequences of failure to treat Kawaski disease?

QUESTIONS FOR REVIEW

1. Describe how blood flows through the venous system. What happens when flow is interrupted?
2. What is the difference between a thrombus and an embolus? What is an infarct?
3. What factors predispose to arterial thrombosis?
4. What are the causes and effects of intracardiac thrombi?
5. What conditions predispose to thrombosis by increasing the coagulability of the blood?
6. What genetic factors lead to increased risk of atherosclerosis?
7. What tests are used to diagnose diseases of the circulatory system?
8. What is the usual cause of an aortic aneurysm? How is an aneurysm treated?
9. What is the difference between an arteriosclerotic aneurysm of the aorta and a dissecting aneurysm of the aorta?

SUPPLEMENTARY READINGS

Lilly, L. S. 2010. *Pathophysiology of Heart Disease: A Collaborative Project of Medical Students and Faculty*. 5th ed. Baltimore, MD: Lippincott Williams & Wilkins.

▶ The area of circulatory disease is so broad (and so detailed) that no set of readings can fully do it justice. This text presents a readable and somewhat technical overview aimed at medical and advanced undergraduate students. It is an excellent single source for additional background for diseases of blood circulation. It is particularly strong on therapy and has a good discussion of atherosclerosis.

American Heart Association. http://www.heart.org/HEARTORG/

American Heart Association. http://www.heart.org/HEARTORG/HealthcareResearch/Healthcare-Research _UCM_001093_SubHomePage.jsp

Stone, N. J. 2013. *ACC/AHA guidelines on the treatment of blood cholesterol to reduce atherosclerotic cardiovascular risk in adults*. http://circ.ahajournals.org/content/129/25_suppl_2/S1

▶ The American Heart Association website is an essential resource for any area of cardiovascular disease. The first entry is the introductory page, and the second entry is the portal for scientific information. AHA statements and guidelines (which can be accessed from this page) are authoritative and carefully reviewed by all health care professionals. The third article provides current guidelines issued by the ACC/AHA joint panels. This is must reading in the area and remains controversial.

American College of Cardiology. www.acc.org

American College of Cardiology. *LDL: Address the risk*. http://www.acc.org/tools-and-practice-support/quality -programs/ldl-address-the-risk?w_nav=MN

▶ As is the case with the AHA website, that of the American College of Cardiology has much available material, which is updated immediately. It also acts as a gateway to a wealth of scientific publications of extremely high quality, much of which is publically available. The second article explains a current initiative to improve patient outcomes in hyperlipidemia and acts as a portal for additional information.

Alagona, P., and Ahmad, T. A. 2015. Cardiovascular disease risk assessment and prevention: Current guidelines and limitations. *Medical Clinics of North America 99*:711–31.

Ezzati, M., et al. 2015. Contributions of risk factors and medical care to cardiovascular mortality trends. *Nature Reviews Cardiology 12*:508–30.

McBride, P., Stone, N. J., and Blum, C. B. 2014. Should family physicians follow the new ACA/AHA cholesterol treatment guidelines? Yes [Editorial]. *American Family Physician 90*:213.

Hayward, R. A. 2014. Not completely [Editorial]. *American Family Physician 90*:223.
   ▶ A set of four readings that summarize current information about risk factors in cardiovascular disease and the effect of the new ACA/AHA guidelines.

Krintus, M., et al. 2014. Critical appraisal of inflammatory markers in cardiovascular risk stratification. *Critical Reviews in Clinical Laboratory Sciences 51*:263–79.
   ▶ The reading reviews the evidence that C-reactive protein is an independent risk factor for cardiovascular disease.

Ouellette, D. R. 2015. *Pulmonary embolism.* http://emedicine.medscape.com/article/300901-overview
   ▶ A useful overview of current background on the pathophysiology and etiology of pulmonary embolic disease. It has an excellent collection of diagnostic images.

American College of Rheumatology. *Vasculitis.* http://www.rheumatology.org/I-Am-A/Patient-Caregiver /Diseases-Conditions/Vasculitis

Jennette, J. C., and Falk, R. J. 2014. Pathogenesis of antineutrophil cytoplasmic autoantibody-mediated disease. *Nature Reviews Rheumatology 10*:463–73.
   ▶ Vasculitis is an important pathogenetic mechanism not discussed in detail in the chapter but covered in the case supplemental readings and in the two above. The first article is a good general overview into the etiology and classification of the vasculitides. ANCA disease discussed in the second article is of particular interest because of the singular mechanisms involved in its pathogenesis. The reading is by two of the world's experts.

Shulman, S. T., and Rowley, A. H. 2015. Kawasaki disease: Insights into pathogenesis and approaches to treatment. *Nature Reviews Rheumatology 11*:475–82.
   ▶ An excellent overview of current ideas about the etiology, pathogenesis, and therapy of Kawasaki disease. A primary source for the case.

The Hematopoietic and Lymphatic Systems

The Hematopoietic System

COMPOSITION AND FUNCTION OF HUMAN BLOOD

Blood is a tissue with both fluid and cellular components. Plasma, the fluid component of blood, contains proteins, nutrients, waste products, vitamins, and inorganic salts and also serves to transport the cellular components of the blood—red cells (**erythrocytes**), white cells (**leukocytes**), and platelets—to all parts of the body via the circulatory system. Erythrocytes are essential for the transport of oxygen to tissues and most CO_2 to the lung (10 percent of CO_2 is also dissolved in the plasma). Leukocytes are critical for host defense, a function they serve primarily after transiting into tissue at the site of injury. Platelets are critical for hemostasis, the termination of bleeding. The proteins carried by plasma serve a variety of functions. Those proteins present in greatest concentration are **albumin**, providing the colloid osmotic pressure

Erythrocyte Red cell.

Leukocyte Collective term for white cells.

Albumin Blood protein providing colloid osmotic pressure in blood.

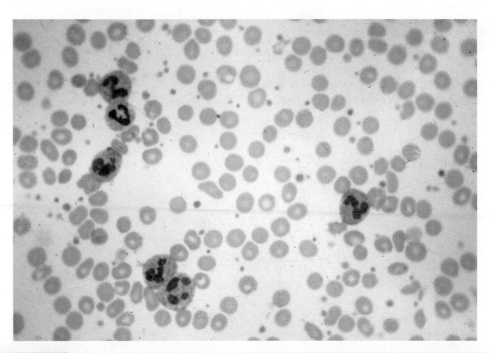

FIGURE 13-1 Stained blood film. Red cells appear as biconcave disks. Several neutrophils can be identified (*center*). Small dark structures are platelets.

Courtesy of Leonard V. Crowley, MD, Century College.

Immunoglobulins Blood proteins forming antibodies.

Fibrinogen Blood protein forming a key element in clotting.

Pluripotential hemopoietic stem cell Precursor for all blood cells.

Lymphoid stem cell Precursor for all lymphocytes.

Progenitor cell Precursor of red cells, nonlymphoid white cells, and platelets.

(oncotic pressure) that helps keep fluid within the blood vessels; **immunoglobulins** (antibodies), which are critical in the adaptive immune response; and **fibrinogen**, a key element in hemostasis that forms the hemostatic plug (clot) that stops bleeding. The volume of blood, which varies with the size of the individual, is about five quarts (five liters) in the average man.

Almost half of the blood consists of cellular elements (**FIGURE 13-1**). All blood cells arise from a common precursor cell within the bone marrow called the **pluripotential hemopoietic stem cell**, which undergoes further differentiation in the marrow to form a **lymphoid stem cell**, the source of lymphocytes critical in the immune response; and a series of **progenitor cells**, which in turn differentiate in the marrow to form the precursors of red cells, nonlymphoid white cells, and platelets that are ultimately released into the bloodstream. The numbers of circulating red cells, white cells, and platelets are expressed as the number per microliter (μl) of blood (1 ml = 1,000 μl). This same quantity can also be expressed as the number per cubic millimeter (mm^3) of blood. The terms are equivalent because 1 μl is the same as 1 mm^3.

Red cells, which are concerned primarily with oxygen transport, are the most numerous cells, averaging about 5 million per microliter of blood. A mature red cell is an extremely flexible biconcave disk measuring about 7 micrometers (microns) in cross-section diameter. Its biconcave configuration is responsible for its characteristic central pallor and more intensely stained periphery, as seen in a stained blood smear. The biconcave configuration also provides the red cell with a large surface area relative to its volume, which facilitates rapid uptake of oxygen as blood flows through the pulmonary capillaries, and a rapid release of oxygen to body cells as blood is delivered to the tissues. The red cell shape also contributes to its extreme flexibility, which allows red cells to squeeze through small blood capillaries less than half the diameter of the red cells. Red cells normally survive for about four months in the circulation.

Leukocytes are much less numerous, averaging about 7,000 per microliter. The following types of leukocytes are recognized: neutrophils, eosinophils, basophils,

TABLE 13-1   Summary of Blood Cells

Name	Light micrograph	Description	Concentration (Number of cells/mm^3)	Life span	Function
Red blood cells (RBCs)		Biconcave disk; no nucleus	4 to 6 million	120 days	Transports oxygen and carbon dioxide
White blood cells (WBCs) Neutrophil		Approximately twice the size of RBCs; multi-lobed nucleus; clearstaining cytoplasm	3,000 to 7,000	6 hours to a few days	Phagocytizes bacteria
Eosinophil		Approximately same size as neutrophil; large pink-staining granules; bilobed nucleus	100 to 400	8 to 12 days	Phagocytizes antigen-antibody complex; attacks parasites
Basophil		Slightly smaller than neutrophil; contains large, purple cytoplasmic granules; bilobed nucleus	20 to 50	Few hours to a few days	Releases histamine during inflammation
Monocyte		Larger than neutrophil; cytoplasm grayish-blue; no cytoplasmic granules; U- or kidney-shaped nucleus	100 to 700	Lasts many months	Phagocytizes bacteria, dead cells, and cellular debris
Lymphocyte		Slightly smaller than neutrophil; large, relatively round nucleus that fills the cell	1,500 to 3,000	Can persist many years	Involved in immune protection, either attacking cells directly or producing antibodies
Platelets		Fragments of megakaryocytes; appear as small dark-staining granules	250,000	5 to 10 days	Play several key roles in blood clotting

monocytes, and lymphocytes. The first three types are collectively called **granulocytes** (because of the characteristic granules in their cytoplasm) or polymorphonuclear leukocytes (because of the multiple lobes of their nuclei). Neutrophils are therefore sometimes called **polymorphonuclear neutrophils (PMNs)**. The last two cell types are collectively called mononuclear cells (because their nuclei do not have multiple lobes). Although all **lymphocytes** are derived from a bone marrow stem cell, those destined to be B lymphocytes continue to mature in the bone marrow until released into the circulation. Precursors of T lymphocytes further mature in the thymus prior to entering the circulation (see discussion on immunity, hypersensitivity, allergy, and autoimmune diseases). Properties of blood cells are summarized in **TABLE 13-1**. In contrast to the relatively long survival of red cells, most white cells have a short

Granulocytes Collective name for neutrophils, eosinophils, and basophils.

Polymorphonuclear neutrophils (PMN) A leukocyte having a multilobed nucleus whose cytoplasm is filled with fine granules.

survival time within the circulation, varying from several hours to several days, and must be replenished continually. In contrast, lymphocytes that have not yet played a role in host defense (naïve lymphocytes) survive for one to three months, and lymphocytes that have been exposed to a foreign substance may survive for years as memory lymphocytes.

The proportions of the various leukocytes vary with the age of the individual. The most numerous in the adult are neutrophils, constituting about 70 percent of the total circulating white cells. Neutrophils are actively phagocytic and predominate in acute inflammatory reactions. Lymphocytes are the next most common type of white cells in adults and are the predominant leukocytes in the blood of children. The lymphocytes in the peripheral blood constitute only a small fraction of the total lymphocytes, most being located in the lymph nodes, spleen, and other lymphoid tissues. Lymphocytes continually recirculate from the bloodstream into lymphoid tissues. They leave the lymphoid tissue through the lymphatic channels and the thoracic duct, returning to the circulation and becoming reestablished for a time in a different site of lymphoid tissue. Lymphocytes take part in cell-mediated and humoral defense reactions.

Small numbers of eosinophils, basophils, and monocytes also are normally present in the blood. **Eosinophils** play a role in allergic reactions and in the defense against parasites. They increase in allergic diseases, in the presence of worm or other animal–parasite infections, and in a few other conditions. **Basophils** contain granules of histamine and an anticoagulant called **heparin**. **Monocytes** are actively phagocytic and are important in chronic inflammation and the response to certain types of chronic and viral infections. Monocytes are the circulating precursors of tissue macrophages, which play an important role in host defense in many body organs. A monocyte/macrophage–lymphocyte interaction is necessary in the initial phase of response to a foreign antigen; it also plays a role in the cell-mediated immune reaction.

Blood **platelets**, which are essential for normal blood coagulation, are much smaller than leukocytes. They represent pieces of the cytoplasm of megakaryocytes, large precursor cells present in the bone marrow. Platelets have a short survival time, comparable to that of most leukocytes.

Normal Hematopoiesis

The bone marrow replenishes the blood cells that are continually being worn out and removed from the circulation and responds to stressors such as infection, or in the case of red cells to bleeding or low oxygen levels, by increasing the number of cells released into the circulation. The rate of release of blood cells from the marrow is controlled by circulating hormonelike proteins (cytokines) that can stimulate blood cell production. Efficient production of blood cells requires a sufficient supply of the pluripotent stem cells. Lack of these cells results in bone marrow failure and decreased levels of all circulating blood cells (**pancytopenia**). Vitamins B_{12} and folic acid, which are required for DNA synthesis in the dividing and maturing red cell precursors, and iron, required for the synthesis of the heme portion of hemoglobin, are necessary for hematopoiesis. Extreme protein deficiency, which may be seen in malnourished children, can result in decreased levels of blood cell production.

Red cells develop from large precursor cells in the bone marrow that are called **proerythroblasts** (*pro* = *before* + *erythro* = red + *blast* = a primitive cell). As the red cell precursors mature, the cells go through different stages during which the nucleus shrinks and increasing amounts of hemoglobin are synthesized. Finally when about 80 percent of the hemoglobin has been synthesized, the red cells lose their nucleus, but retain their ability to produce proteins in the cytoplasm. At this stage,

---

Lymphocyte A mononuclear blood cell produced in lymphoid tissue that takes part in cell-mediated and humoral immunity.

Eosinophil A cell whose cytoplasm is filled with large, uniform granules that stain intensely red with acid dyes. See also *basophil*.

Basophil A cell that contains numerous variable-sized granules that stain intensely purple with basic dyes. See also *eosinophil*.

Heparin An anticoagulant obtained from the liver.

Monocyte A leukocyte having a kidney-shaped nucleus and light blue cytoplasm; a phagocytic cell that forms part of the reticuloendothelial system.

Platelet A component of the blood; a roughly circular or oval disk concerned with blood coagulation.

Pancytopenia Decrease in number of all circulating blood cells.

Proerythroblast Precursor cells in the bone marrow that give rise to red blood cells.

the **reticulocytes** leave the marrow and travel into the circulation, where they rapidly complete differentiation into mature red cells (erythrocytes), losing their ability to synthesize proteins. Reticulocytes may sometimes be detectable in circulation and are distinguished by the use of special stains that detect residual RNA and DNA and by being slightly larger and appearing more blue than a mature red cell. A high reticulocyte count is an indicator that the bone marrow is working particularly hard to produce cells; this might occur with severe blood loss.

Red cell production is regulated by the oxygen content of the arterial blood. A decreased oxygen supply to the tissues stimulates erythropoiesis synthesis by cells in the kidney, which elaborate a hormonelike erythrocyte-stimulating material called **erythropoietin**. For this reason, kidney disease may result in a low level of red cells being synthesized and reduced red cell levels in the blood, a condition termed **anemia**.

The red cell derives its energy only from the enzymatic breakdown of glucose using a process called anaerobic glycolysis, which does not use the oxygen being transported by the cells. Because the red cell lacks a nucleus, it cannot synthesize new enzyme molecules to replace those that gradually wear out. After about four months, the cell is no longer able to function. The worn-out red cell is then removed by the mononuclear phagocyte system, primarily in the spleen, and its **hemoglobin** is degraded. The globin chains are broken down, and their component amino acids are used to make other proteins. The iron is extracted and saved to make new hemoglobin. The porphyrin ring, however, cannot be salvaged. It is degraded and is excreted by the liver as bile pigment.

The factors regulating the production of white blood cells and their delivery into the circulation are complex. Infection, inflammation, and physiologic processes such as exercise and stress can increase the number of white cells in the blood either because of increased marrow synthesis or the release of preformed pools of cells stored in the marrow. A number of protein hormonelike cytokines and growth factors are responsible.

Structure and Function of Hemoglobin

Hemoglobin, the oxygen-carrying protein formed by the developing red cells, is composed of four separate protein subunits termed **globins**, which in turn fit together to form a four-chain molecule called a tetramer (*tetra* = four). Each subunit consists of two parts: the globin chain and a heme group. Heme is a complex nitrogen-containing ring structure (called a porphyrin ring) containing an iron atom. The heme and globin components that make up normal hemoglobin are synthesized separately within the erythroblast. The porphyrin ring is produced by the mitochondria. Then the iron, brought to the cell by an iron transport protein called transferrin, is inserted into the molecule (**FIGURE 13-2**).

Several types of globin chains, differing in their amino acid composition, are formed at varying times and in differing proportions in the embryo, the fetus, and the adult. The chains are designated by Greek letters—alpha (α), beta (β), gamma (γ), delta (δ), and epsilon (ε)—and come in pairs consisting of two identical alpha (α)-like chains and two identical beta (β)-like chains. In the normal adult, about 98 percent of hemoglobin is called hemoglobin A, in which two subunits of the tetramer contain alpha chains and two contain beta chains. The hemoglobin can also be designated by the shorthand notation $\alpha_2\beta_2$. (The chain is designated by the Greek letter and the number of subunits by the subscript.) The remaining 2 percent is called hemoglobin A_2, a tetramer composed of two alpha and two delta chains ($\alpha_2\delta_2$) in which delta chains substitute for beta chains.

Reticulocytes A young red blood cell identified by special staining techniques.

Erythropoietin A humoral substance made by the kidneys that regulates hematopoiesis.

Anemia A decrease in hemoglobin or red cells or both.

Hemoglobin An oxygen transport protein within red cells composed of an iron-porphyrin complex (heme) combined with a protein chain (globin).

Globins Protein with globin fold, a series of eight alpha helical segments. Part of hemoglobin.

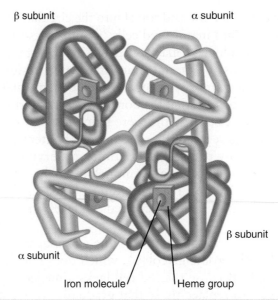

β subunit   α subunit

α subunit

β subunit

Iron molecule   Heme group

FIGURE 13-2 The hemoglobin molecule. The heme groups containing the porphyrin ring are shown as squares.

Fetal hemoglobin A type of hemoglobin containing two alpha and two gamma chains that is able to take up and release oxygen at much lower PO_2 (oxygen partial pressure) than in adult hemoglobin.

In the embryo and fetus, hemoglobin containing different globin chains is produced at various times in the course of prenatal development. Betalike epsilon chain production predominates in the embryo but is soon superseded in the fetus by production of alpha- and beta-like gamma globin chains. Beta chain production does not occur until relatively late in prenatal development. Consequently, the predominant hemoglobin in the fetus is a tetramer of alpha and gamma chains ($\alpha_2\gamma_2$) that is termed **fetal hemoglobin** (hemoglobin F). Fetal hemoglobin is able to take up and release oxygen more efficiently than adult hemoglobin when the oxygen partial pressure (PO_2) of the blood is low, as it is in the fetus as compared to adults. Late in pregnancy, fetal production of beta chains replaces gamma chains, and adult hemoglobin (hemoglobin A) begins to replace fetal hemoglobin in the red cells as the fetus prepares for life outside of the uterus.

The hemoglobin of a newborn infant contains 50 to 95 percent fetal hemoglobin, the rest being the adult type. Normally, no significant fetal hemoglobin synthesis occurs after birth. As new red cells are produced by the infant, the new "replacement" red cells contain essentially only hemoglobin A. Consequently, the concentration of hemoglobin A rises in the infant's blood as hemoglobin F falls. By about six months of age, the hemoglobin is almost entirely hemoglobin A.

OXYGEN TRANSPORT BY HEMOGLOBIN

The heme component gives hemoglobin the ability to reversibly combine with oxygen. For hemoglobin to transport and release oxygen effectively, the heme iron must be in the ferrous (Fe^{2+}) state, and its binding site must be available to pick up and release oxygen. In the lungs where the oxygen partial pressure is high, hemoglobin combines with oxygen to form oxyhemoglobin. In the tissues where oxygen partial pressure is much lower, the oxygen is released and reduced hemoglobin is formed. Two important conditions impair the ability of hemoglobin to transport oxygen: (1) oxidation of the heme iron to form a different type of hemoglobin called methemoglobin, and (2) attachment of carbon monoxide to the heme iron to form carboxyhemoglobin.

IRON METABOLISM AND HEMATOPOIESIS

The body contains about 4 g of iron, of which about 75 percent is contained in hemoglobin. Most of the rest is a reserve supply stored in the liver, bone marrow, and spleen, which is combined with an iron-binding protein called apoferritin, forming an iron–protein complex called ferritin. A small amount of iron also circulates in the blood bound to a protein called transferrin, which is the iron being transported from place to place in the body.

The usual diet of an adult contains from about 10 to 20 mg of iron, but men absorb merely 1 mg per day, and only slightly more iron is absorbed by women and children. Women need more iron to make up for menstrual losses because 1 ml of blood contains about 0.5 mg of iron. Additional iron is also required during pregnancy to supply the needs of the developing fetus. Children require greater amounts of iron to synthesize more hemoglobin during periods of growth when the blood volume is increasing. Because there is no mechanism for iron elimination other than menstruation in women and excessive iron is toxic, iron uptake, which occurs predominantly via the mucosal cells in the duodenum, is carefully regulated.

Hepcidin is a protein synthesized by the liver that blocks dietary iron uptake by the duodenal cells and interferes with the transport of iron to developing erythrocytes. In the case of sufficient iron stores, hepcidin levels are increased. Synthesis of hepcidin is decreased when iron stores are low. From the duodenal mucosa, the iron is transported by transferrin to the bone marrow for hemoglobin synthesis and to the liver and other storage sites where it is available for later use. **FIGURE 13-3** summarizes how iron is handled in the body.

As red cells wear out and are destroyed, the iron from the hemoglobin is recycled, transported by transferrin back to the bone marrow, and used to make new hemoglobin. If sufficient recycled iron is not available for hemoglobin synthesis, additional iron is mobilized from storage sites.

Hepcidin Protein synthesized by the liver that blocks dietary iron uptake; part of the control mechanism for iron metabolism.

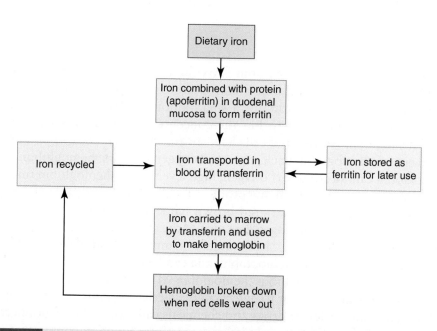

FIGURE 13-3 Iron uptake, transport, storage, and utilization for hemoglobin synthesis. Most of the iron used for hemoglobin synthesis is recycled from worn-out red cells. Chronic blood loss removes iron-containing cells from the circulation, and the iron contained in the red cells can no longer be recycled to make hemoglobin, which leads to iron deficiency anemia.

Iron Overload: Hemochromatosis

Because iron excretory pathways are lacking, any excess iron entering the body cannot be eliminated, causing an overload of iron, which accumulates in the body's tissues and organs. Eventually, the accumulation leads to organ damage, followed by scarring, leading to permanent derangement in the functions of the affected organs.

The usual cause of iron overload is a genetic disease called **hemochromatosis**, which is transmitted as an autosomal recessive trait. The gene occurs in about 10 percent of the white population, but the disease only occurs in homozygous carriers of the gene, who absorb an excessive amount of iron. The disease may result from mutations in several genes controlling iron metabolism, but classic type 1 hemochromatosis is by far the most common and most often results from mutations in a gene called *HFE*. Manifestations of the disease take years to develop as iron accumulates in the body and causes organ damage. Patients with untreated hemochromatosis often have rather typical manifestations of iron accumulation: tan to brown skin caused by iron accumulation in the skin; diabetes caused by damage to the insulin-producing cells of the pancreas; diffuse scarring of the liver (cirrhosis), which interferes with blood flow through the liver (discussed in abnormalities of the liver); and heart failure caused by heart muscle damage and associated scarring, resulting from the iron deposits.

Early recognition and treatment prevents progression of the disease and arrests organ damage. Treatment consists of repeated withdrawal of blood (phlebotomy) to remove iron, often combined with drugs that bind (chelate) iron to remove it from the body.

The excessive iron absorption and storage characteristic of hemochromatosis can be identified by the same type of laboratory tests used to measure iron storage and transport in subjects with iron deficiency anemia: serum ferritin, serum iron, and serum iron-binding capacity. When the body is overloaded with iron, serum ferritin is very high, reflecting the greatly increased iron stores that can be as much as 15–20 g or more instead of the normal amount of about 1 g. Serum iron is also much higher than normal, and the iron-binding protein transferrin is completely loaded (saturated) with iron. These tests all point to increased uptake and storage of iron.

> **Hemochromatosis**
> An autosomal recessive genetic disease characterized by excessive iron absorption, leading to accumulation of excessive amounts of iron in the body, causing organ damage.

METHEMOGLOBIN

If the iron in the heme of hemoglobin is oxidized from the normal ferrous (Fe^{2+}) to the ferric (Fe^{3+}), the hemoglobin is converted to methemoglobin and is no longer able to carry oxygen. Normally, a small amount of hemoglobin is oxidized to methemoglobin continuously, but the concentration is less than 1 percent of the total hemoglobin because red cells have an enzyme (*methemoglobin reductase*) that converts methemoglobin back to normal oxygen-carrying hemoglobin. Because methemoglobin cannot transport oxygen, high levels of methemoglobin (methemoglobinemia) are associated with symptoms related to ischemia (lack of oxygen to tissue). Methemoglobin has a dark red-brown "chocolate" color. A 15 to 20 percent concentration in the blood changes the color of the skin. Higher levels will result in headache, confusion, delirium, cardiovascular symptoms, and ultimately (at levels above 70 percent) death. Methemoglobinemia can be caused by hereditary diseases that result in a type of hemoglobin (hemoglobin M) particularly susceptible to the formation of methemoglobin or to defects in the methemoglobin reductase enzyme. Unfortunately, many different drugs and chemicals can oxidize hemoglobin to methemoglobin, including nitrates and nitrites (sometimes found in contaminated well water), some frequently used local anesthetics such as benzocaine contained in topical anesthetics, and several nonprescription drug products. The preferred treatment of severe methemoglobinemia is methylene blue given intravenously. The compound increases the activity of the red cell methemoglobin reductase enzyme, which speeds the conversion of methemoglobin (Fe^{3+}) back to normal hemoglobin (Fe^{2+}), thereby restoring the oxygen-carrying capacity of the blood to normal.

CARBOXYHEMOGLOBIN

In the presence of adequate oxygen, carbon compounds are converted to carbon dioxide and water by combustion. However, incomplete combustion forms carbon monoxide, which is a potentially hazardous compound because it has more than 200 times the ability of oxygen to combine with hemoglobin. Consequently, carbon monoxide combines preferentially with hemoglobin to form carboxyhemoglobin, which blocks the ability of the hemoglobin to transport oxygen. Exposure of even a low concentration of carbon monoxide for a long time is harmful and may be fatal as progressively larger quantities of hemoglobin are converted to carboxyhemoglobin. If a person exposed to a sublethal concentration of carbon monoxide is removed from the source of the exposure, the carbon monoxide dissociates slowly from its combination with hemoglobin and the oxygen-carrying capacity of the blood slowly returns to normal.

Manifestations of exposure to carbon monoxide depend on the concentration to which the person has been exposed. A concentration of 3 percent or higher in a nonsmoker, and 10 percent or more in smokers (who have a higher concentration caused by the carbon monoxide in cigarette smoke), indicate significant exposure. A high concentration of carboxyhemoglobin in the blood may lead to serious long-term cardiovascular and neurologic problems resulting from the exposure and, if exposure is acute and not corrected, death. An affected person should be removed from the source of exposure and given a high concentration of oxygen by mask to help replace the carbon monoxide with oxygen.

It is easier to prevent carbon monoxide poisoning than to treat it. Many communities now require carbon monoxide detectors in private homes to call attention to any undetected malfunction of the home heating system. Indoor kerosene heaters or open poorly vented fires used as heat sources present a continuing problem, as do auto exhaust fumes in nonventilated spaces. Both types of exposure not uncommonly result in accidental deaths.

Anemia

Anemia, literally "without blood," refers to a decrease in red cell number or to subnormal hemoglobin levels in circulating red cells. Anemia is classified either by etiology (factor causing anemia) or by morphology (the size and appearance of the red blood cells determined by microscopic examination of a stained blood smear and automated blood analyzers).

ETIOLOGIC CLASSIFICATION OF ANEMIA

Anemia can be classified as being caused either by inadequate production of red cells or by an excessive loss or destruction of cells. Inadequate production may result from an insufficiency of stem cells or other factors (such as iron and vitamins) required for red cell maturation. Examples of the former would be genetic defects in stem cells, marrow damage, or replacement of marrow by abnormal cells. Excessive loss of red cells may be caused either by external blood loss or by accelerated destruction of the cells (and hence shortened survival) in the circulation. **TABLE 13-2** presents a classification of the various causes of anemia.

TABLE 13-2 Etiologic Classification of Anemia
Inadequate production of red cells
Caused by inadequate "raw materials"
Iron deficiency
Vitamin B$_{12}$ deficiency
Folic acid deficiency
Caused by impaired function of bone marrow factory
Anemia of chronic disease
Bone marrow damaged or destroyed (aplastic anemia)
Bone marrow replaced by foreign or abnormal cells (bone marrow replacement anemia)
Excessive loss of red cells
Caused by external blood loss (hemorrhage)
Caused by shortened survival of red cells in the circulation
Defective red cells (hereditary hemolytic anemia)
Abnormal red cell shape
Abnormal hemoglobin within red cells
Defective hemoglobin synthesis within red cells
Deficient red cell enzymes
"Hostile environment"
Anti-red cell antibodies
Mechanical trauma to circulating red cells

Normocytic/macrocytic/microcytic Classification of anemia by red cell size, normal, increased, or decreased.

Hypochromic Pale red cell color due to reduced hemoglobin content.

Anemias may be **normocytic**, **macrocytic**, or **microcytic**; that is, characterized by red cells that are normal, increased, or decreased in size. If microcytic cells also have a reduced hemoglobin content, they appear pale and the term **hypochromic** microcytic anemia is used. The appearance of the cells provides a clue to the etiology. Iron deficiency anemia is a hypochromic microcytic anemia. Anemia caused by vitamin B$_{12}$ or folic acid deficiency is a macrocytic anemia. Most other types of anemia are normocytic. Changes in cell shape may also offer clues to the nature of the anemia.

IRON DEFICIENCY ANEMIA

Iron deficiency anemia is the most common anemia worldwide and is frequently encountered in clinical practice, most commonly in children, women of child-bearing age, and in cases of chronic blood loss. Iron deficiency anemia may result from either insufficient intake or failure of absorption of iron from the diet, hemorrhage, or chronic blood loss (sometimes associated with undiagnosed cancer of the gastrointestinal or genitourinary tract).

Iron deficiency caused by inadequate dietary intake may occur in infants during periods of rapid growth. A normal, full-term infant has a reserve supply of iron that was transferred to the fetus from the mother during the last part of pregnancy. Consequently, the newborn infant generally has an adequate short-term supply of iron available for hematopoiesis during the neonatal period when the production of red cells accelerates to supply the needs of an increasing blood volume. A premature infant, however, may not get its full component of iron stores and may not have enough reserve to supply its postnatal needs. Even in full-term infants, the reserve supply of iron for hematopoiesis is limited and must be supplemented by iron from the diet. Breast milk contains very little iron, although the amount available is well absorbed. If the diet is not supplemented by cereals, fruits, vegetables, other foods containing iron, or some type of iron supplement, iron stores will become rapidly exhausted, and iron deficiency anemia will develop in the first year of life. For this reason, many physicians gradually add supplementary foods containing additional sources of iron to infants' diets. Adolescents and pregnant or lactating females also have an increased requirement for iron, and individuals subsisting on an inadequate or poorly balanced diet may develop iron deficiency anemia.

Most cases of iron deficiency anemia in adults in industrialized countries result from a failure to recapture the iron present in red cells for hemoglobin synthesis as a result of chronic blood loss. The iron contained in red cells that are lost from the circulation by bleeding is no longer available to the body for the production of new red cells. Because each milliliter of blood contains 0.5 mg of iron, a loss of 500 ml of blood represents a loss of 250 mg of iron, equivalent to one-fourth of the body's entire iron reserves. Unless dietary intake of iron is extremely liberal, iron stores soon become exhausted and iron deficiency anemia develops.

Iron deficiency anemia is a hypochromic microcytic anemia (**FIGURE 13-4**). The cells are pale because they contain less hemoglobin than normal. The cells are also

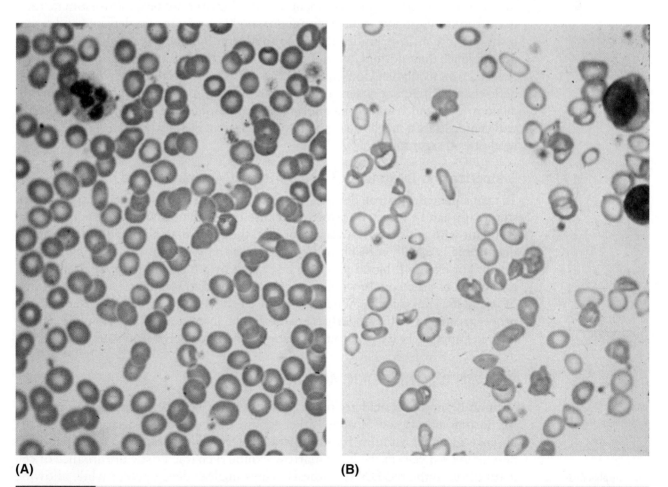

(A) **(B)**

FIGURE 13-4 **(A)** Normal red cells. **(B)** Cells showing hypochromic microcytic anemia caused by chronic iron deficiency (original magnification ×400).

Courtesy of Leonard V. Crowley, MD, Century College.

abnormally small because the body apparently attempts to "scale down" the size of the cell to conform to the reduced hemoglobin content.

ANEMIA OF CHRONIC DISEASE

Persons who suffer from chronic inflammatory conditions such as ongoing microbial infections, immune diseases and certain malignant neoplasms may develop an anemia which, if severe, is hypochromic and microcytic in nature. Chronic inflammation results in the production of cytokines (such as IL-6) which result in the liver synthesizing increased hepcidin. As noted above, hepcidin blocks uptake of iron from dietary sources but also interferes with the transport of iron from body stores to the developing red cell resulting in a disease which is similar to that seen in iron deficiency anemia.

Laboratory Tests to Evaluate Iron Metabolism in Iron Deficiency Anemia

Laboratory tests that measure iron stores, iron transport, and iron metabolism can be used as diagnostic tests in patients with suspected iron deficiency anemia. These include measurements of serum ferritin, serum iron, and total serum iron-binding capacity.

A very small amount of ferritin (about 100 µg per liter) is normally present in blood serum, in an amount proportional to the total amount of ferritin stored in the body. Consequently, measurement of serum ferritin can be used to estimate total body iron stores. In iron deficiency anemia, body iron stores are depleted and serum ferritin is low, as is serum iron, but the total iron-binding capacity in the serum is much higher than normal, apparently reflecting the body's attempt to capture the reduced iron available. Consequently, the characteristic laboratory profile of iron deficiency anemia is low serum ferritin and serum iron. Although the serum will demonstrate a much higher than normal serum iron-binding capacity, the transferrin will demonstrate a much lower than normal percentage of iron bound to it (a lower level of iron saturation).

Evaluation and Treatment of Iron Deficiency Anemia

To treat a patient with iron deficiency anemia, the cause of the anemia must be known so therapy can be directed toward the cause rather than toward the symptoms. In an infant with a history of a very poor diet, the cause may be obvious. In an adult, the anemia is usually a result of blood loss, so the source of the bleeding must be found. For example, blood loss may be caused by a bleeding ulcer or an ulcerated carcinoma of the colon. In women, excessive menstrual bleeding is a common cause of iron deficiency anemia. When the cause of the blood loss has been determined, proper treatment of the underlying cause can be instituted. In addition, the patient is given supplementary iron to replenish the body's depleted iron stores.

VITAMIN B$_{12}$ AND FOLIC ACID DEFICIENCY

Vitamin B$_{12}$ and folic acid are required not only for normal hematopoiesis but also for normal maturation of many other types of bone marrow derived cells. In the absence of either vitamin B$_{12}$ or folic acid, DNA synthesis is impaired, and the developing red cells in the bone marrow exhibit a characteristic disturbance of cell maturation. Impaired DNA synthesis delays nuclear development while allowing for normal cytoplasmic development, resulting in large abnormal cells that do not survive normally in the circulation. The developing red cells, which are larger than normal, are called **megaloblasts** (*megalos* = large). The abnormal red cell maturation is

Megaloblast An abnormal red cell precursor resulting from vitamin B$_{12}$ or folic acid deficiency.

called megaloblastic erythropoiesis. The mature red cells derived from the abnormal maturation also are larger than normal, vary in size, and some may have an oval shape. Therefore, the anemia is classified morphologically as a macrocytic anemia. The development of white cell precursors and megakaryocytes is also abnormal. Consequently, patients with megaloblastic anemia usually also have **leukopenia** (low white cell count) and **thrombocytopenia** (low platelet count) as well as a macrocytic anemia. Vitamin B_{12}, but not folic acid, is also required to maintain the structural and functional integrity of the nervous system (although by a mechanism not believed to involve DNA synthesis); thus, a deficiency of this vitamin also may be associated with pronounced neurologic disturbances. Vitamin B_{12} is found in meat, milk, liver, and other foods rich in animal protein, but not in vegetable products. Strict vegetarians who do not eat meat or dairy products must rely on vitamin B_{12}-fortified cereals or other nonprotein vitamin B_{12}-fortified foods as their source of the vitamin. However, normal body stores of vitamin B_{12} take years to be depleted. The sudden convert to a vegan diet will not develop vitamin B_{12} deficiency rapidly (if at all). Folic acid is widely distributed in nature, being found in abundance in green leafy vegetables as well as in many foods of animal origin.

Anemia as a Result of Folic Acid Deficiency

The body has very limited stores of folic acid, which rapidly become depleted if not replenished continually. Deficiency caused by inadequate dietary intake is found in people subsisting on inadequate diets and is encountered frequently in chronic alcoholics because of their typically deficient diet and, possibly, impaired absorption of folic acid compared with nondrinkers. People with chronic intestinal diseases may become folic acid deficient because of an impaired ability to absorb the vitamin. Pregnant and lactating women also are at risk because pregnancy greatly increases folic acid requirements. Folic acid deficiency anemia in pregnancy is uncommon because physicians routinely prescribe folic acid supplements to pregnant women. Several drugs including methotrexate (an antimetabolite used in the treatment of cancer and rheumatoid arthritis) and the antiepileptic agent phenytoin can interfere with the action of folic acid.

Anemia as a Result of Vitamin B_{12} Deficiency/Pernicious Anemia

Efficient absorption of vitamin B_{12} ingested in food requires a protein called intrinsic factor, secreted by gastric mucosal cells along with hydrochloric acid and digestive enzymes. After the intrinsic factor combines with the vitamin B_{12}, the B_{12}–intrinsic-factor complex is absorbed from the distal small intestine. The absorbed vitamin is stored in the liver and made available to the bone marrow and other tissues as required for cell growth and maturation.

A common cause of vitamin B_{12} deficiency is **pernicious anemia,** in which atrophy of the gastric mucosa is often associated with autoantibodies directed against gastric mucosal cells and intrinsic factor. The atrophic mucosa fails to secrete intrinsic factor, acid, and digestive enzymes, and consequently, vitamin B_{12} is not absorbed. The vitamin B_{12} deficiency causes impaired hematopoiesis as well as various neurologic disturbances.

Pernicious anemia is not the only cause of vitamin B_{12} deficiency. People who have had most of their stomach surgically removed because of ulcer or gastric cancer or who have had a gastric bypass procedure to control obesity may not be able to secrete enough intrinsic factor. People who have had a small bowel resection of the distal ilium, where the vitamin B_{12}–intrinsic factor complex is absorbed, may not be able to absorb enough vitamin to supply their needs. Similarly, an individual with chronic intestinal disease affecting the vitamin B_{12}–absorbing area (such as Crohn

Leukopenia An abnormally small number of leukocytes in the peripheral blood.

Thrombocytopenia A deficiency of platelets.

Pernicious anemia A macrocytic anemia caused by inability to absorb vitamin B_{12} as a result of inadequate secretion of intrinsic factor by gastric mucosa.

disease, which frequently involves the terminal ileum, described in the discussion on the gastrointestinal tract) also may be unable to absorb the vitamin adequately.

Pernicious anemia and other vitamin B_{12} deficiencies are treated with intramuscular administration of vitamin B_{12}. Parenteral administration avoids the problem of poor absorption of the vitamin although very high oral doses may also be effective.

Suppression of Bone Marrow Stem Cell Function/Aplastic Anemia

Many conditions can depress bone marrow function including chronic infection or suppression of marrow stem cells. As noted previously, chronic diseases may impair hematopoiesis and lead to mild or moderate anemia (the anemia of chronic disease). White blood cell and platelet production are usually not disturbed.

The anemia of chronic disease usually causes only a relatively mild suppression of bone marrow function and improves when the disease that caused it is identified and treated. In contrast to the anemia of chronic disease, much more serious and sometimes irreversible damage to the bone marrow results from destruction of the bone marrow stem cell precursors of mature blood cells and platelets. This type of anemia is called **aplastic anemia** (*a* = without + *plasia* = growth), although this term is not strictly accurate because the stem cell damage leads to leukopenia and thrombocytopenia as well as anemia. The anemia is classified as a normocytic anemia because the red cells are normal in size and shape although inadequate in number. Many agents can cause aplastic anemia. Radiation, anticancer chemotherapy drugs, and various toxic chemicals (benzene being a prime example) may cause severe marrow damage. Other drugs, including some antibiotics, anti-inflammatory drugs, and anticonvulsant drugs, may damage marrow stem cells in susceptible individuals. In many cases, however, it is the body's own immune system that is responsible for the aplastic anemia, a manifestation of an autoimmune disease in which the body's own cytotoxic T lymphocytes attack and destroy the marrow stem cells. A type of viral disease (parvovirus B19 infection) results in pure red cell aplasia in which only red cell precursors are affected.

Aplastic anemia is treated initially by blood and platelet transfusions to maintain an adequate volume of circulating blood cells while the cause of the bone marrow failure is being investigated. If the marrow damage is caused by a toxic drug or chemical and is not too severe, marrow function may recover; however, in severe aplastic anemia other methods of treatment are required to restore marrow function. Many patients respond to immunosuppressive agents that act against the destructive (cytotoxic) T lymphocytes responsible for stem cell destruction.

Hematopoietic stem cell transplantation using bone marrow, cord blood, or stem cells isolated from the circulation may be required (see discussion of neoplastic disease therapy).

> **Aplastic anemia** Lack of mature blood cells and platelets caused by stem cell damage.

ACUTE BLOOD LOSS

A normocytic anemia may result from an episode of acute blood loss, as from a massive hemorrhage from the uterus or gastrointestinal tract. Provided that iron stores are adequate, the lost blood is rapidly replaced by the bone marrow, and the newly formed red cells are normal. This is in contrast with the anemia of chronic blood loss, in which the red cells are hypochromic and microcytic because prolonged bleeding has depleted the body's iron stores.

ACCELERATED BLOOD DESTRUCTION

Normal red cells survive for about four months, but their survival can be considerably shortened if the regenerative capacity of the marrow is not sufficient to keep up with the accelerated destruction. This type of anemia is called hemolytic anemia and may be a result of either an intrinsic defect in red cells or an extrinsic condition that shortens the circulating life of the red cells. Hemolytic anemias caused by an inherited defect in red cell structure are called hereditary hemolytic anemias. Those resulting from damage to normal red cells by antibodies or other injurious agents are called acquired hemolytic anemias.

HEREDITARY HEMOLYTIC ANEMIAS

The genetically determined abnormalities of red cells that may shorten their survival fall into four major groups: abnormally shaped cells, abnormal hemoglobins, defective hemoglobin synthesis, or enzyme deficiencies (**TABLE 13-3**).

Shape Abnormalities

The most common abnormality of red cell shape in Caucasians is **hereditary spherocytosis**, which has two distinct genetic forms: a dominant or a recessive inherited pattern of inheritance. In hereditary spherocytosis, the structural framework (cytoskeleton) of the red cell membrane is defective and not properly linked to the lipid membrane of the cell; this reduces the cell's stability and flexibility. New red cells produced by the bone marrow and released into the circulation have a normal biconcave disk configuration, but bits of their unstable cell membranes become detached from the cells as they squeeze through extremely small capillaries in the spleen during their travel through the bloodstream, progressively reducing the surface area of the red cell membranes. The red cells adapt to their reduced surface area relative to their cell volume by gradually changing from biconcave disks to spherical cells, which is the only way the smaller cell membrane can surround the comparatively

Hereditary spherocytosis Cause of abnormally shaped red cells, either spherical or elliptical.

TABLE 13-3	Inheritance and Manifestations of Some Hereditary Hemolytic Anemias		
Anemia	**Inheritance**	**Characteristics of red cells**	**Manifestations**
Hereditary spherocytosis	Dominant or recessive	Spherocytic	Mild-to-moderate chronic hemolytic anemia
Hereditary ovalocytosis	Dominant	Oval	Usually asymptomatic; may have mild anemia
Sickle cell anemia	Codominant	Normocytic; cells sickle under reduced oxygen tension	Marked anemia
Hemoglobin C disease	Codominant	Normocytic	Mild-to-moderate anemia
Sickle cell hemoglobin C disease	Codominant	Normocytic; cells sickle under reduced oxygen tension	Moderate anemia
Thalassemia minor	Dominant (heterozygous)	Hypochromic microcytic; total number of red cells usually increased	Mild anemia
Thalassemia major	Dominant (homozygous)	Hypochromic microcytic	Severe anemia; usually fatal in childhood
Glucose-6-phosphate dehydrogenase deficiency	X-linked recessive	Normocytic; enzyme-deficient cells	Episodes of acute hemolytic anemia precipitated by drugs or infections

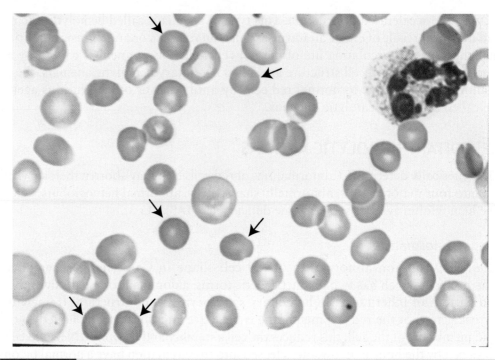

FIGURE 13-5 A stained blood film from a person with hereditary spherocytosis. The many small dark cells with little or no central pallor are spherocytes (*arrows*). The larger, more normal-appearing red cells are young red cells that have the same cell membrane defect but have not been circulating long enough to acquire a spherical shape. The relative large, faintly blue-staining red cell in the center of the field is a reticulocyte.

large volume of the red cell (**FIGURE 13-5**). Unfortunately, the spherical shape puts the red cells at a disadvantage that greatly shortens their survival in the bloodstream. As blood flows through the spleen, normal, flexible disk-shaped red cells can "work their way" through the splenic pulp and into the thin-walled veins (sinusoids) that carry the blood out of the spleen, but spherocytes are not thin enough or flexible enough to get through the spleen. They become trapped in the spleen and are destroyed by the phagocytic cells in the splenic pulp. The bone marrow increases red cell production to compensate for the shortened survival of the spherocytes, resulting in chronic hemolytic anemia. Splenectomy cures the anemia by removing the main site of red cell destruction, but it has no effect on the basic red cell defect.

A somewhat similar condition, which is also transmitted as an inherited dominant trait, is called **hereditary elliptocytosis**. As the name indicates, the red cells are oval rather than round. Most affected individuals are not inconvenienced by the abnormality, but some have a mild hemolytic anemia that can be cured by splenectomy.

Abnormal Hemoglobins/Sickle Cell Disease

If a gene coding for the globin chain gene is abnormal, the amino acids forming the globin chains will be altered, leading to the formation of an abnormal hemoglobin. Genes directing the synthesis of the various types of hemoglobin are codominant. If an abnormal gene is present, the abnormal hemoglobin appears in the red cells. Many different abnormal hemoglobins can be identified and characterized by various laboratory tests. Some of the structurally abnormal hemoglobins function normally, but others have unusual properties that impair their function.

Hemoglobin S (**sickle hemoglobin**) is one of the more important abnormal hemoglobins. Its formation results from a change in a single amino acid in the beta chain of hemoglobin. When the oxygen tension of the blood falls, as in venous blood, the hemoglobin S molecules aggregate and form rigid fibers, a process somewhat like

Hereditary elliptocytosis Cause of abnormally shaped red cells, either spherical or elliptical.

Sickle hemoglobin Abnormal hemoglobin causing red cells to change shape.

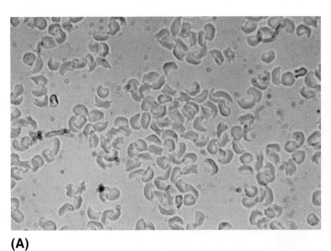
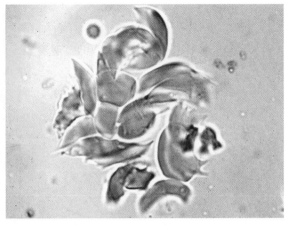

(A)　　　　　　　　　　　　　　　　**(B)**

FIGURE 13-6 Distortion of red cells containing sickle hemoglobin when incubated under reduced oxygen tension. **(A)** Overview of cells under low magnification (×100). **(B)** Higher magnification view of red cell distortion caused by sickle hemoglobin.
Courtesy of Leonard V. Crowley, MD, Century College.

crystallization (**FIGURE 13-6**). This leads to a shape change in the circulating red cells termed *sickling*, which describes their sickled (comma shaped) appearance. The "crystallization" is largely reversible, and the hemoglobin becomes soluble again when the oxygen tension rises as the blood is oxygenated in the lungs. The hemoglobin S gene is common in parts of the world where falciparum malaria is (or was) common because heterozygous carriers of the gene are relatively resistant to this disease. This includes people of African and also Middle Eastern and Indian origin. In Europe the gene is found in populations living around the Mediterranean region (**FIGURE 13-7**). Ten percent of the American black population are heterozygous carriers of the sickle cell gene and have **sickle cell trait**. Their erythrocytes contain both hemoglobin S and hemoglobin A. People with the sickle cell trait usually do not experience any problems related to the sickle hemoglobin in their red cells unless they engage in high-intensity physical activity or spend time at high altitude. In these cases, the oxygen content of their blood falls to a very low level, which may lead to a shape change (sickling) of their cells. Severe dehydration also may further sickling, and sickling may lead to sudden death if clumps of sickled red cells plug coronary arteries. Although these incidents are uncommon, they do occur. Screening for the sickle cell trait is suggested prior to many high-stress athletic and other activities for individuals who do not know their sickle cell status. However, it is important to remember that carriers of the trait do *not* have sickle cell disease and are very unlikely to suffer ill effects from their carrier status. They may, however, transmit the gene to their offspring who, with two carrier parents, have a 25 percent chance of developing sickle cell anemia.

The homozygous state, **sickle cell anemia**, is a serious disease. The cells of affected individuals contain no hemoglobin A, and they become sickled within the capillaries where the oxygen partial pressure is lower than in arterial blood. The clumps of sickled red cells plug blood vessels, obstruct blood flow, and cause progressive damage to the heart, kidneys, spleen, and other organs due to impaired circulation. Anemia develops because the cells containing sickle hemoglobin have a shortened survival time in the circulation. Consequently, the bone marrow must greatly increase its production of red cells (demonstrated by an elevated peripheral blood reticulocyte count) to compensate for the shortened red cell survival.

Newborn infants with sickle cell anemia do not have problems initially because their red cells also contain a large amount of fetal hemoglobin. This fetal hemoglobin

Sickle cell trait/sickle cell anemia Condition in individuals heterozygous for the sickle hemoglobin gene.

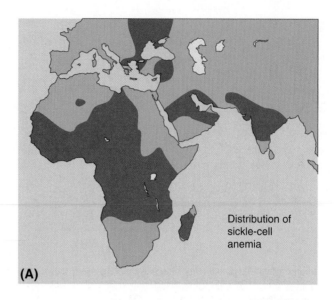

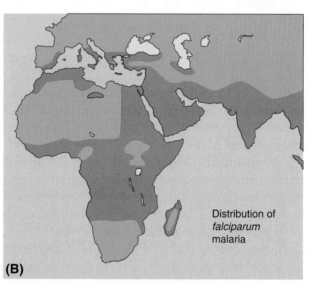

FIGURE 13-7 **(A)** Geographic distribution of sickle cell anemia. **(B)** *Falciparum* malaria in the 1920s before extensive malaria control programs were launched.

Vaso-occlusive crisis
Serious consequence
of sickle cell anemia
characterized by severe
pain when blood vessels
are blocked by sickled cells.

"dilutes" the concentration of sickle hemoglobin in the red cells, allowing these cells to function more like the red cells of a person with sickle cell trait. Symptoms usually do not appear until the infant is about six months old, when the red cells containing both fetal and sickle hemoglobin have been replaced by red cells containing almost entirely sickle hemoglobin.

A serious consequence of sickle cell disease is the occurrence of a **vaso-occlusive crisis**. Such episodes occur periodically in about half of patients and are characterized by severe and debilitating pain that may occur in many different areas, including the bones and abdomen. Vaso-occlusive crises may lead to infarction and damage to many organs, including the liver, kidney, and spleen. Eventual destruction of the spleen is associated with serious bacterial infections. There are many triggers for such episodes, including low oxygenation of the blood and changes in body core temperature (related to fever or environmental heat or cold). Even outside of crisis, individuals often suffer from chronic bone and joint pain. Anemia is always present but is generally compensated although individuals may lack stamina. An aplastic crisis may occur as a result of Parvovirus B19 infection. Splenic sequestration can result in life-threatening anemia in which the spleen becomes enlarged rapidly and blood cell count drops rapidly. There are many other serious and potentially life-threatening effects of the disease, including central nervous system involvement and stroke, which may affect as many as 30 percent of children.

Although there is no cure for sickle cell anemia, advances in treatment have improved survival, and many affected persons now live forty to fifty years. Affected individuals are quite susceptible to infections and should receive pneumococcal vaccine and other immunizing agents to reduce their infection risk. Because the hyperactive bone marrow requires abundant folic acid to promote red cell production, folic acid supplements are recommended to assure that supplies are adequate. Drugs such as hydroxyurea can be given to stimulate the bone marrow to produce fetal hemoglobin, which lowers the concentration of sickle hemoglobin in the red cells and thereby reduces the severity of the disease manifestations. The patient may also receive erythropoietin along with drugs to stimulate fetal hemoglobin production. Hematopoietic stem cell transplantation can result in a cure for sickle cell disease. The procedure has a high success rate (over 80 percent) and a mortality rate of 6 percent or less in selected patients. However, the pool of sickle cell disease patients for whom the risk/benefit ratio is favorable is very small (5 percent) as the prospective candidate must have full siblings who have identical **histocompatibility (HLA)** types to minimize the chances of rejection and potentially fatal side effects from the transplant (**graft versus host disease**). To be eligible, the patient must also have severe disease and be under fifteen years of age.

Simple, readily available tests can detect sickle cell trait in affected individuals, and genetic counseling is recommended for couples who are at risk of having a child with sickle cell anemia. DNA analysis of fetal cells can determine whether the fetus carries the sickle cell gene and, if present, whether the fetus is homozygous or heterozygous for the gene. Screening for sickle cell trait is mandatory in newborns in the United States.

Another common abnormal hemoglobin, called hemoglobin C, also is found predominantly in blacks. Heterozygous individuals, whose cells contain both hemoglobin A and hemoglobin C, are normal clinically. People homozygous for the hemoglobin C gene have a mild hemolytic anemia.

Some people possess genes for two abnormal hemoglobins. This may occur, for example, if one parent carries the hemoglobin S gene and the other carries the hemoglobin C gene, and each parent transmits the abnormal gene. In this case, the red cells of the affected person contain both abnormal hemoglobins in approximately equal amounts, and a hemolytic anemia results.

Defective Hemoglobin Synthesis/Thalassemia

Thalassemias are inherited anemias in which reduced amounts of otherwise normal hemoglobin chains are synthesized. This genetically determined condition is transmitted as a Mendelian-dominant trait although heterozygous carriers are only mildly affected and may be asymptomatic (hence, some authorities consider the disease to be recessive!). The defective synthesis may be of either the alpha chains (alpha thalassemia) or the beta chains (beta thalassemia). The frequency of the two forms of thalassemia differs greatly in different populations. Beta thalassemia is relatively common in people of Greek and Italian ancestry. (The term *thalassemia* comes from the Greek word *thalassa*, meaning sea, and derives from the high incidence of the condition in people who live in regions surrounding the Mediterranean.) Alpha thalassemia is considered to be the most common single gene defect in the world. Either silent carriers or mildly affected individuals are common among individuals of

Histocompatibility (HLA) Genetic locus controlling self-recognition.

Graft versus host disease Condition where a graft of immunologically active cells mounts a response to the host.

African descent. (There is about a 15 percent rate of silent carriers among American blacks although severe disease is rare.) Alpha thalassemia is also common in Southeast Asian (and less frequently in Mediterranean) populations, where it occurs in a more severe or even lethal form. Both thalassemias provide some degree of protection from malaria in the heterozygous state, which explains the distribution of the disease (similar to that of sickle cell anemia).

In beta thalassemia, the production of beta chains is reduced; however, alpha chain production is not, so the synthesis of the two types of chains is unbalanced. An excess of alpha chains accumulates and precipitates within the red cells, which shortens their survival. Because hemoglobin synthesis is reduced, the red cells appear hypochromic and microcytic, somewhat like the appearance of the cells in iron deficiency anemia. In thalassemia, however, the hypochromia is the result of deficient hemoglobin production because of inadequate beta chain synthesis rather than deficient production caused by iron deficiency. Usually, the cells also contain an increased amount of hemoglobin A_2, which does not contain beta chains, to compensate in part for the reduced synthesis of hemoglobin A. The level of residual fetal hemoglobin (having a gamma rather than a beta chain) varies from patient to patient, and those with high levels of fetal hemoglobin have milder disease.

If a person is heterozygous for beta thalassemia, the anemia is mild and the condition is called thalassemia minor. The red cells are hypochromic and microcytic, but there is no additional morbidity or mortality associated with the disease. The homozygous condition, which is called beta thalassemia major, occurs if both parents have thalassemia minor and each transmits the abnormal gene. The affected individual has a severe chronic hemolytic anemia associated with excess compensatory erythropoiesis sometimes outside of the marrow (extramedullary hematopoiesis). Iron overload related to both excess absorption and required transfusion therapy leads to iron deposition in tissues and associated liver disease. Chelation therapy to remove excess iron is critical, and splenectomy may be helpful.

The inheritance of alpha thalassemia is more complex because two functional alpha chain genes are present in tandem on the normal chromosome. A normal individual has four (rather than two) alpha chain genes. Silent alpha thalassemia results when a single alpha chain gene on one chromosome is deleted (or defective), leaving three functioning genes. This condition is asymptomatic and very difficult to diagnosis. Alpha thalassemia trait results when there is loss of two alpha chain genes (and two functional chains remain). This can occur in two forms. Both genes may be lost from a single chromosome (a cis configuration), or one gene may be defective on each chromosome (a trans configuration). In either case, the clinical condition is the same. There is a mild microcytic anemia and a somewhat elevated red blood cell count, but patients are clinically normal. However, a mating between two people having the cis configuration can result in offspring with no functional alpha chain genes, a condition termed homozygous alpha thalassemia (also called **hydrops fetalis** and alpha thalassemia major). Hydrops fetalis patients die at birth or soon after from heart failure and have a very enlarged liver related to severe anemia. Most of their hemoglobin is called hemoglobin Bart's and consists of four gamma chains. This form of hemoglobin does not efficiently deliver oxygen to tissues. Hemoglobin H disease results when there is a single functioning alpha chain gene, and it is named for the presence of the four-beta-chain-containing hemoglobin seen in such patients. Disease symptoms range from very mild in some patients to those who have severe microcytic and hemolytic anemia and require repeated transfusions. Iron overload from repeated hemolysis and therapeutic transfusions may occur with increasing age.

Hydrops fetalis Fatal condition occurring in a fetus with no functional hemoglobin alpha chain genes.

Red Cell Enzyme Deficiencies

Red cells derive energy by metabolizing glucose in a series of chemical reactions catalyzed by various enzyme systems. These same energy-producing reactions also indirectly help prevent oxidation of the hemoglobin, thereby protecting the hemoglobin from the potentially harmful effects of oxidizing drugs or other agents that can damage it. This protective function is compromised if certain red cell enzymes are deficient. Under such circumstances, exposing the red cells to an oxidizing agent causes denaturation and precipitation of the protein chains of hemoglobin, as well as the cell-membrane proteins.

One of the most common red cell enzyme defects is a deficiency of an enzyme called glucose-6-phosphate dehydrogenase. In this condition, which is transmitted as an X-linked recessive trait, the enzyme is unstable and does not function normally. (X-linked inheritance is considered in the discussion on chromosomes, genes, and cell division.) About 10 percent of black men are affected, and 30 percent of black women carry the abnormal gene on one of their X chromosomes. The abnormal gene occurs with high frequency in some white populations as well and is more common in areas with endemic malaria because (as is the case with sickle cell trait and thalassemia) the mutation offers some protection against malaria. The enzyme-deficient cells are highly susceptible to injury by drugs that do not affect normal red cells and to various bacterial and viral infections. More than forty drugs are known to induce an acute hemolytic anemia in susceptible individuals, including such commonly used drugs as sulfonamides, aspirin, some diuretics, some antibiotics, and some vitamins. The disease is also called **favism** because ingestion of fava beans (common in the Mediterranean and Middle Eastern diet) results in hemolysis in affected individuals. Hemolysis begins soon after exposure to the drug or infectious agent and continues for about a week. Considerable red cell destruction results, followed by red cell regeneration and return of red cell levels to normal in about four or five weeks.

Because the mutant gene is carried on the X chromosome, affected males do not produce any normal enzyme, and all of their red cells are subject to hemolysis. Females who carry the mutant gene on one of their X chromosomes are also at risk of drug-induced hemolysis. However, because of random inactivation of one of the X chromosomes in the female (as described in the discussion on chromosomes, genes, and cell division), the normal red cells and enzyme-deficient red cells are present in approximately equal proportions, which results in less intense hemolysis.

Favism Condition in which ingestion of fava beans can result in red cell hemolysis.

ACQUIRED HEMOLYTIC ANEMIA

Sometimes the red cells are normally formed but are unable to survive normally because they are released into a "hostile environment." For example, antibodies that attack and destroy the red cells may be present in the circulation. Some of the autoimmune diseases, such as lupus erythematosus, and some diseases of the lymphatic system may be associated with a hemolytic anemia caused by autoantibodies.

Some drugs also cause a hemolytic anemia by inducing formation of antibodies that damage red cells. Three different immunologic mechanisms have been identified. The most common mechanism results from the effect of the drug on the body's immune system, leading to the formation of an autoantibody directed against the red cell membrane. Other mechanisms include formation of drug–protein complexes. In some cases, the drug combines with a plasma protein, forming a drug–protein complex that is antigenic and induces antibody formation. The antigen and antibody interact within the circulation, forming complexes that attach to the red cells and cause their destruction. In other cases, the drug binds to the red cell membrane, forming an antigenic drug–membrane complex. An antibody against the complex then forms, attacks the cell membrane, and damages the red cells.

In another type of acquired hemolytic anemia, red cells may be destroyed by mechanical trauma. Some diseases are characterized by significant enlargement of the spleen. Red cells passing through a greatly enlarged spleen may be subject to considerable mechanical trauma, accelerating their destruction. Occasionally, a hemolytic anemia may follow insertion of an artificial heart valve because the red cells are injured by contact with some part of the artificial valve. In thrombotic microangiopathic hemolytic anemia, red cells are damaged by contact with fibrin deposited as microthrombi within small vessels. Disseminated intravascular coagulation (see discussion on abnormalities of blood coagulation) is frequently associated with this type of anemia. Fragmented blood cells (**schistocytes**) are found in blood smears from such patients.

DIAGNOSTIC EVALUATION OF ANEMIA

The evaluation of a patient with anemia consists of a careful medical history and physical examination along with a complete blood count to assess the degree of anemia and to determine whether leukopenia and thrombocytopenia also are present. Microscopic examination of a blood smear is used to determine whether the anemia is hypochromic microcytic, normocytic, or macrocytic. The rate of production of new red cells can be estimated by determining the percentage of reticulocytes in the circulation. An increased percentage of reticulocytes indicates rapid regeneration of red cells, as would be encountered after acute blood loss or hemolysis. The use of automated optical instruments simplifies the characterization of circulating red cells, providing data on their number, volume, and hemoglobin content. In some patients, tests that measure iron stores, iron transport, and iron metabolism may be useful. A bone marrow biopsy may also be used. In this procedure, a small amount of bone marrow is removed from the pelvic bone, sternum, or other site and examined microscopically. Characteristic abnormalities in the maturation of the marrow cells are seen in pernicious anemia and in anemia caused by folic acid deficiency. Bone marrow examination also detects interference with bone marrow functions secondary to infiltration by leukemic cells or metastatic tumor. If chronic blood loss from the gastrointestinal tract is suspected, stools are examined for blood, and x-ray studies of the gastrointestinal tract are frequently performed to localize a site of bleeding.

Polycythemia

An increase of red cells and hemoglobin above normal levels, called **polycythemia**, is usually secondary to an underlying disease that produces decreased arterial oxygen saturation (secondary polycythemia), or less frequently may represent a manifestation of a leukemia-like overproduction of red cells for no apparent reason (primary polycythemia).

SECONDARY POLYCYTHEMIA

Any condition associated with a reduced amount of oxygen transported in the bloodstream (low arterial PO_2, see discussion on respiratory system) leads to increased erythropoietin production by the kidney and to increased numbers of circulating red cells. The condition may accompany pulmonary emphysema, pulmonary fibrosis, or some other type of chronic lung disease that impairs the oxygenation of the blood.

Schistocytes Fragmented red cells.

Polycythemia An increase of red cells and hemoglobin above normal levels.

Rarely, polycythemia may be the result of overproduction of erythropoietin by a renal tumor or other tumor.

PRIMARY POLYCYTHEMIA

Primary polycythemia, also called polycythemia vera (true polycythemia), is a manifestation of a diffuse hyperplasia of the bone marrow almost always related to a particular somatic mutation of the *JAK* gene, which results in a gain of function and growth advantage to the clone of cells bearing the mutation. As the erythroid progenitor cells with this mutation mature, they no longer require erythropoietin for growth. Polycythemia vera is characterized by overproduction, predominantly of precursors to red cells but also of white blood cells and platelet precursors. However, the peripheral blood shows only a mild to moderate increase in white cells and platelets. The disease has many features of a neoplastic process and is classified as a **myelodysplastic syndrome**. The disease can be considered as a "pre-leukemia" because some patients with polycythemia vera eventually develop acute myelogenous (granulocytic) leukemia.

COMPLICATIONS AND TREATMENT OF POLYCYTHEMIA

The symptoms of polycythemia are related to the increased blood volume and increased blood viscosity. Many patients with polycythemia develop thromboses because of the increased blood viscosity and elevated platelet levels. Polycythemia vera is usually treated by drugs that suppress the bone marrow overactivity. Secondary polycythemia is sometimes treated by periodic removal of excess blood.

Myelodysplastic syndrome Marrow disease with features of a "pre-leukemia."

Petechia/ecchymoses Small pinpoint hemorrhage or larger hemorrhage caused by decreased platelets, abnormal platelet function, or capillary defect.

Purpura Skin or mucous membrane bleeding.

Thrombocytopenia

Blood platelets are fragments of the cytoplasm of megakaryocytes that are released into the bloodstream. These small structures serve a hemostatic function, sealing small breaks in capillaries and interacting with plasma factors in the initial stages of blood clotting (see discussion of abnormalities of blood coagulation). A significant reduction in the numbers of platelets in the blood leads to numerous small, pinpoint hemorrhages from capillaries in the skin and mucous membranes, called **petechiae**, and to larger areas of hemorrhage, called **ecchymoses**. This type of skin and mucous membrane bleeding is called **purpura**, and the disease entity is called thrombocytopenic purpura. The number of platelets may be reduced by bone marrow disease, which impairs platelet production, or by accelerated destruction of platelets in the circulation.

Many cases of thrombocytopenic purpura develop when drugs, chemicals, or other substances damage the bone marrow. Others develop when the bone marrow is infiltrated by leukemic cells or metastatic carcinoma. These conditions are called secondary thrombocytopenic purpura because the purpura results from an underlying disease of the bone marrow and is often associated with leukemia-like disease of lymphocytic cells (chronic lymphocytic leukemia [CLL]).

Sometimes the bone marrow produces platelets normally, but the platelets are rapidly destroyed in the circulation. Autoantibodies directed against platelets can often be detected in the blood of affected individuals. Cases of this type, in which no underlying disease can be detected, are called idiopathic (or immune) thrombocytopenic purpura (ITP). Idiopathic thrombocytopenic purpura is often found in children, sometimes following a mild viral disease, and subsides spontaneously within a short time. When the disease develops in adults, it tends to be more chronic and is not treated when the number of platelets in the bloodstream (platelet count) is only moderately reduced. However, treatment is essential if the platelet count is so low that the patient is at risk of severe life-threatening bleeding, such as a cerebral hemorrhage. The initial treatment usually consists of corticosteroid hormones that raise the platelet count by suppressing the immune system, which is the source of the autoantibodies that are destroying the platelets. Patients who do not respond to initial treatment are usually treated by removal of the spleen (splenectomy), the site where the antibody-coated platelets are removed from the circulation.

The Lymphatic System

The lymphatic system consists of the lymph nodes and spleen, together with various organized masses of lymphoid tissue elsewhere throughout the body such as the tonsils, the adenoids, the thymus, and the lymphoid aggregates in the intestinal mucosa, respiratory tract, and bone marrow. The primary function of the lymphatic system is to provide immunologic defenses against foreign material by means of cell-mediated and humoral defense mechanisms. The lymph nodes, which constitute a major part of the system, form an interconnected network linked by lymphatic channels.

Lymph nodes are small, bean-shaped structures that vary from a few millimeters to as much as 2 cm in diameter. They are interspersed along the course of lymphatic channels, where they act somewhat like filters. Frequently, they form groups at locations where many lymphatic channels converge, such as around the aorta and inferior vena cava, in the mesentery of the intestine, in the axillae (armpits) and groin, and at the base of the neck. Each node consists of a mass of lymphocytes supported by a meshwork of reticular fibers, which are scattered phagocytic cells of the mononuclear phagocyte system (reticuloendothelial system). As the lymph flows through the nodes, the phagocytic cells filter out and destroy any microorganisms or other foreign materials that have gotten into the lymphatic channels. The lymphocytes and mononuclear phagocytes within the node also interact with the foreign material and initiate an immune response. The functions of the various lymphoid cells and their role in immunity are considered in the discussion on immunity, hypersensitivity, allergy, and autoimmune diseases.

The spleen is specialized to filter blood rather than lymph. Much larger than lymph nodes, it is about the size of a man's fist and is located under the ribs in the left upper part of the abdomen. It consists of compact masses of lymphocytes and a network of sinusoids (capillaries having wide lumens of variable width) within a supporting framework composed of reticular fibers and numerous phagocytic cells. As the blood flows through the spleen, worn-out red cells are removed from the circulation by the phagocytic cells, and the iron that they contain is salvaged for reuse. Abnormal red cells, such as those that are damaged by disease, are abnormal in shape, or contain a large amount of an abnormal hemoglobin, also are destroyed by the splenic phagocytes, which accounts for their shortened survival in the circulation.

In addition to removing worn-out or abnormal red cells, the spleen is an efficient blood filtration system. Any bacteria or other foreign material that gain access to the bloodstream are promptly removed by the splenic phagocytes as the blood flows through the spleen. In addition, the spleen manufactures antibodies that facilitate prompt elimination of pathogenic organisms.

Sometimes it is necessary to remove the spleen. Splenectomy may be required to prevent fatal hemorrhage if the spleen has been lacerated in an automobile accident or other injury. Splenectomy is also frequently performed on patients with blood diseases characterized by excessive destruction of blood cells within the spleen, such as thrombocytopenic purpura and some types of hereditary hemolytic anemia.

Splenectomized individuals are less able to eliminate bacteria that gain access to the bloodstream and do not produce antibodies as well as before removal of the spleen. Consequently, they are likely to develop serious bloodstream infections caused by pathogenic bacteria. These infections may respond poorly to antibiotics. To reduce this risk, splenectomized patients are often immunized with bacterial vaccines because high levels of antibacterial antibodies facilitate removal of bacteria from the circulation, and this can substitute for splenic function to some extent. Many physicians also recommend that a splenectomized individual either take antibiotics continuously or begin taking antibiotics at the first sign of a respiratory infection or other febrile illness.

The thymus is a bilobed lymphoid organ overlying the base of the heart. It is a large structure during infancy and childhood but gradually undergoes atrophy in adolescence. Only a remnant persists in the adult. The thymus plays an essential role in the prenatal development of the lymphoid system and in the formation of the body's immunologic defense mechanisms.

DISEASES OF THE LYMPHATIC SYSTEM

The principal diseases affecting the lymphatic system are infections and neoplasms.

Benign Lymphocytosis

Benign lymphocytosis, an increase in the number of circulating lymphocytes, is most often a reflection of viral disease. The circulating lymphocytes may be enlarged and atypical looking. **Infectious mononucleosis**, a relatively common viral disease, is the most common cause of benign lymphocytosis, particularly in children and adolescents (where it is transmitted by close contact). The disease is caused by a herpes virus (as are fever blisters) named the **Epstein-Barr virus** (usually simply called EBV). The virus causes an acute, debilitating, febrile illness associated with a diffuse hyperplasia of lymphoid tissue throughout the body, particularly the lymph nodes and spleen, which may double or triple in size. The lymphocytes circulating in the peripheral blood show distinctive morphologic abnormalities, being larger than normal with abundant deep blue cytoplasm and an irregularly shaped nucleus (**FIGURE 13-8**). The atypical lymphocytes are cytotoxic (CD8+) T lymphocytes, which destroy B cells infected by EBV. Enlargement and ulceration of lymphoid tissue in the throat is responsible for the sore throat often accompanying the disease.

The disease diagnosis is most often based on clinical symptoms and detection of antibodies using a monospot test. EBV infection results in both antibodies directed toward the virus but also an unusual class of **heterophile antibodies**, that react with unrelated substances (sheep and horse red cells). The monospot test detects such antibodies and is very specific for the disease.

Generally, the disease is self-limited, and no specific treatment is required. However, it may be several weeks before the patient feels well again, and the spleen may be sensitive to trauma while it remains enlarged. Contact sports should be avoided during this time.

Inflammation of the Lymph Nodes (Lymphadenitis)

Lymph nodes draining an area of infection may become enlarged and tender, resulting from spread of bacterial or fungal infection through the lymphatic channels and the resulting acute inflammation in the node. This is called **lymphadenitis**.

Infectious mononucleosis A common viral disease, the most common cause of benign lymphocytosis.

Epstein-Barr virus A virus that causes infectious mononucleosis.

Heterophile antibodies Antibodies that react with substances unrelated to the immunizing antigen.

Lymphadenitis Inflammation of the lymph node.

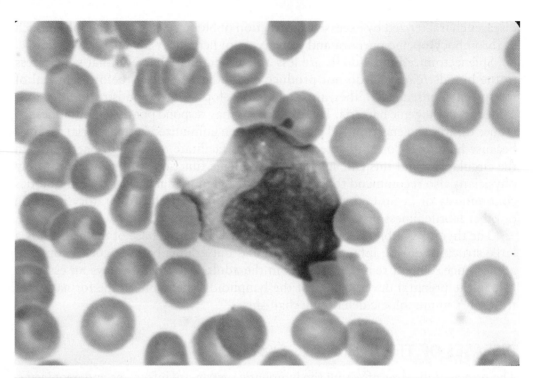

FIGURE 13-8 Large lymphocyte from individual with infectious mononucleosis, illustrating characteristic morphologic abnormalities (original magnification ×1,000).

Courtesy of Leonard V. Crowley, MD, Century College.

Leukemia

Leukemia A neoplasm of hematopoietic tissue.

Lymphoma A neoplasm of lymphoid cells limited to lymph nodes and sometimes spleen.

Myeloid/lymphoid Classification of leukemia by hematopoietic tissue of origin.

The term **leukemia** refers to a neoplasm of hematopoietic tissue. In contrast to solid tumors, which form nodular deposits, leukemic cells diffusely infiltrate the bone marrow and lymphoid tissues, spill over into the bloodstream, and infiltrate the various organs of the body. The leukemic cells may be mostly mature, or they may be extremely primitive. The overproduction of white cells in leukemia may be revealed in the peripheral blood by a very high white blood count. In some cases of leukemia, however, the proliferation of the white cells is largely confined to the bone marrow, and there is no significant increase in the number of white cells in the bloodstream. At times there is some degree of overlap with **lymphoma** in which the neoplastic cells are predominantly found in lymph nodes but may also occur in essentially any tissue. Lymphomas can be "leukemia-like" and be found in the blood and bone marrow.

CLASSIFICATION OF LEUKEMIA

Leukemia is classified on the basis of both the cell type and the maturity of the proliferating cells. Any type of hematopoietic cells can give rise to leukemia, but the most common types are **myeloid** and **lymphoid**. Leukemia developing from stem cells that would normally give rise to the leukocytes containing specific granules (neutrophils, eosinophils, basophils) is called myeloid leukemia. Likewise, leukemia developing from precursor cells that give rise to monocytes is termed monocytic leukemia (often myelomonocytic leukemia); lymphocytic leukemia is derived from lymphoid precursor cells. Various complex subclassifications have been established within these major groups on the basis of the characteristics of the cell membranes, the enzymes present within the leukemic cells, and genetic changes, as determined by highly specialized techniques.

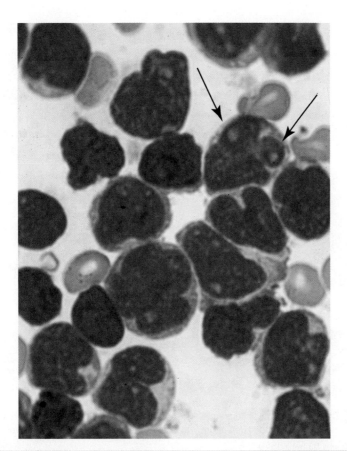

FIGURE 13-9 A photomicrograph of a blood smear from a patient with acute leukemia. The nuclei of the white cells have fine chromatin structure and prominent nucleoli indicating immaturity (*arrows*). Nuclei are irregular in size and configuration.

Courtesy of Leonard V. Crowley, MD, Century College.

If the leukemia cells are mostly primitive forms, the leukemia is classified as acute leukemia (**FIGURE 13-9**). Such leukemias have rapid onset, are clinically aggressive, and are characterized by the presence of blasts (poorly differentiated cells). If the cells are more mature-appearing, the leukemia is classified as chronic leukemia. Chronic leukemias have an insidious onset and are usually less aggressive and may be compatible with relatively long survival.

Myelogenous Leukemias

Chronic myelogenous leukemias are classified as myeloproliferative disorders of which chronic myelogenous leukemia (CML) and polycythemia vera (discussed previously) are common examples. Myeloproliferative disorders are characterized by highly cellular bone marrows containing an abundance of precursors for the leukemic cell (myeloid precursors in the case of CML). The elevated number of circulating cells may range from mature granulocytes to immature forms (**FIGURE 13-10**). Almost all cases of CML are associated with the presence of a **Philadelphia chromosome**, which represents a translocation between two chromosome (9 and 22). This results in the formation of BCR-ABL fusion protein (kinase) with inappropriately increased activity, which is responsible for the leukemic process (see discussion on neoplastic disease). Specific drugs such as imatinib are available to inhibit this inappropriate enzymatic activity. The drug is initially effective in greater than 90 percent of patients, but resistance occurs with time, requiring either another inhibiting drug or other forms of therapy. With time and failure of drug therapy, CML tends to progress to

Philadelphia chromosome Chromosome translocation common in neoplastic cells of chronic myelogenous leukemia.

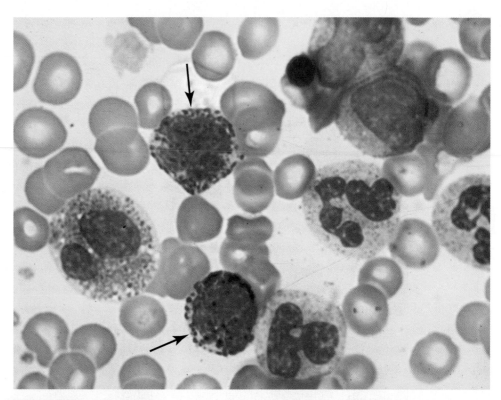

FIGURE 13-10 Chronic granulocytic leukemia. Most of the cells in the photomicrograph are mature. Note the basophils (*arrows*), the eosinophil (*left of arrows*), and the two neutrophils (*right of arrows*).

Courtesy of Leonard V. Crowley, MD, Century College.

an acute blast phase, and increased numbers of such cells appear in the bone marrow and blood. Blast cells show additional mutations, become resistant to drug therapy, and the prognosis is poor.

As well as being the result of a myeloproliferative disorder, acute myeloid leukemia (AML) may arise de novo, or less frequently as a side effect of radiation or cytotoxic therapy. In AML greater than 20 percent of undifferentiated myeloblasts are found in the bone marrow where they crowd out normal hematopoietic cells, resulting in leukopenia, thrombocytopenia, and anemia. AML cells harbor many mutations (Figure 13-9). There are many types of AML, and specific forms of chemotherapy are available for several of them. However, the overall prognosis for the disease is very poor; chemotherapy is only temporarily effective and is followed by relapse. In such cases, bone marrow transplantation is considered for therapy.

Lymphocytic Leukemias

In chronic lymphocytic leukemia (CLL), the circulating cells are mostly small, mature lymphocytes (**FIGURE 13-11**). The most common type of CLL is mature **B cell** leukemia, which is equivalent to small cell lymphocytic lymphoma (SLL). The two differ only in whether the disease is predominantly based in the bone marrow or in the lymph node and blood. B-cell CLL/SLL is the most common type of adult leukemia in the Western world. The disease is most commonly indolent and is often discovered as an incidental finding. Patients without symptoms may not require therapy and often survive more than ten years. However about 30 percent of patients will experience progression of the disease to other forms of leukemia/lymphoma with worsening symptoms. Patients with CLL may develop hypogammaglobulinemia and

B cell A lymphocyte that differentiates into plasma cells and is associated with humoral immunity.

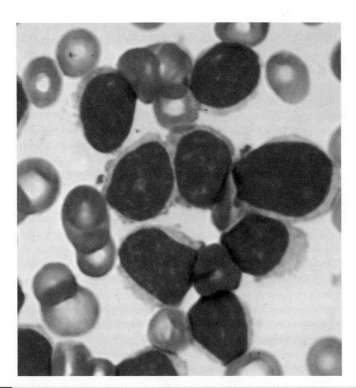

FIGURE 13-11 Chronic lymphocytic leukemia. The dense nuclear chromatin structure indicates that the lymphocytes are mature (compare with Figure 10-26). The total white count is elevated.

Courtesy of Leonard V. Crowley, MD, Century College.

susceptibility to infection and autoimmune hemolytic anemia. Although the disease may be kept in check using chemotherapy, it generally cannot be cured.

Precursor B cell acute lymphoblastic leukemia (Precursor B cell ALL, often incorrectly referred to simply as ALL) is the most common malignancy of childhood, accounting for about a quarter of all pediatric cancer. It generally occurs in children between two and five years of age, with more than half of cases occurring in children younger than six. The cause is unknown, but there is an increased incidence in several genetic diseases (such as Down syndrome). At times the disease predominantly involves lymph nodes and is referred to as lymphoblastic lymphoma. Small to medium-size lymphoblasts, which are similar to very early precursors of mature B cells, replace much of the bone marrow and can be found in the blood. This results in anemia, neutropenia, and thrombocytopenia because precursors for these cell lines are lost from the marrow. The disease may disseminate into the CNS and organs. Occasionally, however, the marrow may be crowded with abnormal cells, but the number of white blood cells in the blood is normal or decreased, a variant termed leukemic leukemia. Many different chromosomal abnormalities can found in precursor B cell ALL (including the BCR-ABL fusion protein), and the particular abnormalities have an impact on prognosis. Therapeutic advances now allow for a 90-percent total remission rate using chemotherapy, and in refractory disease, hemopoietic stem cell transplantation. As in B cell derived ALL, **T cell** derived disease also occurs and has a worse prognosis than does B cell disease. T cell ALL frequently presents as a soft tissue mass outside the marrow (often in the mediastinal space, the central area of the chest cavity).

Many additional forms of neoplastic diseases of lymphoid cells are characterized depending on the cell type (B cell versus T cell) and stage of maturity of the neoplastic cell involved. As a single example, **multiple myeloma** is a neoplasm of plasma cells, with

T cell A type of lymphocyte associated with cell-mediated immunity.

Multiple myeloma A neoplasm of plasma cells characterized by production of M-protein.

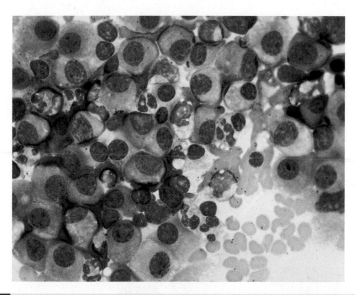

FIGURE 13-12 Photomicrograph illustrating aspirated bone marrow from a patient with multiple myeloma. Almost all cells are immature plasma cells containing large eccentric nuclei and abundant cytoplasm.

Courtesy of Leonard V. Crowley, MD, Century College.

the highly differentiated B cell responsible for the production of immunoglobulins. For this reason, multiple myeloma is often characterized by the production of an M-protein (myeloma protein or monoclonal gammopathy). The uniform immunoglobulin produced by the neoplastic plasma cells, which are monoclonal (derived from a single transformed neoplastic cell precursor), can be detected in the blood. In many ways, multiple myeloma resembles leukemia, but the neoplastic plasma cell proliferation is generally confined to the bone marrow (**FIGURE 13-12**). The malignant cells produce "punched-out" lesions of the bones, which may lead to bone destruction and fractures characteristic of the disease (**FIGURE 13-13**). At times an M-protein

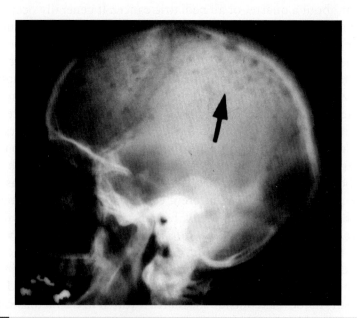

FIGURE 13-13 A skull x-ray from a patient with multiple myeloma. Multiple punched-out areas in skull bones (*arrow*) result from bone destruction caused by nodular masses of neoplastic plasma cells growing in bone marrow.

Courtesy of Leonard V. Crowley, MD, Century College.

may be detected in the blood prior to the detection of abnormal plasma cells in the bone marrow. This is termed a monoclonal gammopathy of unknown significance (MGUS). Although an MGUS is not associated with symptomatic disease, it is a precursor lesion that indicates a risk of developing multiple myeloma.

Precursors of Leukemia: The Myelodysplastic Syndromes

Acute leukemia in older patients may not have an abrupt onset but can be preceded by a period lasting from several months to several years. During that time, affected patients have only a refractory anemia, sometimes associated with reduced white cells (leukopenia) and low blood platelets (thrombocytopenia). Examination of the bone marrow of these patients reveals variable degrees of disturbed growth and maturation of red cells, white cell precursors, and megakaryocytes, but not leukemia. The condition is termed myelodysplastic syndrome (*myelo* = marrow + *dysplasia* = disturbed growth). Several different types have been described that differ somewhat in their clinical and hematologic manifestations. In general, the more severe the maturation disturbance in the bone marrow, the greater likelihood that leukemia will eventually occur. Nearly half of patients with myelodysplastic syndrome will develop AML. Unfortunately, there is no specific treatment available for most patients with these conditions, although some patients with severe "preleukemic" changes in their bone marrow have been treated successfully by bone marrow transplantation.

LYMPHOMAS

All neoplasms of lymphoid tissue are called lymphomas although, as noted previously, there may be considerable overlap between leukemias and lymphomas depending on the major precursor of the malignant cells. Over 80 percent of lymphomas arise from B cells. Most of the rest come from T cells, and a few originate from NK cells (natural killer cells) or histiocytes. The neoplastic cells of most lymphomas arise from early precursor stages in the development of mature B and T cells. The abnormal proliferation of lymphoid cells often also disrupts the normal functions of the immune system, which may be manifested either as an impairment of the body's immune defenses resulting in increased susceptibility to infection or as an abnormal immune response manifested as some type of autoimmune disease.

Lymphomas are subdivided into two major groups: Hodgkin lymphoma, sometimes called **Hodgkin's disease**, and non-Hodgkin lymphoma. Hodgkin lymphoma has several features that are quite different from other lymphomas. The disease frequently occurs in young adults, in contrast to non-Hodgkin lymphoma, which usually affects much older people. The disease often starts in a single lymph node or small group of nodes and then spreads to adjacent nodes before eventually spreading to other parts of the body. The tumor has a variable histologic appearance, consisting of large atypical B cells called **Reed-Sternberg cells** intermixed with lymphocytes, plasma cells, eosinophils, and fibrous tissue. The Reed-Sternberg cells make up only a small proportion of the total cells in the tumor, but they secrete cytokines that attract the other cells, which become intermixed with the Reed-Sternberg cells and are the neoplastic cells responsible for the disease. The typical Reed-Sternberg cell is a large cell that characteristically contains either a single nucleus or two nuclei that appear as mirror images of each other. Each nucleus contains a large nucleolus surrounded by a clear halo (**FIGURE 13-14**). Several different histologic types of Hodgkin disease are recognized that differ somewhat in their clinical behavior and prognosis. A person

Hodgkin's disease A form of lymphoma that occurs in young adults with Reed-Sternberg cells mixed with other cell types.

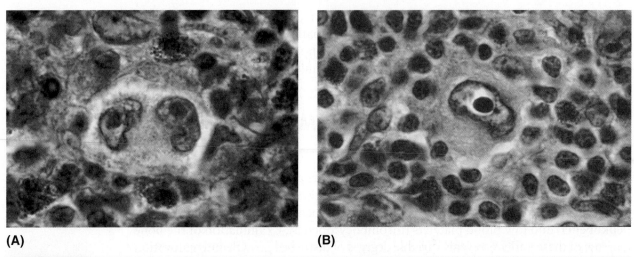

(A)   **(B)**

FIGURE 13-14 Characteristic appearance of Reed-Sternberg cells. **(A)** Binucleate cell. Note the mirror image nuclei with prominent nucleoli. **(B)** Cell with single nucleus illustrating prominent nucleolus and perinuclear halo (original magnification ×400).

Courtesy of Leonard V. Crowley, MD, Century College.

with Hodgkin lymphoma usually first becomes aware of a painless enlargement of a single lymph node or group of nodes. In more advanced cases, several groups of nodes may be involved. Most patients are treated with courses of chemotherapy consisting of four drugs (doxorubicin, bleomyxin, vinblastine, and dacarbazine) as well as radiotherapy to the involved areas. The combined therapy approach has been very successful.

All other lymphomas are grouped together under the general term of non-Hodgkin lymphomas. Most are B cell lymphomas that are quite variable in their appearance, behavior, and prognosis depending on the particular developmental stage and function of the lymphocyte that gave rise to the neoplastic cells that form the lymphoma. The disease is often widespread by the time the lymphoma is diagnosed, so it is difficult to cure the lymphoma because the tumor cells have already spread throughout the body. The prognosis depends on the particular type of lymphoma, some being very aggressive, others less so.

The variable appearance and sometimes poor correlation between histologic appearance and biologic behavior have created difficulties in classifying lymphomas. Lymphomas can also be classified into prognostic groups based on their histologic appearance. Currently lymphomas are divided into four large groups based on the type of cells giving rise to the tumor (T cells, B cells, NK cells, or histiocytes) and the developmental stage and functional origin of the cell. There are many subgroups within each of the four major groups, and sophisticated determination of the cell surface characteristics of the lymphoma cell as measured using immunological tests are used to aid the physician in determining the specific type of non-Hodgkin lymphoma affecting the patient, which also helps determine the prognosis and the appropriate type of treatment.

METASTATIC TUMORS IN LYMPH NODES

Lymph nodes may be affected by the spread of metastatic tumor from malignant tumors arising in the breast, lung, colon, or other sites. The nodes first affected lie in the immediate drainage area of the tumor. The tumor may then spread to other more distant lymph nodes through lymphatic channels and may eventually gain access to the circulatory system through the thoracic duct.

The Enlarged Lymph Node as a Diagnostic Problem

The patient who visits a physician because one or more lymph nodes is enlarged (**lymphadenopathy**) can present a difficult diagnostic problem. Lymph node enlargement may be a manifestation of a localized infection in the area drained by the node, a systemic infection with initial manifestations in the node, a metastatic tumor in the node, or an early manifestation of leukemia or malignant lymphoma. Often, the cause of the lymphadenopathy can be determined by the physician from the clinical evaluation of the patient in conjunction with laboratory studies, including an examination of the peripheral blood. If the cause cannot be established, the physician must perform a lymph node biopsy to determine the reason for the enlargement. The enlarged lymph node may be surgically excised or a needle used to take a small biopsy of the node. The tissue is submitted to the pathologist for microscopic and immunological examination. In some cases, the histologic pattern of the node can be used to determine if lymphoma is present. In difficult cases, it may be necessary to determine whether a lymphocyte proliferation within a lymph node arose from a single abnormal lymphocyte that formed a clone of identical cells (a monoclonal proliferation), indicating a lymphoid neoplasm, or from many different lymphocytes that formed multiple clones of cells (a polyclonal proliferation), which is characteristic of a benign lymphocyte proliferation. Generally, the pathologist can make a specific diagnosis on the basis of such studies.

PRINCIPLES OF TREATMENT

The goal of the physician treating leukemia or lymphoma is to produce a durable (long-lasting) cure. This (at least in theory) requires destruction of all the neoplastic lymphoid cells that could resume division at some future time and allow the disease to reoccur, but it is a difficult goal to obtain. More often the abnormal proliferation of the leukemic cells can be stopped for a variable period of time by various anti-cancer drugs, and the patient appears to have completely recovered and is said to be in **remission**. In many cases, however, the disease returns (the patient undergoes a **relapse**) and may ultimately prove fatal. The type of therapy is dependent on many clinical variables including the age of the patient, severity of the disease when diagnosed, and the specific type of leukemia or lymphoma. Some patients with CLL may require no therapy at all, whereas others may progress to a more aggressive disease that requires therapy to control symptoms. Other forms of leukemia and lymphoma always require aggressive chemotherapy. For example, ALL of children was nearly uniformly fatal in the mid-1960s with an overall cure rate of <10 percent. By the mid-1980s, following advances in the treatment of CNS disease associated with ALL, cure rates approached 50 percent. Currently, modern chemotherapy protocols lead to a cure rate of 90 percent. This rate, however, comes at the cost of extensive and complex therapy and associated clinical support. A similar increase in survival has occurred with Hodgkin lymphoma; cure rates using chemotherapy, often combined with limited x-ray therapy, now result in a 98-percent cure rate. Unfortunately, as was noted in the discussion of CML, specific drugs that target the abnormal gene product directly responsible for the neoplastic disease are already in use, but only limited agents are available to deal with relapse related to resistance. Many forms of leukemia and lymphoma may be resistant to therapy or relapse after initially successful therapy, but these otherwise intractable diseases sometimes can be treated by hematopoietic stem cell transplantation.

Lymphadenopathy Enlargement of one or more lymph nodes.

Remission Patient appears to be completely recovered from neoplastic disease with no cancer cells present.

Relapse Return of cancer cells after a period of remission.

HEMATOPOIETC STEM CELL THERAPY (BONE MARROW TRANSPLANTATION)

Hematopoietic stem cells (HSC) for transplantation may be obtained from several sources. The best known is bone marrow although cord blood harvested at delivery provides a very rich source of HSC. Increasingly, HSC may be harvested from peripheral blood taken from donors using sophisticated apheresis machines able to "sort out" circulating HSC based on their cell surface properties and return the unneeded cells to the donor. This allows processing of a large volume of blood from a donor with little or no side effects. Each source of HSC has advantages and disadvantages associated with it, and the choice depends on available donor material and the needs of the patient.

A major concern in HSC transplantation is the necessity that the transplanted cells not be rejected by the host (patient) and that the transplanted (grafted) cells not result in overly severe graft versus host disease (GVH). GVH occurs because the donor lymphocytes in the transplant are immunologically active and can recognize the patient's cells as antigenically different. The transplanted cells attempt to destroy host tissue leads to various clinical manifestations, including skin rash, liver injury, gastrointestinal symptoms, and, in severe cases, death. This is the reverse of the usual situation in which the patient's immune system tries to reject the transplant. Although physicians try to control the level of GVH, the condition is also beneficial in that the transplanted cells are effective in destroying the remaining neoplastic cells in the host. Thus the clinician tries to maintain a delicate balance where the beneficial effects of GVH outweigh the detrimental.

HSC may be derived from the patients themselves (autologous transplant). Clinicians may give the patient levels of chemotherapy that in themselves would be lethal because they would totally destroy the patient's bone marrow. Prior to such therapy (and usually when the patient is in remission and has a low level of leukemic of lymphoma cells) the physician harvests bone marrow or peripheral blood HSC and stores the harvest to be reinfused into the patient to "rescue" the patient from the chemotherapy. The goal is to totally destroy any neoplastic cells by the aggressive chemotherapy. The harvested HSC can also be treated to remove any residual tumor cells in the restored HSC. This type of HSC therapy has no concern about rejection or GVH because the cells are the patient's own.

Most transplants are not autologous and come from either a related (generally a sibling) or unrelated donor. Such transplants are termed **allogeneic** (not from self). One fortuitous special case is when a patient (host) has an identical twin. Such donors are termed **syngeneic** and are antigenically identical to the patient. The transplant will not be rejected, and any GVH is relatively mild. (For this reason, syngeneic transplants tend to have a higher risk of recurrence of disease.) The tissue from an identical twin is completely histocompatible; that is, it will be recognized as self and not rejected. In the likely absence of an identical twin, the next best source of donors is a sibling (full brother or sister). Matching is done by testing for antigens controlled by the HLA gene complex, which controls the synthesis of those cell surface proteins (antigens) most critical in telling the immune system what is self and what is foreign. Three sets of HLA antigens (HLA-A, HLA-B, and HLA-DRB1) are most critical in determining how compatible transplanted tissue will be. The three sets of antigens are (almost always) inherited as blocks, and the antigens inherited from the maternal and paternal chromosomes are both expressed on tissue. Because siblings inherit one set of antigens from the mother and one from the father, there is a 25-percent chance that any two full siblings will share the antigens inherited from both parents. This is called a six-antigen match (HLA-A, HLA-B, and HLA-DRB1 are identical from both parents) and provides the best, most histocompatible match

Allogeneic/syngeneic/ autologous Terms used to classify the relationship of donor cells to the patient, not from self/from an identical twin/from self.

and best results in HSC transplants. However, many other factors (antigens) not likely to be identical in siblings also are important in determining histocompatibility. For this reason, even when a six-antigen sibling donor is available, patients must be prepared (primed) before transplantation using potent immunosuppressive drugs to prevent graft rejection because some degree of GVH is likely to occur.

In the absence of a six-antigen sib-match, large data banks of volunteer, previously HLA typed, unrelated donors may be searched to find identical donors. These donors are not as effective as matched siblings and are more likely to be rejected. Sometimes unmatched or partially matched siblings may also be considered as donors. Banks of stored cord bloods are also available, but the number of HSC available from these is a major limitation in use to transplant adults.

Five-year survival rates following sibling donor HSC transplantation depend on the particular leukemia or lymphoma being treated and the clinical status of the patient. Overall survival rates are at least 50 percent when a sibling donor is used, with unrelated donors providing a somewhat lower survival rate. Although marrow/HSC transplantation is an important advance, it is not always successful. Patients may develop life-threatening infections related to the immunosuppression required to maintain the transplant, and in some patients, the leukemia recurs, arising from the patient's surviving leukemic cells that were not destroyed by the prior chemotherapy and radiation.

CASE 13-1

Candy is a four-year-old female who has been feeling poorly for the past several weeks. She has complained of bone pain and has started to limp while playing outside. Her mother notes that she tires easily, appears pale, and comes in to take naps. Candy now has a moderate fever in the evening (38.5°C, 101.3°F oral). More alarming, Candy has had repeated nose bleeds (epistaxis) and has developed small purple spots (petechiae) on her arms and legs. Concerned that Candy may have a "summer virus," her mother brings her to the family pediatrician.

On physical examination, the pediatrician determines that Candy has enlarged lymph nodes and possibly an enlarged spleen. Noting the patient's pallor and signs of a bleeding tendency and fatigue, the pediatrician suspects any of several diseases involving the blood and bone marrow, including anemia, idiopathic thrombocytopenic purpura (ITP, possibly postviral), or a leukemia. An in-office CBC (complete blood count) reveals a very elevated white cell count (30,000 per microliter with below 10,000 considered normal) with a low red cell and platelet count. A peripheral blood smear discloses multiple abnormal cells with very little cytoplasm, which the pediatrician believes are lymphoblasts (neoplastic, immature lymphocytes) (FIGURE 13-15A). The pediatrician refers Candy to a pediatric hematologist at a regional hospital center for further evaluation.

The hematologist suspects that Candy has acute lymphoblastic leukemia of childhood and orders several additional tests. These include a bone marrow aspiration (FIGURE 13-15B and C). Candy's bone marrow has a predominance of lymphoblastic cells and a great reduction of the other cell lineages (developing granulocytes, platelets, and red cells) in the marrow. A normal marrow is provided for comparison. A lumbar puncture is performed to evaluate whether leukemic cells are present in the cerebrospinal fluid. No such cells are found. A chest x-ray shows no abnormality. Immunological studies of Candy's leukemic cells indicate they are of B cell origin and have cell surface antigens characteristic of immature cells. A karyotypic (chromosome) study of the leukemic cells show the cells are hyperdiploid (have greater than the normal 46 chromosomes, a good prognostic sign).

(continues)

CASE 13-1 *(Continued)*

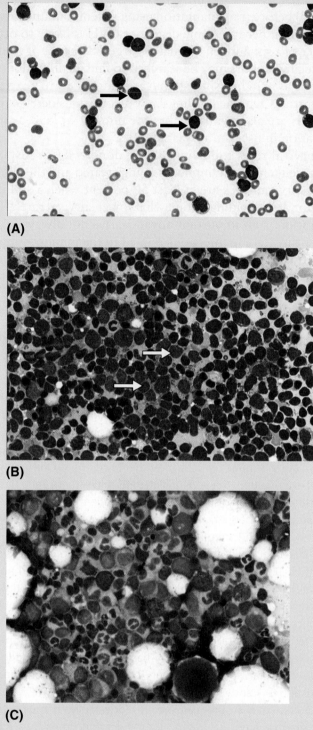

(A)

(B)

(C)

FIGURE 13-15 **(A)** Peripheral blood smear from patient. Two examples of lymphoblastic cells are indicated *(arrows)*. **(B)** Bone marrow sample from patient. The majority of marrow cells are lymphoblasts *(arrows)*. **(C)** Normal bone marrow demonstrating multiple lineages of developing cells. The clear spaces are fat found in normal marrow.

Courtesy of Department of Pathology and Laboratory Medicine, University of North Carolina at Chapel Hill.

CASE 13-1 *(Continued)*

Candy begins a long course of chemotherapy. Her initial evaluation (based on age, cell number, cell type, and chromosome number) would place her in a standard (not high risk) group; this classification helps determine the particular chemotherapy to be used. Although therapy will continue for at least two years, Candy has an excellent chance of a cure. The five-year survival rate with no evidence of further disease is 95 percent for similar patients, and overall a cure rate of greater than 80 percent is expected.

Discussion

The evaluation of childhood leukemia and therapy of the disease is complex and depends on several variables, including the age of the patient, the severity of the disease at diagnosis, and the nature of the leukemic cell and the molecular abnormalities present in those cells. For example, T cell leukemia in children has a worse prognosis. The chest x-ray is performed because T cell leukemia often occurs in the mediastinum (chest) and can compromise cardiac function. Hence the x-ray is part of standard workup. A small percentage of children with ALL have a Philadelphia chromosome and a BCR-ABL fusion gene, as discussed under chronic myelogenous leukemia. These patients have a worse prognosis, but treatment with kinase inhibitors has much improved survival.

Chemotherapy for childhood ALL is a multistep process. Initial therapy (remission induction) usually takes place for about four weeks, with some time initially in a hospital setting, and involves the use of several chemotherapeutic agents in combination. Almost all (95 percent) patients have success in achieving remission initially. This is followed by the consolidation phase, with the aim of eliminating any residual disease, which involves continuing outpatient chemotherapy for as long as six to nine months. This is followed by a prolonged maintenance phase with continuing less intense chemotherapy with antimetabolites given orally for up to three years. In addition, therapy against leukemia in the CNS is always included and is started during remission induction. This includes intrathecal medication (administration of drugs within the membranes of the spinal cord) to ensure the drug enters the cerebrospinal fluid. Up to 20 percent of patients will suffer a relapse, which is often treated by redoing the initial remission induction therapy. All of the drugs used have toxic side effects.

Five percent of children treated with these agents will get a secondary cancer (AML). A number of other chronic long-term effects including impairment of fertility, learning problems, and heart and lung disease may also occur. For this reason, long-term follow-up of childhood cancer survivors is critical.

Etiology and Pathogenesis

B cell acute lymphoblastic leukemia of childhood.

Questions

1. Are there known predisposing environmental or genetic factors for acute lymphoblastic leukemia?

2. What are some of the potential risks and side effects of the chemotherapy used in the treatment of acute lymphoblastic leukemia?

3. No evidence of leukemic cells were found in Candy's cerebrospinal fluid. Nevertheless, therapy for CNS disease was performed. Why is such therapy always done in these cases?

4. What psychosocial effects might Candy's illness have on both her and her family?

5. Can you estimate the economic cost of Candy's therapy? What would happen if Candy were not covered by medical insurance?

QUESTIONS FOR REVIEW

1. What types of cells are found in the circulating blood, and what are their major functions?

2. What is anemia?

3. What is an iron deficiency anemia? How does it arise? How is it treated? What is the morphologic appearance of the red cells?

4. What is the effect of vitamin B_{12} and folic acid on blood cell maturation? What type of anemia results from deficiency of these vitamins?

5. What is the difference between an aplastic anemia and a hemolytic anemia? What is the difference between polycythemia and thrombocytopenia? What is hemochromatosis? What are its manifestations? How is the condition diagnosed and treated?

6. What is the lymphatic system? How is it organized? What are the major cells of the lymphatic system? What are the major functions of the lymphatic system? What are the functions of the spleen? What are the adverse effects of splenectomy?

7. What is the EB virus? What is its relationship to infectious mononucleosis? What are the clinical manifestations of infectious mononucleosis? How is the disease treated? What are some possible complications of the infection?

8. A patient has an enlarged lymph node. What types of diseases could produce lymph node enlargement? How does the physician arrive at a diagnosis when the patient presents with enlarged lymph nodes?

9. What types of altered immune reaction are sometimes encountered in diseases of the lymphatic system?

10. Compare and contrast leukemia, lymphoma, and myelodysplastic syndrome.

SUPPLEMENTARY READINGS

Valdez, R., et al. Chapter 26, "Hematopathology." 2014. In *Rubin's Pathology*, edited by D. S. Strayer and E. Rubin. Philadelphia, PA: Lippincott Williams & Wilkins, Wolters Kluwer.

▶ It is difficult to provide pertinent and useful supplementary readings for the introductory reader in the area of hematology because it encompasses an extremely wide range of physiological processes and diseases. Many recent changes in the classification of and suggested therapies for hematological disease are based on an increased understanding of the molecular basis of these diseases. This chapter in a recent pathology textbook aimed at medical education is a good place to start. Additional readings provide recent in-depth reviews of selected topics.

Bain, B. J. 2005. Diagnosis from the blood smear. *New England Journal of Medicine 353*:498–507.

▶ This reading never goes out of date. Although digital technology has improved the ability to transmit images to consultants for interpretation or second opinions, the blood smear remains a valuable diagnostic tool. Examination of a well-stained blood smear is essential whenever the results of a complete blood count indicate an abnormality.

Heinig, K., Sage, F., Robin, C., and Sperandio, M. 2015. Development and trafficking function of hematopoietic stem cells and myeloid cells during fetal ontogeny. *Cardiovascular Research* (Epub ahead of print, May 17).

Sankjaran, V. G., and Weiss, M. J. 2015. Anemia: Progress in molecular mechanisms and therapies. *Nature Medicine 21*:221.

▶ Both references explore the details of hematopoietic stem cell development in the fetus. The second article extends this to discuss the role of genetic disorders in the pathogenesis of anemia.

Brittenham, G. M. 2011. Iron-chelating therapy for transfusional iron overload. *New England Journal of Medicine 364*:146–56.

Silva, B., and Faustino, P. 2015. An overview of molecular basis of iron metabolism regulation and the associated pathologies *Biochemica et Biophysica Acta 1852*:1347–59.

▶ The first article describes why iron chelation therapy is still the mainstay of therapy for hematological diseases that require repeated transfusions to prevent iron overload. The second article presents an updated view of the molecular details of iron metabolism and some of diseases associated with defects in iron metabolism pathways.

Weaver, L. K. 2009. Clinical practice. Carbon monoxide poisoning. *New England Journal of Medicine 360*:1217–25.

▶ An excellent article on the pathogenesis, manifestations, and treatment of this condition, which is often called the "silent killer." The prevalence tends to increase when economic difficulties prevent families from having safe and effective means of providing heat during the winter. The advantages of administering oxygen under increased pressure in a hyperbaric chamber are described, although this facility may not be available in all communities.

ACSM and NCAA Joint Statement on Sickle Cell Trait and Exercise. 2013. http://www.ncaa.org/health-and-safety/medical-conditions/acsm-and-ncaa-joint-statement-sickle-cell-trait-and-exercise

Yawn, B. P., Buchanan, G. R., Afenyi-Annan, A. N., et al. 2014. Management of sickle cell disease. Summary of the 2014 evidence-based report by expert panel members. *JAMA 312*(10):1033–48.

▶ There is still both controversy and misunderstanding about the health effects of being a sickle cell disease carrier. The first reading presents a well-thought-out discussion of the effect of being a carrier on athletic participation. The second reading provides a definitive discussion of approaches to the management of sickle cell disease.

Piel, F. B., and Weatherall, D. J. 2014. The alpha thalassemias. *New England Journal of Medicine 371*:20.

Kuymar, R., Sagar, C., Sharma, D., et al. 2015. Beta-globin genes: Mutation hot-spots in the global thalassemia belt. *Hemoglobin 39*:1–8.

▶ The thalassemias have been early and continuing models for the use of molecular biology to explain human pathophysiology. Dr. Weatherall, a coauthor of the first reading, is a world authority in the area. This is an excellent introduction to the molecular biology of globin chains. The second article provides a concise summary of the current state of knowledge about beta globin gene mutations and beta thalassemia.

Odenike, O., Onida, F., and Padron, E. 2015. Myelodysplastic syndromes and myelodysplastic/myeloproliferative neoplasms: An update on risk stratification, molecular genetics and therapeutic approaches including allogeneic hematopoietic stem cell transplantation. *American Society of Clinical Oncology Education Book 35*:e398–412.

▶ The reading details approaches to myelodysplasia, "preleukemia," looking in detail at the question of when to consider therapy.

Azzato, E. M., and Bagg, A. 2015. Molecular genetic evaluation of myeloproliferative neoplasms. *International Journal of Laboratory Hematology 37*(Supp 1):61–71.

Talati, C., Ontiveros, E. P., Griffiths, E. A., et al. 2015. How we will treat chronic myeloid leukemia in 2016. *Blood Reviews 29*:137–42.

Jabbour, E., Kantarjian, H., and Cortes, J. 2015. Use of second and third generation tyrosine kinase inhibitors in the treatment of chronic myeloid leukemia: An evolving treatment paradigm. *Clinical Lymphoma, Myeloma and Leukemia 15*:323–34.

▶ The first and second articles review the molecular genetics of and current therapeutic approaches to chronic myelogenous (myeloid) leukemia. The third article looks at the continuing development of "mutation specific" therapy directed toward the BCR-ABL gene product. A good overview of what "personalized therapy" can, and cannot, do in the treatment of leukemia.

Strefford, J. C. 2015. The genomic landscape of chronic lymphocytic leukaemia: Biological and clinical implications. *British Journal of Haematology 169*:14–31.

Thompson, P. A., Shpall, E. J., and Keating, M. J. 2015. Shifting paradigms in the treatment of chronic lymphocytic leukemia. *Future Oncology 11*:641–57.

▶ Together the two readings provide a detailed overview of the current state of knowledge regarding chronic lymphocytic leukemia. CLL is generally considered uncurable, and the second reading examines this question and suggests potential new approaches to therapy.

Bhojwani, D., Yang, J. J., and Pui, C-H. 2015. Biology of childhood acute lymphoblastic leukemia. *Pediatric Clinics of North America 62*:47–60.

Cooper, S. L., and Brown, P. A. 2015. Treatment of pediatric acute lymphoblastic leukemia. *Pediatric Clinics of North America 62*:61–73.

    ▶   The treatment of childhood acute lymphoblastic leukemia is one of the great success stories of modern oncology. Increasing knowledge of the immunology and molecular biology of ALL discloses the presence of several variants that differ in prognosis and therapy. The two readings provide an overview of the current state of the art regarding the disease.

Blombery, P. A., Wall, M., and Seymour, J. F. 2015. The molecular pathogenesis of B-cell non-Hodgkin lymphoma. *European Journal of Haematology*. doi: 10.111/ejh.12589

Venkataraman, G., Mirza, M. K., Eichenauer, D. A., et al. 2014. Current status of prognostication in classical Hodgkin lymphoma. *British Journal of Haematology 165*:287–99.

    ▶   The area of lymphoma biology could, in itself, fill a book. These two readings have been selected to provide an introduction. The first reading presents an interesting overview of changing ideas about the pathogenesis of Hodgkin lymphoma and presents the modern classification scheme used in describing disease subtypes (not covered in the text).

Moore, T., and Ikeda, A. K. 2014. *Bone marrow transplantation*. http://emedicine.medscape.com/article/1014514-overview

    ▶   An excellent brief introduction to the area with a good selection of additional readings.

Abnormalities of Blood Coagulation

LEARNING OBJECTIVES

1. Contrast hemorrhage with thrombosis, describing functions and processes.
2. Describe the functions of blood vessels and platelets in controlling bleeding.
3. Explain primary hemostasis and secondary hemostasis and list the coagulation factors involved.
4. Describe the clotting cascade, including the extrinsic and intrinsic pathways.
5. Describe how to stop clotting using drug therapy.
6. List the most common clinically significant disturbances of hemostasis and describe their clinical manifestations and therapy.
7. Describe the laboratory tests used to evaluate hemostasis.

Description of Hemostasis

Hemostasis (blood clotting) is central to the tissue response to injury. Rupture of larger veins and arteries often occurs after vascular injury resulting from trauma, inflammatory or neoplastic damage, erosion of a vessel wall, or occasionally with congenital malformations of the vasculature. All may lead to **hemorrhage**, uncontrolled movement of blood into tissues, body spaces, and the gastrointestinal or urinary tract. The term **hemorrhagic diathesis** refers to a variety of clinical disorders, some congenital, some acquired, in which usually insignificant (or even unapparent) injury leads to unusual bleeding.

Normal hemostasis must accomplish two seemingly contradictory functions: the maintenance of blood in a fluid, **thrombus** (clot) free state in normal vessels and at the same time have the ability to form a localized hemostatic plug at the site of an injury. Such hemostatic plugs are referred to as thrombi, when within the body, and clots when they occur outside the body. The overall process is usually referred to as blood clotting or coagulation. **Thrombosis** is the opposite of hemorrhage, the pathologic activation of hemostasis under inappropriate conditions.

The proper functioning of the hemostasis system depends on the integrated functioning of four major components. These include integrity of the small blood vessels and their lining cells (endothelium), adequate numbers of structurally and functionally normal platelets, normal levels of humoral coagulation factors (proteins found in the blood plasma), and normal levels of coagulation inhibitors to control,

Hemostasis Process of blood clotting.

Hemorrhage Release of blood into surrounding tissue.

Hemorrhagic diathesis Variety of clinical disorders in which small injuries lead to unusual bleeding.

Thrombus Clot.

Thrombosis The pathologic activation of hemostasis under inappropriate conditions.

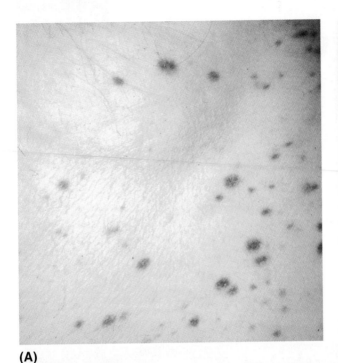

(A)

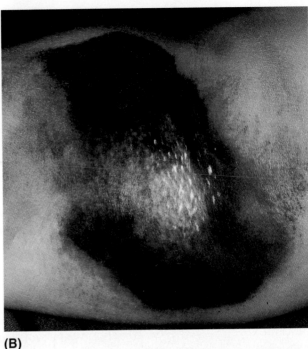

(B)

FIGURE 14-1 Characteristics of bleeding in patients with disturbed hemostatic function. **(A)** Petechial hemorrhages indicative of thrombocytopenia or defective platelet function. **(B)** A large hemorrhage (hematoma) associated with a deficiency of plasma coagulation factors.

Courtesy of Leonard V. Crowley, MD, Century College.

Hematoma Accumulation of blood within tissue.

Ecchymosis Bruise.

Hemarthrosis Hematoma within joint.

Hemothorax Hematoma within the chest.

Hemopericardium Hematoma between the heart and its pericardial lining.

Cardiac tamponade Accumulation of blood adjacent to the heart prevents normal cardiac function.

Petechia A small pinpoint hemorrhage caused by decreased platelets, abnormal platelet function, or capillary defect.

Purpura Larger hemorrhages in the skin.

localize, and terminate the hemostatic process to prevent pathologic thrombosis. Adequate concentration of calcium ions in the blood is also necessary for appropriate hemostasis (although hypocalcemia is not commonly associated with hemorrhagic symptoms).

Some specialized terminology is associated with the description of hemorrhagic processes. A **hematoma** is the accumulation of blood within tissue. It may be insignificant such as a bruise (**ecchymosis**) on a limb or life-threatening should it occur within the skull. A large accumulation of blood within a body space is a **hemarthrosis** (if within joints), **hemothorax** (within the chest), and **hemopericardium** (between the heart and its pericardial lining). Such accumulations are likely to lead to compromise of normal function. For example, a hemopericardium may lead to **cardiac tamponade**, a condition in which the accumulation of blood adjacent to the heart prevents normal cardiac function. **Petechiae** are small 1 to 2 mm pinpoint hemorrhages in the skin, mucous membrane, or serosa that are often indicative of a failure of platelet function and of capillary bleeding. **Purpura** are similar but larger (**FIGURE 14-1**).

Blood Vessels and Their Endothelial Lining

The small blood vessels are the body's first line of defense. If a vein or artery is injured, it automatically contracts (reflex vasoconstriction), facilitating closure of the vessel by a blood clot. In a normal vessel, the endothelium (the cells that line blood vessels and are in intimate contact with the blood) acts as an anticoagulant surface by secreting a variety of agents that prevent the adherence and activation of platelets. In addition, the surface of uninjured endothelium is rich in inhibitors of humoral coagulation. Injury to the vessel also leads to disruption of the endothelium, exposing the underlying connective tissue. Platelets accumulate and adhere to the subendothelium at the site

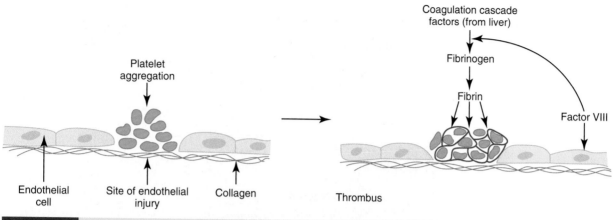

FIGURE 14-2 Platelets aggregate and stick to collagen at the site of endothelial injury.

of injury, where they plug the defect in the vessel wall, liberate vasoconstrictors and compounds that cause platelets to aggregate, and release substances (phospholipids) that initiate the process of blood coagulation (**FIGURE 14-2**).

ABNORMALITIES OF THE VESSEL WALL AND ENDOTHELIAL CELLS

In addition to physical damage (as in trauma to a vessel), other forms of injury to either the vessel or the endothelium can lead to hemorrhage and activation of hemostasis. An uncommon autosomal dominant genetic disorder, **Osler-Weber-Rendu disease (OWRD)** (also called **hereditary hemorrhagic telangiectasia [HHT]**), leads to defects in blood vessels in the body expressed as **telangiectases** (spiderlike dilations of capillaries and other small vessels) in the skin and mucous membrane as well as venous and arterial malformations that can occur in any body system. The result is the occurrence of severe spontaneous nosebleeds (**epistaxis**), gastrointestinal bleeding, and a variety of arteriovenous defects in the liver and lung. The disease tends to progress with age.

After injury, the normally anticoagulant endothelial cells can become procoagulant in function. The cells may express **tissue factor**, a protein that is a major trigger for humoral coagulation, and secrete **von Willebrand Factor (vWF)**, a very large protein that acts as a "glue" to adhere platelets to collagen in the subendothelial layer exposed on loss of endothelial cells. Lack of functional vWF, von Willebrand disease (vWD), is most commonly inherited as an autosomal dominant condition with symptoms that range from mild (often observed in female patients as excessive bruising and menstrual bleeding) to a severe hemorrhagic condition similar to hemophilia. vWD in its mildest form is perhaps the most commonly observed genetic disease associated with bleeding. Disorders in endothelial function may also be acquired as a result of vitamin C deficiency (scurvey), inflammation of the vessels (vasculitis), and as a result of infectious disease. **Rocky Mountain spotted fever** (most common in the southeastern United States) is a result of rickettsial infection of endothelial cells (**FIGURE 14-3**).

The rash and severe headache characteristic of the disease are both a result of loss of normal endothelial function and leakage of blood out of capillaries. The dreaded hemorrhagic fever viruses (such as Ebola) produce systemic hemorrhagic effect and subsequent shock by damaging the endothelium. Release of a number of substances into the circulation can lead to widespread intravascular coagulation, a life-threatening condition termed **disseminated intravascular coagulation (DIC)**, which results in paradoxical bleeding as a result of consumption of factors needed for coagulation.

Osler-Weber-Rendu disease (OWRD)/ hereditary hemorrhagic telangiectasia (HHT) Disease caused by hereditary defects in blood vessels leading to spontaneous bleeding.

Epistaxis Severe spontaneous nosebleed.

Tissue factor Protein that is a trigger for extrinsic coagulation.

von Willebrand Factor (vWF) A large protein that acts to adhere platelets to collagen.

Rocky Mountain spotted fever Disease caused by rickettsial infection of endothelial cells.

Disseminated intravascular coagulation (DIC) A disturbance of blood coagulation as a result of the uncontrolled activation of the coagulation mechanism.

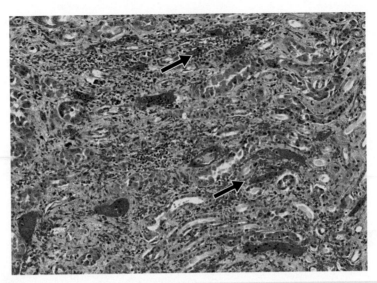

FIGURE 14-3 Kidney from a patient who died of Rocky Mountain spotted fever. There are multiple areas of hemorrhage from damaged vasculature into the renal parenchyma (*arrows*).

Courtesy of Department of Pathology and Laboratory Medicine, University of North Carolina at Chapel Hill.

Blood Vessels and Platelets

Platelets, which play an essential role in blood coagulation, are very small anucleate fragments of the cytoplasm from large precursor cells in the bone marrow called mega-karyocytes. They have an average survival in the circulation of about ten days, after which they are removed by macrophages in the spleen. Platelets contain contractile proteins and two types of granules with a variety of bioactive mediators of coagulation essential for normal platelet functions. Immediately after vessel injury, platelets adhere to the wall of the injured vessel to form a temporary "patch" at the site of injury, a process in which vWF is critical. Adhesion of platelets provokes **platelet activation** and the release reaction resulting in secretion of a number of active components. Serotonin (a histamine-like substance) causes vasoconstriction. In addition, several **platelet agonists** (substances that promote platelet function), including ADP and thromboxane A2 (a lipid derived prostaglandin-like substance), are released. These substances promote platelet–platelet aggregation (in part by binding to the plasma protein fibrinogen that forms bridges between platelets) and recruit additional platelets from the circulation. In addition, platelets dramatically change their shape, much increasing their surface area. This mass of aggregated platelets is termed the **primary hemostatic plug**, which initially controls bleeding but can be reversed or washed away. The formation of the primary hemostatic plug defines what is often termed **primary hemostasis**, that part of the hemostatic process that does not involve the humoral coagulation factors.

Aggregated platelets express negatively charged phospholipids on their surface. Such phospholipids are critical surfaces on which **secondary hemostasis** is carried out. This process involves the plasma coagulation factors, a series of inactive enzymes and cofactors that assemble in the presence of the phospholipid surface and calcium ions to produce active enzymes. Early in this process, the enzyme **thrombin** is produced from its precursor prothrombin. Thrombin plays a critical role in secondary hemostasis (humoral coagulation). However, some of the earliest thrombin produced binds to a specific receptor on the aggregated platelets, resulting in platelet contraction and formation of an irreversibly fused collection of platelets and fibrinogen. This mass forms the stable **secondary hemostatic plug**, which along with the adhesive fibrous protein **fibrin** (formed from fibrinogen by the action of thrombin) are the major components of the mature thrombus. But note that formation of the mature thrombus requires the interaction of humoral coagulation factors.

Platelet activation Release of active clotting components after adhesion of platelets.

Platelet agonists Substances promoting platelet function.

Primary hemostatic plug Mass of aggregated platelets at site of injury.

Primary hemostasis Part of hemostatic process that is mostly platelet dependent.

Secondary hemostasis Process involving plasma coagulation factors.

Thrombin A coagulation factor formed by activation of prothrombin in the process of blood coagulation.

Secondary hemostatic plug Formation of mature thrombus along with fibrin.

Fibrin The meshwork of protein threads that form during the clotting of blood.

ABNORMALITIES OF PLATELET NUMBERS OR FUNCTION

A decrease in platelets, called **thrombocytopenia** (*thrombus* = clot + *cyte* = cell + *penia* = deficiency), may be a result of injury or disease of the bone marrow that damages the megakaryocytes in the marrow, the precursor cells of the platelets. Thrombocytopenia may also occur because the bone marrow has been infiltrated by leukemic cells or by cancer cells that have spread to the skeletal system, crowding out the megakaryocytes, or because antiplatelet autoantibodies destroy the platelets in the peripheral blood (as seen in some autoimmune diseases). The most common cause of thrombocytopenia is **iatrogenic** (medically caused) as a result of cytotoxic therapy used in cancer treatment, which damages the bone marrow. Use of non-steroidal anti-inflammatory drugs (such as aspirin) blocks the synthesis of thromboxane and interferes with platelet function. Sometimes platelets are normal in quantity but abnormal in function and cannot initiate the clotting process. Bleeding associated with defective or inadequate platelets is generally manifested by small petechial hemorrhages rather than by large areas of hemorrhage; however, a major diminution of platelet number and function can result in severe hemorrhage and may be treated by platelet transfusions.

Plasma Coagulation Factors

The blood plasma contains a number of different proteins called coagulation factors, now designated by Roman numerals (and occasionally by historical names). The process of blood coagulation resembles a chain reaction or cascade in which each component of the chain is formed from an inactive precursor in the blood, and each activated component in turn activates the next member of the chain. Critical to the process is the presence of a negatively charged phospholipid surface (mostly platelet derived) on which the reactions take place, and the calcium ion that "anchors" certain of the factors to the surface. The process of humoral coagulation is most often divided into two pathways of activation that come together into a common pathway. This is presented in a simplified and abbreviated manner to clarify a complex process (**FIGURE 14-4**). Humoral coagulation can be activated via either an **extrinsic pathway** (so named because it was believed to need substances outside the vascular system for activation) or an **intrinsic pathway** (because all the substances necessary for activation were felt to be "intrinsic" to the vessels). Activation of the extrinsic pathway is now considered to be the key step in triggering humoral coagulation.

Factor VII (F.VII) is normally present in the plasma as an inactive enzyme. However, in the presence of tissue factor (normally present in the tissue surrounding the blood vessel or turned on in a damaged endothelial cell), F.VII becomes active and in turn activates another proenzyme, F.X, to an active enzyme, F.Xa. F.Xa in turn activates **prothrombin** (also called F.II) to release the critical enzyme thrombin (sometimes called F.IIa). This is the same thrombin molecule described earlier in relation to its role in platelet activation, but the protease has several other critical functions. Thrombin removes small peptides from the **fibrinogen** molecule (a soluble protein synthesized in the liver), converting it into the insoluble fibrous protein fibrin, which forms the bulk of the mature clot. Plasma F.XIII, which must be activated by thrombin, acts on the fibrin clot by forming bonds between the fibrin molecules, increasing the strength and stability of the clot. Another critical function of thrombin is to activate two nonprotease "cofactors" critical in humoral coagulation, F.V and F.VIII. When activated by thrombin, the cofactors speed up the coagulation process by many thousandfold. For example, active F.V (F.Va) "orients" F.Xa and prothrombin on the phospholipid surface in the presence of the calcium ion, which speeds up the enzymatic reaction producing thrombin.

Thrombocytopenia
A deficiency of platelets.

Iatrogenic Condition that is medically caused.

Extrinsic pathway Clotting process needing substances outside the vascular system for activation.

Intrinsic pathway Clotting process needing only substances within the blood vessels.

Prothrombin Clotting factor activated by factor X to release thrombin/F.IIa.

Fibrinogen A precursor in plasma converted into fibrin by thrombin during blood coagulation.

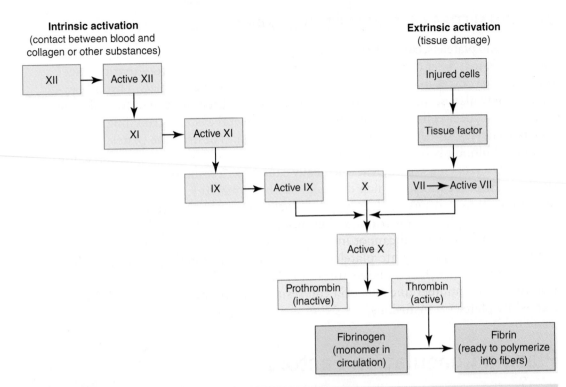

Intrinsic activation
(contact between blood and
collagen or other substances)

Extrinsic activation
(tissue damage)

FIGURE 14-4 A simplified view of the clotting cascade. Note that Factors VIII and V are not shown although critical for normal hemostasis.

The intrinsic pathway is an alternative (and critical) second method of generating F.Xa (and hence thrombin). The exact steps in intrinsic pathway activation are complex, but basically the inactive protease F.XII becomes active XIIa in the presence of collagen and other surfaces. FXIIa activates F.XI to F.XIa, which in turn activates the protease F.IX to F.IXa. In a manner analogous to F.Xa activating prothrombin (in the presence of F.Va), F.IXa activates F.X to F.Xa in the presence of the cofactor F.VIIIa. Once again, the cofactor F.VIIIa is critical to speed up the reaction. This part of the intrinsic pathway is associated with two relatively common serious hemorrhagic diseases. Lack of active F.VIII causes **hemophilia A**; lack of active F.IX causes **hemophilia B**.

Coagulation Inhibitors and Fibrinolysis

Coagulation factors are counterbalanced by various coagulation inhibitors that restrict the clotting process to a limited area. Coagulation inhibitors protein C and protein S function together to inactivate two coagulation factors (Va and VIIIa). Another important member of this group is antithrombin III, which inhibits not only thrombin but also several other activated coagulation factors generated in the clotting process.

An equally important control system is one that digests fibrin after it has formed. A precursor compound in blood plasma called **plasminogen** is activated to form **plasmin**, which dissolves fibrin in blood clots. The **fibrinolytic system** is activated at the same time that the coagulation process is initiated, and thrombin produced in the coagulation process also activates this system. Another important plasminogen activator is a substance called tissue plasminogen activator (TPA), which is released from endothelial cells in the region where the clot is forming. As described in the discussion on cardiovascular system, tissue plasminogen activator or another plasminogen activator called streptokinase, produced by streptococci, is administered intravenously to dissolve blood clots in the coronary arteries of patients who have had a recent heart attack. Administration of one of these plasminogen activators within

Hemophilia A Bleeding disease caused by lack of active F.VIII.

Hemophilia B Bleeding disease caused by lack of active F.IX.

Plasminogen Precursor compound of plasmin in the blood.

Plasmin Blood enzyme that degrades blood plasma proteins including fibrin clots.

Fibrinolytic system Process of breaking down clots.

a few hours after onset of symptoms dissolves the clot and restores flow through the artery, which minimizes heart muscle damage resulting from the blockage.

Calcium and Blood Coagulation

Adequate amounts of calcium ions (Ca^{2+}) are required in all phases of blood coagulation because blood will not clot in the absence of calcium. Calcium levels sufficiently low to affect blood coagulation are most often incompatible with life.

Deficiency of Plasma Coagulation Factors

Deficiencies of factors concerned with the humoral phase of coagulation are usually hereditary and are relatively rare. Only three hereditary bleeding diseases occur with any frequency.

Hemophilia A (F.VIII deficiency) and B (F.IX deficiency), X-linked hereditary diseases affecting males and only rarely females, are the most common and best known hereditary bleeding diseases. The inheritance of these conditions is considered in the discussion on congenital and hereditary diseases. Clinically, the diseases are characterized by episodes of hemorrhage in joints and internal organs after minor injury and at times life-threatening intracerebral bleeds. Both Hemophilia A and B have the same clinical manifestations. Serious symptoms occur in patients when the levels of the proteins fall below 5 percent of normal. Mild forms of the disease are only detected by chance. The most common, hemophilia A or classic hemophilia, is characterized by a decrease in coagulation factor VIII (also called antihemophilic factor). The less common form of hemophilia is hemophilia B, or Christmas disease. It is caused by a deficiency of coagulation factor IX, which is also called Christmas factor (named after an affected patient, not the holiday). Factor IX, is synthesized by hepatocytes within the liver in the liver. F.VIII is synthesized in several organs but predominantly in the liver by a population of endothelial cells.

A third previously mentioned hereditary bleeding disease, vWD, is important in both primary and secondary hemostasis. The disease when severe also is characterized by excessive bleeding after a minor injury, but usually the bleeding is not in the joints, as is characteristic of hemophilia. The protein is synthesized in endothelial cells and released into the bloodstream where it forms a complex in the circulation with factor VIII, which is required to maintain a normal level of factor VIII in the blood. For this reason, the level of factor VIII is often low in patients with von Willebrand disease, although synthesis of F.VIII is normal.

Patients with hemophilia A, hemophilia B, and von Willebrand disease who have bleeding episodes can be treated by administration of factor concentrates prepared from human blood plasma or using recombinant DNA technology. Early studies using gene therapy to cure or ameliorate hemophilia B have shown some preliminary promise.

A number of coagulation factors, including F.II, VII, IX, and X and the inhibitor of coagulation protein C (called vitamin K–dependent factors), are produced in the liver. Vitamin K, required for the synthesis of these factors in an active form, is synthesized by intestinal bacteria and also can be obtained from foods, especially green leafy vegetables. It is a fat-soluble vitamin, requiring bile for its absorption. The vitamin is required for a secondary, postsynthetic modification of certain glutamic acid residues (gamma carboxylation), which is necessary for calcium ion binding, and the lack or deficiency in this vitamin can result in a bleeding disease. Inadequate synthesis of vitamin K may occurs if the intestinal bacteria have been eradicated by prolonged antibiotic therapy, as sometimes occurs in seriously ill, hospitalized patients. Another cause of inadequate uptake of vitamin K is blockage of the common bile duct by a gallstone or tumor, preventing bile from entering the intestine to promote absorption of the vitamin. Yet another vitamin K–deficient group is newborn infants who lack the intestinal bacteria to make the vitamin and are not yet eating foods that contain the vitamin. They are at risk for serious bleeding called hemorrhagic disease of the newborn. To prevent this condition, all newborn infants routinely receive a vitamin K injection to prevent spontaneous bleeding caused by lack of the vitamin.

Patients with severe liver diseases have deficiencies and may have a bleeding tendency because the liver is so badly damaged that it can no longer synthesize adequate amounts of coagulation factors.

Anticoagulant drugs such as Coumadin, warfarin, and similar compounds are sometimes used to treat patients with an increased tendency to develop blood clots in their leg veins, such as patients having a total hip or total knee replacement procedure or other surgical procedures that increase their risk of forming leg vein clots. The drug is also given to patients with some types of heart disease in which blood clots tend to form within the cardiac chambers and to patients with some types of artificial heart valves to prevent clot formation within the artificial valve, which would disrupt the function of the valve. The amount of warfarin or related anticoagulant given to the patient must be monitored closely to reduce blood coagulability sufficiently to prevent unwanted blood clots forming in the heart chambers, leg veins, or other locations without reducing the coagulation factors to such an extent that spontaneous bleeding occurs. Warfarin-like anticoagulant drugs act by inhibiting the synthesis of biochemically active vitamin K–dependent factors. Intramuscular administration of vitamin K corrects coagulation disturbances resulting from such anticoagulants, inadequate synthesis of vitamin K, or insufficient absorption of the vitamin. The coagulation disturbance associated with severe liver disease does not respond because the diseased liver is no longer capable of synthesizing sufficient coagulation factors to provide efficient hemostasis.

Heparin, a sulfated glycosaminoglycan, is also a commonly used antithrombotic drug that functions by complexing with the inhibitor protein antithrombin III, potentiating its ability to inhibit F.X and thrombin. A major drawback is that heparin must be injected and may be associated with serious thrombotic side effects. A number of other anticoagulant drugs are available that may have advantages over warfarin-like drugs in specific clinical situations. Some newer anticoagulant drugs act by interfering with thrombin or factor X in the humoral phase of blood coagulation. Such anticoagulants can be given as a standard daily dose without requiring laboratory tests, which simplifies the patient's treatment.

Liberation of Procoagulant Material into The Circulation

In a number of diseases associated with shock, overwhelming or toxin producing bacterial infection, products of tissue necrosis and other substances (such as amniotic fluid postpartum) are liberated into the circulation, leading to widespread intravascular coagulation of the blood. This may result because the direct procoagulant activity of the material in circulation activates intrinsic coagulation or because the inciting agent damages endothelial cells causing them to express tissue factor and activating extrinsic coagulation (**FIGURE 14-5**). Because clotting uses platelets and the various plasma coagulation factors, the levels of these components in the blood drop precipitously, resulting in a hemorrhagic state.

To defend itself against widespread intravascular clotting, the body activates the fibrinolytic system, which dissolves clots and reduces the potential for obstruction of

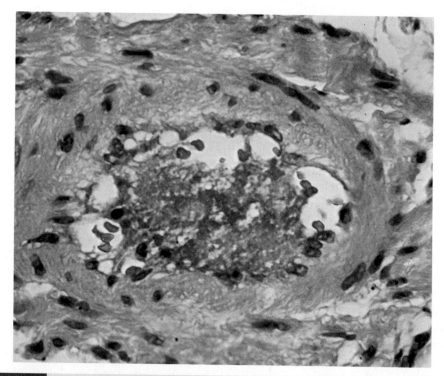

FIGURE 14-5 Fibrin thrombus in small blood vessel of a patient with disseminated intravascular coagulation syndrome (original magnification ×400).

Courtesy of Leonard V. Crowley, MD, Century College.

the circulatory system by massive intravascular coagulation. The breakdown products produced during degradation of the fibrin (fibrinopeptides) act as additional inhibitors of the clotting process.

The net effect of this abnormal bleeding state is called disseminated intravascular coagulation syndrome, or **consumption coagulopathy**. The latter term alludes to consumption of the clotting factors as a result of the pathogenic coagulation process. **FIGURE 14-6** summarizes the pathogenesis of this bleeding syndrome. Although

Consumption coagulopathy See disseminated intravascular coagulation.

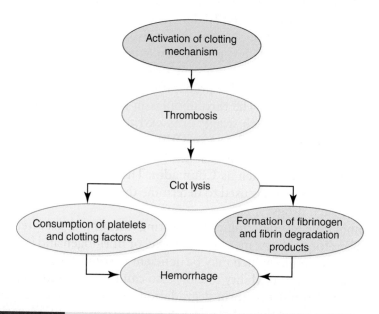

FIGURE 14-6 Pathogenesis of disseminated intravascular coagulation syndrome.

expressed as a hemorrhagic state, the inciting cause is the widespread intravascular triggering of thrombosis.

Laboratory Tests to Evaluate Hemostasis

Several laboratory tests can evaluate the overall efficiency of the coagulation process, detect the presence of inhibitors of coagulation, and estimate the number and function of the platelets. These tests include the blood smear, bleeding time, and tests of the time it takes for plasma to clot.

The number of platelets in the blood can be estimated by examining the blood smear, and more precise data can be obtained by using automated blood cell counting devices. Special tests (platelet aggregometry) also are available to evaluate the ability of platelets to aggregate in the presence of agonists such as thromboxane and thrombin. The function of both capillaries and vWF in the hemostatic process is evaluated by measuring the time it takes for a small, standardized skin incision to stop bleeding, a test termed the **bleeding time**. Both platelet function tests and the bleeding time are extremely sensitive to the use of NSAIDs (such as aspirin), and patients must refrain from their use for a period of time prior to testing.

Several tests are used to evaluate the various proteins concerned with blood coagulation (coagulation factors) and to monitor the efficacy of anticoagulant therapy by warfarin-like drugs such as Coumadin. The tests, performed on plasma obtained from blood collected in tubes containing the anticoagulant citrate (which functions by binding calcium ion), are the **partial thromboplastin time (PTT)**, or more often the activated partial thromboplastin time (aPTT), the **prothrombin time (PT)**, and the **thrombin time**. Each test measures a different part of the coagulation process. When the tests are used together, the location of the coagulation factor deficiency can be identified if any of the tests yield an abnormal result.

The activated partial thromboplastin time (aPTT) test measures the time it takes for blood plasma to clot after a lipid substance and an activating agent such as silica is added to the plasma along with calcium to start the clotting process. The lipid added is similar to the lipid material released from platelets to initiate secondary hemostasis, and the activating agent substitutes for the activation that occurs in intrinsic coagulation. The aPTT is most often used to measure defects in the intrinsic pathway of coagulation (F.IX and F.VIII deficiency in particular) and to monitor the effect of heparin anticoagulation, but the test is also sensitive to defects in the common part of the pathways (F.X, F.V, prothrombin, and fibrinogen).

The prothrombin time test measures the time it takes for blood plasma to clot after adding a commercially available preparation (thromboplastin) along with calcium to start the coagulation. The thromboplastin added mimics the tissue factor and platelet derived lipid, which triggers the extrinsic pathway of coagulation. A prolonged PT is indicative of a defect in F.VII or the above-mentioned factors in the common pathway. However, the real utility of the PT is measuring the effect of warfarin-like anticoagulants such as Coumadin. The PT test is designed by manufacturers for this purpose and is used to determine the INR, a standardized measure of the efficacy of such drugs.

The thrombin time test determines the clotting time of plasma after the addition of thrombin. Therefore, the test measures the level of fibrinogen and its ability to clot in the presence of thrombin, which may be deficient in some conditions. The level of fibrinogen (irrespective of its ability to clot) also can be measured directly by other tests, and one can also test for fibrin degradation products, which are increased if fibrinolysis is excessive and thrombosis is occurring such as in DIC. A variety of tests

---

Bleeding time Time needed for a small standardized skin incision to stop bleeding.

Partial thromboplastin time (PTT) test A test that measures the overall efficiency of the blood coagulation process. Detects defects in intrinsic coagulation and is used to monitor heparin therapy.

Prothrombin time (PT) test A test that detects defects in extrinsic coagulation and is used to monitor warfarin-like anticoagulant therapy.

Thrombin time test A laboratory test measurement that determines the concentration of fibrinogen in the blood by determining the clotting time of the blood plasma after addition of thrombin.

can be used to measure the activity of specific coagulation factors. For example, the plasma of patients suspected of having hemophilia with an abnormally prolonged aPTT can be tested for specific levels of F.VIII and F.IX to determine whether they have hemophilia A or B, an important distinction for choosing appropriate therapy. Uncommonly, some individuals (such as hemophiliacs lacking a particular coagulation factor and occasionally otherwise normal individuals) may produce antibodies (termed inhibitors) against the therapeutically infused replacement factor (or as part of an autoimmune response to an endogenous coagulation factor). Laboratory tests for such inhibitors involve mixing patient and normal plasma prior to aPTT testing to determine whether the patient plasma will reduce the activity of coagulation factors in the normal plasma.

CASE 14-1

John is a four-year-old child who goes with his family on a trip to visit a farm. During the trip, he drinks a glass of raw (unpasteurized) milk fresh from the cow. His father objects, but his mother, noting that the farm is "organic," encourages him to drink. Late in the next day John complains to his mother that he feels warm. She notes an oral temperature of 102°F (38.9°C) and treats him with acetaminophen. John develops diarrhea and complains of stomach pain. His pediatrician diagnosis gastroenteritis (believing it to be reovirus, which was currently affecting children in John's day care) and suggests food restriction, fluid replacement, and alternating ibuprofen and acetaminophen for fever control.

John's parents become increasing concerned. There are traces of blood in the child's stool, and he is becoming lethargic. On day four of John's illness, his parents note that he is pale, his face has become puffy, and he seems to be urinating very little, if at all (is becoming **anuric**). Alarmed, John's pediatrician has him admitted to a local hospital.

At the local hospital John is found to be hypertensive, and tests of kidney function disclose acute renal failure with elevated levels of serum creatinine. Blood studies are abnormal with a low platelet count, decreased levels of several coagulation factors including fibrinogen, and elevated levels of fibrin degradation products. A peripheral blood smear shows that several percent of the red cells are **schistocytes** (fragmented irregular cells). Stool culture shows *E. coli O157:H7*. John remains hospitalized for several days, and his blood electrolyte levels, renal function, and platelet count are carefully monitored. His hydration status is checked to maintain normal fluid volume. He is treated with an antihypertensive drug (a calcium channel blocker). Renal dialysis is considered, but John slowly begins to recover renal function. He is discharged with frequent follow-up visits to monitor his continuing renal function.

Discussion

The case is a classic presentation of Shiga toxin producing *E. coli* induced **hemolytic uremic syndrome (STEC-HUS)**, predominantly a pediatric disease usually occurring in children between one and four years of age. This is most frequently caused by *E. coli* 0157:H7, an **enterohemorrhagic** strain of the bacteria that produces an enterotoxin (a bacterial secreted toxin that targets the gastrointestinal tract). A similar toxin is produced by the *Shigella* species of bacteria responsible for types of bacterial dysentery (hence the term "shiga toxin"). The bacteria *E. coli* 0157:H7 is very resistant and may contaminate the environment for months. Most cases of STEC-HUS are related to meat or milk products contaminated with animal waste, and cattle are the major reservoir. Contaminated raw milk would be a likely source in this case. About 10 percent of children infected with *E. coli* 0157:H7 will develop STEC-HUS. The disease presents with three sets of abnormalities: (1) **microangiopathic anemia**, a type

Anuric Forms little or no urine.

Microangiopathic anemia A type of anemia related to mechanical damage of red cells as they pass through thrombosed or otherwise damaged small blood vessels.

(continues)

CASE 14-1 *(Continued)*

of anemia related to mechanical damage of red cells as they pass through thrombosed or otherwise damaged small blood vessels, (2) thrombocytopenia, and (3) acute renal failure.

The abnormalities are all related to the effect of the Shiga toxins produced by the bacteria. The toxin is produced by bacteria that adhere to the gut wall and is absorbed from the inflamed colon. Subsequently, the toxin binds to vascular endothelial cells predominantly in the gut and kidney. The toxin damaged endothelial cells become prothrombotic, leading to platelet adhesion and aggregation and the formation of microthrombi within the vasculature of the kidney. The damaged endothelium and adherent fibrin thrombi shear red cells as they flow through, resulting in the microangiopathc anemia characterized by the presence of damaged red cells (schistocytes). The disseminated intrarenal thrombosis leads to consumption of platelets (hence thrombocytopenia) and also of coagulation factors. Fibrinolysis of the microthrombi leads to the presence of fibrin degradation products. The vascular damage to the kidney results in acute renal failure (**FIGURE 14-7**).

Etiology and Pathogenesis

Infection with a shiga toxin producing strain of bacteria *E. coli* 0157:H7 resulting in STEC hemolytic uremic syndrome. STEC-HUS can be seen as a renal/gut limited form of disseminated intravascular coagulation.

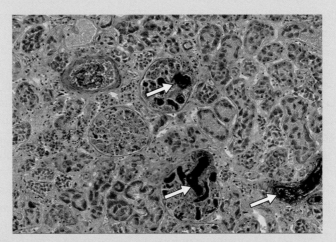

FIGURE 14-7 Kidney from a patient suffering from bacterial hemolytic uremic syndrome. A special stain to highlight fibrin has been used. Thrombi are visible in renal (glomerular) capillaries and small vessels (*arrows*).

Courtesy of Department of Pathology and Laboratory Medicine, University of North Carolina at Chapel Hill.

Questions

1. What preventative measures should be undertaken to prevent infection by food-borne enteropathic bacteria?

2. Some advocates suggest that the production of antibiotic-free beef will lower the incidence of *E. coli* 0157:H7 infections. Do you believe there is any potential validity to the claim?

3. STEC-HUS may be seen as a localized form of DIC. Support this contention.

4. STEC-HUS initially can be diagnosed using a simple blood-based test that can be done in many doctors' offices. What is the test, and how is it used to make the diagnosis?

QUESTIONS FOR REVIEW

1. How does blood clot?

2. What are some of the common disturbances of blood coagulation?

3. What is thrombocytopenia? What type of bleeding is produced when platelets are markedly reduced? What types of diseases are associated with thrombocytopenia?

4. What types of diseases produce abnormalities in primary hemostasis?

5. What is the consequence of liberation of procoagulant material into the circulation?

6. What laboratory tests are used to evaluate the coagulation of blood?

7. A patient with a bleeding tendency has a prolonged activated partial thromboplastin time (aPTT) with a normal prothrombin time. In what phase of the clotting process is the disturbance located? What is one possible disease that could produce these findings?

8. What are the effects of Coumadin anticoagulants on the clotting mechanism? How do they work? What laboratory test can be used to monitor the effect of the anticoagulant?

SUPPLEMENTARY READINGS

Kumar, V., Abbas, A. K., Fausto, N., et al. 2014. *Robbins and Cotran Pathologic Basis of Disease.* 9th ed. Philadelphia, PA: Elsevier Saunders.

www.practical-haemostasis.com
- ► Few resources do a good job of explaining the complexities of hemostasis. The first entry is a classic that has particularly well-detailed figures to complement the text. The second entry is an excellent website that provides details on laboratory testing for hemostatic disorders.

James, P. D., and Lillicrap, D. 2013. The molecular characterization of von Willebrand disease: Good in parts. *British Journal of Hematology 161*:166–76.
- ► This reference provides a clear introduction to the complexities of von Willebrand disease, a far more complex disease than the discussion in this chapter suggests.

Funk, D. M. 2012. Coagulation assays and anticoagulant monitoring. *American Society of Hematology* (Education Book) *2012*:460–65. http://asheducationbook.hematologylibrary.org/content/2012/1/460.long
- ► An introduction to the many new drugs used in anticoagulant and how their effect is measured in the laboratory.

High, K. H., et al. 2014. Current status of haemophilia gene therapy, *Haemophilia Supplement 4*:43–49.
- ► A recent review by leaders in the field.

The Respiratory System

1. Explain the basic anatomic and physiologic principles of ventilation and gas exchange.
2. Describe the physiological basis and use of pulmonary function tests.
3. Describe the causes, clinical effects, complications, and treatment of pneumothorax and atelectasis.
4. Describe the clinical symptoms, complications, and treatment of pneumonia.
5. Describe the histologic characteristics of a tuberculous infection. Explain the possible outcome of an infection. Describe methods of diagnosis and treatment.
6. Differentiate between bronchitis and bronchiectasis.
7. List the anatomic and physiologic derangements in chronic obstructive lung disease. Explain its pathogenesis. Describe the clinical manifestations and methods of treatment.
8. Describe the pathogenesis and manifestations of bronchial asthma and respiratory distress syndrome.
9. Explain the causes and effects of pulmonary fibrosis. Describe the special problems associated with asbestosis.
10. List the major types of lung carcinoma. Describe the clinical manifestations of lung carcinoma and explain the principles of treatment.

Oxygen Delivery: A Cooperative Effort

Normal life processes require that an adequate supply of oxygen be delivered to the tissues and that the volatile waste products of cell metabolism be removed. These functions are carried out by a cooperative effort of the respiratory and circulatory systems. The respiratory system oxygenates the blood and removes carbon dioxide. The circulatory system transports these gases in the bloodstream.

Structure and Function of the Lungs

The lungs consist of two distinct components: a system of tubes whose chief function is to conduct air into and out of the lungs and the **alveoli** (singular, alveolus), where oxygen and carbon dioxide are exchanged between air and the pulmonary capillaries. Just as a tree branches progressively and ends in a foliage of leaves, so the conducting tubes branch repeatedly and terminate in clusters of pulmonary alveoli. The lung is divided into several large segments called lobes. Each lobe in turn consists of a large number of smaller units called lobules. The architecture and structural features of a normal lung

> **Alveoli/alveolus** One of the terminal air sacs of the lung.

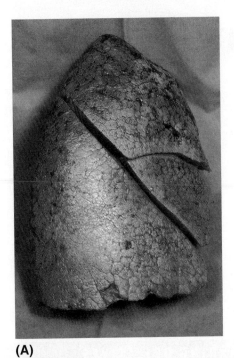
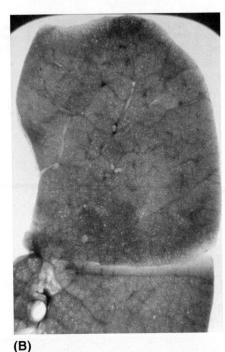

(A) **(B)**

FIGURE 15-1 Normal lung that has been inflated and air dried so that the structure of the lobes and lobules can be visualized and the fine structure of the alveoli can be studied. **(A)** External surface illustrating lobes and fissures. The faint cobblestone-like pattern of the pleural surface defines the individual lung lobules. **(B)** A backlighted section of lung illustrating the fine, sponge-like pattern produced by the respiratory units where gas exchange occurs.

Courtesy of Leonard V. Crowley, MD, Century College.

can be studied to best advantage when the lung is inflated and air dried (**FIGURE 15-1A**). The individual lobes, fissures, and pleural surfaces are well defined. The poorly defined cobblestone-like pattern of the pleural surface defines the location of the individual lung lobules, which frequently are accentuated by environmental carbon pigment deposited in the connective tissue that surrounds and circumscribes the individual lobules, a process termed **anthracosis**. When sections of normal air-dried lung are examined against an illuminated background, the spongelike, fine structure of a normal lung, which is essential for normal gas exchange (**FIGURE 15-1B**), can be examined.

BRONCHI, BRONCHIOLES, AND ALVEOLI

The largest conducting tubes are called **bronchi** (singular, bronchus). Tubes less than about 1 mm in diameter are called **bronchioles** (little bronchi), and the smallest bronchioles, which function only for conduction of air, are called terminal bronchioles. The tubes distal to the terminal bronchioles are called respiratory bronchioles because they have alveoli in their walls and not only transport air but also participate in gas exchange. Each terminal bronchiole gives rise to several respiratory bronchioles, which branch to form alveolar ducts. The alveolar ducts in turn subdivide into alveolar sacs, and multiple alveoli open into each alveolar sac (**FIGURE 15-2A** and **FIGURE 15-2B**).

Each alveolus is a small air space surrounded by a thin wall, the alveolar septum, which consists of thin-walled capillaries supported by a few connective tissue fibers and lined by a layer of epithelial cells (**FIGURE 15-2C**). Hence, the air in the alveolus is closely apposed to the circulation by a single layer of cells lining the alveolus, a basement membrane, and the endothelial cells lining the alveolus. Each alveolus

Anthracosis Carbon pigment deposited in the connective tissue around the individual lobules of lung.

Bronchi/bronchus One of the large subdivisions of the trachea.

Bronchiole One of the small terminal subdivisions of the branched bronchial tree.

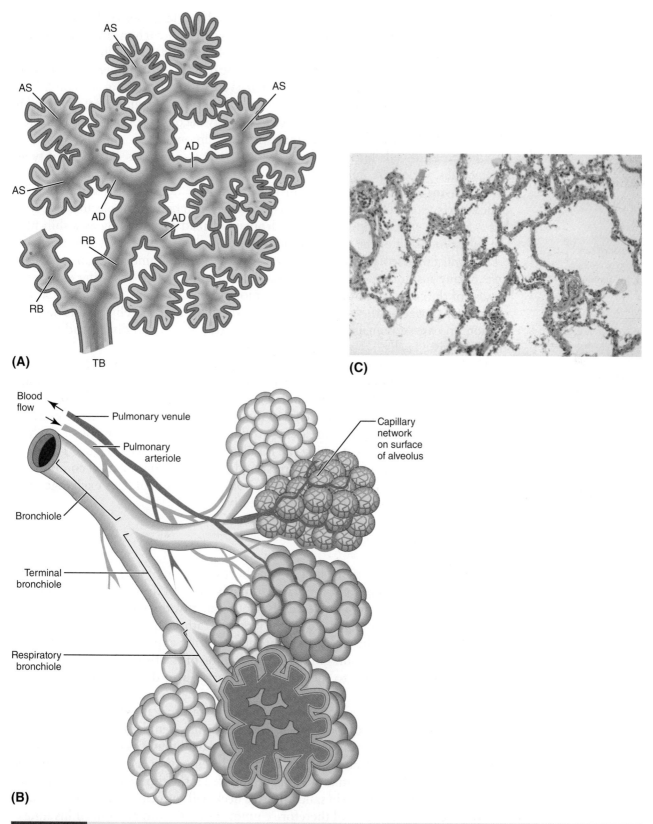

FIGURE 15-2 **(A)** Structure of a respiratory unit. Representative terminal bronchiole are designated TB. Respiratory bronchiole (RB) has alveolar sacs projecting from the wall of the bronchiole. Alveolar ducts are designated AD, and alveolar sacs are designated AS. Multiple alveoli (not labeled) open into each alveolar sac. **(B)** Structure of terminal air passages. The interior of one alveolar duct is illustrated in cutaway view. **(C)** Histologic structure of the lung illustrating alveoli and thin alveolar septa containing pulmonary capillaries (original magnification ×100).

Courtesy of Leonard V. Crowley, MD, Century College.

contains a relatively small volume of air surrounded by a large network of capillaries, conditions that promote rapid diffusion of oxygen and carbon dioxide between alveolar air and pulmonary capillaries as the blood flows through the lung. Any condition that enlarges the pulmonary alveoli or reduces the number of pulmonary capillaries impedes the efficiency of pulmonary ventilation. Under normal conditions, the connective tissue supporting the alveolar capillaries is insignificant; however, in some diseases, this interstitial connective tissue may become prominent and interfere with gas exchange, for example, in interstitial pneumonia.

Two types of cells line the alveoli. Most are flat squamous cells termed **type I pneumocytes**, which are important in gas exchange. A few are larger cuboidal **type II pneumocytes**, secretory cells that produce a lipid material called **surfactant** that reduces surface tension. Surface tension is the attraction between molecules of a fluid that causes the fluid to aggregate into droplets instead of spreading as a thin film. The surface tension of the molecules in the fluid lining the alveoli would normally tend to pull the alveolar walls together. This effect would hinder expansion of the lungs during inspiration and would cause the alveoli to collapse during expiration because of the cohesive force of the water molecules. Surfactant acts somewhat like a detergent, lowering the surface tension of the fluid and thereby facilitating respiration. In case of damage to type I pneumocytes, type II can divide and produce additional type I cells.

The functional unit of the lung is called a **respiratory unit**. It is formed by the cluster of respiratory bronchioles, alveolar ducts and sacs, and alveoli derived from a single terminal bronchiole. A **lung lobule** consists of a small group of terminal bronchioles and the respiratory units that arise from them. Lobules are partially circumscribed by connective tissue septa and are easiest to identify just beneath the pleura, where the connective tissue septa defining the lobules can be easily seen (Figure 15-1A).

Respiration has two functions, corresponding to the two structural components of the lungs, ventilation and gas exchange. Both ventilation and gas exchange must function normally if respiration is to be effective.

Type I pneumocytes/type II pneumocytes Cells lining the alveoli.

Surfactant A lipid material secreted by type II pneumocytes that facilitates respiration by decreasing the surface tension of the fluid lining the pulmonary alveoli.

Respiratory unit A functional unit of the lung consisting of a cluster of respiratory bronchioles, alveolar ducts, and alveoli derived from a single terminal bronchiole. Another term for acinus.

Lung lobule A small group of terminal bronchioles and their subdivisions.

VENTILATION

Air is moved into and out of the lungs by the bellows action of the thoracic cage. During inspiration, the ribs become more horizontal because of the action of the intercostal muscles, and the diaphragm descends. Consequently, the volume of the thoracic cage increases. The lungs expand to fill the larger intrathoracic space, and air is drawn into the lungs through the trachea and bronchi. During expiration, the ribs become more vertical, and the diaphragm rises. The volume of the thoracic cage is reduced. The lungs, which conform to the size of the thorax, also decrease in volume, and air is expelled.

Normal respiratory movements require that respiratory muscles, innervation of the muscles, and mobility of the thoracic cage be normal. Ventilation is impaired if the nerve supply to the respiratory muscles is damaged by disease, as in poliomyelitis, or if the respiratory muscles undergo atrophy and degeneration, as in some uncommon types of muscle disease. Ventilation is also impaired if the thoracic cage is immobile. For example, a person buried in sand up to his neck will suffocate because he is unable to move his thoracic cage and therefore cannot move air into and out of his lungs.

GAS EXCHANGE

Oxygen and carbon dioxide, along with nitrogen and water vapor, are in the atmospheric air that we breathe, in the air within the pulmonary alveoli, and in the blood.

At sea level, the atmospheric pressure exerted by the mixture of all the gases is 760 mm Hg. Each gas exerts a proportionate part of the total atmospheric pressure, depending on its concentration in the mixture of gases. For example, the concentration of oxygen in atmospheric air is 20 percent. Therefore, the pressure exerted by oxygen is 20 percent of the total pressure exerted by all the gases ($0.20 \times 760 = 152$ mm Hg). The part of the total atmospheric pressure exerted by a gas is called the partial pressure of the gas. Partial pressure is usually expressed by the letter "P" preceding the chemical symbol for the gas as, for example, PO_2 152 mm Hg.

Gases diffuse between blood, tissues, and pulmonary alveoli because of differences in their partial pressures. Venous blood returning from the tissues is low in oxygen (PO_2 40 mm Hg) and high in carbon dioxide (PCO_2 47 mm Hg). This blood is pumped through the pulmonary capillaries, where it comes into contact with the air in the pulmonary alveoli. Alveolar air has a much higher concentration of oxygen (PO_2 105 mm Hg) but a lower concentration of carbon dioxide (PCO_2 35 mm Hg). Therefore, oxygen diffuses from alveolar air into pulmonary capillaries, and carbon dioxide diffuses from pulmonary capillaries into the alveoli. The situation is reversed in the tissues. The tissue oxygen concentration is much lower (PO_2 about 20 mm Hg), and the carbon dioxide concentration is much higher (PCO_2 about 60 mm Hg); so oxygen diffuses into the tissues from the blood, and carbon dioxide diffuses in the opposite direction.

Carbonic acid represents physically dissolved carbon dioxide in plasma. This is in equilibrium with the carbon dioxide in the pulmonary alveoli. Hyperventilation lowers the alveolar carbon dioxide partial pressure (PCO_2) and leads to a rapid decrease in the concentration of carbon dioxide and carbonic acid in the plasma. Decreased or inadequate pulmonary ventilation results in elevation of alveolar PCO_2, which in turn raises plasma carbon dioxide and carbonic acid as described in the discussion of acid base balance and the urinary system.

Exchange of gases between alveolar air and pulmonary capillaries is accomplished by diffusion across the alveolar membrane. Efficient gas exchange requires (1) a large capillary surface area in contact with alveolar air, (2) unimpeded diffusion of gases across the alveolar membrane, (3) normal pulmonary blood flow, and (4) normal pulmonary alveoli. The spongy structure of the lungs, in which each tiny air sac is surrounded by a large network of capillaries, provides the large surface area required for efficient gas exchange (**FIGURE 15-3A**). Destruction of alveolar septa leads to coalescence of alveoli and a reduction in the size of the capillary network surrounding the alveoli, resulting in less efficient gas exchange (**FIGURE 15-3B**).

If the alveolar septa are thickened and scarred, the diffusion of gases across the thickened alveolar membranes is impeded (**FIGURE 15-3C**). Gas exchange is also impaired if pulmonary blood flow to a portion of the lung is obstructed, as might be caused by a pulmonary embolus obstructing a large pulmonary artery or by blockage of pulmonary capillaries by fat emboli or foreign material (**FIGURE 15-3D**). If the pulmonary alveoli become filled with fluid or inflammatory exudate, inspired air cannot enter the diseased alveoli, and pulmonary gas exchange is impeded (**FIGURE 15-3E**).

The Pleural Cavity

The lungs are covered by a thin membrane called the **pleura**, which also extends over the internal surface of the chest wall. Because the lungs fill the thoracic cavity, the two pleural surfaces are in contact. The potential space between the lung and the chest wall is the pleural cavity. Normally, the apposing pleural surfaces move smoothly over one another. In disease, however, the pleural surfaces may become roughened because of inflammation and may become adherent. Inflammatory exudate may accumulate in the pleural cavity and separate the two pleural surfaces.

Pleura The mesothelial covering of the lung (visceral pleura) and chest wall (parietal pleura).

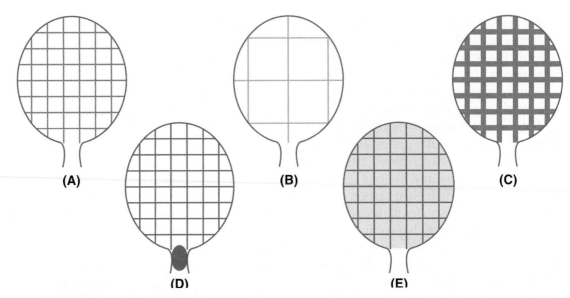

FIGURE 15-3 Types of structural and functional abnormalities that adversely affect pulmonary gas exchange. **(A)** Normal alveoli and pulmonary blood flow. **(B)** Destruction of alveolar septa, leading to coarsening of alveolar structure with corresponding reduction in size of pulmonary capillary bed. **(C)** Fibrous thickening and scarring of alveolar septa, impeding diffusion of gasses across alveolar membrane. **(D)** Obstruction of pulmonary blood flow to a part of the lung. **(E)** Alveoli filled with fluid or inflammatory exudate.

The lungs are held in an expanded position within the pleural cavity because the pressure within the pleural cavity (intrapleural pressure) is less than the pressure of the air within the lungs (intrapulmonary pressure). The pressure differences develop when the thoracic cavity enlarges after birth. When respirations are initiated, the size of the thoracic cavity increases. The lungs become filled with air at atmospheric pressure and expand to fill the enlarged thoracic cavity, stretching the elastic tissue within the lungs. The tendency of the stretched lung to pull away from the chest wall and return to its original contracted state creates a slight vacuum within the pleural cavity. Because the intrapleural pressure is slightly less than atmospheric pressure, it is often called "negative pressure."

Pulmonary Function Tests

Pulmonary function tests can be used to evaluate the efficiency of pulmonary ventilation and pulmonary gas exchange. Pulmonary ventilation is usually tested by measuring the volume of air that can be moved into and out of the lung under standard conditions. Two commonly used measurements are **vital capacity**, which measures the maximum volume of air that can be expelled after a deep inspiration, and the **one-second forced expiratory volume (FEV₁)**, which measures the maximum volume of air that can be expelled in one second. If the bronchioles are narrowed by inflammation or spasm, impeding the movement of air out of the lungs, FEV_1 is often reduced. Specialized tests can measure the total volume of air in the lungs and the volume of air remaining in the lungs after a maximum expiration.

The concentrations of oxygen and carbon dioxide (O_2 and CO_2) in the patient's arterial blood can also be measured to determine the efficiency of gas exchange in the lungs. In chronic pulmonary disease, oxygenation of the blood is inefficient. Oxygen concentration is reduced, and arterial oxygen saturation is decreased correspondingly. Often, the arterial PCO_2 also is higher than normal because carbon dioxide is inefficiently eliminated by the lungs. Arterial blood for analysis is

Vital capacity The maximum volume of air that can be forcefully expelled after a maximum inspiration.

One-second forced expiratory volume (FEV₁) The maximum volume of air that can be expelled from the lungs in one second.

usually collected by inserting a small needle into the radial artery in the wrist and withdrawing a small amount of blood. One can also determine how effectively the lungs are oxygenating the blood (arterial oxygen saturation) using a device called a pulse oximeter. A fingertip is inserted into the device, which measures photoelectrically the changes in light absorption of the hemoglobin in the fingertip capillaries at various wavelengths during systole and diastole. Then the data are used to automatically calculate the oxygen saturation of the arterial blood, and the device promptly displays the result.

Pneumothorax

Because the intrapleural pressure is below that of the atmosphere, air flows into the pleural space if the lung or chest wall is punctured. When this occurs, the negative pressure that holds the lung in the expanded position is lost, and the lung collapses because the elastic tissue within the lung contracts. This condition, which is called a **pneumothorax** (*pneumo* = air), may follow any type of lung injury or pulmonary disease that allows air to escape from the lungs into the pleural space. It also may result from a stab wound or some other penetrating injury to the chest wall that permits atmospheric air to enter the pleural space (**FIGURE 15-4**).

> **Pneumothorax**
> Accumulation of air in the pleural cavity.

Occasionally, a pneumothorax occurs without apparent cause. This is called spontaneous pneumothorax. Most cases occur in young healthy people, usually as a result of rupture of a small, air-filled, subpleural bleb at the apex of the lung.

The sudden escape of air into the pleural cavity that is associated with any type of pneumothorax usually causes chest pain and often some shortness of breath. The breath sounds, which normally can be heard with a stethoscope when the air moves in and out of the lung during respiration, are diminished on the affected side. A chest x-ray reveals partial or complete collapse of the lung and the presence of air in the pleural cavity (**FIGURE 15-5**).

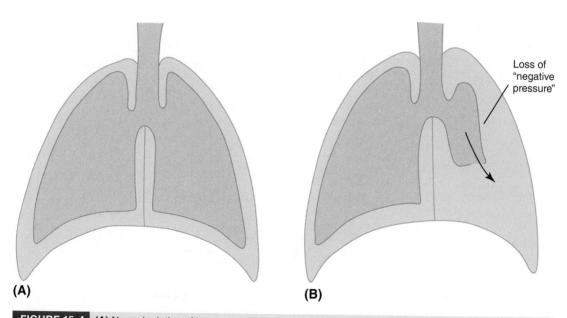

Loss of "negative pressure"

(A)   **(B)**

FIGURE 15-4 **(A)** Normal relation of lung to chest wall. Pleural space is exaggerated, and surfaces are normally in contact. "Negative pressure" is primarily a result of the tendency of the stretched lung to pull away from the chest wall. **(B)** Pneumothorax caused by a perforating injury of lung, allowing the air under atmospheric pressure to escape into the pleural cavity.

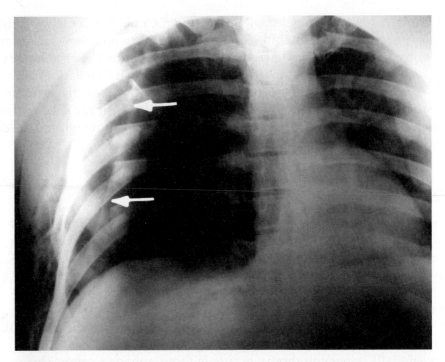

FIGURE 15-5 X-ray illustrating pneumothorax secondary to multiple rib fractures in which broken ends of fractured ribs have torn through the pleura and torn the underlying lung. The surface of the lung is no longer in contact with chest wall (*arrows*).

Courtesy of Leonard V. Crowley, MD, Century College.

The development of a positive (higher than atmospheric) pressure in the pleural cavity, called tension pneumothorax, may accompany any type of pneumothorax. This dangerous complication may occur if the lung has been perforated in such a way that the pleural tear acts as a one-way valve (**FIGURE 15-6**). With each inspiration, more air enters the pleural cavity but cannot escape. Eventually, the pleural cavity becomes

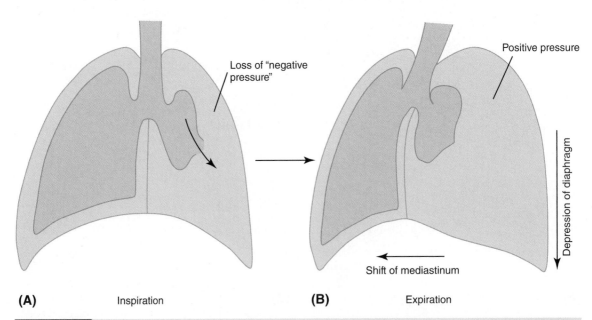

(A) Inspiration

(B) Expiration

FIGURE 15-6 Pathogenesis of tension pneumothorax. **(A)** Air enters the pleural cavity during inspiration as intrapleural pressure falls. **(B)** Rising intrapleural pressure on expiration closes the pleural tear, trapping air within the pleural space. The diaphragm on the affected side is displaced downward. The trachea and mediastinal structures are shifted away from the side of pneumothorax and encroach on the opposite pleural cavity.

overdistended with air under pressure, and the affected lung collapses completely. As the pressure builds up in the pleural cavity, the heart and mediastinal structures are displaced away from the side of the pneumothorax and encroach on the opposite pleural cavity, impairing the expansion of the opposite lung (**FIGURE 15-7**). A tension pneumothorax can be fatal if it is not recognized and treated promptly by evacuating the trapped air to relieve the pressure.

A pneumothorax is usually treated by inserting a tube into the pleural cavity through an incision in the chest wall. The tube prevents accumulation of air in the pleural cavity and aids reexpansion of the lung. The tube is connected to an apparatus that permits the air to be expelled from the pleural cavity during expiration but prevents the air from being sucked back into the pleural cavity during inspiration. The tube is left in place until the tear in the lung heals and no more air escapes. Any air remaining in the pleural cavity is gradually reabsorbed into the bloodstream, and the lung reexpands as the air is absorbed. Sometimes a slight vacuum is applied to the tube to evacuate the air more rapidly and hasten reexpansion of the lung.

Atelectasis

Atelectasis literally means incomplete expansion of the lung (*ateles* = incomplete + *ectasia* = expansion). It refers to a collapse of parts of the lung. There are two types of atelectasis: obstructive and compression. A special form of atelectasis may occur

> **Atelectasis** Collapse of the lung, either caused by bronchial obstruction (obstructive atelectasis) or external compression (compression atelectasis).

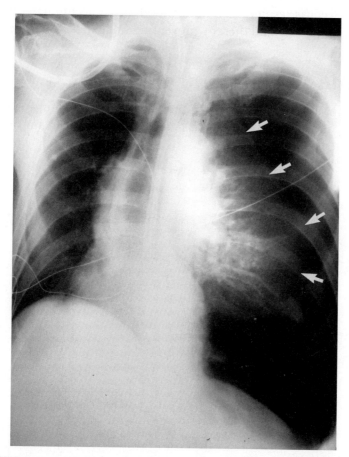

FIGURE 15-7 An x-ray of tension pneumothorax showing the surface of the collapsed lung (*arrows*). Note the low diaphragm on the affected side and displacement of mediastinal structures.

Courtesy of Leonard V. Crowley, MD, Century College.

in neonates who have not synthesized sufficient surfactant to allow for lung expansion. This may result in a condition termed neonatal respiratory distress syndrome.

OBSTRUCTIVE ATELECTASIS

Complete blockage of a bronchus by thick mucous secretions, by a tumor, or by an aspirated foreign object prevents air from entering or leaving the alveoli supplied by the blocked bronchus, and the air already present is gradually absorbed into the blood flowing through the lungs. As a result, the part of the lung supplied by the blocked bronchus gradually collapses as the air is absorbed. The volume of the affected pleural cavity also decreases correspondingly, causing the mediastinal structures to shift toward the side of the atelectasis and the diaphragm to elevate on the affected side (**FIGURE 15-8** and **FIGURE 15-9**). If the bronchial obstruction is relieved promptly, the lung reexpands normally.

Atelectasis sometimes develops as a postoperative complication. Because of postoperative pain, the patient does not cough or breathe deeply, and mucous secretions accumulate in the bronchi. To prevent this problem, the physician encourages the postoperative patient to breathe deeply and cough frequently to keep the respiratory passages clear of secretions. A device called an incentive spirometer allows the patient to monitor his breathing and work to prevent the problem.

COMPRESSION ATELECTASIS

Compression atelectasis results when fluid, blood, or air accumulates in the pleural cavity, reducing its volume and thereby preventing full expansion of the lung.

Pneumonia

Pneumonia Inflammation of the lung.

Pneumonia is an inflammation of the lung characterized by the same type of vascular changes and exudation of fluid and cells as that of inflammation in any other location.

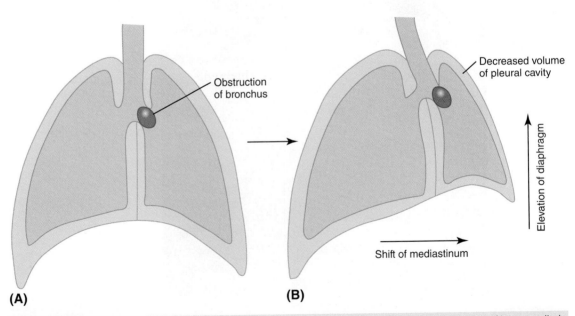

Obstruction of bronchus

Decreased volume of pleural cavity

Elevation of diaphragm

Shift of mediastinum

(A)   **(B)**

FIGURE 15-8 Atelectasis caused by bronchial obstruction. **(A)** Blockage of bronchus prevents aeration of lung supplied by obstructed bronchus. **(B)** Absorption of air causes collapse of the lung and a corresponding reduction in size of the pleural cavity. The diaphragm rises, and the mediastinum shifts toward the affected side.

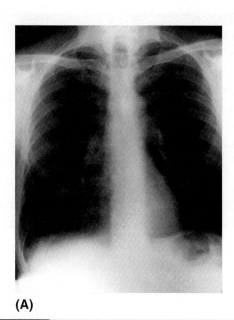
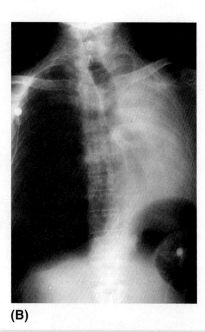

(A)   **(B)**

FIGURE 15-9 Complete atelectasis of the left lung caused by obstruction of left, main bronchus **(A)** Chest x-ray before development of atelectasis. **(B)** Atelectasis of entire left lung. The collapsed lung appears dense because the air has been absorbed. The left half of the diaphragm is elevated. Trachea and mediastinal structures are shifted toward the side of the collapse.

Courtesy of Leonard V. Crowley, MD, Century College.

However, the inflammatory process is influenced by the spongy character of the lungs. In the case of most bacterial infections, the inflammatory exudate spreads unimpeded through the lung, filling the alveoli, and the affected portions of lung becomes relatively solid (termed consolidation) (**FIGURE 15-10**). The inflammatory exudate may reach the pleural surface in some areas, causing irritation and inflammation of the pleura; sometimes inflammatory exudate accumulates in the pleural space.

CLASSIFICATION OF PNEUMONIA

Pneumonia may be classified in several ways including etiology, anatomic distribution, or predisposing factors.

The etiologic classification is the most important because it serves as a guide to treatment. Pneumonia may be caused by bacteria, chlamydiae, mycoplasmas, rickettsiae, viruses, or fungi. Whenever possible, the pneumonia is classified in greater detail by designating the exact organism responsible for the infection, such as the pneumococcus, staphylococcus, mycoplasma, or coronavirus. The most common type of bacterial pneumonia is caused by infection with *Streptococcus pneumoniae*. Pneumonia as a result of infection by this organism is a common cause of death in debilitated elderly individuals. A variety of bacteria can cause community acquired pneumonia. Pneumococcal pneumonia generally occurs in adolescent to middle-aged individuals, often following an infection of the upper respiratory tract such as influenza when host defense barriers are compromised. Antibiotic resistant strains of agents are a serious problem in hospitalized patients or those likely to have recurrent pneumonias.

The anatomic classification describes what part of the lung is involved (Figure 15-10). Lobar pneumonia refers to an infection of an entire lung lobe. Bronchopneumonia describes an infection involving only parts of one or more lobes (lung lobules) adjacent to the bronchi. Lobar pneumonia and bronchopneumonia are infections caused by pathogenic bacteria. The classic example of lobar pneumonia

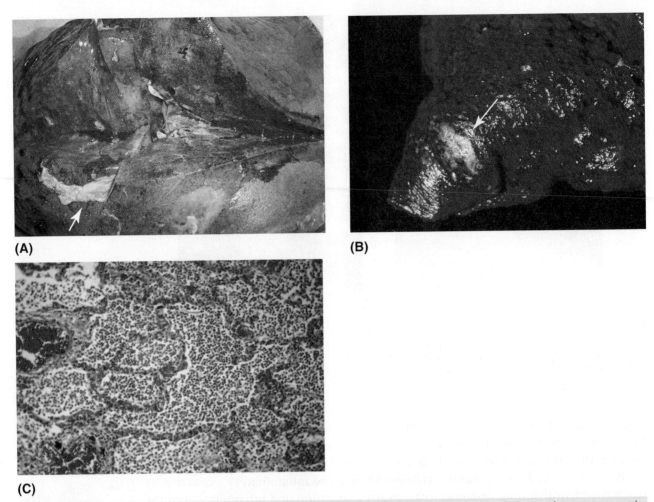

(A)

(B)

(C)

FIGURE 15-10 **(A)** Consolidation of lung lobe caused by lobar pneumonia. The lung has been incised, and cut surfaces are exposed. There is a deposit of fibrin (*arrow*) on pleura. **(B)** Bronchopneumonia. Inflammation involves lung lobules rather than an entire lobe. The most severely involved lobules (*arrow*) are shown. **(C)** Histologic appearance of pneumonia. Alveoli are filled with neutrophils, and no air can enter the affected alveoli (original magnification ×100).

Courtesy of Leonard V. Crowley, MD, Century College.

Interstitial pneumonia
Characterized by thickening of supporting tissues between the air sacs of the lungs.

is that caused by *Streptococcus pneumoniae*; however, with antibiotic therapy many cases are expressed as bronchopneumonias. A third anatomic classification is **interstitial pneumonia**, or primary atypical pneumonia, and is usually caused by a virus or mycoplasma (*Mycoplasma pneumoniae*). This type of pulmonary infection involves the pulmonary alveolar septa rather than the alveoli, and the inflammatory cells infiltrating the septa are primarily lymphocytes, monocytes, and plasma cells rather than neutrophils (**FIGURE 15-11**).

Classification of pneumonia by predisposing factors is common. Any condition associated with poor lung ventilation and retention of bronchial secretions predisposes an individual to the development of pneumonia. Postoperative pneumonia is a pulmonary inflammation that develops in the postsurgical patient who is unable to cough or breathe deeply because of pain; the resultant poor ventilation and retention of secretions predisposes to atelectasis of lung lobules, which is followed by secondary bacterial invasion leading to bronchopneumonia. Aspiration pneumonia occurs when a foreign body, food, vomit, or other irritating substance is aspirated into the lung. Obstructive pneumonia develops in the lung distal to an area where a bronchus is narrowed or obstructed. Blockage of a bronchus by a tumor or foreign body leads to poor aeration and to retention of bronchial secretions in the obstructed part of the lung, which predisposes to infection.

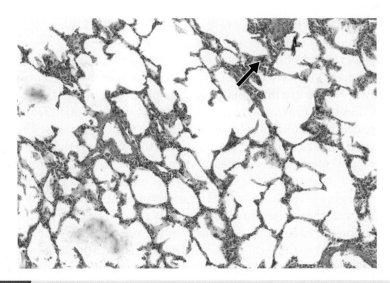

FIGURE 15-11 Interstitial pneumonia caused by a viral (measles) infection. The multiple fused cells (*arrow*) are characteristic of measles pneumonia, hence the alternate name of giant cell pneumonia.

Courtesy of Department of Pathology and Laboratory Medicine, University of North Carolina at Chapel Hill.

CLINICAL FEATURES OF PNEUMONIA

The signs and symptoms of pneumonia are those of any systemic infection. The patient is ill and has an elevated temperature, and the number of white blood cells in the peripheral blood is frequently higher than normal. Bronchial inflammation is evident, manifested by cough and purulent sputum. If the inflammatory process involves the pleura, the patient experiences pain on respiration because the inflamed pleural surfaces rub against each other. The patient may also have symptoms related to partial loss of lung function caused by consolidation of part of the lung, resulting from the accumulation of inflammatory cells within the alveoli. Oxygenation of the blood is impaired, and the patient may become quite short of breath. Pneumonia is treated by correcting any predisposing factors that contributed to the development of the pulmonary infection and administering appropriate antibiotic therapy.

Legionnaires' disease is a type of pneumonia caused by a gram-negative, rod-shaped bacterium called *Legionella pneumophila* that is widely distributed in the environment: in the soil and in freshwater ponds, lakes, and streams. The organism thrives in moist environments, such as air-conditioning ducts, shower heads, and humidifiers. People become infected by inhaling airborne organisms in aerosolized water droplets. The infection is not transmitted directly from person to person. The disease was first recognized in 1976 among people attending an American Legion convention in Philadelphia. After the infectious agent was identified, it was determined in retrospect that this same organism had in the past caused other outbreaks of pneumonia, but the infectious agent was not identified at the time. Clinically, the disease is characterized by the usual symptoms of a pulmonary infection and often abdominal pain. The chest x-ray reveals characteristic evidence of pneumonia. The infection responds to appropriate antibiotics.

Legionnaires' disease
A type of pneumonia caused by an airborne bacterium called *Legionella pneumophila*.

Additional Lung Infections: SARS and MERS

These conditions, severe acute respiratory syndrome (SARS) and Middle Eastern respiratory syndrome (MERS are highly communicable, serious pulmonary infections caused by unusual coronaviruses that have spread rapidly through several countries since each was first identified (SARS in late 2002, MERS in 2012). SARS was last reported in 2004; MERS infections are still occurring in 2015. No effective antiviral drugs are available that can influence the course of the disease.

Coronaviruses are ribonucleic acid (RNA) viruses that received their name from the crownlike spikes projecting from the viruses as seen by electron microscopy (*corona* = crown). There are three major groups of coronaviruses that cause disease in animals and humans. Previously, most of the infections in humans caused by coronaviruses were common colds, not lower respiratory tract infections. The SARS- and MERS-associated viruses, however, are unique in that they are the first ones known to cause severe, potentially lethal disease in people. Precautions to prevent infection when dealing with patients include gloves, gowns, masks, and eye protection.

The illness begins with chills and fever, sometimes mild respiratory symptoms, and occasionally diarrhea. After three to seven days, manifestations of lower respiratory tract infection appear: cough, shortness of breath, and evidence of pneumonia demonstrated by chest x-ray examination. The severity of the illness is quite variable. The lungs of severely affected patients show the characteristic features of adult respiratory distress syndrome, and patients require mechanical ventilation using an increased oxygen concentration to improve the diffusion of oxygen across the thickened edematous alveolar septa, as well as other measures to improve pulmonary function. Although current cases in the recent outbreak of MERS are a result of human-to-human spread, animal reservoirs for the virus are likely. The disease started in the Middle East and has spread to Korea. Bats and camels are suspected to harbor the MERS virus; bats, civet cats, and possibly other small mammals harbor SARS.

PNEUMOCYSTIS PNEUMONIA

Humans harbor *Pneumocystis jiroveci*, a small parasite of low pathogenicity in immunocompetent individuals, which is now classified as a fungus. The parasite does not affect normal people but may cause serious pulmonary infections in susceptible individuals. Those at risk include adults whose immune defenses have been impaired by communicable disease, such as by AIDS, or by administration of immunosuppressive drugs, and premature infants in whom immune defenses are poorly developed.

The life cycle of the parasite is complex. The most easily recognized form is a round or cup-shaped cyst about the size of a red blood cell that cannot be identified by routine (hematoxylin and eosin) stains but can be demonstrated by means of special stains containing silver compounds. The parasites, intermixed in the alveolar exudate but unstained by routine stains, appear as pale areas within the brightly stained exudate, imparting a foamy, "soap-bubble" appearance to the exudate. Special stains, however, demonstrate that the soap bubbles represent *Pneumocystis* cysts and may also reveal central clusters of sporozoites, which appear as dark dots in the centers of the cysts (**FIGURE 15-12**).

Clinically, pneumocystis pneumonia is characterized by progressive shortness of breath and cough in a person whose immunologic defenses are impaired and who is at high risk of developing the disease. The infection is always very serious and is often life-threatening because it affects people whose ability to respond to infection is greatly impaired. Treatment consists of administering antibiotic drugs that inhibit the growth of the organism.

Tuberculosis

Pulmonary tuberculosis is a special type of pneumonia caused by an acid-fast bacterium, the tubercle bacillus *Mycobacterium tuberculosis*. Because the tubercle

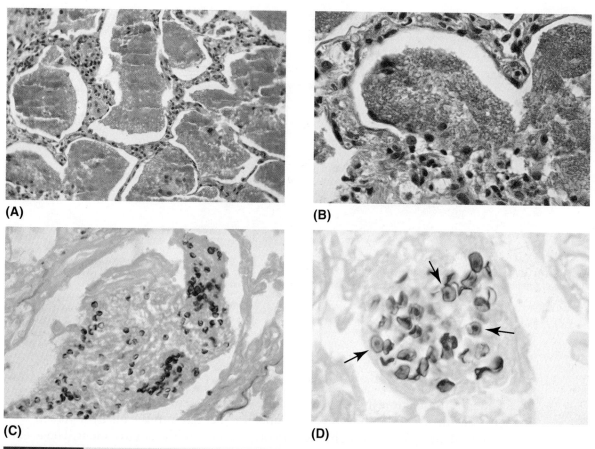

FIGURE 15-12 Pneumocystis pneumonia. **(A)** Pulmonary alveoli filled with dense protein exudate (original magnification ×100). **(B)** Higher magnification, illustrating the foamy "soap-bubble" appearance of the alveolar exudate. The clear areas in the alveolar exudate are *Pneumocystis* organisms that are not stained by routine stains (original magnification ×400). **(C)** Demonstration of *Pneumocystis jiroveci* cysts within the alveolar exudate by means of silver-containing stains (original magnification ×400). **(D)** High-magnification view of the organisms demonstrated by silver stains. Central dark dots within the cysts are clusters of sporozoites (original magnification ×1,000).

Courtesy of Leonard V. Crowley, MD, Century College.

bacillus has a capsule composed of waxes and fatty substances, it is more resistant to destruction than many other organisms. The body's response to the tubercle bacillus also differs from the usual acute inflammatory reaction. **Epitheliod macrophages**, characterized by their flat, epithelial appearance, accumulate around the bacteria; many of them fuse, often forming large, multinucleated cells called giant cells. Lymphocytes and plasma cells also accumulate, and fibrous tissue proliferates around the central cluster of epitheliod macrophages and giant cells. The central portion of the cellular aggregation usually becomes necrotic. Because of its gross appearance, the necrotic center is described as **caseous** (derived from the German word for cheese). This characteristic nodular mass of cells with central necrosis is called a caseating granuloma, and the inflammatory process is called a granulomatous inflammation (**FIGURE 15-13**). The granulomatous response to the tubercle bacillus and the necrosis within the granulomas indicate the development of cell-mediated immunity against the organism, which is the primary immune defense against the tubercle bacillus. Caseating granulomas (sometimes called tubercules) are highly characteristic of tuberculosis infection. Other disease processes can result in granulomatous inflammation, but in those cases the granulomas do not have caseating centers.

Epitheliod marcophages Appearance of macrophages around the tubercle bacillus.

Caseous Necrotic center of nodule characteristic of tuberculosis.

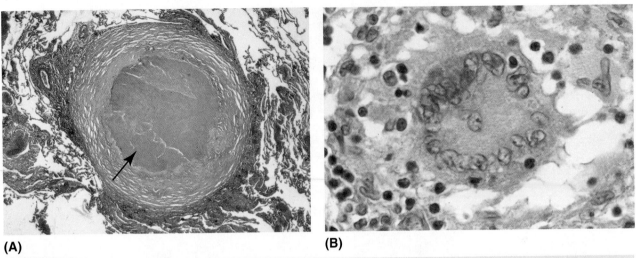

(A)

(B)

FIGURE 15-13 **(A)** Granuloma as a result of tuberculosis. The central part (*arrow*) consists of necrotic tissue (original magnification ×40). **(B)** Multinucleated giant cell characteristic of tuberculosis infection (original magnification ×400).

Courtesy of Leonard V. Crowley, MD, Century College.

COURSE OF A TUBERCULOUS INFECTION

Primary tuberculosis Initial infection of tuberculosis.

Ghon complexes Inactive tubercular lesions.

Latent tuberculosis Arrested tuberculosis infection containing viable organisms.

Progressive primary tuberculosis Initial tubercular infection that does not go into remission.

The initial infection (**primary tuberculosis**) is acquired from organisms inhaled in airborne droplets that have been coughed or sneezed into the air by a person with active tuberculosis who is discharging organisms into the environment. The organisms lodge within the pulmonary alveoli, where they proceed to multiply. Initially, the organisms introduced into the lungs do not elicit a marked inflammatory reaction because they do not produce any toxins or destructive enzymes that damage the tissues. Macrophages phagocytose the bacteria but are unable to destroy them; they may even carry the organisms to other parts of the lung and into the regional lymph nodes. After several weeks, however, a cell-mediated immunity develops. Sensitized lymphocytes attract and activate macrophages, which acquire a greatly enhanced phagocytic and destructive capability. The activated macrophages attack and destroy many of the organisms, forming characteristic granulomas containing areas of necrosis surrounded by a rim of fibrous tissue. In the majority of cases, the infection is arrested; the granulomas in the lung and regional lymph nodes heal with scarring and calcification, often followed by development into inactive lesions called **ghon complexes** (**FIGURE 15-14**). In most cases, the infection does not cause any symptoms, and the person may be unaware of the infection. Sometimes the granuloma in the lung is large enough to be identified in a chest x-ray, but often the area of infection is too small to be detected in an x-ray. A positive skin test (Mantoux test) reveals a hypersensitivity to the proteins of the tubercle bacillus and may be the only evidence of recent infection.

Cell-mediated immunity generally controls the infection, and the arrested infection may never cause any further problems. This condition is **latent tuberculosis** because the healed granulomas contain small numbers of viable organisms. Although these individuals are not infectious, the disease may become reactivated, leading to secondary (cavitary) progressive pulmonary tuberculosis if the body's cell-mediated immunity declines.

Not all primary infections respond as favorably. If a large number of organisms are inhaled or if the body's defenses are inadequate as in patients with AIDS, the inflammation may progress, a condition termed **progressive primary tuberculosis**,

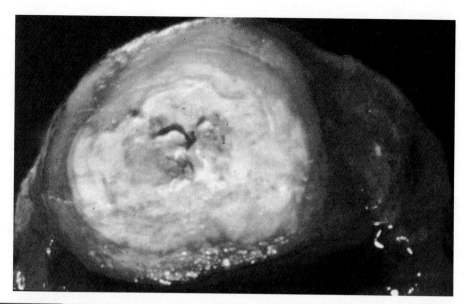

FIGURE 15-14 Ghon complex from a healed pulmonary granuloma as a result of primary tuberculosis. The central part consists of necrotic tissue containing calcium deposits surrounded by a rim of dense fibrous tissue.

Courtesy of Leonard V. Crowley, MD, Century College.

which occurs in less than 10 percent of primary TB exposures. In these cases, there is extensive destruction of lung tissue (**FIGURE 15-15**) and potentially spread of the infection throughout the body. Organisms are often carried in lymphatic channels from the lung into the peribronchial lymph nodes, leading to a tuberculous inflammation in

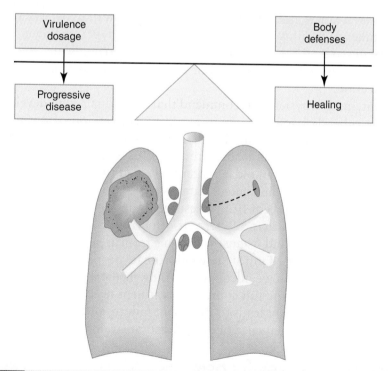

FIGURE 15-15 Possible outcome of a tuberculosis infection in relation to virulence and dosage of the organism and resistance of the body. The frequent involvement of the regional lymph nodes is indicated. *Left*, progressive disease with formation of cavity within lung, caused by infection by a large number of organisms or inadequate body defenses. *Right*, healing with scarring as a result of small numbers of organisms or a high degree of resistance to infection.

the regional lymph nodes. Systemic spread of disease is associated with the formation of multiple small granulomas in many organs, a condition termed **miliary tuberculosis** (because of the resemblance of the small granulomas to millet seeds).

Ninety percent of cases of active progressive pulmonary tuberculosis do not result from the initial infection but rather reactivation of latent TB leading to active progressive disease or occasionally reinfection. If the resistance of the individual is lowered by AIDS or other debilitating diseases, by treatment with adrenal corticosteroids, or by other factors, an apparently healed focus of tuberculosis may flare up and lead to active progressive tuberculosis. In these cases, the granulomatous inflammatory process makes contact with a bronchus, and the necrotic inflammatory tissue is discharged into it. A cavity then forms within the lung, surrounded by granulomatous inflammatory tissue containing masses of tubercle bacilli (**FIGURE 15-16**). People who have active progressive tuberculosis with a tuberculous cavity can infect others because they discharge large numbers of tubercle bacilli in their sputum, which can lead to additional cases of both primary and secondary TB.

EXTRAPULMONARY TUBERCULOSIS

Sometimes tuberculosis develops in the kidneys, bones (particularly the spine where it is termed Pott's disease), uterus, fallopian tubes, or other extrapulmonary location. The infection results from hematogenous spread of tubercle bacilli from a focus of tuberculosis in the lung. Sometimes, the secondary focus of infection may progress even though the pulmonary infection has healed, leading to an active extrapulmonary tuberculous infection without clinically apparent pulmonary tuberculosis.

DIAGNOSIS AND TREATMENT OF TUBERCULOSIS

Tuberculous infection is associated with the development of hypersensitivity to proteins in the tubercle bacillus, as discussed in immunity, hypersensitivity, allergy, and autoimmune diseases. A positive skin test (Mantoux test) indicates that the person was at one time infected with the tubercle bacillus; it does not necessarily indicate an active infection.

At present, many physicians recommend that individuals who develop an infection with the tubercle bacillus, as manifested by conversion of a negative into a positive skin test reaction, be treated with antituberculosis drugs. Treatment is also recommended for patients with inactive tuberculosis who have an increased risk of developing a reactivation of an old, apparently healed tuberculous infection.

The incidence of TB in the United States is currently at an all-time low, having decreased more than 60 percent from a resurgence in the 1990s (related in part to the AIDS epidemic). More than 60 percent of current cases occur in immigrants (predominantly Hispanics and Asians) who come from areas where the prevalence of tuberculosis is much higher. Many of these unfortunate people with active tuberculosis or latent disease do not receive adequate ongoing medical care; they also may not be motivated to complete the full course of treatment needed to arrest the disease. Failure to complete treatment leads to treatment failure, and premature cessation of treatment promotes the emergence of drug-resistant strains of the organism.

DRUG-RESISTANT TUBERCULOSIS

Effective drug treatment of tuberculosis has transformed the infection from a potentially fatal chronic disease to one that could be treated effectively by a number of antibiotics and chemotherapeutic agents, but now drug-resistant tuberculosis (TB)

Miliary tuberculosis
Multiple foci of tuberculosis throughout the body as a result of bloodstream dissemination of tubercle bacilli from a primary focus in the lung or peribronchial lymph nodes.

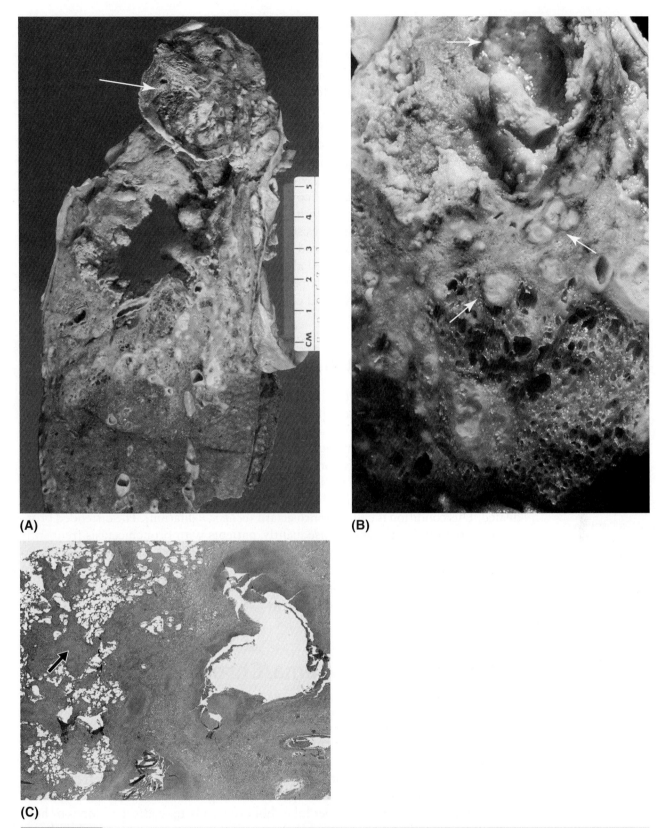

(A)

(B)

(C)

FIGURE 15-16 Far-advanced pulmonary tuberculosis. **(A)** The upper lobe (*arrow*) has been completely destroyed by tuberculosis, and there is extensive tuberculosis in the lower lobe with a large cavity in the lung that communicates with a bronchus. Only the lower part of the lobe is free of disease (*extreme bottom*). **(B)** A closer view of tuberculosis. A large cavity (*upper arrow*) surrounded by nodular and diffuse granulomatous inflammation. Several discrete granulomas (*lower arrows*) can be seen below the cavity. **(C)** Low-power photomicrograph. The large cavity is on the right side of the figure. Numerous small granulomas (*arrow*) are present on the left side.

(A, B) Courtesy of Leonard V. Crowley, MD, Century College; (C) Courtesy of Department of Pathology and Laboratory Medicine, University of North Carolina at Chapel Hill.

is becoming a major problem. Tuberculosis caused by organisms resistant to at least two of the most commonly used antituberculosis drugs is designated multiple drug-resistant tuberculosis (MDR-TB), which is more difficult to treat. Currently the rate of MDR-TB is low in the United States (less than 1.5 percent, with most cases occurring in the foreign born). However, rates may be as high as 20 percent in some parts of the world. Recently, the drug-resistance problem has become even more threatening. Some strains have become "super resistant." They no longer respond to a large number of antituberculosis drugs, and an infection by these organisms is designated extremely drug-resistant tuberculosis (XDR-TB). Although XDR-TB is uncommon in the United States, with less than seventy cases reported to date, it is a major public health risk. Several countries have reported XDR-TB resistant to all currently available drugs. People with XDR-TB need to obtain treatment at a facility accustomed to dealing with these resistant organisms, and the patients' activities need to be restricted so they cannot spread the infection. The World Health Organization has become increasingly concerned about the spread of XDR-TB cases. Most have been concentrated in Eastern Europe, South Africa, and Asia, but as noted, cases do appear in the United States, and control measures to prevent further spread are considered essential.

Bronchitis and Bronchiectasis

Acute inflammation of the tracheobronchial mucosa is common in many upper respiratory infections. The raw throat and cough associated with many respiratory infections are a result of the associated acute bronchitis. Chronic bronchitis also is common; often, it results from constant irritation of the respiratory mucosa by smoking cigarettes or breathing air containing large amounts of atmospheric pollution.

Sometimes the bronchial walls in parts of the lung become weakened as a result of severe inflammation or other factors, and the affected bronchi become markedly dilated. This condition is called **bronchiectasis** (*ectasis* = dilation). The distended bronchi tend to retain secretions. Consequently, patients with bronchiectasis frequently have a chronic cough associated with production of large amounts of purulent sputum. Often, they suffer repeated bouts of pulmonary infection. Brochiectasis is not curable, but symptoms may respond to drug and exercise therapy. Oxygen therapy may be required in severe disease. Bronchiectasis can be recognized by means of lung function tests and radiography.

Bronchiectasis Dilatation of bronchi caused by weakening of their walls as a result of infection.

Emphysema Disease in which the air spaces in the lung are enlarged and their walls destroyed.

Chronic obstructive pulmonary disease (COPD) Combination of emphysema and chronic bronchitis.

Pulmonary Emphysema/Chronic Obstructive Lung Disease

Pulmonary **emphysema** is a disease in which the air spaces distal to the terminal bronchioles are enlarged and their walls are destroyed. The disease is an important cause of disability and death and in the United States is strongly associated with smoking. In emphysema, the normally fine alveolar structure of the lung is destroyed, and large, cystic air spaces form throughout the lung (**FIGURE 15-17**). The destructive process usually begins in the upper lobes but eventually may affect all lobes of both lungs. Usually, there is an associated chronic inflammation of the terminal bronchioles. Emphysema and chronic bronchitis occur together so frequently that they are usually considered a single entity, designated **chronic obstructive pulmonary disease (COPD)**. The chief clinical manifestations of any type of chronic pulmonary disease are dyspnea and cyanosis. Dyspnea is a sensation of shortness of breath. Cyanosis is a

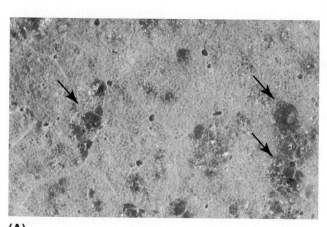

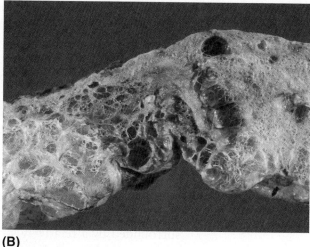

(A)

(B)

FIGURE 15-17 Sections of air-dried lung preparations illustrating the gross appearance of emphysema. **(A)** Mild emphysema. Beginning breakdown of lung tissue to form cystic spaces (*arrows*). Most of the alveoli appear normal. **(B)** Advanced emphysema with multiple confluent cystic spaces within lung. Very little normal lung tissue remains. The dark color is a result of accumulation of carbon pigment in the emphysematous lung from inhaling "dirty" air.

Courtesy of Leonard V. Crowley, MD, Century College.

blue tinge of the skin and mucous membrane that results from an excessive amount of reduced hemoglobin in the blood. Reduced hemoglobin is dark purplish red, in contrast with normally oxygenated blood, which is bright red. The chief symptom of emphysema is shortness of breath. Initially, this is noted only on exertion, but later it may be present even at rest. The patient usually also has a chronic cough with purulent sputum, owing to the associated chronic bronchitis. Eventually, severely affected patients may die because they lack enough functionally normal lung tissue to sustain life or because of a superimposed pulmonary infection. Emphysema is also a frequent cause of respiratory acidosis, one of the common disturbances of acid–base balance presented in the discussion of the kidney.

The three main anatomic derangements in chronic obstructive pulmonary disease are (1) inflammation and narrowing of the terminal bronchioles, (2) dilatation and coalescence of pulmonary air spaces, and (3) loss of lung elasticity. These derangements in turn cause severe disturbances in pulmonary function.

DERANGEMENTS OF PULMONARY STRUCTURE AND FUNCTION IN EMPHYSEMA

Chronic inflammation of the bronchioles probably initiates the destructive process. Chronic inflammation causes swelling of the bronchial mucosa, which reduces the caliber of the bronchi and bronchioles and stimulates increased bronchial secretions. Because a tube's resistance to air flow varies with the fourth power of its diameter, a slight reduction in the caliber of the bronchioles greatly restricts the flow of air. Normally, the bronchi and bronchioles dilate slightly during inspiration and become smaller during expiration. Consequently, air can enter the lungs more readily than it can be expelled through the narrowed bronchioles; so air tends to become trapped in the lungs during expiration. The lungs cannot empty completely, and they become chronically overinflated. As a result, the amount of additional air that can be inspired when the subject takes a deep breath is much reduced, and the subject is unable to increase his or her ventilation adequately in response to increased demand.

The bronchiolar obstruction also disturbs pulmonary function by causing unequal air flow to various parts of the lung. Some alveoli are overventilated; others are inadequately supplied, reducing the overall efficiency of pulmonary ventilation. The excess air supplying the overventilated alveoli is "wasted" because more is provided than is needed to completely oxygenate the blood flowing through the surrounding pulmonary capillaries. Conversely, the blood flowing to the poorly ventilated alveoli does not become fully oxygenated. When it mixes with normally oxygenated blood flowing from other parts of the lungs, the oxygen content of the blood delivered to the tissues is reduced.

The destruction of the alveolar septa leads to enlargement of the air spaces and at the same time reduces the number of pulmonary capillaries available for gas exchange. Diffusion of gases is much less efficient from large cystic spaces because the spaces contain a much larger volume of air than does a normal alveolus and are surrounded by a relatively sparse network of capillaries. Moreover, the movement of air into and out of the enlarged spaces is impeded by the bronchiolar obstruction (**FIGURE 15-18**).

Destruction of the alveolar septa also leads to loss of the elastic tissue in the septa that forms the structural framework of the lungs, and so the lungs no longer "recoil" normally after they have been stretched during inspiration. Expiration is no longer a passive process. The air must be actively forced out of the lungs by contraction of the intercostal muscles. Breathing requires more effort that in turn requires a greater oxygen consumption. The pressure required to actively force air out of the lungs during expiration also raises the intrapleural pressure and compresses the lungs, which causes further problems with pulmonary ventilation. The bronchi and bronchioles have lost their normal structural support because of loss of lung elasticity and tend to collapse during expiration, obstructing the outflow of air and trapping more air within the lungs.

PATHOGENESIS OF CHRONIC OBSTRUCTIVE PULMONARY DISEASE

Cigarette smoking is by far the major factor responsible for COPD in the United States. In developing countries, women exposed to fumes produced by cooking with biomass fuels (wood, crop wastage, etc.) are also at increased risk. Exactly how the destructive effect on the lung occurs is not completely understood. **FIGURE 15-19** summarizes one concept of the pathogenesis of this serious and disabling disease.

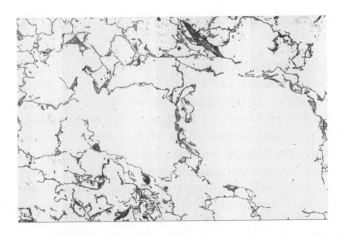

FIGURE 15-18 Photomicrograph of emphysematous lung. Note the large cystic airspaces that have resulted from the destruction of the alveolar walls.

Courtesy of Department of Pathology and Laboratory Medicine, University of North Carolina at Chapel Hill.

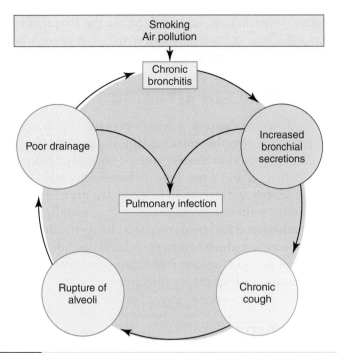

FIGURE 15-19 A concept of the pathogenesis of chronic obstructive pulmonary disease.

Smoking and lung irritants expose the bronchial mucosa to chronic irritation, eventually producing chronic bronchitis associated with a chronic cough and increased bronchial secretions. The inflammatory swelling of the mucosa narrows the smaller bronchioles, increasing their resistance to expiration and causing air to be trapped within the lung.

The leukocytes that accumulating in the bronchioles and alveoli contribute to the lung damage by releasing proteolytic (protein-digesting) enzymes, principally elastase, that attack the elastic fibers making up part of the lung's structural framework. The body produces an intrinsic antielastase (alpha$_1$ antitrypsin), but the inflammatory infiltrate produced by smoking overwhelms this natural defense mechanism.

Repeated bouts of coughing, with consequent extreme elevations in intrabronchial pressure, cause the alveolar septa to rupture, gradually converting the alveoli into large, cystic air spaces. The lungs become overdistended and lose their normal elasticity. The patient cannot expel air normally from the overdistended lungs because normal lung elasticity is lost and the bronchioles are obstructed; difficulty expectorating the excessive bronchial secretions also is apparent. Retention of secretions and poor drainage of secretions from the bronchi tend to perpetuate the chronic bronchitis, and a vicious circle is created. The diseased lungs are also more susceptible to infection because of impaired pulmonary ventilation, bronchial inflammation, bronchiolar obstruction, and excessive bronchial secretions. Therefore, patients with COPD frequently have repeated bouts of pneumonia, further damaging the lung tissue.

PREVENTION AND TREATMENT

For the most part, COPD can be prevented by refraining from smoking and avoiding inhalation of other substances known to be injurious to the lungs. Atmospheric air pollution contributes to the increasing incidence of emphysema, and various measures are being undertaken to control this serious public health problem. However, after emphysema has developed, the damaged lungs cannot be restored to normal. Several measures can be employed to promote the drainage of bronchial secretions, to improve pulmonary ventilation, and to decrease the frequency of superimposed pulmonary infections. These measures, along with cessation of smoking, will retard or arrest further progression of the disease.

EMPHYSEMA AS A RESULT OF ALPHA₁ ANTITRYPSIN DEFICIENCY

Blood and other body fluids contain a serum protein called alpha$_1$ antitrypsin, a normally occurring antineutrophil elastase, and its concentration in the blood is genetically determined. Most individuals produce normal amounts of this molecule; others are severely deficient, and a third group has subnormal levels of this protein.

Individuals with severe antitrypsin deficiency are prone to develop an uncommon type of progressive pulmonary emphysema that usually becomes manifest in adolescence or early adulthood and tends to affect chiefly the lower lobes of the lungs. People with only moderately reduced antitrypsin levels do not develop severe emphysema at an early age but are quite susceptible to lung damage from cigarette smoking, atmospheric air pollution, or respiratory infections.

Bronchial Asthma

Bronchial asthma is characterized by periodic recurring bronchial hyperresponsiveness and recurring brochoconstriction of the smooth muscle in the walls of the smaller bronchi and bronchioles in response to a number of different agents. It is also associated with increased secretions by the bronchial mucous glands. Asthmatic attacks cause shortness of breath, and wheezing respirations occur caused by restricted movement of air through the tightly constricted air passages. The physiologic derangements in asthma result from narrowing of the bronchioles and are similar to those in patients with COPD. Bronchiolar spasm exerts a greater effect on expiration than on inspiration because the caliber of the bronchioles varies with the phase of respiration. Consequently, air flow is impeded more on expiration than on inspiration, which leads air being trapped in the lungs and overinflation of the lungs. The disease is most commonly diagnosed in the young (most before the age of eighteen) and often becomes milder (or disappears) with increasing age.

Many cases of asthma have an allergic basis although other factors such as cold and exercise may contribute to the disease. The attacks are precipitated by inhalation of dust, pollens, animal dander, or other allergens, which interact with mast cells coated with IgE antibody. This leads to release of chemical mediators that induce the bronchospasm. Acute attacks are treated by administering drugs such as epinephrine or short acting beta2 adrenergic agonists such as albuterol, which relaxes the bronchospasm, combined with an antisecretory drug. Often, attacks can be prevented by administering drugs that block the release of mediators from mast cells (cromolyn sodium), corticosteroids, and long-acting theophylline. Therapy is complex and generally undertaken by a specialist in the disease, often a pediatric allergist. (Allergic diseases are considered in the discussion on immunity, hypersensitivity, allergy, and autoimmune diseases.)

Respiratory Distress Syndrome

RESPIRATORY DISTRESS SYNDROME OF NEWBORN INFANTS

Respiratory distress syndrome of newborn infants is characterized by progressive respiratory distress that occurs soon after birth, leading to serious problems in oxygenation of the blood. The condition occurs most often in premature infants, infants delivered by cesarean section, and infants born to mothers with diabetes. The basic cause is an inadequate quantity of surfactant in the lungs of the affected infants. As a result, the alveoli do not expand normally during inspiration and tend to collapse during expiration. The permeability of the pulmonary capillaries also is increased, and protein-rich fluid leaks from the pulmonary capillaries. The fluid, which is rich in fibrinogen, tends to clot and form adherent membranes that line the air passages. These membranes contribute to respiratory distress by impeding the diffusion of gases between the air passages and the pulmonary capillaries. The presence of these prominent acellular red-staining membranes lining the alveoli was the basis for the older name given to this condition, hyaline membrane disease (**FIGURE 15-20**).

If delivery of a premature infant with immature lungs cannot be avoided, adrenal corticosteroid hormones administered to the mother within twenty-four hours of anticipated delivery will stimulate increased production of surfactant by the fetal lungs, thereby reducing the risk of respiratory distress syndrome. Infants who have developed respiratory distress syndrome after delivery are treated with supplementary oxygen and instillation of a surfactant-type material that resembles natural surfactant. The material is instilled by means of a tube inserted into the infant's trachea (endotracheal tube), and the surfactant treatments are continued for several days after delivery. **TABLE 15-1** compares the respiratory distress syndrome in infants with a somewhat similar condition in adults, which has a different pathogenesis and method of treatment, although the histologic changes in both conditions are quite similar.

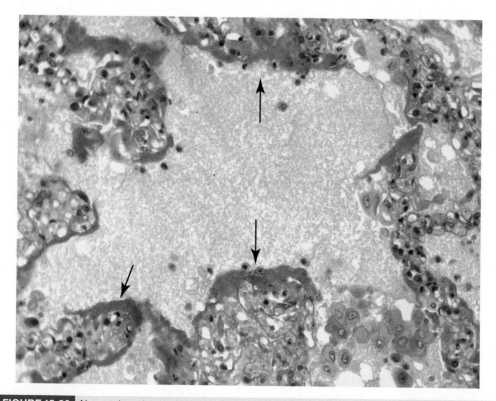

FIGURE 15-20 Neonatal respiratory distress syndrome. Eosinophilic hyaline membranes (*arrows*) composed of coagulated protein cover alveolar septa, impeding gas exchange between alveoli and pulmonary capillaries.

Courtesy of Leonard V. Crowley, MD, Century College.

TABLE 15-1 Comparison of Neonatal and Adult Respiratory Distress Syndrome

	Neonatal	Adult
Groups affected	Premature infants Delivery by cesarean section* Infant born to diabetic mother**	Adults who have sustained direct or indirect lung damage
Pathogenesis	Inadequate surfactant	*Direct damage:* lung trauma, aspiration, irritant or toxic gasses *Indirect damage:* reduced pulmonary blood flow caused by shock or sepsis *Associated condition:* surfactant production reduced
Treatment	Corticosteroids to mother before delivery Endotracheal surfactant Oxygen	Support circulation and respiration Endotracheal tube and respirator Positive pressure oxygen

*Labor increases surfactant synthesis, which is lacking in cesarean delivery.

**High insulin blood level in the fetus of a mother with diabetes suppresses surfactant synthesis.

ADULT RESPIRATORY DISTRESS SYNDROME

Adult respiratory distress syndrome (ARDS) is referred to as **diffuse alveolar damage (DAD)** by pathologists and is sometimes called "shock lung" because shock may be associated with the syndrome. ARDS may result from any process that disturbs the alveolar capillary permeability barrier with resultant movement of fluid into the alveolar space. Damage to either the capillary endothelium or the alveolar epithelium may be involved. The most common risk factors are sepsis and related septic shock, bacterial infection, trauma, burns, fractures, near drowning, and aspiration of vomitus; sometimes no cause is evident. In many of instances, reduced blood flow to the lung (shock) may occur and result in alveolar damage.

Whatever the predisposing cause of the alveolar damage, the pathophysiologic derangements are the same as in neonatal respiratory distress syndrome: damage to alveolar capillaries and alveolar lining cells, impaired formation of surfactant, leakage of protein-rich fluid from the injured capillaries into the alveolar septa with formation of intra-alveolar hyaline membranes, and impaired diffusion of oxygen across the swollen, thickened alveolar septa. Later in the disease course, fibrosis of the damage lung tissue may occur and further compromise respiration (**FIGURE 15-21**).

Treatment is directed toward correcting the shock, treating the underlying condition that initiated the respiratory distress, and improving the oxygenation of the blood by means of a ventilator capable of delivering an increased concentration of oxygen to the lungs under slightly increased pressure, thereby facilitating diffusion of oxygen across the swollen alveolar septa. Even with therapy, about a third of cases result in death.

Adult respiratory distress syndrome (ARDS)/ diffuse alveolar damage (DAD) Result of process disturbing the alveolar capillary permeability barrier.

Pulmonary Fibrosis

The lungs are continually exposed to a number of injurious substances, such as irritant gases discharged into the atmosphere and many kinds of airborne organic and inorganic particles. As noted previously, severe pulmonary injury and ARDS may lead to pulmonary fibrosis. Fibrous thickening of alveolar septa makes the lungs increasingly rigid, restricting normal respiratory excursions. Diffusion of oxygen and carbon dioxide

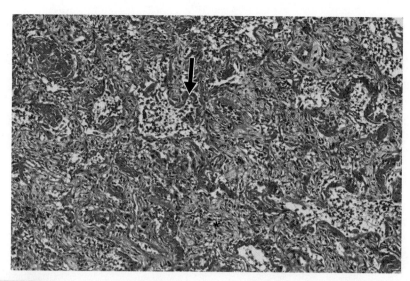

FIGURE 15-21 Late diffuse alveolar damage (DAD). Most alveoli are filled with fibroblasts preventing oxygenation of blood (*). Hyaline membranes remain present along alveolar walls (*arrow*).

Courtesy of William Funkhouser Department of Pathology and Laboratory Medicine, University of North Carolina at Chapel Hill.

between alveolar air and pulmonary capillaries also is hampered because of the increased thickness of the alveolar septa. Pulmonary fibrosis causes progressive respiratory disability similar to that encountered in pulmonary emphysema.

Some types of diseases characterized by injury to connective tissue, may have as their major manifestation injury to the connective tissue framework of the lung, leading to pulmonary fibrosis. Other fibrotic lung diseases may be idiopathic (with no known cause) or be related to inherited disease.

Certain occupational diseases are recognized as being caused by inhalation of injurious substances. The general term **pneumoconiosis** (*pneumo* = lung + *konis* = dust + *osis* = condition) is used to refer to lung injury produced by inhalation of injurious dust or other particulate material. The best known of the pneumoconioses are silicosis and asbestosis. **Silicosis** is a type of progressive nodular pulmonary fibrosis caused by inhalation of rock dust and other materials containing silica. Recent cases have occurred in workers installing silica containing kitchen countertops. **Asbestosis** is a diffuse pulmonary fibrosis caused by inhalation of asbestos fibers. Within the body, the fibers become coated with a protein having a high content of iron to form characteristic structures called asbestos bodies. Sometimes these can be identified in the sputum of patients with asbestosis (**FIGURE 15-22**). Inhalation of coal dust, cotton fibers, certain types of fungus spores, and many other substances associated with certain occupations also may cause pulmonary fibrosis.

Patients with asbestosis have other problems as well because asbestos fibers appear to be carcinogenic. These patients have a higher incidence of lung carcinoma than the general population, and some develop an unusual type of malignant tumor (malignant mesothelioma) arising from pleural mesothelial cells.

Pneumoconiosis An occupational lung disease caused by inhalation of injurious substances such as rock dust.

Silicosis A type of occupational lung disease caused by inhalation of silica rich rock dust.

Asbestosis A type of pneumoconiosis caused by inhalation of asbestos fibers.

Lung Carcinoma

Lung carcinoma is another important disease related to cigarette smoking. Lung carcinoma was once uncommon. Now lung cancer is the chief cause of cancer deaths, which kills 160,000 people annually. It is a common malignant tumor in men, and the mortality in women caused by lung carcinoma now far exceeds that of breast carcinoma. The tumor is uncommon in nonsmokers. Because the neoplasm often arises

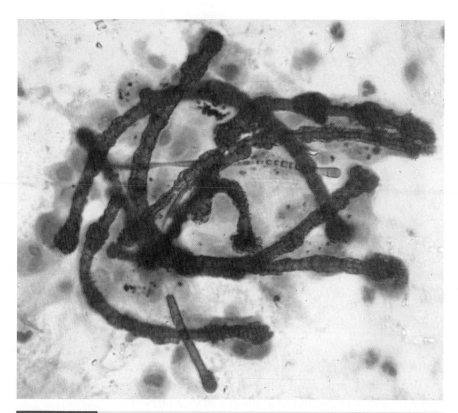

FIGURE 15-22 Cluster of asbestos bodies in sputum (original magnification ×1,000).
Courtesy of Leonard V. Crowley, MD, Century College.

from the bronchial mucosa, the term bronchogenic carcinoma is often used when referring to lung cancer. There are several different histologic types. Squamous cell carcinoma and adenocarcinoma are two of the more common (**FIGURE 15-23**). A third type composed of large, bizarre, epithelial cells is referred to as large cell carcinoma.

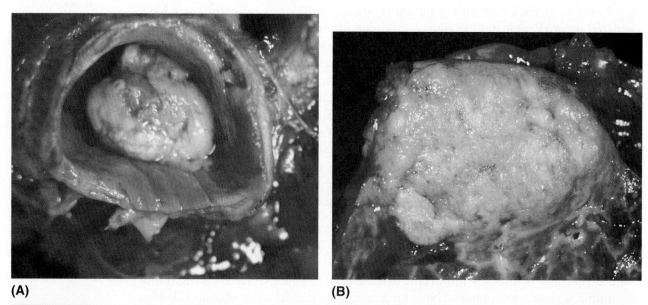

(A)   **(B)**

FIGURE 15-23 Gross appearance of lung carcinoma. **(A)** A squamous cell carcinoma partially obstructing a major bronchus. **(B)** An adenocarcinoma arising from smaller bronchus at the periphery of the lung.

Courtesy of Leonard V. Crowley, MD, Century College.

A fourth type is composed of small, irregular, dark cells with scanty cytoplasm that look somewhat like lymphocytes. This small cell carcinoma carries a very poor prognosis (**FIGURE 15-24**). Until recently it was sufficient for the pathologist to classify lung cancer as being of small cell type or "other non–small cell lung cancer (NSCLC)" because disseminated small cell lung cancer, although having a very poor long-term prognosis (2 percent five year survival), is susceptible to chemotherapy and radiation, which provide short-term relief. Currently, a limited number of adenocarcinomas of the lung have been characterized as having defined somatic mutations of the *EGFR* gene, which can be treated with drugs that block the kinase activity of the mutated gene (oncogene) as discussed in neoplastic disease. Although only a limited number of adenocarcinoma patients have the "drugable" mutation (predominantly Asiatic, female nonsmokers) this targeted form of chemotherapy may slightly prolong life (at best providing several months of disease progress free survival).

Because of the rich lymphatic and vascular network in the lung, the neoplasm readily gains access to lymphatic channels and pulmonary blood vessels and soon spreads to regional lymph nodes and distant sites. Treatment usually consists of surgical resection of one or more lobes of the lung. Radiation therapy in combination with anticancer chemotherapy rather than surgery is used to treat small cell carcinoma and is also used to treat tumors that are too far advanced for surgical resection. Results of treatment are disappointing because the disease is often widespread by the time it is recognized.

Chest x-rays for lung carcinoma have not been very effective in reducing lung carcinoma mortality because, often, the detected tumor has already spread beyond the lungs and is no longer curable. Specialized CT examination can pick up tumors

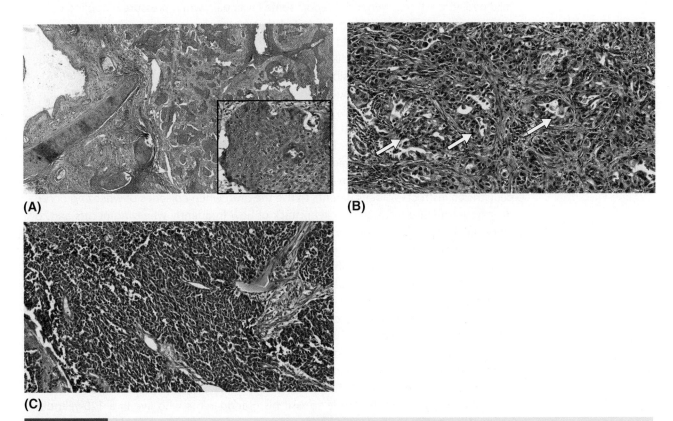

(A)

(B)

(C)

FIGURE 15-24 Histologic appearance of three common types of lung carcinoma. **(A)** Squamous cell carcinoma arising adjacent to bronchus (*left*). Inset shows carcinoma at high power. **(B)** Adenocarcinoma showing formation of gland-like structures (*arrows*). **(C)** Small cell carcinoma (same magnification as B). Area of tumor cell necrosis is at upper left.

Courtesy of William Funkhouser Department of Pathology and Laboratory Medicine, University of North Carolina at Chapel Hill.

earlier, which provides a better chance of survival, but repeated CT procedures for screening are expensive and expose the individual to significantly more radiation than chest x-ray exams. Because 87 percent of lung cancers are caused by smoking, many physicians believe that the longer term goal should be to eliminate the cause of most lung cancers by not smoking.

CASE 15-1

Wilber is a five-year-old male child of two upper-middle-class parents who live in Spotless Dell Community in a recently built home. Wilber has previously been healthy with only an occasional upper respiratory tract infection. About a month ago, Wilber complained of facial pain along with a case of the "sniffles." He began to cough at night (generally in the early a.m.) and also when he played outside with other children. Because the coughing was mild and tended to stop on its own and was not accompanied by production of sputum (was "nonproductive"), Wilber's parents were not concerned and assumed he had a "cold." About two weeks ago, Wilber's parents purchased a robotic vacuum cleaner (a Roomba™). Wilber enjoyed following it around his bedroom but started to complain about feeling "funny" in his chest. His mother noticed that he made an odd "whistling" sound as he breathed out (expired). Wilber's complaints were occasional but tended to occur when the vacuum cleaner was being used or when Wilber's mother fluffed up the duvet or changed the sheets on Wilber's bed. Concerned that Wilber might be developing an "allergy," his parents brought Wilber to see his pediatrician.

Wilber's pediatrician was concerned that the child's symptoms might indicate very mild pediatric asthma. Wilber did report some facial pain when pressure is applied to his maxillary area, and the pediatrician noted that his conjunctiva were slightly inflamed, suggesting the possibility of mild allergic rhinitis. His physical examination was otherwise normal. Still concerned, the pediatrician asks Wilber to imagine he is trying to "blow out birthday candles as hard as possible." With forced expiration, she notices a distinct wheeze (whistling sound due to air turbulence on expiration, suggesting some degree of pulmonary obstruction). Because the symptoms are mild, the pediatrician elects to forgo additional testing and suggests that Wilber's parents should not use the vacuum cleaner in Wilber's presence and that they buy special impermeable bed covers for his room. The pediatrician also prescribes a rapid acting beta-2 agonist as an inhaler (albuterol). The drug causes smooth muscle relaxation in the respiratory system, acting as a bronchodilator. The pediatrician instructs Wilber's parents to use the drug when episodes of wheezing occur. His parents are also instructed to keep track of how frequently wheezing occurs and to immediately report back if symptoms worsen or if the wheezing is not relieved.

The medication initially controls Wilber's wheezing attacks, but after a time they appear to increase in frequency. Wilber complains of increased chest discomfort and interacts less with his playmates. Wilber's pediatrician is now more concerned about the presence of asthma and prescribes the use of an inhaled corticosteroid (beclomethasone), which both acts as an inhibitor of and relaxer for bronchoconstriction and as an anti-inflammatory reducing the sensitivity of the airway to agents inducing the asthma attacks. She instructs the parents to use the albuterol inhaler only when Wilber suffers from sudden discomfort. Wilber does much better on the inhaled corticosteroid for several months, and his parents decide to taper the medication, noting no change in Wilber's health.

Wilber and his parents decide to visit his grandparents who live in a 120-year-old house on a ranch in Dusty Gulch. Wilber's parents pack the albuterol inhaler because they are somewhat concerned about the presence of "dust and germs" triggering an attack. At his grandparents' house, Wilber sleeps in a room with heavy hand-woven carpets on

CASE 15-1 (Continued)

the floor and antique loomed fabrics on the walls. He wakes up in the early morning and calls his parents, complaining of difficulty breathing. He says his chest feels tight, and his parents note a very loud wheeze as Wilber attempts to exhale. They note that his chest muscles seem to be "working hard" as he attempts to breath. They have Wilber use the albuterol inhaler, but it has little effect. Panicked, they rush Wilber to the local hospital's urgent care center. At the center the on-call resident notes that Wilber has a very increased respiratory rate (over 30 breaths per minute), an increased heart rate (130 beats per minute), and a markedly reduced oxyhemoglobin saturation (determined using a pulse oxymeter to be 92 percent saturation). Concerned with the inability of a moderate dose of a rapid acting brochodilator to afford relief, the resident increases the dose of this drug and begins IV therapy with corticosteroids. He also has Wilber inhale oxygen via a face mask. After an hour, Wilber's oxyhemoglobin saturation begins to climb, and after six hours Wilber is feeling much better with improved breathing and lack of wheezing. He is scheduled for an intensive workup by a pediatric allergist in the next few days.

Discussion

Asthma is a complex chronic disease in which symptoms result from an obstruction of air flow, which is often periodic and triggered by an inciting agent. The most common inciting agent is an environmental allergen that triggers immune-mediated brochospasm, mucosal edema, and excess mucous production, which plug the airways. With time this leads to structural changes in the airway that include the continued presence of inflammatory cells (often eosinophils), basement membrane thickening, mucous gland hyperplasia, and mucoid plugging of airways (FIGURE 15-25). The immunopathology of asthma is complex and is discussed in the presentation on immunology, hypersensitivity, allergy, and autoimmune diseases. In brief, IgE antibodies reactive with the allergen bind to mast cells in the respiratory tree. In the presence of allergen, the IgE antibodies trigger the mast cells to immediately release a number of inflammatory mediators (including histamine, prostaglandins, and leukotrienes) that mediate bronchoconstriction. With time the activated mast cells also will release additional mediators that promote the migration of numerous inflammatory cells into the tissues of the airway, notably eosinophils. These cells promote additional airway damage.

Many environmental allergens can trigger allergic asthma. At the top of the list are dust mites, other household insects such as roaches, and animal dander. The **hygiene hypothesis** suggests that current increases in the rate of childhood asthma are a result of child rearing in an excessively clean environment. Studies have suggested that children raised in farm environments have fewer cases of asthma than those raised in nonrural environments. In Wilber's case, the association of symptoms with exposure to vacuuming, disturbed bedding, and textiles suggests that household dust mites are a likely trigger.

The treatment of asthma is complex and far more extensive than discussed in the Case. Treatment involves pulmonary function tests, determination of the allergic trigger, and evaluation of multiple potential therapeutic interventions. However, it is important to understand that asthma is a serious disease affecting at least 10 percent of the population. There has been a surprising increase in incidence (some accounts report increases of over 75 percent in recent years). Asthma is the most common reason for admission to pediatric hospitals and accounts for more school absences than any other chronic disease. In addition, unrelieved asthma (status asthmaticus) results in 5,000 deaths per year. Figure 15-25 is taken from such a lethal case.

Hygiene hypothesis
Theory that lack of early childhood exposure to infectious agents, symbiotic microorganisms (such as the gut flora or probiotics), and parasites increases susceptibility to allergic diseases by suppressing the natural development of the immune system.

(continues)

CASE 15-1 (Continued)

Etiology and Pathogenesis

Allergic asthma triggered by the presence of environmental allergens, possibly dust mites, resulting in inflammation of the respiratory tree, airway hypersensitivity, bronchospasm, excess mucous production, and inflammation-induced changes in the respiratory tree.

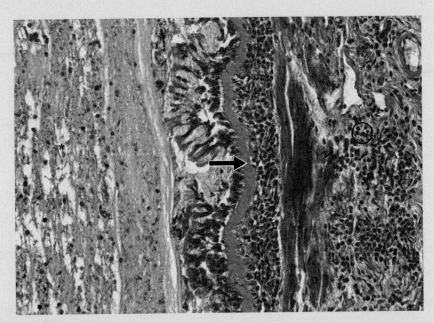

FIGURE 15-25 Histopathology of respiratory tissue from a case of status asthmaticus (detailed view) demonstrating a mucous plugged bronchus (*left*). Note the entrapped ciliary columnar epithelial cells. The epithelial basement membrane is much thickened (*arrow*). The tissue demonstrates influx of inflammatory cells. A group of eosinophils with characteristic red granules are within the circle.

Courtesy of Department of Pathology and Laboratory Medicine, University of North Carolina at Chapel Hill.

Questions

1. In addition to dust mites, insects, and animal dander, what are other common triggers for allergic asthma?

2. What are common nonallergic triggers for asthma?

3. Can you think of any additional studies that would help to prove (or disprove) the hygiene hypothesis of asthma susceptibility?

4. Allergic asthma is an example of type 1 hypersensitivity. What are the major characteristics of this type of hypersensitivity reaction?

5. How could Wilber's parents alter their household environment to prevent additional asthmatic attacks in Wilber?

6. How can the allergen(s) responsible be identified?

QUESTIONS FOR REVIEW

1. How do the lungs function? What is the difference between ventilation and gas exchange? How is pulmonary function disturbed if the alveolar septa are thickened and scarred?

2. What is pneumothorax? How does it develop? What is its effect on pulmonary function?

3. What is pneumonia? How is pneumonia classified? What are its major clinical features?

4. How does the tubercle bacillus differ in its staining reaction from other bacteria? What type of inflammatory reaction does it cause? What factors determine the outcome of a tuberculous infection? How does a cavity develop in lungs infected with tuberculosis? Is a person with a tuberculous cavity infectious to other people? What is miliary tuberculosis?

5. A patient has tuberculosis of the kidney, but no evidence of pulmonary tuberculosis is detected by means of a chest x-ray. How did this happen?

6. What is meant by the term "inactive tuberculosis"? Under what circumstances may an old inactive tuberculous infection become activated? What type of patients are susceptible to reactivation of a tuberculous infection?

7. What is the difference between bronchitis and bronchiectasis?

8. What is pulmonary emphysema? What factors predispose to its development? How may it be prevented? What is the difference between pulmonary emphysema and pulmonary fibrosis?

9. What is the relationship between carcinoma of the lung and cigarette smoking? How is lung carcinoma treated?

SUPPLEMENTARY READINGS

Funkhouser, W. K., Chapter 12, "Pulmonary Pathology." 2015. In *Pathology: A Modern Case Study*, edited by H. M. Reisner. New York: McGraw Hill Lange.

▶ A brief introduction to the pathology of pulmonary disease that is strong on overviews and case studies. It covers additional important diseases of the lung not included in the chapter.

Zarogoulidis, P., Kioumis, I., Pitsiou, G., et al. 2014. Pneumothorax: From definition to diagnosis and treatment. *Journal of Thoracic Disease* 6(Suppl 4):S372–76.

Restrepo, R. D., and Braverman, J. 2015. Current challenges in the recognition, prevention and treatment of perioperative pulmonary atelectasis. *Expert Review of Respiratory Medicine* 9:97–107.

▶ The first entry presents an overview of the physiology, pathology, and therapy of pneumothorax. The second entry concentrates on the problem of atelectasis occurring in the perioperative period.

Centers for Disease Control and Prevention. *Tuberculosis (TB)*. http://www.cdc.gov/tb/

Centers for Disease Control and Prevention. *Find TB resources*. http://findtbresources.cdc

Munoz, L., Stagg, H. R., and Abubaker, I. 2015. Diagnosis and management of latent tuberculosis infection. *Cold Spring Harbor Perspectives in Medicine* June 8, 5(11). doi: 10.1101/cshperspect.a017830

Centers for Disease Control and Prevention. *Middle East respiratory syndrome (MERS)*. http://www.cdc.gov/coronavrus/mers/

▶ The first two entries present an up-to-date overview of the status of TB infection in the United States, with the second entry providing a gateway to an extensive list of additional resources. The third entry discusses the ongoing problem of latent TB. How do you treat, diagnose, and manage individuals who may (for the moment) be asymptomatic yet represent a potential risk? The final entry provides the latest information on the MERS outbreak in the Middle East and currently in Korea. The site is updated frequently.

Kamangar, N. 2015. *Bacterial pneumonia*. Medscape. http://emedicine.medscape.com/article/300157-overview

Mosenifar, Z. 2015. *Viral pneumonia*. Medscape. http://emedicine.medscape.com/article/300455-overview

▶ The amount of material on bacterial and viral pneumonia is enormous and highly specialized. These two e-medicine references do a very nice job of summarizing these important areas and provide many additional resources for those interested.

Skalski, J. H., Kottom, T. J., and Limper, A. H. 2015. Pathobiology of pneumocystis pneumonia: Life cycle, cell wall, and cell signal transduction. *FEMS Yeast Research* (Epub June 12). doi: 10.1093/femsyr/fov046

▶ For a long time Pneumocystis infection was a leading cause of death in AIDS patients, and it remains a major problem for immunodeficient individuals. The organism is widespread and has an interesting life cycle and pathobiology, which are reviewed in this article.

Sharma, G. D., Bye, M. R., et al. 2014. *Pediatric asthma: Practice essentials, background, pathophysiology*. http://emedicine.medscape.com/article/1000997-overview

Saaden, C. K., Byrd, R. P., et al. 2014. *Status asthmaticus*. http://emedicine.medscape.com/article/2129484-overview

▶ These two references were most helpful in Case construction. They provide an overview of the diagnosis, pathophysiology, and therapy of asthma.

Modrykamien, A. M., and Gupta, P. 2015. The acute respiratory distress syndrome. *Baylor University Medical Center Proceedings* 2:163–71.

▶ Acute respiratory distress syndrome (diffuse alveolar damage to the pathologist) is a major cause of acute respiratory failure and mortality associated with many forms of injury to the lung. This review covers definition risk factors and pathophysiology of what is an often misunderstood condition.

Norbet, C., Joseph, A., Rossi, S. S., et al. 2015. Asbestos-related lung disease: A pictorial review. *Current Problems in Diagnostic Radiology* 44(4):371–82.

▶ Pulmonary asbestosis, although becoming uncommon with our better understanding of risk, presents a serious burden to people previously exposed to asbestos-related dusts. This article covers the diagnosis and radiology of the condition.

Franks, T. J., and Galvin, J. R. 2015. Smoking-related "interstitial" lung disease. *Archives of Pathology & Laboratory Medicine* 139(8):974–77.

Woodruff, P. G., et al. 2015. Current concepts in targeting chronic obstructive pulmonary disease pharmacotherapy: Making progress toward personalized management. *Lancet* 385:1789–98.

McGary Houghton, A. 2015. Matrix metalloproteinases in destructive lung disease. *Matrix Biology* 44–46:167–74.

Craig, T. J. 2015. Suspecting and testing for alpha-1 antitrypsin deficiency—An allergist's and/or immunologist's perspective. *Journal of Allergy and Clinical Immunology Practice* 3(4):506–11.

▶ The set of four references covers the pathology associated with smoking: emphysema, COPD, and other forms of lung damage. The fourth article provides accurate information on the clinical features associated with alpha-1 antitrypsin deficiency, a condition that synergizes with smoking to promote early onset emphysema.

Woods, S. L., et al. 2015. Molecular histology of lung cancer: From targets to treatments. *Cancer Treatment Reviews* 41:361–75.

▶ A review of the molecular analysis of lung cancer and its use in potential therapeutic approaches.

The Breast

Courtesy of Leonard V. Crowley, MD, Century College

Structure and Physiology of the Breast

The female breasts are each composed of about twenty lobes of glandular tissue embedded in fibrous and adipose tissue (**FIGURE 16-1**). The lobes are arranged circumferentially much as petals on a flower. Each lobe consists of clusters of glands (terminal ductules or acini) in which milk is made during pregnancy, and a series of intralobular ducts connecting the acini and the stromal tissue in which the acini and ducts are located. Taken together these three components are called the **terminal duct lobular unit (TDLU)**. The ducts of the TDLU converge to form large ducts that extend to the nipple. The ductules and ducts of the lobular system are bilayered. The luminal epithelial cells lining the ducts are the source of milk during lactation and also of much breast pathology, the most important being carcinoma. The outer layer is myoepithelial in nature and characteristically is lost in invasive breast cancer (**FIGURE 16-2**). Preservation versus loss of the bilayered nature of the lobular system is an important diagnostic criterion in separating benign from malignant breast disease.

The breasts are modified sweat glands that have become specialized to secrete milk. Before puberty, breast tissue in both sexes consists only of branching ducts and fibrous tissue without glandular tissue or fat. In the female, the breasts enlarge at puberty in response to estrogen and progesterone produced by the ovaries, whereas the unstimulated male breasts retain their prepubertal form. Postpubertal changes in

Terminal duct lobular unit (TDLU) Lobe of female breast including the cluster of milk gland ducts and stromal tissue.

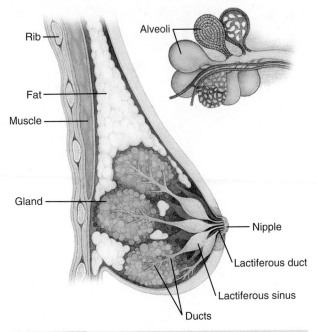

FIGURE 16-1 Anatomy of the breast ducts and lobules.

the female include proliferation of glandular and fibrous tissue and accumulation of adipose tissue within the breasts. Variations in the size of the postpubertal breasts of nonpregnant women are primarily the result of variations in the amount of fat and fibrous tissue in the breasts rather than differences in the amount of glandular tissue.

The breasts are fixed to the chest wall by bands of fibrous tissue called suspensory ligaments, which extend from the skin of the breast to the connective tissue covering the muscles of the chest wall. The breasts have an abundant blood supply and a rich lymphatic drainage. Lymphatic channels drain from each breast into groups of lymph nodes located in the armpit, or axilla (axillary lymph nodes), above the clavicle (supraclavicular lymph nodes), and beneath the sternum (mediastinal lymph nodes).

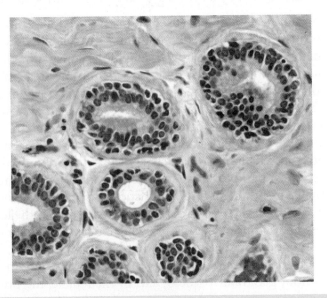

FIGURE 16-2 Breast glands. Each gland is lined by two layers of cells: an inner epithelial layer and an outer layer of myoepithelial cells.

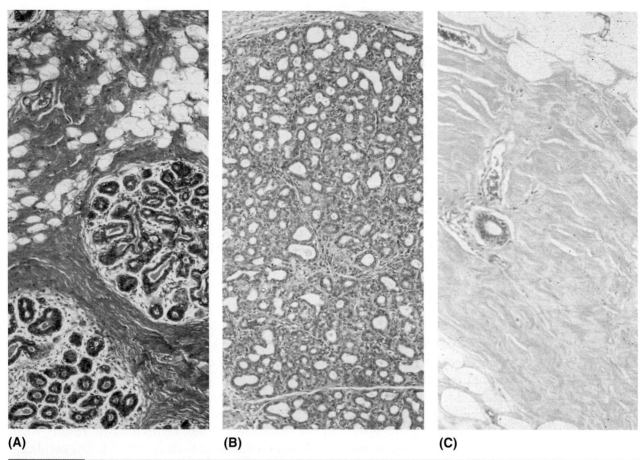

FIGURE 16-3 Photomicrographs illustrating the appearance of breasts under varying hormonal conditions (original magnification ×40). **(A)** Normal nonpregnant breast. Two lobules of glandular tissue appear in the lower half of the photograph. **(B)** Glandular hyperplasia in pregnancy. **(C)** Postmenopausal atrophy.

Courtesy of Leonard V. Crowley, MD, Century College.

The breasts are extremely responsive to hormonal stimulation. Mild cyclic hyperplasia followed by involution of breast tissue occurs normally during the menstrual cycle. The glandular and ductal tissues of the breast become markedly hypertrophic under the hormonal stimulus of pregnancy and lactation, and the breast undergoes regression in the postpartum period. After menopause, sex hormone levels decline, and the breasts gradually decrease in size. **FIGURE 16-3** illustrates the histologic appearance of breast tissue under varying hormonal conditions.

Abnormalities of Breast Development

ACCESSORY BREASTS AND NIPPLES

Embryologically, the breasts develop from columns of cells called **mammary ridges**, which extend along the anterior body wall from the armpits to the upper thighs. Most of the ridges disappear in the course of prenatal development except for the parts in the midthoracic region, which give rise to the breasts and nipples. Sometimes people have extra breasts or nipples. These are most commonly found in the armpits or on the lower chest below and medial to the normal breasts, but they may appear anywhere along the course of the embryonic mammary ridges (the milk line). Extra nipples and breast tissue may be a source of embarrassment to the individual, but usually they do not cause other problems.

Mammary ridges
Location of embryonic cells that develop into breasts.

UNEQUAL DEVELOPMENT OF THE BREASTS

The fully developed breasts are usually similar in size and shape but are not identical. Occasionally, one breast may fail to develop as much as its counterpart and may be significantly smaller than the opposite breast. Moreover, any condition that causes the breasts to enlarge may accentuate the disproportion.

BREAST HYPERTROPHY

At puberty, one or both, commonly both, female breasts may overrespond to hormonal stimulation and enlarge excessively. True breast hypertrophy is primarily caused by overgrowth of fibrous tissue, not glandular tissue or fat. The person may experience considerable back and shoulder discomfort caused by the excessive weight of the breasts. If symptoms are severe, the excessive breast tissue may be surgically resected, after which the breasts may be reconstructed so that they have a more normal size and shape.

GYNECOMASTIA

Gynecomastia Excessive development of the male breast.

Fibrocystic change (FCC) Common benign cystic change in breast tissue.

Occasionally, at puberty, the ductal and fibrous tissue of the adolescent male breast begin to proliferate, forming a distinct nodule of breast tissue under the nipple. This condition, which is called **gynecomastia** (*gyne* = woman + *mastos* = breast), may affect one or both breasts. It appears to result from a temporary physiological imbalance of male and female hormones that sometimes occurs in the male at puberty. Normally, the male secretes both male and female hormones, but male hormones predominate and "cancel out" the effects of the female hormones. Gynecomastia results when there is a temporary increase in estrogen relative to male hormones. The condition is not serious but may cause considerable emotional distress to the affected youth. Nonphysiological gynecomastia may occur in males who use certain drugs and may result be the result of hormone producing tumors of the testes. Unilateral breast masses or enlargement in males must be examined to rule out cancer, which does occur in males although it is uncommon.

NONPROLIFERATIVE FIBROCYSTIC CHANGE IN THE BREAST

Nonproliferative (benign) cystic changes in breast tissue, often called benign cystic disease or benign **fibrocystic change (FCC)**, is a common condition that bears no increased risk for development of cancer. FCC occurs in about one-third of women from the age of twenty to the menopausal period, after which the condition recedes. It is characterized by focal areas of proliferation of glandular and fibrous tissue in the breast associated with localized dilatation of ducts, resulting in the formation of various-sized cysts within the breast. Cystic change appears to be caused by irregularities in the response of the breast tissue to the normal cyclic variations of each menstrual cycle. Clinically, a breast cyst may feel very firm and may appear to be a solid tumor. Ultrasound examination of the breast is often helpful in distinguishing a cystic from a solid mass in the breast (**FIGURE 16-4**). Often, if the physician believes the mass to be a cyst rather than a solid tumor, an attempt is made to aspirate the cyst. A needle is introduced into the breast under local anesthesia. If a cyst is present, the fluid is aspirated and the mass disappears. If no fluid can be obtained, surgical excision is performed.

FIBROADENOMA

Fibroadenoma is the most common benign tumor of the female breast. It occurs most frequently in the third and fourth decades but also may present in a juvenile

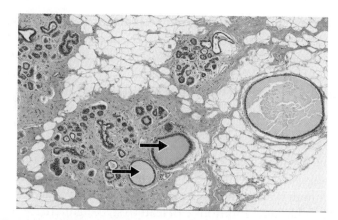

FIGURE 16-4 Nonproliferative cystic change in a breast. The biopsy demonstrates multiple localized dilated ducts forming cysts varying in size (*arrows*).

Courtesy of Department of Pathology and Laboratory Medicine, University of North Carolina at Chapel Hill.

(adolescent) form. The tumors have both an epithelial (glandular) and surrounding stromal component. They are painless, well circumscribed, and slow growing but may increase in size during pregnancy. Tumors are usually solitary and often are detected during routine mammography. Although the tumor is benign, it may, in some cases, be excised to distinguish it from a potentially malignant tumor (phylloides tumor), which is similar in appearance but generally larger and more rapid in growth (**FIGURE 16-5**).

Carcinoma of the Breast

Breast carcinoma occurs in both sexes. It is a rare tumor in men, whose breast tissue is not subjected to stimulation by ovarian hormones, but it is the most frequently diagnosed cancer in women and ranks second as a cause of cancer deaths (exceeded only by lung cancer). Breast cancer incidence rates declined drastically in the early part of the 21st century with the recognition that combined estrogen-progesterone

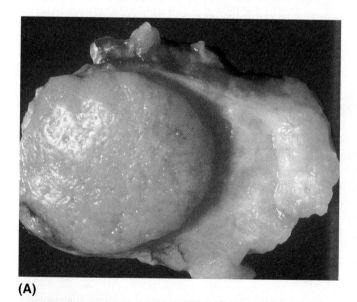

(A)

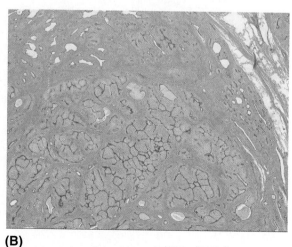

(B)

FIGURE 16-5 Benign fibroadenoma of the breast. The tumor is well circumscribed and readily separates from the breast. **(A)** Gross specimen. **(B)** Photomicrograph (low power); the fibrous stromal component and compressed glands and ducts are visible.

(A) Courtesy of Leonard V. Crowley, MD, Century College; (B) Courtesy of Department of Pathology and Laboratory Medicine, University of North Carolina at Chapel Hill.

Menarche Onset of menses.

Ductal carcinoma in situ (DCIS) The precursor lesion to most breast cancer.

therapy to reduce the symptoms associated with menopause (hormone replacement therapy) was a major risk factor for breast cancer. Additional modifiable risk factors include being overweight, physically inactive, consuming alcohol, or being a heavy smoker. Hormonal factors also influence the risk of breast carcinoma. Women who have never borne children or had their first child after age thirty are at increased risk, as are women who have had early onset of menses (**menarche**) or late menopause (that is, have had a long menstrual history). High breast tissue density (increased glandular relative to fat tissue) as measured on mammography also may indicate increased risk, but this may be due to the difficulty of early detection in such breasts rather than to heightened risk. There is some tendency for breast carcinoma to run in families, and a woman is at higher than normal risk if her mother or sister has had a breast carcinoma. Inherited mutations can lead to striking increases in breast cancer susceptibility. Two genes (*BRCA1* and *BRCA2*), although rare in the population (less than 1 percent), account for up to 10 percent of all female breast cancer and up to 20 percent of breast cancer that occurs in families. In summary, the etiology of breast cancer is multifactorial and involves genetic background, hormonal status, and poorly defined environmental factors. Significant differences in breast cancer frequencies are found in different populations and socioeconomic groups. Mammography has led to the understanding that breast cancer originates in "in situ disease," which is restricted to the ducts and lobular system and is not (yet) capable of metastasis. **Ductal carcinoma in situ (DCIS)**, the precursor lesion to most breast cancers, is now diagnosed with fivefold greater frequency as a result of screening mammography. With time, in situ disease leads to populations of neoplastic cell that can traverse the ductal basement membrane, invade the surrounding tissue, and metastasize to distant sites. Because it is unclear which cases of DCIS will progress to invasive disease, DCIS is treated aggressively with excision and sometimes radiation and hormonal therapy. The process of progression is accompanied by loss of the myoepithelial cell layer surrounding the ducts and lobules of the TLDU (**FIGURE 16-6**).

BREAST CARCINOMA SUSCEPTIBILITY GENES

A small proportion of breast carcinomas are hereditary and can be traced to inheritance of mutant breast cancer susceptibility genes. The two most important

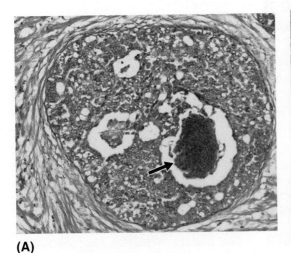
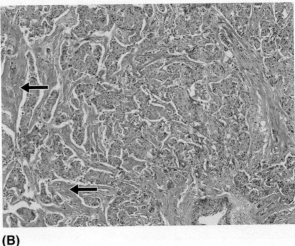

(A)   **(B)**

FIGURE 16-6 Ductal carcinoma. **(A)** Ductal carcinoma in situ (DCIS). This high-grade lesion demonstrates intraductal necrosis (*arrow*) characteristic of the lesion. The lesion is confined by the basement membrane. **(B)** Invasive ductal carcinoma infiltrates breast tissue and is associated with a fibrotic reaction of surrounding tissue (*arrows*).

Courtesy of Department of Pathology and Laboratory Medicine, University of North Carolina at Chapel Hill.

susceptibility genes are *BRCA1* and *BRCA2*, both involved in the process of DNA repair. The *BRCA1* gene is a very large gene, and a large number of different mutations have been described. A woman who inherits a mutant *BRCA1* gene has a 40 to 80 percent chance of developing breast carcinoma during her lifetime and an approximately 20 to 40 percent lifetime risk of ovarian carcinoma as well. A woman who inherits a mutant *BRCA2* gene has a 30 to 60 percent lifetime risk of breast carcinoma, but the lifetime risk of ovarian carcinoma is only about 10 to 20 percent, which is significantly lower than the ovarian carcinoma risk associated with a *BRCA1* mutation. (The role of tumor suppressor genes on cell functions and the effects of inherited mutations are considered in the neoplastic disease discussion.) Although the frequency of *BRCA1/BRCA2* mutations are low in the general population (0.2 percent or less), the frequency is up to tenfold higher in some populations (notably Ashkenazi Jews). Individuals who come from certain cancer families, those who have had early onset or bilateral breast cancer, and those of Ashkenazi Jewish background are suggested candidates for genetic testing for mutations in *BRCA1/BRCA2*. There is no simple way to reduce the risk of breast, ovarian, and several other cancers in carrier individuals. Hence, intensive screening tests every six months are recommended to identify and treat any newly detected carcinomas in this high-risk group. Unfortunately, early-stage carcinomas detected by screening tests do not guarantee a successful response to treatment. It is difficult to detect an ovarian carcinoma in its early stage, and many breast carcinomas in affected women are aggressive, rapidly growing tumors that may already have spread by the time they are detected. Consequently, many high-risk women carrying *BRCA1* or *BRCA 2* mutations have chosen to have their fallopian tubes and ovaries removed or have a bilateral mastectomy; often both procedures are performed to avoid the risk of both breast and ovarian carcinoma.

CLASSIFICATION OF BREAST CARCINOMA

Breast cancers are classified according to the site of origin, the presence or absence of invasion, the degree of differentiation, and more recently the molecular characteristics (nature of genes expressed) of the tumor cells. More than 90 percent of carcinomas arise from the epithelium of the ducts and are called **ductal carcinomas**. The rest arise from the lobules and are designated **lobular carcinomas**. As previously noted, a precursor in situ lesion for ductal carcinoma (DCIS) has been defined. Lobular carcinoma in situ (LCIS) occurs but is usually not considered an in situ carcinoma requiring surgical excision. However, certain specific types of LCIS may be an in situ precursor for forms of lobular carcinoma and require excisional therapy.

The therapy and prognosis for invasive breast carcinoma depend on many variables, but current practice focuses on the molecular characteristics of the carcinoma cells, which differ from case to case. The characteristics examined include the presence of several cell surface receptors including **estrogen receptors (ER)** and **progesterone receptors (PR)**, which are almost always present or absent together, and the **human epidermal growth factor receptor 2 (HER-2)**. ER positivity is a favorable prognostic indicator and suggests that the cancer cells may still respond to hormonal stimulation. Patients with these cancers are excellent candidates for drugs that block the effects of estrogens (such as tamoxifen) and slow the growth of the cancer cells. Some breast carcinomas overexpress (make excessive amounts of) the HER-2 protein and other genes associated with HER-2. These carcinomas are aggressive and have a poor prognosis. However, they are candidates for therapy using antibodies that target the HER-2 receptor (the monoclonal antibody trastuzumab and others) or for a drug that blocks the pathway stimulated by HER-2 (lapatinib, a tyrosine kinase

Ductal carcinoma Tumor arising from the epithelium of the ducts.

Lobular carcinoma Tumor of the breast arising from the lobules.

Estrogen receptors (ER)/ progesterone receptors (PR) Breast cell surface receptors.

Human epidermal growth factor receptor 2 (HER-2) Breast cell surface receptor.

Gene expression profile
List of proteins synthesized by breast cancer cells.

Luminal A/ Luminal B
Specific types of gene expression profiles found in breast cancer cells.

Basal-like tumors Type of breast cancer cell demonstrating a specific gene expression profile.

Triple-negative Breast cancer cell lacking ER, PR, and HER-2.

Mammography/ mammogram
Technique of an x-ray of the breast used to detect tumors and other abnormalities within the breast.

inhibitor). Tests that determine the **gene expression profile** of breast carcinomas have been devised recently. These tests determine which sets of proteins are produced by the carcinomas and divide the disease into subtypes that have particular prognostic characteristics. **Luminal A** carcinomas make up about 50 percent of cases and are most like the normal (non-neoplastic) breast epithelial cells. Luminal A cancers are low grade; that is, they are most similar to the normal cells they originate from and are generally ER positive. Individuals with these carcinomas have an excellent prognosis and are treated with hormonal therapy. **Luminal B** tumors (15 to 20 percent of cases) have a higher grade than Luminal A tumors but usually still express some level of ER. Individuals with these carcinomas have a poorer prognosis and are treated with both hormonal and other forms of chemotherapy. Individuals with **basal-like tumors** (15 to 20 percent of cases) have a poor prognosis. Their pattern of gene expression is most similar to the myoepithelial cells that line breast TLDUs. These tumors are commonly of the **triple-negative** type, lacking in ER, PR, and HER-2. Most tumors in *BRCA1*-positive individuals are of this type. Although the tumors are sensitive to chemotherapy, patients have a high relapse rate, and the tumors tend to metastasize to the viscera and brain. HER-2-positive tumors (10 percent of cases) are extremely aggressive. These tumors contain multiple copies of the gene responsible for the HER-2 protein and have large amounts of the HER-2 receptor on their surface. Like basal-cell-type tumors, they have very high rates of cell division but can be treated using anti-HER-2 therapy. Another important factor in deciding on the likely prognosis of breast carcinoma (and choosing a therapy) is the stage of the tumor at detection.

EVOLUTION OF BREAST CARCINOMA

In its early stages, a breast carcinoma is too small to be detected by breast examination but can often be demonstrated by **mammography**, sometimes as early as two years before it becomes large enough to form a palpable lump within the breast. Frequently, focal areas of necrosis occur within the proliferating tumor cells, and calcium salts diffuse from the bloodstream into the areas of necrosis (**FIGURE 16-7**). These small focal calcium deposits often can be identified in mammograms, which raises a suspicion of calcium deposits within a ductal carcinoma. Calcium deposits

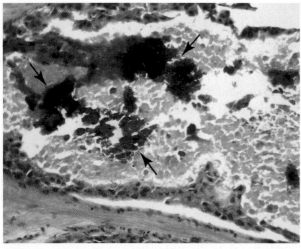

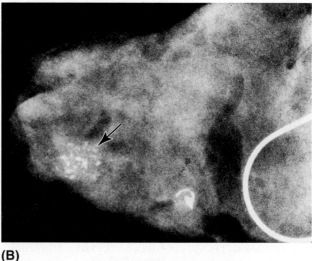

(A) **(B)**

FIGURE 16-7 **(A)** Ductal carcinoma of the breast, showing necrosis and calcification (*arrows*) within the tumor. **(B)** Characteristic appearance of stippled calcification within the tumor (*arrow*) that can be identified by mammograms.

Courtesy of Leonard V. Crowley, MD, Century College.

are not conclusive evidence of breast carcinoma, however, because calcium deposits also accumulate in some benign breast lesions.

Many breast carcinomas induce fibrosis in the surrounding normal breast tissue that is being invaded by the tumor cells, as though the body were trying to defend itself by laying down fibrous tissue to contain the tumor (see Figure 16-6B). Consequently, many breast cancers are very firm and have a puckered, scarred appearance with irregular margins that blend into the surrounding breast tissue. This appearance is caused more by the proliferation of fibrous tissue in response to the tumor than by the tumor cells themselves. Nevertheless, this appearance is quite characteristic of many breast cancers and aids in identifying a carcinoma by mammography. Not all breast carcinomas have such a characteristic appearance. In many instances, the mammogram identifies an abnormal or suspicious area within the breast that could be an early carcinoma but is not conclusive, and a biopsy is necessary to establish the exact diagnosis. As a breast tumor continues to grow, it infiltrates the breast tissues more extensively and, left untreated, eventually metastasizes to regional lymph nodes and distant sites. Hence, early diagnosis allows prompt treatment and much improves the cure rate. For this reason, routine screening mammography is recommended for all women starting at age forty (and earlier in selected individuals). Breast self-examination to detect early changes in the breast should be a regular practice for all women twenty years old and older.

MAMMOGRAMS

A **mammogram** is a special type of x-ray examination that allows the physician to visualize the internal structure of the breast and recognize abnormalities that may not be detected by clinical examination. In a mammogram, the fibrous and glandular tissue of the breast appear as interlacing white strands. The less dense fatty tissue, which transmits x-rays readily, appears dark (**FIGURE 16-8** and **FIGURE 16-9**). Cysts and tumors within the breast appear as dense white masses surrounded by the less

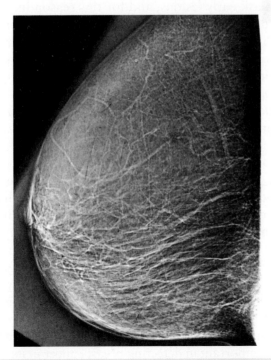

FIGURE 16-8 A normal mammogram.

Courtesy of Leonard V. Crowley, MD, Century College.

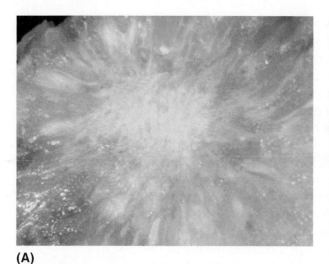

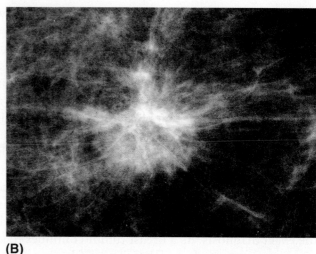

(A) **(B)**

FIGURE 16-9 Breast carcinoma. **(A)** Cross section of a breast biopsy. The tumor appears as a firm, poorly circumscribed mass that infiltrates the surrounding fatty breast tissue. **(B)** The appearance of breast carcinoma in a mammogram. The tumor appears as a white area with infiltrating margins. Note that the same criteria used to identify breast carcinoma on gross examination are used to recognize malignancy in the mammogram.

Courtesy of Leonard V. Crowley, MD, Century College.

dense dark tissue of the adjacent normal breast. Cysts and benign tumors appear well circumscribed, whereas malignant tumors often have irregular margins that indicate infiltration of the tumor into the surrounding breast tissue. These same criteria are used to distinguish between benign and malignant tumors on gross examination when a biopsy specimen is examined. Malignant tumors also frequently contain fine flecks of calcium that indicate calcification within the carcinoma. This is another feature suggestive of malignancy when seen on the mammogram.

The density of breasts (the ratio of glands and connective tissue to fat) differs from woman to woman as does the degree of benign fibrocystic change. Dense and cystic breasts may mask early lesions, and for this reason improvements in breast screening have been devised. Digital mammography (electronic imaging is substituted for photographic film) has become standard and provides better resolution for small lesions. Recently, ultrasound has been used as an adjunct to mammography and is of particular utility in evaluating dense and cystic breasts.

Periodic mammograms are recommended for all women as a screening procedure. Mammograms can detect early breast cancers much sooner than they could be felt by physical examination of the breasts, and early detection followed by prompt treatment while a tumor is still small greatly increases the woman's chance of survival. The current American Cancer Society recommendations are for an initial baseline mammogram at age forty, followed by repeat mammograms every year as long as the women is in good health. Mammography can pick up small tumors before they can be detected by breast examination, but the procedure has limitations and yields both false-positive and false-negative results. The procedure may not always identify a small carcinoma in the dense breast tissue of younger women, which obscures the tumor. Despite its limitations, the value of screening mammography appears to be well established. Screening has reduced breast cancer mortality 20 to 30 percent in women fifty to sixty-nine years of age, and slightly less in women forty to forty-nine years of age who have denser breast tissue and faster growing tumors. Mammography is sensitive in detecting changes, so routine examination carefully comparing prior and current results is important in detecting breast cancer in its earliest state. In very limited cases in which there is a high lifetime risk of developing breast cancer, the use of MRI technology is also recommended.

CLINICAL MANIFESTATIONS

The most common initial manifestation of breast carcinoma is a lump in the breast. It may be detected by the patient herself or by a routine mammogram. A more advanced carcinoma may cause secondary changes in the overlying skin or the nipple. The neoplasm may infiltrate the suspensory ligaments, exerting traction on the ligaments and causing them to shorten. Because the ligaments attach to the skin of the breast, shortening of the ligaments causes the overlying skin to retract as well. Consequently, skin or nipple retraction generally indicates the presence of an infiltrating carcinoma deeper within the breast.

If the tumor infiltrates and plugs the lymphatic vessels that drain lymph from the skin, the overlying skin may become edematous. (Lymphatic obstruction as a cause of edema is considered in the circulatory disturbances discussion.) Skin edema produces a rather characteristic appearance in which the normal cutaneous hair follicles stand out sharply as multiple small depressions within the edematous skin. The appearance has been compared with the skin of an orange and is usually called the orange-peel (peau d'orange) sign (**FIGURE 16-10**). Unfortunately, this finding indicates an advanced carcinoma that has already invaded lymphatic vessels and has probably also metastasized to regional lymph nodes. The likelihood of curing the cancer is much reduced at this stage.

If the patient delays in consulting her physician and a breast cancer is not treated, the tumor will eventually infiltrate the entire breast and will become fixed to the chest wall. The tumor will also metastasize widely. Although a far-advanced cancer often can be controlled for a time by various methods of treatment, there is no longer a possibility of cure.

TREATMENT

There are several ways to treat breast carcinoma, depending on the stage, prognostic characteristics, and desire of the patient. These decisions are extremely complex and involve discussions between the clinical oncologist, radiologist, surgeon, pathologist, and the patient. Decisions will be guided by the grade (possibly using gene expression analysis), receptor status, and stage of disease at the time of diagnosis.

Surgery is the mainstay for breast cancer therapy. Although in theory some in situ cancers (DCIS in particular) might not progress, there is currently no way to predict the behavior of such lesions, so these lesions are treated surgically. In some

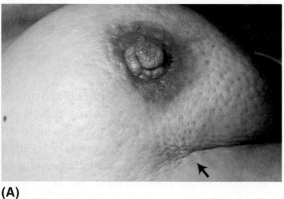

(A)

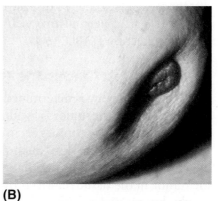

(B)

FIGURE 16-10 Changes in the breast caused by advanced carcinoma. **(A)** Skin retraction (*arrow*) and orange-peel appearance of the skin. **(B)** Nipple retraction.

Courtesy of Leonard V. Crowley, MD, Century College.

TABLE 16-1   Breast Cancer Stage Groupings and Corresponding Survival Rates

Stage	Simplified description	5-Year survival
Stage 0	Carcinoma in situ	100%
Stage IA	Tumor less than 2 cm	100%
Stage IB	Tumor less than 2 cm, with microscopic foci* of cancer in lymph nodes	
Stage IIA	Tumor less than 2 cm with spread to 1–3 axillary lymph nodes** OR Tumor between 2 and 5 cm without spread to lymph nodes	86%
Stage IIB	Tumor between 2 and 5 cm with spread to 1–3 axillary lymph nodes OR Tumor larger than 5 cm without extension to lymph nodes	
Stage IIIA	Tumor no more than 5 cm, with spread to 4–9 axillary lymph nodes or enlarged internal thoracic lymph nodes, OR Tumor larger than 5 cm with spread to up to 9 axillary lymph nodes	57%
Stage IIIB	Tumor of any size that has grown into chest wall or skin, with or without nodal spread	
Stage IIIC	Tumor of any size that has spread to 10 or more axillary lymph nodes, to axillary and internal thoracic lymph nodes, or to infra- or supraclavicular lymph nodes	
Stage IV	Cancer of any size with any degree of lymph node involvement, with spread to distant sites	20%

*Microscopic foci are tumor deposits less than 2 mm in diameter.

**Regional lymph nodes include both axillary and internal thoracic lymph nodes. Axillary lymph nodes are easily accessible to the surgeon, but internal thoracic (mammary) ones are usually sampled only when they are highlighted by the sentinel lymph node procedure. Involvement of internal thoracic lymph nodes imparts a slightly worse prognosis than involvement of axillary lymph nodes.

cases of cancer detected early in its course, surgery can be curative. In more advanced cases, surgery may remove the bulk of the lesion and enable the surgeon to stage the cancer. Is the cancer small and localized, or has it spread outside the breast? The TNM scores (see below) are grouped to determine the stage. Similar stages tend to have the same prognosis. The system is complicated, but the higher the stage, the poorer the prognosis. For example, stage I disease has small tumors and either no or very minimal spread to lymph nodes, whereas stage IV disease is defined by having distant metastases. Stage I disease has a 100-percent five-year survival rate; stage IV disease has a 22-percent five-year survival rate, which emphasizes the importance of early detection (**TABLE 16-1**).

Staging of Breast Cancer: The TNM System

Breast cancer staging is determined using the TNM system. "T" represents the tumor size and whether the tumor is localized to the breast or has spread into adjacent tissue. For example, T1 are tumors 2 cm (3/4 inch) across or less. T4 tumors have grown into the chest wall or skin. Such determinations are made by the surgeon (guided by mammographic and other data) and the pathologist who evaluates the extent of the tumor in the tissue removed by the surgeon. In the TNM system "N" represents nearby lymph nodes. This too is evaluated by the surgeon, most often guided by a technique called **sentinel lymph node** analysis. The invasion of nearby lymph nodes by cancer cells negatively affects prognosis and depends on the number of nodes involved (and in some cases, how many cancer cells have invaded the node). Finally,

Sentinel lymph node The lymph node in a group of lymph nodes that is located closest to a malignant tumor, which is examined to determine whether the tumor has spread to the node. If the sentinel node is not involved, additional lymph node dissection is not required.

the "M" represents invasion of distant sites by cancer cells (metastases) and has a serious impact on the likelihood of five-year survival. This is determined using both physical examination and a number of radiographic procedures (such as CT). The histologic grade, a measure of how similar the breast carcinoma cells appear to their normal tissue counterparts, also has prognostic value, and low-grade tumors (more similar to normal) having a better prognosis. As previously discussed, gene expression profiling correlates, in part, with grade.

Examination of Axillary Lymph Nodes: The Role of the Sentinel Node

Although cancer that has invaded lymph nodes may be detectable based on node size and texture, small numbers of cancer cells are detected through microscopic analysis of the node by a pathologist. Many lymph nodes, primarily in the axillary area, are located near and drain the lymphatic channels of the breast. In addition, internal mammary nodes found near the breast bone also drain the breast and may be a site for cancer cell invasion. Because the nodes that receive drainage from the breast are interconnected, the lymph from the breast is filtered through several lymph nodes before being returned to the venous circulation via the thoracic duct or right lymphatic duct. If one or more axillary lymph nodes contain metastatic carcinoma, the tumor already has spread beyond the breast, and the greater the number of involved lymph nodes, the less favorable the prognosis.

Surgical dissection of axillary lymph nodes may at times be complicated by edema of the arm, resulting from disruption of the lymphatic drainage channels in the axilla, and may also be associated with temporary limitation of shoulder mobility and axillary discomfort. Often it is possible to avoid such dissection while still obtaining information about the presence or absence of metastases. This is accomplished using a technique to identify the first lymph node in the chain of nodes that receives drainage from the tumor. This node is called the sentinel lymph node. If the sentinel node does not contain metastatic tumor, it is very unlikely that any of the other axillary nodes will contain tumor, and a more extensive axillary dissection is avoided. The surgeon injects either a dye or radiotracer into the tumor and detects the first lymph node (or nodes) to be marked either by the dye or radioactive compound. The sentinel node (or nodes) is removed and examined for the presence of cancer cells. When cancer is found in the sentinel node, more extensive analysis of additional nodes is necessary (**FIGURE 16-11** and **FIGURE 16-12**).

Surgical Techniques in Breast Cancer Therapy

Surgical treatment of breast cancer can be divided into two general approaches. The first, **breast conserving surgery** (sometimes called a "lumpectomy") attempts to remove the minimal amount of breast tissue while still removing all of the cancer and nearby tissue. The degree of tissue removed will depend on the size and location of the lesion. The surgeon, working closely with the pathologist, will examine the removed tissue during surgery to ensure that the cancer is removed with adequate margins of healthy tissue on all sides of the removed tissue. This surgery is followed by radiation therapy directed toward the site of the tumor or, in some cases, chemotherapy to suppress any residual cancer cells. In cases of low stage breast cancer, breast conserving surgery accompanied by radiation therapy results in as good a prognosis as **mastectomy** (removal of the breast and sometimes underlying tissue). However, patients with low stage disease sometimes decide against radiation therapy (for example, in cases of pregnancy) and elect a less conservative surgical approach.

When the cancer is large or has spread (higher stage cancers), total mastectomy may be required. There are many variations in surgical approach. In **simple mastectomy** (total mastectomy) the breast and nipple are removed (but not axillary lymph nodes

> **Breast conserving surgery** Surgery designed to remove the minimal amount of breast tissue.
>
> **Simple mastectomy/ radical mastectomy** Surgery to remove the breast and sometimes underlying tissue. May be simple mastectomy (only breast tissue) or radical mastectomy (breast and underlying tissue).

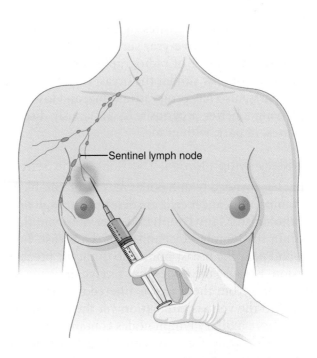

FIGURE 16-11 Schematic diagram of sentinel lymph node biopsy.

or muscle from under the breast). This can be done in such a way as to spare breast skin, which allows for immediate breast reconstruction. There is some concern that skin-sparing surgery (particularly if the nipple is spared) may present a greater risk of recurrence. In a modified **radical mastectomy,** the axillary lymph nodes are also removed. Most invasive is a radical mastectomy in which lymph nodes and chest wall muscles are removed. Such surgery is currently rarely done except in cases where the tumor is large and has penetrated the muscle. The choice between breast conserving and more extensive procedures is complex and depends both on the nature of the cancer and patient preferences.

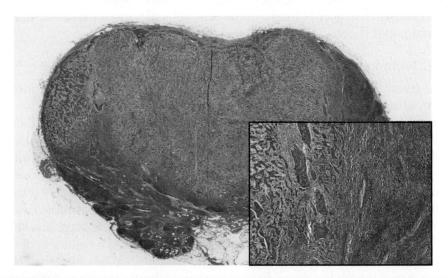

FIGURE 16-12 Axillary lymph node with metastatic tumor. Inset: Breast tumor cells on right are effacing the normal lymphatic tissue on left (high power).

Courtesy of Department of Pathology and Laboratory Medicine, University of North Carolina at Chapel Hill.

Adjuvant Therapies in Breast Cancer

In addition to surgical and radiation therapy, a number of systemic forms of drug therapy (**adjuvant therapy**) may be used to reduce the risk of cancer recurrence. The term *neoadjuvant therapy* is used when therapy is started prior to surgery, often in an attempt to reduce tumor mass and render surgery more effective. As noted, about two-thirds of breast cancer cells have estrogen or progesterone receptors that promote cancer cell growth in the presence of these hormones. Drugs that block the effect of estrogen (such as tamoxifen) help to prevent cancer recurrence in receptor positive cancer (and for women treated for DCIS such treatment tends to prevent the occurrence of invasive cancer). A second class of drugs called **aromatase inhibitors** blocks production of estrogen by fat cells in postmenopausal women. (These drugs do not block ovarian estrogen production and cannot be used in premenopausal patients.) Aromatase inhibitors may be more effective (and have fewer side effects) than tamoxifen, and these drugs are often recommended for use for at least five years postsurgery.

About 20 percent of breast cancer patients make an excess of the HER-2 protein on the surface, and drugs that target this protein (either monoclonal antibodies such as Herceptin or nonantibody drugs such as Lapatinib) can be used as adjuncts in therapy of early and more advanced cancers. A number of more "traditional" chemotherapeutic drugs (such as doxorubicin and paclitaxel) can be used either as adjuvant therapy postsurgery or in advanced cases of cancer that have metastasized.

> **Adjuvant therapy** Drug therapy used along with surgery and radiation.

> **Aromatase inhibitor** A drug that inhibits the conversion of adrenal androgenic steroids to estrogens, used as postresection adjuvant therapy to treat postmenopausal women with estrogen-positive breast carcinoma.

TREATMENT OF RECURRENT AND METASTATIC CARCINOMA

A significant number of patients treated for breast carcinoma develop recurrent or metastatic carcinoma, which may appear many years after the original tumor had been resected. The methods selected to treat patients with recurrent carcinoma depend on many factors, including the hormone receptor status of the tumor, the location of the metastases, the age of the patient, and the length of time that has elapsed between the initial treatment and the appearance of metastases. Although the tumor is no longer curable, treatment can control tumor growth, relieve symptoms, and improve the patient's quality of life.

Risks Related to Hormone Treatment

Hormones have been used in the past to treat menopausal symptoms. Treatment consists of either estrogen or estrogen along with a progestin (a synthetic compound with progesterone activity). Long-term hormone use increases the risk of breast carcinoma, and the magnitude of the risk depends on what hormones are taken and how long they are used. Estrogen–progestin use poses the greatest risk. Estrogen plus progestin increases the risk of breast carcinoma, and the tumors are more likely to have spread to the regional lymph nodes by the time they are recognized, which is associated with a less favorable prognosis and higher mortality. Currently, hormone treatment is recommended only to relieve menopause-related hot flashes and other disturbing menopausal symptoms, using only the lowest effective dose for as short a time as possible.

CASE 16-1

Jane is a thirty-three-year-old concerned about the possibility of breast disease. A maternal aunt was diagnosed with invasive breast cancer at the age of forty-eight. Jane's mother (age sixty-two) has been biopsied on several occasions for suspicious breast lesions that were diagnosed as benign cysts, and twice as a fibroadenomas. Because of her concern, Jane is careful to practice breast self-examination and has elected to have yearly mammography starting at age thirty. Jane paid to be tested for *BRCA1* and *BRCA2* and was found to be negative. She has been diagnosed as having mild fibrocystic disease but otherwise had a normal mammogram six months ago. On self-examination, Jane now notes a single hard mass in the upper inner quadrant of her left breast. The mass appeared to be adherent to the skin. Jane's physician confirmed a 3 cm mass that was tender to firm palpation. The physician noted a slight skin retraction over the mass and was concerned about the possibility of a rapidly growing carcinoma. Mammography revealed an irregular mass with some architectural distortion and calcification, supporting the concern for malignancy. Because of this concern, Jane elected to have an excisional biopsy in which the entire mass was removed. The surgeon noted the mass was yellow in color, appeared to be fibrotic with areas of calcification, and had several small cystic regions. Microscopic analysis of the tissue (**FIGURE 16-13**) demonstrates a process consistent with **fat necrosis** of the breast. This is a specific form of necrosis associated with damage to areas of the body rich in lipid-containing cells. Fat necrosis in the breast is a benign process that requires no therapy. However, the process may be difficult to differentiate from cancer and requires biopsy for diagnosis. A much relieved Jane is carefully questioned about possible trauma to her breast. About three months before noting the mass, Jane remembers that she came to a very sudden stop while driving. She noted some bruising and pain along the area of her breast crossed by the seatbelt.

Discussion

Fat necrosis (also termed **enzymatic fat necrosis**) is a sterile form of inflammation that occurs after trauma (or other damage) to areas of the body rich in lipid. In fat necrosis, lipid released from damaged fat cells is saponified (converted to soap) by tissue lipases in the presence of calcium. The lipid may form cysts in the tissue and provokes a chronic inflammatory response. Macrophages ingest the lipid (foamy macrophages) and fuse to form **giant cells** in response to the irritant material. Ultimately, healing occurs accompanied by fibrosis (scarring), deposition of calcium in the tissue, and potentially residual lipid cysts. Pathologists usually think about the area around the pancreas when they consider fat necrosis because it is common in this region in response to pancreatitis. (In this setting fat necrosis has serious medical consequences.) However, fat necrosis is not uncommon in the breast and buttocks. Fat necrosis accounts for about 3 percent of benign breast lesions. Seatbelt induced injury and trauma related to breast surgery are common causes. Most cases of fat necrosis in the breast are easy to diagnosis based on the presence of radiolucent cysts (using mammography often combined with ultrasound) and may not require biopsy. With time, continuing inflammation, fibrosis, and calcification may present in a manner similar to cancer and require biopsy. For this reason, a careful patient history that discloses possible breast trauma is important in the clinical decision-making process. Although it was understandable for Jane to be concerned about breast cancer given her history, it is important to realize that the majority of breast lesions biopsied are not cancer (**FIGURE 16-14**).

Fat necrosis A sterile form of inflammation that occurs after trauma (or other damage) to areas of the body rich in lipid.

Enzymatic fat necrosis See fat necrosis.

CASE 16-1 (*Continued*)

Etiology and Pathogenesis

Fat necrosis of the breast as a result of seatbelt induced tissue trauma.

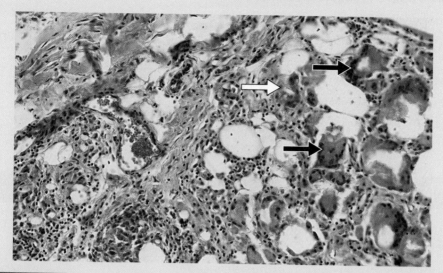

FIGURE 16-13 Excisional biopsy of breast demonstrating fat necrosis (photomicrograph). Examples of giant cells (*black arrows*) and lipid filled (foamy) macrophages (*white arrow*). Lymphocytes and numerous small oil cysts are scattered through the tissue. Fibrosis is present on the upper left margin.

Courtesy of Department of Pathology and Laboratory Medicine, University of North Carolina at Chapel Hill.

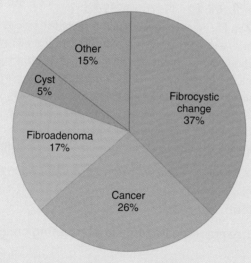

FIGURE 16-14 Relative frequency of lesions of the breast that are biopsied out of concern for cancer.

Questions

1. Given Jane's family history, were her concerns about early onset breast cancer justified?

2. The American Cancer Society suggests routine mammography begin at age forty. Other expert opinions suggest starting later. What drawbacks would there be to recommending routine mammography very early (at age twenty or thirty, for example)?

3. Suppose Jane's mammogram disclosed a cystic area. Do you believe she would have been wise to proceed to a biopsy?

QUESTIONS FOR REVIEW

1. What are the common diseases of the breast that may be manifested as a lump in the breast? How are they distinguished from one another by a physician?

2. What is a mammogram? How is it used by a physician?

3. What are estrogen receptors in tumor cells? How is an estrogen receptor analysis used in management of patients with breast carcinoma?

4. What is gynecomastia?

5. What methods are used to treat breast carcinoma?

6. What is an aromatase inhibitor, and how is it used?

SUPPLEMENTARY READINGS

Livasy, C. Chapter 16, "Breast Pathology." 2015. In *Pathology: A Modern Case Study*, edited by H. Reisner. New York: McGraw Hill Lange.

American Cancer Society. http://www.cancer.org/cancer/breastcancer/

National Institutes of Health. http://www.cancer.gov/cancertopics/types/breast

World Health Organization. 2014. *WHO position paper on mammography*. Geneva: World Health Organization.

Ehsani, S., et al. 2015. Screening magnetic resonance imaging recommendations and outcomes in patients at high risk for breast cancer. *The Breast Journal*. doi: 10.1111/tbj.12396

▶ The literature about breast cancer is immense and at times controversial. This set of five articles has been selected as an overview. The first entry provides a brief recent review of the pathology of breast cancer aimed at undergraduate medical students. It presents a readable and case-rich introduction to the area for anyone interested in background to the diagnosis of breast disease, including infection and inflammation. The Case in the chapter was suggested in part by this reference. Entries two and three provide excellent overviews and additional references to breast cancer screening and therapy. Many of the clinical guidelines in this chapter are those given by the American Cancer Society. The fourth entry presents an international perspective on the area of mammographic screening with an emphasis on economic issues. MRI has been suggested as an important aid in breast cancer screening, and the fifth entry presents an expert overview of the utility of the technique.

Arteaga, C. L. 2013. Progress in breast cancer: Overview. *Clinical Cancer Research 19*:6353–59.

▶ This article provides an overview of recent advances in the field of breast cancer translational (clinically oriented) research. An introduction to important new areas of research.

Elmore, J. G., et al. 2015. Diagnostic concordance among pathologists interpreting breast biopsy specimens. *JAMA 313*:1122–32.

Davidson, N. E., and Rimm, D. L. 2015. Expertise vs evidence in assessment of breast biopsies. An atypical science (Editorial). *JAMA 313*:1109–10.

▶ Breast biopsy by highly trained surgical pathologists represents the mainstay in clinical decision making with respect to both diagnosis and therapy. How good is the pathologist's eye? These two entries explore a much discussed study, answering questions and suggesting the need for new approaches.

Van de Vijver, M. J. 2014. Molecular tests as prognostic factors in breast cancer. *Virchows Archiv 464*:283–91.

▶ An introduction to how molecular-based tests are used in guiding breast cancer therapy and suggesting prognosis.

Abramson, V. G., et al. 2014. Subtyping of triple-negative breast cancer: Implications for therapy. *Cancer 121*:8–16.

Dietze, E. C., et al. 2015. Triple-negative breast cancer in African-American women: Disparities versus biology. *Nature Reviews Cancer 4*:248–54.

▶ Triple-negative breast cancer is most common in BRCA1 patients and has a very poor prognosis. For this reason, the area is now a target for sophisticated molecular studies with the goal of improving therapy and prognosis. The first article provides a good review of cancer molecular subtyping. The second article addresses the question of why triple-negative cancer disproportionately affects young African American women, and why clinical outcomes are worse for them than for women of European origin. Is it genetics or social disparities?

Roy, R., Chun, J., and Powell, S. N. 2012. BRCA1 and BRCA2: Different roles in a common pathway of genome protection. *Nature Reviews Cancer 12*:68–78.

Rich, T. A., et al. 2015. Hereditary breast cancer syndromes and genetic testing. *Journal of Surgical Oncology 111*:66–80.

▶ The role of BRCA1 and BRCA2 as risk factors for breast and other cancers is explored in the first article. The second article explores the use of "next generation" technology in testing for inherited breast cancer syndromes in addition to BRCA1 and BRCA2.

Ottini, L. 2014. Male breast cancer: A rare disease that might uncover underlying pathways of breast cancer. *Nature Reviews Cancer 14*:643–44.

▶ Although uncommon, male breast cancer has a very poor prognosis and is often ignored.

Tan, P. H., et al. 2006. Fat necrosis of the breast: A review. *The Breast 15*:313–18.

▶ All breast disease is not cancer. This review was useful in constructing the Case. The condition is becoming increasingly frequent in cases of breast reconstruction and aesthetic modification.

The Female Reproductive System

LEARNING OBJECTIVES

1. Describe the anatomy of the female reproductive tract.
2. Outline the menstrual cycle.
3. Describe the common infections of the genital tract and relate them to sexually transmitted diseases.
4. Explain the pathogenesis, clinical manifestations, and treatment of toxic shock syndrome.
5. Describe the common diseases of the vulva, cervix, and uterus.

6. List the common causes of irregular uterine bleeding.
7. Describe the clinical manifestations and complications of endometriosis.
8. List the common cysts and tumors of the ovary.
9. Categorize the common methods of artificial contraception, explain how they prevent conception, and describe their possible side effects.

Anatomy of the Female Genital Tract

The female genital tract consists of the ovaries, the uterus, the Fallopian tube; the vagina, and the vulva. The ovaries are divided into a cortex that supports follicular development and a medulla containing blood vessels and loose connective tissue. With each menstrual cycle one follicle develops into a corpus luteum following ovulation. Mature ova travel from the ovaries, through the Fallopian tube, to the uterus. The uterus has three regions: the cervix, the body or corpus, and the fundus (which forms the top of the uterus, opposite the cervix). The cervix is further divided into the vaginal portion and the endocervix (**FIGURE 17-1**). The corpus consists of the endometrium surrounded by the myometrium. Changes in the endometrium that occur during the menstrual cycle are keyed to the rise and fall in the levels of ovarian hormones. The cervix opens into the vagina. The external female genitalia (the vulva) consists of the mons pubis and clitoris along with the labia majora and minora.

The Menstrual Cycle

The uterine lining undergoes a cyclic change approximately every thirty days in response to hormones secreted by the ovaries. The proliferation of the endometrial cells lining the uterus is mediated by increases in estrogen produced by the developing ovarian graafian follicle, corresponding to an increase in follicle stimulating hormone

FRONT VIEW   SIDE VIEW

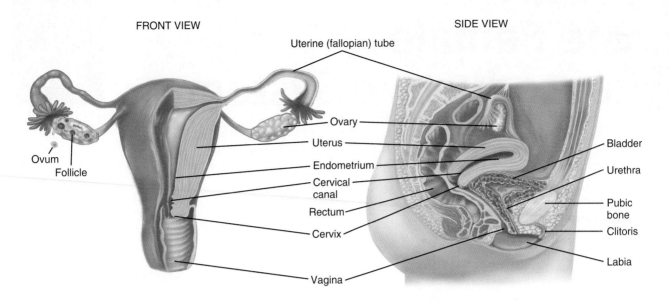

FIGURE 17-1 Anatomy of the female genital organs.

produced by the anterior pituitary gland (**proliferative phase**). Ovulation occurs at the end of this phase at about day fourteen in response to a surge of luteinizing hormone. The graafian follicle, having discharged the ovum, becomes a corpus luteum. Cells of the corpus luteum secrete progesterone, which starts the secretory phase of the menstrual cycle. In the absence of embryo implantation, the corpus luteum degenerates, progesterone levels fall, and the menses start at day twenty-eight. Menses last three to seven days, resulting in stromal hemorrhage. This material is discharged through the vagina, and the uterine endometrium begins to regenerate (**FIGURE 17-2**).

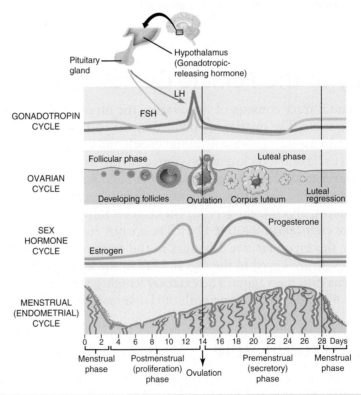

FIGURE 17-2 The menstrual cycle. Temporal relationship of changes in the endometrium, maturation of an ovum, and levels of hormone through one cycle.

Infections of the Female Genital Tract

Infections of the genital tract are common. Frequently involved sites are the vagina, the cervix, and the fallopian tubes. In addition, certain virus infections of the genital tract cause highly characteristic lesions, called **condylomas**. Most of the infectious agents of the female genital tract are sexually transmitted and are discussed in the presentation on those diseases.

VAGINITIS

Vaginal infections are common. They frequently cause vaginal discharge, together with vulvovaginal itching and irritation. These infections are caused by the fungus *Candida albicans*, the protozoan parasite *Trichomonas vaginalis*, or a small gram-negative bacterium called *Gardnerella (Haemophilus) vaginalis*, in conjunction with various anaerobic vaginal bacteria.

Candida vaginitis is described along with other fungal infections in the discussion on pathogenic microorganisms. The protozoan parasite *Trichomonas vaginalis* is considered with the parasitic infections in the discussion on animal parasites. The third common type of vaginitis, often called nonspecific vaginitis, is usually associated with a profuse, foul-smelling vaginal discharge. So-called nonspecific vaginitis often results from *Gardnerella* infection. Highly specific methods of treatment are available for each type of vaginitis. Unlike *Trichomonas* and *Gardnerella* infection, candidiasis is not sexually transmitted but often occurs with diabetes, antibiotic use, or pregnancy.

CERVICITIS

Mild chronic inflammation of endocervical glands is very common in women who have had children. Cervicitis causes few symptoms and is of little clinical significance. More severe cervical inflammation may result from a gonococcal infection discussed in communicable diseases or a chlamydial infection in diseases caused by pathogenic microorganisms. Both infections are sexually transmitted and may be followed by the spread of the infection into the fallopian tubes and adjacent tissues.

SALPINGITIS AND PELVIC INFLAMMATORY DISEASE

Salpingitis means an inflammation of the fallopian tube (*salpinx* = tube). The more general term **pelvic inflammatory disease (PID)** refers to any infection that affects the fallopian tubes and adjacent tissues. Sometimes the ovaries are infected along with the fallopian tubes. Most cases are secondary to the spread of a cervical gonorrheal or chlamydial infection through the uterus into the fallopian tubes and surrounding tissues. Less commonly, other pathogenic organisms are involved. An acute pelvic infection causes severe lower abdominal pain and tenderness, together with elevated temperature and leukocytosis.

Both gonorrheal and nongonorrheal salpingitis respond to appropriate antibiotic therapy; healing of the inflammation, however, may be associated with scarring and obstruction of the tubal lumen. Sterility may result if the tubal obstruction is bilateral (**FIGURE 17-3**). Sometimes, even if the tubes are not completely occluded, the scarring may delay the transport of a fertilized ovum through the tube and lead to implantation of the ovum in the fallopian tube rather than in the endometrial cavity. This condition is called an **ectopic pregnancy** and is considered in prenatal development and diseases associated with pregnancy and also as a case in the discussion of sexually transmitted diseases

Condyloma A warty tumorlike overgrowth in the squamous epithelium of the anorectal or genital tract, caused by a virus that is spread by sexual contact.

Salpingitis Inflammation of the fallopian tubes.

Pelvic inflammatory disease (PID) A general term for an infection affecting the fallopian tubes and adjacent pelvic organs.

Ectopic pregnancy A pregnancy outside the endometrial cavity.

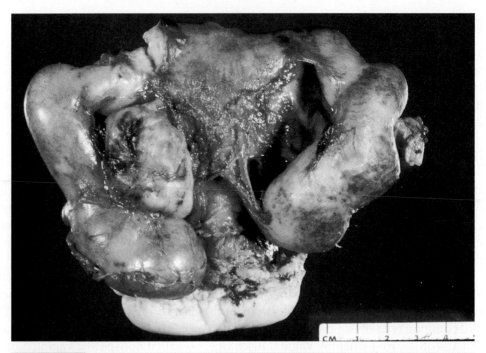

Toxic Shock Syndrome

Toxic shock syndrome (TSS) was first recognized thirty-five years ago in menstruating women who used high-absorbency tampons for prolonged periods of time, but its frequency has declined as other menstrual products replaced them, although no tampon is entirely free from risk. Currently half of the cases of TSS are not associated with menstruation, but barrier contraception still is a risk factor. Cases are also associated with nongynecologic infections involving surgery and burns, often of a serious nature. A quarter of cases occur in men.

Clinically, the disease is characterized by elevated temperature, vomiting and diarrhea, muscular aches and pains, a fall in blood pressure (often to shock levels), and various other systemic manifestations. A characteristic feature of the disease is an erythematous (sunburnlike) skin rash that is followed by flaking and peeling of the affected skin (somewhat like the peeling that occurs after a severe sunburn).

The clinical manifestations of toxic shock syndrome are caused by toxins (TSST-1 and enterotoxin-B) produced by *Staphylococcus aureus*. The toxins act as **superantigens**, causing widespread activation of T cells and the release of cytokines (T cell products) that cause shock and tissue damage. Although TSS from any cause is not common (1 case per 10,000), the overall mortality rate is high (over 30 percent). Menstrual-related TSS has a much lower case fatality rate of about 2 percent.

Condylomas of the Genital Tract and HPV Infection

Condylomas, sometimes called venereal warts, are benign, warty, tumorlike overgrowths of squamous epithelium caused by **human papillomavirus (HPV)**. Infection

Toxic shock syndrome (TSS) Disease characterized by elevated temperature, vomiting and diarrhea, muscular aches, and a fall in blood pressure.

Superantigens Toxins produced by *Staphylococcus aureus* in toxic shock that cause widespread activation of T cells and release of cytokines.

Human papillomavirus (HPV) A virus that stimulates epithelial cell proliferation. Causes warts and genital tract condylomas.

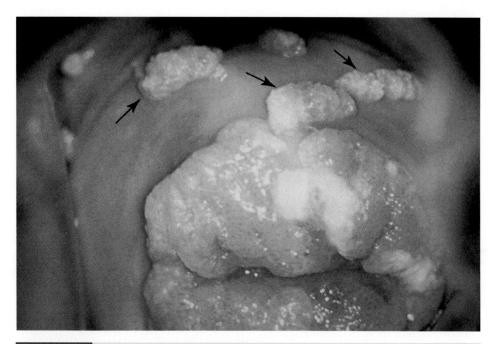

FIGURE 17-4 Cervical and vaginal mucosa viewed through vaginal speculum, revealing multiple condylomas (*arrows*) arising from mucosa.

Courtesy of Leonard V. Crowley, MD, Century College.

with HPV is the most common sexually transmitted disease in the United States, with 30–40% of women between the ages of twenty and thirty being infected. HPV occurs as different strains termed **serotypes**, two of which (6 and 11) are responsible for most cases of condylomas. However, other serotypes (16, 18, and other high-risk types) are major risk factors for **squamous intraepithelial lesions (SILs)** and invasive squamous cell cancers in regions of the female genital tract including the vulva and cervix.

Condylomas vary in size from a few millimeters to more than 1 cm in diameter and are frequently multiple. Condylomas develop most often on the vulvar mucosa, on the mucosa of the cervix and vagina (**FIGURE 17-4**), around the vaginal opening, and around the anus. Treatment consists of destroying the lesions; this may be accomplished by applying a strong chemical (podophyllin), by electrocoagulation, by freezing (cryocautery), or by surgical excision. Condylomas caused by HPV types 6 and 11 rarely become malignant. However, other condyloma-like skin lesions are associated with high-risk HPV types and may present a risk for becoming malignant.

Diseases of the Vulva

VULVAR INTRAEPITHELIAL NEOPLASIA

There are two different forms of **vulvar intraepithelial neoplasia (VIN)**, either of which can progress to invasive squamous cell carcinoma if untreated. The first (classic or usual VIN UVIN) comprises about 40 percent of cases and is caused by infection with high-risk HPV serotypes (usually HPV16, sometimes 18, or others). It has the same risk factors as condylomas and tends to occur in younger women (forty to fifty years of age) with multiple sexual partners and young age at first intercourse. Whereas condylomas are classed as squamous intraepithelial lesions of low risk (LSIL), untreated UVIN have about a 10-percent risk of becoming invasive and are

Serotype Immunologically detected pathogen strains.

Squamous intraepithelial lesions (SILs) Precancerous results of infection with some HPV serotypes.

Vulvar intraepithelial neoplasia (VIN) Cancer of the vulva.

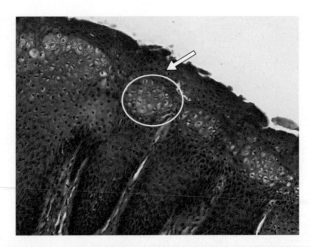

FIGURE 17-5 UVIN lesion of the vulva (flat, basaloid type). The lesion has a thickened keratinized layer and is hyperkeartotic (*arrow*). Many cells show koilocytosis; they have enlarged and irregular nuclei surrounded by a perinuclear halo (*circled area*). This is indicative of infection with HPV.

Courtesy of Department of Pathology and Laboratory Medicine, University of North Carolina at Chapel Hill.

classified as high-risk lesions (HSIL). The lesion may be multifocal and associated with lesions of other areas of the genitalia such as the cervix that are also related to high-risk HPV serotypes and are classed as HSIL. Lesions may be warty (condyloma-like) or flat (basaloid) (**FIGURE 17-5**).

The more common form of VIN, called differentiated VIN (DVIN), occurs in older, usually postmenopausal women in the seventh decade. DVIN is not associated with HPV but tends to occur in the setting of chronic vulvar inflammatory/ dermatological conditions. The epithelium of the vulva may exhibit irregular areas of thickening and inflammation that appear as white patches. Histologically, the affected epithelium is heavily keratinized, and the epithelial cells show variable abnormalities of maturation. Clinically, the condition is associated with intense itching and tenderness of the affected areas. The nonspecific descriptive term leukoplakia (*leuko* = white + *plakia* = patch) is sometimes applied to this lesion. Untreated DVIN has an appreciable frequency of progression to invasive cancer (33 percent). Various types of local treatment are frequently effective, but if significant precancerous changes are present in the epithelium, the affected areas are generally removed surgically. As noted, vulvar carcinoma (invasive squamous cell carcinoma) may occur in both pre- and postmenopausal women (**FIGURE 17-6**). Treatment consists of resection of the vulva (vulvectomy) along with the inguinal lymph nodes, which receive lymphatic drainage from the vulva.

Conditions of the Cervix

CERVICAL POLYPS

Occasionally, benign polyps arise from the cervix. Usually, they are small and do not cause symptoms, but some may be quite large. Sometimes the tip of the polyp becomes eroded and causes bleeding. Treatment consists of surgically removing the polyp.

CERVICAL INTRAEPITHELIAL LESIONS (CIN)

In the past, cervical cancer was the number one cause of cancer death in American women. Although worldwide it remains the second most common cancer in women,

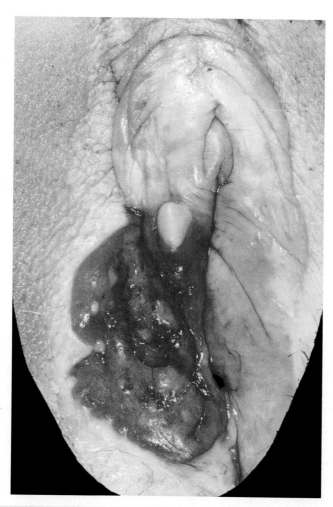

FIGURE 17-6 A large carcinoma of the vulva. The white appearance of the skin adjacent to the carcinoma is caused by preexisting vulvar dystrophy.

Courtesy of Leonard V. Crowley, MD, Century College.

mortality has fallen drastically in the United States as a result of cytological screening of cervical cells (PAP smear). Cervical cancer is the ultimate result of untreated, high-risk squamous intraepithelial lesions (HSIL) of the cervix. As is the case with UVIN, CIN is related to infection with HPV and bears the same risk factors. Low-risk squamous intraepithelial lesions (LSIL) are classified as CIN I or mild dysplasia and are related to infection with low-risk HPV serotypes (6 and 11), which may be expressed as genital warts on the cervix. Such lesions rarely progress and may disappear spontaneously. Low-risk HPV does not become integrated into host cell DNA but remains as an **episome**. Virus accumulates in the infected cell, eventually killing it. High-risk squamous intraepithelial lesions (HSIL) are classified as CIN II moderate dysplasia or CIN III severe dysplasia or carcinoma in situ, and are associated with infection by high-risk HPV serotypes (16, 18, and many others) and do not regress spontaneously. Such HPV serotypes integrate into the host cell DNA and synthesize viral proteins that allow for tumor progression into invasive disease. Although rates of infection with HPV are substantial (30 percent of twenty- to thirty-year-olds were found to be infected with high-risk serotypes in family planning and primary care settings), the incidence of cancer is far lower. Only the small proportion of women infected with a cancer-causing HPV type who are unable to eliminate the virus are at risk of cervical dysplasia and cervical carcinoma.

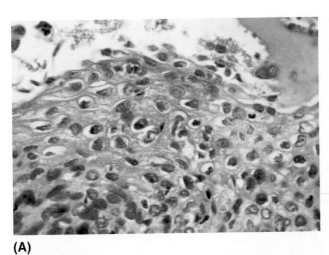
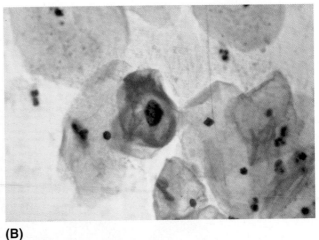

(A) **(B)**

FIGURE 17-7 **(A)** Cervical epithelial dysplasia (CIN III carcinoma in situ) caused by papilloma virus. **(B)** Dysplastic epithelial cell identified in Papanicolaou smear (original magnification ×400).

Courtesy of Leonard V. Crowley, MD, Century College.

Abnormal growth and maturation of cervical squamous epithelium is called cervical dysplasia and is discussed in the presentation on cells and tissues, their structure and function in health and disease. Dysplastic changes range from mild disturbances of epithelial maturation (CIN I) to severe cellular abnormalities (CIN II and CIN III). Severe dysplasia does not regress and progresses to in situ carcinoma and eventually to invasive carcinoma after a variable period of time (**FIGURE 17-7**).

HPV testing of cervical material obtained when a routine Pap test is performed can be helpful when the cytologic changes in the Pap smear are inconclusive (classified as atypical squamous cells of undetermined significance or ASCUS). If the HPV test is negative, the cytologic changes are probably not significant, and no further studies are required. On the other hand, if the HPV test is positive, further evaluation of the patient is required. Routine Pap smear combined with HPV testing is now recommended for all women over age thirty as older women may have difficulty clearing HPV infections.

HPV VACCINE

Two anti-HPV vaccines are available. Both are prepared from virus proteins and do not contain live virus. The first vaccine, which was licensed in 2006, provides immunity against four HPV types: 6 and 11 (low risk), and 16 and 18 (high risk). The second vaccine, licensed in 2009, only protects against the cancer-causing types 16 and 18. Unfortunately, the vaccines are not effective against any of the HPV types in the vaccine to which the subject has already been infected but will still provide protection from the other viruses covered by the vaccine. The vaccines are recommended primarily for girls eleven to twelve years old before they become sexually active because they are unlikely to have been infected with the HPV types covered by the vaccines and would get the most protection from the vaccines. Even in immunized females, regular gynecologic care and Pap smears are required because other carcinogenic serotypes not covered by the vaccine may still cause papillomas, dysplasia, and cervical cancer. The vaccines are not 100 percent effective.

DIAGNOSIS AND TREATMENT OF CERVICAL DYSPLASIA

The cellular abnormalities indicative of CIN (dysplasia and carcinoma in situ) develop first in the cells at the junction between the squamous epithelium covering the exterior of the cervix and the columnar epithelium lining the cervical canal. This region is called the squamocolumnar junction, or transition zone, and is usually located at the external opening (external os) of the cervix. During a Pap smear, cells are collected both from the area of the transition zone and from the endocervical canal because adenocarcinoma of the endocervical canal can result from HSIL occurring in that area.

An abnormal Pap smear requires further evaluation, which is usually accomplished by means of a binocular magnifying instrument called a **colposcope**. This instrument provides the physician with a greatly magnified view of the cervix and endocervical canal. In cervical dysplasia and carcinoma, characteristic abnormalities in the cervical epithelium and underlying blood vessels can be identified that define the location and extent of the abnormal epithelium. Multiple biopsy specimens are then taken from the abnormal-appearing areas, and material is also obtained from the endocervical canal. Treatment depends on the results of the biopsies. CIN II and CIN III lesions (HSIL) are usually treated by destruction of the abnormal epithelium by freezing (cryocautery), by laser light, by surgical excision of the abnormal area, or sometimes by removal of the uterus (hysterectomy).

HSIL lesions can be cured by proper treatment and carry an excellent prognosis. These lesions may remain localized within the epithelium of the cervix for as long as ten years before eventually becoming invasive. After invasion has occurred, however, the neoplasm is much harder to treat, and the results are less satisfactory. The tumor may extend through the cervix into the adjacent tissues and may infiltrate the rectum and bladder. The ureters, which lie on each side of the cervix, may also be invaded and obstructed by the neoplasm. Metastatic spread to regional lymph nodes and distant sites also is common. Invasive carcinoma is treated either by radiation or by resection of the uterus, fallopian tubes, ovaries, and adjacent tissues (radical hysterectomy).

Other Sites of HPV Infection

In addition to HPV-caused cervical cancer, HPV has also been identified in association with carcinoma of the vulva, penis, rectum, oral cavity, and pharynx where it may have been transmitted from a cervical infection.

Conditions of the Uterus

BENIGN PROLIFERATIVE CHANGES IN THE UTERUS

An excess of estrogen outside the usual menstrual cycle may result from a variety of causes, including anovulatory cycles, estrogenic drug therapy, obesity, and polycystic ovary syndrome, and will result in persistent proliferative uterine changes. With continuing stimulation, increased glandular hyperplasia occurs, a condition called **nonatypical endometrial hyperplasia**, which is characterized by irregular areas of increasing gland density throughout the uterus (**FIGURE 17-8**). These glands are often dilated and show a tubular ciliated structure similar to the proliferative phase of the menstrual cycle. Although in itself a benign condition, long-term nonatypical endometrial hyperplasia may develop areas of atypical hyperplasia (**endometrial intraepithelial neoplasia [EIN]**), a precursor lesion to cancer. Continued presence of estrogens will result in irregular uterine bleeding, and a sudden lack of estrogen can result in extremely heavy menses.

Benign polyps in the endometrium are also common. An endometrial polyp may cause uterine bleeding if the tip becomes inflamed or ulcerated.

Colposcope A binocular magnifying instrument used to view the cervix and endocervical canal.

Nonatypical endometrial hyperplasia Uterine condition characterized by irregular areas of increasing gland density in the uterus.

Endometrial intraepithelial neoplasia (EIN) Result of long-term nonatypical endometrial hyperplasia; a precursor lesion to cancer.

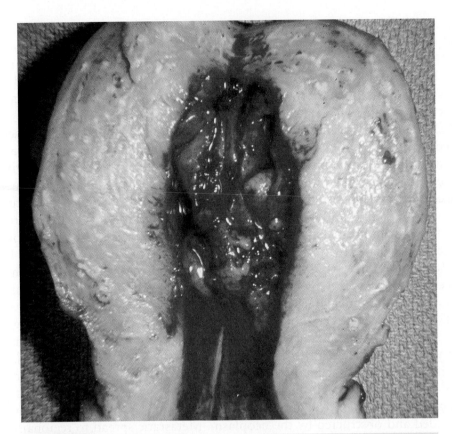

FIGURE 17-8 Nonatypical endometrial hyperplasia (benign endometrial hyperplasia). The uterus opened to reveal polypoid masses of hyperplastic endometrium filling endometrial cavity.

Courtesy of Leonard V. Crowley, MD, Century College.

UTERINE LEIOMYOMAS

Benign, smooth muscle tumors called **leiomyomas** (myomas or fibroids) arise in the wall of the uterus (**FIGURE 17-9**). They are frequently encountered and are said to occur in approximately 30 percent of women over thirty years of age. Occasionally, leiomyomas may be responsible for excessive or irregular uterine bleeding or may produce symptoms related to pressure on the adjacent bladder or rectum. When symptomatic, myomectomy (removal of the leiomyoma) or hysterectomy (removal of the uterus) may be required.

Leiomyomas Benign, smooth muscle tumors.

Neoplastic Proliferative Changes in the Uterus

Endometrial intraepithelial neoplasia (EIN) is the precursor lesion to endometrial adenocarcinoma, the most common gynecologic cancer (comprising 3 percent of all cancers in women). Levels of endometrial cancer have fallen precipitously with the realization that estrogen treatment to alleviate menopausal symptoms was a major risk factor in the development of uterine cancer. Uterine cancer has two major types. Type I disease is endometroid; that is, it resembles the proliferative glands seen in nonatypical endometrial hyperplasia in its earliest stages (grade 1 lesions). Increasingly advanced disease (grades 2 and 3) is poorly differentiated, with loss of glandlike structures showing increasing degrees of cellular atypia including increased

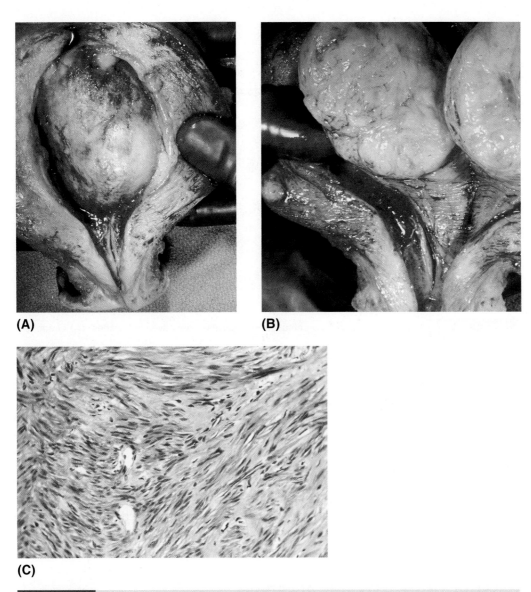

(A)

(B)

(C)

FIGURE 17-9 Uterine myoma. **(A)** A uterus opened to reveal a large spherical myoma protruding into endometrial cavity. **(B)** A cross section of myoma illustrating well-circumscribed tumor without evidence of necrosis, features suggesting a benign neoplasm. **(C)** Histologic appearance, revealing interlacing bundles of mature smooth muscle cells that resemble the normal muscle cells from which the tumor arose (original magnification ×100).

Courtesy of Leonard V. Crowley, MD, Century College.

and abnormal mitosis (**FIGURE 17-10**). Type I carcinoma has its origin in continued unopposed estrogen stimulation of the uterus. It comprises about 80 percent of cases and tends to occur either in older premenopausal women or at the time of menopause. The disease usually has a favorable course and is detected at a low grade while confined to the uterus. Type II endometrial carcinoma occurs in older women and has a much more serious course with a poor prognosis because the cancer is invasive and often discovered at a late stage. The most common form of type II disease (serous adenocarcinoma) may spread through the fallopian tubes and invade the peritoneal surface. The disease is not related to estrogen induced hyperplasia. Endometrial cancer is not reliably detected by Pap smears but is suspected when abnormal uterine bleeding occurs in older (peri- or postmenopausal women). Transvaginal ultrasound is helpful in diagnosis. Type I disease confined to the endometrium may be treated

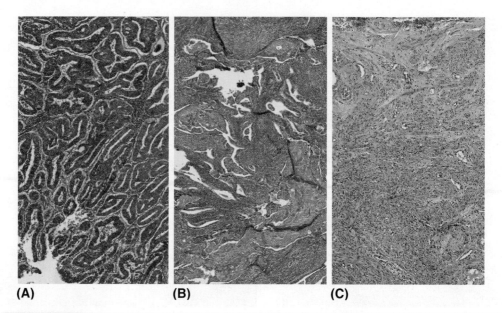

(A)   **(B)**   **(C)**

FIGURE 17-10　Uterine adenocarcinoma demonstrating increasingly advanced grades. **(A)** Grade 1. **(B)** Grade 2. **(C)** Grade 3.

Courtesy of Department of Pathology and Laboratory Medicine, University of North Carolina at Chapel Hill.

by hysterectomy (sometimes accompanied by radiation). Type II disease is often accompanied by metastases to the lung and lymph nodes associated with the aorta.

Irregular Uterine Bleeding

Excessive or irregular uterine bleeding is a common gynecologic problem. Most cases in younger women result from a disturbance in the normal cyclic interaction of estrogen and progesterone on the endometrium. This is usually called dysfunctional uterine bleeding. In older women, bleeding can be the result of many causes, including neoplastic disease.

DYSFUNCTIONAL UTERINE BLEEDING

Dysfunctional uterine bleeding refers to cases in which the cause lies outside the uterus and in the network of endocrine glands that control uterine function. Most cases of dysfunctional uterine bleeding occur because the follicle fails to mature to the point of ovulation and, consequently, no corpus luteum forms. As a result, the endometrium is subjected to continuous estrogen stimulation and responds by shedding in an irregular way instead of shedding all at once as in a normal period. This condition is also called anovulatory bleeding (*ana* = without + ovulation). It tends to arise at both extremes of reproductive life: when normal menstrual cycles are being established at puberty and near menopause when ovarian function is declining. Less commonly, irregular bleeding is the result of continuous secretion of progesterone from a corpus luteum that fails to involute. This prolongs the secretory phase of the endometrium, which sometimes sheds irregularly.

　　Dysfunctional uterine bleeding is treated by administering hormones to restore the proliferative-secretory sequence in the endometrium that is characteristic of a normal menstrual cycle. In one common treatment, the patient is given a synthetic steroid hormone having progesterone activity. The hormone induces secretory changes in the endometrium and stops the bleeding. The hormone treatment is then stopped, and the endometrium sheds as in a normal period. Frequently, the next cycle is normal and usually no further treatment is required. Multiple recurrent episodes of dysfunctional bleeding that lead to anemia resulting from excessive blood loss may require more aggressive treatment such as uterine ablation, destruction of the endometrium by a variety of physical methods including heat, cold, or microwave radiation. Because the technique has serious consequences (including likely loss or compromise of fertility), medical treatment is preferred when feasible.

Disease intrinsic to the uterus is not considered dysfunctional. This includes benign endometrial hyperplasia, endometrial and cervical polyps, uterine leiomyomas, EIN, and uterine carcinoma. For this reason, abnormal uterine bleeding (particularly in peri- and postmenopausal women) must be clinically evaluated with dispatch.

DIAGNOSIS AND TREATMENT

Irregular bleeding is always a cause for concern when it occurs in an older woman nearing the end of her reproductive years or after menopause because it may be the result of an endometrial carcinoma. Bleeding in older women is usually treated by dilating the cervix with various metal dilators and then scraping out the lining of the uterus with a long-handled scooplike instrument called a curette. This procedure is called **dilatation and curettage** or simply abbreviated as **D&C**. The tissue removed is examined microscopically by the pathologist. If the endometrial tissue is not malignant, no further treatment is needed. If endometrial carcinoma is detected on histologic examination, further treatment is required, usually consisting of hysterectomy, sometimes preceded by a course of radiation therapy.

Endometriosis

Endometriosis refers to the presence of uterine endometrium in any location outside the endometrial cavity (**FIGURE 17-11**). Ectopic deposits (*ecto* = outside) of endometrium occasionally may be encountered most commonly in the ovary (**FIGURE 17-12**), in the wall of the uterus, or elsewhere in the pelvis. Sometimes endometrial tissue is found in the appendix or in the rectum. Endometriosis is a common problem, occurring in about 10 to 15 percent of women, and results in pelvic pain, irregular menses, or dysmenorrhea. Endometriosis results in infertility in as many as 30 percent of patients. Often, the condition appears to occur in families, and a woman is more likely to develop endometriosis if her mother had it. Ectopic endometrial deposits respond to normal hormonal stimuli and therefore undergo cyclic menstrual desquamation and regeneration. Because the misplaced endometrial tissue does not communicate with the endometrial cavity, the "menses" tissue is not discharged through the vagina. Old blood and desquamated material are retained in the ectopic sites, leading to considerable scarring and causing crampy pain during menstrual periods. With time, ectopic foci become inflamed and fibrotic. Obstruction of the fallopian tubes by scarring may cause sterility.

The reason endometrial deposits occur in unusual locations is unknown, although many theories have been proposed. Some cases seem to be caused by reflux of bits of shed endometrium along with menstrual blood through the fallopian tubes into the peritoneal cavity during menstruation (retrograde menstruation), which then implant and grow in the pelvis. This does not provide a complete explanation as endometriosis is occasionally found in the lungs and lymph nodes, suggesting transport through the blood or lymph.

Diagnosis of endometriosis is usually established by visualizing the ectopic deposits within the pelvis with a lighted tubular instrument called a **laparoscope**,

Dilatation and curettage (D&C) Procedure involving scraping the lining of the uterus; used to treat irregular bleeding.

Endometriosis Presence of endometrial tissue in abnormal locations, such as in the ovary or pelvis.

Laparoscope A long tubular telescope-like instrument passed through the abdominal wall to examine structures within the peritoneal cavity.

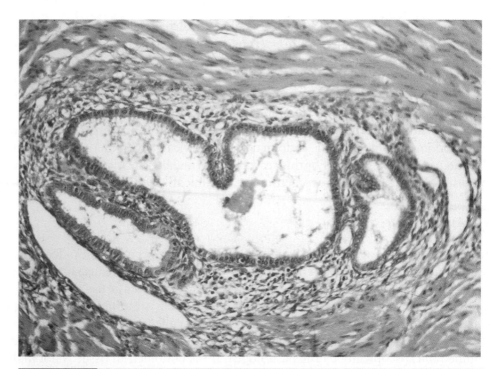

FIGURE 17-11 A photomicrograph of endometriosis in the uterine wall. Normal endometrial glands and stroma are surrounded by uterine muscle (original magnification ×100).

Courtesy of Leonard V. Crowley, MD, Century College.

discussed on general concepts of disease, principles of diagnosis. Treatment consists of removing or destroying the deposits surgically or impeding the progression of endometriosis by administering drugs or hormones. Hormone treatments commonly used include synthetic hormones having progesterone activity that completely suppress the menstrual cycles or birth-control pills that suppress ovulation so the endometrium becomes thin and atrophic, and menstrual periods are very light. The endometriosis is similarly suppressed, retarding its progression and associated scarring.

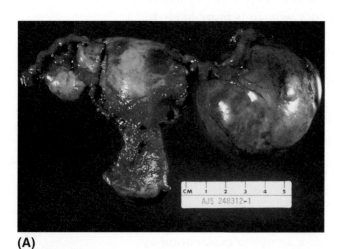

(A)

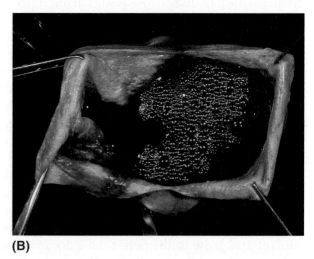

(B)

FIGURE 17-12 **(A)** Endometriosis of the ovary. An accumulation of blood and debris within the ovarian endometriosis has led to formation of an endometrium-lined cyst filled with old blood and desquamated endometrial tissue within the right ovary (*right*). **(B)** Endometrial cyst opened, revealing cyst contents consisting of old blood and debris derived from the endometrium lining the cyst.

Courtesy of Leonard V. Crowley, MD, Century College.

Another treatment is to administer drugs that suppress the output of gonadotropins from the pituitary gland. This, in turn, leads to a decline in ovarian function, similar to that occurring in menopause. The deposits of endometriosis, deprived of cyclic estrogen–progesterone stimulation, undergo regression.

Dysmenorrhea

Dysmenorrhea means painful menstruation. There are two types: primary dysmenorrhea, in which the pelvic organs are normal, and secondary dysmenorrhea, which results from various diseases of the pelvic organs, such as endometriosis.

Primary dysmenorrhea is the more common type. The pain is crampy, begins just prior to menstruation, and lasts for one or two days after onset of the menstrual flow. Usually, menstrual periods are painless for the first year or two after onset of menses during adolescence because early menstrual cycles are usually anovulatory, and primary dysmenorrhea does not occur unless ovulation occurs. Dysmenorrhea does not usually become a problem until regular ovulatory menstrual cycles are established.

Crampy menstrual pain is caused by a class of compounds called **prostaglandins**. Prostaglandins are synthesized within the endometrium under the influence of progesterone produced by the ovary during the secretory phase of the cycle. When the endometrium breaks down during menstruation, the prostaglandins are released and diffused into the myometrium, where they cause the spasmodic myometrial contractions that are responsible for the crampy menstrual pain. Dysmenorrhea does not occur if cycles are anovulatory because no corpus luteum forms and no progesterone is produced to stimulate prostaglandin synthesis.

Treatment consists of aspirin or another anti-inflammatory drug such as ibuprofen, which is administered before the onset of menses. These drugs suppress the synthesis of prostaglandins within the endometrium. Primary dysmenorrhea can also be treated very effectively with oral contraceptive pills, which prevent dysmenorrhea by suppressing ovulation.

Dysmenorrhea Painful menstruation.

Prostaglandin A complex derivative of a fatty acid (prostanoic acid) that has widespread physiologic effects.

Endometrial cyst An ovarian cyst lined by endometrium and filled with old blood and debris. A manifestation of endometriosis.

Polycystic ovary syndrome (PCOS) Common endocrine disorder and common cause of anovulatory infertility; associated with obesity, diabetes, and hirsutism.

Cysts and Tumors of the Ovary

NONNEOPLASTIC LESIONS

The ovary gives rise to a wide variety of cysts and tumors, and only the more common ones are considered here. Benign ovarian cysts arise either from ovarian follicles or from corpora lutea (**FIGURE 17-13**) that have failed to regress normally and instead become converted into fluid-filled cysts. Follicle cysts and corpus luteum cysts are often called functional cysts because they represent a derangement of the normal maturation and involution of a follicle or corpus luteum. Functional cysts do not usually become very large, and most regress spontaneously. Endometrial deposits in the ovary resulting from endometriosis may form cysts lined by endometrium and filled with old blood and debris. These are called **endometrial cysts**.

POLYCYSTIC OVARY SYNDROME

Polycystic ovary syndrome (PCOS), also known as Stein-Leventhal syndrome, is a common endocrine disorder affecting 10 percent of women in the United States. It is often diagnosed in the second to third decade because PCOS is a very common cause of anovulatory infertility. The disease is also associated with obesity, diabetes, hirsutism (excess body hair), and other virilizing signs such as acne. Ovaries are enlarged and contain multiple cysts related to high levels of circulating gonadotrophins. The

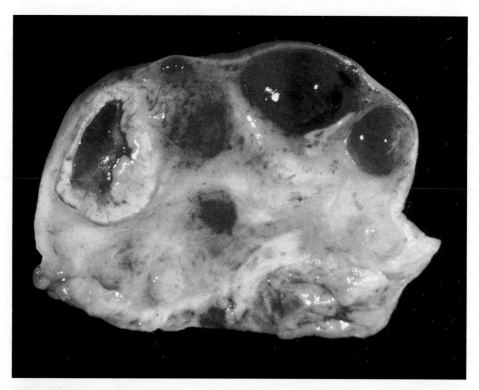

FIGURE 17-13 Section of normal ovary. There are two follicles beneath the capsule (*right side*) and a corpus luteum (*left side*).

Courtesy of Leonard V. Crowley, MD, Century College.

disease is associated with hyperandrogenism (excess production of male hormones) most likely in the ovary. Some of these androgens are converted to estrogens in the ovary, resulting in excess estrogen production. PCOS occurs with hyperinsulinemia and resistance of insulin targets to its effect (insulin resistance), the cause of which is uncertain. The defect in insulin function appears to result in the hormonal imbalance that occurs.

OVARIAN NEOPLASMS

Although ovarian tumors are the second most common gynecologic cancer, they account for the greatest number of deaths. Because they are difficult to detect, most patients present with high stage (disseminated) disease. Ovarian cancer is predominantly a disease of older women and is most often diagnosed around age sixty with an increasing frequency of occurrence through the eighth decade. Although rare, the disease can occur in the very young. The disease has a strong genetic component, with about 10 percent of cases being familial. In these cases, the disease appears a decade earlier. Mutations in a number of genes are associated with common types of ovarian cancer, notably *BRCA1* and *BRCA2*. Individuals harboring these mutations have risks as high as 45 percent and 20 percent for the respective genes. Because of the difficulty in early diagnosis, patients may elect to undergo oophorectomy (removal of the ovaries).

Ovarian neoplasms may arise in one or both ovaries. They may be either benign or malignant, cystic or solid, and derive from several cell types including the surface epithelium, germ cells, or stromal cells. Of these, epithelial tumors are the most common. The epithelial cells on the surface of the ovary, and the epithelium of the tumor cells, may resemble the cells found in other parts of the genital tract. If the tumor epithelium resembles the cells lining the fallopian tube, the tumor is classified as a **serous tumor**. At least some of these tumors may, in fact, derive from cells of the fallopian tube. If the tumor epithelium resembles the mucus-secreting epithelium of the endocervix, it is called a **mucinous tumor**; if the tumor epithelium resembles endometrium, it is termed an **endometrioid tumor**. Many of the serous and mucinous tumors are cystic, and the term serous cystadenoma or, when of high grade (either borderline or clearly malignant), serous cystadenocarcinoma is used. In many of these serous tumors, the neoplastic epithelium may extend onto the external surface of the tumor (**FIGURE 17-14**). When this occurs, small pieces of the projecting tumor may break off and implant elsewhere in the pelvis, peritoneal cavity, and omentum, where they continue to grow. Tumors manifesting this behavior may be difficult to remove completely. A mucinous tumor is designated as either a mucinous cystadenoma or a mucinous cystadenocarcinoma. Mucinous tumors generally consist of multiple small cysts and may be very large (**FIGURE 17-15**). The distinction between benign, borderline (tumors of low malignant potential), and malignant cystadenomas/adenocarcinomas depends on degree of cell proliferation and nuclear atypia. Any tumor demonstrating invasion into the ovarian stroma is suggestive of malignancy.

Most of the ovarian tumors with endometrium-like epithelium are malignant and are called endometrioid carcinomas. Less common are **clear cell carcinoma**, glycogen-rich tumors similar to the endometroid carcinoma, and **transitional cell (Brenner) tumors**, which are benign tumors containing nests of urothelial-like cells (those lining the bladder) surrounded by a fibrous stroma. Malignancy is most common in the high-grade serous category (70 percent), followed by endometroid and clear cell carcinomas (10 percent).

About 25 percent of ovarian tumors derive from germ cells and, in adults, almost all are benign (although in children they are most often malignant). Ovarian tumors are very similar to testicular germ cell tumors discussed in the presentation on the male reproductive system as both derive from germ cells. The most common of these, **mature teratomas** (also known as mature cystic teratoma, **dermoid cysts**), arise from unfertilized ova that have undergone neoplastic change. The haploid cells develop by parthenogenesis to yield 46,XX cells. The teratomas often contain skin, hair, teeth,

Serous tumor Ovarian tumor resembling cells in the fallopian tube.

Mucinous tumor Ovarian tumor made of cells resembling the mucus-secreting epithelium of the endocervix.

Endometrioid tumor Tumor epithelium resembles endometrium.

Clear cell carcinoma Glycogen-rich tumors similar to endometroid carcinoma.

Transitional cell tumor/ Brenner tumor Benign tumor containing nests of urothelial-like cells.

Mature teratomas/ dermoid cyst A common type of benign cystic teratoma that commonly arises in the ovary.

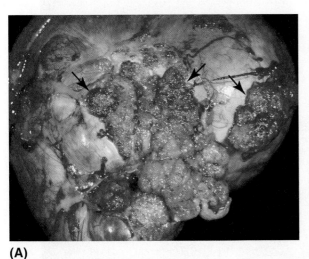

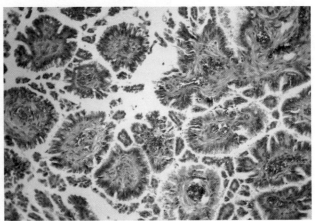

(A) **(B)**

FIGURE 17-14 **(A)** A resected serous tumor of the ovary measuring 10 cm in diameter. Several masses of tumor (*arrows*) project from the surface. **(B)** Histologic appearance of the tumor, which forms papillary processes covered by well-differentiated epithelial cells (original magnification ×100).

Courtesy of Leonard V. Crowley, MD, Century College.

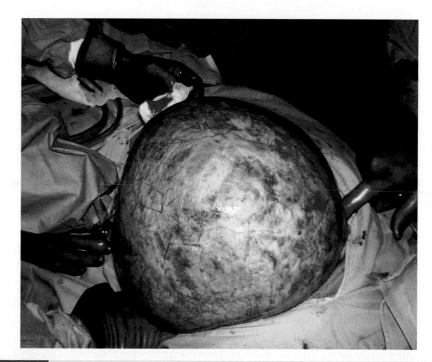

FIGURE 17-15 A large benign cystic ovarian tumor removed from a pregnant woman. The tumor weighed 35 lbs.

Courtesy of Leonard V. Crowley, MD, Century College.

bone, parts of gastrointestinal tract, thyroid, and other tissues growing in a jumbled fashion (**FIGURE 17-16**). A dermoid cyst apparently represents an abortive attempt of an unfertilized ovum to realize its potential by producing diverse tissues like those in a fetus. In contrast with the frequency of benign ovarian teratomas, malignant teratomas of the ovary are quite rare.

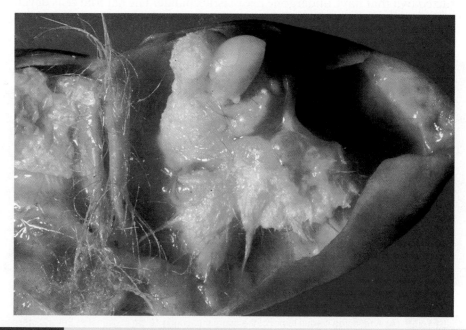

FIGURE 17-16 Opened dermoid cyst of ovary (benign cystic teratoma) with contents removed. The cyst contains a well-formed jawbone with two teeth (*center*). Note the hair arising from the skin that lines the cyst.

Courtesy of Leonard V. Crowley, MD, Century College.

The last group of ovarian tumors derive either from the fibrous connective tissue of the ovary (**fibromas**) and are almost always benign or from the developing sex cords and may produce female or, rarely, male sex hormones. One type arises from the estrogen-producing cells lining the follicles (granulosa cells) and the closely associated cells adjacent to the follicle cells (theca cells). These cells produce estrogen and so does a tumor arising from these cells, which is called a **granulosa cell tumor** or a **thecoma**. The former may be fibroma-like and benign, the latter are of low-grade malignant potential. The tumors may induce endometrial hyperplasia caused by excessive endometrial stimulation from the estrogen produced by the tumor. A granulosa cell tumor in a postmenopausal woman may induce irregular uterine bleeding. A few rare types of ovarian tumor (Sertoli-Leydig cell tumors) produce male sex hormones instead of estrogen and may induce masculinization.

Fibromas Benign tumor arising from the fibrous connective tissue of the ovary.

Granulosa cell tumor-thecoma An estrogen-producing ovarian tumor arising from the estrogen-producing granulose cell of an ovarian follicle.

Contraception

Methods of contraception fall into two major groups: "natural" methods and artificial methods. Natural family planning methods attempt to prevent pregnancy by avoiding intercourse around the time of ovulation when pregnancy is most likely to occur. A number of methods are available to help women determine when they ovulate. For example, the temperature method relies on the finding that basal temperature goes up slightly after ovulation. Unprotected intercourse must be avoided from the start of menstruation until three days after ovulation. Charts for monitoring temperature daily and special sensitive basal thermometers are available. However, great care must be taken regarding when in the day and how the temperature is determined. In addition, factors outside the menstrual cycle can affect basal temperature. These methods have no side effects or medical complications (other than undesired pregnancies) but require a high degree of motivation and are less effective than artificial methods. In contrast, artificial methods act by preventing the union of sperm and egg (barrier methods), preventing ovulation, or preventing implantation of the fertilized ovum. Many of these methods are highly effective, but some have potentially serious side effects.

Diaphragms, cervical caps, vaginal sponges, and condoms are mechanical devices that usually are used in conjunction with a spermicidal foam or jelly. Functioning by preventing the union of sperm and egg, they are highly effective when used correctly and have no serious side effects. These methods require proper use prior to intercourse and vary in effectiveness from person to person. Condoms, if always used, have about a 2-percent failure rate as opposed to about 6 percent for diaphragms.

Most contraceptive pills (combination pills), a very popular contraceptive method, consist of a synthetic estrogen combined with a compound having progesterone activity (progestin). "The pill" prevents ovulation by suppressing release of the pituitary gonadotropic hormones that regulate ovarian follicle growth, maturation, and ovulation and causes changes in the cervical mucus and endometrial lining that also discourage pregnancy. When taken properly, contraceptive pills are almost 100-percent effective, but there are potential side effects. The estrogen in the pill promotes increased synthesis of blood coagulation factors, predisposing individuals to formation of blood clots within the circulatory system. Women who smoke cigarettes and women over thirty-five years of age are at especially high risk. Some women on the pill develop high blood pressure. The elevated pressure probably results from an increased synthesis of a blood protein (called angiotensinogen) induced by the estrogen in the pill, which interacts with rennin produced by the kidney to yield angiotensin, a potent blood pressure–raising compound described in the urinary system.

Several birth control pills (Yaz, Yasmin, Ocella, and others) containing a synthetic progesterone (drospirenone) may have slightly higher risk of thrombosis, but the magnitude of the additional risk is disputed. These pills claim to be useful in managing premenstrual behavioral problems such as mood shifts, managing premenstrual physical discomfort (the premenstrual dysphoric disorder), and in controlling acne. Another less frequently used type of pill, progestin-only birth control pills, act by thickening cervical mucous and avoid some of the more serious potential thrombotic risks associated with combination pills. However they have a much higher failure rate (as high as 13 percent) and are sometimes used by nursing mothers (where the risk of unprotected conception is reduced).

For women who do not like to take pills, other methods are available that provide the same type of estrogen and progestin formulations used in contraceptive pills: either incorporated in a very small (54 mm diameter) ring inserted into the vagina, where the estrogen and progestin are slowly released from the ring and absorbed from the vagina into the bloodstream; provided as injections lasting several months; or provided as implants placed under the skin that can last for up to three years.

An intrauterine device (IUD) is a small, T-shaped flexible plastic structure that is inserted into the uterine cavity by a physician or nurse practitioner (**FIGURE 17-17**). IUDs are used less frequently now by women in the United States and Canada, but worldwide they are used widely as an effective and relatively inexpensive contraceptive method that does not require much attention from the user. A string attached to the device extends through the cervix into the vagina. The string serves two purposes. The woman can assure herself that the device is still within the uterine cavity by feeling the string. It also facilitates removal of the IUD by the physician when it is no longer needed.

Intrauterine devices most likely work by affecting the ability of sperm to fertilize the egg. Two types of IUD are available. Copper containing IUDs secrete small

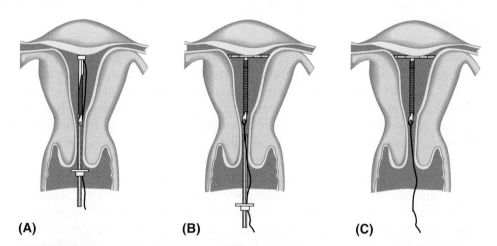

(A)   **(B)**   **(C)**

FIGURE 17-17 Technique of inserting intrauterine device. **(A)** The device is retracted into the insertion tube, and the tube is introduced through the cervix to the fundus of the uterus. **(B)** The tube is retracted, allowing the plastic device to resume its original configuration. **(C)** The tube is withdrawn. A string attached to the IUD protrudes through the cervix into the vagina.

amounts of copper, which acts as a spermicide. Hormone secreting IUDs thicken the cervical mucous, preventing fertilization and may also prevent implantation. Either type is 98 to 99 percent effective and lasts for three to ten years depending on the type.

Serious problems associated with IUDs are uncommon. There is the potential for uterine and tubal infections, which tend to occur within several weeks of insertion. If untreated, the infection may be followed by tubal scarring and impaired fertility. A second potential problem relates to tubal pregnancies. Because an IUD prevents implantation only within the uterus and does not prevent either ovulation or fertilization, implantation may occur within the tube in the unlikely event a women became pregnant while using an IUD. (The discussion on prenatal development and diseases associated with pregnancy describes tubal pregnancy and the significance of previous tubal infection as a predisposing factor.)

EMERGENCY CONTRACEPTION

Many unintended pregnancies occur each year. Most result from failure to use effective contraception, but some result from failure of the method being used, such as a broken condom, or from a sexual assault. These pregnancies could be prevented by the use of emergency contraception. The likelihood of pregnancy after unprotected intercourse can be greatly reduced by a postcoital (after intercourse) contraceptive. Several potential approaches are available. Copper containing IUDs provide highly effective contraception if used up to five days after unprotected sex. They have the advantage of continuing to provide contraception for a prolonged period. However, insertion can be costly and a trained individual is required.

The best known emergency contraceptive pill (morning after pill) is a progestin-only 1.5 mg levonorgestrel pill (marketed under several names), which is available without a prescription and should be taken regardless of the cycle day when unprotected intercourse occurred. The progestin may inhibit ovulation, and also impairs tubal motility, which slows transport of the ovum through the fallopian tube, effects that reduce the likelihood of conception. Finally, the progestin changes the endometrium so that it becomes unsuitable for implantation even if fertilization should occur, and the progestin-mediated change in the endometrium occurs before a fertilized ovum can complete its seven-day journey into the endometrium. When the pill is taken within twelve hours after unprotected intercourse, the pregnancy risk is less than 1 percent, and is about 3 percent when taken within seventy-two hours, but some protection is still provided for as long as five days. The pill is less effective for women with a body mass index over 25 and may not work if it is over 30.

Another alternative marketed as Ella One is a 30 mg tablet of ulipristal acetate, a synthetic steroid hormone. Ulipristal acts by delaying or preventing ovulation and also changes the endometrium so that it becomes unsuitable for implantation, much like a progestin-only contraceptive. Ella One is effective for as long as five days after unprotected intercourse, and its effectiveness does not decrease if there is a time delay between intercourse and the time that the pill is taken. It is also more effective in women with an elevated body mass index. The pill requires review by a licensed physician prior to provision, but this can be done using an online questionnaire.

CASE 17-1

Fifteen-year-old Janice was becoming increasingly depressed by the constant teasing of her female friends. Breast development started normally at age eleven, followed by menarche (first menstrual period) at age twelve and a half. Now, three years later, Janice had experienced only three additional menstrual periods. This concerned her because her friends were all "regular" with their menstrual cycles. She had annoying outbreaks of acne, and her skin was very oily. When she was thirteen, her mother took her to their family physician concerned about irregular periods. At that time, the physician explained that menstrual cycles often take a long time to regulate. He also explained that acne and some facial hair were not unusual during early adolescence and tended to decrease with time.

Currently, Janice's major complaint was how hairy she had become. She had noticeable coarse dark hair above her upper lip, on her chin, and around her nipples. She would not wear a two-piece bathing suit at the beach because she had a streak of dark hair running from her pubis up the center of her abdomen. Her thighs and lower back also grew dark hair. Her friends who had seen her undressed said she had hair "like a boy," and the teasing increased. She also began to put on weight. Janice visited her physician again. The physician carefully examined Janice and confirmed that she had an unusual amount of hair that was distributed in a male pattern (hirsutism). Janice had persistent oligomenorrhea (few menstrual periods) and had remained amenorrheic for over three months. The physician was also concerned about Janice's weight gain and referred her to a gynecologist who specialized in endocrine and developmental problems.

The gynecologist confirmed a diagnosis of hirsutism. This finding, along with acne, prolonged amenorrhea, and increasing weight gain, suggested that Janice was suffering from an excess of androgens (male hormones), which could be responsible for her symptoms. A very common endocrine disorder, polycystic ovary syndrome (PCOS), occurs in up to 10 percent of females and is associated with hyperandrogenism. PCOS is often diagnosed during adolescence. The gynecologist ordered a series of additional tests for Janice to rule out other possible causes of hyperandrogenism. These included determination of blood testosterone levels (and a number of other endocrine hormone level determinations), ovarian ultrasound, insulin levels, and glucose tolerance testing. Test results disclosed an abnormally high androgen levels without an indication of adrenal or thyroid dysfunction. Janice had high levels of circulating insulin and an abnormal glucose tolerance test, suggesting the early onset of insulin resistance. Abdominal ultrasound suggested increased ovarian volume (but this is a common finding in adolescents). Janice underwent transvaginal ultrasound and was found to have an excess of cystic areas on her ovaries, consistent with PCOS. Janet's gynecologist diagnosed PCOS based on the findings of hyperandrogenism and ovulatory dysfunction (in the absence of other factors), polycystic ovaries, and the suggestion of early onset type 2 diabetes with obesity.

Janice was treated with combination birth control pills (containing both estrogen and progesterone) and an androgen blocking agent (spironolactone). This regularized her menses and reduced the hirsutism. She was counseled regarding a healthy lifestyle, including exercise and weight control. The drug metformin was also prescribed because of increasing concern about her diabetes.

Discussion

One might imagine that PCOS would be relatively easy to diagnose in an adolescent considering the distinctive signs and symptoms. This is incorrect. Normal body hair distribution varies greatly from person to person, dependent upon both degree of sexual development and, in particular, ethnic origin. For example, what might be considered as an abnormal amount of hair in a person of Chinese (Han) origin might be quite normal in a white or black female.

CASE 17-1 *(Continued)*

The semiquantitative Ferriman-Gallwey score can be used in the clinical assessment of hair, but half of women with isolated hirsutism are found not to have excess androgens. For this reason, only moderate to extreme excess of hair (particularly in a male growth pattern) is suggestive of PCOS.

Laboratory testing for levels of circulating androgens (testosterone) is difficult to perform and interpret. There is no universally accepted "normal" level, particularly in developing female adolescents. Another complicating factor is that much of the testosterone in circulation is bound to steroid, hormone-binding globulin and thus is not hormonally active. Hence, determination of androgen level must be done by a reliable laboratory that has established accurate and appropriate normal controls for both sexes at different ages. In the absence of other symptoms, a single high androgen level should be interpreted with caution. In addition, abnormally high androgen levels in a female can be caused by ovarian and adrenal tumors and adrenal hyperplasia.

Primary ovarian failure (not related to excess androgen levels) can result from a variety other hormonal abnormalities. Determining whether the ovaries show a polycystic morphology is most commonly accomplished using transvaginal ultrasound, but there is no widely accepted definition for an "abnormal" polycystic ovarian morphology in adolescents. A large number of adolescent females without hyperandrogenism show evidence of such an ovarian morphology. It is accepted that there is a high level of insulin resistance and obesity associated with PCOS in adolescents. Hence, the diagnosis of PCOS requires multifactorial evaluation coupled with clinical expertise to avoid errors in diagnosis.

The etiology of PCOS remains uncertain. Clearly, abnormally high androgen levels, produced in the ovary and adrenals, are central in pathogenesis. There is a clear genetic component to PCOS and suggestions of association with a variety of genes in the population. The relation of high insulin level, insulin resistance, and obesity to hyperandrogenism remains speculative but clearly contributes to the hormonal abnormality. To date, the exact cause-effect relationship between PCOS and the associated metabolic disturbances is undefined.

Etiology and Pathogenesis

Polycystic ovary syndrome and associated insulin resistance and obesity resulting in hyperandrogenism and hyperandrogen induced ovarian disease.

Questions

1. What are the milestones in the development of sexual maturity in the female; at what age are they expected to occur?

2. How much variation is considered normal in the menstrual cycle at the start of menarche? after five years?

3. How might a clinician distinguish hyperandrogenism resulting from PCOS from that resulting from other causes (such as a tumor)?

4. What are the differences in distribution of body hair in a normal male and female?

QUESTIONS FOR REVIEW

1. What controls the menstrual cycle?

2. What are the possible results of HPV infection?

3. A patient consults her physician because of irregular uterine bleeding. What are some of the diseases of the genital tract that can cause this bleeding?

4. What is endometriosis? What symptoms does it produce? What are some complications that may be associated with endometriosis?

5. What is the difference between in situ and invasive cervical carcinoma? How is the Pap smear used in the diagnosis of carcinoma?

6. What is a dermoid cyst?

7. What is toxic shock? What role do staphylococci play?

8. How do contraceptive pills and IUDs exert their contraceptive effects? What medical problems may be associated with their use?

SUPPLEMENTARY READINGS

Boston Women's Health Book Collective. 2011. *Our Bodies, Ourselves*. New York: Touchstone.

Boston Women's Health Collective. http://www.ourbodiesourselves.org/health-information

Planned Parenthood. http://www.plannedparenthood.org/

▶ The book referenced in the first entry covers a wide range of subjects dealing with sexual anatomy, physiology, and pathology in a clear and concise manner. The second entry is an excellent source of additional health information for women and has links to many other useful sites. The third entry has extensive information on birth control, emergency contraception, and STDs.

Banet, N., and Lininger R. A., Chapter 17, "The Female Reproductive Tract." 2015. In *Pathology: A Modern Case Study*, edited by H. Reisner. New York: McGraw Hill Lange.

Shors, T. 2013. *Understanding Viruses*. 2nd ed. Burlington, MA: Jones & Bartlett Learning.

Tan, H. H., and Chan, R., Chapter 22, "Genital Warts." 2012. In *Sexually Transmitted Infections: Diagnosis, Management, and Treatment*, edited by J. M. Zenilman and M. Shamanesh. Burlington, MA: Jones & Bartlett Learning.

▶ The three recommended texts contain useful additional background information relating to diseases discussed in this chapter. The first entry has many additional short cases and illustrations of gynecological pathology. It provides a brief overview aimed at undergraduate medical students. Several chapters on HPV in the second reference provide additional information on the role of HPV in human cancer. The third entry is specifically cited for the chapter on genital warts, but other chapters have useful background on many sexually transmitted diseases.

Thaxton, L., and Waxman, A. G. 2015. Cervical cancer prevention: Immunization and screening. *Medical Clinics of North America* 99:469–77.

Dillner, J. 2014. Prevention of human papillomavirus-associated cancer. *Seminars in Oncology* 42:272–83.

▶ The first article reviews the efficacy of HPV immunization schemes and the role of the addition of HPV testing to routine Pap tests used alone. The second article reviews details on the many serotypes of HPV and their relationship to cervical cancer. Both provide up-to-date information.

De Joliniere, B., et al. 2014. Endometriosis: A new cellular and molecular genetic approach for understanding the pathogenesis and evolutivity. *Frontiers in Surgery* (Epub May 27). doi: 10.3389/fsurg

Brown, J., and Farquhar, C. 2014. Endometriosis: An overview of Cochrane Reviews. *Cochrane Library* (Epub March 10). doi:10.1002/14651858.CD009590.pub2
▶ The etiology of endometriosis is controversial, but there is evidence for a genetic component. The first article is a recent overview of possible genetic components of the disease that summarizes cellular abnormalities found in endometriotic tissue. The second article provides thoughtful statistical meta analysis of previously published articles; in this case proposed interventions for pain relief and infertility associated endometriosis. Of particular interest is a review of claimed benefits of Chinese herbal therapy.

Le Gallo, M., and Bell, D. W. 2014. The emerging genomic landscape of endometrial cancer. *Clinical Chemistry* 60:98–110.

Setiawan, V. W., et al. 2013. Type I and Type II endometrial cancers: Have they different risk factors? *Journal of Clinical Oncology* 31:2607–18.
▶ Both references detail significant advances in the understanding of endometrial cancer. The first article presents evidence for distinct subgroups of the disease based on molecular analysis. The second article suggests that types I and II endometrial cancer may not be as distinct as previously believed.

Lim, D., and Oliva, E. 2013. Precursors and pathogenesis of ovarian carcinoma. *Pathology* 45:229–42.

Nezhat, F. R., et al. 2015. New insights in the pathophysiology of ovarian cancer and implications for screening and prevention. *American Journal of Obstetrics and Gynecology* (Epub March 25). doi: http://dx.doi.org/10.1016/j.ajog.2015.03.044
▶ Both references suggest a dualistic model of ovarian carcinogenesis and discuss the controversial subject of the cellular origin of such cancers. The relationship of endometriosis to endometrioid ovarian cancer is considered.

Reyes, M. C., and Cooper, K. 2014. An update on vulvar intraepithelial neoplasia: Terminology and a practical approach to diagnosis. *Journal of Clinical Pathology* 67:290–94.
▶ A brief review of current terminology and differential diagnosis.

Lucidi, R. S. *Polycystic ovarian syndrome.* Medscape. http://emedicine.medscape.com/article/256806-overview#aab6b2b3

Witchel, S. F., et al. 2015. The diagnosis of polycystic ovary syndrome during adolescence. *Hormone Research in Paediatrics* 83:376–89.
▶ These two references were used in the Case construction. The first article provides a recent summary of the etiology, pathogenesis, diagnosis, and treatment of PCOS. The second article is an attempt to standardize clinical diagnostic practice in adolescents.

Prenatal Development and Conditions Associated with Pregnancy

LEARNING OBJECTIVES

1. Explain the processes of fertilization, implantation, and early development of the ovum, including the origin of the decidua, fetal membranes, and placenta.

2. Describe how amnionic fluid is formed and eliminated. Identify the conditions leading to abnormal amounts of amnionic fluid.

3. Explain the causes and effects of spontaneous abortion and ectopic pregnancy.

4. Describe the mechanism and clinical manifestations of the problems associated with abnormal attachment of the placenta within the uterus and abnormal attachment of the umbilical cord.

5. Differentiate between identical and fraternal twins. Describe how zygosity can be determined from examination of the placenta.

6. Classify the types of gestational trophoblast disease. Explain their prognoses, and describe the methods of treatment.

7. Explain the pathogenesis, clinical manifestations, diagnostic criteria, and methods used to treat hemolytic disease of the newborn.

8. Understand the causes and effects of gestational diabetes and pregnancy-associated toxemia.

Fertilization and Prenatal Development

DEVELOPMENT OF GAMETES AND FERTILIZATION

The development of mature sperm begins at the start of puberty in the male within the seminiferous tubules of the testes. The primordial spermatogonia undergo a complicated maturation process that results in the production of four immature haploid spermatids. A number of changes occur as the spermatid matures into a mature spermatozoon (sperm). The nucleus condenses as the DNA associates with a specialized protein (protamine) that is synthesized during spermatogenesis. The cytoplasm leaves the nuclear region, and the golgi apparatus is converted into the **acrosome**, which contains enzymes necessary for penetration of the ovum by the sperm (**fertilization**) to occur. The condensed nucleus and acrosome form the head of the sperm, which is covered by an acrosomal (or head) cap. The centriole, on the opposite side of the nucleus from the acrosome, generates the flagellum, which is characteristic of the sperm and provides for motility in the genital tract. The middle portion of the sperm between the head and the flagellar tail is the mitochondrial sheath containing the mitochondrial energy generating apparatus of the sperm (**FIGURE 18-1A**). The process

Acrosome Previously the sperm golgi apparatus; contains enzymes necessary for penetration of the ovum.

Fertilization Penetration of the ovum by the sperm.

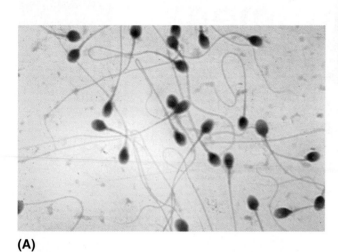

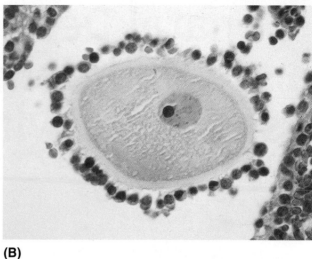

(A)

(B)

FIGURE 18-1 **(A)** Normal sperm in vaginal secretions. The darkly staining head containing the genetic material is covered by a lightly staining head cap that contains the enzymes needed to penetrate the ovum during fertilization. The long narrow tail provides propulsion (original magnification ×1,000). **(B)** Mature ovum with adherent granulosa cells. The nucleus is seen near the center of the cell. The homogeneous band surrounding the ovum is the zona pellucida (original magnification ×400).

Courtesy of Leonard V. Crowley, MD, Century College.

Zona pellucida A layer of acellular material surrounding the ovum.

Corona radiata Crownlike structure composed of layers of granulosa cells.

Capacitation Process in which the surface of the sperm is altered.

of maturation takes several weeks and continues during the adult reproductive period. During spermatogenesis, a significant number of aberrant sperm with visible structural defects (such as malformed flagella) are produced, but they are ineffective in fertilization. Sperm can travel several millimeters per minute by their own propulsive efforts, and they also are passively transported by rhythmic contractions of the uterine muscles, which aspirate them upward into the fallopian tubes (sometimes called the oviduct or uterine tube) and the uterus. Further details of the process of gametogenesis are discussed under cell division.

The ovum, expelled from the follicle at ovulation, is surrounded by a thin layer of acellular material called the **zona pellucida** to which are attached clusters of **granulosa cells** from the follicle (**FIGURE 18-1B**). The layers of granulosa cells form a crownlike structure called the **corona radiata**. The ovary is positioned adjacent to the open funnel-like end of the fallopian tube (the infundibulum). Projections from the infundibulum, termed fimbriae, guide the released ovum into the fallopian tube. The ovum is swept into and along the fallopian tube by the beating of the cilia covering the tubal epithelium and is propelled down the tube by the peristaltic contractions of the smooth muscle in the tubal wall. Fertilization is possible when intercourse occurs reasonably close to the time of ovulation. However, the likelihood of a successful conception is related primarily to the survival time of the ovum, about twelve to twenty-four hours, rather than the sperm, which can survive in the genital tract and fertilize an ovum for as long as six days. The likelihood of a successful conception increases as intercourse occurs closer to the time of ovulation, but no conceptions occur the day after ovulation because of the ova's short life. In many successful conceptions, the sperm were already "lying in wait" for the ovum in the fallopian tube. The sperm "waiting" in the fallopian tube undergo a process called **capacitation**, which is mediated by tubal secretions. During this process the surface properties of the sperm are altered, and components of semen adhering to the sperm surface are removed. Only capacitated sperm are active in fertilization. The ovum spends four days in the fallopian tube moving toward the upper third of the tube where fertilization usually occurs by waiting capacitated sperm (**FIGURE 18-2**). After fertilization, the ovum moves into the uterus, implants, and develops further. If the ovum is not fertilized, it degenerates in the uterus.

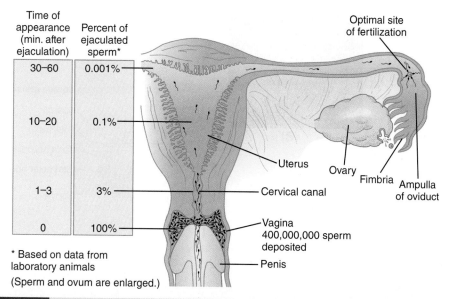

Time of appearance (min. after ejaculation)	Percent of ejaculated sperm*	
30–60	0.001%	
10–20	0.1%	
1–3	3%	
0	100%	

* Based on data from laboratory animals
(Sperm and ovum are enlarged.)

Optimal site of fertilization

Uterus

Ovary

Fimbria

Ampulla of oviduct

Cervical canal

Vagina
400,000,000 sperm deposited

Penis

FIGURE 18-2 Sperm transport in the female reproductive system. Sperm move rapidly up the female reproductive tract in humans principally as a result of contractions in the muscular walls of the uterus and uterine tubes. Notice the rapid decline in sperm numbers along the way.

The enzymes in the acrosome of the sperm disperse the cluster of granulosa cells in the corona radiata and permit the sperm head to penetrate the zona pellucida. After the sperm has penetrated, the ovum completes its second meiotic division and forms the female pronucleus (oogenesis is described in the discussion on chromosomes, genes, and cell division). Sperm penetration causes the zona pellucida to become impermeable to penetration by other sperm, assuring that only one sperm can enter the egg. Fusion of the cell membrane of the sperm and oocyte occurs (**FIGURE 18-3**). Within the cytoplasm of the egg, the sperm tail degenerates and the sperm nucleus enlarges, forming a male pronucleus. Fusion of the male and female pronuclei (each containing twenty three chromosomes) restores the genetic component of the cell to forty-six chromosomes; the fertilized ovum is now termed a **zygote**.

EARLY DEVELOPMENT OF THE FERTILIZED OVUM

As the fertilized ovum passes along the fallopian tube, it undergoes a series of mitotic divisions. The first cell division is completed about thirty hours after fertilization. Subsequent divisions occur in rapid succession and convert the zygote into a small, mulberry-shaped ball of cells (blastomeres) called a **morula** containing twelve to thirty-two blastomeres, enclosed within the zona pellucida. The morula reaches the endometrial cavity by about the third day. Soon fluid begins to accumulate in the center of the morula, and a central cavity forms. At this stage of development, the structure is called a **blastocyst**. The cells of the blastocyst begin to differentiate into two groups: the **inner cell mass**, which will form the embryo, and the **trophoblast**, a peripheral rim of cells that give rise to the fetal membranes and contribute to the formation of the placenta.

The blastocyst lies free within the endometrial cavity for several days. Then the zona pellucida degenerates, exposing the trophoblast. The blastocyst begins to burrow into the endometrium by the end of the first week after fertilization and soon becomes completely embedded (**FIGURE 18-4**).

Soon after implantation, the inner cell mass becomes a flat structure called the **germ disk**, which differentiates into the three germ layers: ectoderm, mesoderm, and

Zygote The fertilized ovum.

Morula A mulberry-shaped solid cluster of cells formed by division of the fertilized ovum.

Blastocyst A stage of development of the fertilized ovum (zygote) in which a central cavity forms within the cluster of developing cells.

Inner cell mass A group of cells derived from the fertilized ovum that is destined to form the embryo.

Trophoblast Cell derived from the fertilized ovum that gives rise to the fetal membranes and contributes to the formation of the placenta.

Germ disk A three-layered cluster of cells that will eventually give rise to an embryo.

Amnionic sac The fluid-filled sac surrounding the embryo. One of the fetal membranes.

Yolk sac A sac formed adjacent to the germ disk that will form the gastrointestinal tract and other important structures in the embryo.

Mesoderm The middle germ layer of the embryo, which gives rise to specific organs and tissues.

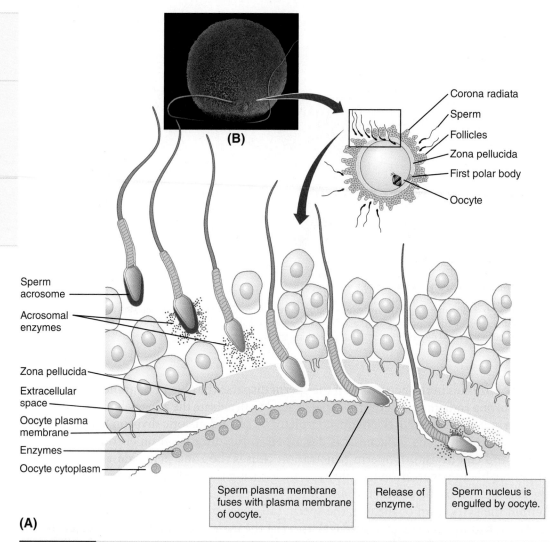

FIGURE 18-3 Fertilization. **(A)** The plasma membrane of the sperm and the outer membrane of the acrosome fuse and the membrane breaks down, releasing enzymes that allow the sperm to penetrate the corona radiata. Sperm digest their way through the zona pellucida via enzymes associated with the inner acrosomal membrane. Sperm are engulfed by the oocyte plasma membrane. Cortical granules are released when the sperm contacts the membrane. These granules cause other sperm in contact with the membrane to detach. **(B)** Although many sperm gather around the egg, only one will enter.

Chorion The layer of trophoblast and associated mesoderm that surrounds the developing embryo.

Chorionic vesicle The chorion with its villi and enclosed amnion, yolk sac, and developing embryo.

Chorionic villi Fingerlike columns of cells extending from the chorion that anchor the chorionic vesicle in the endometrium.

entoderm. Each of the layers will give rise to specific tissues and organs as described in the discussion on cells and tissues. A fluid-filled sac called the **amnionic sac** forms between the ectoderm of the germ disk and the surrounding trophoblast, and a second sac called the **yolk sac** forms on the opposite side of the germ disk. The interior of the blastocyst cavity then becomes lined by a layer of primitive connective tissue cells (**mesoderm**) that also covers the external surfaces of the amnionic sac and yolk sac. After the blastocyst cavity acquires a connective tissue lining, it is called the chorionic cavity, and its wall is called the **chorion**. The entire sac with its enclosed amnion, yolk sac, and developing embryo is called the **chorionic vesicle**. Fingerlike columns of cells called **chorionic villi** extend from the chorion and anchor the chorionic vesicle in the endometrium (**FIGURE 18-5**).

The chorionic cavity continues to enlarge, and the chorionic vesicle increases in size and complexity. By the end of the second week after fertilization, the small germ disk with its surrounding amnion and yolk sac projects into the chorionic cavity,

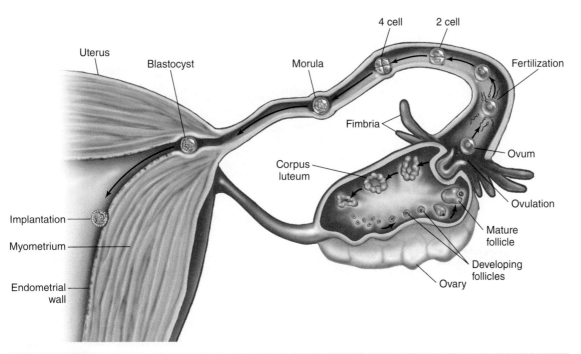

FIGURE 18-4 Summary of the maturation of the ovum, fertilization, and early development of the fertilized ovum.

suspended from the wall of the chorion by a mass of connective tissue called the **body stalk** (**FIGURE 18-6**).

By the fourth week after fertilization, the organ systems begin to form, and the embryo, which had been flat, becomes cylindrical. The central part of the germ disk grows more rapidly than the periphery as the nervous system begins to form. As a result, the germ disk flexes and bulges into the amnionic cavity. The amnionic sac, which is attached to the lateral margins of the germ disk, follows the changing contour of the embryo and is reflected around the embryo. Part of the yolk sac also becomes enfolded within the embryo when flexion occurs (**FIGURE 18-7**). The enclosed part will give rise to the intestinal tract and other important structures. The lateral

Body stalk The structure connecting the embryo to the chorion. Eventually develops into the umbilical cord.

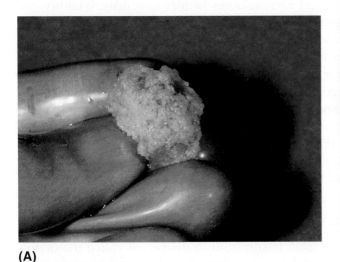

(A)

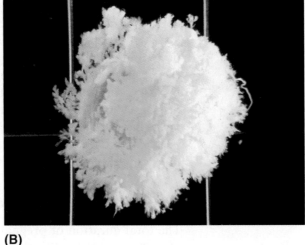

(B)

FIGURE 18-5 **(A)** Spontaneously aborted chorionic vesicle about six weeks after conception. **(B)** Closer view of a chorionic vesicle illustrating frondlike chorionic villi projecting from the chorion.

Courtesy of Leonard V. Crowley, MD, Century College.

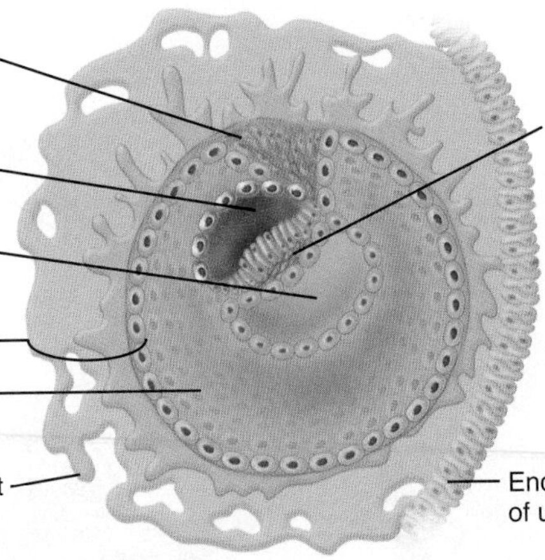

FIGURE 18-6 Appearance of the chorionic vesicle at the end of the second week after ovulation, illustrating the relation of the germ disk to the amnion, chorion, body stalk, and chorionic cavity.

margins of the germ disk fuse in the midline to form the ventral (anterior) body wall. The fusion is incomplete in the middle of the body wall where the umbilical cord is attached, and part of the yolk sac that was not included within the embryo protrudes through this defect. It persists for a time but soon degenerates.

STAGES OF PRENATAL DEVELOPMENT

It is customary to subdivide prenatal development into three main periods: the preembryonic, the embryonic, and the fetal period. The first three weeks after fertilization are the preembryonic period. During this time, the blastocyst becomes implanted and the inner cell mass differentiates into the three germ layers that will eventually form specific tissues within the embryo.

The embryonic period extends from the third through the seventh week. This is the time when the developing organism begins to assume a human shape and is called an **embryo**. This is also the time when all the organ systems are formed, and it is a critical period of development. At this stage, drugs ingested by the mother, radiation, some viral infections, and various other factors may disturb embryonic development and lead to congenital abnormalities (described in the discussion on congenital and hereditary diseases).

The fetal period extends from the eighth week until the time of delivery. The developing organism is no longer called an embryo; the term **fetus** is now applied. As the fetus grows, it becomes larger and heavier, but there are no major changes in its basic structure comparable to those in the embryonic period. Initially, the fetal head is disproportionately large, and the body appears quite scrawny because subcutaneous fat has not yet been deposited (**FIGURE 18-8**). Shortly before delivery, subcutaneous fat begins to accumulate and the body begins to fill out. **FIGURE 18-9** illustrates the progressive changes in the size of the fetus in relation to the duration of the gestation.

DURATION OF PREGNANCY

The total duration of pregnancy from fertilization to delivery is called the period of **gestation**, approximately thirty-eight weeks when dated from the time of ovulation. Usually, however, the actual date of ovulation is not known, and the length of gestation is calculated from the beginning of the last normal menstrual period. Expressed in this way, the duration of pregnancy is forty weeks because the first

Embryo The developing human organism from the third to the seventh week of gestation.

Fetus The unborn offspring after eight weeks' gestation.

Gestation Duration of pregnancy from fertilization to delivery.

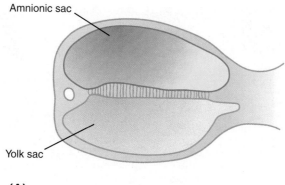

Amnionic sac

Yolk sac

(A)

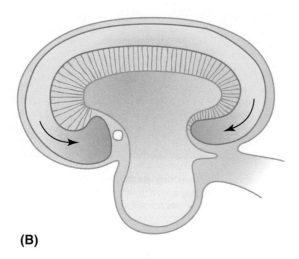

(B)

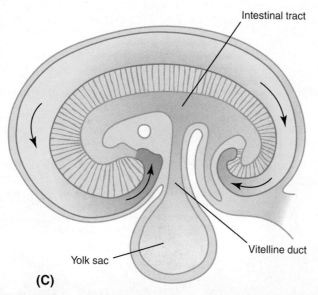

Intestinal tract

Yolk sac

Vitelline duct

(C)

FIGURE 18-7 Changes in the shape of the embryo resulting from more rapid growth of the germ disk. **(A)** The flat germ disk with the amnionic sac above and the yolk sac below. **(B)** The embryo begins to bulge into the amnionic sac. **(C)** Flexion completed. Part of the yolk sac is included in the body of the embryo and will form the intestinal tract. The embryo now has a cylindrical configuration. Part of the yolk sac remains connected to the embryo by a narrow vitelline duct.

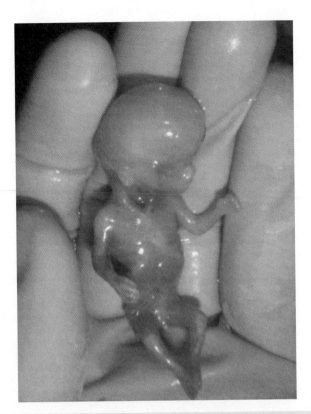

FIGURE 18-8 Small, well-formed, spontaneously aborted fetus near the end of the first trimester. At this stage, this fetus weighs only 10 g and measures 5 cm from head to buttocks. Its small size can be appreciated by comparing the fetus with the gloved hand that holds it.

Courtesy of Leonard V. Crowley, MD, Century College.

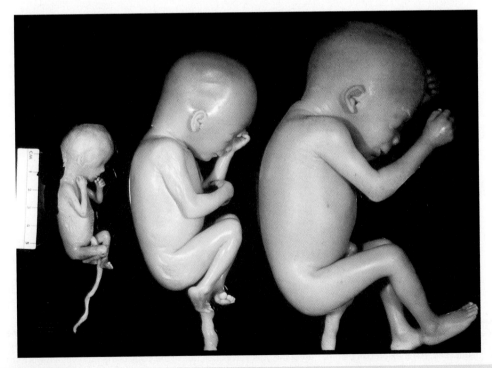

FIGURE 18-9 Progressive changes in the size of the fetus at various stages of gestation: (*left*) three and one-half months (32 g), (*center*) four and one-half months (230 g), (*right*) five and one-half months (420 g).

Courtesy of Leonard V. Crowley, MD, Century College.

day of the calculation is actually about two weeks before the date of conception. The gestation calculated in this way may also be expressed as 280 days, as ten lunar (twenty-eight-day) months, or nine calendar (thirty-one-day) months. Often the nine calendar months are subdivided into three periods called trimesters, each of three months' duration.

Decidua, Fetal Membranes, and Placenta

THE DECIDUA

The endometrium of pregnancy is called the **decidua**. **FIGURE 18-10** demonstrates the relationship of the embryo to the surrounding amnionic sac and chorion about seven weeks after fertilization. **FIGURE 18-11** diagrammatically illustrates these relationships in both early and late pregnancy.

> **Decidua** The endometrium of pregnancy.

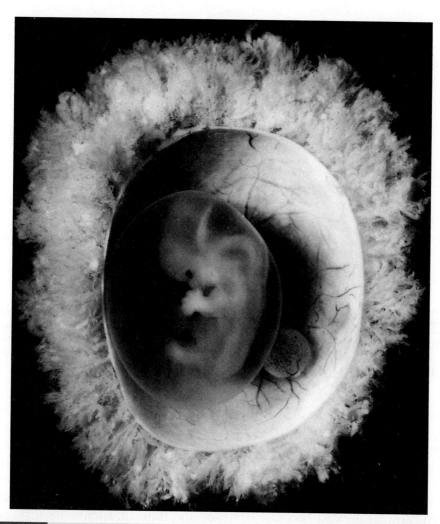

FIGURE 18-10 Relationship of the embryo to the amnionic sac, yolk sac, and chorionic cavity at about seven weeks after conception. The chorionic sac has been bisected. At this stage, villi still arise from the entire periphery of the chorion, and the amnionic sac surrounding the embryo does not completely fill the chorionic cavity. The embryo is attached to the chorion by the umbilical cord (not shown). The yolk sac is located to the right of the amnionic sac, between the amnionic sac and the chorion (photograph courtesy of the Carnegie Institution of Washington).

Courtesy of the Carnegie Institute of Washington.

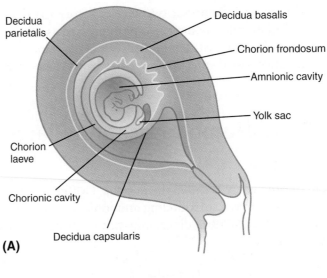

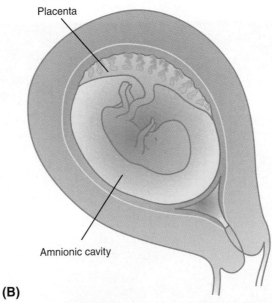

FIGURE 18-11 **(A)** Relationship of the fetus to the decidua, fetal membranes, and chorion in early pregnancy. The part of the yolk sac not incorporated within the fetus lies between the amnionic sac and the chorion. **(B)** relationship in late pregnancy. The amnionic sac envelops the fetus and now completely fills the chorionic cavity. The amnionic membrane lies against the chorion. The decidua capsularis has fused with the chorion laeve and has become adherent to the decidua parietalis on the opposite wall of the uterus.

Special names are applied to the parts of the decidua in which the chorionic vesicle is embedded, as indicated in Figure 18-11. The part beneath the chorionic vesicle is called the decidua basalis and forms the maternal portion of the placenta. The part that is stretched over the vesicle is called the decidua capsularis, and the part that lines the rest of the endometrial cavity is called the decidua parietalis (*parietes =* wall). As the embryo and its surrounding amnionic sac continue to increase in size, the thin capsular decidua becomes stretched and thinned. Eventually, it fuses with the decidua parietalis on the opposite wall of the uterus.

THE CHORION AND CHORIONIC VILLI

The chorion contains the fetal blood vessels that extend into the chorionic villi. The villi arising from the deeper portion of the chorion adjacent to the decidua basalis proliferate actively. These villi project into the large blood-filled spaces within the decidua basalis through which the maternal blood flows. Some of the villi also function as anchoring villi, which attach the chorion to the basal decidua, as well as sending extensions into the maternal blood-filled spaces in the basal decidua. Blood vessels that form within the villi as they grow become connected with blood vessels in the chorion and the body stalk, as well as within the body of the embryo. As soon as the embryo's heart begins to beat, blood begins to flow through this developing network of vessels.

THE AMNIONIC SAC

The amnionic sac is enclosed within the chorion. At first the sac is much smaller than the chorionic cavity (see Figure 18-10), but the enlarging sac expands into the chorionic cavity. Eventually the amnionic sac completely fills the chorionic cavity, and the amnionic membrane lies against the chorion. The sac functions as a buoyant, temperature-controlled environment that protects the fetus throughout pregnancy and assists in opening the cervix during childbirth.

THE YOLK SAC

In the human being, the yolk sac never contains yolk but performs other important functions, serving as the source of hematopoietic cells and the primordial germ cells that eventually form sperm and eggs in the developing gonads. Part of the yolk sac becomes incorporated into the body of the embryo to form the intestinal tract. The part that is not included within the embryo persists for a time but usually atrophies. In a small number of adults, a remnant persists as a Meckel diverticulum (discussed further with the intestinal tract).

THE PLACENTA

The **placenta** is a flattened, disk-shaped structure weighing about 500 g. It has a dual origin, both fetal and maternal (**FIGURE 18-12**). The chorion and the villi are formed from the trophoblast, which is of fetal origin, and the decidua basalis in which the villi are anchored is derived from the endometrium. Incomplete partition of decidua extends into the villi and divides them into areas called **cotyledons**, which impart a vague cobblestone appearance to the maternal surface of the placenta. The amnion and chorion extend from the margins of the placenta to form the fluid-filled sac that encloses the fetus and that ruptures at the time of delivery. The fetus is connected to the placenta by the umbilical cord, which contains two arteries. On the surface of the placenta, the artery divides into multiple branches, each supplying an individual cotyledon. Blood returning from the cotyledons is collected into large veins on the surface of the placenta to form the umbilical vein, which returns the blood to the fetus.

Placenta Flat, disk-shaped structure that maintains the developing organism within the uterus.

Circulation of Blood in the Placenta

The placenta has a dual circulation of blood (**FIGURE 18-13**). The fetoplacental circulation delivers arterial blood low in oxygen from the fetus to the chorionic villi through the umbilical artery and returns oxygenated blood to the fetus through the single umbilical vein. The uteroplacental circulation delivers oxygenated arterial blood from the mother into the large placental blood spaces located between the villi called the intervillous spaces. The blood flows into the intervillous spaces from the many uterine arteries that penetrate the basal portion of the placenta. Blood flows back into the maternal circulation through veins that penetrate the basal part

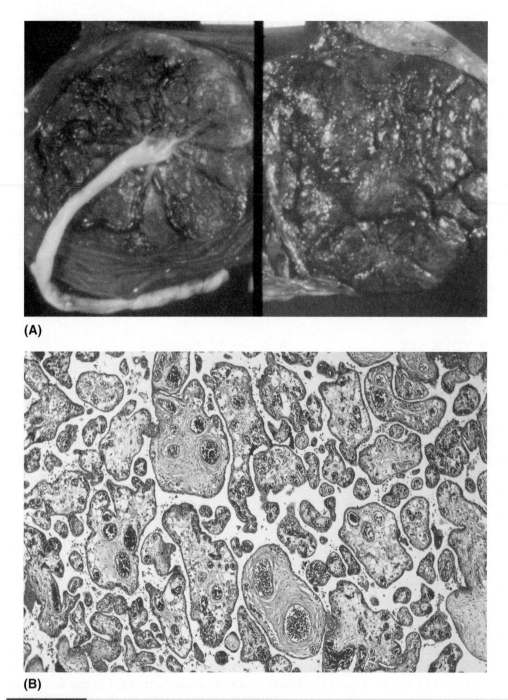

FIGURE 18-12 **(A)** Normal placenta. The fetal surface (*left side*) shows the umbilical cord and cord vessels that subdivide on the placental surface to supply chorionic villi. The cobblestone appearance of the maternal surface of the placenta (*right side*) is caused by the cotyledons, which are clusters of villi separated by decidual partitions extending between the villi. **(B)** Histologic section of placenta revealing chorionic villi viewed in cross section. Blood vessels in villi contain fetal cells. When the placenta is within the uterus, the spaces between the villi are filled with maternal blood (original magnification ×100).

Courtesy of Leonard V. Crowley, MD, Century College.

of the placenta. The arrangement of the two circulations in the placenta brings the maternal and fetal blood into close approximation. In this way, oxygen and nutrients can be exchanged between the maternal and fetal circulations, but there is no actual intermixing of fetal and maternal blood although very small amounts of fetal blood sometimes enter maternal circulations through small defects in the placental membrane.

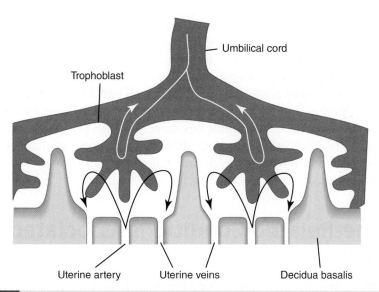

FIGURE 18-13 Dual circulation of blood in the placenta. Fetal blood circulates through the villi, and maternal blood flows around the villi, but circulations do not intermix.

Endocrine Function of the Placenta

The placenta synthesizes two steroid hormones, estrogen and progesterone, and two protein hormones called **human chorionic somatomammotropin (HCS)** (also called human placental lactogen) and **human chorionic gonadotropin (HCG)**. HCS stimulates maternal metabolic processes acting as an anti-insulin, increasing maternal glucose levels. HCG is quite similar to the gonadotropic hormones produced by the pituitary gland that suppresses the onset of menstruation. Pregnancy tests detect HCG. The newer, more sensitive tests performed on blood or urine become positive as early as ten to twelve days after fertilization, even before the woman misses her first period.

Amnionic Fluid

The quantity of amnionic fluid, produced both by filtration and by excretion, varies with the stage of pregnancy. During the early part of pregnancy, the amnionic fluid is formed chiefly by filtration of fluid into the amnionic sac from maternal blood as it passes through the uterus and from fetal blood passing through the placenta. Additional fluid diffuses directly through the fetal skin prior to its maturation and keratin formation from the fetal respiratory tract. Later, when the fetal kidneys begin to function at about the eleventh week, the fetus urinates into the amnionic fluid, and fetal urine becomes the major source of this fluid. By late pregnancy, up to half a quart (500 ml) of urine is contributed by the fetus. Both filtration and fetal urine continually add to the volume of fluid, but the additions are counterbalanced by losses of amnionic fluid into the fetal gastrointestinal tract. Normally, the fetus swallows as much as 400 ml of fluid per day. This fluid is absorbed from the fetal intestinal tract into the fetal circulation, transferred across the placenta into the mother's circulation, and eventually excreted by the mother in her urine. Excess fluid also contributes to fetal urine and is recirculated into the amniotic fluid.

Polyhydramnios and Oligohydramnios

Polyhydramnios is a condition in which the volume of amnionic fluid is markedly increased. This can be caused by congenital maldevelopment of the fetal brain called

Human chorionic somatomammotropin (HCS) One of the hormones produced by the placenta that has properties similar to pituitary growth hormone. Also called human placental lactogen.

Human chorionic gonadotropin (HCG) A hormone made by the placenta in pregnancy having actions similar to pituitary gonadotropins. Same hormone is made by neoplastic cells in some types of malignant testicular tumors.

Polyhydramnios An excess of amnionic fluid.

Anencephaly A congenital malformation: absence of brain, cranial vault, and scalp as a result of defective closure of the neural tube.

Oligohydramnios An insufficient quantity of amnionic fluid.

Hyperemesis gravidum Excess vomiting associated with pregnancy.

anencephaly (see discussion on the nervous system), which disturbs the normal swallowing mechanism, so that the fetus is unable to swallow amnionic fluid, or a congenital obstruction of the fetal upper intestinal tract blocks the entry of swallowed fluid into the small intestine where it can be absorbed. **Oligohydramnios** is a marked reduction in the volume of amnionic fluid that occurs either because the fetal kidneys have failed to develop and no urine is formed or because a congenital obstruction blocks the urethra so that urine cannot be excreted. When preterm rupture of membranes occurs too early to allow for immediate delivery, those neonates who survive suffer from oligohydramnios and developmental abnormalities associated with it (as discussed in the Case) and have a high incidence of intrauterine infection.

Hormone-Related Conditions Associated with Pregnancy

The hormones produced by a woman's endocrine glands and by her placenta during pregnancy maintain the pregnancy and sustain the fetus, but some have undesirable effects on the pregnant woman. Nausea and vomiting during early pregnancy is related to the rapidly increasing levels of estrogen in early pregnancy; nausea and vomiting often occur in the morning (morning sickness) and usually subside by the end of the first trimester (first three months of pregnancy). **Hyperemesis gravidum** literally means excessive vomiting of pregnancy; it probably has the same hormonal basis as morning sickness but is more prolonged and severe. Weight loss and dehydration may require treatment with intravenous fluids.

Gestational Diabetes

EFFECTS OF HYPERGLYCEMIA ON PREGNANCY

In all pregnancies during the second three months (second trimester) the high placental hormone levels cause the body to become less responsive to insulin (called insulin resistance), which tends to raise blood glucose. Most often the pregnant woman compensates by secreting more insulin, and the blood glucose remains normal.

Any elevated blood glucose concentration in the maternal blood (hyperglycemia), as in diabetes (described in the discussion on the pancreas and diabetes mellitus), is harmful to the developing fetus. In early pregnancy when the organ systems are developing, the hyperglycemia may cause congenital malformations or even lead to fetal death. Later in the pregnancy, the extra glucose crossing the placenta into the fetal bloodstream causes the fetal pancreas to release more insulin, and the extra glucose is metabolized to promote fetal growth. As a result, the fetus becomes larger than average size; the larger fetal kidneys secrete more urine, which contributes to the volume of amnionic fluid and causes its volume to increase. Delivery of the oversized fetus may be more difficult, possibly requiring a cesarean section. After delivery, the infant's blood glucose may fall precipitously (hypoglycemia) because the newborn infant's pancreas has been accustomed to dealing with a much higher intrauterine blood glucose concentration and has not had time to compensate for the lower post-delivery blood glucose. The infant also faces neonatal respiratory distress problems caused by inadequate surfactant, as described in the discussion on the respiratory system. For these reasons, recognition and treatment of hyperglycemia in pregnancy are in the best interest of both the mother and her baby.

Some women who were considered nondiabetic before becoming pregnant may not be able to produce enough insulin to maintain a normal glucose concentration during pregnancy because of the insulin resistance caused by the high hormone levels in pregnancy. The condition is called **gestational diabetes** because the blood glucose is likely to return to normal after the pregnancy, although women with gestational diabetes may be at higher risk of developing type 2 diabetes in later years.

Gestational diabetes occurs in about 2 percent of pregnancies and is much higher in older women, in obese women, and in women from ethnic groups having a high frequency of diabetes. It is important to identify pregnant women with gestational diabetes so they can be treated by diet and additional insulin if necessary to maintain a normal blood glucose during pregnancy, which avoids the hazards of hyperglycemia on her fetus.

Pregnant women should be evaluated on their initial visit for any risk factors—such as obesity, gestational diabetes in a previous pregnancy, a family history of diabetes, and any other factors that might predispose her to gestational diabetes—and some type of screening test should be performed. The usual screening test consists of 50 g of glucose solution given orally without regard to fasting status, followed by determining the concentration of glucose in the patient's blood one hour later. If the result exceeds a predetermined concentration, more comprehensive studies are performed to confirm the diagnosis of gestational diabetes, and a course of treatment is begun.

Spontaneous Abortion

Most spontaneous abortions (miscarriage) occur early in pregnancy, generally within the first twelve weeks or earlier. Ten to 20 percent of pregnancies result in a spontaneous abortion that is noted. However, studies of early preimplantation blastocysts undertaken as part of in vitro fertilization indicate that between 40 and 60 percent of these early zygotes have detectable chromosomal abnormalities (i.e., are aneuploid). In some cases, these aneuploid zygotes show detectable structural abnormalities and, of those, 75 percent have abnormal chromosomes. This is consistent with estimates that that up to 50 percent of zygotes fail to develop into blastocysts and implant. In such cases, the affected woman is unlikely to realize she was pregnant. In most cases, the cause of spontaneous abortion in early pregnancy cannot be determined, but it is likely to result from lethal chromosomal abnormalities. Many embryos recovered from spontaneous abortions show a variety of serious developmental defects.

Intrauterine fetal deaths that occur later in pregnancy (after twenty weeks, defined as **stillbirths**) are not common, occurring in about 0.6 percent of pregnancies. Stillbirths are generally caused by partial detachment of the placenta from the wall of the uterus, which is called placental **abruption**, or by obstruction of the blood supplied through the umbilical cord. Compression of the blood vessels in the umbilical cord, shutting off the blood supply to the fetus, may occur if the cord becomes knotted or wrapped tightly around the infant's neck or limbs (**FIGURE 18-14**). If the placenta becomes separated or the cord becomes obstructed, the fetus no longer receives oxygen and nutrients from the mother, and dies. Drug abuse during pregnancy is also associated with stillbirths (about 4 percent). Cocaine use is of particular note because the vasoactive effects may lead to placental abruption. A dead fetus is usually expelled promptly, but occasionally it is retained within the uterine cavity for several weeks or months.

If a dead fetus is retained for some time within the uterine cavity, products of degenerated fetal tissue diffuse into the maternal circulation. This material has thromboplastic activity and may induce a hemorrhagic disease in the mother because of depletion of maternal blood coagulation factors, which occurs when the coagulation mechanism is activated by the thromboplastic material. A retained dead fetus is one

Gestational diabetes Diabetes during pregnancy.

Stillbirth Spontaneous abortion after twenty weeks' gestation.

Abruption Partial detachment of the placenta.

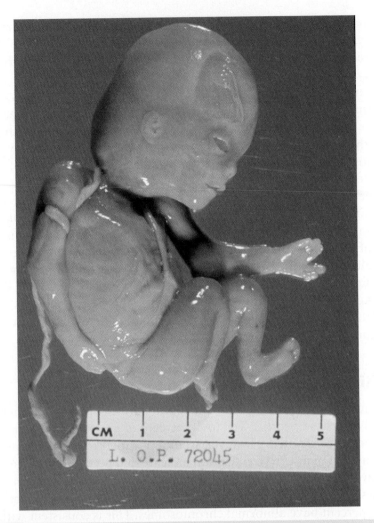

FIGURE 18-14 Fetus spontaneously aborted late in pregnancy because of interruption of blood supply through the umbilical cord. The cord extended around the back of neck and had become tightly wrapped around the upper arm, shutting off circulation and leading to intrauterine death.

Courtesy of Leonard V. Crowley, MD, Century College.

Disseminated intravascular coagulation syndrome (DIC) A disturbance of blood coagulation as a result of activation of the coagulation mechanism.

cause of the **disseminated intravascular coagulation syndrome (DIC)**, which is discussed in the abnormalities of blood coagulation.

Ectopic Pregnancy

An ectopic pregnancy (*ecto* = outside) is the development of an embryo outside its normal location within the uterine cavity. Most ectopic pregnancies occur in the fallopian tubes, but on rare occasions a fertilized ovum develops in the ovary or abdominal cavity. Implantation can take place in the fallopian tube if transport of the ovum is delayed. A previous infection in the fallopian tubes may cause failure of the tubal muscle contractions and can predispose a woman to this condition. Fallopian tube infections often are followed by scarring and fusion of tubal folds, which retards the passage of the fertilized egg through the tube. Frequently, the conditions that predispose to a tubal pregnancy affect both fallopian tubes. Consequently, a woman who has had one tubal pregnancy is more likely to develop an ectopic pregnancy in the opposite tube. The consequences of ectopic pregnancy associated with gynecologic infection are explored in the Case discussion of sexually transmitted disease.

Because of the potential life-threatening risk of a ruptured tubal pregnancy, a physician always considers the possibility any woman of reproductive age who exhibits any suggestive symptoms. A pelvic examination reveals an area of tenderness adjacent to the uterus and may also reveal a fullness or mass caused by the swollen tube. A positive pregnancy test confirms the pregnancy, and an ultrasound examination demonstrates that the chorionic vesicle indicative of pregnancy is not within the uterus. Laparoscopic examination is performed, allowing the physician to visualize the fallopian tubes and ovaries and to identify the unruptured pregnancy within the fallopian tube. Both surgical and nonsurgical approaches are used to remove the ectopic fetus. A single oral dose of an antimetabolite drug called methotrexate can destroy the tubal pregnancy, eliminating the need for a surgical procedure in which the tube is incised and the pregnancy is evacuated.

Abnormal Attachment of the Umbilical Cord and Placenta

VELAMENTOUS INSERTION OF THE UMBILICAL CORD

If the umbilical cord vessels are not gathered together normally, the cord attaches to the membranes attached to the placenta (fetal membranes) rather than to the placenta itself. When this occurs, the umbilical vessels must travel for a distance within the fetal membranes before reaching the placenta (**FIGURE 18-15**). This is called a **velamentous insertion of umbilical cord** (*velum* = veil). The abnormality may be hazardous to the

Velamentous insertion of umbilical cord Attachment of the umbilical cord to the fetal membranes rather than to the placenta.

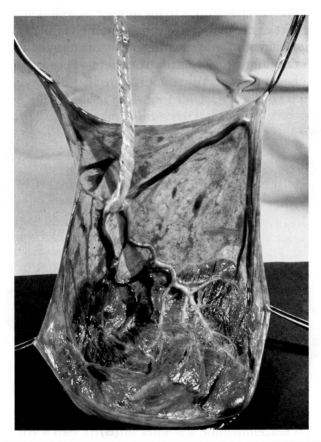

FIGURE 18-15 Velamentous insertion of umbilical cord. Note the vessels traversing the membranes to reach the placenta.

Courtesy of Leonard V. Crowley, MD, Century College.

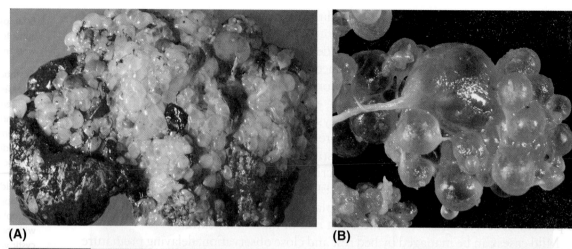

(A) **(B)**

FIGURE 18-20 Hydatidiform mole. **(A)** Placenta converted into a large mass of cystic villi. **(B)** Closer view of cystic villi.
Courtesy of Leonard V. Crowley, MD, Century College.

Less commonly a hydatidiform mole results from fertilization of a normal ovum by two sperm, resulting in a fertilized ovum containing three sets of chromosomes, one maternal and two paternal, for a total of sixty-nine chromosomes resulting from the fertilization of a haploid ovum by two haploid sperm (or a single sperm that has not undergone meiosis). An embryo forms but does not survive, and the trophoblastic tissue consists of a mixture of normal and cystic villi. This type of mole, which does not exhibit aggressive growth, is called a partial mole.

A hydatidiform mole is a relatively common complication of pregnancy occurring about once in 1,500 pregnancies in the United States and Canada, but is encountered ten times more frequently in women from the Far East and Southeast Asia. It occurs more frequently in girls under fifteen years of age. Risk then increases for women over age forty.

Because of the increased volume of the placenta caused by the multiple cystic villi, the patient with a mole experiences an enlargement of the uterus that is much greater than would be expected in relationship to the duration of the pregnancy. Erosion of maternal blood vessels by the mole may cause irregular uterine bleeding. The overdistension of the uterus caused by the mole may precipitate uterine contractions leading to expulsion of pieces of the mole.

Diagnosis of a mole is based on the clinical features of the pregnancy, by identifying cystic villi covered by proliferating trophoblast expelled from the uterus, or by ultrasound examination, which reveals a characteristic appearance caused by the cystic villi that fill the uterine cavity. Because complete moles occasionally progress to choriocarcinoma, chemotherapy is required if hCG levels do not normalize after removal of the mole. Disseminated disease rarely occurs after therapy.

An invasive mole resembles a complete hydatidiform mole but exhibits a much more marked trophoblastic proliferation and a much more aggressive behavior. Although trophoblastic tissue may invade deeply into the uterine wall and cause considerable bleeding, it does not metastasize.

CHORIOCARCINOMA

Choriocarcinoma is the most aggressive form of gestational trophoblast disease and behaves like a malignant tumor. Masses of abnormal actively proliferating trophoblast may extend into the vagina and may metastasize to the lungs, brain, and other

circulations is disrupted, and some of the Rh positive fetal cells within the villi may be expressed into the uterine blood vessels and may enter the mother's circulation After sensitization has occurred, Rh hemolytic disease will develop in any subsequent pregnancy in which the fetus is Rh positive.

Rh hemolytic disease now occurs only rarely because the formation of Rh antibodies by an Rh negative mother can be prevented by treating the mother with Rhogam, an immune globulin containing a high concentration of human anti Rh D antibodies given at twenty-eight to thirty weeks antepartum and at the time of birth. Rhogam is also given to Rh negative mothers who have an abortion or miscarriage or who may have inadvertently received a transfusion with incompatible Rh D+ blood. Such therapy is extremely successful in preventing hemolytic disease of the newborn and is routinely offered to all pregnant Rh D negative women. Combined antepartum and postpartum administration reduces the incidence of sensitization to about 0.5 percent.

When administered to an unsensitized Rh negative mother, the anti Rh D antibody in the immune globulin coats the Rh antigen sites on the surface of any fetal red cells that have entered the mother's circulation, leading to rapid removal of the antibody-coated red cells so that they do not persist long enough to induce sensitization. It is of no value if the mother has already formed antibodies. The incidence of Rh hemolytic disease has been greatly reduced by the routine use of Rh immune globulin, but the disease has not been completely eliminated. A very small number of Rh negative women form Rh antibody in their first pregnancy, apparently because of prior contact with Rh antigen from an unrecognized abortion, transfusion of Rh positive blood, or another cause.

TREATMENT OF HEMOLYTIC DISEASE

Although hemolytic disease caused by Rh incompatibility was formerly a more common problem than it is now, it still does occasionally occur (occasionally because of poor prenatal care). In these cases, an **exchange transfusion** may be undertaken to provide the infant with a population of cells that will not be destroyed by the antibody. In the case of hemolytic disease caused by Rh incompatibility, a transfusion of Rh negative blood is given. At the same time, exchange transfusion provides the infant with bilirubin-free plasma to replace the jaundiced plasma, thereby helping to prevent severe elevation of potentially toxic, unconjugated bilirubin. It should be emphasized that the exchange transfusion has no effect on the infant's own blood type. The transfused Rh negative cells will be gradually eliminated and replaced by the infant's own Rh positive cells. The purpose of the exchange transfusion is to tide the infant over during an acute, life-threatening situation. This is accomplished by decreasing the rate of red cell destruction through transfusion of cells not subject to hemolysis and by lowering the concentration of potentially toxic unconjugated bilirubin in the infant's plasma.

The elevated level of unconjugated bilirubin that causes kernicterus can also be somewhat reduced by exposing the unclothed jaundiced infant to fluorescent lights continuously for several days. The light exposure acts by converting the toxic unconjugated bilirubin into less toxic compounds that are not as hazardous to the infant. This procedure, called **phototherapy**, has reduced the need for exchange transfusions. The level of unconjugated serum bilirubin normally rises after delivery even in normal infants, usually reaching a peak of about 6 mg/dl or sometimes even higher within the first few days after delivery and then falls toward normal. In hemolytic disease, unconjugated bilirubin levels rise faster, and levels are often much higher than in a normal newborn infant. Levels exceeding 20 mg/dl are potentially hazardous, put the infant at risk of kernicterus, and require treatment to lower the serum bilirubin level. Phototherapy is

Exchange transfusion Partial replacement of blood of infant with hemolytic disease by blood lacking the antigen responsible for hemolytic disease, as when transfusing Rh negative blood to an Rh positive infant. Performed to reduce intensity of hemolytic jaundice.

Phototherapy Fluorescent light treatment of jaundiced babies to reduce the concentration of unconjugated bilirubin in their blood.

sometimes used in neonates who have high levels of unconjugated bilirubin because of delays in liver maturation rather than immune destruction of red cells.

ABO HEMOLYTIC DISEASE

ABO hemolytic disease
A mild hemolytic disease in group A or B infants or group O mothers as a result of maternal anti-A and anti-B antibodies.

With the decline in the frequency of Rh hemolytic disease, now most cases of hemolytic disease result from ABO blood group differences between the mother and infant. In this condition, called **ABO hemolytic disease,** the mother is group O (and has anti-A and anti-B antibodies in her serum), and the infant is either group A or group B. In many women, the A or B fetal antigens stimulate the production of IgG maternal ABO antibodies, which can cross the placenta. The disease occurs in a first ABO-incompatible pregnancy because it is caused by preexisting anti-A and anti-B antibodies in the mother. ABO hemolytic disease is a much less severe disease than Rh incompatibility and is generally only detected antepartum when hyperbilirubinemia occurs. Generally, the elevated bilirubin responds well to fluorescent light phototherapy although a few unusual cases requiring exchange transfusion have been reported.

CASE 18-1

Sarah and Sidney had one child, a healthy two-year-old female. The couple was delighted when Sarah became pregnant with a male child. Unfortunately, the pregnancy did not turn out well. An ultrasound of the developing fetus at eighteen weeks' gestation detected a possible abnormality of the child's urinary system, and Sarah's developing fetus was now subject to frequent careful examination. At twenty-four weeks, an MRI study of the developing fetus disclosed definite swelling of the fetal bladder, ureters (hydroureter), and swelling and abnormalities of the developing kidneys (hydronephrosis). Continued monitoring of fetal development confirmed the problem. The fetal abnormalities were accompanied by a reduced amount of amniotic fluid (oligohydramnios).

Sarah and Sidney discussed the findings with their obstetrician. They were told that the chances of the child surviving to birth were low. Even if the fetus survived, death soon after birth was extremely likely. Although many parents in such circumstances would elect to undergo a therapeutic abortion, Sarah and Sidney elected to continue the pregnancy. At thirty-two weeks, the child was found to be in an abnormal position (breech) and a uterine infection was suspected. The child was delivered by C-section but expired shortly after birth. Heartbroken, the couple agreed to a complete autopsy in an attempt to understand what went wrong with the pregnancy and to help them understand the risk of such an event occurring in a subsequent pregnancy.

Autopsy Results

At birth the child had an abnormal facial appearance (facies). The facial features (nose, chin, forehead) appeared to be compressed and flattened as if they had developed pressed against the uterine wall. One leg was malrotated (a club foot). Internal examination disclosed severe pulmonary hypoplasia. The two lungs together weighed 6 g, normal lungs would have weighed about 37 g (**FIGURE 18-23**). The lungs were collapsed and could not function to provide oxygen at birth. The kidneys were fluid filled and had cysts the pathologist described as being consistent with an obstruction in the urinary system (obstructive nephropathy). The ureters were fluid filled and dilated, as was the bladder. Examination showed that the outlet from the bladder was defective, and the urethra (which normally would carry urine from the bladder to the opening in the penis) was malformed. This lack of a urinary outlet caused fetal urine to "back up" into the bladder, ureters, and kidney. The pathologist diagnosed **Potter sequence.**

CASE 18-1 *(Continued)*

Discussion

Potter sequence is also called Potter syndrome but "sequence" is the more accurate term. A *syndrome* is often defined as a group of signs and symptoms that occur together and are characteristic of a disease. The term *sequence* is used by physicians who study developmental abnormalities to define the secondary consequences of a defect in development. The defect could be the result of **dysplasia** (an intrinsic disruption of the proper development of an organ such as might be cause by a genetic defect), of a **disruption** (an environmental disruption of proper development not intrinsic to the fetus), a **deformation** (a secondary defect of development related to some other primary cause), or, as in the case of Potter sequence, a combination of all three.

At the heart of Potter sequence is oligohydramnios, a lack of the proper amount of amniotic fluid. Why should this occur? The simplest explanation is early disruption of fetal membranes causing chronic physical leakage. Usually, however, the cause of oligohydramnios is more complex. Starting at about sixteen weeks' gestation, the source of the bulk of amniotic fluid is fetal urine. The fetus swallows the amniotic fluid (mostly fetal urine) and recycles it through the kidneys. Any interruption in this cycle will result in oligohydramnios. One common cause is failure of the fetal kidneys to develop (bilateral renal dysplasia), which is invariably fatal. With no kidneys, no fetal urine is produced. A second cause is a blockage in the urinary tract, which may happen at the level of the urethra (urethral valves, a blockage within the lumen of the urethra) or because of more complex failures of development of the urinary tract (as was the case here). If there is no outlet for urine into the amniotic fluid, the urine

> **Dysplasia** Abnormal maturation of cells. Localized areas of dysregulated growth.

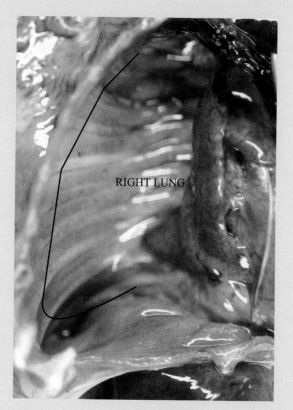

FIGURE 18-23 Hypoplastic right lung in a case of Potter sequence. Line indicates expected extent of normal lung.

Courtesy of Vincent Moylan Jr. MS PA (ASCP) Department of Pathology and Laboratory Medicine University of North Carolina at Chapel Hill.

(continues)

CASE 18-1 *(Continued)*

backs up, swelling the bladder and the ureters and leading to pressure damage to the developing kidneys. The lack of amniotic fluid has other serious consequences. Pulmonary development in the fetus requires the breathing in of amniotic fluid into the developing lung. If this does not occur, pulmonary hypoplasia results. Finally, amniotic fluid protects and cushions the developing fetus. When the protective fluid is absent, the fetus tends to be pressed against the uterine wall, which results in "flattened" facial features and malpositioned and malrotated limbs. Thus, many of the seemingly unconnected defects in Potter sequence are related to the lack of amniotic fluid, which may be caused by a number of mechanisms. Because of the multiple potential causes, the exact frequency of Potter sequence is unclear. Although about 1 in 5,000 births have Potter sequence related to renal agenesis (sometimes called *classic Potter*), the overall frequency is perhaps five times higher. Risk is higher in males. Many mutations are associated with renal agenesis, but in the absence of a family history or the occurrence of multiple affected pregnancies, the risk of recurrence is low.

Etiology and Pathogenesis

Potter sequence caused by complex maldevelopment of the lower urinary tract leading to total urinary obstruction.

Questions

1. Certain types of Potter sequence might be amenable to intrauterine therapy. Which causes of Potter sequence might be corrected; for which causes would this be unlikely?

2. Injection of fluid into the uterus has been suggested as a potential intervention for Potter sequence. What are some potential problem with this approach?

3. What other developmental abnormalities are frequently detected using fetal ultrasound?

4. Fetal DNA can be recovered from maternal circulation and sequenced to detect mutations. Would this approach aid in the early diagnosis of Potter sequence?

5. Potter sequence is a consequence of a combination of dysplasia, disruption, and deformation. How are each of these related to the findings in the case?

QUESTIONS FOR REVIEW

1. Why do spontaneous abortions occur? What are the consequences of prolonged retention of a dead fetus within the uterine cavity?

2. What is an ectopic pregnancy? What factors predispose to development of an ectopic pregnancy in the fallopian tube? What are the consequences of a tubal pregnancy?

3. What is the difference between a hydatidiform mole and a choriocarcinoma?

4. In infants with hemolytic disease, why does jaundice increase after delivery? Why does anemia become more severe after delivery?

5. How does the physician make a diagnosis of hemolytic disease? How is the disease treated?

6. What structures contribute to the formation of the placenta? What are the main functions of the placenta?

7. Describe some of the important abnormalities of the placenta and umbilical cord that may have an unfavorable effect on pregnancy.

8. What is the source of amnionic fluid? What factors regulate the total volume of amnionic fluid?

9. What are the possible causes and the significance of polyhydramnios? of oligohydramnios?

SUPPLEMENTARY READINGS

Chiras, D. D., Chapter 22, "Human Development and Aging." 2012. In *Human Biology*. 7th ed. by D. D. Chiras. Sudbury, MA: Jones & Bartlett Learning.

Moore, K. L., Persaud, T. V. N., and Torchia, M. G. 2016. *The Developing Human*. 10th ed. Philadelphia, PA: Elsevier.
  ► Human development and pregnancy is a complex and well-documented area. Those wishing for additional details should start with the chapter listed in the first entry, which provides an excellent overview of the area. The figures are of particular use. The second entry is a recent text much used in medical education that provides clinically relevant details.

Martin, J. A., et al. 2015. Births: Final data 2013. *National Vital Statistics Report 64*(1).

Dunson, D. B., et al. 1999. Day-specific probabilities of clinical pregnancy based on two studies with imperfect measures of ovulation. *Human Reproduction 14*:1835–39.

Orzack, S. H., et al. 2015. The human sex ratio from conception to birth. *PNAS* (online March 30). doi:10.1073 /pnas.1416546112
  ► These three papers provide a statistical overview of birth. The first entry is for the standard U.S. report on current birth statistics including maternal age, live-birth order, and much else. The second entry is a classic paper on the probability of conception. It is still much quoted and provides the information basis for "natural" methods of birth control. The third article describes an extensive current study looking at the sex ratio from time of conception to birth; it presents data that differs from what currently is often quoted.

Stillbirth Collaborative Research Network Writing Group. 2011. Causes of death among stillbirths. *JAMA 306*:2469.
  ► The number of stillbirths is 1/160 pregnancies, a number equal to the number of expected infant deaths. Shockingly, U.S. rates are significantly higher than those in other countries. The paper looks not only at causes but at racial disparities. This is must reading for those interested in the social aspects of prenatal care.

Capalbo, A., et al. 2014. Correlation between standard blastocyst morphology, euploidy and implantation: An observational study in two centers involving 956 screened blastocysts. *Human Reproduction 29*:1173–81.

de CassiaSavio Figueira, R., et al. 2015. Blastocyst morphology holds clues concerning the chromosomal status of the embryo. *International Journal of Fertility and Sterility 9*:215–20.
  ► The growing popularity of assisted reproductive technology (in vitro fertilization and related techniques) has allowed the gathering of new information relating to the frequency of chromosomal abnormalities in preimplantation zygotes and the role of these abnormalities in very early embryo development. These two papers discuss the most "pre" of prenatal screening.

Cain, M. A., Bornick, P., and Whitemen, V. 2013. The maternal, fetal and neonatal effects of cocaine exposure in pregnancy. *Clinical Obstetrics and Gynecology 56*:124–32.

▶ Illicit drug use during pregnancy presents a serious risk to both mother and fetus. Of abused drugs, cocaine presents a unique series of risks because of its physiological effects.

Basu, S., Kaur, R., and Kaur, G. 2011. Hemolytic disease of the fetus and newborn: Current trends and perspectives. *Asian Journal of Transfusion Science 5*:3–7.

▶ Although less of a problem in the United States, hemolytic disease of the newborn is still a frequent problem in the developing world. A good overview by a well-published author in the field of transfusion medicine.

Mol, B. W. J., et al. 2015. Pre-eclampsia. *Lancet* (online September 3). doi: 10.1016/s0140-6736(15)00070

▶ A *Lancet* seminar review covering both clinical and physiological aspects of a condition that is still a major contributor to morbidity in pregnancy.

Grijseels, E. W., et al. 2011. Outcome of pregnancies complicated by oligohydramnios or anhydrmnios of renal origin. *Prenatal Diagnosis 31*:1039–45.

Gupta, S., et al. 2015. Potter syndrome. *EMedicine*. http://emedicine.medscape.com/article/983477-overview

▶ These two sources were used in constructing the Case.

Acid-Base Balance and the Urinary System

1. Describe the role of the kidneys in maintaining water and electrolyte balance in the body.

2. Describe the role of the kidneys in the regulation of blood pressure and blood pH.

3. Describe the normal structures of the kidneys and their functions with special emphasis on the nephron.

4. Explain the pathogenesis of glomerulonephritis, nephrosis, and nephrosclerosis. Describe the clinical manifestations of each of these disorders.

5. Describe the clinical manifestations and complications of urinary tract infections.

6. Explain the mechanism for formation of urinary tract calculi. Describe the complications of stone formation. Explain the manifestations of urinary tract obstruction.

7. Differentiate the major forms of cystic disease of the kidney and their prognoses.

8. Name the more common kinds of tumors affecting the urinary tract.

9. Describe the causes, clinical manifestations, and treatment of renal failure.

10. Describe the principles and techniques of hemodialysis and renal transplantation.

11. Describe the techniques used to evaluate kidney disease.

Role of the Kidneys

The amount of water and electrolytes in the body represents a balance between the amounts ingested in food and fluids and the amounts excreted in the urine, through the gastrointestinal tract, in perspiration, and as water vapor excreted by the lungs. The kidneys are important in controlling the concentration of body water and electrolytes. Under the influence of adrenal cortical and posterior pituitary hormones (discussed in the presentation on the endocrine glands), the kidneys regulate the internal environment of the body by selectively excreting or retaining water and electrolytes as required to maintain a uniform composition of the body fluids.

The kidneys are also important excretory organs, functioning along with the lungs in excreting the waste products of food metabolism including carbon dioxide and water. Protein metabolism produces urea, as well as various acids, which only the kidneys can excrete. The kidneys also play an important role in regulating mineral and water balance by excreting minerals and water that have been ingested in excess of the body's requirements and conserving minerals and water as required. In a sense, the environment of the body is determined not by what a person ingests but rather by what the kidneys retain.

MANAGEMENT OF WATER, ELECTROLYTES, AND WASTE IN THE BODY

About 60 percent of the body consists of water, about two-thirds of which is within cells as intracellular water. The remainder, called extracellular water, is within the interstitial tissues surrounding the cells and in the blood plasma. The body water contains dissolved mineral salts (**electrolytes**) that dissociate in solution, yielding positively charged ions (**cations**) and negatively charged ions (**anions**). The fluid within the cells is separated from the interstitial fluid by the cell membrane, which is freely permeable to water but relatively impermeable to sodium and potassium ions. The principal extracellular ions are sodium (Na^+), chloride (Cl^-), and bicarbonate (HCO_3^-), whereas the principal intracellular ions are potassium (K^+), magnesium (Mg^{2+}), and phosphate (PO_4^{3-}).

The differences in the concentration of the ions on different sides of the cell membrane are a result of the metabolic activity of the cell. Energy provided by ATP is used to power a Na^+ K^+ exchange pump, which moves Na^+ from the intracellular compartment to the extracellular and moves K^+ from the extracellular to intracellular compartment, thus maintaining the difference in ion concentrations on each side of the cell membrane. The overall electrical charge in each fluid compartment is neutral: the total number of anions times the negative charge of each anion equals the total number of cations times the positive charge of each cation. The amount of an ion in body fluids is most often measured as **milliequivalents (mEq)**, which is equal to the **millimolar** concentration of the ion times the charge of the ion. This is convenient because equal concentration in mEq of cations will balance the charge of an equal concentration in mEq of anions.

DISTURBANCES OF WATER/ELECTROLYTE BALANCE

The most common disturbance of water balance is dehydration, which may be caused by inadequate water intake or excess water loss. Most cases of dehydration seen in medical practice result from excessive loss of fluid from the gastrointestinal tract as a consequence of vomiting or diarrhea. Fluid intake in these circumstances is usually decreased, contributing to the dehydration.

Overhydration is less common than dehydration. Sometimes overhydration results from administering too much fluid intravenously, but it also may occur when a person with impaired renal function drinks a large amount of fluid and the kidneys are unable to excrete it efficiently. Drinking a large amount of water may also change the concentration of the electrolytes in the extracellular fluid, even in a person with normal renal function. As the ingested water is absorbed into the circulation, the water increases the volume of the extracellular fluid, which lowers its sodium ion concentration (**hyponatremia**) as the fluid becomes more dilute. Marked hyponatremia may have serious and sometimes life-threatening consequences.

Most electrolyte disturbances result from depletion of body electrolytes. Depletions of sodium and potassium generally occur together, often because of loss of electrolytes along with water from the gastrointestinal tract as a result of vomiting or diarrhea. Large amounts of sodium and potassium also may be lost in the urine as a result of prolonged use of diuretics. Diuretics are substances that promote excretion of salts and water by the kidneys by impairing reabsorption of these substances from the glomerular filtrate; they are often administered to patients with heart failure, cirrhosis of the liver, and some types of kidney diseases. Loss of large amounts of electrolytes may also accompany excessive excretion of water in the urine in uncontrolled diabetes, as a result of the diuretic effect of the excreted glucose (see discussion on the pancreas and diabetes mellitus), or in renal tubular disease, in

---

Electrolytes Dissolved mineral salts.

Cations Positively charged ions in electrolytes.

Anions Negatively charged ions in electrolytes.

Milliequivalents (mEq) Measurement of the amount of an ion in body fluids.

Millimolar Concentration of one thousandth of a mole per liter.

Hyponatremia Lower concentration of sodium ions in extracellular fluid as it becomes diluted.

which the regenerating renal tubules are unable to conserve electrolytes and water (see discussion on the urinary system).

Renal Regulation of Blood Pressure, Blood Volume, and Blood pH

Along with water/electrolyte balance, the kidneys play a major role in regulating blood pressure and blood volume. The kidneys regulate both the blood pressure and blood volume by secreting **renin**, which is released into the bloodstream from the juxtaglomerular cells in the walls of the afferent glomerular arterioles. Renin is an enzyme that interacts with a blood protein called angiotensinogen and splits off a short peptide fragment called angiotensin I. Then, as the blood flows through the lungs, the newly formed angiotensin I is almost immediately converted to angiotensin II by an enzyme called angiotensin converting enzyme (ACE), which is present in the endothelium of the pulmonary capillaries.

Angiotensin II is a powerful vasoconstrictor that raises the blood pressure by causing the peripheral arterioles to constrict and also stimulates the adrenal cortex to secrete a steroid hormone called aldosterone, which increases reabsorption of sodium chloride and water by the kidneys. As a result, after the blood volume is increased by the greater volume of salt and water entering the circulation, the blood pressure rises because there is more fluid within the vascular system. Thus, renin regulates blood pressure both by controlling the degree of arteriolar vasoconstriction and by regulating the volume of fluid within the circulation. The system is self-regulating because renin secretion declines as blood pressure, volume, and sodium concentration are restored to normal (**FIGURE 19-1**).

> **Renin** A humoral substance secreted by the kidneys in response to a fall in blood pressure, blood volume, or sodium concentration.

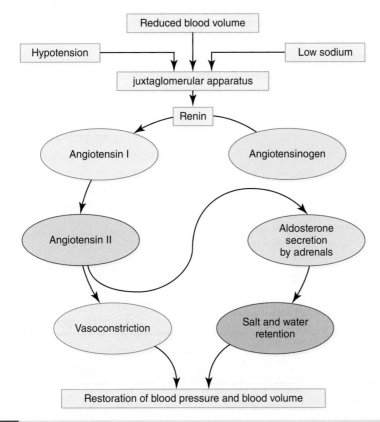

FIGURE 19-1 The role of the kidneys in the regulation of blood pressure and blood volume.

REGULATION OF BLOOD pH

The major mechanism for the control of blood pH is the sodium bicarbonate–carbonic acid buffer system. A buffer system is a solution containing a weak acid and related base that resists a change in pH. The concentration of carbonic acid (dissolved carbon dioxide), the weak acid, is controlled by the lungs, and the concentration of bicarbonate (the related base) is controlled by the kidneys. Respiratory control of pH is rapid, whereas renal control is relatively slow and may occur over days.

Carbonic acid represents physically dissolved carbon dioxide in plasma. This is in equilibrium with the carbon dioxide in the pulmonary alveoli. (The concentration of a gas in a mixture is expressed in terms of its partial pressure. This is a hypothetical measure of what the pressure of the gas would be if it were the only component and occupied the same volume.) Increased respiration lowers the alveolar carbon dioxide partial pressure (PCO_2) and leads to a rapid decrease in the concentration of carbon dioxide and carbonic acid in the plasma. This makes the blood more alkaline (less acid) and is called **respiratory alkalosis**. Decreased or inadequate pulmonary ventilation results in elevation of alveolar PCO_2, which in turn raises plasma carbon dioxide and carbonic acid. This makes the blood more acidic and is called **respiratory acidosis**. The relative degree of acidity/alkalinity of the blood is measured in terms of pH units (a measure of the concentration of hydrogen ions) and is normally under careful regulation to fall between pH 7.37 and 7.42. A pH of 7.0 is neutral (neither acidic or alkaline). Hence, blood is normally slightly alkaline (**FIGURE 19-2**).

The kidneys play two important roles in regulating the pH of the blood. Under normal circumstances, the kidneys reabsorb almost all of the bicarbonate that otherwise would be lost in the urine, and the kidneys excrete acids that are the products of cellular metabolism. The kidneys regulate bicarbonate concentration in the plasma by selectively reabsorbing filtered bicarbonate as necessary to meet the body's requirements. In addition, the kidneys can manufacture bicarbonate to replace the amounts lost in buffering acids produced as a consequence of normal metabolic processes. Failure of the kidneys to excrete acidic products of metabolism or produce sufficient bicarbonate results in **metabolic acidosis**. **Metabolic alkalosis** can result from disease of the endocrine system, loss of chloride ions, and several other causes. These two (lung/kidney) bicarbonate-regulating functions depend on the secretion of hydrogen ions by

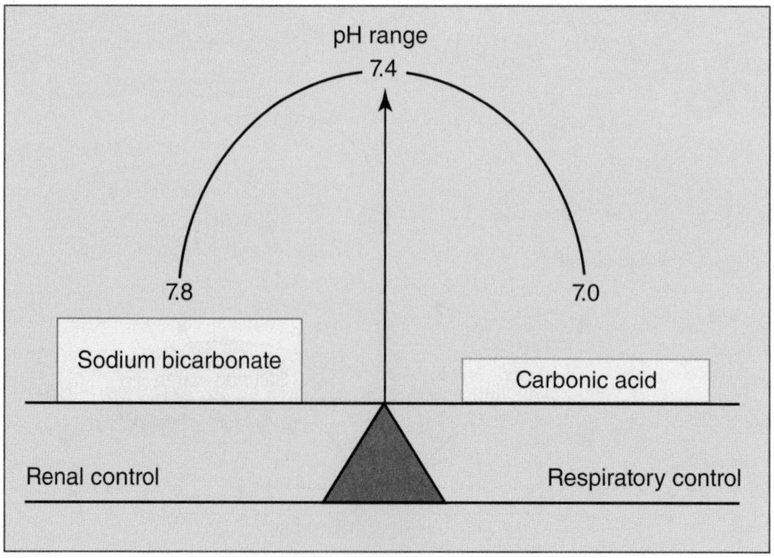

Respiratory alkalosis
A disturbance in the body's acid–base balance in which the pH of the extracellular fluids is shifted toward the alkaline side of normal.

Respiratory acidosis
A disturbance in the body's acid–base balance in which the pH of the extracellular fluids is shifted toward the acidic side of normal.

Metabolic acidosis
Condition resulting from increase in serum bicarbonate often associated with loss of acidic gastric contents, overuse of certain diuretics or endocrine disease.

Metabolic alkalosis
Condition resulting from disease of the endocrine system or loss of chloride ions.

FIGURE 19-2 "Board-and-fulcrum" concept of normal bicarbonate–carbonic acid relationships.

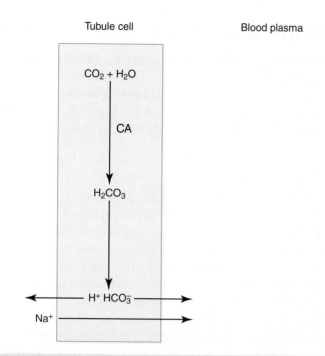

Tubular filtrate   Tubule cell   Blood plasma

FIGURE 19-3 Formation and excretion of hydrogen ions by renal tubular epithelial cells in exchange for sodium. CA indicates carbonic anhydrase.

the renal tubules in exchange for sodium ions that are simultaneously reabsorbed from the tubular filtrate into the circulation as illustrated in **FIGURE 19-3** and **TABLE 19-1**. Under the influence of the enzyme carbonic anhydrase, carbonic acid (H_2CO_3) is formed from carbon dioxide (CO_2) and water (H_2O) within the tubular epithelial cells and dissociates into hydrogen (H^+) and bicarbonate (HCO_3^-) ions. The hydrogen ions enter the tubular filtrate in exchange for sodium ions (Na^+). The bicarbonate ions enter the bloodstream along with the sodium ions that have been absorbed from the filtrate.

TABLE 19-1   Comparison of Common Acid–Base Disturbances

Disturbance	Primary abnormality	Compensation	Usual causes
Metabolic acidosis	Excess endogenous acid depletes bicarbonate	Hyperventilation lowers PCO_2; kidney excretes more hydrogen ions and forms more bicarbonate	Renal failure; ketosis; overproduction of lactic acid
Respiratory acidosis	Inefficient excretion of carbon dioxide by lungs	Formation of additional bicarbonate by kidneys	Chronic pulmonary disease
Metabolic alkalosis	Excess plasma bicarbonate	None	Loss of gastric juice; chloride depletion; excess corticosteroid hormones; ingestion of excessive bicarbonate or other antacids
Respiratory alkalosis	Hyperventilation lowers PCO_2	Increased excretion of bicarbonate by kidneys	Severe anxiety with hyperventilation; stimulation of respiratory center by drugs; central nervous system disease

Structure and Function of the Urinary System

The urinary system (**FIGURE 19-4A**) consists of the kidneys, a transport system for the urine, the bladder, and the urethra. The kidneys also serve an endocrine function. Specialized cells in the kidneys elaborate a hormone called erythropoietin, which regulates red blood cell production in the bone marrow, and as discussed previously, the protease renin, which takes part in the regulation of the blood pressure.

THE KIDNEYS

The kidneys are paired, bean-shaped organs located along the dorsal body wall below the diaphragm and adjacent to the vertebral column. Their structure is illustrated in **FIGURE 19-4B**. The region where the blood vessels enter and leave and where the ureter exits to descend to the bladder is called the **hilus** of the kidney. The expanded upper end of the ureter is the **renal pelvis**, which divides into several large branches called the **major calyces** (singular, calyx). Further subdivision forms the minor calyces. The renal substance is divided into an outer **cortex** and an inner **medulla**. The cone-shaped masses of renal tissue in the medulla that project into the minor calyces are called the renal pyramids, with the renal papilla at the tip facing the renal pelvis. Columns of cortical tissue that extend into the medulla between the pyramids are called the renal columns.

The calyces and pelvices convey the urine into the ureters, which extend downward to enter the posterior wall of the bladder near its base in an area called the **trigone** (illustrated in Figure 19-4A). Each ureter enters the bladder at an angle; when the bladder contracts, its muscular wall compresses the ureters as they run obliquely through it, somewhat like a one-way valve. This prevents backflow of urine into the ureters during voiding (urination). The ureteral openings into the bladder also appear to have a valvular function preventing backflow.

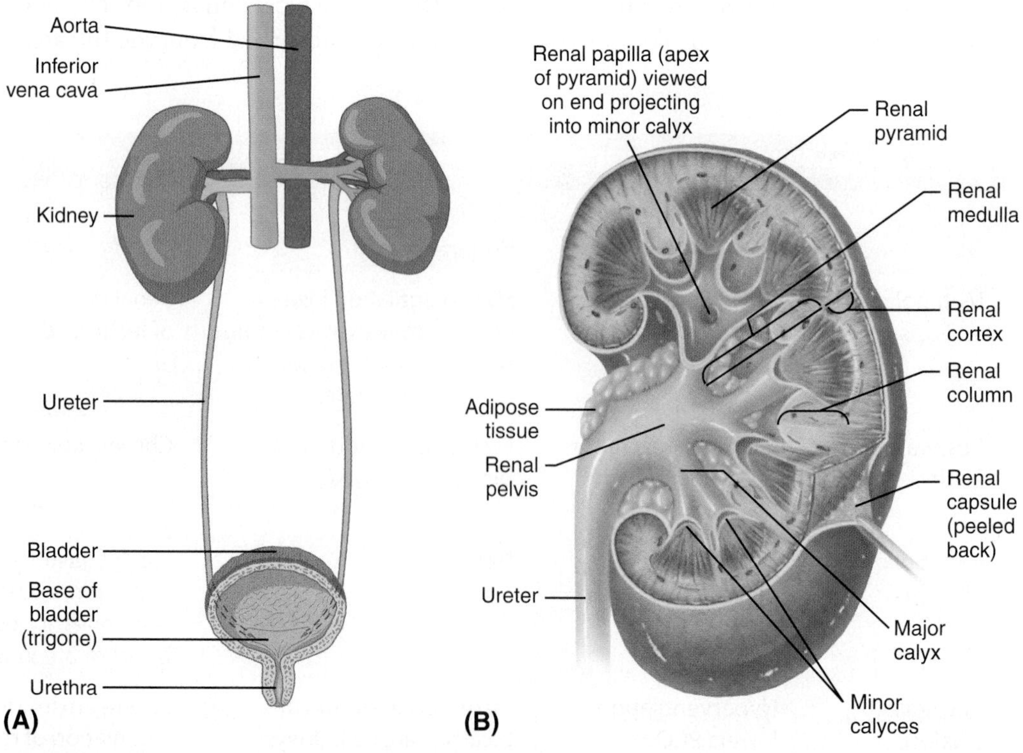

Hilus Region of kidney where blood vessels enter.

Renal pelvis/major calyces Expanded upper end of the ureter and divisions of the renal pelvis.

Cortex Outer part of the kidney.

Medulla Inner part of the kidney.

Trigone Triangular area at the base of the bladder.

FIGURE 19-4 (A) Components of the urinary system. (B) Structure of the kidney in longitudinal section.

THE URETERS

The ureters are muscular tubes that propel the urine into the bladder by wavelike contractions of their muscular walls (**peristalsis**). Urine is discharged into the bladder in spurts. It does not drain by gravity.

THE BLADDER AND URETHRA

The urinary bladder is the distensible reservoir for urine lined by transitional epithelium continuous with the lining of the remainder of the urinary tract. The opening of the urethra is located at the base of the bladder, with the ureteral openings on either side and behind the urethral opening. The triangular area at the base of the bladder bounded by the two ureteral orifices posteriorly, and the urethral orifice anteriorly, is called the trigone of the bladder (*tri* = three).

The Nephron

The basic structural and functional unit of the kidney is the nephron, with about one million nephrons in each kidney. Each nephron consists of a glomerulus and a renal tubule. The glomerulus is a tuft of capillaries supplied by an afferent glomerular arteriole. The capillaries of the glomerulus then recombine into an efferent glomerular arteriole, which in turn breaks up into a network of capillaries that supplies the renal tubules, which ultimately conduct urine to the renal calyces. The site where the afferent arteriole enters the glomerulus and the efferent arteriole exits is called the **vascular pole** of the glomerulus.

The histologic structure of the glomerulus and related structures is illustrated schematically in **FIGURE 19-5**. The expanded proximal end of the tubule is called **Bowman's capsule**. The tuft of capillaries that make up the glomerulus is pushed into Bowman's capsule much as one would push a fist into a balloon. The layer of Bowman's capsule cells, which is pushed in (invaginated), becomes closely applied to the capillaries of the glomerulus and is called the visceral layer of Bowman's capsule or simply the **glomerular epithelium**. The cells of this layer have long, footlike cytoplasmic processes and are usually called **podocytes** (*podos* = foot). The outer layer of Bowman's capsule is called the parietal layer of Bowman's capsule, or simply the **capsular epithelium**. The space between the two layers, into which the urine filters, is called Bowman's space.

The capillary tuft is held together and supported by groups of highly specialized cells called mesangial cells (*meso* = middle + *angio* = vessel). In addition to their support function, they are also contractile cells that play a role in regulating glomerular filtration by varying the caliber of the capillaries, and they are also phagocytic cells. Also located at the vascular pole is a specialized cluster of cells called the **juxtaglomerular apparatus** (*juxta* = near to), which regulates blood flow through the glomerulus (Figure 19-5B). It also plays a role in regulating blood pressure by producing renin.

Water and soluble material filter from the blood through the glomerular capillaries into Bowman's space. When visualized by electron microscopy, the membrane through which the filtrate passes can be seen to consist of three layers, as depicted in **FIGURE 19-6**. The inner layer is formed by the endothelium of the glomerular capillaries. The cytoplasm is very thin and is perforated by many small holes called fenestrations (*fenestra* = window). This layer is freely permeable to water and to many large molecules. The middle layer is the basement membrane, which supports the capillary endothelium. The basement membrane has a negative charge and tends to exclude substances that are anionic while allowing cationic and neutral substances

Peristalsis The wavelike contractions of the wall of a tubular anatomic structure such as the alimentary tract or ureter which propel luminal contents forward.

Vascular pole Site where the afferent arteriole enters the glomerulus and the efferent arteriole exits.

Bowman's capsule The cuplike expanded end of the nephron that surrounds the tuft of glomerular capillaries.

Glomerular epithelium Layer of Bowman cells closely applied to the capillaries. It is also termed the visceral layer of Bowman's capsule.

Podocytes Cells with highly branched cytoplasmic processes covering the glomerular capillaries of the kidneys.

Capsular epithelium Outer layer of cells of Bowman's capsule. It is also termed the parietal layer of Bowman's capsule.

Juxtaglomerular apparatus A specialized group of cells at the vascular pole of the glomerulus that regulates blood flow through the glomerulus of the kidneys.

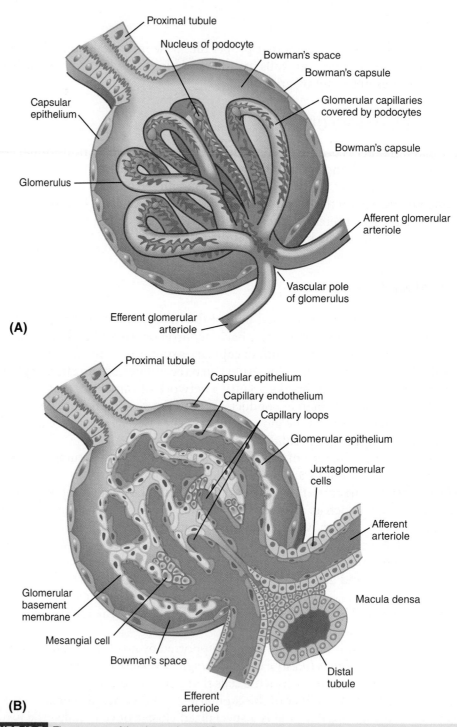

(A)

(B)

FIGURE 19-5 The structure of the glomerulus and Bowman's capsule. **(A)** Anterior half of Bowman's capsule removed to reveal capillary tuft covered by podocytes (schematic). **(B)** Cross section through glomerulus to reveal structure of glomerular filter and juxtaglomerular apparatus.

to pass. Filtration is also based on molecular size, with selective passage for lower molecular weight substances. The outer layer is composed of the podocytes. Their highly branched cytoplasmic processes are called foot processes, which are attached to the basement membrane and interdigitate with others from the same cell or adjacent cells. The narrow spaces between adjacent interdigitating pedicels are called filtration slits. Each slit is covered by a thin membrane called a slit diaphragm, which is

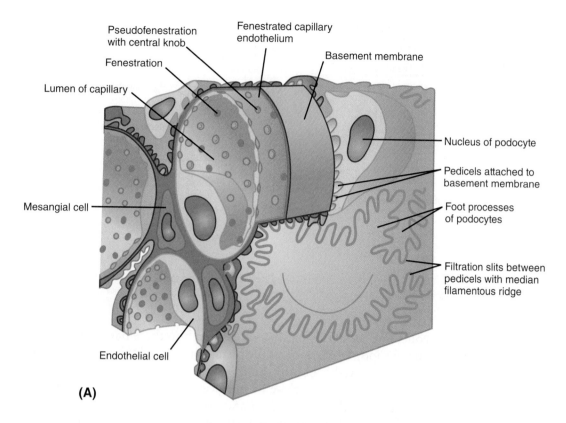

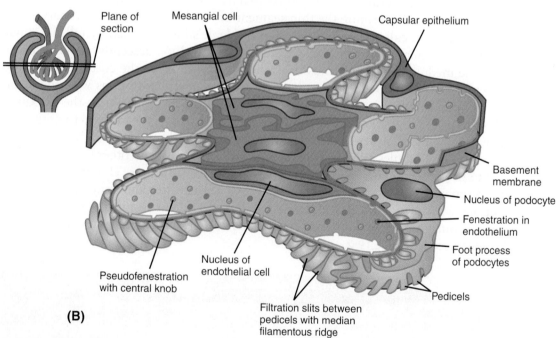

FIGURE 19-6 A schematic representation of the fine structure of the glomerular filter as visualized by electron microscopy. **(A)** Segment of glomerular capillaries. **(B)** Cross section through the center of the glomerulus, including part of Bowman's capsule.

less porous than the other layers of the glomerular filter and is the major barrier to protein loss from the circulation.

The renal tubules are long tubes that measure as much as 4 cm in length. The proximal end of the tubule is invaginated by the glomerulus, and its distal end

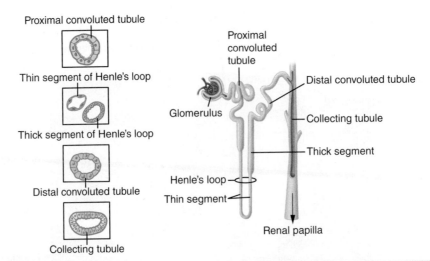

FIGURE 19-7 The structure of the renal tubule illustrating its relationship to the glomerulus and the collecting tubule. The epithelium characteristic of each part of the renal tubule and the collecting tubule are also illustrated.

empties into a collecting tubule. The tubule is divided into three parts: the proximal convoluted tubule, the loop of Henle, and the distal convoluted tubule (**FIGURE 19-7**).

The proximal convoluted tubule is the greatly coiled first part of the tubule, its convolutions being located very close to the glomerulus. The loop of Henle is a U-shaped segment composed of descending and ascending limbs joined by a short segment. The descending limb and proximal half of the ascending limb are lined by flat epithelial cells, forming the thin segment of Henle's loop. The distal part of the ascending limb, called the thick segment of Henle's loop, is lined by tall columnar epithelium similar to that lining the distal tubule. The loop descends from the cortex into the medulla and then bends back sharply, returning to the cortex close to the vascular pole of its own glomerulus, where it becomes continuous with the distal convoluted tubule. The distal convoluted tubule, much shorter than the proximal tubule, empties into a collecting tubule that passes through the medulla to drain into one of the minor calyces at the apex of a renal pyramid (renal papilla).

The renal tubules selectively reabsorb water, minerals, and other substances that are to be conserved and excrete unwanted materials, which are eliminated. Urine is the glomerular filtrate that remains after most of the water and important constituents have been reabsorbed by the renal tubules and other substances excreted by the renal tubules have been added. The functions of the components of the nephron are summarized in **TABLE 19-2**.

TABLE 19-2	Functions of the Nephron and the Collecting Duct
Structure	**Function**
Renal corpuscle	
Glomerulus	Filters water and dissolved substances from plasma
Glomerular capsule	Receives glomerular filtrate
Renal tubule	
Proximal convoluted tubule	Reabsorbs glucose, amino acids, creatine, acids, and ions by active transport; reabsorbs water by osmosis; reabsorbs chloride and other negative ions by electrochemical attraction; actively secretes penicillin, histamine, creatinine, and hydrogen ions

TABLE 19-2 Functions of the Nephron and the Collecting Duct *(Continued)*	
Structure	**Function**
Descending limb of nephron loop	Reabsorbs water by osmosis
Ascending limb of nephron loop	Reabsorbs sodium, potassium, and chloride ions by active transport
Distal convoluted tubule	Reabsorbs sodium ions by active transport, reabsorbs water by osmosis, and secretes hydrogen and potassium ions by electrochemical attraction
Collecting duct	Reabsorbs water by osmosis

Disturbances of Normal Renal Function

The functions of the two kidneys reflect the sum of the functions of their individual nephrons. Derangement of any of these functions results in kidney disease.

For a nephron to function normally, there must be free flow of blood through the glomerular capillaries, the glomerular filter must function normally, the tubules must be able to selectively reabsorb/excrete substances as needed, and the urine formed by the nephron must be able to flow freely from the kidney into the bladder.

DEVELOPMENTAL DISTURBANCES

The urinary system develops from several different components. The kidneys form from masses of primitive connective tissue (mesoderm) located along the back body wall of the embryo. The bladder develops as an offshoot of the lower end of the intestinal tract. The ureters, renal pelves, renal calyces (the urinary drainage system), and the renal collecting tubules derive from paired tubular structures called ureteric buds. Each bud grows upward from the developing bladder and connects with the kidney that is forming on the corresponding side. The kidneys begin their development within the pelvis. Later, as the embryo grows, the kidneys and their excretory ducts come to occupy a higher location, until eventually they ascend to reach their final positions in the upper lumbar region (**FIGURE 19-8A**).

Sometimes this developmental process is disturbed, and congenital malformations result. Three of the more common developmental abnormalities are failure of one or both kidneys to develop (renal agenesis), formation of extra ureters and renal pelves, or malpositions of one or both kidneys.

Renal agenesis (*a* = without + *genesis* = formation) may affect one or both kidneys, but bilateral renal agenesis is uncommon. Agenesis, which often accompanies other congenital malformations, is incompatible with postnatal life. In contrast, unilateral renal agenesis (**FIGURE 19-8B**) is a relatively common condition with an incidence of about 1 in 1,000 persons, about the same frequency as cleft palate. When one kidney is absent, the other kidney enlarges and is able to carry out the functions of the missing kidney. The recognition of this condition, however, is of great importance to the clinician who is treating an individual with kidney disease because one can never assume that the patient has two kidneys. Before a surgeon performs a kidney operation, diagnostic studies must be performed to ascertain that the patient has two kidneys.

Duplications of the urinary tract may be unilateral or bilateral. Sometimes a kidney has an extra renal pelvis and ureter that drains separately into the bladder

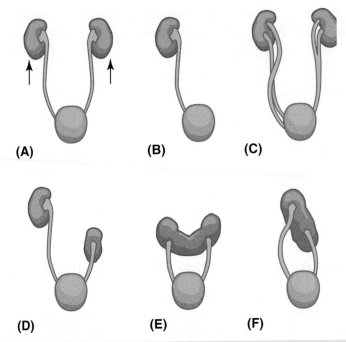

FIGURE 19-8 Common congenital abnormalities of kidneys and urinary tract. **(A)** Normal ascent of kidneys. **(B)** Unilateral renal agenesis. **(C)** Various types of duplications of ureters and renal pelves resulting from formation of an extra ureteric bud (*left*) or premature splitting of a single ureteric bud (*right*). **(D)** Failure of one kidney to ascend to normal position. **(E)** Horseshoe kidney resulting from fusion of lower poles of kidneys. **(F)** Fusion of the lower pole of one kidney to the upper pole of opposite kidney, which has failed to ascend normally.

(complete duplication). Sometimes double ureters draining the kidney unite to form a single ureter just before entering the bladder (partial duplication). Duplications result from abnormal prenatal development of the ureteric buds. A complete duplication results when an extra ureteric bud develops and gives rise to a separate excretory system draining the kidney on the affected side. If the ureteric bud branches after it has formed, only the upper part of the excretory system is duplicated; the lower part of the ureter is not duplicated and enters the bladder normally (**FIGURE 19-8C**).

Abnormalities of position and fusion of the kidneys may occur if both kidneys remain in the pelvis where they began their development or if they ascend only part way (**FIGURE 19-8D**). Kidneys that fail to ascend normally are in very close approximation as they develop and may become fused. One of the more common fusion abnormalities is a union of the lower poles of the two kidneys to form a U-shaped mass of renal tissue called a horseshoe kidney (**FIGURE 19-8E**). In other cases, when the kidneys ascend abnormally, the upper pole of one kidney may become fused to the lower pole of the other (**FIGURE 19-8F**).

Renal duplications, malpositions, and fusions often are of little clinical significance. At times, however, drainage of urine may be impeded by the abnormalities, causing the urine to stagnate and predisposing the patient to urinary infections. Another important developmental abnormality called congenital polycystic kidney disease is considered in the section on renal cysts.

Nephropathies: An Introduction

Interruption of normal function in the kidneys that are related to glomerular malfunction include glomerulonephritis, nephrotic syndrome, and diabetic nephropathy. Renal hypertensive disease results in hypertensive nephrosclerosis associated with vascular injury. Damage to the renal tubules and interstitium of the kidney may result in acute tubular injury and pyelonephritis associated with bacterial infections, which generally have ascended the urinary tract to reach the kidney. End stage renal disease (ESRD) occurs when renal failure is so severe that either dialysis or transplantation is required to sustain life. The most common causes of ESRD are diabetic nephropathy and hypertensive nephrosclerosis.

Glomerular renal disease that is associated with extreme proteinuria (loss of protein into the urine greater than 3 g/24 hr) defines **nephrosis** (nephrotic syndrome) and is often associated with edema, which can be widespread and severe (termed **anasarca**). Nephrotic patients also may have hyperlipidemia and secrete lipids in their urine as **fatty casts**, aggregated lipids that maintain the cylindrical shape of the tubule where they were formed.

GLOMERULONEPHRITIS

Glomerulonephritis, an inflammation of the glomeruli caused by an immune reaction within the glomerulus (including the glomerular capillaries and mesangium), will result in an inflammatory influx of leukocytes and injury to the glomerulus, which, if severe, will result in glomerular necrosis. The signs and symptoms of glomerulonephritis are related to the changes within the glomeruli. Because many glomeruli are damaged or destroyed by inflammation, less blood is filtered and less urine is excreted. As urinary output is reduced, waste products are retained and accumulate in the blood. Other glomeruli, damaged by lysosomal enzymes, are no longer able to function as efficient filters. Protein and red cells leak through the damaged glomerular capillary walls and are excreted in the urine. Frequently, masses of red cells and protein accumulate within the tubules and become molded to the shape of the renal tubules before finally being excreted. These structures, which are called urinary casts, are an important indication of glomerular injury. Patients with glomerulonephritis are often hypertensive and have some degree of renal failure. Depending on the severity of disease, they may also show proteinuria (but not as severe as that in nephritic syndrome). In some cases, glomerulonephritis may progress so rapidly that dialysis is needed within months to sustain life, a condition called rapidly progressive glomerulonephritis (RPGN).

The glomerular inflammation can be the result of the formation of antigen–antibody complexes either within the glomerular capillaries or deposited within the glomerulus from the circulation. The interaction of antigen and antibody activates complement and liberates mediators that attract polymorphonuclear leukocytes to the glomerulus. The actual glomerular injury is caused by destructive lysosomal enzymes that are released from the leukocytes that have accumulated within the glomeruli. In some cases (antineutrophil cytoplasmic antibody [ANCA] glomerulonephritis), antibodies bind directly to the surface of the leukocytes and cause them to release the destructive mediators within the glomerulus.

The antigen–antibody reaction within the glomeruli may take place in two ways. Either immune complexes are deposited on the walls of the glomerular capillaries or an autoantibody can react with the capillary basement membrane. **FIGURE 19-9** illustrates the histologic appearance of these two types of glomerulonephritis compared with the appearance of a normal glomerulus. In ANCA glomerulonephritis there is no deposition of antibody within the glomerulus (but rather direct activation of inflammatory cells).

Poststreptococcal Immune-Complex Glomerulonephritis

Immune-complex glomerulonephritis may develop as a complication about two weeks after infection by certain beta streptococci, the same type of organism that

Nephrosis Renal disease resulting from excessive protein loss in the urine, caused by various types of renal injury. Also referred to as nephrotic syndrome.

Anasarca Widespread edema.

Fatty casts Aggregated lipids that maintain the cylindrical shape of the tubule.

Glomerulonephritis An inflammation of the glomeruli caused by either antigen–antibody complexes trapped in the glomeruli or by antiglomerular basement membrane antibodies.

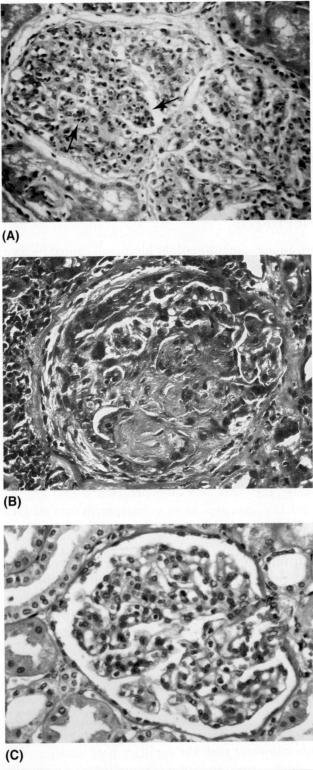

(A)

(B)

(C)

FIGURE 19-9 **(A)** Immune complex glomerulonephritis. Two glomeruli contain large numbers of neutrophils (*arrows*). **(B)** Anti-GBM glomerulonephritis, revealing severe glomerular injury and scarring. **(C)** Normal glomerulus for comparison (original magnifications ×400).

Courtesy of Leonard V. Crowley, MD, Century College.

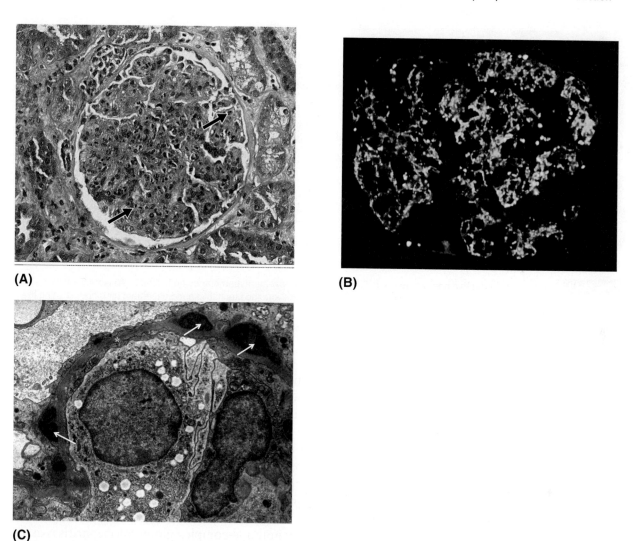

FIGURE 19-10 **(A)** Glomerulus from a patient with poststreptococcal glomerulonephritis. Several inflammatory cells (neutrophils) are indicated (*arrows*) on trichrome stain of biopsy specimen (blue color highlights connective tissue). Compare with Figure 19-9C. **(B)** Biopsy from same case stained with a fluorescent antibody that detects human IgG. The "bumpy" green color indicates deposited immune complexes. **(C)** Electron micrograph of biopsy from the same case showing immune complexes (*arrows*) trapped beneath the basement membrane (*star*). Lumen of capillary is filled with inflammatory cells.

Courtesy of Drs Singh & Nickeleit Department of Pathology and Laboratory Medicine, University of North Carolina at Chapel Hill.

causes the familiar streptococcal sore throat. Fortunately glomerular inflammation occurs only in a small percentage of patients with streptococcal infections and usually resolves spontaneously. In affected individuals (most often children), the body responds to the streptococcal infection by forming antistreptococcal antibodies that interact in the bloodstream with soluble antigens from the streptococci to form immune complexes. Some of the antigen–antibody complexes are small enough to pass completely through the walls of the glomerular capillaries and be excreted in the urine. Larger complexes, however, pass through the endothelium and basement membranes of the glomerular capillaries but become trapped between the filtration slits of the glomerular epithelial cells in a subepithelial position, where they induce an inflammatory reaction. **FIGURE 19-10** demonstrates a case of this disease. (The patient recovered slowly, and a biopsy was necessary to confirm the diagnosis.)

Acute glomerulonephritis may at times follow other bacterial or viral infections. **Type I membranoproliferative glomerulonephritis** is a more severe form of the disease associated with infections of the heart, bone, and chronic hepatitis C. In this condition,

Type I membranoproliferative glomerulonephritis
A more severe form of glomerulonephritis associated with infections of the heart, bone, and chronic hepatitis C.

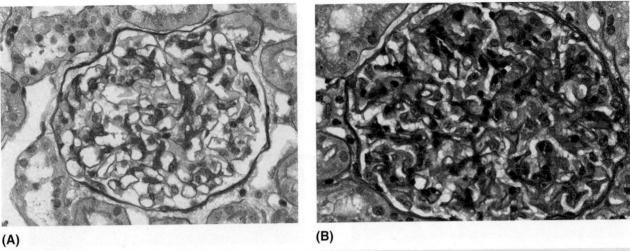

(A)　　　　　　　　　　　　　　　　　　　**(B)**

FIGURE 19-11 The two glomeruli have been stained with PAS to highlight basement membranes (in fuschia). **(A)** Normal glomerulus. **(B)** Glomerulus from a patient with membranoproliferative glomerulonephritis. Note the much thickened basement membranes lining the capillaries.

Courtesy of Drs Singh & Nickeleit Department of Pathology and Laboratory Medicine, University of North Carolina at Chapel Hill.

immune complexes are also found in the mesangium, which results in the influx of inflammatory cells to this location and proliferation of mesangial cells. The basement membrane of the glomerular capillaries becomes markedly thickened (**FIGURE 19-11**). The mechanism of glomerular injury is similar to that of poststreptococcal glomerulonephritis in that immune complexes play a critical role. Elimination of the infection sometimes results in a cure, whereas in other cases the glomerulonephritis never heals completely. Although poststreptococcal glomerulonephritis is usually acute and self-limited, type I membranoproliferative glomerulonephritis often becomes chronic, progresses slowly, and eventually causes renal failure.

Another relatively common type of immune-complex glomerulonephritis is associated with proliferation of mesangial cells and accumulation of immune complexes containing immunoglobulin A (IgA) within the cells. Because of the type of immunoglobulin associated with the disease, it is often called IgA nephropathy (or Berger disease). Unfortunately, this type of glomerulonephritis becomes chronic in many patients and is slowly progressive.

Immune-complex glomerulonephritis may also occur in association with auto-immune diseases in which autoantibody-containing immune complexes become trapped in renal glomeruli, as in lupus erythematosus (see discussion on immunity, hypersensitivity, allergy, and autoimmune diseases). Several classes of glomerular disease occur with SLE, and some may be rapidly progressive.

Anti-GBM Glomerulonephritis

Glomerulonephritis caused by autoantibodies directed against glomerular basement membranes (anti-GBM glomerulonephritis) is a relatively uncommon autoimmune disease. In some patients, the anti-GBM antibodies may also injure the basement membranes of the pulmonary capillaries and may cause intrapulmonary hemorrhage as well as acute glomerulonephritis (Goodpasture syndrome).

Special studies on biopsy tissue can distinguish immune-complex glomerulonephritis from anti-GBM glomerulonephritis. Immune-complex glomerulonephritis is characterized by large, irregular, lumpy deposits composed of antigen, antibody, and complement. These deposits form along the outer surface of the glomerular basement membranes, where the complexes have been trapped between the filtration slits of the glomerular epithelial cells. In contrast, anti-GBM nephritis is characterized by

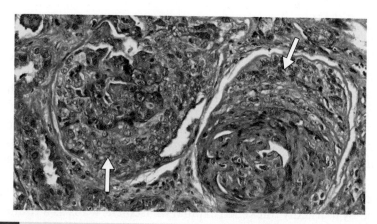

FIGURE 19-12 Rapidly progressive glomerulonephritis from a patient with ANCA glomerulonephritis. Two glomeruli are trichrome stained to emphasize connective tissue/scarring (in blue). The glomerulus on the right is necrotic. Both demonstrate crescent formation (*arrows*).

Courtesy of Drs Singh & Nickeleit Department of Pathology and Laboratory Medicine, University of North Carolina at Chapel Hill.

a relatively uniform layer of antibody and complement deposited along the inner surface of the glomerular basement membranes. Anti-GBM disease is severe and rapidly progressive, leading to end stage renal disease if immunosuppressive therapy is ineffective. Patients with anti-GBM disease almost always have **crescentic glomerulonephritis** in which Bowman's space (surrounding the glomerular capillary tuft) becomes filled with proliferating cells derived from the parietal epithelium of Bowman's capsule, possibly as a result of inflammatory cytokines that leak into the space from the damaged glomerular capillaries (**FIGURE 19-12**).

ANCA Glomerulonephritis

ANCA associated glomerulonephritis is the result of autoimmune ANCA antibodies that react with cytoplasmic components of neutrophils. When ANCA antibodies react with their target antigens (which transiently are expressed on the surface of neutrophils), the cells become activated and provoke an inflammatory reaction that destroys the glomerular capillary endothelial cells. ANCA disease is very severe and may progress rapidly, resulting in crescentic glomerulonephritis (Figure 19-12). In the absence of effective immunosuppressive therapy, ESRD will occur in most patients within five years. Many patients with ANCA glomerulonephritis also have small vessel vasculitis (inflammation of capillaries and venules), which results in disease in many additional organ systems.

NEPHROTIC SYNDROME

Nephrotic syndrome refers to a group of abnormalities characterized by a severe loss of protein in the urine. Urinary excretion of protein is so great that the body is unable to manufacture protein fast enough to keep up with the losses, resulting in the concentration of protein in the blood plasma decreasing. This, in turn, causes significant edema owing to the low plasma osmotic pressure (presented in the discussion on circulatory disturbances). Nephrotic syndrome may be produced by a number of different types of renal diseases. The basic cause is injury to the glomerulus, which allows proteins to leak through the damaged basement membrane. Because the albumin molecule is much smaller than the globulin molecule, a disproportionately large amount of albumin is lost in the urine. The osmotic pressure of the plasma falls to such an extent that excessive amounts of fluid leak from the capillaries into the interstitial tissues and body cavities. Patients with the nephrotic syndrome have marked leg edema, and fluid often collects in the

Crescentic glomerulonephritis Form of glomerulonephritis in which Bowman's space (surrounding the glomerular capillary tuft) becomes filled with proliferating cells derived from the parietal epithelium of Bowman's capsule.

Nephrotic syndrome Characterized by severe loss of protein.

abdominal cavity (called ascites); sometimes fluid also accumulates in the pleural cavities (called hydrothorax).

When the nephrotic syndrome occurs in children, it is usually caused by extensive loss of the foot processes (termed effacement) of the glomerular epithelial cells. Because no abnormality is seen in the glomerulus by light microscopy, this is termed **minimal change nephropathy**. Nephrotic syndrome caused by this type of glomerular abnormality responds to corticosteroid therapy, and most children recover completely.

In contrast to the favorable outcome in children, the nephrotic syndrome in adults is usually a manifestation of progressive, more serious renal disease in which there are marked structural changes in the glomeruli. The most common nephritic disease in Caucasian and Asiatic adults is **membranous glomerulopathy**. The disease is characterized by markedly thickened capillary basement walls as a result of immune complex formation. In many cases, the immune complexes form within the glomerulus as a result of circulating autoantibodies that react with a component of podocytes. The disease is very variable, sometimes remitting with time, sometimes progressing. In adult blacks, **focal segmental glomerulosclerosis (FSGS)** is most common. The name derives from the fact that only some glomeruli show abnormalities, and often only a portion of a given glomerulus is affected. Sclerosis refers to the production of collagen containing scars within the glomerulus. The disease is not related to immune complex formation but is associated with a variety of etiologic agents including viruses, familial mutations, drugs, and "overwork" and is seen in people with obesity or in people with only a single functioning kidney. The disease prognosis depends on the cause and is usually slowly progressive (**FIGURE 19-13**).

ARTERIOLAR NEPHROSCLEROSIS

Arteriolar nephrosclerosis (sometimes called simply **nephrosclerosis**) is a complication of severe hypertension. Because of the extreme elevation of the systemic blood pressure, the small arterioles and arteries throughout the body are called on to carry blood at a much higher pressure than normal. As a result, the blood vessels undergo severe degenerative changes characterized by thickening and narrowing of the lumens, which reduces blood flow through the narrowed arterioles. The name of the disease, which means literally "sclerosis of the arterioles of the nephrons," refers to these characteristic renal vascular changes. Glomerular filtration is reduced

Minimal change nephropathy Common kidney disease of young children that is generally idiopathic.

Membranous glomerulopathy A slowly progressive disease of the glomeruli most often found in Caucasian and Asian patients between the ages of thirty and fifty.

Focal segmental glomerulosclerosis (FSGS) Scar tissue in the filtering unit of the kidney.

Nephrosclerosis Thickening and narrowing of the afferent glomerular arterioles as a result of disease.

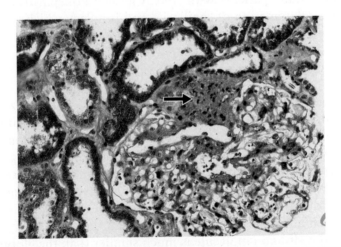

FIGURE 19-13 Renal biopsy from a patient with focal segmental glomerulosclerosis (FSGS), stained with trichrome stain. The glomerulous (on the edge of the biopsy) shows focal sclerosis (scarring) (*arrow*).
Courtesy of Drs Singh & Nickeleit Department of Pathology and Laboratory Medicine, University of North Carolina at Chapel Hill.

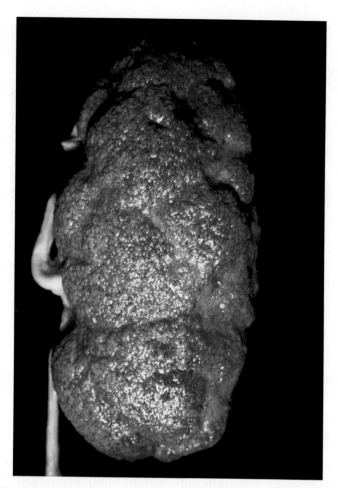

FIGURE 19-14 Irregular scarring of kidney as a result of nephrosclerosis.
Courtesy of Leonard V. Crowley, MD, Century College.

because the arterioles are greatly narrowed. The renal tubules, which also are supplied by the glomerular arterioles, undergo degenerative changes as well. Eventually, the kidneys become shrunken and scarred as a result of reduction of their blood supply (**FIGURE 19-14**). Patients with severe nephrosclerosis may die from renal insufficiency, as well as from the effects of severe hypertension.

DIABETIC NEPHROPATHY

People with long-standing diabetes mellitus often develop progressive renal damage. The glomerular basement membranes exhibit characteristic nodular and diffuse thickening called **diabetic glomerulosclerosis** (**FIGURE 19-15**), which disturbs glomerular function. Usually there is severe sclerosis of the glomerular arterioles, impairing the flow of blood to the glomeruli and tubules. Sometimes the general term diabetic nephropathy (*nephros* = kidney + *path* = disease) is used when referring to both the glomerular and the arteriolar lesions.

Clinically, the condition is characterized by progressive impairment of renal function that may eventually lead to renal failure. Protein leaks through the diseased glomeruli and is lost in the urine. In some patients, so much protein is lost that the nephrotic syndrome develops. No specific treatment can arrest the progression of the disease. A renal transplant may be required if the patient develops renal failure.

> **Diabetic glomerulosclerosis** Diffuse and nodular thickening of glomerular basement membranes, a common occurrence in patients with long-standing diabetes mellitus.

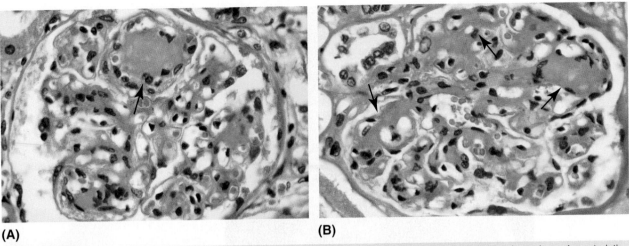

FIGURE 19-15 **(A)** Nodular glomerulosclerosis. Nodular areas of glomerular basement membrane thickening (*arrow*) are characteristic of diabetes. **(B)** Diffuse glomerulosclerosis. Diffuse glomerular basement membrane thickening (*arrows*) also occurs in diabetes, but it may occur in other types of glomerular disease as well.

Courtesy of Leonard V. Crowley, MD, Century College.

(Diabetes mellitus and its complications are considered in the pancreas and diabetes mellitus discussion.)

ACUTE RENAL TUBULAR INJURY

The blood supply to the renal tubules is derived from the efferent glomerular artery, and minor degrees of tubular injury are seen in many diseases affecting the renal glomeruli. Renal tubular injury in the absence of glomerular disease may be encountered in two situations: tubular injury as a result of impaired renal blood flow or tubular injury caused by toxic drugs and chemicals. Any condition associated with shock and a marked drop in blood pressure leads to impaired blood flow to the kidneys, which often causes damage and flattening of proximal tubular epithelial cells. Edema in the interstitium of the kidney and debris within the tubular lumens also occurs. Many drugs (such as aminoglycoside antibiotics) and chemicals that are ingested or absorbed by the body are excreted by the kidneys. Thus, they may cause direct toxic injury to the tubular epithelium, which may be associated with necrosis of the epithelial cells (**FIGURE 19-16**).

Acute tubular injury causes severe impairment of renal function characterized by a marked decrease in urine output (oliguria) or complete suppression of urine formation (anuria). This condition is called acute kidney injury (or sometimes acute renal failure). The reason urine output is reduced is not well understood. Apparently, marked constriction of renal arterioles reduces blood flow to the kidneys and decreases glomerular filtration. Other factors also may contribute to the reduction of urine output. Many of the tubules are blocked by casts and necrotic debris. The damaged tubular epithelium also has lost its capacity for selective tubular reabsorption, and the glomerular filtrate diffuses back through the damaged tubular epithelium into the adjacent peritubular blood vessels. After a period of several weeks, tubular function is slowly restored by regeneration of the damaged epithelium, but several months may be required before renal function returns completely to normal. During the period of acute renal injury, waste products must be removed from the blood by means of dialysis until tubular function has been restored.

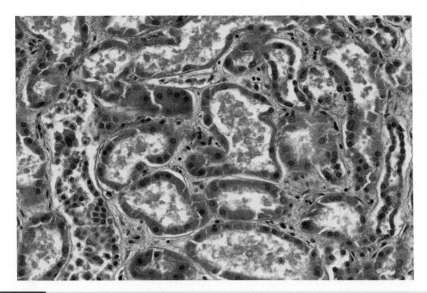

FIGURE 19-16 Acute tubular injury. Most of the tubules demonstrate flattening of epithelial cells and cellular necrosis shown by loss of nuclei and detachment from basement membranes. The tubules are filled with cellular debris and detached epithelial cells.

Courtesy of Department of Pathology and Laboratory Medicine, University of North Carolina at Chapel Hill.

Infections of the Urinary Tract

Urinary tract infections are common and may be either acute or chronic. An infection that affects only the bladder is called **cystitis** (*cystis* = bladder). If the upper urinary tract is infected, the term is **pyelonephritis** (*pyelo* = pelvis + *nephros* = kidney + *itis* = inflammation). Most infections are caused by gram-negative intestinal bacteria. These organisms often contaminate the perianal and genital areas and gain access to the urinary tract by ascending the urethra.

Free urine flow, large urine volume, and complete emptying of the bladder protect against urinary tract infections because any bacteria that enter the bladder are soon flushed out during urination instead of being retained to multiply in the bladder urine. An acid urine is an additional defense against infection because most bacteria grow poorly in an acid environment. On the other hand, several conditions predispose to urinary tract infections including impaired free urine drainage, injury to the mucosa, or introduction of a catheter. Any condition that impairs free drainage of urine increases the likelihood of infection because stagnation of urine favors multiplication of any bacteria that enter the urinary tract. Injury to the mucosa of the urinary tract, as by a kidney stone (calculus) or foreign body, disrupts the protective epithelium, permitting bacteria to invade the deeper tissues and set up an infection. Introduction of a catheter or instrument into the bladder may carry bacteria into the urinary tract when the catheter or instrument is introduced and may also injure the bladder mucosa.

CYSTITIS

Cystitis is more common in women than in men, probably because the short female urethra allows infectious organisms to enter the bladder more easily. Young, sexually active women are especially predisposed because sexual intercourse promotes transfer of bacteria from the distal urethra into the bladder and may cause minor injury to the mucosa at the base of the bladder (trigone). Cystitis is also common in older men who cannot empty their bladders completely because of an enlarged prostate

Cystitis/pyelonephritis
Urinary tract infections affecting only the bladder or upper urinary tract.

gland (see discussion on the male reproductive system). The urine remaining in the bladder after voiding favors multiplication of bacteria and may lead to infection.

The manifestations of cystitis result from congestion and inflammation of the bladder (vesical) mucosa. The patient complains of burning pain on urination and a desire to urinate frequently. The urine contains many bacteria and leukocytes. Cystitis is not usually a serious problem and generally responds promptly to antibiotics. Sometimes, however, the infection may spread into the upper urinary tract to affect the renal pelvis and kidney.

PYELONEPHRITIS

Most cases of pyelonephritis are secondary to the spread of infection from the bladder (ascending pyelonephritis), but occasionally the organisms are carried to the kidneys through the bloodstream (hematogenous pyelonephritis). The symptoms of pyelonephritis are those of an acute infection, together with localized pain and tenderness over the affected kidney. Histologically, the infected portion of the kidney is infiltrated by masses of leukocytes and bacteria, and many of the renal tubules in the inflamed area are filled with leukocytes (**FIGURE 19-17**). Because cystitis and pyelonephritis are

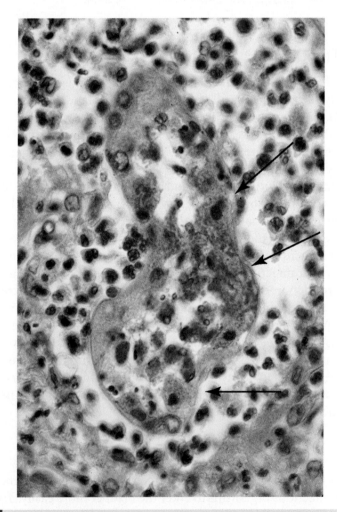

FIGURE 19-17 Acute pyelonephritis. The tubule in the center of field contains masses of bacteria that extend through wall of tubule (*middle arrow*). Some tubule cells are necrotic (*upper and lower arrows*). Many neutrophils surround the tubules (original magnification ×400).

Courtesy of Leonard V. Crowley, MD, Century College.

frequently associated, the patient also experiences urinary frequency and pain on urination; the urine contains many bacteria and leukocytes. Treatment is with appropriate antibiotics, together with measures directed at correcting any abnormalities in the lower urinary tract that may impede drainage of urine and predispose to infection.

Most episodes of pyelonephritis respond promptly to treatment. If part of the kidney is severely damaged by the infection, the injured area heals by scarring. The main danger of pyelonephritis lies in the tendency of the disease to become chronic and recurrent. With each subsequent attack, more kidney tissue may be destroyed and healed by scarring. After many episodes of infection, the kidneys may become markedly scarred and shrunken, until the patient eventually exhibits manifestations of renal insufficiency.

VESICOURETERAL REFLUX AND INFECTION

Normally, effective mechanisms prevent urine from flowing upward from the bladder into the ureters during urination. Sometimes, however, these mechanisms are defective, permitting urine to flow retrograde (reflux) into one or both ureters when the bladder contracts during urination. This condition is called **vesicoureteral reflux**. It predisposes to urinary tract infection by preventing complete emptying of the bladder. The urine forced into the ureters during voiding flows back into the bladder at the completion of urination, so residual urine remains in the bladder. Bacteria also may be carried into the upper urinary tract by the reflux of urine; this predisposes to pyelonephritis.

UROLITHIASIS

Stones may form anywhere in the urinary tract. They are usually called **calculi** (singular, calculus), which is a Latin word meaning "little stone" or "pebble." Nephrolithiasis refers to stone formation in the kidney; urolithiasis is a more general term for stone formation at any location in the urinary tract. Most calculi are composed either of uric acid or of a mixture of calcium salts. Three factors predispose to stone formation: increased concentration of salts in the urine most often due to low fluid intake, infection of the urinary tract, and urinary tract obstruction.

A greatly increased excretion of salts in the urine causes the urine to become supersaturated, and the salts may precipitate to form calculi, especially if the urine is concentrated. For example, in the disease called **gout** (presented in the discussion on the musculoskeletal system), excretion of uric acid is often greatly increased, which may cause uric acid to precipitate from the urine and form uric acid calculi. However, many individuals with urate stones have neither gout nor elevated urate levels. In conditions characterized by hyperfunction of the parathyroid glands, which regulate calcium metabolism (presented in the discussion on the endocrine glands), or other conditions where excessive calcium is excreted in the urine, subsequent formation of urinary tract calculi composed of calcium salts is common. Infection predisposes to calculi primarily by reducing the solubility of the salts in the urine. Clusters of bacteria also serve as sites where urinary salts may crystallize to form the stone.

Most calculi are small, but occasionally they may gradually increase in size to form large branching structures that adopt the contour of the renal pelvis and calyces where they have formed. This kind of structure is called a staghorn calculus because it vaguely resembles the antlers of a male deer (**FIGURE 19-18**). Smaller stones sometimes pass into the ureter. The smooth muscle of the ureter contracts spasmodically to propel the stone along the ureter, causing renal colic—paroxysms of intense flank pain radiating into the groin. Frequently, the rough edges of the stone injure the lining of the ureter, causing red blood cells to appear in the urine. Many stones can

Vesicoureteral reflux Retrograde flow of urine from the bladder into the ureter during voiding.

Calculi Stones formed within the body, as in the kidney or gallbladder.

Gout A disorder of nucleoprotein metabolism characterized by elevated uric acid and deposition of uric acid in and around joints.

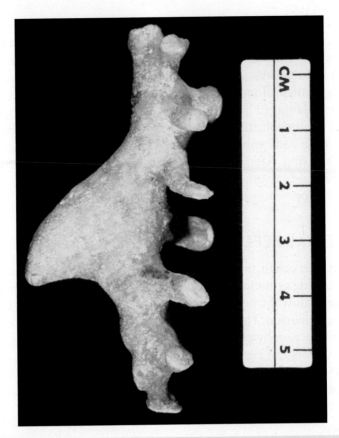

FIGURE 19-18 Large staghorn calculus of kidney.

Courtesy of Leonard V. Crowley, MD, Century College.

be passed through the ureter and excreted in the urine, but some become impacted in the ureter and must be removed. A stone lodged in the distal ureter can usually be removed by inserting a cystoscope into the bladder and then passing a specially designed catheter-like instrument through the cystoscope into the ureter. The instrument is constructed to snare the stone, which is then pulled through the ureter into the bladder and extracted through the cystoscope. A stone lodged in the proximal ureter may be broken into fragments by **shock wave lithotripsy**, a procedure that can break a large stone too big to pass through the ureter into small fragments that can be excreted in the urine instead of requiring a surgical procedure to remove the stone. The usual method for fragmenting a calculus involves positioning the recumbent patient on a specially designed table. Above the table is x-ray equipment capable of visualizing the location of the stone within the kidney. Below the table is a device called a lithotriptor, which can generate electrically produced shock waves capable of fragmenting the stone. When the exact location of the stone has been determined by x-ray examination, the shock wave–generating equipment is focused very precisely on the kidney stone, and shock waves directed at the stone fragment the stone into fine particles that are excreted in the urine. The success of the technique depends on the size and composition of the stone and, to some degree, the size of the patient. In a large sized patient, the shock wave may be prevented from impacting on the stone.

Sometimes stones form in the bladder. Usually, this stone formation is secondary to the combined effect of infection and stasis of urine, which decrease the solubility of dissolved salts in the urine. Sometimes bladder calculi can be removed through the bladder by means of a cystoscope. The stones are first broken up by an instrument passed through the cystoscope into the bladder and are then flushed out.

OBSTRUCTION

For urine to be excreted normally, the urinary drainage system that transports the urine must permit free flow of urine. Obstruction or marked narrowing of the system at any point (stricture) causes the system proximal to the blockage to dilate progressively because of the pressure of the retained urine. Dilatation of the ureter is called **hydroureter**. Dilatation of the renal pelvis and calyces is called **hydronephrosis** (*hydro* = water + *nephros* = kidney + *osis* = condition) (**FIGURE 19-19**). The distention of the calyces and pelvis in turn causes progressive atrophy of the kidney on the affected side because of the high pressure of the urine within the obstructed drainage system. Eventually, if the obstruction is not relieved, the affected kidney is reduced to a thin shell of atrophic parenchyma covering the overdistended pelvis and calyces.

Which part of the drainage system is affected by the obstruction depends on the location of the block. Obstruction to the outflow of urine from the bladder, as by an enlarged prostate gland or stricture in the urethra, leads to bilateral hydronephrosis and hydroureter, as well as causing overdistention of the bladder (**FIGURE 19-20A**). Hydronephrosis and hydroureter are unilateral if the obstruction is located low in the ureter, as might be caused by an obstructing calculus impacted in the ureter or an obstructing tumor of the ureter (**FIGURE 19-20B**). If the obstruction is located at the junction of the renal pelvis and ureter, as might be caused by scarring of the ureter

> **Hydroureter** A dilatation of the ureter secondary to obstruction of the urinary drainage system, often associated with coexisting dilatation of the renal pelvis and calyces (hydronephrosis).
>
> **Hydronephrosis** A dilatation of the urinary drainage tract proximal to the site of an obstruction.

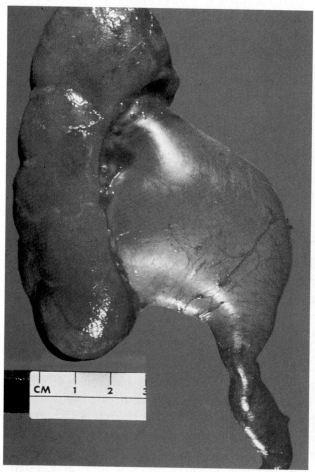

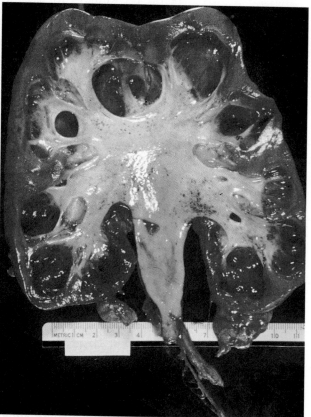

(A)　　　　　　　　　　　　　　　**(B)**

FIGURE 19-19 **(A)** Marked hydronephrosis and hydroureter. **(B)** Bisected hydronephrotic kidney, illustrating enlargement of calyces with atrophy of the renal parenchyma caused by the increased pressure exerted by the urine within the distended renal pelvis and calyces.

Courtesy of Leonard V. Crowley, MD, Century College.

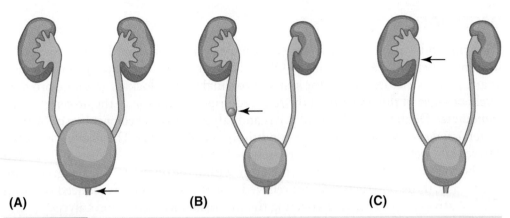

(A)   **(B)**   **(C)**

FIGURE 19-20 Possible locations and results of urinary tract obstruction. The *arrows* indicate sites of obstruction. **(A)** Bilateral hydronephrosis and hydroureter with distention of the bladder caused by urethral obstruction. **(B)** Unilateral hydroureter and hydronephrosis caused by obstruction of the distal ureter. **(C)** Unilateral hydronephrosis caused by obstruction at the ureteropelvic junction.

in this area, a unilateral hydronephrosis develops, but the ureter on the affected side is of normal caliber (**FIGURE 19-20C**).

Diagnosis of urinary tract obstruction is usually made by means of a pyelogram or by CT scan (procedures described in the discussion on general concepts of disease, principles of diagnosis). These procedures demonstrate the dilatation of the urinary tract. Treatment is directed toward relieving the obstruction by appropriate means before the kidneys are irreparably damaged.

Renal Cysts

SOLITARY CYSTS

Solitary cysts of the kidney are relatively common. They vary in diameter from a few millimeters to about 15 cm. They are not associated with impairment of renal function and are of no significance to the patient.

CONGENITAL POLYCYSTIC KIDNEY DISEASE

Although several different conditions are associated with the formation of kidney cysts, the most common (affecting as many as 1 in 400 people) and clinically most important of these conditions is autosomal (adult) dominant polycystic kidney disease (ADPKD). Two different genes, designated *PKD1* and *PKD2* (for Polycystic Kidney Disease), located on separate chromosomes are involved. About 85 percent of cases result from mutation of *PKD1*. In most of the others, the mutation involves *PKD2*, which is associated with later onset and slower progression of the disease. A few unfortunate people have mutations of both *PKD1* and *PKD2*, which causes severe and rapidly progressive disease. The disease is characterized by disturbed proliferation of tubular epithelial cells, leading to the formation of cysts that become detached from the tubules. The epithelium lining the cysts secretes fluid that accumulates within the cysts and causes them to enlarge. As the cysts gradually increase in size, they cause progressive enlargement of both kidneys, where they compress and destroy adjacent renal tissue. Eventually, almost no normal kidney tissue remains, and renal failure supervenes (**FIGURE 19-21**). Sometimes small numbers of cysts also form in the liver, but usually they do not disturb liver function. Some affected people also have small cystlike outpouchings extending from the cerebral arteries at the base

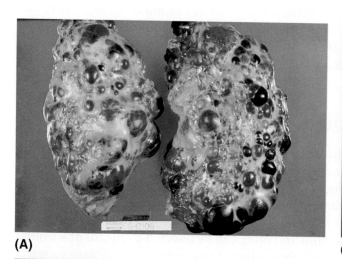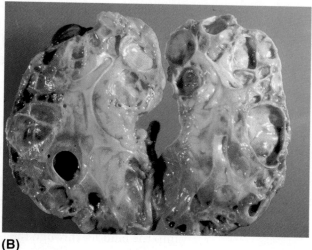

(A)   **(B)**

FIGURE 19-21 **(A)** Greatly enlarged abnormal kidneys characteristic of congenital polycystic kidney disease. **(B)** Cut surfaces of diseased kidneys, illustrating multiple large cysts. No normal renal tissue remains.

Courtesy of Leonard V. Crowley, MD, Century College.

of the brain, which are called congenital cerebral aneurysms. Because congenital cerebral aneurysms may rupture and cause a brain hemorrhage, some physicians have advocated routine magnetic resonance screening of all patients with autosomal dominant polycystic kidney disease. Congenital aneurysms and their complications are described in the discussion on the nervous system.

Because renal tissue is destroyed slowly, renal insufficiency does not usually occur until the patient reaches middle age, and some patients do not experience problems until they are in their forties. Many individuals with congenital polycystic kidney disease are free of symptoms until the disease has markedly progressed, but some experience hypertension, periodic urinary tract infections, or episodes of bloody urine (hematuria) caused by bleeding into one of the enlarging cysts. Some patients also develop hypertension, which often accompanies renal failure.

Polycystic kidney disease can often be suspected by physical examination, which reveals the greatly enlarged kidneys and can be confirmed by ultrasound or CT examination. There is no specific treatment. When the kidneys fail, dialysis treatments or a kidney transplant may be required. A much less common congenital polycystic disease of the kidney (autosomal recessive polycystic disease) occurs in infants, many of whom die in the neonatal period.

Tumors of the Urinary Tract

Tumors may arise from the epithelium of the renal tubules in the cortex of the kidney, from the transitional epithelium lining the urinary tract, or rarely from remnants of embryonic tissue within the kidney.

RENAL CORTICAL TUMORS

Benign tumors called renal cortical adenomas sometimes arise within the kidney. Usually, a benign adenoma is small, well circumscribed, located within the renal cortex, and can be removed by a limited resection. Unfortunately, much more common are malignant tumors, renal cell carcinoma being the most common. Less well-differentiated carcinomas are larger, grow more rapidly, extend into the renal medulla, and exhibit aggressive behavior. Often, the first manifestation of an aggressive carcinoma is blood in the urine (hematuria) as a result of ulceration of the epithelium of the pelvis or calyces caused by the growing tumor. The tumor eventually invades the renal vein and gives rise to distant metastases. The use of tobacco products is a well-established risk factor.

TRANSITIONAL CELL TUMORS

Almost all tumors arising from the transitional epithelium of the urinary tract are malignant and are called transitional cell carcinomas. Most arise from bladder epithelium, are of low-grade malignancy, and carry a good prognosis. The tumors are often quite vascular, and they tend to bleed; hematuria may be the first manifestation of the neoplasm. Bladder tumors can be visualized by means of a cystoscope inserted into the bladder through the urethra and often can be resected by means of a similar type of instrument inserted through the urethra. Sometimes it is necessary to resect part of the bladder to remove the tumor completely.

NEPHROBLASTOMA (WILMS TUMOR)

An unusual highly malignant tumor composed of primitive cells sometimes arises in the kidney of infants and young children. Histologically, the tumor bears some resemblance to the structure of an embryonic kidney and is called a nephroblastoma, or Wilms tumor. The neoplasm often metastasizes widely. Treatment is by nephrectomy followed by radiotherapy and chemotherapy.

Renal Failure (Uremia)

Renal failure is an inability of the kidneys to adequately perform their normal regulatory and excretory functions. Function may decline rapidly, which is called acute renal injury, or slowly but progressively, which is called chronic renal injury.

Uremia is the end stage of many different types of kidney disease. Metabolic acidosis occurs because the failing kidneys are unable to efficiently excrete the various acid waste products produced by the body's normal metabolic processes. **Ketosis** results from overproduction of the acid ketone bodies, acetoacetic acid and beta-hydroxybutyric acid, which are derived from the metabolism of fat.

ACUTE KIDNEY INJURY

Acute kidney injury (AKI) (sometimes called acute renal failure) can be defined as prerenal AKI when caused by a disturbance "prior" to the kidney. An example would be severe hemorrhage or dehydration. Postrenal AKI is related to causes distal to the kidney such as urinary tract obstruction. Renal AKI relates to injury to any part of the kidney, glomeruli, tubules, or the renal vasculature.

CHRONIC RENAL FAILURE

In contrast to acute renal failure, this condition is a gradual deterioration of renal function resulting from chronic renal disease. Approximately 50 to 75 percent of all cases of chronic renal failure result from diabetes and hypertension. Chronic pyelonephritis, congenital polycystic renal disease, chronic glomerulonephritis, and autoimmune diseases involving the kidney account for most of the remainder.

Uremia An excess of urea and other waste products in the blood, resulting from renal failure.

Ketosis Results from overproduction of products of fat metabolism.

Acute kidney injury (AKI) Injury to any part of the kidney. May also be defined as prerenal or postrenal.

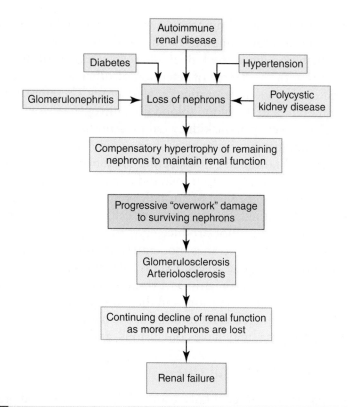

FIGURE 19-22 Self-perpetuating progression of chronic kidney disease.

A normal kidney contains about one million nephrons. In chronic renal failure, renal function declines as the population of nephrons decreases, although relatively normal renal function can be maintained until the number of functioning nephrons falls below 20 to 30 percent of normal. Unfortunately, all types of chronic renal disease tend to progress because of the way the surviving nephrons respond to the declining renal function (**FIGURE 19-22**). The surviving nephrons are forced to "work harder" to accomplish the functions previously performed by a full complement of nephrons. Each of the remaining nephrons receives a larger volume of blood to process at a higher than normal pressure. The high blood volumes and pressures damage the arterioles and glomerular capillaries, which leads to thickening of the walls of glomerular arterioles with narrowing of their lumens (arteriolosclerosis) along with glomerular capillary injury followed by scarring (glomerulosclerosis). The tubules are also damaged because the blood vessels that supply the glomeruli also supply the tubules. Consequently, a vicious cycle is created in which the reduced number of functioning nephrons indirectly damages the overworked surviving nephrons, many of which become scarred and cease to function. As more nephrons are lost, an additional burden is placed on those that still survive, which eventually causes many of them to fail. As this process continues, progressively more nephrons are lost at an increasing rate, until eventually renal function deteriorates to the point where the kidneys are no longer able to perform their regulatory and excretory functions. The patient experiences severe derangements of fluid, electrolyte, and acid–base balance. Various acids that would normally be excreted by the kidneys are retained, which disturbs the normal pH of body fluids, leading to a condition called metabolic acidosis (described in the earlier discussion on water, electrolyte, and acid–base balance). The failing kidneys cannot produce erythropoietin to stimulate bone marrow function, and the patient becomes anemic. As noted previously, renal failure is sometimes called uremia. This term refers to the characteristic retention of urea in the blood when

Urea Normal by-product of protein metabolism excreted in the urine.

the kidneys fail. **Urea** is a normal by-product of protein metabolism and is excreted in the urine. It is not a toxic compound and is only one of many substances that accumulates in the blood when the kidneys fail. The amount of urea in the blood, however, correlates with the degree of retention of other waste products and with the clinical manifestations of deteriorating renal function. Therefore, measurement of the concentration of urea in the blood (blood urea nitrogen test or BUN) provides a rough estimate of the severity of the kidney failure. Another commonly used measure of renal functional impairment is the level of creatinine in the blood.

Symptoms of renal failure are nonspecific. They begin to appear when about 80 percent of renal function has been lost and are quite pronounced by the time renal function has fallen to 5 percent of normal. Symptoms include weakness, loss of appetite, nausea, and vomiting. Production of red cells by the bone marrow decreases because the failing kidneys cannot produce erythropoietin to stimulate bone marrow function, and the patient becomes moderately anemic. Waste products are not eliminated and increase to toxic levels. Excess salt and water are retained by the failing kidneys, resulting in weight gain as a result of retained fluid. The blood volume increases because of fluid retention, and the blood pressure also tends to rise as the intravascular volume increases. If untreated, the patient in chronic renal failure eventually lapses into coma, may have convulsions, and eventually dies.

TREATMENT FOR RENAL FAILURE

The outlook for patients with renal failure and ESRD has improved dramatically in recent years because of two effective methods of treatment: hemodialysis and renal transplantation. Hemodialysis and peritoneal dialysis remove waste products from the patient's blood. Both methods are equally effective, and each has advantages and disadvantages. Every year, many new patients with advanced renal disease begin dialysis. Some will continue on dialysis indefinitely. Others will rely on dialysis until a kidney becomes available for transplantation. Renal transplantation, using kidneys from living related donors or recently deceased persons (cadaveric donors), is the most desirable option; however, kidneys for transplantation are in very short supply.

HEMODIALYSIS

Hemodialysis substitutes for the functions of the kidneys. Waste products from the patient's blood diffuse across a semipermeable membrane into a solution (the dialysate) on the other side of the membrane. The rate of diffusion is determined by several factors: the concentration of the substances on the two sides of the membrane, the rate of blood flow and flow of the dialysate through the dialyzer, and the characteristics of the dialyzer membrane. Waste products, which are present in high concentrations in the patient's blood, diffuse from the blood into the dialysate because of differences in the concentration on the two sides of the membrane. Usually, the patient's blood is dialyzed by an "artificial kidney" machine. This type of hemodialysis is called extracorporeal hemodialysis (*extra* = outside + *corpus* = body) because the blood is transported outside the patient's body for dialysis in the artificial kidney and then returned by means of a system of tubes connected to the patient's circulatory system.

Hemodialysis is usually performed in an outpatient dialysis center three times per week for three or four hours during each dialysis session, but it can be performed at home by the patient with the assistance of a family member who has been given special training. The patient's blood flows along one side of a synthetic semipermeable membrane that restricts the passage of blood cells and protein but permits the passage of water and small molecules. The dialysate flows on the other side of the membrane in a direction opposite to the flow of blood. This type of flow pattern, which is called countercurrent dialysis (*counter* = against + *current* = blood flow), promotes more efficient removal of waste products than when dialysate and blood flow in the same direction.

During dialysis, plastic tubes connect the patient's circulation to the dialyzer in the artificial kidney machine. One tube transmits blood to the dialyzer unit where the blood is cleansed and excess fluid is removed, and the other tube conveys the blood from the dialyzer back to the patient's circulation. Before dialysis begins, the coaguability of the patient's blood is reduced by administration of heparin to prevent the blood from clotting as it flows through the dialyzer.

To perform hemodialysis on a regular basis, one of the patient's arteries and a large vein must be easily accessible so that the tubes that transport blood to and from the dialyzer unit can easily and repeatedly be connected to the patient's blood vessels. Although several methods have been devised to gain access to the patient's circulation, the preferred method consists of surgically interconnecting the radial artery in the wrist and an adjacent vein, forming an artificial communication called an arteriovenous fistula (**FIGURE 19-23A**). After the fistula has been created, arterial blood is short-circuited directly into the vein instead of flowing through the peripheral capillaries. The vein, which now receives blood directly under high pressure, becomes much larger and develops a thick wall over a several month period. When the vein has become suitable for use, dialysis treatments are begun. Two needles are inserted through the skin directly into the vein. One needle is attached to the tube that delivers blood to the dialyzer, and the second needle is attached to the tube that returns the blood to the patient. Less commonly, other procedures are used to gain access to the patient's circulation for dialysis.

There are many types of artificial kidney machines. Many are quite compact, and portable units are available. Improvements in the design and operation of the machines are being made continually. The essential component of the artificial kidney machine is the dialyzer. Attached to it are the tubes that carry blood to and from the patient and the tubes that carry dialysate to and from the unit. A hollow fiber dialyzer, which is quite compact and efficient and is the most commonly used type, consists of a bundle of hollow synthetic fibers through which the blood passes. The dialysate circulates around the outside of the fibers in the opposite direction (**FIGURE 19-23B**).

Peritoneal Dialysis

Peritoneal dialysis uses the patient's own peritoneum as the dialyzing membrane. To perform peritoneal dialysis, a large plastic tube must first be inserted into the patient's abdominal (peritoneal) cavity and fixed in position by suturing it to the skin. The dialysis procedure consists of instilling several liters of dialysis fluid through the tube into the peritoneal cavity and allowing the fluid to remain within the peritoneal cavity for a variable time. During this time, waste products diffuse across the peritoneum from the underlying blood vessels into the dialysis fluid that fills the peritoneal cavity. Dialysis fluid is then withdrawn and fresh fluid is instilled. Peritoneal dialysis can be performed by means of an automated system in which the machine automatically fills and drains the peritoneal cavity at night while the patient is asleep. Another similar method is called continuous ambulatory peritoneal dialysis. In this procedure, 2 liters of fluid remain within the peritoneal cavity all the time. The patient replaces the fluid with fresh dialysis fluid four or five times a day. Patients carry out their usual activities when they are not draining and refilling their peritoneal cavities.

Peritoneal dialysis is used less frequently than extracorporeal hemodialysis. Not all patients requiring dialysis are suitable candidates for peritoneal dialysis, but the procedure offers an advantage to patients who wish to continue working full time or part time, as they do not have to spend several daytime hours three days each week at a dialysis center, and many patients who choose peritoneal dialysis are quite

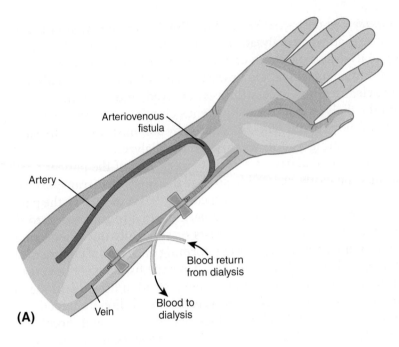

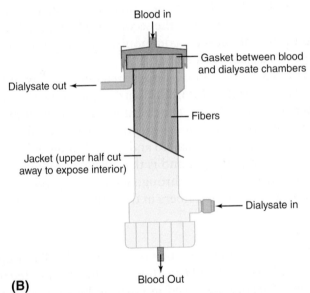

FIGURE 19-23 **(A)** Arteriovenous fistula created between radial artery and adjacent vein. **(B)** Hollow fiber dialyzer.

satisfied with their choice. However, peritoneal dialysis has disadvantages. It is less efficient at removing waste products and carries some risk of peritonitis, which can result if bacteria gain access to the peritoneal cavity around the tube that extends from the skin surface directly into the peritoneal cavity.

RENAL TRANSPLANTATION

When the kidneys fail, a normal compatible kidney sometimes can be transplanted from a close relative, an unrelated volunteer donor, or a recently deceased person (cadaveric donor). The best results are obtained from a living kidney donor even when such donors are not completely compatible.

In any kidney transplantation, an attempt is made to match the transplanted kidney as closely as possible with the donor to give the transplant the best chance of survival in the recipient. Unless the transplanted kidney comes from an identical twin, the transplant will invariably contain foreign antigens that the patient lacks. Consequently, the patient's immunologic defenses will respond to the foreign antigens and attempt to destroy (reject) the foreign kidney unless the patient's immune system is suppressed by drugs or other agents (presented in the discussion on immunity, hypersensitivity, allergy, and autoimmune diseases).

The ABO blood group antigens of the proposed donor must be compatible with the blood group antibodies in the blood of the proposed recipient because the ABO blood group antigens are present in body tissues (including the kidney) as well as on red cells. For example, one could not give a kidney from a group A donor to a group O recipient because the recipient's blood contains anti-A and anti-B antibodies that would attack and destroy the donor kidney. The principles are the same as when selecting blood for a blood transfusion.

The next group of important antigens are the HLA antigens (discussed in the presentation on the hematopoietic and lymph system). The best results are obtained from siblings who have identical HLA antigens; however, transplants with a totally HLA mismatched donor have the same level of success as a transplant from a completely matched cadaveric donor. More than 90 percent of transplanted kidneys survive for five years when the transplanted kidney is obtained from a close relative whose HLA antigens very closely resemble those of the patient. The use of potent immunosuppressive drugs has much improved the overall survival rate of transplanted kidneys even with donors who are not closely matched. The overall one-year survival rate for transplants may be as high as 90 percent, and the ten-year survival rate is over 50 percent. Some patients, however, reject the transplant despite intensive immunosuppressive therapy. Most rejections occur within the first few months after transplantation. Should this occur, the patient resumes dialysis treatments until another kidney suitable for transplantation becomes available.

Although a well-functioning transplanted kidney permits the patient to lead a relatively normal life, the patient with a renal transplant may have other problems. Immunosuppressive drugs may need to be continued indefinitely to prevent rejection of the foreign kidney, and adverse side effects sometimes result from these drugs. The immunosuppressed patient is also more susceptible to infection because the body's immune defenses have been weakened so the transplant can survive. Occasionally, the disease that destroyed the patient's own kidneys, such as glomerulonephritis, also destroys the function of the transplanted kidney.

Diagnostic Evaluation of Kidney and Urinary Tract Disease

A variety of methods are used to detect disease of the kidneys and urinary tract, to evaluate the degree to which renal function is disturbed, and to define the type of disease present.

URINALYSIS

The most widely used diagnostic test is an examination of the urine called **urinalysis**. The examination is useful for detecting whether urinary tract disease is present and for detecting other systemic diseases that alter renal function. The examination includes determinations of urine pH (acidity) and specific gravity (a measure of urine concentration) and simple tests for glucose and protein. The urinalysis may also include tests for bile pigment, acetone, and other constituents that may appear in the urine

Urinalysis A commonly performed chemical and microscopic analysis of the urine.

in association with various diseases. A sample of the urine is also centrifuged, and the sediment is examined microscopically. If the urinalysis is normal, renal disease is unlikely. Alternatively, the presence of red cells and protein in the urine may indicate that damage to the glomerular filter has permitted these substances to leak into the glomerular filtrate or that bleeding is occurring somewhere in the urinary tract. Renal casts, which are collections of protein and cells molded into the shape of the kidney tubules, are an indication of glomerular or tubular disease. Leukocytes and bacteria in the urinary sediment indicate urinary tract infection.

Additional tests may be performed on the urine as indicated by the patient's clinical condition. If a urinary tract infection is suspected, for example, the urine is cultured for pathogenic bacteria and sensitivity tests are performed if bacteria are present. Measurement of urine albumin levels is an accurate determination of the function of the glomerular filtration barrier. The value is usually expressed as the **albumin to creatinine ratio (ACR)** and is often used to monitor kidney damage in type 2 diabetes. Urine levels of the protein beta 2 microglobulin (B2M) increase in the case of renal tubular damage because the renal tubules normally resorb this protein. For this reason, an elevated B2M level suggests a tubular rather than a glomerular defect.

KIDNEY FUNCTION TESTS

Impairment of renal function can be recognized by measuring the concentration in the blood of various substances, such as urea (BUN or blood urea nitrogen) and serum creatinine, which are waste products excreted by the kidneys. Elevated levels indicate impaired renal function, and the degree of elevation is a measure of the degree of impairment.

The efficiency of the glomerular filtration apparatus can be an early indicator of impaired renal function, even before elevated levels of waste products are present in the blood. The **glomerular filtration rate (GFR)** is a measure of the volume of body fluid cleared by the kidneys per unit of time. This is generally reported in milliliter/minute. The GFR is usually measured by the ability of the kidney to clear creatinine using the **creatinine clearance test**. This test calculates how much blood plasma must flow through the kidney each minute and be completely cleared of creatinine to provide the quantity of creatinine that appears in the urine within the same period of time. Clearance tests provide a rough estimate of the degree of kidney damage, and periodic clearance tests can be used to follow the progress of renal disease. A gradual fall in the renal clearance of a substance means that renal function is declining. The test requires a cumbersome twelve- or twenty-four-hour collection and measurement of urine volume as well as measuring the creatinine level and the serum creatinine level. Often the GFR is calculated based solely on the patient's serum creatinine level, age, gender, and race. The calculated value has some limitations but is easier to obtain and is often used to follow kidney function in chronic renal disease.

ADDITIONAL TECHNIQUES

Many other specialized procedures can be used to study the kidneys and urinary tract, including various x-ray examinations, ultrasound examinations, and cystoscopy. These examinations are described in the discussion on general concepts of disease, principles of diagnosis. Their specific diagnostic applications also have been considered in conjunction with the various renal and urinary tract diseases for which they provide useful information. X-ray examination of the abdomen, for example, can identify the size and location of the kidneys and can detect radiopaque calculi in the kidneys or urinary tract. CT scans and intravenous pyelograms can detect anatomic

Albumin to creatinine ratio (ACR) Measurement of urine albumin levels compared to amount of creatinine.

Glomerular filtration rate (GFR) Measure of the volume of body fluid cleared by the kidneys per unit of time.

Creatinine clearance test A test of renal function that measures the ability of kidneys to remove (clear) a substance from the blood and excrete it in the urine.

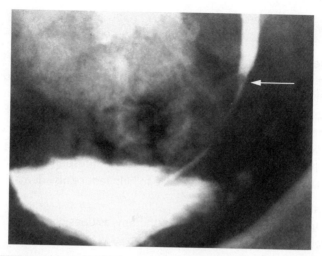

FIGURE 19-24 Intravenous pyelogram. Contrast material fills the bladder at the bottom of the image and the proximal portion of the right ureter. A stone (*arrow*) is lodged in the ureter causing dilation of the ureter above the stone and preventing urine from filling the distal portion. The dye in the bladder comes from urine passing through the opposite ureter.

abnormalities within the kidneys, such as cysts and tumors, and many abnormalities of the urinary drainage system, such as hydronephrosis (**FIGURE 19-24**). Renal arteriograms, using techniques similar to those used to study the coronary arteries, can determine the caliber of the renal arteries, can detect segmental areas of narrowing in the renal arteries, and can identify areas of increased vascularity within the kidney, which often occur when a tumor is present.

Sometimes the clinician cannot make an exact diagnosis concerning the type of renal disease without resorting to biopsy of the kidney. This can be accomplished without undue difficulty or serious risk to the patient by introducing a small biopsy needle through the skin of the flank directly into the substance of the kidney. A small bit of kidney tissue is removed for histologic study. Examination of the biopsy material by the pathologist is often necessary to allow the pathologist to provide an exact diagnosis as to the nature and extent of the renal disease, which serves as a guide to proper treatment.

CASE 19-1

Antoine is a three-year-old male child of African American parents. He had just recovered from a mild upper respiratory infection when his parents noticed that his face appeared "swollen." On closer examination, they noted that his legs and scrotum also appeared to be "puffy" (a physician would say edematous). Antoine also seems tired and has little appetite. Concerned, his parents take him to the family pediatrician. The pediatrician confirms marked facial and dependent edema (accumulation of fluid in tissue predominantly below the heart, such as the legs). Careful examination of the patient's fingernails shows a pattern of horizontal lines (Muehrcke lines) in the bed of the nails, which blanch when the nail is pressed. The physician remembers that such lines are sometimes associated with vascular changes that occur when plasma albumin levels are very low, and he orders urinalysis.

Antoine's urine shows extreme proteinuria. The albumin to creatinine ratio is 6 and the urine has a very high specific gravity. These findings would be consistent with loss of protein in the urine because of impaired urinary filtration. The patient's serum albumin is

(continues)

CASE 19-1 (Continued)

2.3 g/dl (dl is the abbreviation for deciliter or 100 ml), which is abnormally low. These findings taken together are consistent with the diagnosis of nephrotic syndrome. Because at least 90 percent of nephrosis in children of Antoine's age is minimal change disease, no invasive investigation of the kidney (such as a renal biopsy) is undertaken. Even if that were done, light microscopy would not be expected to disclose any changes in the glomerulus.

The physician decides to try corticosteroid therapy using prednisone because about 90 percent of children with minimal change disease will respond within two weeks. His parents are told to reduce Antoine's salt intake to help reduce his edema.

The Happy Ending

Antoine's proteinuria clears after ten days of therapy, as does his edema. Drug therapy is continued for four weeks at a reduced dose, and no relapse is noted.

The Not-So-Happy Ending

No change is noted in the degree of nephrosis after two weeks of therapy. Antoine complains of increasing abdominal pain, and his blood pressure begins to increase. Therapy with diuretics and antihypertensive medication becomes necessary. His disease is now classified as **steroid-resistant nephrotic syndrome (SRNS).** Because of his continuing disease, the nephrologist in charge of Antoine's case decides to request a needle biopsy of Antoine's kidney. Light microscopic analysis of the glomerular disease is consistent with focal segmental glomerulosclerosis (FSGS) (see Figure 19-13). This was not surprising because 70 percent of children with SRNS have FSGS. Aggressive treatment with increased doses of prednisone and immunosuppressive agents was ineffective. Ultimately Antoine developed end stage renal disease and required a kidney transplant.

Discussion

Minimal change disease is thought to be related to an increased level of a number of cytokines that cause T cells to release an agent that damages the function of the epithelial cell foot processes; however, the exact mechanism is unclear. Although no changes to affected glomeruli are noted by light microscopy, damage to the foot processes (fusion or effacement), as disclosed in EM studies, is characteristic of the disease (**FIGURE 19-25**). The etiology of the disease remains obscure (although it may occur following an upper respiratory tract infection or allergic reaction). Ninety percent of children with minimal change disease respond to prednisone therapy. Failure of response (SRNS) is an indicator of the likelihood of a different disease process, and as noted about 70 percent of children with SRNS have focal segmental glomerulosclerosis. FSGS is significantly increasing in frequency in Caucasian and, notably, in African American populations, where it is the most common cause of adult nephrosis. FSGS is associated with diverse etiologies and diagnostic subclassifications, including primary (idiopathic) disease or secondary disease related infection (HIV), drugs, reduced renal mass and hereditary defects in podocyte genes, and (particularly in African Americans) a circulating protein apolipoprotein L1. The frequency of the variant of the *apoL1* gene associated with FSGS susceptibility is more than ten times higher in African Americans than in Caucasians and is associated with an increased risk of FSGS and hypertensive end stage renal disease. The presence of two high-risk alleles of *apoL1* is responsible for nearly 20 percent of FSGS. The high-risk alleles of *apoL1* are associated with the ability to lyse trypanosomes associated with African sleeping sickness. Individuals with a single high-risk allele are relatively resistant to this parasitic disease, whereas inheritance of two high-risk alleles is associated with a much higher risk of kidney disease. This pattern of heterozygous advantage (versus homozygous disadvantage) is analogous to that seen with sickle cell trait and disease (discussed under diseases of blood circulation) The lack of response by Antoine to steroids and immunosuppressive therapy is consistent with a hereditary condition, but no additional family history

CASE 19-1 *(Continued)*

or genetic studies are available. However, it is clear that African Americans are at increased risk of FSGS, and hypertensive renal disease is likely to be related in part to hereditary factors.

Etiology and Pathogenesis

Minimal change disease of unknown etiology or steroid resistant nephrosis associated with focal segmental glomerulosclerosis, possibly of hereditary origin involving *apoL1* high-risk alleles or podocyte protein defects.

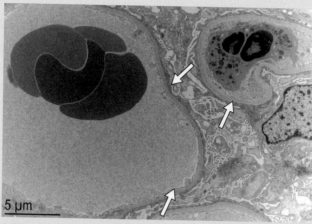

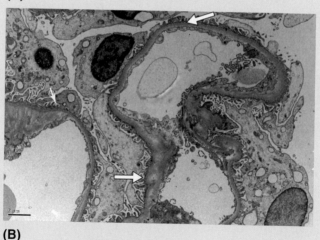

FIGURE 19-25 Electron micrograph images: **(A)** Glomerular capillaries in minimal change disease. Both capillaries show effacement (flattening) of podocytes (*arrows*). One capillary has red cells in the lumen, the other a neutrophil. **(B)** Normal glomerular capillaries demonstrating podocytes (*arrows*).

Courtesy of Drs Singh & Nickeleit Department of Pathology and Laboratory Medicine, University of North Carolina at Chapel Hill.

Questions

1. There is much discussion about the appropriate role of racial identification of patients. When do you think doing so is appropriate?

2. Clearly distinguish between nephrosis and nephritis. Which is this Case a good example of and why?

3. Why would immediate renal biopsy of a child with nephrosis be inappropriate? When would this be appropriate?

4. Correlate the laboratory findings in this Case with the disease process.

5. Correlate the EM findings in this Case with the disease process.

QUESTIONS FOR REVIEW

1. What is the difference between glomerulonephritis and pyelonephritis? What is the relationship between glomerulonephritis and beta-streptococcal infection? What factors predispose to urinary tract infection?

2. What is the difference between nephrotic syndrome and nephrosclerosis? Why does edema develop in a patient with nephrosis?

3. What are the common causes of urinary tract obstruction? What are the effects on the kidneys and lower urinary tract?

4. What conditions lead to renal tubular necrosis? What are its clinical manifestations?

5. What is uremia? What are its manifestations? How is it treated? What is the role of urea in producing the clinical manifestations of uremia?

6. What methods does the clinician use to establish a diagnosis of renal disease?

7. What is congenital polycystic kidney disease? What are its clinical manifestations? What is its pattern of inheritance? How is it treated?

8. What is the difference between acute and chronic renal failure?

9. What is the difference between hemodialysis and peritoneal dialysis? How is the patient's circulation connected to the artificial kidney for hemodialysis?

10. Why does a kidney transplant from a donor who is a close relative usually have a greater likelihood of survival than does a cadaver transplant?

11. How does diabetes affect the kidneys? What are the clinical manifestations? How does gout affect the kidneys?

SUPPLEMENTARY READINGS

Jennette, J. C., and Gasim, A. M. H. Chapter 12, "Pathology of Medical Renal Disease." 2015. In *Pathology: A Modern Case Study*, edited by H. M. Reisner. New York, NY: McGraw Hill Lange.

▶ A brief introduction to the pathology of renal disease that is strong on overviews and case studies.

Wouters, O. J., et al. 2015. Early chronic kidney disease: Diagnosis, management and models of care. *Nature Reviews Nephrology* 11:491–502.

Coresh, J., et al. 2014. Decline in estimated glomerular filtration rate and subsequent risk of end-stage renal disease and mortality. *JAMA* 311:2518–31.

▶ The first entry is a recent review that includes a discussion of the social costs, epidemiology, and diagnosis of chronic renal disease. The second entry describes the use of a common clinical laboratory test as a strong estimator of the risk of end stage renal disease. Also discusses how to estimate the progression of chronic renal disease.

Saigusa, T., and Bell, P. D. 2015. Molecular pathways and therapy in autosomal dominant polycystic kidney disease. *Physiology* 30:195–207.

▶ An excellent article on the important concepts regarding this disease, including pathogenesis, genetics, associated conditions, complications, clinical manifestations, monitoring disease progression, and treatment.

Merchant, A. A., Quinn, R. R., and Perl, J. 2015. Dialysis modality and survival: Does the controversy live on? *Current Opinion in Nephrology and Hypertension* 24:276–83.

▶ A recent review of the status of a long-standing controversy over the relative utility of conventional hemodialysis versus peritoneal dialysis.

Morrissey, P. E., and Monaco, A. P. 2014. Donation after circulatory death: Current practices, ongoing challenges, and potential improvements. *Transplantation* 97:258–64.

Maggiore, U., et al. 2015. Strategies to increase the donor pool and access to kidney transplantation: An international perspective. *Nephrology Dialysis Transplantation* 30:217–22.

Matas, A. J. 2014. Transplantation: Increased ESRD and mortality risk for kidney donors? *Nature Reviews Nephrology* 10:130–31.

> ▶ Renal transplantation, although the optimal solution for most patients with ESRD, is associated with several major problems. Donor access is limited and kidneys from donors who have undergone circulatory death may (or may not) be as likely to function as well as those from living donors. Are living donors at increased risk of kidney disease? These three papers review important areas of the discussion.

Arora, P. 2015. *Chronic kidney disease.* http://emedicine.medscape.com/article/238798-overview

National Kidney Foundation. https://www.kidney.org/

Meyer, T. W., Hostetter, T. H. 2014 Approaches to uremia. *Journal of the American Society of Nephrology* 25:2151–58.

> ▶ Current concepts and discussion of the pathophysiology of chronic renal failure and the complexities of treating uremia. The second entry provides an excellent, easy-to-read approach to both chronic renal failure and many other aspects of renal disease.

Fisang, C., et al. 2015. Urolithiasis—An interdisciplinary diagnostic, therapeutic and secondary preventive challenge *Deutsches Ärzteblatt International* 112:83–91.

> ▶ A detailed overview of the causes and therapy of urolithiasis that includes lithotripsy and many newer endoscopic techniques. Although the journal is published in Germany, the article is freely available online.

Kumar, S., Dave, A., and Wolf, B. 2015. Urinary tract infections. *Disease-a-Month* 61:45–59.

> ▶ A clinically oriented detailed review of this very common medical condition.

Kruzel-Davila, E., et al. 2015. APOL1 nephropathy: From gene to mechanism of kidney injury. *Nephrology Dialysis Transplantation* (Epub January 5).

Rood, I. M., Deegens, J. K. J., and Wetzels, J. F. M. 2012. Genetic causes of focal segmental glomerulosclerosis: Implications for clinical practice. *Nephrology Dialysis Transplantation* 27:1–9.

> ▶ These two references were used in the Case construction. The first entry highlights an exciting new finding in genetic risk factors for serious renal disease in African Americans that has similarities to sickle cell disease. The second article reviews other inherited diseases associated with FSGS.

The Male Reproductive System

Courtesy of Department of Pathology and Laboratory Medicine, University of North Carolina at Chapel Hill

1. Name the anatomic structures of the male reproductive system. Describe their functions as they relate to the diseases affecting them.

2. Differentiate between benign prostatic hyperplasia and prostatic carcinoma. Describe clinical manifestations and methods of treatment.

3. Discuss symptoms and treatment for erectile dysfunction.

Structure and Function of the Male Reproductive Organs

The components of the male reproductive system are the penis, the prostate and certain other accessory glands (including the seminal vesicles and the bulbourethral and urethral glands), the two testes, and a paired duct system for transporting sperm from the testes to the urethra. The transport duct system begins as the epididymis, which is closely applied to the testes, and continues as the vas deferens. The vas deferens extends upward in the spermatic cords, is joined by the seminal vesicles, and enters the prostatic urethra as the ejaculatory ducts. The urethra is divided into a short segment traversing the prostate gland (the prostatic urethra) and a long penile urethra. The distal penile urethra is known as the anterior urethra, and the prostatic urethra and adjacent proximal part of the penile urethra is the posterior urethra. **FIGURE 20-1** illustrates the anatomy of the male reproductive system. A working knowledge of how these structures are interrelated is necessary to understand the spread of inflammatory disease in the male reproductive tract and the various complications that may result.

The prostate is a spherical gland about 5 cm in diameter that surrounds the urethra just below the base of the bladder (**FIGURE 20-2A**). It is composed of numerous branched glands arranged in two major groups intermixed with masses of smooth muscle and fibrous tissue (**FIGURE 20-2B**). The inner group of glands form the **transition zone**, which surrounds the urethra as it passes through the prostate and includes the periurethral area; the **central zone** surrounds the ejaculatory ducts; and the **peripheral zone** surrounds the other zones and forms the outer boundary of the gland, making

Transition zone Part of the prostate that surrounds the urethra.

Central zone Part of the prostate that surrounds the ejaculatory ducts.

Peripheral zone Part of the prostate that surrounds the other zones.

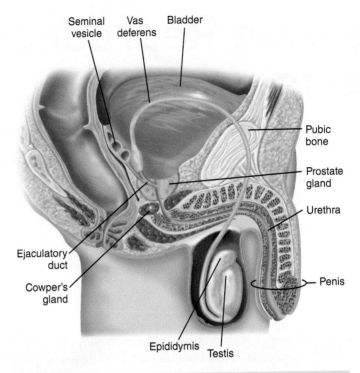

Seminal vesicle · Vas deferens · Bladder · Pubic bone · Prostate gland · Urethra · Penis · Ejaculatory duct · Cowper's gland · Epididymis · Testis

FIGURE 20-1 A side view of the male reproductive system. Seminal fluid consists of sperm mixed with secretions of seminal vesicles, prostate gland, and bulbourethral glands. The testes, excretory ducts, seminal vesicles, and bulbourethral glands are paired structures.

up the bulk of prostatic glandular tissue. The gland is capped with an aglandular fibromuscular zone (**FIGURE 20-2C**). The anatomic zones are of significance because hyperplasia of the prostate occurs predominantly in the transition zone, and cancer occurs in the peripheral zone. The prostate secretes a thin alkaline fluid containing a high concentration of an enzyme secreted by prostatic epithelial cells. The prostatic secretions are discharged into the urethra during ejaculation through very fine ducts that open near the orifices of the ejaculatory ducts. These secretions mix with sperm and the secretions of the seminal vesicles to form the seminal fluid. The urethral glands discharge into the penile urethra and contribute a mucouslike component to semen.

The two testes (also called testicles), which originally developed within the abdomen, occupy separate compartments within the scrotum. In the fetus, the testes descend through the inguinal canals into the scrotum, bringing their blood vessels, nerves, and excretory ducts with them as the spermatic cords. The testes usually have completed their descent about one month before birth. To guide descent of the testes, a band of fibrous tissue called a gubernaculum (a Latin word meaning rudder or guide) extends from the inferior surface of each testis through the inguinal canal into the scrotum where it attaches. As the gubernaculum shortens, it guides each testis into the scrotum, where a fibrous remnant of the gubernaculum (scrotal ligament) remains to anchor each testis within its scrotal compartment. Normally, a broad band of connective tissue attaches each testis within the scrotum, which allows the testis some mobility, but the broad attachment prevents rotation of the testis on its axis, which would also twist the spermatic cord and obstruct the blood vessels supplying the testis.

As the testes descend, fingerlike projections of peritoneum called vaginal processes project from the peritoneal cavity into the scrotal compartments, and the testes descend into the scrotum posterior to the vaginal processes. After the testes

by irradiation rather than surgery. Radical prostatectomy alone or combined with radiation therapy appears to improve survival in many patients. There is considerable controversy, however, about the effectiveness of radical surgery or radiation therapy in older men with localized well-differentiated carcinoma of the prostate. Many physicians believe that treatment does not improve survival in this group of patients, that the treatment causes more disability and complications than the tumor, and that a slowly growing prostatic carcinoma in an older man is best left alone.

When a prostatic carcinoma has advanced to the stage that it has spread beyond the prostate, it is often possible to induce regression of the tumor by altering the level of male sex hormones in the body. Most prostatic carcinomas are initially dependent on the male sex hormone for their continued growth. Therefore, many advanced prostatic tumors can be treated effectively by surgical removal of the testes, eliminating the source of the male sex hormone. Alternatively, drugs that suppress output of pituitary gonadotropic hormone can be administered, thereby inhibiting testicular testosterone secretion. Either surgical or hormone-induced castration or hormone treatment usually causes a temporary regression of the tumor. Widespread metastatic disease to lymph nodes, bones, liver, and lungs is often accompanied by hormone independent tumor growth, and traditional chemotherapy and local radiation are used palliatively.

CARCINOMA OF THE TESTIS

Although testicular tumors are uncommon, they most frequently develop between the ages of thirty and forty. Testicular tumors are rare in prepubertal males (but both benign and malignant tumors occur infrequently). Most tumors arise from the germinal epithelium of the testicular tubules and are malignant. There are several different types. The type with the most favorable prognosis is called a **seminoma**. (This is an exception to standard terminology, as the term refers to a malignant neoplasm that resembles spermatogonia rather than to a benign tumor.) The tumor, which is detectable as a growing scrotal mass, is highly sensitive to radiation therapy; a greater than 90 percent cure rate is possible using orchiectomy and radiation and, in the case of large tumors, chemotherapy.

Some testicular tumors are derived from undifferentiated embryonal cells and are called **embryonal carcinomas**. More differentiated embryonal cells give rise to **teratocarcinomas** (**malignant teratomas**), which are composed of many different types of malignant tissues, some of which demonstrate the characteristics of a variety of somatic or extraembryonic cells of the developing embryo (described in the discussion on neoplastic disease). Some other testicular tumors resemble placental trophoblastic tissue. An example is **choriocarcinoma**, which is the same kind of tumor that arises from trophoblastic tissue in the uterus (described in the discussion on prenatal development and diseases associated with pregnancy).

The neoplastic cells of many testicular tumors produce **human chorionic gonadotropin (hCG)**, which is the same hormone made by the placenta in pregnancy. Consequently, a pregnancy test given to a man with testicular cancer may be positive. Some testicular tumors also produce **alpha fetoprotein (AFP)**, which is a protein produced by the fetus early in prenatal development but not normally found in the adult. If a testicular carcinoma produces these substances, the concentrations fall after successful treatment of the tumor and rise again if the tumor recurs. Consequently, the physician can monitor the response of the testicular tumor to treatment by serial determinations of hCG and AFP in the same way that carcinoembryonic antigen analyses are used to evaluate the response to treatment of other malignant tumors (described in the discussion on neoplastic disease). Nonseminoma tumors are not as sensitive to radiation and often require the use of chemotherapy in management.

Seminoma One type of malignant tumor of the testis.

Embryonal carcinoma A malignant testicular tumor in which the malignant cells have features resembling rapidly growing trophoblastic tissue.

Teratocarcinomas/malignant teratomas A malignant testicular tumor composed of many different types of malignant tissues.

Choriocarcinoma A malignant proliferation of trophoblastic tissue.

Human chorionic gonadotropin (hCG) A hormone made by the placenta in pregnancy that has actions similar to pituitary gonadotropins. The same hormone is made by neoplastic cells in some types of malignant testicular tumors.

Alpha fetoprotein (AFP) Protein produced by fetal liver early in gestation. Sometimes produced by tumor cells. Level is elevated in amnionic fluid when fetus has neural tube defect.

CARCINOMA OF THE PENIS

Carcinoma of the penis is uncommon and is almost never encountered in a circumcised male. It is possible that the secretions that accumulate under the foreskin of the penis are carcinogenic and that this accumulation is prevented by circumcision. However, other factors also may account for the low incidence of carcinoma in circumcised males. Carcinogenic strains of the papilloma virus, the same virus that appears related to cervical dysplasia and carcinoma in women, may play a major role in causing penile cancer. The papilloma virus may grow well beneath an intact foreskin but does not grow if the foreskin has been removed. Treatment usually consists of partial or complete resection of the penis.

Developmental Abnormalities

CONGENITAL DISORDERS OF THE URETER

Obstructions to the lower urinary tract are not uncommon developmental abnormalities in neonatal males. **Posterior urethral valves (PUV)** is the most frequent obstruction, occurring in about 1 in 8,000 male births. During gonadogenesis, the defect occurs when an embryological structure that normally recedes during male development leaves a remnant in the prostatic urethra, termed the verumontanum; when this occurs, it can partially or completely block the fetal urethra. This can lead to failure of normal development of the fetal kidney, which may lead to chronic renal failure, end stage renal disease, and the necessity for renal transplantation. Early detection and repair via cystoscopy is indicated. Severe cases may lead to total renal dysplasia, failure of pulmonary development (dependent on fetal renal function), and death in utero or shortly after birth.

CONGENITAL DISORDERS OF PENILE DEVELOPMENT

Hypospadias, a congenital abnormality of penile development, occurs when the urethral opening is located on the ventral side of the penis rather than at the tip of the glans. The abnormal location of the urethra may occur near the tip (leading to an abnormal urethral meatus) or further down the shaft (more proximal) near the scrotum. The defect results from abnormal fusion of the genital folds, which during the twelfth to sixteenth week of development form the shaft of the penis, and labioscrotal folds, which fuse to form the scrotum. (In the female, the process leads to formation of the clitoris and the nonfused labioscrotal folds form the labia minora and majora.) The condition is very common, occurring in about 1 in 250 male births. Surgical repair is generally done for both cosmetic and functional reasons. **Epispadias**, opening of the urethra on the dorsum of the penis, is far less common (about 1 in 25,000 births) and also occurs in females (as a bifid clitoris). The condition is most often associated with serious malformations of the bladder (extrophy, eversion of part of the bladder onto the abdominal wall).

Phimosis, the inability to retract the prepuce (foreskin) over the glans of the penis, is a physiologic condition occurring normally in newborn males. The condition is the result of adhesion between the epithelium of the foreskin and the glans and usually disappears with continued retraction and erection. The condition may persist in a small percentage of males over the age of sixteen and occasional requires corrective surgery, usually circumcision. Infection of the prepuce and head of the penis (balanitis) can also result in a secondary form of phimosis.

Posterior urethral valves (PUV) Most frequent developmental abnormality in the lower urinary tract of males.

Hypospadias A congenital abnormality of penile development.

Epispadias Opening of the urethra on the dorsum of the penis.

Phimosis The inability to retract the foreskin in newborn males.

CRYPTORCHIDISM

Cryptorchidism (*crypto* = hidden + *orchis* = testis), failure of descent of one or both testes, occurs in about 5 percent of term infants and persists through the first year in 20 percent of these infants. Most commonly the undescended testes is located in the inguinal or upper scrotal region. Surgical repair of the condition (orchioplexy) is critical because the condition is associated with oligospermia (a low sperm count), if one testis is affected, and complete lack of sperm (azoospermia), if both testes are undescended. Abnormalities of testicular development begin as early as two years of age, and early repair (between six months and one year) is recommended. In addition to infertility, a twenty to fortyfold increase in the rate of testicular cancer is associated with cryptorchidism. Surprisingly, a contralateral, normally descended testis is also at a fourfold increased risk. It is unclear if early surgical repair reduces the rate of such cancers. In contrast, the testosterone-producing interstitial cells of the cryptorchid testis are unaffected and will function normally at puberty when stimulated by gonadotropic hormones even though sperm production is no longer possible because the germ cells have been destroyed (**FIGURE 20-8**).

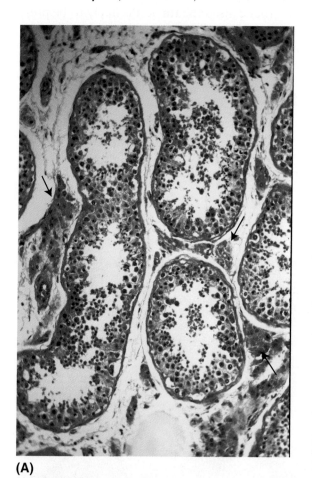
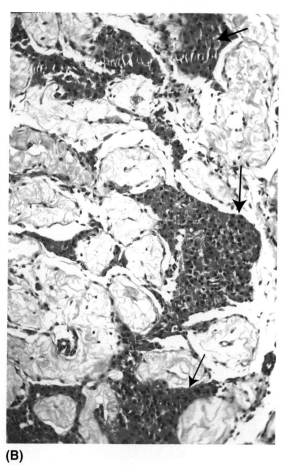

(A) **(B)**

FIGURE 20-8 Photomicrographs comparing a normal scrotal testis with an intra-abdominal testis. **(A)** Normal testis showing active spermatogenesis within testicular tubules. The clusters of cells between the tubules are interstitial cells (*arrows*). **(B)** Intra-abdominal testis, showing marked atrophy and fibrosis of testicular tubules. The large clusters of cells between the hyaline atrophic tubules (arrows) are interstitial cells, which function normally at body temperature. They appear quite prominent because of the marked tubular atrophy (original magnification ×160).

Courtesy of Leonard V. Crowley, MD, Century College.

TESTICULAR TORSION

If the fibrous tissue derived from the gubernaculum that attaches the testis to the scrotum is a relatively long and narrow band rather than a short broad attachment, the testis may undergo a rotary twist on its axis, which also twists the spermatic cord and interrupts the blood supply to the testis (**FIGURE 20-9A**). The thin-walled veins in the cord are compressed first, which impedes return of venous blood from the testis, but flow through the arteries continues for a time, leading to marked engorgement of the testis with blood, which is soon followed by complete hemorrhagic necrosis of the testis called a hemorrhagic infarction (**FIGURE 20-9B**). The condition may occur in the neonatal period (either in the fetus or soon after birth) where it is not associated with an anatomic defect. Adult testicular torsion is most common in adolescents but may occur at any age. A testicular torsion is characterized by an acute onset of severe testicular pain associated with swelling of the involved testis and is an acute surgical emergency. If the torsion can be untwisted and the testis is properly anchored in the scrotum within a few hours after onset of the torsion, the testis probably can be salvaged. The longer the delay, the less likely is the possibility that the testis will survive. Adult testicular torsion is associated with **bell-clapper defect**, an anatomic abnormality responsible for increased testicular mobility. Because the abnormal mobility of the testis within the scrotum that caused the torsion is likely to be present in the other testis as well, the other testis generally is surgically anchored in the scrotum so that it cannot undergo torsion.

Bell-clapper defect Anatomic abnormality responsible for increased testicular mobility.

Scrotal Abnormalities

HYDROCELE

Normally the saclike tunica vaginalis contains only a very small amount of fluid (**FIGURE 20-10A**), but when a much larger amount of fluid accumulates in the sac, a

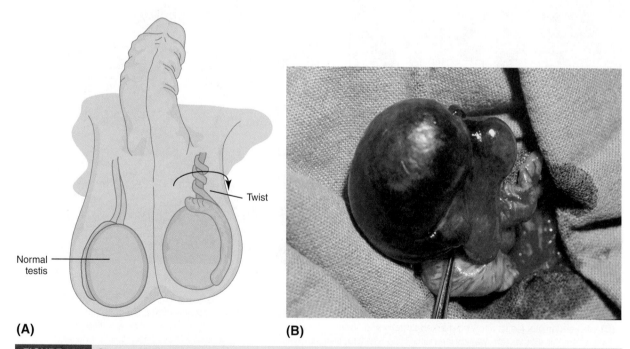

(A)   **(B)**

FIGURE 20-9 Cause and effect of testicular torsion. **(A)** Rotary twist of testis also twists spermatic cord, interrupting blood supply to the testis. Normally, the epididymis is located along the posterior surface of the testis, but the torsion has rotated the testis and also rotated the epididymis anteriorly. **(B)** Hemorrhagic infarction of testis caused by torsion.

Courtesy of Leonard V. Crowley, MD, Century College.

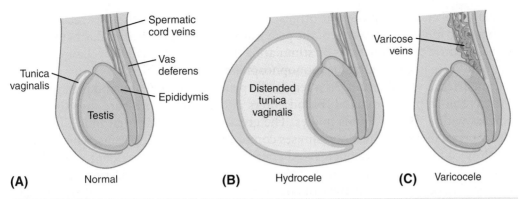

FIGURE 20-10 **(A)** Normal tunica vaginalis containing a small amount of fluid. **(B)** Hydrocele. **(C)** Varicocele.

hydrocele (*hydro* = water + *cele* = swelling) results (**FIGURE 20-10B**). The condition may be congenital or result from trauma, infection, or other causes. Although this usually does not require therapy, the scrotal swelling may be uncomfortable. Long-standing hydrocele can cause testicular atrophy and may require surgical excision of the sac. When a physician examines a patient believed to have a hydrocele, a careful examination of the testis and scrotum is also performed, which may be supplemented by an ultrasound examination to exclude the possibility of a testicular tumor or some other condition associated with the hydrocele.

> **Hydrocele** An accumulation of excess fluid within the tunica vaginalis of the testis.
>
> **Varicocele** Varicose veins that develop within the spermatic cord veins.

VARICOCELE

The term **varicocele** (*varix* = dilated vein + *cele* = swelling) refers to varicose veins that develop within the spermatic cord veins that drain blood from the testis, caused by failure of the vein valves to function properly and allowing for backflow, pooling of blood, and veinous dilation (**FIGURE 20-10C**). Varicose veins form in a similar fashion in other locations, as described in the cardiovascular system. When the scrotum is examined while the patient is standing, the scrotal varicose veins located above the testis are sometimes described as "feeling like a bag full of worms." When the patient lies down, blood drains easily from the veins and the varicocele can no longer be felt. Generally, a varicocele does not cause symptoms. However, varicoceles may occasionally reduce fertility by impairing spermatogenesis, possibly as result of the higher scrotal temperature caused by warm venous blood pooling in the varicose scrotal veins. A varicocele can be treated surgically if it causes scrotal discomfort or impairs fertility. Otherwise no treatment is required.

Erectile Dysfunction

PHYSIOLOGY OF PENILE ERECTION

The penis consists primarily of three cavernous bodies, which are cylinders of extremely vascular erectile tissue; two laterally placed corpora cavernosa; and the midline corpus spongiosum that surrounds the penile urethra. Each cylinder, surrounded by a thick fibrous tissue capsule, is composed of a spongy meshwork of endothelium-lined blood sinuses supported by trabeculae (partitions) composed of connective tissue and smooth muscle. The blood sinuses of the erectile tissue are supplied by arteries and drained by veins. Normally, the arteries are constricted and very little blood flows into the cavernous bodies, and the vascular sinuses are collapsed. During sexual excitement parasympathetic nerve impulses arising from the sacral part of the spinal cord release the neurotransmitter nitric oxide, which causes relaxation of the smooth muscle in the walls of the penile arteries and in the trabeculae between the sinuses. Nitric oxide functions by stimulating the enzyme guanylate cyclase, resulting in an increase in cyclic guanine monophosphate (cGMP), which plays an important role in arterial vasodilation. As a result, the penile arteries dilate, and the sinuses in the cavernous bodies expand. Blood enters under arterial pressure into the blood sinuses within the cavernous bodies. The greatly increased arterial blood flow and rising pressure within the blood sinuses compresses the draining veins, which retards outflow of blood from the penis and contributes to the engorgement of the blood sinuses. The penis rapidly becomes rigid and erect (**FIGURE 20-11**). Detumescence (loss of erection) occurs by activation of adrenergic nerves producing vasoconstriction of penile vessels Additionally, phosphodiesterases hydrolyse the cGMP to an inactive form and plays a role in detumescence.

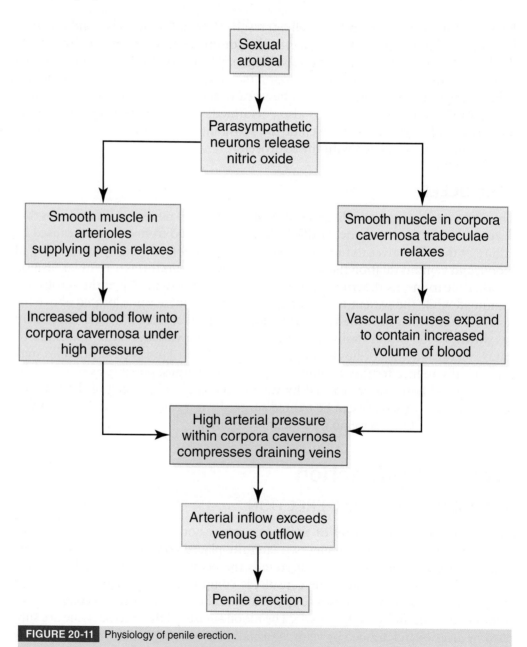

FIGURE 20-11 Physiology of penile erection.

Erectile dysfunction is an inability to achieve and maintain a penile erection of sufficient rigidity to penetrate the vagina and maintain the erection during sexual intercourse. This is a relatively common problem that increases in frequency with advancing age. Penile erection is a complex process. First, sexual desire is required to initiate the physiologic events that increase blood flow to the penis. Second, the arteries supplying the cavernous bodies must dilate enough to deliver a large volume of blood to the penis. Third, the pressure of the blood within the cavernous bodies must be sufficiently high to compress the draining veins. Blood must flow into the penis faster than it drains out, or an erection cannot be maintained.

CAUSES OF ERECTILE DYSFUNCTION

To achieve and sustain a penile erection, the sensory, motor, and autonomic nerve supply to the penis must be normal, and the blood vessels supplying the penis must be able to deliver an adequate volume of blood to the penis. Various factors may disturb these physiologic processes. These include a low testosterone level, which inhibits sexual desire and arousal; damage to the nerves supplying the penis, resulting from radical prostate surgery or neurologic diseases; impaired blood supply to the penis, resulting from arteriosclerosis of the blood vessels that deliver blood to the penis; effect of drugs used to treat hypertension that target the autonomic nervous system, which also affects the autonomic nerves supplying the penis; or effect of stress, emotional factors, or chronic illnesses, which may impair the person's quality of life and also adversely affect sexual performance.

TREATMENT

Both medical and surgical procedures can be used to treat erectile dysfunction, depending on the cause and patient's preference. One well-known treatment involves the use of drugs that inhibit phosphodiesterase and promote increased blood flow to the penis. Several phosphodiesterase inhibiting drugs are available (sildenafil, vardenafil, tadalafil) and differ primarily in their duration of action. They are relatively safe drugs when used properly, but rarely may be associated with serious complications. The best known of these drugs is sildenafil, better known by its trade name Viagra.

CASE 20-1

The patient is an eighteen-year-old male who visits his physician at the urging of his girlfriend. She has noted bilateral enlargement of his breasts and is concerned that he might have breast cancer. The physician confirms nontender gynecomastia (breast enlargement in a male). The patient states that he has had mild dyspnea (shortness of breath) for about a month. On questioning he notes that he has had a painless mass in the right testis in the last several months. His history is also pertinent; he had cryptorchidism that was surgically repaired at twenty-four months. He does not know which testis was cryptorchid. The physician confirms a painless hard right testicular mass by palpation with otherwise normal male genitalia showing obvious distortion visible through the scrotum. Questionable supraclavicular lymphadenopathy (enlargement of the lymph nodes above the clavicle) is also noted. The physician orders laboratory tests for hCG (chorionic gonadotrophin) and AFP (alpha fetoprotein), both of which are positive. The physician refers the patient to a urologist who performs testicular ultrasound and notes that a "fluffy" density has replaced much of the right testis. The left testis appears normal. A chest x-ray shows multiple lesions consistent with metastatic disease. The patient undergoes orchiectomy of the right testis.

(continues)

CASE 20-1 *(Continued)*

Histopathological examination of the testis discloses a nonseminomatous germ cell tumor (NSGCT) described as a teratocarcinoma (malignant teratoma). The patient has high stage disease with pulmonary metastases. After undergoing several cycles of chemotherapy using platinum-based agents, he has been disease free for three years.

Discussion

About 50 percent of all germ cell tumors of the testes are NSGCTs, and about two-thirds of these are teratocarcinomas. The tumors are believed to derive from embryonal carcinoma cells that have differentiated into a mixture of mature looking tissues normally found in a variety of organs (**FIGURE 20-12**). These tumors are often "mixed" and also contain embryonal cells that are not differentiated and maintain malignant potential.

It is of interest that the mature appearing cells (as shown in Figure 20-12) may survive chemotherapy, whereas the malignant embryonal component forming metastases is eliminated. In fact, there is an excellent potential for cure even in advanced stage disease. The presence of gynecomastia can be physiological and is a common transient finding in pubertal boys. However, the occurrence of gynecomastia should prompt examination for testicular tumors. Between 5 and 10 percent of testicular germ cell tumor patients will show gynecomastia. Over 70 percent of NSGCTs secrete hCG or AFP. The hCG molecule shares components with a number of other human hormones. hCG tends to increase the level of the female hormone estrogen more than that of testosterone, and the increased ration of the former to the latter results in gynecomastia.

Etiology and Pathogenesis

Nonseminiferous germ cell tumor (NSGCT) of the subclass containing mixed differentiated tissue components (malignant teratoma) with metastatic disease to lymph nodes and lungs. Gynecomastia related to production of hCG by the tumor.

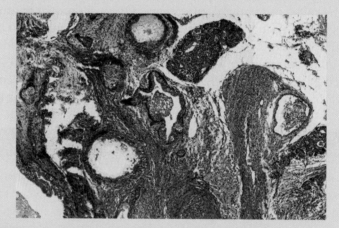

FIGURE 20-12 Nonseminomatous germ cell tumor (NSGCT) of teratocarcinoma type. Tumor shows a mixture of mature appearing tissue elements.

Courtesy of Department of Pathology and Laboratory Medicine, University of North Carolina at Chapel Hill.

Questions

1. Considering that testicular cancer is uncommon and quite curable, propose a simple screening protocol for early detection of this disease.

2. Propose a likely mechanism for the secretion of hCG by embryonal tumors.

3. Assume you are a male of forty years of age with no prior family history of prostatic cancer. Your doctor suggests screening for this disease. (A) What tests is your doctor likely to perform? (B) Your test results are of "borderline significance" for the presence of prostatic cancer. What tests is your physician likely to suggest? (C) Would you agree to the testing procedure? Support the logic of your answer.

QUESTIONS FOR REVIEW

1. What are the components of the male reproductive system?
2. What is benign prostatic hyperplasia? What are its clinical manifestations? How is it treated?
3. How does administration of female sex hormones affect prostatic carcinoma? What is the effect of castration on prostatic carcinoma?
4. A young man has a positive pregnancy test. Under what circumstances could this occur?
5. What factors predispose to the development of carcinoma of the penis? How may the disease be prevented?
6. What is cryptorchidism? What are the clinical manifestations? How is the condition treated? Why should it be treated?
7. What is a testicular torsion? What are its manifestations and complications? How is the condition treated?
8. A young man has an undescended testis within the abdomen. How does this affect testicular function? What complications may result from this condition?

SUPPLEMENTARY READINGS

Loeffler, A. G., and Hart, M. N. 2015. *Introduction to Human Disease*. 6th ed. Burlington, MA: Jones & Bartlett Learning.
▶ Those interested in the detailed study of male reproductive disease should consult a work on human pathology aimed at the undergraduate medical curriculum. However, a good place to start at a less advanced level is by reading Chapter 16 in this book.

Simmons, M. N., Berglund, R. K., and Jones, S. J. 2011. A practical guide to prostate cancer diagnosis and management. *Cleveland Clinic Journal of Medicine 78*:321–31.

Ilic, D., Neuberger, I. D., Djulbegovic, M., and Dahm, P. 2013. Screening for prostate cancer (Review). Wiley Online Library. The Cochrane Collaboration. doi: 10.1002/14651858.CD004720.pub3

Hayes, J. H., and Barry, M. J. 2014. Screening for prostate cancer with prostate-specific antigen test. A review of current literature. *JAMA 311*:1143–49.
▶ One of the more controversial areas in urology is the appropriate role of prostate cancer screening. The first reference represents a conservative point of view for both diagnosis and therapy. The second entry provides a book-length review (see pages 1–9 for a brief review aimed at nontechnical readers). Both the second and third entries provide exhaustive of the literature with results that suggest little or no benefit for most groups of men (as measured in reduced deaths as a result of prostate cancer) using current approaches to screening.

Presner, J. R., et al. 2012. Beyond PSA: The next generation of prostate cancer biomarkers. *Science Translational Medicine 4*:(127).
▶ This article provides is an excellent overview of current prospects in the field of prostate cancer research.

Hanna, N. H., and Einhorn, L. H. 2014. Testicular cancer—Discoveries and updates. *New England Journal of Medicine 371*:2005–16.
▶ This article provides a recent overview of testicular cancer emphasizing therapy.

Lin, K., and Sharangpani, R. 2010. Screening for testicular cancer: An evidence review for the U.S. Preventive Service Task Force. *Annals of Internal Medicine 153*:396–99.
▶ Screening for testicular cancer would seem to be a "no-brainer," but somewhat surprisingly that may not be so. This is a thought-provoking reading.

Crawford, P., and Crop, J. A. 2014. Evaluation of scrotal masses. *American Family Physician 89*:723–27.

▶ This review covers multiple medical aspects of the diagnosis of scrotal masses.

Bing, Z., and Bai, S. 2012. Gynecomastia: An uncommon but important clinical manifestation for testicular tumors. *Open Journal of Pathology 2*:6–13.

▶ This reading reviews gynecomastia in relation to testicular tumors and was useful in constructing the Case for this chapter.

The Liver and the Biliary System

LEARNING OBJECTIVES

1. Describe the normal structure and function of the liver, and explain how they relate to major liver diseases.

2. List the major causes of liver injury, and describe their effects on hepatic function.

3. Compare the three major types of viral hepatitis in terms of their pathogenesis, incubation period, incidence of complications, and frequency of carriers. Explain the diagnostic tests used to

identify each type of viral infection, and describe methods of prevention.

4. Explain the adverse effects of excess alcohol intake on liver structure and function.

5. Explain how gallstones are formed, and describe their causes and effects.

6. Compare the three major causes of jaundice.

Structure and Function of the Liver

The liver, the largest organ in the body, has a roughly triangular shape and is located beneath the diaphragm in the upper abdomen (**FIGURE 21-1**). Its many functions include the following:

- Storage of glycogen, iron, copper, triglycerides, and lipid-soluble vitamins such as B_{12}.
- Synthesis of certain serum proteins including albumin, proteins important in coagulation and inflammation, and binding proteins for many of the substances stored.
- Metabolism of glucose and free fatty acids.
- Catabolism of both endogenous substances such as hormones and exogenous toxic agents. The liver also removes ammonia derived from amino acid breakdown.
- Excretion and production of bile.

The liver has a double blood supply. About 70 percent of the blood flow is provided by the portal vein, which drains the spleen and gastrointestinal tract. Portal blood is rich in nutrients absorbed from the intestines but low in oxygen content. The rest of the blood, which comes from the hepatic artery, has a high oxygen content but is low in nutrients. Blood flowing from the hepatic artery and the portal vein travel

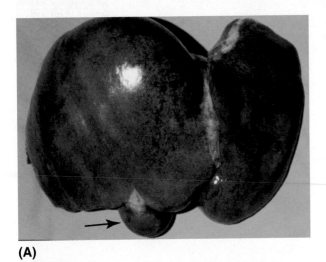

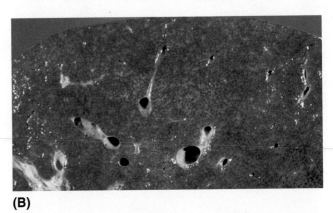

(A)

(B)

FIGURE 21-1 **(A)** A normal liver viewed from above to show its superior and anterior surfaces. The gallbladder is located on the undersurface of the liver, and the fundus of the gallbladder projects slightly beyond the anterior edge of the liver (*arrow*). **(B)** Section of liver illustrating the uniform appearance of the hepatic parenchyma and the large blood vessels (branches of the portal vein) transporting blood into the liver from the gastrointestinal tract.

Courtesy of Leonard V. Crowley, MD, Century College.

Portal tract/triad Branch of hepatic artery, portal vein, and bile duct located at periphery of liver lobule.

Liver lobule A histologic subdivision of the liver in which columns of liver cells converge toward a central vein and portal tracts are located at the periphery.

Bile canaliculi Small terminal bile channels located between liver cords.

together and mixes as the blood flows through the liver and is eventually collected into the right and left hepatic veins, which drain into the inferior vena cava.

The liver cells are arranged in the form of long, wide plates interconnected at angles to form a lattice. The hepatic sinusoids occupy the spaces between the plates (**FIGURE 21-2A**). Branches of the hepatic artery, portal vein, bile ducts, and lymphatic vessels travel together within the liver and are called the **portal tracts**, or **triads** (**FIGURE 21-2B**). The terminal branches of both the hepatic artery and the portal vein discharge their blood into the hepatic sinusoids (**FIGURE 21-2C**). In histologic sections, the liver plates appear as cords surrounded on each side by sinusoids that converge toward the central veins. The portal tracts appear at the periphery. This anatomic configuration, which is called a **liver lobule**, is illustrated diagrammatically in **FIGURE 21-3A**.

Blood flow in the liver is from portal tracts through the sinusoids into central veins (**FIGURE 21-3B**). Consequently, the liver cells nearest the portal tracts receive the most oxygen and nutrients, with those nearest the central veins much less well supplied. Because of their relatively poor nutritional state and lower degree of oxygenation, the liver cells nearest the central veins are more vulnerable to injury from toxic agents or circulatory disturbances, as occurs in shock and heart failure, than are the cells nearer the portal tracts.

The small terminal bile channels, called **bile canaliculi**, are located between adjacent liver cords and drain into the bile ducts traveling in the portal tracts. The direction of the bile flow is opposite that of the blood flow in the sinusoids (Figure 21-3B). The bile ducts gradually converge to form larger ducts, which finally unite as the large right and left hepatic ducts. The two hepatic ducts join to form the common hepatic duct. The gallbladder joins the common hepatic duct by means of the cystic duct to form the common bile duct that enters the duodenum (**FIGURE 21-4**).

Causes and Effects of Liver Injury

The liver is vulnerable to injury by many agents including viral infection, excess consumption of alcohol, and many toxic agents and drugs. Histologically, liver injury

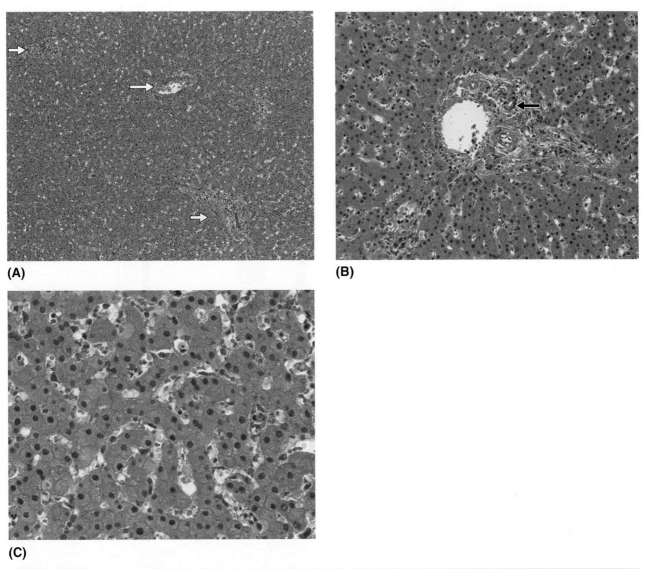

(A)

(B)

(C)

FIGURE 21-2 Photomicrographs showing the cellular structure of a normal liver. **(A)** Low-magnification photomicrograph illustrating plates of liver cells, which appear as cords in histologic sections, and sinusoids between cords, which drain into central veins (*arrows*). Short arrow indicates portal triads. **(B)** Higher magnification illustrating portal tract. Branch of hepatic artery is below the bile duct (*arrow*), and branch of portal vein is left and below bile duct. **(C)** High magnification of liver cell cords and hepatic sinusoids. Sinusoids show some residual blood cells.

Courtesy of Department of Pathology and Laboratory Medicine, University of North Carolina at Chapel Hill.

may be manifested by necrosis or apoptosis of liver cells, by accumulation of fat within the liver cell cytoplasm, or by a combination of the two. Some injurious agents primarily cause cell necrosis or apoptosis, whereas others chiefly induce fatty change in liver cells.

Many times, the exact cause and extent of liver disease in a given patient is difficult to determine. In such cases, a biopsy of the liver can be performed by inserting a needle through the skin directly into the liver and extracting a small bit of liver tissue. This can be examined microscopically by the pathologist to diagnose the nature and severity of the liver disease.

The effect of hepatic injury depends on the extent of damage induced by the injurious agent. If liver injury is mild, the liver cells will regenerate and recover, restoring liver function to normal. Fortunately, this is the usual outcome. If the injury is extremely severe, large amounts of liver tissue are completely destroyed, and not

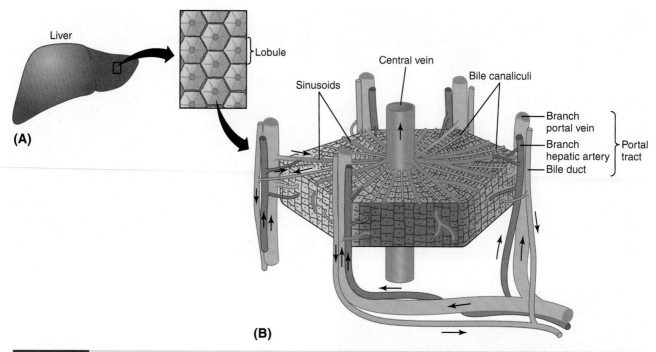

FIGURE 21-3 **(A)** Concept of liver lobule, consisting of cords of cells radiating toward central vein with portal tracts at periphery. Lobules are outlined in diagram. **(B)** Blood flow in sinusoids toward central vein; flow of bile toward portal tract.

enough liver may remain to sustain life. If the patient does survive, healing of the severe injury may be associated with severe scarring (postnecrotic scarring), and liver function may never return to normal. Multiple episodes of relatively mild liver injury may have a cumulative effect, leading to scarring (fibrosis) and permanent

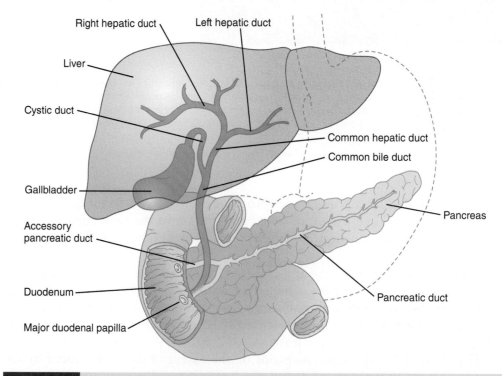

FIGURE 21-4 Anatomy of the biliary duct system. Right and left hepatic ducts form the common hepatic duct, which is joined by the cystic duct to form the common bile duct, which opens into the duodenum along with the pancreatic duct through a common channel.

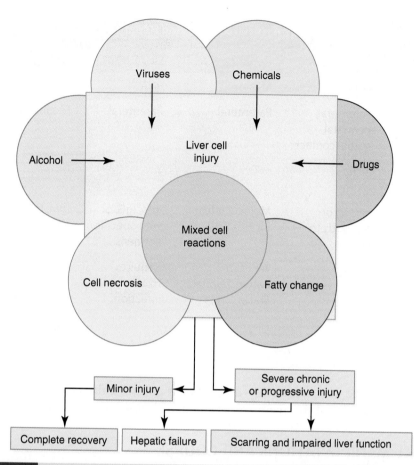

FIGURE 21-5 Summary of causes and effects of liver injury. Many agents can cause injury to liver cells, manifested either as fatty change, necrosis, or a combination of both. Mild injury is followed by complete recovery. Severe, chronic, or progressive injury may lead to hepatic failure or diffuse scarring with impaired hepatic function.

impairment of liver function. Similarly, any chronic or progressive injury may cause scarring and impairment of function (**FIGURE 21-5**).

Clinically, the most common types of liver disease characterized by injury to liver cells are viral hepatitis or injury associated with consuming excessive amounts of alcoholic beverages (**alcoholic liver disease**). Nonalcoholic fatty liver disease (NAFLD) associated with obesity and impaired glucose metabolism and insulin resistance (termed the **metabolic syndrome**) has become the most common cause of chronic liver disease as a result of increasing levels of obesity in the Western population. Chronic liver cell injury from any cause may in turn be followed by diffuse scarring throughout the liver, which is called **cirrhosis of the liver**.

Viral Hepatitis

The term viral **hepatitis** applies to several clinically similar infections that result in inflammation and necrosis. Hepatitis A, B, and C (HAV, HBV, and HCV) account for almost all cases of viral hepatitis in the United States and Europe. Two additional types of viral hepatitis also have been identified: hepatitis D or delta hepatitis, which occurs in people already infected with the hepatitis B virus, and hepatitis E, which is found primarily in developing countries and is infrequently encountered in North America. HBV and HCV can lead to chronic infection, which is associated with cirrhosis and liver cancer. It is estimated that half a billion people have these chronic infections, which result in 60 percent of cirrhosis and 75 percent of primary liver

Alcoholic liver disease Injury associated with excessive amounts of alcohol.

Nonalcoholic fatty liver disease (NAFLD) Fatty liver without significant inflammation or scarring within the liver, which usually occurs in insulin-resistant obese people with lipid abnormalities.

Metabolic syndrome A syndrome characterized by obesity and insulin resistance often associated with nonalcoholic fatty liver disease.

Cirrhosis of the liver A disease characterized by diffuse intrahepatic scarring and circulatory disturbance within the liver.

Hepatitis Inflammation of the liver.

TABLE 21-1   Comparison of Viruses Most Commonly Associated with Viral Hepatitis

Virus	Hepatitis A	Hepatitis B	Hepatitis C	Hepatitis D	Hepatitis E
Type	RNA	DNA	RNA	RNA	RNA
Route of transmission	Fecal–oral	Parenteral, perinatal, sexual contact	Parenteral	Parenteral	Fecal–oral
Chronic liver disease	Never	10%	~80%	5%	Never
Diagnosis	IgM	HBsAg or antibody to HBcAg	Molecular test for HCV RNA	IgM, IgG, or viral-specific antigens	IgM, IgG, or viral-specific antigens
Highest prevalence	Rural areas with poor sanitation and hygiene	Asia	Western nations, United States	Requires HBV for infection	Zoonotic reservoir; India
Fatality	<1%				Highest in pregnant women

cancer cases. Hence, viral hepatitis is a significant public health concern worldwide. The overall properties of the agents of viral hepatitis are summarized in **TABLE 21-1.**

CLINICAL MANIFESTATIONS AND COURSE

All of the hepatitis viruses produce similar histologic changes in the liver, characterized by diffuse inflammation throughout the liver lobules associated with liver cell swelling and necrosis of scattered individual liver cells or cells in small groups. Apoptotic cell death characterized by cell shrinkage and dark red color (termed **Councilman** or **apoptotic bodies**) is also seen (**FIGURE 21-6A**). When the acute disease is

Councilman/apoptotic bodies Cell shrinkage/apoptotic cell death in inflammation of the liver.

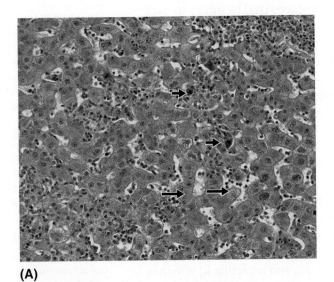

(A)

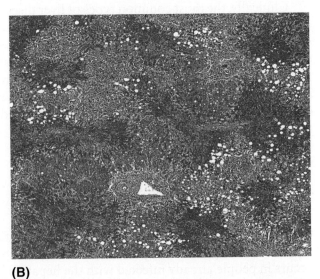

(B)

FIGURE 21-6 **(A)** Acute viral hepatitis. Cords of liver cells have lost their orderly arrangement and appear disrupted by swelling of liver cells (*arrows*), necrosis of individual cells, and scattered aggregates of inflammatory cells throughout the liver lobules. Apoptotic bodies are visible as condensed intensely red cells (*short arrows*). **(B)** Confluent hepatic necrosis showing geographic areas of hemorrhage and necrosis throughout the liver.

Courtesy of Department of Pathology and Laboratory Medicine, University of North Carolina at Chapel Hill.

severe (most commonly in HBV infection), confluent areas of the liver may undergo necrosis that may result in destruction of essentially all hepatocytes and collapse of the liver (**FIGURE 21-6B**). The clinical manifestations of acute viral hepatitis are variable and correlate with the degree of liver cell injury and associated inflammation. Some affected individuals experience loss of appetite, feel ill, become jaundiced, and have abnormal laboratory tests. Others become ill, and their laboratory tests are abnormal, but they never become jaundiced. This condition is called **anicteric hepatitis** (*ana* = without + *icterus* = jaundice). Still others have few symptoms and do not seek medical attention, but laboratory tests reveal liver injury. Their infection, which could easily escape detection, is sometimes called **subclinical hepatitis**. Despite the absence of symptoms, these individuals can transmit the infection to others.

The outcome of viral hepatitis depends primarily on which virus caused the infection. Many cases of hepatitis caused by the hepatitis A virus (HAV) are quite mild, and patients recover completely without complications. An unfavorable outcome occurs in only a very small percentage of cases. In contrast, people infected with hepatitis B virus (HBV) or hepatitis C virus (HCV) may become chronic carriers of the virus and develop chronic progressive hepatitis that eventually leads to cirrhosis and liver failure.

HEPATITIS A

Hepatitis A virus (HAV) is an RNA-containing virus measuring 27 nm (1 nanometer, abbreviated nm, equals one-billionth of a meter). Hepatitis A has a relatively short incubation period that varies from two to six weeks. The virus is excreted in oropharyngeal (nose and throat) secretions and in the stools during the late-incubation period and for about two weeks after the onset of symptoms. Transmission is by direct person-to-person contact or by fecal contamination of food or water. Food- or waterborne infections may occur in epidemics. The infection is self-limited, and there are no chronic carriers of the virus.

Antibodies to hepatitis A virus, which appear in the blood after recovery, provide immunity against hepatitis A virus but not against other hepatitis viruses. Hepatitis A is a common infection in the United States, and almost half the adult population has antibodies against the virus. A highly effective inactivated hepatitis A vaccine has been available since 1995 and is recommended to immunize people at relatively high risk of becoming infected, such as health care workers who have frequent contact with infected patients or people traveling in foreign countries where there is a high incidence of hepatitis A in the population. Although not universally required, many physicians recommend routine immunization of children (often given in combination with vaccination for hepatitis B). Increased levels of immunization have led to a marked decrease in hepatitis A in the United States. If an unvaccinated individual is exposed to hepatitis A (as may occur if a restaurant worker is found to have the disease), hepatitis immune globulin containing antibodies to HAV can prevent infection if given within two weeks of exposure.

HEPATITIS B

Hepatitis B virus (HBV) is a DNA-containing virus measuring 42 nm, somewhat larger than the hepatitis A virus, and is composed of an inner core and an outer surface envelope. The core contains a partially double stranded circle of DNA and an enzyme (DNA polymerase) enclosed within a protein shell. The inner protein shell forms the **hepatitis B core antigen (HBcAg)**. The same gene that codes for the core antigen also produces a somewhat longer protein that forms the **hepatitis E antigen (HBeAg)**. Continued presence of HBeAg in the blood of an infected person is a marker

Anicteric hepatitis Symptoms of hepatitis without appearance of jaundice.

Subclinical hepatitis Liver inflammation resulting in few symptoms.

Hepatitis B core antigen (HBcAg) The antigen contained in the core of the hepatitis B virus.

Hepatitis E antigen (HBeAg) Antigen associated with active hepatitis B virus proliferation.

for continued viral replication and indicates continued infectivity and likely chronic infection. The outer surface envelope is composed of lipid and glycoproteins, the latter of which constitutes the **hepatitis B surface antigen (HBsAg)**. The viral core and surface envelope together form the complete virus particle, which is often called the Dane particle after the pathologist who first described it.

The clinical features of HBV infection are indistinguishable from those of HAV although HBV has a longer incubation period, which varies from two weeks to six months. Also, unlike hepatitis A, HBV disease can progress in several patterns. Initial HBV infection may be asymptomatic in 50 percent of cases or can produce an acute hepatitis that may end in viral clearance and recovery or may (uncommonly) result in fulminant hepatitis with liver necrosis. Acute hepatitis may not result in viral clearance but rather in a chronic disease state that may, in turn, progress to cirrhosis. Some chronic carriers may be asymptomatic but nevertheless are infectious. Also HBV-induced chronic liver disease is associated with the development of liver cancer (hepatocellular carcinoma).

The host immune response to HBV is the major factor in the course of disease. The virus does not directly cause hepatocyte injury. In chronic disease, the host T cell response to virally infected cells does not eliminate the virus but continually damages host liver cells, resulting in scarring and cirrhosis (**FIGURE 21-7**).

When an individual becomes infected, the virus invades the liver and multiplies within the hepatic cells. The core of the virus is produced in the cell nucleus, and the surface antigen is produced in the cytoplasm. For some unexplained reason, much more surface antigen is produced within the infected cells than is necessary to coat the virus particles, and the large excess is released into the bloodstream, where it can be detected by laboratory tests. Such blood is called surface-antigen (HBsAg) positive. Although the laboratory tests detect only the surface antigen, HBsAg-positive blood is infectious because it also contains complete virus particles.

Serological testing of blood is critical in the diagnosis of HBV infection and in charting the progress of the disease. In the course of an infection, HBsAg appears during the incubation period and can be detected during the first few weeks. It is

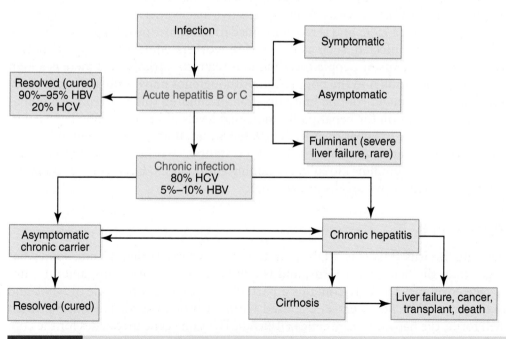

FIGURE 21-7 Natural history of hepatitis B and C infections.

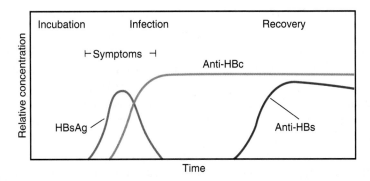

FIGURE 21-8 Acute HBV infection and recovery, illustrating serial changes of major antigens and antibodies used to aid in the diagnosis of HBV infection and monitor its course. Serial changes in HBeAg and anti-HBe are not shown. HBeAg rises along with HBsAg during active infection, and anti-HBe appears along with anti-HBc during recovery.

a marker for the infectious state of the patient. Normally, it does not persist in the blood for more than two or three weeks and disappears during convalescence. Antibody to the surface antigen (anti-HBs) then begins to appear and provides lifelong immunity to future infections. Antibody to the viral core (anti-HBc) appears early in the course of infection and does not provide future immunity. Antibody to HBe generally indicates clearance of the virus and recovery. However, some patients with these antibodies have persistent chronic infection (**FIGURE 21-8**). Many people possess antibodies against the virus as a result of deliberate immunization or as a result of prior infection. Unlike infection, immunization results only in antibodies to HBsAg (not HBc or HBe) because the vaccine contains a recombinant form of pure HBsAg.

Most infected individuals eliminate the virus from the bloodstream in a few weeks and recover completely, but about 10 percent become chronic carriers of the virus. Some of the carriers develop chronic hepatitis, which results in progressive liver damage. About 0.5 percent of the U.S. population are asymptomatic chronic carriers of the virus although the rate may be as high as 20 percent in some areas of the world. In these areas, the high rate is a result of maternal transmission to the infant at birth. Overall, it is estimated that more than 350 million people worldwide are infected with the hepatitis B virus, and about 1 million people die each year of complications of the disease. Although the availability (and often mandatory nature) of childhood immunization to HBV has drastically cut the number of cases seen in the United States, it is estimated that more than 20,000 acute cases of the disease occur per year and that about 1 million individuals have chronic disease.

The highest levels of hepatitis B virus are found in blood with lower levels being present in semen and saliva. The virus is not excreted in stool, tears, sweat, and urine. Consequently, transmission does not occur by means of contaminated food or water. HBV infections result only from mucosal or parenteral contact with the blood or body fluids of HBsAg-positive individuals. In the United States, the most common route of transmission is by heterosexual or homosexual (MSM) contact. Presumably the MSM population acquire the disease from virus-bearing semen in contact with abraded rectal mucosa. Infection via direct deliberate therapeutic infusion of contaminated blood products (blood transfusions, for example) no longer occurs as a result of careful donor blood screening procedures. However, health care workers are still at risk as a result of accidental contact with contaminated material or surfaces as are intravenous drug abusers. High-risk sexual behavior and intravenous drug use accounts for 80 percent of all new cases of hepatitis B in the United States. One year of IV drug use results in a 40-percent risk of infection; ten years of use brings the risk to 80 percent. In areas of the world with high levels of chronic infection, perinatal infection is the most common mechanism for transmission. Over 70 percent of infants born to mothers who are HBsAg- and HBeAg-positive become infected, and almost all of these infections will be chronic. Immediate treatment of these children at birth with vaccine and antibody containing hepatitis B immune globulin reduces the risk to under 15 percent. Pretreatment of the mother with antiviral agents or immune globulin may further reduce the risk.

As noted previously, hepatitis B immune globulin provides good protection if administered promptly after exposure to the virus. Several antiviral drugs are available that can suppress viral multiplication and slow disease progression in people with chronic disease. These drugs are used in combination with a type of interferon that helps the immune system clear the virus. However, vigorous use of childhood vaccination provides the best way of reducing the population burden of the disease.

HEPATITIS C

The hepatitis C virus is an 80-nm RNA virus that is transmitted by infected blood and body fluids, as is HBV. There are six serologic types and a number of subtypes, which differ in their response to treatment. Type 1 is both the most common (infecting 50 to 60 percent of U.S. patients) and the most resistant to treatment and is associated with more severe liver disease and a higher risk of chronicity. In many ways, HCV infection is an even more serious problem than HBV infection. HCV is the major cause of chronic liver disease in the United States, accounting for 40 percent of reported cases. It has surpassed AIDS/HIV as a cause of death. Seventy-five percent of HCV-infected individuals are unable to eliminate the virus and become chronic carriers; of these, between 20 percent and 50 percent will develop cirrhosis with a potential result of liver failure. Between 10 percent and 20 percent of patients will develop hepatocellular carcinoma. It is estimated that over 1 percent of the population are chronic carriers of the virus with infectious blood and body fluids. In some countries, the rate of infection is higher, over 6 percent in Africa and over 20 percent in Egypt.

There are no agents like immune globulin that can protect an uninfected person who has been exposed to the virus, for example, from an accidental needle stick when drawing blood from an infected person. The HCV uses an RNA-dependent RNA polymerase during replication, which is prone to making errors. This results in a high rate of natural mutation. One of the envelope proteins of the virus (E2) is particularly prone to mutating, most likely because of selective pressure from antibodies developed by the infected host to the virus. The virus changes rapidly enough that the immune system cannot effectively eliminate it. Thus, no immunizing agent is available that can be used to establish an active immunity against the virus, and none is likely to be developed in the near future.

HCV-infected persons may experience symptoms of hepatitis, as previously described, but most infected individuals have few symptoms of infection and those that occur are often not related to the liver. For example, joint and muscle aches, itching, and paresthesias (unusual sensations such as "pins and needles" relating to peripheral nerve damage) are common, and some may not even know that they have become infected. Infected people develop antibodies against HCV, usually within two months of infection, that remain during the chronic phase of the disease. Viral RNA, a measure of virus particles in the circulation, is an indication of continuing infection, and the amount of viral RNA can be measured in the blood of infected people to monitor the course of the disease. In addition to liver disease, individuals with chronic HCV infection suffer from a wide variety of extrahepatic diseases, many of which are believed to be autoimmune in nature and possibly related to the chronic but ineffective immune response to the virus.

In the past, many HCV infections followed transfusion of HCV-infected blood or blood products. Modern ultrasensitive molecular testing techniques reduce the risk to about 1 in 100,000 units. However, many of those currently suffering chronic disease were infected prior to this testing. Currently, most new HCV infections are acquired from infected blood or body fluids in much the same ways that HBV is acquired. The Centers for Disease Control and Prevention estimates that about 60 percent of HCV infections occur in injection drug users who share virus-contaminated needles. In 20 percent of cases, the infection was acquired by sexual contact, although HCV is not as readily transmitted sexually as HBV. About 10 percent of cases result from other types of blood and body fluid exposures, such as household contacts, infections associated with hemodialysis treatment, occupational exposures of health care workers, and virus transmission from mother to infant during childbirth. In another 10 percent of cases, the source of infection could not be determined. Recently the U.S. Preventative Services Task Force has recommended that all baby-boomers (those born between 1945 and 1965) should been screened a single time for HCV infection.

Because of the potential late complications of HCV infection, all HCV-positive individuals are considered for therapy to reduce viral load and to eliminate the virus. Acute HCV infection responds well to prolonged interferon therapy. Those who have chronic hepatitis, as demonstrated by abnormal liver function tests, viral RNA in their blood, and any liver biopsy demonstrating chronic inflammation in the liver are treated with drugs that inhibit viral multiplication and hence prevent progression to cirrhosis. Therapy significantly reduces the risk of progression of disease and of death. The preferred treatment is an antiviral compound called ribavirin, combined with interferon or a modification of interferon (called pegylated interferon) that has a more prolonged antiviral action. This mode of therapy is effective less than half the time with HCV type 1 infections. Fortunately, treatment has improved with the addition of several protease and viral polymerase inhibitors that may be given along with ribavirin and interferon. These new combinations have greatly improved the response to treatment of type 1 HCV along with the other types and require a relatively short period of therapy.

HEPATITIS D (DELTA HEPATITIS)

This type of hepatitis is caused by a small defective RNA virus that can only infect people who are already infected with the hepatitis B virus, either chronic carriers of HBV or those with an acute HBV infection (termed superinfection). The delta virus is always associated with an HBV infection because the virus is unable to produce its own outer viral coat and can reproduce itself only by coating itself with HBsAg produced by HBV, thereby forming complete but hybrid virus particles composed of a delta virus core and an HBsAg outer layer. Delta virus superinfection increases the probability HBV will become chronic and increases the severity of already chronic HBV disease. Delta hepatitis is uncommon in the United States, and most cases are found among intravenous drug abusers. The disease is more common in regions where rates of HBV infection remain high, such as in developing nations.

HEPATITIS E

Hepatitis E is caused by an RNA virus that is transmitted by the fecal–oral route. As is the case with hepatitis A virus, most cases are in developing countries where outbreaks have been traced to contaminated water supplies. Only a few cases have been reported in North America, and the infected individuals acquired the disease while traveling outside the United States. A diagnostic test has been developed to detect anti-HEV antibodies as an indication of HEV infection. Although the disease is often acute and self-limited, it is a particular danger to pregnant women where mortality rates may reach 40 percent. A vaccine has been developed but is not licensed for use in the United States.

OTHER HEPATITIS VIRUSES

Yellow fever virus causes a severe hepatitis and is still a serious risk in tropical areas. A vaccine is available for travelers visiting areas where the disease is endemic. Other viruses may, at times, cause a mild hepatitis. These include the **Epstein-Barr (EB) virus**, which causes infectious mononucleosis (see discussion in the hematopoietic and lymphatic systems), and another somewhat similar virus called **cytomegalovirus**, which may also cause an infection resembling infectious mononucleosis. **GB virus C** (once called hepatitis G virus [HGV]) is now not believed to cause clinical disease in humans.

Fatty Liver

The liver performs many important functions related to the metabolism of food, including an important role in fat metabolism, so conditions that disturb liver functions can lead to accumulation of fat in liver cells. Fatty liver is a particular type of liver injury (**FIGURE 21-9**) associated with a number of injurious agents capable of increasing the synthesis or decreasing oxidation of free fatty acids by the liver or impairing the release of lipids bound to carrier proteins (lipoproteins). All of these derangements can result in fat accumulation in the organ leading to an accumulation of fat globules within the liver cell cytoplasm (**steatosis**) (**FIGURE 21-10**). Diffuse fatty change within the liver can be demonstrated by ultrasound examination, by

Epstein-Barr (EB) virus A virus that causes infectious mononucleosis.

Cytomegalovirus One of the herpes viruses. Causes an infectious mononucleosis-like syndrome in adults; may cause congenital malformation in fetus.

GB virus C Once called hepatitis G virus; does not cause clinical disease in humans.

Steatosis Abnormal storage of fat in the liver. Can result from alcoholic damage or some other cause.

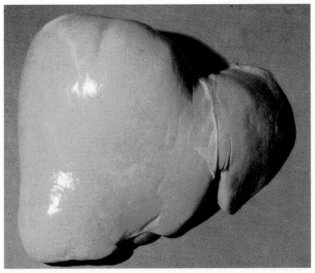

(A)

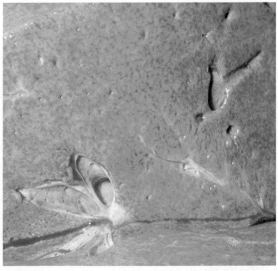

(B)

FIGURE 21-9 Fatty liver. **(A)** The liver appears yellow because of a large amount of fat within liver cells, but otherwise appears normal. **(B)** A section of liver that appears normal except for the yellow color caused by the fat.

Courtesy of Leonard V. Crowley, MD, Century College.

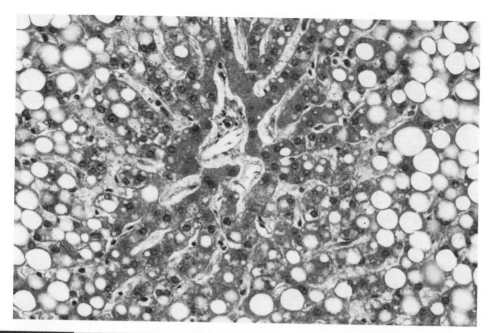

FIGURE 21-10 Photomicrograph of fatty liver. Liver cord cells (*center*) appear relatively normal. Other cells contain large fat globules that appear as clear spherical vacuoles within the liver cells. Processing of tissue for microscopy dissolves the fat.

Courtesy of Leonard V. Crowley, MD, Century College.

computed tomography (CT) scans, or by magnetic resonance imaging (MRI). Liver biopsy can determine whether there is any liver cell damage associated with the fatty change. In the United States, the most common cause of fatty liver is excessive alcohol ingestion (alcoholic fatty liver disease or alcoholic steatosis), but a number of volatile solvents, drugs, chemicals, and some poisons can also cause fat accumulation in liver cells, as can obesity and type 2 diabetes.

Alcoholic Liver Disease

Alcoholic liver disease refers to a group of structural and functional changes in the liver resulting from excessive alcohol consumption. The severity of the liver injury and its rate of progression are determined not only by how much alcohol is consumed but also by how long the person has been drinking excessively. It is convenient to subdivide alcoholic liver disease into three stages of progressively increasing severity: (1) alcoholic fatty liver, (2) alcoholic hepatitis, and (3) alcoholic cirrhosis.

Alcoholic fatty liver is the mildest form of alcoholic liver disease. If the person stops drinking, the liver function gradually returns to normal, and the fat globules in the liver cells disappear as the liver cells process the accumulated fat.

Alcoholic hepatitis is the next stage in the progressive liver injury caused by alcohol. In this case, the term "hepatitis" refers to the inflammatory cell infiltration secondary to liver cell necrosis and does not imply an infection, as in viral hepatitis. Heavy alcohol intake not only promotes fatty change in liver cells but causes other degenerative changes as well and may actually induce liver cell necrosis. A characteristic feature of severe alcoholic liver injury is the accumulation of irregularly shaped, pink deposits within the cytoplasm of the liver cells. These structures, which are called **Mallory bodies** or alcoholic hyalin, indicate that the cell has been irreparably damaged. Neutrophilic leukocytes also accumulate in response to the liver cell necrosis, and the injury is followed by progressive fibrous scarring throughout the

Mallory body An irregular, red-staining structure in the cytoplasm of injured liver cells, usually resulting from alcohol-induced liver injury.

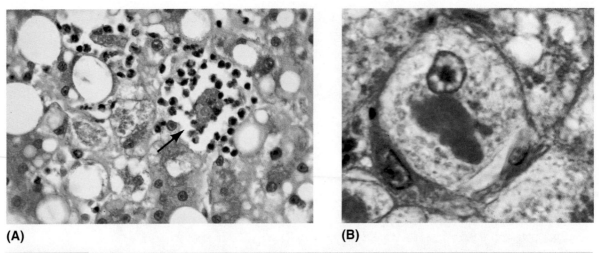

(A)   **(B)**

FIGURE 21-11 A photomicrograph illustrating hepatic cellular structure in alcoholic hepatitis. **(A)** Many cells contain fat vacuoles. Others are swollen and contain Mallory bodies. One necrotic cell (*arrow*) is surrounded by cluster of neutrophils. **(B)** A high-magnification photomicrograph of Mallory body in swollen liver cell.
Courtesy of Leonard V. Crowley, MD, Century College.

liver. Alcoholic hepatitis refers to this type of liver injury, which is characterized not only by fatty change but also by liver cell degeneration with Mallory bodies and leukocyte infiltration (**FIGURE 21-11**).

Alcoholic cirrhosis, the third and most advanced stage of alcoholic liver injury, is characterized by diffuse scarring throughout the liver, which disturbs liver function and impedes blood flow through the liver. In the United States, a large number of cases of cirrhosis are related to heavy alcohol ingestion and follow repeated episodes of alcoholic hepatitis. Although there is considerable individual variation in susceptibility to alcoholic liver injury, in general a person must drink more than 1 pint of whiskey daily, or its equivalent in other alcoholic beverages, for ten to fifteen years to develop alcoholic cirrhosis. Occasionally, the disease develops more rapidly, and it may been seen in teenagers and young adults.

Nonalcoholic Liver Disease

Obese individuals and many people with diabetes also accumulate excess fat in the liver unrelated to excess alcohol consumption, a condition of increasing importance referred to as nonalcoholic fatty liver disease (NAFLD). Usually, the affected individuals have a higher than normal blood glucose or type 2 diabetes related to obesity, which causes the body cells to become less responsive to insulin (metabolic syndrome). The fatty change in the liver cells is called nonalcoholic fatty liver to distinguish it from the fatty liver of alcoholic patients. Heavy fat infiltration may impair liver function and cause mild liver injury, but the liver cell damage usually is reversible. However, prolonged and severe fatty infiltration can cause significant liver cell damage associated with inflammation and scarring similar to the liver cell damage encountered in alcoholic patients (nonalcoholic steatohepatitis, NASH), which can progress to cirrhosis and eventually to liver failure in a manner similar to the condition that occurs in alcoholic liver disease. Unfortunately, NAFLD and its complications are becoming more frequent because of the increasing frequency of obesity and diabetes in our population. NASH is now the leading cause of chronic liver disease in the United States, and some estimate that up to 20 percent of the population have nonalcoholic steatohepatitis.

Cirrhosis of the Liver

Cirrhosis of the liver, regardless of cause, refers to obliteration of the normal architecture of the liver and replacement of the parenchyma by regenerating nodules of hepatocytes surrounded by bands of collagen (fibrosis) (**FIGURE 21-12**). Any substance capable of injuring the liver may cause cirrhosis under certain conditions. The most common cause of cirrhosis is chronic hepatitis caused by HBV or HCV infections, followed in frequency by alcoholic liver disease resulting from repeated episodes of alcoholic hepatitis. NAFLD is also increasing in frequency.

Less common causes of cirrhosis include use of drugs and chemicals that damage liver cells, genetic diseases that directly or indirectly lead to liver damage such as hemochromatosis (discussion on the hematopoietic and lymphatic systems) alpha$_1$ antitrypsin deficiency, which also causes some types of pulmonary emphysema (discussion on the respiratory system), or long-standing bile duct obstruction, which causes a special type of cirrhosis called **biliary cirrhosis**.

In cirrhosis, the liver is converted into a mass of scar tissue containing nodules of degenerating and regenerating liver cells, proliferating bile ducts, and inflammatory cells (**FIGURE 21-13**). The normal architectural pattern of the liver is completely disorganized, and the intrahepatic branches of the hepatic artery and portal vein are constricted by scar tissue and ultimately isolated from the vascular outflow tract (central vein). This results in **portal hypertension** characterized by increased resistance to blood outflow and impaired liver function followed by hepatic encephalopathy as a possible sequela.

IMPAIRED LIVER FUNCTION

As a result of liver cell damage, scarring, and impairment of blood supply to the liver caused by scarring, the number of functioning liver cells is greatly reduced and function is impaired. Eventually, a patient with cirrhosis may die of liver failure. Clinical manifestations commonly found in men with advanced cirrhosis are testicular atrophy, loss of sex drive, and breast hypertrophy. These manifestations result from impaired liver function and appear to be the result of an excess of estrogen.

> **Biliary cirrhosis** Diffuse liver cell damage and scarring with distortion of liver cell structure and function (cirrhosis) caused by obstruction of bile ducts.
>
> **Portal hypertension** Characterized by increased resistance to blood outflow and impaired liver function.

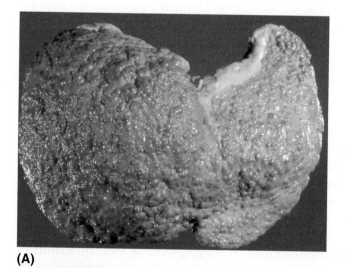
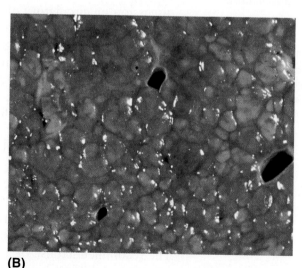

(A)   **(B)**

FIGURE 21-12 Advanced hepatic cirrhosis illustrating elevated nodules of liver tissue surrounded by depressed areas of scar tissue. **(A)** Exterior of liver. **(B)** A closer view of the liver in cross section.
Courtesy of Leonard V. Crowley, MD, Century College.

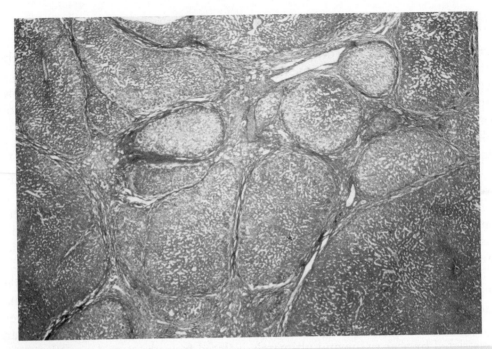

FIGURE 21-13 A low-magnification photomicrograph of cirrhotic liver illustrating nodules of liver cells circumscribed by dense scar tissue (blue-green stain). The normal architectural pattern is lost. The number of functioning liver cells is reduced and replaced by scar tissue, and the scar tissue disrupts blood flow through the liver. Compare with Figure 21-2.

Courtesy of Leonard V. Crowley, MD, Century College.

Normally, men produce not only the male sex hormone (testosterone) but also small amounts of estrogen. The estrogen is normally inactivated by the liver and exerts little effect. The cirrhotic liver, however, is unable to accomplish this function efficiently; consequently, estrogen accumulates and produces these associated clinical manifestations.

Albumin, which is produced by the liver, is reduced in cirrhosis. This can result in **ascites** because albumin is crucial to maintaining the normal colloid osmotic pressure of the blood, which is the force that tends to hold fluid in the capillaries (see discussion on circulatory disturbances). Because most proteins important in blood coagulation are produced in the liver, individuals with impaired liver function may be susceptible to hemorrhage.

In addition to liver impairment from alcohol ingestion, other diseases can result from liver impairment. An example is **Reye's syndrome** (rhymes with "eye"), now an extremely uncommon acute illness that develops in infants and children after a mild viral infection and is characterized by both marked swelling of the brain with neurologic dysfunction and accumulation of fat within the cytoplasm of liver cells associated with impaired liver function. In severely affected patients, the mortality rate is about 25 percent, and some of the survivors may be left with neurologic abnormalities or psychiatric disturbances. There is no specific treatment.

Current evidence suggests that Reye's syndrome is related in some way to acetylsalicylic acid (aspirin) given to treat the fever and discomfort associated with the viral infection and likely also with otherwise undiagnosed inborn errors of metabolism. The recommended use of acetaminophen to treat symptoms of viral infections in infants and children has lead to a much diminished frequency of the condition, with two cases or less being reported per year in the United States. However, it should be noted that acetaminophen overdose can be associated with severe acute liver disease, which may require transplantation (see Case).

Ascites Fluid accumulating in body cavities due to low albumin.

Reye's syndrome Acute illness following mild viral infection in children, characterized by brain swelling associated with aspirin consumption.

PORTAL HYPERTENSION

Normally, the portal vein blood passes through sinusoids into the hepatic veins and then into the inferior vena cava. In cirrhosis, venous return through the portal system and liver sinusoids is impaired because of scar tissue leading to portal hypertension. The high pressure affects the portal capillaries, contributing to excessive leakage of fluid. Eventually, the abdomen becomes distended by ascites, fluids that accumulate within the abdominal cavity (**FIGURE 21-14**).

Because of the obstruction of portal venous return, a collateral circulation develops in response to increased portal pressure in an attempt to bypass the intrahepatic obstruction and deliver portal blood directly into the systemic circulation. Anastomoses develop where tributaries of portal and systemic veins are closely associated, and they shunt blood from the portal system of veins where the pressure is high into the veins of the systemic circulation where the pressure is much lower. The communications that are most important clinically are the anastomoses developing between veins around the stomach and spleen, which drain into the portal vein, and the esophageal veins that eventually drain into the superior vena cava by way of

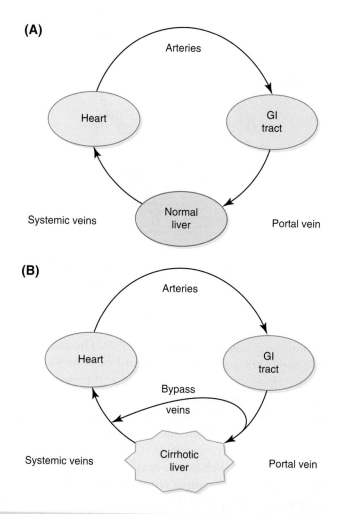

FIGURE 21-14 A comparison of normal blood flow pathways with those in cirrhosis. **(A)** Normal flow pattern. The heart pumps blood through the aorta to the gastrointestinal tract from which blood collects in the portal vein and flows through hepatic sinusoids into hepatic veins, then into vena cava, and finally, back to the heart to be repumped. **(B)** The flow pattern in cirrhosis. Blood pumped to the gastrointestinal tract is collected in portal vein; however, flow through hepatic sinusoids is interrupted by intrahepatic scarring, and portal vein pressure rises. Bypass channels shunt blood into superior or inferior vena cava to return blood to the heart. Bypass veins cannot handle increased blood flow under increased pressure and become dilated.

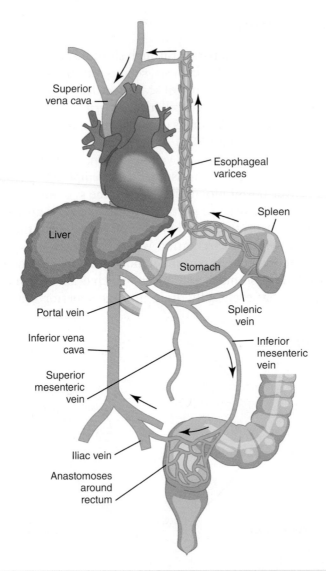

FIGURE 21-15 Formation of collateral venous channels that return blood to the systemic circulation when portal blood flow is impeded by cirrhosis. The arrows indicate direction of blood flow.

the intercostal veins and azygos veins (**FIGURE 21-15**). The esophageal veins are not equipped to handle the increased blood flow and high pressure. In 90 percent of patients with cirrhosis, these veins become dilated and form varicose veins (**esophageal varices**). Esophageal varices are thin-walled vessels covered by a thin layer of esophageal epithelium (**FIGURE 21-16**) and frequently rupture, leading to profuse and often fatal hemorrhage in chronic alcoholics (who, in addition, often have diminished levels of circulating coagulation proteins, thereby exacerbating the problem). The blood flow through the collateral channels may somewhat reduce the engorgement of the abdominal organs that has resulted from the portal hypertension, but it is not sufficient to return the pressure to normal.

The extent of the communications between the portal and systemic vein branches in patients with advanced cirrhosis is not always obvious. Special photographic techniques, however, can demonstrate the dilated veins extending in the subcutaneous tissues of the chest and abdominal wall that are shunting blood around the scarred liver. More direct measurement of hepatic vein pressure may be accomplished using pressure-sensing catheters placed in the terminal hepatic

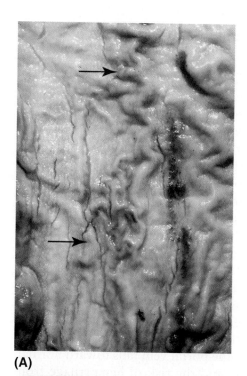

(A)

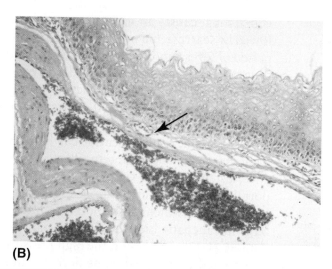

(B)

FIGURE 21-16 **(A)** Mucosal surface of esophagus illustrating varices, which appear as tortuous elevations of the mucosa (*arrows*). **(B)** A photomicrograph of a varix. The very thin vein wall (*arrow*) is covered only by a thin layer of esophageal squamous epithelium and is very susceptible to rupture.

Courtesy of Leonard V. Crowley, MD, Century College.

vein. Although this chapter has focused on **sinusoidal** (intrahepatic) causes of portal hypertension, occlusive disease of the portal vein can result in **presinusoidal portal hypertension**, and thrombosis of the hepatic vein (**Budd Chiari syndrome**) can lead to **postsinusoidal portal hypertension**.

HEPATIC ENCEPHALOPATHY

The cirrhotic liver is not able to detoxify or excrete toxic substances that accumulate in the bloodstream. Hepatic encephalopathy (*encephalon* = brain + *pathy* = disease) is a deterioration of brain function characterized by impaired consciousness, confusion, disorientation, and eventually coma. Not all of the toxic products have been identified, but many of them are products of protein digestion, especially ammonia, which comes from deamination of amino acids and other products derived from bacterial decomposition of material in the colon. In a person with advanced liver disease, any event that further compromises liver function may precipitate hepatic encephalopathy. This includes such events as an episode of binge drinking in a person with alcoholic liver disease; a hemorrhage into the gastrointestinal tract, which drops blood pressure and reduces hepatic blood flow; or a systemic infection with a fever that reduces hepatic blood flow and increases liver cell metabolism. Even a portal–systemic vein bypass procedure, which diverts some of the portal vein blood directly into the systemic circulation in an attempt to lower portal pressure, may precipitate hepatic encephalopathy in some patients because the procedure also bypasses whatever remaining detoxification function the diseased liver still possesses, delivering blood and its toxins directly into the systemic venous circulation. Many bypass patients can tolerate the diversion, but some cannot.

Sinusoid The modified blood vessel between the sheets of hepatocytes, forming the bulk of the liver.

Presinusoidal portal hypertension Portal hypertension resulting from occlusions in portal vein.

Budd Chiari syndrome/ postsinusoidal portal hypertension Hypertension resulting from thrombosis of the hepatic vein.

Procedures to Treat Manifestations of Cirrhosis

If a patient has developed esophageal varices and is acutely bleeding, a variety of endoscopic treatment procedures are available at the level of the esophagus. The varices may be endoscopically ligated (EVL procedure), or an attempt may be made to obliterate them by injecting them with a sclerosing solution. The solution, which is irritating, causes an inflammation in and around the dilated veins, which is followed by scarring and eventual obliteration of the varices. Multiple injections over a period of several months are usually required. The vasoconstrictive somatostatin-like drug octreotide is often combined with endoscopic esophageal therapy, but control is often temporary at best. To achieve a more permanent solution, endoscopic or surgical procedures are available that attempt to shunt the portal to the veinous systemic circulation, thereby bypassing the liver and reducing portal pressure. A nonsurgical portal–systemic communication can be accomplished by means of a procedure called a **transjugular intrahepatic portosystemic shunt** (the TIPS procedure). Under x-ray guidance, a stent is placed via the jugular and inferior vena cava within the liver to join portal and systemic circulation. The shunt is used to artificially connect one of the hepatic veins (which drain blood from the liver into the inferior vena cava) with a large intrahepatic branch of the portal vein, thus bypassing the hepatic sinusoids (**FIGURE 21-17**). As a result, the high pressure in the portal vein falls toward normal. The dilated esophageal veins decrease in size, and the risk of hemorrhage from

Transjugular intrahepatic portosystemic shunt
A nonsurgical method used to lower portal vein pressure in a person with cirrhosis by connecting an intrahepatic branch of the portal vein to a hepatic vein branch.

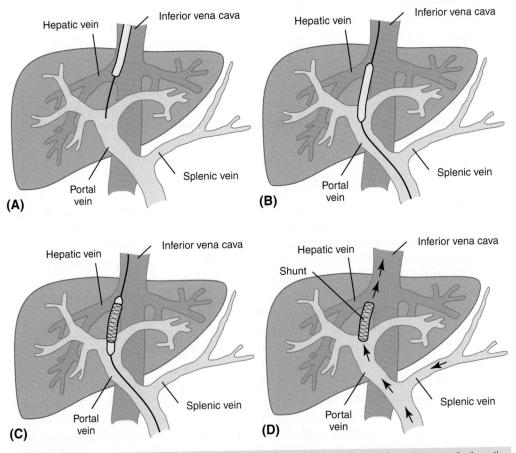

FIGURE 21-17 The TIPS procedure. **(A)** Intrahepatic communication (tract) established between the hepatic and portal vein. **(B)** Angioplasty balloon dilates tract. **(C)** Expandable metal stent inserted into tract and dilated by angioplasty balloon. **(D)** Completed shunt between hepatic artery and portal vein lowers portal vein pressure. Esophageal varices become smaller as portal vein pressure falls.

varices is greatly reduced. The shunt also may improve the patient's ascites because the lower portal pressure resulting from the shunt lowers the venous pressure in the capillaries draining into the portal system, and less fluid is forced from the capillaries to accumulate in the abdominal cavity.

In the case of continued bleeding, surgical shunting procedures such as connecting the splenic vein to the renal vein side-to-side (**splenorenal shunt**) or making a side-to-side connection between the portal vein and the inferior vena cava (**portacaval shunt**) are available. A shunt decompresses the portal system by permitting portal blood to flow directly into the inferior vena cava. In the case of a patient with advanced liver disease, liver transplantation may be considered as an alternative.

Bile

FORMATION AND EXCRETION

Bile is an aqueous solution excreted by the liver that contains various dissolved substances including conjugated bilirubin, bile salts, lecithin, cholesterol, water, minerals, and other materials that have been detoxified by liver cells and excreted. **Cholesterol** is a lipid with a complex ring structure that is classified as a sterol. **Bile salts**, the major constituent of bile, are derivatives of cholesterol and certain amino acids. They function as detergents because of their molecular structure, which contains both a lipid-soluble (hydrophobic) and a water-soluble (hydrophilic) part. **Lecithin** is a phosphorous-containing lipid (phospholipid) that has detergent properties similar to bile salts. Bile is secreted continually and is concentrated and stored in the gallbladder. During digestion, the gallbladder contracts, squirting bile into the duodenum. Bile does not contain digestive enzymes but functions as a biologic detergent. Bile salts emulsify fat into small globules, increasing the surface area so that the fat can be acted on more readily by pancreatic enzymes. Digestion of fat is much less efficient in the absence of bile.

The excretion of bile, a product of the breakdown of red blood cells, is an important function of the liver. Red cells normally survive for about four months. The worn-out erythrocytes are broken down by the mononuclear phagocytes (reticuloendothelial cells) predominantly in the spleen liver and bone marrow. The iron derived from the hemoglobin is conserved by the body and reused to synthesize new hemoglobin. The iron-free heme pigment forms **bilirubin**. Because the breakdown of red cells proceeds in mononuclear phagocytes in several locations, small quantities of bile pigment are continually present in the blood complexed to albumin. When the blood passes through the liver, the bilirubin is removed from the albumin and taken up by the hepatocytes. Excretion is accomplished by combining the bilirubin with glucuronic acid (which has a structure similar to glucose). This process, termed conjugation, requires certain specific enzymes (uridine diphosphate-glucuronyl transferase, UGT). Most of the bilirubin is conjugated with glucuronic acid and excreted as bilirubin glucuronide. The **conjugated bilirubin** is much more water soluble and less toxic than the unconjugated material. **Gilbert syndrome** is a very common inherited condition, occurring in 5 to 10 percent of the population, related to a mild lack of sufficient levels of synthesis of UGT. The condition is most often not associated with disease. However, a complete lack or severe deficiency of UGT (**Crigler-Najjar syndrome**) causes severe disease in early childhood related to the effects of unconjugated bilirubin on the brain (kernicterus). After the bile pigment is excreted into the small bile channels between the liver cell cords, it is collected into large ducts at the periphery of the lobules, which eventually unite to form the major bile ducts. Figure 21-4 summarizes the basic anatomy of the biliary duct system.

Splenorenal shunt Surgically created anastomosis between splenic vein and renal vein, performed to lower portal pressure in the treatment of esophageal varices.

Portacaval shunt Surgically created anastomosis between the portal vein and the vena cava, performed to lower portal pressure in the treatment of esophageal varices.

Bile A secretion of the liver containing bile salts, cholesterol, and other substances.

Cholesterol A complex lipid (sterol) containing several ring structures.

Bile salts Derivatives of bile acids present in bile that act as emulsifiers to promote fat digestion and absorption.

Lecithin A phosphorus-containing lipid (phospholipid) having detergent properties similar to bile salts.

Bilirubin One of the bile pigments derived from the breakdown of hemoglobin.

Conjugated bilirubin A more soluble form of bilirubin produced by the addition of two molecules of glucuronic acid to the bilirubin molecule.

Gilbert syndrome Common inherited condition related to a mild lack of uridine diphosphate-glucuronyl transferase (UGT).

Crigler-Najjar syndrome Lack of UGT, which causes a severe disease of early childhood.

Jaundice

Jaundice, a yellow discoloration of the skin and the sclerae (whites of the eyes) that results from accumulation of bilirubin in the tissues and body fluids, can have several causes. Jaundice is generally classified on the basis of the disturbance responsible for the retention of bile pigment, either hemolytic, hepatocellular, or obstructive. Jaundice can usually be classified correctly on the basis of certain laboratory tests in conjunction with clinical features. Physiological neonatal jaundice occurs transiently in up to 70 percent of newborns and is related to a low level of liver UGT in the newborn in combination with normally increased red cell destruction. In severe cases or in premature infants, phototherapy by exposure of the neonate to selected wavelengths of visible light converts unconjugated bilirubin to several water soluble forms.

HEMOLYTIC JAUNDICE

Under conditions associated with the accelerated breakdown of red cells, excessive bile pigment is delivered to the liver beyond the liver's ability to conjugate and excrete the pigment. Therefore, unconjugated bile pigment accumulates in the blood. Hemolytic jaundice is sometimes seen in adults with hemolytic anemia and in the case of certain congenital disorders of red blood cells such as sickle cell disease, but it is encountered most frequently in newborn infants with hemolytic disease as a result of blood group incompatibility between mother and infant (discussion on prenatal development and diseases associated with pregnancy).

HEPATOCELLULAR JAUNDICE

If the liver is severely damaged, as in hepatitis or cirrhosis, conjugation of bilirubin is impaired. This may be related to a number of congenital genetic conditions that interfere with the mechanism of bilirubin conjugation or that prevent transport of conjugated bilirubin into the bile canaliculi, which lead to the bile ducts. Moreover, the excretion of conjugated bilirubin may be hampered because of injury to liver cells and disruption of the canaliculi that lie between liver cell cords. As a result, conjugated bilirubin leaks back into the blood through the ruptured intrahepatic bile channels. **Cholestasis** refers to decreased bile flow and bile stasis in the liver, which may result from intrahepatic or extrahepatic obstruction of bile flow. This leads to local damage to hepatocytes and ultimately to cirrhosis. As serum bile acids increase, intense itching may result.

OBSTRUCTIVE JAUNDICE

In obstructive jaundice, the extraction and conjugation of bilirubin by liver cells are not impaired, but jaundice develops because the bile duct is obstructed, preventing delivery of bile into the duodenum. Often, the obstruction is caused by an impacted stone in the common duct. Carcinoma of the head of the pancreas is another common cause of common bile duct obstruction. The common duct passes very close to the head of the pancreas as it enters the duodenum (**FIGURE 21-18**). Therefore, a pancreatic tumor frequently compresses and invades the common duct. As previously described, long-standing common bile duct obstruction leads to obstructive biliary cirrhosis.

Biliary Cirrhosis

In some types of cirrhosis, the initial target of the liver damage is the epithelium of the bile ducts rather than the functional cells (hepatocytes) of the liver lobules. This type of cirrhosis is called **biliary cirrhosis** to distinguish it from the more common type

---

Jaundice Yellow discoloration of skin and white of eyes resulting from an accumulation of bilirubin in the body.

Cholestasis Decreased bile flow and bile stasis.

Biliary cirrhosis Liver damage of the epithelium of the bile ducts.

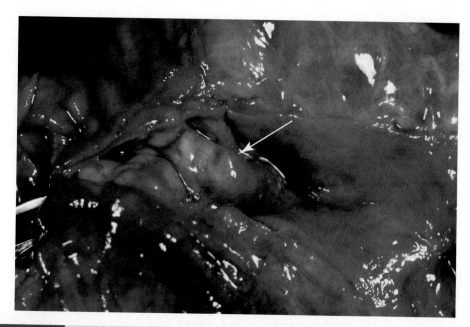

FIGURE 21-18 Carcinoma arising from common bile duct (*arrow*) blocking outflow of bile into duodenum. Common bile duct has been opened and is distended, a result of the increased pressure of the bile within the common duct caused by the duct obstruction.

Courtesy of Leonard V. Crowley, MD, Century College.

of cirrhosis in which hepatocyte injury is the primary event. The cirrhotic component of the disease is a late complication representing secondary damage to hepatocytes. There are two main types of biliary cirrhosis. The first, which is called primary biliary cirrhosis, is an autoimmune disease that targets the small intrahepatic bile ducts. The second, called secondary biliary cirrhosis or obstructive biliary cirrhosis, results from long-standing obstruction of the large extrahepatic bile ducts.

PRIMARY BILIARY CIRRHOSIS

This is a slowly progressive, chronic disease found almost exclusively in women and is characterized by inflammation and destruction of the small intrahepatic bile ducts. Bile excretion is disrupted and is followed by scarring, which begins in the portal tracts and eventually spreads into the liver lobules. The disease appears to be caused by autoantibodies that are directed against bile duct epithelial cells. Antinuclear autoantibodies and antimitochondrial antibodies can usually be demonstrated in the blood of affected patients.

Because excretion of bile is impeded, products accumulate in the blood that are normally excreted in the bile, including bile pigment (bilirubin), bile salts, and cholesterol. Accumulation of bile pigment in the blood results in jaundice and pruritus (itching). As a result of the high blood cholesterol, masses of cholesterol accumulate in the skin and form small yellow skin nodules called xanthomas. Unfortunately, there is no effective treatment for this condition, which progresses slowly over many years and eventually leads to liver failure. Ultimately, a liver transplant may be required.

SECONDARY (OBSTRUCTIVE) BILIARY CIRRHOSIS

This condition is caused by long-standing blockage of the large extrahepatic bile ducts associated with obstructive jaundice. The bile duct obstruction leads to stasis of bile within the ducts. The pressure within the ducts rises, and the larger ducts become dilated. The elevated intraductal pressure is transmitted back into the smaller intrahepatic bile ducts and from there into the small bile channels (bile canaliculi) that carry bile from the liver lobules into the bile ducts within the portal tracts at the periphery of the lobules. The elevated intraductal pressure and bile stasis damage the intrahepatic bile ducts, which is followed by portal tract inflammation and scarring.

The clinical manifestations of the extrahepatic bile duct obstruction are much the same as those caused by primary biliary cirrhosis. Treatment consists of various surgical procedures to unblock the obstructed bile duct. If this is not possible, some type of surgical procedure is used to bypass the obstruction and reestablish bile flow into the duodenum.

Cholelithiasis (Gallstones)

FACTORS AFFECTING THE SOLUBILITY OF CHOLESTEROL IN BILE

Because cholesterol is a lipid, it is not soluble in an aqueous solution such as bile but is brought into solution by bile salts and lecithin, which aggregate in clusters called **micelles**. In a micelle, the lipid-soluble (hydrophobic) parts of the bile salt molecules are oriented toward the center of the cluster, and the opposite water-soluble (hydrophilic) ends face outward. Cholesterol becomes soluble by dissolving in the hydrophobic center of the micelles, and the cholesterol-containing micelles dissolve in the bile because the peripheral hydrophilic parts of the bile salt molecules are water soluble. Lecithin participates in the formation of the micelles by fitting between the molecules of the bile salts (**FIGURE 21-19**).

Approximately seven molecules of bile salts interspersed between lecithin molecules in a micelle are required to dissolve one molecule of cholesterol. Consequently,

Micelle An aggregate of bile salt and lecithin molecules by which cholesterol is brought into solution in bile.

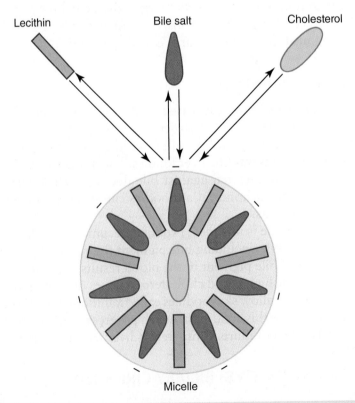

FIGURE 21-19 The manner in which cholesterol dissolves in micelles composed of bile salts and lecithin. If the bile salt concentration is insufficient relative to that of cholesterol, cholesterol will precipitate and form gallstones.

the solubility of cholesterol in bile depends not only on its cholesterol content but also on its content of bile salts and lecithin, because these substances are needed to hold the cholesterol in solution. Cholesterol remains soluble provided its concentration is not excessive in relation to the amounts of available bile salts and lecithin.

FORMATION OF GALLSTONES

Whenever bile contains a relative excess of cholesterol, it becomes supersaturated with cholesterol, and under proper conditions, the cholesterol may precipitate to form the beginnings of gallstones. The formation of stones within the gallbladder is called **cholelithiasis** (*chole* = bile + *lith* = stone) (**FIGURE 21-20**). This situation may arise because of an increased excretion of cholesterol in the bile, a reduced excretion of bile salts and lecithin, or a combination of both factors. As long as the bile remains supersaturated, cholesterol crystals continue to accumulate around those that have already precipitated, and the gallstones slowly increase in size. Eventually, the gallbladder may become filled with gallstones, the end stage of a process that began several years earlier. This process often leads to **cholecystitis**, inflammation of the gallbladder.

Some people are known to have an increased risk of forming gallstones. The incidence of gallstones is higher in women than in men, higher in obese women, and higher in multipara than in childless women. It is also twice as high in women who use contraceptive pills as in women who use other types of contraception, all conditions that lead to increased cholesterol secretion.

Higher estrogen levels are likely to account for the increased risk to women as well as for the association with multiple pregnancies and the use of oral contraceptives. Obesity predisposes to gallstones because extremely overweight individuals have a higher blood cholesterol and excrete more cholesterol in their bile than do people of normal weight. Less commonly, gallstones form as a result of infection of the gallbladder. Infection predisposes to "brown pigment" gallstones by deconjugating bilirubin and thereby reducing its solubility.

Cholelithiasis Formation of gallstones.

Cholecystitis Inflammation of the gallbladder.

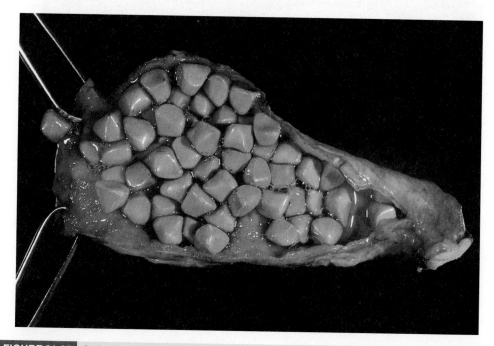

FIGURE 21-20 Opened gallbladder filled with gallstones composed of cholesterol.
Courtesy of Leonard V. Crowley, MD, Century College.

COMPLICATIONS OF GALLSTONES

Gallstones that remain in the gallbladder rarely cause symptoms. Unfortunately, gallstones are sometimes extruded into the cystic duct or common bile duct when the gallbladder contracts after a fatty meal, and they may become impacted within the biliary ducts. This event causes severe abdominal pain called **biliary colic**. The pain results from spasm of the smooth muscle in the ducts combined with forceful contractions of the gallbladder that attempt to propel the stone through the ducts. Sometimes a stone can be passed through the ducts into the duodenum, but often it becomes impacted. If the stone lodges in the cystic duct, bile can neither enter nor leave the gallbladder, but flow of bile from the liver into the duodenum is not disturbed. However, if the stone blocks the common duct, bile can no longer be excreted into the duodenum, and it accumulates in the bloodstream. This condition is called **obstructive jaundice**. Such blockage is also a common cause of acute pancreatitis, a serious and painful inflammatory condition of that organ (discussed in the section on the pancreas). Blockage of the cystic duct by a stone can lead to bacterial infection, distension of the gallbladder, compromise of blood flow and ultimately inflammation, ischemia, and necrosis of the mucosa. In addition, concentrated bile within the gallbladder may lead to mucosal injury. The result is **acute calculous cholecystitis** (**FIGURE 21-21**). If there is no underlying gallbladder infection, the bile trapped within the gallbladder by the impacted stone is gradually absorbed into the bloodstream, and eventually the contents of the gallbladder consist only of mucus that has been secreted by the epithelial cells lining the gallbladder. A small number of cases are **acalculous cholecystitis** not related to gallstones but rather to infection (not associated with gallstones), prolonged fasting, or trauma. **Chronic cholecystitis** is generally associated with gallstones but is also likely to involve chronic ongoing irritation of the gallbladder by repeated bouts of acute disease. Uncomplicated cholecystitis related to gallstones may be treated with antibiotics and analgesics. Recurrent or severe, intractable disease is treated by laparoscopic surgical removal of the diseased gallbladder (cholecystectomy). In some cases, an acute bout

Biliary colic Abdominal pain that results when a gallstone enters the biliary duct system.

Obstructive jaundice Symptom from a blocked common bile duct.

Acute calculous cholecystitis Mucosal injury from concentrated bile within gallbladder.

Acalculous cholecystitis Results from infection, prolonged fasting, or trauma.

Chronic cholecystitis Ongoing irritation of the gallbladder by repeated bouts of acute disease.

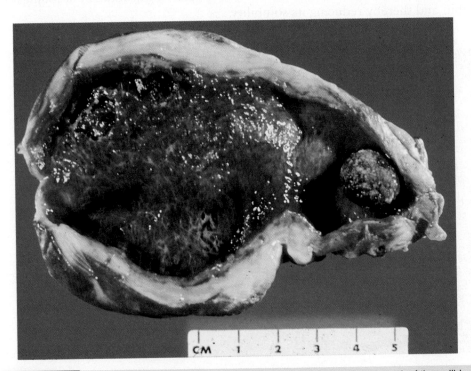

FIGURE 21-21 An inflamed, thick-walled gallbladder with a stone impacted in the neck of the gallbladder.

Courtesy of Leonard V. Crowley, MD, Century College.

of obstructive jaundice may be treated by endoscopic removal of the stone blocking the duct. Adenocarcinoma of the gallbladder is associated with cholelithiasis and is an incidental finding in about 2 percent of surgically removed organs.

Tumors of the Liver

The most common primary malignant tumor of the liver, **hepatocellular carcinoma (HCC)**, may be the most common human cancer when viewed worldwide. Almost 90 percent of HCC cases occur in countries with high levels of HBV carriers. As noted, HCC is associated with cirrhosis in such patients (**FIGURE 21-22**). Once rare in industrialized countries, an increasing incidence of HCV carriers has led to a doubling of HCC in

Hepatocellular carcinoma (HCC) Most common liver cancer.

(A)

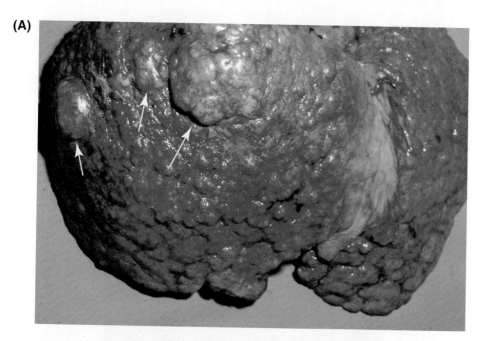

(B)

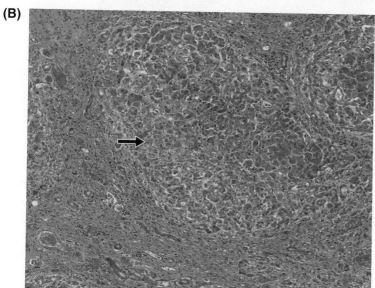

FIGURE 21-22 **(A)** Cirrhosis of liver complicated by hepatocellular carcinoma (*arrows*). **(B)** Hepatocellular carcinoma in a cirrhotic liver (*arrow*) (microscopic view).

(A) Courtesy of Leonard V. Crowley, MD, Century College; (B) Courtesy of Department of Pathology and Laboratory Medicine, University of North Carolina at Chapel Hill.

(A)

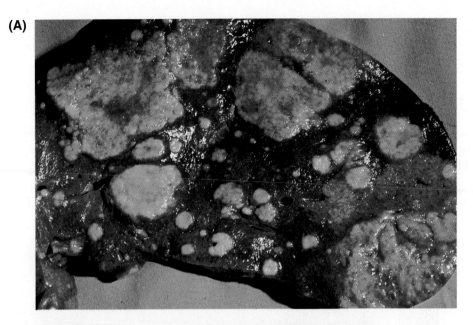

(B)

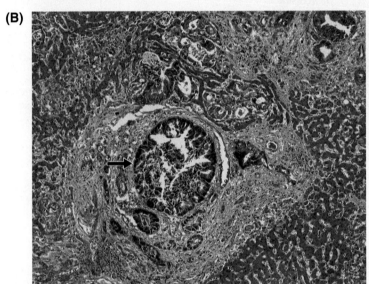

FIGURE 21-23 **(A)** A cross section of liver containing multiple nodules of metastatic carcinoma. **(B)** Nodules of metastatic adenocarcinoma in the liver (*arrow*). The likely source was colonic adenocarcinoma (microscopic view).

(A) Courtesy of Leonard V. Crowley, MD, Century College; (B) Courtesy of Department of Pathology and Laboratory Medicine, University of North Carolina at Chapel Hill.

the past several decades. HCC occurs in some areas of Africa as a result of fungal contamination of ground nut meal, corn, and sorghum by a fungus that produces a potent carcinogen, aflatoxin B. This carcinogen produces a specific mutation in the *TP53* gene, which is associated with HCC that occurs in these areas. Aflatoxin contamination may occur in agricultural products in parts of the United States. For example, fungal contaminated corn in bovine feeds results in aflatoxin levels in milk. Mandatory monitoring of milk and other products is carried out to reduce risk.

The liver is a common site of metastatic carcinoma (**FIGURE 21-23**). Carcinoma arising in the gastrointestinal tract may spread to the portal venous blood. Tumors from the breast, lung, and other sites also often spread to the liver. The tumor cells are carried in the blood delivered to the liver by the hepatic artery. Various diagnostic procedures, such as guided needle biopsy, can be used to identify tumors in the liver.

CASE 21-1

John is a sixteen-year-old high school student who is interested in trying out for the school wrestling team. One week before tryouts he badly sprains his back playing touch football. He is in considerable pain and is concerned that he will not be able to make the team. He visits his physician who confirms that the injury is not serious but quite painful. To relieve John's discomfort, the physician prescribes a mild opiate anti-inflammatory medication (Endocet™ 7.5/500, 24 pills). John is instructed to take two pills three times a day for pain relief. Concerned about his ability to compete for the team, John takes the pills four times a day until he runs out. In addition, he self-medicates with extra strength acetaminophen (Tylenol™), taking three pills every four hours in combination with the Endocet™. On the weekend previous to his injury, John attended a party and overindulged in drinks containing alcohol. Four days after seeing his physician, John becomes severely nauseated, sweaty, and "flulike." John's mother notes that he seems sluggish and confused and brings her son to the local emergency room.

In the emergency room, the physician carefully reviews John's history of medication. John's liver is noted to be tender and mildly enlarged on physical examination. The physician is concerned about possible drug toxicity. John has consumed 4 grams of acetaminophen (from the Endocet™) and 6 grams of acetaminophen by self-medication per day. Thus, John has consumed 10 grams of acetaminophen per day for three days. The maximum recommended dose of acetaminophen is 3 grams per day for an adult. Concerned about hepatic toxicity, the physician orders liver function tests that indicate acute liver failure. A serum acetaminophen assay discloses a potentially toxic amount of the drug. John is treated on an emergency basis with oral N-acetylcysteine and medication to control nausea. He recovers with normalization of liver function tests over the period of several weeks. He does not make the wrestling team.

Discussion

Acetaminophen (better known by its trade name Tylenol™) has gained popularity as an over-the-counter pain medication and aspirin replacement over the last several decades, in part because of the association of Reye's syndrome with aspirin in children and the reduced level of gastric side effects. Although acetaminophen is generally a safe medication, with a toxic dose (generally considered to be above 8 grams per 8 hours or less) far above the recommended maximum therapeutic dose of 3 grams per day, it is often abused. This is related to a lack of knowledge about potential toxicity and the widespread availability of the drug, which is often combined with other medications and hence is not obvious to the user. It may surprise individuals to learn that acetaminophen is responsible for over half of all cases of drug-induced liver injury, almost 80,000 ER visits, and more than 30,000 hospitalizations per year in the United States. Acetaminophen overdose was responsible for more than 300 deaths in 2010—half accidental, half suicidal and is the second most common cause of acute liver failure requiring transplantation.

Ninety-five percent of ingested acetaminophen is detoxified and chemically modified in the liver and ultimately excreted in the urine. About 5 percent of acetaminophen is modified by the cytochrome P-450 enzymes to a toxic intermediate called NAPQI. NAPQI binds to mitochondrial proteins and leads to the formation of reactive oxygen species, which result in hepatocyte death and, if levels are high enough, acute hepatic necrosis. Two factors influence the degree of toxicity. Cytochrome P-450 enzymes are increased by alcohol consumption, leading to the formation of more of the toxic metabolite NAPQI. Liver cells have a detoxifying chemical GSH (reduced glutathione), which binds to NAPQI and renders it harmless. However, large amounts of NAPQI can deplete available glutathione. The drug used to treat John (N-acetylcysteine) replenishes stores of GSH, reducing the toxic effects of NAQPI.

(continues)

CASE 21-1 (Continued)

Etiology and Pathogenesis

Drug-induced acute liver injury resulting from acetaminophen overdose.

Questions

1. What metabolic factors influence the toxicity of ingested acetaminophen?

2. What over-the-counter drugs are likely to contain "hidden" acetaminophen? It would be instructive to read the contents of the drugs found in your own medicine cabinet.

3. Given the potential toxicity of acetaminophen, what additional controls on its sales (if any) might be reasonable to control accidental overdosing?

QUESTIONS FOR REVIEW

1. What are some of the principal functions of the liver? How does the blood supply to the liver differ from that to the other organs? Why does severe liver disease cause disturbances in blood clotting?

2. What is the difference between hemoglobin and bilirubin? How does conjugated bilirubin differ from unconjugated bilirubin? What is the difference between bilirubin and bile? What role does bile play in digestion?

3. What are the possible causes and effects of liver injury (see Figure 21-5)? What is the usual outcome of a liver injury?

4. What is viral hepatitis? What are its major symptoms? How is hepatitis transmitted?

5. What is the difference between hepatitis A and hepatitis B? What is anicteric hepatitis? What is subclinical hepatitis?

6. What effect does alcohol have on the liver? What types of liver disease are associated with excessive alcohol ingestion?

7. What is cirrhosis? What liver diseases may lead to cirrhosis? Why does portal hypertension develop in patients with cirrhosis? Why does ascites develop in patients with cirrhosis? Why do esophageal varices develop?

8. What is jaundice? How is jaundice classified? Under what circumstances do gallstones cause jaundice?

9. What factors predispose to the development of gallstones?

10. What is the difference between viral hepatitis and alcoholic hepatitis?

SUPPLEMENTARY READINGS

Loeffler, A. G., and Hart, M. N. 2015. *Introduction to Human Disease*. 6th ed. Burlington, MA: Jones & Bartlett Learning.
▶ Those interested in the detailed study of liver disease should consult a work on human pathology aimed at the undergraduate medical curriculum. However, a good place to start at a less advanced level is by reading Chapter 15 of this book.

Centers for Disease Control and Prevention. http://www.cdc.gov/hepatitis/
▶ The CDC has an extensive online compilation of information about all forms of viral hepatitis.

Shors, T. 2015. *Understanding Viruses*. 2nd ed. Burlington, MA: Jones & Bartlett Learning.
▶ A thorough discussion of infectious viral hepatitis with an emphasis on molecular aspects of the infectious agents is presented in Chapter 17.

Tsochatzis, E. A., Bosch, J., and Burroughs, A. K. 2014. Liver cirrhosis. *Lancet* 383:1749–61.
▶ An in-depth recent review covering the development and therapy of cirrhosis.

Gravitz, L. 2014. Liver cancer (Nature|Outlook). *Nature* 516:s1–s17.
▶ An up-to-the minute set of reviews of liver disease with an emphasis of fatty liver disease and liver cancer.

Heuman, D. M. 2015. *Gallstones (Cholelithiasis)*. http://emedicine.medscape.com/article/175667-overview
▶ Current information on the pathophysiology, etiology, and medical aspects of Gallstones (Cholelithiasis).

McGill, M. R., and Jaeschke, H. 2013. Metabolism and disposition of acetaminophen: Recent advances in relation to hepatotoxicity and diagnosis. *Pharmaceutical Research* 30:2174–87.
▶ Additional information on the mechanism of acetaminophen toxicity with an emphasis on pharmacology.

The Pancreas and Diabetes Mellitus

1. Describe the pathogenesis and treatment of acute pancreatitis.
2. Describe the pathogenesis, manifestations, complications, and prognosis of pancreatic cystic fibrosis.
3. Differentiate between the two principal types of diabetes mellitus with respect to pathogenesis, incidence, manifestations, complications, and treatment.
4. Compare and contrast diabetes with metabolic syndrome.

Structure and Function of the Pancreas

The pancreas is actually two glands in one: a digestive exocrine gland and an endocrine gland. The exocrine tissue of the pancreas, which is concerned solely with digestion, secretes an alkaline pancreatic juice rich in digestive enzymes into the duodenum through the pancreatic duct. The powerful digestive enzymes break down proteins (trypsin and chymotrypsin), carbohydrates (amylase), and fats (lipase). The protein-digesting (proteolytic) enzymes are secreted in an inactive form and are activated after they are discharged into the duodenum. Exocrine pancreatic tissue makes up more than 80 percent of the pancreas and consists of enzyme-secreting **acini** arranged around ductules that ultimately drain into the pancreatic duct. The endocrine tissue of the pancreas consists of multiple small clusters of cells scattered throughout the gland called the pancreatic islets, or **islets of Langerhans**, which discharge their secretions directly into the bloodstream. Each islet is composed of several different types of cells, including alpha cells, beta cells, and delta cells. Alpha cells secrete a hormone called glucagon. The more numerous beta cells secrete insulin in response to a rise in blood glucose after eating, which restores blood glucose to normal. Both glucagon and insulin regulate the level of glucose in the blood but have opposing effects. Glucagon raises blood glucose; insulin lowers it. Delta cells produce a hormone called **somatostatin**, which inhibits secretion of both glucagon and insulin. Diffuse islets of Langerhans occur in the head of the pancreas as cords between pancreatic **acinar** cells. The diffuse islets contain predominantly beta cells and cells that secrete human pancreatic polypeptide (HPP), which helps regulate both pancreatic and gastrointestinal function and may also play a role in regulating food intake. **FIGURE 22-1** shows the anatomy and cellular structure of the pancreas.

Acini/acinar Acini are small lobules of glands composed of a cavity surrounded by secretory cells. Acinar having the properties of acini.

Islets of Langerhans Cluster of endocrine cells in the pancreas.

Somatostatin Hormone produced by the delta cells of the pancreas.

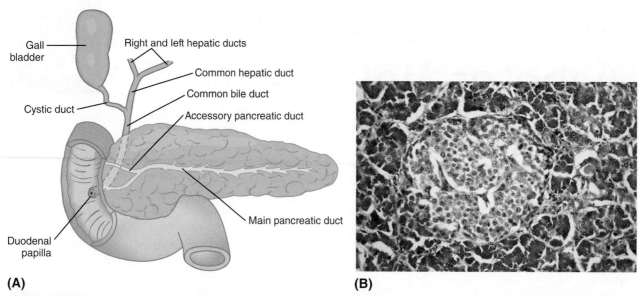

(A)   **(B)**

FIGURE 22-1 **(A)** Duct system of pancreas. The main pancreatic duct usually joins the common bile duct to form a common channel that enters the duodenum by a single opening at the apex of a nipplelike projection called the duodenal papilla (ampulla of Vater). A much smaller accessory pancreatic duct is frequently present and opens into the duodenum by a separate opening proximal to the duodenal papilla. **(B)** A photomicrograph of pancreatic islet surrounded by exocrine pancreatic tissue.

Courtesy of Leonard V. Crowley, MD, Century College.

Pancreatitis

Pancreatitis refers to the inflammation of the pancreas for any reason. It usually presents as either acute or chronic pancreatitis.

ACUTE PANCREATITIS

Acute pancreatitis is caused by escape of pancreatic juice from the ducts into the substance of the pancreas, which leads to destruction of pancreatic acinar and islet tissue by activated pancreatic enzymes, accompanied by acute inflammation of the affected pancreatic tissue. Some of the enzymes leak from the damaged tissue into the bloodstream, where elevated levels of amylase and lipase can be detected by appropriate laboratory tests. The clinical manifestations of acute pancreatitis depend on how much pancreatic tissue has been damaged. Mild episodes are accompanied by abdominal pain with elevated pancreatic enzymes; however, the pain subsides, and the patient recovers. Patients with severe acute pancreatitis have marked abdominal pain and tenderness and are seriously ill. The activated pancreatic enzymes not only destroy much of the pancreas but also damage pancreatic blood vessels, which leads to marked hemorrhage in the damaged tissues. This condition is often referred to as **acute hemorrhagic pancreatitis**, and it may be associated with multiple organ systemic disease, shock, and death (**FIGURE 22-2**).

Acute hemorrhagic pancreatitis Severe pancreatic inflammation with necrosis of pancreatic ducts and release of pancreatic enzymes that damage the pancreas.

The pathogenesis of acute pancreatitis usually involves active secretion of pancreatic juice while the pancreatic duct is obstructed at its entrance into the duodenum. The buildup of obstructed secretions greatly increases the pressure within the duct system, causing the ducts to rupture and the pancreatic juice to escape. Autoactivation of the digestive enzymes occurs within the pancreas and surrounding tissue leading to digestion of the affected areas. Two factors predisposing to acute pancreatitis are disease of the gallbladder and excessive alcohol consumption.

Pancreatitis often develops in patients with gallstones because in most individuals the common bile duct and common pancreatic duct enter the duodenum through a

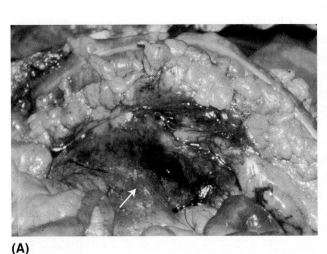

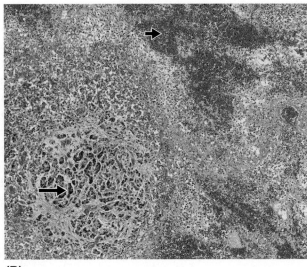

(A)   **(B)**

> **FIGURE 22-2** **(A)** Acute pancreatitis. Transverse colon (*upper part of photograph*) has been elevated to reveal pancreas (*arrow*), which is inflamed and contains large areas of hemorrhage. **(B)** Photomicrograph of acute hemorrhagic pancreatitis. Damaged exocrine gland of pancreas (*arrow*). An area of hemorrhage is visible on the right of the image (*short arrow*).
>
> (A) Courtesy of Leonard V. Crowley, MD, Century College; (B) Courtesy of Department of Pathology and Laboratory Medicine, University of North Carolina at Chapel Hill.

common channel (the **ampulla of Vater**). If a stone becomes impacted in the ampulla, it can obstruct the pancreatic duct and precipitate pancreatitis.

> **Ampulla of Vater**
> Common channel through the pancreas.

Patients who drink excessive amounts of alcohol also are prone to pancreatitis. Alcohol is a potent stimulus of pancreatic secretions, and it may also induce edema and spasm of the pancreatic sphincter in the ampulla of Vater. Pancreatitis develops because alcohol-induced hypersecretion combined with sphincter spasm leads to high intraductal pressure, followed by duct necrosis, and escape of pancreatic juice. In addition, acute pancreatitis may be associated with certain therapeutic drugs, viruses, and trauma related to endoscopic or surgical procedures. A number of cases have no known cause (are idiopathic); other cases relate to inherited defects in the precursor protein for trypsin (trypsinogen) and in otherwise undiagnosed forms of cystic fibrosis. Such inherited lesions often result in chronic disease.

CHRONIC PANCREATITIS

Chronic pancreatitis often results from repeated episodes of mild acute pancreatitis associated with chronic alcoholism or other forms of recurrent pancreatic injury. Each bout of pancreatitis destroys some pancreatic tissue, but the inflammation subsides and the damaged pancreatic tissue is replaced by scar tissue. Eventually, as progressively more pancreatic tissue is destroyed, the affected person has difficulty digesting and absorbing nutrients because there is not enough surviving pancreatic tissue to produce adequate digestive enzymes. The associated destruction of pancreatic islets may also lead to diabetes. Chronic pancreatitis is often accompanied by debilitating pain. Death may occur with recurrent acute attacks.

Cystic Fibrosis of the Pancreas

Cystic fibrosis is the most common potentially lethal autosomal recessive disease in Caucasians. With a disease incidence of 1 in 2,500 births, about 1 in 30 Caucasians are carriers. (The disease is far more infrequent in black and Asian Americans.) Cystic fibrosis is a multisystem disease related to the production of abnormally viscous epithelial cell secretions (mucous). The abnormality results from a mutation of the *CFTR* gene, which stands for cystic fibrosis transmembrane conductance regulator, a rather formidable term meaning that the gene regulates the movement of chloride in most epithelial cells by means of ion channels located on the cell membranes. The *CFTR* gene, localized to the long arm of chromosome 7, has a large number of gene mutations, but about 70 percent of patients have a single mutation. Tests can identify carriers of the gene mutations responsible for most cases of cystic fibrosis. The mutation results in deletion of three bases at position 508 (termed ΔF508), which results in loss of a phenylalanine residue. The mutation blocks maturation of the protein, which is not transported to the cell surface and is degraded. In some individuals, the disease is relatively mild and compatible with survival into adolescence or adult life. However, most affected individuals have severe disease and in the past did not survive childhood. Modern therapy has much improved survival rates; nevertheless, the average (median) life expectancy is only about forty years.

As a result of the gene mutation, there is decreased secretion of chloride and increased reabsorption of sodium from epithelial cells in many organ systems. The defect in ion transport leads to increased cellular uptake of water from the lumen of organs and hence increased viscosity of the mucus secreted by the epithelial cells of the pancreas, bile ducts, mucosa of respiratory tract, and other mucus-secreting cells throughout the body. As a result, the mucus becomes abnormally thick and tends to form dense plugs that obstruct the pancreatic ducts, bronchi and bronchioles, and bile ducts.

Although lung disease characterized by chronic viscid mucous obstructed bronchioles and bronchi leading to repeated bouts of infection is the major cause of illness and death in cystic fibrosis patients, about 85 percent of patients have chronic pancreatitis as well. Mucous plugs in the small pancreatic ducts block the secretion of pancreatic juice, which accumulates under increased pressure within the obstructed ducts. Eventually, the ducts become cystically dilated. The pancreatic secretory cells, unable to discharge their secretions into the duodenum, undergo atrophy and are replaced by fibrous tissue, but the pancreatic islets are unaffected because they discharge their hormones directly into the bloodstream. Eventually, the pancreas becomes converted into a mass of cystically dilated ducts surrounded by dense fibrous tissue (**FIGURE 22-3**). For this reason, many cystic fibrosis patients need to take capsules containing pancreatic enzymes to digest and absorb food properly because their own pancreas has been destroyed by the disease. The name of the disease derives from these characteristic structural abnormalities.

The function of sweat glands also is abnormal in cystic fibrosis. The sweat glands are unable to reabsorb sodium and chloride, so the sweat of affected individuals contains an excessively high salt concentration. This biochemical abnormality has served as the basis of a diagnostic test for cystic fibrosis called a **sweat test**. A small quantity of sweat is collected, and the sodium and chloride concentrations are determined. The salt concentration of the sweat is low in normal persons and high in persons with cystic fibrosis.

The discovery of the *CFTR* gene and its defective counterpart have stimulated active research efforts that recently have led to the development of a drug that improves *CFTR* gene function, as demonstrated by more efficient chloride transport across the cell membrane, which is associated with improved pulmonary function. These encouraging results have stimulated further pharmacologic studies designed to correct the biochemical disturbances resulting from the genetic defects responsible for cystic fibrosis. However, prophylactic use of antibiotics remains critical to impede the occurrence of bacterial lung disease.

Sweat test Diagnostic test for cystic fibrosis.

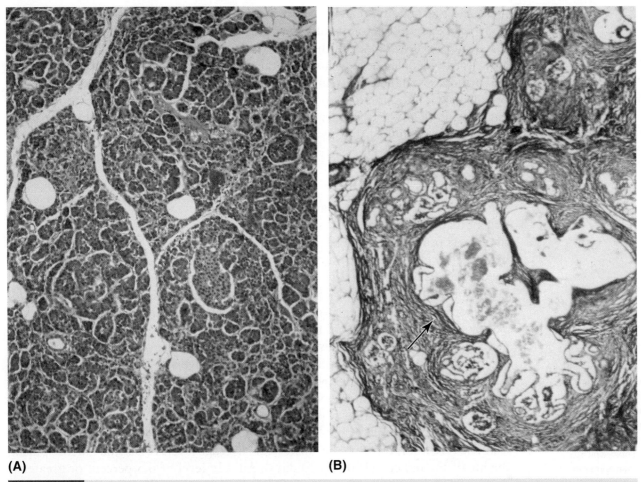

(A)

(B)

FIGURE 22-3 Low magnification photomicrographs comparing normal pancreas **(A)** with pancreas of patient with cystic fibrosis **(B)**. Duct in center of field (*arrow*) exhibits cystic dilatation. Most of pancreatic glandular tissue has undergone atrophy and has been replaced by fibrous tissue.

Courtesy of Leonard V. Crowley, MD, Century College.

Role of Insulin in Metabolism

The insulin made by the pancreas has a number of critical roles in controlling energy metabolism. Insulin is responsible for the movement of glucose transport proteins onto the surface of muscle cells, allowing the importation of glucose from the circulation into the cytoplasm where it can be used in energy production. In addition, insulin stimulates the conversion of hepatic glucose into glycogen while suppressing the conversion of glycogen into glucose. Insulin also plays an important role in stimulating liver lipid synthesis. This enables the liver to "store" excess calories in a more efficient and osmotically inactive form that ultimately is deposited as visceral fat contained in adipocytes. Insulin also promotes entry of amino acids into the cells and stimulates protein synthesis. Insulin stimulates endothelial cells to produce nitric oxide (eNOS) a potent vasodilator increasing blood flow to skeletal muscle. The main stimulus for insulin release is elevation of the level of glucose in the blood, as occurs after a meal. In **diabetes mellitus**, glucose is absorbed normally. However, because of lack of insulin or of insulin insensitivity, which occurs in the various forms of diabetes mellitus, glucose is not used to produce energy and is not stored as glycogen as in a normal person. Consequently, glucose accumulates in the bloodstream, resulting in **hyperglycemia**. The excessive glucose "spills over" in the

Diabetes mellitus
A metabolic disease characterized by hyperglycemia and caused by insufficient insulin secretion or inefficient utilization of insulin.

Hyperglycemia
Excessively high blood glucose concentration.

urine and is excreted. Because glucose must be excreted in the urine in solution, the body loses excessive amounts of water and electrolytes along with the glucose. This may lead to a disturbance in the water balance and the acid–base balance. (Water and electrolyte balance is discussed in the discussion on kidneys, water, electrolyte, and acid–base balance.) Protein synthesis is also compromised, and body protein is broken down into amino acids. The liver converts these amino acids into glucose, augmenting the hyperglycemia and leading to additional losses of glucose, water, and electrolytes in the urine.

Diabetes Mellitus

Diabetes mellitus is a very common and important metabolic disease that results either because of a deficit in the secretion of insulin by the pancreatic islets or because the targets of insulin action become resistant to its effects. The major symptom is a high level of glucose in the blood (hyperglycemia). A normal fasting blood glucose concentration is considered to be 70–100 mg per 100 ml of plasma (abbreviated 70–100 mg/dl). A diagnosis of diabetes requires a fasting glucose of 126 mg/dl or higher, confirmed by repeat testing, or a glucose concentration over 200 mg/dl determined by an oral glucose tolerance test (75 g of oral glucose two hours prior to testing of plasma glucose levels). Fasting blood glucose levels between 110 and 125 mg/dl are considered to be impaired and indicative of a "prediabetic" condition. Another test, called a **glycated hemoglobin test or the hemoglobin A1c test**, is based on the observation that hemoglobin in the blood is non–enzymatically glycated to a degree based on the level of plasma glucose. Fasting plasma glucose or postglucose tolerance testing levels are both "snapshots" of glucose metabolism at the time of the test. The A1c test represents the "historical" average levels of plasma glucose during the life of the red cell (100 to 120 days). An A1c level of 6.5 percent or greater is diagnostic of diabetes; levels between 5.7 and 6.4 percent indicate a prediabetic state.

The hyperglycemia of diabetes affects carbohydrate, fat, and protein metabolism. These derangements may result in acute and life-threatening disease and serious and chronic disturbances of multiple organ systems, notably the cardiovascular system, kidney, retina, and nervous system, leading to significant excess mortality, particularly in relationship to diabetes associated with obesity. More than 9 percent of the U.S. population have diabetes, rising to 26 percent in the population over age sixty-five. The disease is the seventh most common cause of death in the United States. The death rate from cardiovascular disease, heart attack and stroke, is between 1.5 and 1.8 times as high in diabetics. Diabetic kidney disease is responsible for 44 percent of cases of kidney failure. The overall annual cost of diabetes, for 2012, in the United States is almost $250 billion.

Diabetes is divided into two major groups, depending on whether the diabetes results from an autoimmune disease leading to the destruction of beta cells in the pancreas and hence a deficit in insulin production (**type 1 diabetes mellitus [T1DM]**) or from the resistance of target tissue to the effect of insulin and a compensatory over-secretion of insulin by the pancreas (**type 2 diabetes mellitus [T2DM]**). T2DM (formerly noninsulin dependent diabetes mellitus) is the more common form, often associated with obesity and occurring in adults. T1DM accounts for fewer than 10 percent of cases and usually occurs in a population less than twenty years of age. A subtype of T1DM, termed **latent autoimmune diabetes of adults (LADA)**, occurs in older individuals and may be misdiagnosed as T2DM. Because LADA also relates to autoimmune damage to beta cells, the terms "juvenile" and "adult-onset" diabetes are somewhat inaccurate and no longer used. **TABLE 22-1** compares the major features of the two types of diabetes. Diabetes may also occur in association with pregnancy (gestational

Glycated hemoglobin test/ hemoglobin A1c test A test that measures the amount of glucose permanently attached to hemoglobin, which is higher than normal in many people with diabetes.

Type 1 diabetes mellitus (T1DM) Diabetes resulting from a deficit in insulin production.

Type 2 diabetes mellitus (T2DM) Diabetes resulting from the resistance of target tissue to the effect of insulin with a compensatory oversecretion by the pancreas.

Latent autoimmune diabetes of adults (LADA) Subtype of type 1 diabetes first appearing in adults.

TABLE 22-1   Comparison of Two Major Types of Diabetes Mellitus

	Type 1	Type 2
Usual age of onset	Child to Young Adult	Middle age or later
Body build	Normal	Overweight
Plasma insulin	Absent or low	Normal or high
Complications	Ketoacidosis	Hyperosmolar coma
Response to insulin	Normal	Reduced
Response to oral antidiabetic drugs	Unresponsive	Responsive

diabetes) or in association with mutations in single genes (monogenic diabetes). Certain drugs and viral infections may lead to islet destruction independent of auto-immune reactivity.

TYPE 1 DIABETES MELLITUS

Type 1 diabetes is an autoimmune disease in which cytotoxic CD8+ T lymphocytes attack and destroy the pancreatic islets. The production of autoantibodies to beta cell products and components including insulin accompanies beta cell destruction. Such antibodies may be found before there is any evidence of clinical disease. The rate at which islets are destroyed by the immune system and the rate at which insulin secretion declines varies among affected individuals, but the disease usually has a long onset with severe disease being present after about 80 percent of beta cells are destroyed. In some cases, onset may be so slow as to not be noted until adulthood (LADA). However, the peak incidence of T1DM occurs primarily in children and young adults, most often around puberty. There is a clear hereditary predisposition to type 1 diabetes. People who inherit certain HLA-D types are at increased risk of acquiring this type of diabetes as well as other autoimmune diseases of the endocrine system. (HLA types and predisposition to disease are considered in the discussion on immunology.) Other nongenetic factors are also important in the causation of T1DM. More than 80 percent of patients do not have an affected relative, and fewer than half of identical twins both develop the disease. Seasonal variation in frequency and changes in the frequency of T1DM with time in a population suggest that environmental agents (and in particular infectious disease) may have a role in T1DM etiology. Infection with Coxsackie B virus has been noted to precede some cases of the disease.

The pathogenesis of T1DM is clearly related and proportional to the lack of insulin and consequent metabolic changes associated with it. Uncontrolled hepatic glucose output and lack of storage into muscle and fat tissue leads to high blood sugar (hyperglycemia). The osmotic effect (hyperosmolarity) leads to excessive urination (polyuria) with dehydration, increased thirst (polydipsia), and loss of minerals. The person with type 1 diabetes, lacking insulin, is unable to use carbohydrates because insulin is required to promote entry of glucose into the cells where the glucose can be metabolized to yield energy. Metabolism falls into a starvation-like state. Adipose stores are used as an energy source, and the oxidation of fat produces **ketone bodies**, which are released from the liver into the blood, leading to metabolic acidosis (**diabetic ketosis**). Together the acidosis, dehydration, and loss of ions can lead to coma and ultimately death if left untreated by provision of exogenous insulin.

Ketone bodies Various derivatives of acetyl-CoA, resulting from excessive mobilization of fat as an energy source.

Diabetic ketosis A disturbance of the body's acid–base balance (acidosis) caused by an inability to utilize glucose, which requires the body to use fat as an energy source. Fat metabolism generates excessive amounts of acid ketone bodies, which disrupts the normal alkalinity of body fluids.

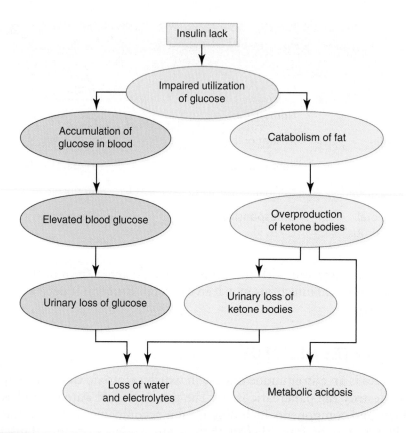

FIGURE 22-4   Major metabolic derangements in type 1 diabetes mellitus.

All these effects can be reversed by supplying insulin, which promotes normal utilization of glucose and storage of glycogen. The disturbances of fat and protein metabolism also are reversed by the action of insulin. **FIGURE 22-4** summarizes the major metabolic disturbances in type 1 diabetes.

TYPE 2 DIABETES MELLITUS

Type 2 diabetes, by far the more common type, is a complex metabolic defect associated with obesity (often in the elderly) in about 80 percent of cases. The pancreatic islets secrete insulin normally, followed by increasing amounts of insulin, but target tissues are relatively insensitive to the action of insulin and are unable to respond appropriately (termed **insulin resistance**). Eventually insulin output becomes unable to meet demand and hyperglycemia ensues. Unlike the case in T1DM, there is no autoimmune destruction of islet cells, although with increasing age fibrosis and deposition of amyloid (abnormally precipitated protein composed of a beta cell secreted protein termed amylin) can occur in the islets (**FIGURE 22-5**). There is increasing evidence that there are reduced numbers of islets/beta cells associated with T2DM, which is related to increased beta cell death. The cause of the loss and its relation to the etiology of T2DM remains unclear.

The reason for the impaired response to insulin is not completely understood, but it is central to the pathogenesis of T2DM. Insulin resistance is related to obesity because weight reduction restores insulin responsiveness and frequently controls the diabetes (although the exact mechanism remains unclear). However, congenital genetic diseases that prevent normal deposition of visceral fat (lipodystrophies) are often associated with severe insulin resistance. Hence, an optimal amount of visceral fat is necessary to buffer excess calories and prevent insulin resistance. The

Insulin resistance
Condition when target tissues are relatively insensitive to the action of insulin.

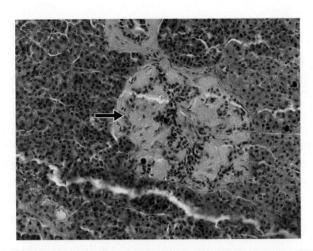

FIGURE 22-5 Amyloid deposition in pancreatic islet in long-standing T2DM. Islet where most cells have been replaced by amyloid (*arrow*) is visible as amorphous pink material.
Courtesy of Department of Pathology and Laboratory Medicine, University of North Carolina at Chapel Hill.

root cause of insulin resistance remains speculative. Excess adipose tissue associated with T2DM may contain inflammatory cells that secrete a number of cytokines, in particular tumor necrosis factor alpha and interleukin-1, which can lead to insulin resistance in experimental animal models. However, the evidence supporting this in T2DM limited.

Early symptoms of type 2 diabetes may be mild, with the disease disclosed only on routine testing (such as by glucose tolerance tests). The early symptoms are similar to that of type 1 diabetes, with polyuria, polydypsia, increased hunger, and sometimes unexplained weight loss. Itchiness and fatigue may also occur. Ketosis does not usually occur as a complication of type 2 diabetes, but affected individuals may develop another complication called **hyperosmolar coma**, which results from the marked hyperglycemia. Of critical concern are the chronic effects of the disease, which are expressed in essentially every organ, and most notably, in the cardiovascular and renal systems. Many of the chronic effects of T2DM relate to the dyslipidemia (increased triglycerides and reduced high-density lipoprotein cholesterol). Dyslipidemia is expressed in essentially every organ system in the body as a chronic disease state. The risk of atherosclerotic vascular disease with an increased incidence of hypertension, heat attack, and strokes; nonalcoholic fatty liver disease, which may progress to steatohepatitis; endocrine disease; renal disease; retinal disease; and an increased risk of cancer are all associated with the chronic dyslipidemia of T2DM.

Type 2 diabetes is a hereditary disease in which genetic factors play an even greater role than in type 1 diabetes. About 50 percent of the risk of type 2 diabetes is heritable although in most cases we do not know the exact mode of inheritance or the genes that predispose for this type of diabetes. Children of parents who both have T2DM have a 70-percent risk of also eventually becoming diabetic, and about one-third of diabetics have a parent who also had the disease. The risk of diabetes occurring in both of a pair of monozygotic (identical) twins is near 100 percent. In some population groups, such as the Pima Indians of Arizona, as many as 40 percent of adults are diabetic, and obesity is common. Although genetics is clearly important in this population, environmental and nutritional factors also play a major role. Pima Indians currently have a sedentary lifestyle with a diet high in fat. Related Indian groups with a more active lifestyle and diet lower in fat have a lower frequency of obesity and T2DM.

More than forty genetic loci are associated with increased risk for type 2 diabetes, but these loci contribute only about 10 percent of the risk attributable to

Hyperosmolar coma
Coma resulting from neurologic dysfunction caused by hyperosmolarity of body fluids as a consequence of severe hyperglycemia.

genetic background. However, variants (polymorphisms) of one gene (*TCF7L2*) are involved in about 20 percent of all cases of type 2 diabetes, and people homozygous for the high-risk allele of the gene have about a twofold increased risk of disease. The biological function of many of these genes in increasing the risk of disease remains unknown. Obesity (central obesity, the accumulation of visceral fat), a clear risk factor for T2DM, also has a strong genetic as well as an environmental component. About 40 to 70 percent of the risk for central obesity relates to multiple genetic factors. Hence, it is not surprising that genes that contribute to the risk of central obesity also may increase the risk of T2DM. The best characterized of these is a set of genes on chromosome 16 located near the gene *FTO* (fat mass and obesity associated). Genetic variants of the *FTO* gene have a marked effect on the risk of adult obesity. The effects are likely to be meditated through a second gene, *Irx3*, whose level of expression is controlled by *FTO*. *Irx3* is expressed in an area of the brain (the hypothalamus) critical in energy regulation. Additional information is available in the discussion of obesity under gastrointestinal issues.

An uncommon autosomal dominant genetic form of diabetes representing 1 to 2 percent of cases is maturity onset diabetes of the young (MODY). The name is a misnomer because the disease is not related to T2DM (generally associated with adult onset) but rather relates to mutations in a number of genes associated with impaired insulin secretion/ beta cell function occurring at an early age. Six genes have been associated with MODY. The most common form of MODY (MODY1) results from mutations in the *HNF1A* gene, which leads to progressive beta cell failure and a reduction in important steps in glucose transport and metabolism. The disease is progressive with age and associated with diabetic complications. The second most common form (MODY2) is associated with mutations in the glucokinase gene (*GCK*). These mutations interfere with the formation of glucose-6 phosphate, which ultimately stimulates the "glucose sensor" on the beta cell, but the beta cells cannot respond appropriately to the degree of glycemia. This disease is mild and does not progress with age.

PREDIABETES

Many people who eventually develop diabetes have blood glucose that is higher than normal but not high enough to establish a diagnosis of diabetes (although the cut-off is arbitrary). This condition is closely associated with visceral obesity, and in particular with deposition of adipose tissue in the abdominal region (as opposed to the hips and buttocks), and is associated with metabolic syndrome. This borderline abnormality in blood glucose and glucose tolerance testing is termed **prediabetes** to indicate that increased beta cell insulin production can no longer completely keep pace with the increasing resistance of insulin targets to the effect of the hormone. Reducing the demands on the pancreas can be accomplished by weight loss and moderate exercise (which reduce the insulin resistance of body cells so less insulin is required) and by healthy eating habits emphasizing fruits, vegetables, and whole grains (called the "Mediterranean-style diet"). Certain medications (such as metformin, which inhibits the production of glucose by the liver) may also be required. All these measures help preserve beta cell function and promote more efficient utilization of glucose so that blood glucose does not rise as high after eating.

Prediabetes Higher than normal blood glucose but not high enough to establish diagnosis of diabetes.

GESTATIONAL DIABETES

The high levels of placental hormones in pregnancy (see discussion on prenatal development and diseases associated with pregnancy) cause the pregnant woman to develop insulin resistance, but most women can compensate by secreting more insulin, and the blood glucose does not rise excessively. Women who are unable to secrete enough additional insulin develop pregnancy-related diabetes caused by their insulin resistance. **Gestational diabetes** is distinct from preexisting T2DM or LADA. Gestational diabetes is not uncommon, affecting nearly 10 percent of pregnancies. The condition is treated in a manner similar to prediabetes, with some physicians preferring supplementary insulin rather than metformin because hyperglycemia is harmful to the developing fetus. Although blood glucose returns to normal after delivery, a woman who has demonstrated significant insulin resistance/gestational diabetes during pregnancy is at risk of developing T2DM in later years. Gestational diabetes should serve as a "wake-up call" to begin taking steps such as weight loss, exercise, and diet modification to avoid T2DM.

> **Gestational diabetes**
> Elevated blood glucose caused by insulin resistance resulting from elevated hormones related to the pregnancy. Blood glucose returns to normal postpartum, but the woman has increased risk of diabetes later in life.

DIABETES AND THE METABOLIC SYNDROME

Metabolic syndrome is defined as abnormal fasting plasma glucose caused by insulin resistance, mild hypertension, and dyslipidemia (elevated plasma triglycerides and low plasma high-density lipoprotein [HDL] cholesterol). The syndrome occurs with abdominal obesity and a sedentary lifestyle. Metabolic syndrome may progress to diabetes-associated complications as well as to cardiovascular disease and its complications.

Overweight people with excess abdominal fat, as indicated by their waist circumference and waist to hip ratio (in men a circumference of over 40 in. or a waist to hip ratio greater than 0.9; in women a circumference of over 35 in. or a waist to hip ratio greater than 0.85), should be screened for the other conditions associated with the syndrome by measuring blood pressure, blood glucose, and blood lipids. If other metabolic syndrome–associated abnormalities are detected, treatment to correct or improve the associated conditions can be undertaken.

MONITORING CONTROL OF DIABETES

The current goal of treatment is to achieve control of blood glucose (glycemic control) that is as close as possible to normal, as close control of hyperglycemia reduces the long-term complications caused by diabetes. It is clear that such stringent management of hyperglycemia is associated with lower risk, increased life expectancy, and reduced vascular complications. As noted previously, two methods are used to assess the degree of glycemic control (i.e., the level of blood glucose). Self-monitoring of blood glucose by the patient (SMBG) is accomplished by the patient using finger-stick blood and portable semiautomated devices. This is generally done before and after eating, before stress (such as exercise), and if the patient recognizes the signs of low blood glucose (which can result in confusion and fainting). Insulin dosage (when used) is carefully tailored to help achieve as near to normal blood glucose levels as possible. Recently the FDA approved devices that continuously monitor interstitial blood glucose levels using a small sensor inserted under the skin. The devices are equipped with an alarm to indicate hypo- or hyperglycemia. These devices are being coupled to glucose pumps to achieve what might be considered an "artificial pancreas." The advantages of continuous glucose monitoring are unclear, but this does help some patients achieve better long-term control.

Tests for the level of glycated hemoglobin (also called hemoglobin A1c and often abbreviated as HbA1c) as an index of long-term control of hyperglycemia are generally done twice a year, or more frequently when therapy is changed. These tests are useful predictors of diabetic complications. Urine tests may be used in special circumstances to check for ketone bodies as an indication of diabetic ketosis in people with type 1 diabetes. The goal of frequent in-home blood glucose testing (or continuous glucose monitoring) is to monitor and control insulin dosage to achieve an optimal level of blood glucose with minimal variation in the face of varying nutrition and stress.

TREATMENT OF DIABETES

Type 1 diabetics require insulin at doses adjusted to control the level of blood glucose as closely as possible to reduce late complications. Most type 1 diabetics require several insulin injections spaced throughout the day to maintain blood glucose within reasonably normal limits. A variety of insulins are used that provide prolonged effects with relatively slow onset (basal insulins) or that act rapidly with shorter periods of action (bolus insulins). The exact dosing regimen optimal for a T1DM patient must be determined individually, but initially a mixture of 50 percent bolus and 50 percent basal is often used as a starting point. Frequent measurements of blood glucose permit better regulation of insulin dosage and improve control of the diabetes.

Insulin pumps are sometimes useful for type 1 diabetics who are difficult to treat because of their need for frequent insulin injections. An insulin pump is a small, battery-operated device that can be attached to the patient's belt. A short length of tubing extends from the pump to a fine (27 gauge) needle inserted into the subcutaneous tissue of the abdominal wall and secured with tape. The pump is programmed to deliver a small, constant infusion of insulin, supplemented by larger doses just before meals, simulating the release of insulin by the pancreas. Despite the convenience, use of an insulin pump requires very close medical supervision because complications can arise from pump malfunction or infections at the site of needle placement. Ultimately the goal is to combine these pumps with continuous blood glucose monitoring in what is described as a "closed-loop" system.

Type 2 diabetic patients can often be managed by diet and weight reduction alone. If they do not respond adequately, oral hypoglycemic drugs are added. Metformin, a biguanidine class drug, is the recommended preferred initial agent. If sufficient control cannot be achieved, either an additional oral agent or insulin is added. There are many additional oral pharmacologic agents other than metformin available, each with potential advantages and disadvantages. The choice is determined by the patient in consultation with the physician and is based on effectiveness, potential side effects, effects on weight, the likelihood of hypoglycemia, and cost. Many of these agents are extremely expensive, and the choice of second agent is often not obvious. (Metformin, the initial suggestion, is low in cost.)

COMPLICATIONS OF DIABETES

Complications of diabetes include increased susceptibility to infection, apparently related to the high levels of blood glucose, or development of diabetic coma as a result either of ketoacidosis or of the greatly increased osmolarity of body fluids resulting from hyperglycemia. Diabetics have a greater incidence of arteriosclerosis and its associated vascular complications such as strokes, heart attacks, and gangrene of the legs and feet as a result of poor circulation. The vascular problems probably result both from abnormalities in fat metabolism associated with diabetes and from the elevated blood lipids frequently found in diabetics. Patients with diabetes are also subject to other late complications, which increase in frequency with the duration of the disease. The small blood vessels supplying the retina of the eye often undergo degenerative changes, which may eventually lead to blindness in some patients. The glomerular arterioles and capillaries within the kidneys also undergo degenerative changes, which impair renal function and may result in renal failure (discussed in the section on the urinary system). The peripheral nerves may undergo degenerative changes, called peripheral neuritis, which cause pain and disturbed sensation in the extremities.

The chronic complications of diabetes including cardiovascular disease, nephropathy, retinopathy, and neuropathy relate in great part to damage to the vascular system. In addition, host responses to infection by bacteria and fungi are also impaired. How high glucose leads to organ damage is not completely understood, but the organ damage is related either directly or indirectly to the hyperglycemia. One concept proposes that the hyperglycemia causes the proteins in the retina, peripheral nerves, and capillary basement membranes to undergo the same type of glycation as hemoglobin. These glycated proteins undergo further interactions with other cell components, leading eventually to the blood vessel and organ damage characteristic of long-standing poorly controlled diabetes.

OTHER CAUSES OF HYPERGLYCEMIA

Other conditions may lead to impaired glucose utilization and hyperglycemia, but they are much less common than true diabetes mellitus. These conditions include chronic pancreatic disease, in which the hyperglycemia results from damage or destruction of pancreatic islets; endocrine diseases associated with overproduction of pituitary or adrenal hormones, which also raise blood glucose; ingestion of certain drugs, such as diuretics or antihypertensive drugs, that impair glucose metabolism as a side effect; and a few rare hereditary diseases in which carbohydrate metabolism is disturbed.

Hypoglycemia

The normal pancreas continually monitors the blood glucose and automatically adjusts its output of insulin to maintain the blood glucose level within the normal range. The type 1 diabetic patient, however, must adjust the dose of insulin to match the amount of carbohydrate to be metabolized. If there is insufficient insulin, the blood glucose is too high. If there is too much insulin, the blood glucose is too low, a condition called **hypoglycemia** (*hypo* = under). Two conditions predispose to hypoglycemia in a diabetic patient taking insulin. The first is a reduced intake of food, such as skipping a meal; blood glucose falls because carbohydrate intake is insufficient in relation to the amount of insulin injected. The second condition is increased activity, such as vigorous exercise, which lowers blood glucose by increasing glucose utilization. As a result, there is a relative excess of insulin. Too much insulin causes a precipitous drop in the level of glucose in the blood and initiates a chain of events called an **insulin reaction** or **insulin shock**. The adrenal medulla responds to the hypoglycemia by discharging epinephrine (adrenaline), which tends to raise blood glucose by converting liver glycogen into glucose. Epinephrine exerts widespread systemic effects as well: rapid heart rate, rise in blood pressure, constriction of cutaneous blood vessels causing the skin to appear pale, stimulation of sweat glands causing a cold sweat, and stimulation of the nervous system leading to increased excitability, anxiousness, hyperactive reflexes, and tremors.

Neurologic manifestations appear if the blood glucose continues to fall because the nervous system requires glucose to carry out its metabolic processes and begins to malfunction when deprived of its energy source. The individual becomes confused, loses consciousness, may have convulsions, and soon lapses into a deep coma. Prolonged severe hypoglycemia may cause permanent brain damage.

Hypoglycemia Lower than normal concentration of glucose in the blood.

Insulin reaction/insulin shock Condition in which there is too much insulin in the blood.

TABLE 22-2   Differentiation of Insulin Shock from Ketoacidosis and Hyperosmolar Coma

Diagnostic feature	Insulin shock	Ketoacidosis	Hyperosmolar coma
Food intake	May be insufficient	Normal or excessive	Normal or excessive
Insulin	Excessive	Insufficient	Normal or increased
Onset of symptoms	Rapid	Gradual (several days)	Gradual (several days)
Skin	Cold sweat, pale	Dry and flushed	Dry and flushed
Respirations	Normal or shallow	Slow and deep	Usually normal
Reflexes	Hyperactive	Depressed	Normal
Heart rate	Rapid	Rapid	Usually normal
Blood pressure	Normal or slightly elevated	Low	Usually normal
Glucose in urine	Absent	Large amount	Large amount
Blood glucose	Very low	High	Extremely high
Blood bicarbonate and pH	Normal	Low	Normal
Acetone in blood and urine	Absent	Present	Absent

If the patient is still conscious and able to swallow, the insulin reaction can be stopped by ingesting a quick-acting carbohydrate, such as a piece of candy or a glucose tablet. The diabetic patient should always have a quick-acting carbohydrate available for such emergencies. If the patient is unconscious, an injection of glucagon can be given; this raises blood glucose by mobilizing glucose from liver glycogen. A concentrated glucose solution may also be given intravenously.

Insulin shock must be distinguished from diabetic ketoacidosis or hyperosmolar nonketotic coma, two other conditions to which the diabetic patient is predisposed (**TABLE 22-2**). Determination of blood sugar level (low in insulin shock) is a first step.

Tumors of the Pancreas

Carcinoma of the pancreas is relatively common and develops most often in the head of the pancreas. In this location, the neoplasm blocks the common bile duct, resulting in obstructive jaundice. Carcinoma elsewhere in the pancreas is usually far advanced when first detected and produces no specific symptoms.

Sometimes, benign tumors arise from the islet cells and produce symptoms as a result of overproduction of hormones. Beta cells give rise to insulin-secreting tumors that cause episodes of severe hypoglycemia similar to those experienced by a diabetic who receives too much insulin.

CASES 22-1

Case 1: Jane is a twelve-year-old female who has begun to have a variety of problems at school. She has been losing weight and is concerned because she has not yet achieved menarche, unlike many of her friends. Her schoolwork has begun to suffer. She is fatigued and has trouble concentrating; she has difficulty participating in athletics, and her vision is occasionally blurred. She is embarrassed because her teacher has noticed that she frequently must ask to go to the rest room and is constantly drinking. While trying to exercise in the gym, she faints and is taken to the hospital by ambulance. Her temperature is normal. Respirations are rapid and deep. Blood pressure is normal. She is comatose but responded to painful stimuli. Her skin is warm and dry. The remainder of the physical signs are normal. The patient's urine contained large amounts of glucose. There was a strongly positive reaction for acetone and other ketone bodies. Blood glucose was 565 mg/dl (normal range 60–100 mg/dl). Other laboratory studies revealed a low blood pH and reduced plasma bicarbonate of 8 mEq/l (normal range 24–28 mEq/l). The patient was considered to have severe diabetic acidosis probably precipitated by stress during exercise. After intensive treatment with intravenous fluids and insulin, her condition gradually improved. The following day she was conscious and oriented and was able to take fluids orally. She continued to improve and was eventually discharged from the hospital. Testing revealed a moderately elevated level of hemoglobin A1c. She was diagnosed with type 1 diabetes mellitus and instructed in the details of a diabetic diet and taught to do frequent self-monitoring for blood glucose levels. She required a minimum of two injections of insulin with occasional supplementation with a rapid-acting inhaled insulin prior to strenuous exercise. She is now doing well in school and is monitored regularly by a physician specializing in diabetes in the young.

Case 2: John is an obese, sixty-eight-year-old man who was diagnosed several years ago as being prediabetic on the basis of a borderline abnormal glucose tolerance test and minimally elevated hemoglobin A1c. He was also been found to be moderately hypertensive at that time, but John has not seen a physician since nor has he modified his sedentary lifestyle. He has experienced increased urinary output and thirst for the last two weeks. He attends the North Carolina State Fair on an extremely warm and humid day and consumes large quantities of sugar-containing soft drinks, cotton candy, and fried chocolate candy bars. He becomes progressively more confused and collapses in a coma. He is brought to the hospital by the local emergency rescue squad with a suspicion of heat exhaustion, but his temperature is only slightly elevated. On admission, he is comatose and dehydrated. His respiratory rate is not increased. Blood pressure is normal. The urine contains a large amount of glucose but no ketone bodies. Blood pH and bicarbonate are normal. Blood glucose is 1,750 mg/dl (normal range 60–100 mg/dl), and the osmolarity of the plasma is 396 mOsm/liter (normal range 280–295 mOsm/liter). A diagnosis of hyperosmolar nonketotic coma is made. He is treated with large volumes of hypotonic (0.45 percent) saline solution and with insulin. His condition gradually improves over the next several days. His blood glucose gradually falls toward normal and eventually reaches 150 mg/dl on the fourth day. Plasma osmolarity also returns to normal as the elevated blood glucose declines. He is diagnosed as having type 2 diabetes mellitus and is instructed to lose weight and begin a moderate exercise program. He is placed on an oral hypoglycemic agent (metformin) but also requires supplemental insulin to control his blood glucose level. He does forswear high-sugar snacks in future visits to the fair.

Discussion

The purpose of these cases is to illustrate some of the typical symptoms of type 1 and type 2 diabetes mellitus and acute medical problems associated with each. It is not uncommon for

(Continues)

CASES 22-1   (*Continued*)

emergency medical responders to be required to diagnose and begin therapy for ketoacidosis, hyperosmolar coma, and insulin shock (the latter not illustrated in the cases). Table 22-2 summarizes the differential signs of each. Type 1 and type 2 diabetes mellitus are both characterized by hyperglycemia, but the etiologies and presentations of the diseases are quite different. Although acute complications of both diseases may differ, the chronic multisystem effects of poorly controlled disease are similar.

Etiology and Pathogenesis

Case 1 is undiagnosed type 1 diabetes mellitus associated with autoimmune destruction of the pancreatic islets and consequent lack of sufficient insulin production. A common acute presentation (diabetic ketoacidosis) relates to the production of acidic metabolic products of excessive lipid metabolism, which exceed the buffering capacity of the plasma. Case 2 demonstrates the progression of prediabetes into symptomatic type 2 diabetes in an individual suffering from uncontrolled metabolic syndrome. In this case, increasing insulin resistance related to obesity and lifestyle progress to the point at which extreme hyperglycemia related to the sudden intake of massive amounts of sugar occurs.

Questions

1. Type 1 diabetes mellitus (unlike type 2 diabetes mellitus) is often discovered when a person suffers from the sudden occurrence of ketoacidosis. Why do the two diseases differ in this respect?

2. Type 1 and type 2 diabetes mellitus both result in hyperglycemia, but the etiologies are distinct. What are the likely etiologies for the two conditions?

3. How are the symptoms and clinical signs of both forms of diabetes related to the pathophysiology of the diseases?

4. The second case description states the patient has metabolic syndrome. What is this syndrome, and how does the description of the patient support this? What is the relationship of metabolic syndrome to type 2 diabetes mellitus?

QUESTIONS FOR REVIEW

1. What is the difference between acute and chronic pancreatitis?
2. What are the major metabolic disturbances in type 1 diabetes? How does insulin correct these disturbances?
3. What are the major complications of diabetes?
4. Which type of diabetes can be treated by diet alone?
5. What is meant by the following terms: *sweat test*, *hyperglycemic coma*, and *insulin resistance*?
6. What is cystic fibrosis of the pancreas? What are its clinical manifestations? What is its pattern of inheritance?
7. What is hypoglycemia? What are its clinical manifestations? How is it treated?
8. What are the major differences between diabetic ketoacidosis and insulin shock?
9. What is gestational diabetes? Why does it occur?
10. Compare and contrast diabetes mellitus and metabolic syndrome.

SUPPLEMENTARY READINGS

Muniraj, T., et al. 2014. Chronic pancreatitis, a comprehensive review and update. Part I: Epidemiology, etiology, risk factors, genetics, pathophysiology and clinical features. *Disease-a-Month* 60:530–50.

Testoni, P. A. 2014. Acute recurrent pancreatitis: Etiopathogenesis, diagnosis and treatment. *World Journal of Gastroenterology* 20:16891–901.

▶ These two entries are recent reviews of the etiology and pathogenesis of the most significant forms of pancreatitis.

Sawczak, V., et al. 2015. Novel approaches for potential therapy of cystic fibrosis. *Current Drug Targets* 16(9): 923–36.

Kumar, S., Tana, A., and Shankar, A. 2014. Cystic fibrosis—What are the prospects for a cure? *European Journal of Internal Medicine* 25:803–7.

▶ These two references review current approaches to the treatment of cystic fibrosis using both pharmacology and molecular biology.

Lin, H. C., et al. 2015. Enterovirus infection is associated with an increased risk of childhood type 1 diabetes in Taiwan: A nationwide population-based cohort study. *Diabetologia* 58:79–86.

▶ Both a detailed investigative study and a recent review of literature supporting a link between viral infection and type 1 diabetes mellitus.

Moodley, N., et al. 2015. Historical perspectives in clinical pathology: A history of glucose measurement. *Journal of Clinical Pathology* 68(4):270–73.

▶ Glucose testing is the key to diabetes diagnosis and therapy. This is a fascinating review of methods for glucose testing in body fluids from ancient Egypt to the present.

Inzucchi, S. E., et al. 2015. Management of hyperglycemia in type 2 diabetes, 2015: A patient-centered approach: Update to a position statement of the American Diabetes Association and European Association for the Study of Diabetes. *Diabetes Care* 38:140–49.

American Diabetes Association. 2014. Standards of medical care in diabetes–2014. *Diabetes Care* 37(Suppl 1):14–80.

American Diabetes Association. 2014. Diagnosis and classification of diabetes mellitus. *Diabetes Care* 37(Suppl 1):81–90.

> ▶ These three references present the current "official" stance on the treatment of diabetes by the American Diabetes Association. Each is an exhaustive overview of all clinical aspects of diabetes with extensive reviews. An excellent and definitive first source for information.

O'Neill, S., and O'Driscoll, L. 2015. Metabolic syndrome: A closer look at the growing epidemic and its associated pathologies. *Obesity Reviews* 16:1–12.

> ▶ A troubling overview of the ever-increasing worldwide prevalence of metabolic syndrome and the pathologies associated with it.

Brunetti, A., Chiefari, E., and Foti, D. 2014. Recent advances in the molecular genetics of type 2 diabetes mellitus. *World Journal of Diabetes* 5:128–40.

Murphy, R., Carroll, R. W., and Krebs, J. D. 2013. Pathogenesis of the metabolic syndrome: Insights from monogenetic disorders. *Mediators of Inflammation* ID 920214.

> ▶ Two recent reviews in what is still a very confusing and quickly changing area of research. Figure 1 in the Brunetti review is a very useful summary of the factors involved in type 2 diabetes mellitus.

The Gastrointestinal Tract

LEARNING OBJECTIVES

1. Identify the major types of cleft lip and cleft palate deformity.
2. Explain the pathogenesis of dental caries and periodontal disease, and describe prevention and treatment.
3. Name and describe the three most common lesions of the esophagus that lead to esophageal obstruction.
4. Describe the common types of gastritis and their clinical manifestations.
5. Explain the pathogenesis of peptic ulcer. Describe the three major complications of peptic ulcer and their treatment. Name the methods of treatment.

6. Differentiate between appendicitis and Meckel diverticulitis in terms of pathogenesis, clinical manifestations, and treatment.
7. Describe the common types of chronic and acute enteritis and their clinical manifestations.
8. Describe the pathogenesis of diverticulitis, and explain the role of diet in the development of lesion.
9. Name the causes, clinical manifestations, and complications of intestinal obstruction, carcinoma of the colon, and diverticulosis of the colon. Explain their treatment.
10. Understand the major eating disturbances and their effects.

Structure and Functions

The gastrointestinal tract, which is concerned with the digestion and absorption of food, reabsorption of water, and elimination of wastes, comprises the oral cavity and related parts of the face, the esophagus, the stomach, the small and large intestines, the rectum, and the anus.

Abnormalities of the Oral Cavity

CLEFT LIP AND CLEFT PALATE

Embryologically, the face and palate are formed by coalescence of masses of cells that merge to form the facial structures and to separate the nasal cavity from the mouth. In the upper part of the face, the areas of coalescence are located on either side of the midline in a line that passes through the upper lip and jaw and extends into each nostril. The palate is formed by two shelf-like masses of tissue that grow medially and fuse in the midline to close the communication between nose and mouth. If these developmental processes are disturbed, defects may result in the upper lip and jaw (**cleft lip**) or in the palate (**cleft palate**).

Cleft lip and cleft palate are common abnormalities that frequently occur in combination. The incidence of these abnormalities is about 1 per 1,000 births. Both cleft lip and cleft palate follow a multifactorial pattern of inheritance (see discussion of congenital and hereditary diseases). Cleft lip with or without cleft palate and cleft palate alone have different epidemiology and risk factors. The incidence of cleft lip with or without cleft palate is much higher among the children of parents who previously gave birth to an infant with cleft lip (but not one with only a cleft palate). The incidence of cleft palate is higher among parents who themselves have a cleft palate (but not with a cleft lip or cleft lip and palate).

Cleft lip may be unilateral or bilateral and may range in severity from a relatively minor defect in the mucosa of the lip to a large cleft extending deeply into the upper jaw. Even very minor defects in the muscular ring around the oral cavity detected only on radiography present an increased familial risk for more severe clefting. In the most severe deformity, the cleft extends completely through the upper jaw into the floor of the nose (complete cleft) and may also extend posteriorly into the palate. Large bilateral clefts extending into the palate completely separate the hard palate from the midline tissue that forms part of the upper jaw, and the separated tissue is often displaced forward (**FIGURE 23-1**). Midline cleft palate may occur as an isolated abnormality, but it is usually associated with unilateral or bilateral cleft lip. Cleft lip and palate may occur as isolated defects or much less frequently as part of developmental syndromes associated with other defects.

There are several potential risks to a child born with a cleft. Aspiration of milk may occur because of communication between the oral and nasal cavity. Airway obstruction may occur because of tongue placement, and feeding difficulties and regurgitation are likely. Cleft lip usually does not cause major difficulties in feeding but might with more severe clefts. Cleft lip and palate frequently occur together but are corrected surgically at different times. Generally, cleft lip is repaired very soon

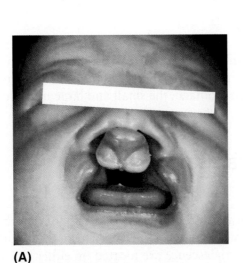
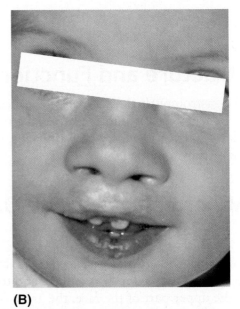

(A)   **(B)**

FIGURE 23-1 **(A)** A complete bilateral cleft lip and cleft palate with anterior protrusion of tissues between clefts. **(B)** The same child at eighteen months of age after surgical correction of the defect.

Courtesy of Leonard V. Crowley, MD, Century College.

after birth. Repair of cleft palate is generally deferred until the child is between one and two years old. After the cleft palate is repaired, speech therapy is begun in early childhood to correct the nasal quality that often results from abnormal palatal function.

ABNORMALITIES OF TOOTH DEVELOPMENT

The teeth are specialized structures developed in the tissues of the jaws. Each tooth consists of a solid portion called **dentine**, which forms the bulk of the tooth; an enamel crown covering the exposed surface of the tooth; and a central pulp cavity containing nerve fibers, lymphatics, and blood vessels. The root of the tooth, which is embedded in the jaw, is covered by a thin layer of bone-like tissue called **cementum**, and the tooth is anchored in the jaw by dense connective tissue fibers (**FIGURE 23-2**).

There are two sets of teeth. The first set, called the temporary or deciduous teeth, consists of a total of twenty teeth (ten in each jaw) that erupt in childhood. Eventually, these temporary teeth are replaced by a second, permanent set of thirty-two teeth. When the permanent teeth begin to grow, they press against the roots of the temporary teeth. This causes resorption of the roots and loosening of the temporary teeth, which eventually fall out and are replaced by the permanent teeth.

Each deciduous and permanent tooth develops from a separate tooth bud. Development of the tooth requires the interaction of the **odontoblasts**, the mesenchymal derived cells that form the dentin, and the epithelial derived **ameloblasts** that form the tooth enamel. Calcium is deposited in the dentine and enamel of the tooth as it is being formed. The deciduous teeth are formed before birth and erupt during childhood. The permanent teeth do not begin to develop until after birth and erupt at various times in late childhood and adolescence.

The absence of one or more teeth is relatively common and is often a familial trait that follows a multifactorial pattern of inheritance resulting from failure of one or more tooth buds to develop. Sometimes an extra tooth bud forms, resulting in an extra tooth.

Enamel forms within the developing teeth at specific times. If the antibiotic tetracycline is administered while enamel is being formed in the teeth, the antibiotic is deposited with calcium in the enamel and causes permanent yellow-gray to brown

Dentine Bony structure of the tooth.

Cementum Bonelike tissue covering the root of the tooth.

Odontoblasts Mesenchymal derived cells that form the dentine.

Ameloblasts Epithelial derived cells that form the tooth enamel.

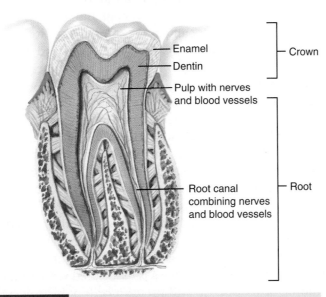

Enamel — Crown
Dentin —
Pulp with nerves and blood vessels
Root canal combining nerves and blood vessels — Root

FIGURE 23-2 The structure of a tooth.

discoloration in the crowns and may disturb enamel formation. Therefore, tetracycline (and similar antibiotics such as doxycycline) should not be given to pregnant women or to infants and children through infancy and childhood to about the age of eight years.

Dental Caries and Its Complications

The oral cavity contains a diverse collection of both aerobic and anaerobic bacteria. Masses of these bacteria intermixed with bacterial products and proteins from saliva form a biofilm called **dental plaque**, which adheres to the teeth and predisposes to tooth decay.

Caries, the term for tooth decay, is a Latin word meaning dry rot. The condition is a decalcification of the tooth structure caused by mouth bacteria acting on bits of retained food material, such as sugar and highly refined, starchy foods. Bacterial fermentation liberates organic acids that erode the covering enamel, exposing the underlying dentine, which is attacked by the acids and invaded by mouth bacteria. The loss of tooth structure that results from the combined acid and bacterial action is called a dental **cavity**. The affected area appears discolored and is quite soft when probed with a dental instrument. Dental x-rays reveal the cavity as an area of decreased density in the affected tooth. Saliva buffers the bacterially produced acid. For this reason, people who lack saliva (have **xerostoma**, a dry mouth) have a high incidence of caries.

If the cavity is not treated and continues to enlarge, the decay eventually reaches the dental pulp. The bacteria invade the pulp and incite an inflammation (**pulpitis**) that causes the throbbing pain characteristic of a toothache. Unchecked, the infection may spread to the apex of the tooth root, which is embedded in the jawbone, and from there spread to the bone surrounding the dental root. The result may be an abscess surrounding the apex of the tooth, which is called a **periapical abscess** (*peri* = around).

The incidence of tooth decay can be reduced by proper mouth hygiene, including frequent brushing of the teeth and use of dental floss to remove food particles that promote bacterial growth. Fluoride added to water supplies and toothpaste helps to prevent cavities by promoting formation of a more acid-resistant tooth structure that resists decay. Dental caries is treated by removing the decayed area and packing the defect with some type of dental filling material. After infection of the pulp and dental root has occurred, more extensive treatment and possibly the use of antibiotics is required. Infection of the root canal is resistant to antibiotics and requires that the pulp cavity along with the root canal be cleaned out and packed with a filling material, a procedure called a **root canal** treatment. Sometimes the tooth cannot be salvaged and must be extracted.

Masses of bacteria and debris accumulating around the base of the teeth may incite an inflammation. Initially, the inflammation affects only the gums surrounding the roots of the teeth, which is called **gingivitis** (*gingiva* = gum). Later, the inflammation extends between the teeth and the adjacent gums, leading to the formation of small pockets of infection between the teeth and gums. This condition is called **periodontal disease** (*peri* = around + *dens* = tooth). If pus is discharged from the margins of the infected gums, the descriptive term pyorrhea (*pyo* = pus + *rhea* = flow) is often used. The infection may spread into the tooth sockets that anchor the teeth in the jawbone, causing the teeth to loosen and eventually fall out. Various methods of treatment to the gums and teeth may control or arrest the condition, which is an important cause of loss of teeth. Chronic peridontal disease is associated with a number of systemic conditions, including heart disease and preterm or low-birth-weight pregnancies; however, this remains an area of controversy.

Dental plaque Masses of bacteria, bacterial products, and salivary proteins adherent to teeth, which predispose to tooth decay.

Caries Tooth decay.

Cavity (dental) A loss of tooth structure caused by the combined action of mouth bacteria and organic acids derived from bacterial fermentation of retained food particles.

Xerostoma Dry mouth which is lacking in saliva.

Pulpitis Inflammation of the dental pulp.

Periapical abscess Infection of the tooth root.

Root canal Replacement of tooth root canal with a filling material.

Gingivitis Gum inflammation.

Periodontal disease Pockets of infection between teeth and gum.

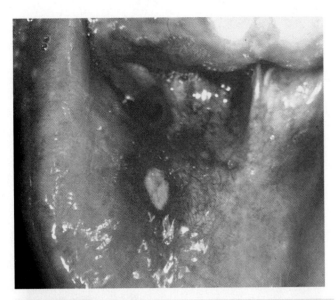

FIGURE 23-3 Superficial shallow ulcer of oral mucosa caused by canker sore.
Courtesy of Leonard V. Crowley, MD, Century College.

INFLAMMATION OF THE ORAL CAVITY

An inflammation of the oral cavity, called **stomatitis** (*stoma* = mouth), may be caused by a number of irritants and infectious agents. Common irritants are alcohol, tobacco, and hot or spicy foods. Infectious agents include the herpes, human papilloma and several other viruses, the fungus *Candida albicans* (which also causes vaginal infections) particularly in immunosuppressed individuals and diabetics, and a combination of two bacteria that cause necrotizing gingivitis called trench mouth or Vincent angina.

Canker sores are another relatively common inflammatory disease involving the oral cavity. A canker sore appears as a small, painful, superficial ulcer of the oral mucosa surrounded by a narrow zone of inflammation that appears as a red border surrounding the ulcer (**FIGURE 23-3**). The cause of the sores is unknown, but an immune reaction to oral bacteria has been suggested as a cause.

TUMORS OF THE ORAL CAVITY

Leukoplakia, the presence of white lesions on the mucosa of the oral cavity, is common, and about 20 percent demonstrate cellular dysplasia, a precursor to oral cancer. **Erythroplakia**, depressed red lesions on the oral mucosa, are of more concern, frequently being associated with dysplasia and even carcinoma in situ. Dentists are careful to search for and evaluate such lesions, often by biopsy. Carcinoma of the oral cavity, which may arise from the squamous epithelium of the lips, cheek, tongue, palate, or back of the throat, is relatively common with about 40,000 cases per year in the United States (**FIGURE 23-4**). Squamous cell carcinoma of the oral cavity is similar to that seen at other sites and frequently metastasizes. The nasal cavity and sinuses also may develop squamous cell carcinomas that may be associated with industrial exposure to nickel and other agents and also may be associated with the HPV.

Both benign and malignant tumors of the salivary glands occur (most frequently in the parotid gland). The most common benign tumor (pleomorphic adenoma) is slow growing and painless, consisting of a mixture of epithelial and duct-like cells, but it can be difficult to completely remove. Malignant salivary gland tumors consist of a number of different carcinomas that require surgery and sometimes radiation therapy.

Stomatitis Inflammation of the oral cavity.

Canker sores Inflammatory disease of the oral cavity.

Leukoplakia White lesions on the mucosa of the oral cavity.

Erythroplakia Depressed red lesions on the oral mucosa.

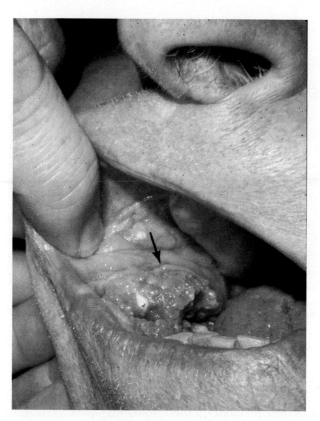

FIGURE 23-4 Squamous cell carcinoma of oral mucosa (*arrow*), which appears as an irregular overgrowth of tissue arising from the mucosa of the cheek.

Courtesy of Leonard V. Crowley, MD, Century College.

Diseases of the Esophagus

The esophagus is a muscular tube extending from the pharynx to the stomach with sphincters at both upper and lower ends. The upper sphincter relaxes to allow passage of swallowed food, which is propelled down the esophagus by rhythmic peristaltic contractions. The lower esophageal sphincter (called the **gastroesophageal or cardiac sphincter**) relaxes when the food reaches the lower end of the esophagus and allows the food to pass into the stomach. Problems with the esophagus include failure of the lower sphincter, tears in the lining, obstruction, inflammation, and neoplasia.

Symptoms of esophageal disease include difficulty swallowing (**dysphagia**) together with variable degrees of substernal discomfort or pain (often called "heartburn"). Complete obstruction of the esophagus leads to an inability to swallow, which is often associated with regurgitation of food into the trachea, causing episodes of choking and coughing. Irregularities in the esophageal mucosa (esophageal webs and rings) may occur as congenital lesions or as the result of disease. Diverticula in the esophagus may occur as a result of motor disturbances. Elderly patients may acquire a **Zenker diverticulum**, which is an outpouching in the upper portion of the esophagus that traps food and causes regurgitation.

CARDIAC SPHINCTER DYSFUNCTION

The two major disturbances of cardiac sphincter function are failure of the cardiac sphincter to open properly, which is called **acalasia (formerly cardiospasm)**, and inability of the sphincter to remain closed properly, which is called an incompetent cardiac sphincter and leads to **reflux esophagitis**.

Gastroesophageal/cardiac sphincter Lower esophageal sphincter.

Dysphagia Difficulty swallowing.

Zenker diverticulum Outpouching in the upper portion of the esophagus.

Acalasia/cardiospasm Inability of the sphincter to relax.

Reflux esophagitis Inflammation of the lining of the esophagus caused by reflux of acidic gastric secretions through an incompetent lower gastroesophageal sphincter.

Achalasia

Sometimes the cardiac sphincter fails to open properly, caused by a malfunction of the nerve plexuses in the esophagus that control its functions. As a result, food cannot pass normally into the stomach, and the smooth muscle in the wall of the esophagus must contract more vigorously to force the food past the constricted sphincter. Eventually the esophageal muscle undergoes marked hypertrophy, and the esophagus becomes dilated proximal to the constricted sphincter because of food retention. This results in dysphagia and sometimes in food regurgitation. A number of drugs are useful in helping to relax the muscle, including endoscopic injection of botulinum toxin, which blocks the transmission of nerve impulses from the nerve plexuses to the muscle fibers for several months. More permanent therapy consists of periodic stretching of the sphincter or by surgically cutting the muscle fibers in the constricted area.

Incompetent Cardiac Sphincter and Its Complications

In this relatively common condition, acid gastric juice leaks back into the esophagus through the improperly closed, incompetent lower esophageal sphincter. The squamous epithelial lining of the esophagus, which was not "designed" to tolerate high-acid secretions, becomes irritated and inflamed, leading to reflux esophagitis. The condition is most commonly found in people after the age of forty and is associated with obesity, smoking, and alcohol consumption. In some patients, the squamous mucosal lining may actually become ulcerated and scarred. Sometimes the squamous lining responds to the acidity by undergoing a change (metaplasia) into a more acid-resistant columnar gastric type mucosa. This condition is called **Barrett esophagus** after the person who first described it. Unfortunately, the metaplastic columnar epithelium is frequently abnormal and poses an increased risk of developing adenocarcinoma arising in the abnormal columnar epithelium (**FIGURE 23-5**). Patients with a significant degree of Barrett esophagus require periodic endoscopic monitoring and biopsy to detect early cancer. The condition may be treated endoscopically by using radiofrequency-induced heating to ablate affected areas. Treatment of reflux esophagitis to prevent progression to Barrett esophagus consists of avoiding lying down soon after eating because the recumbent position promotes reflux, sleeping with the head of the bed elevated to minimize reflux,

> **Barrett esophagus**
> Squamous lining changes to a more acid-resistant columnar mucosa.

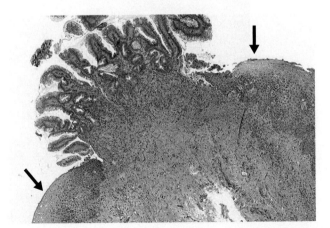

FIGURE 23-5 Barrett esophagus. A biopsy specimen from a patient with Barrett esophagus. The two *arrows* indicate areas of normal squamous mucosa. The area between them demonstrates mucosal metaplasia where the squamous epithelium has been replaced by columnar epithelium.

Courtesy of Department of Pathology and Laboratory Medicine, University of North Carolina at Chapel Hill.

and avoiding alcoholic beverages because alcohol not only stimulates gastric acid secretion but also tends to relax the lower esophageal sphincter, facilitating reflux. Drugs that reduce secretion of gastric acid and antacids that neutralize gastric acid are helpful.

GASTRIC MUCOSAL TEARS

Retching and vomiting may cause linear tears in the mucosa of the gastroesophageal junction where the esophagus passes through the diaphragm or in the lining of the distal esophagus, and these tears can bleed profusely (Mallory Weiss syndrome) (**FIGURE 23-6**). The repetitive, intermittent, vigorous contractions of the abdominal muscles associated with vomiting raise intragastric pressure while lowering the intrathoracic pressure and lead to distension and extremely forceful ejection of stomach contents through the esophagus. The additional stresses resulting from vigorous contractions of the muscular walls of the stomach and esophagus associated with vomiting probably place additional stress on the mucosa, which also plays a role in causing the laceration. This vomiting-related complication is not uncommon and is responsible for up to 10 percent of cases of bloody vomiting (**hematemesis**) and often follows the retching and vomiting related to excess alcohol intake, but it may follow vomiting from any cause, including self-induced vomiting to control weight.

Hematemesis Bloody vomit.

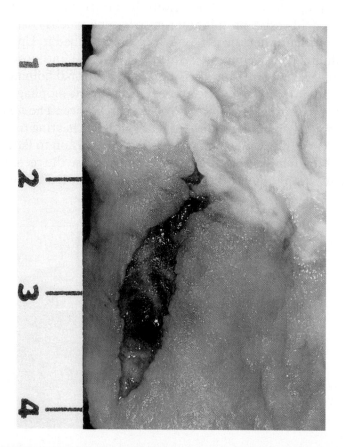

FIGURE 23-6 Gastric mucosal tear caused by retching and vomiting. The opaque mucosa in the upper part of the photograph is the normal stratified squamous mucosa of the esophagus. The 2 cm long tear extends distally from the gastroesophageal junction and caused a fatal gastric hemorrhage.

Courtesy of Leonard V. Crowley, MD, Century College.

ESOPHAGEAL OBSTRUCTION

Carcinoma of the Esophagus

Carcinoma may arise anywhere in the esophagus, either from the squamous epithelium (squamous cell carcinoma) or from the columnar epithelium associated with Barrett esophagus (adenocarcinoma). Worldwide, squamous cell carcinoma is the more common although frequency varies in different geographic areas. The disease is related to alcohol intake, smoking, the consumption of near boiling beverages (often tea), and possibly HPV and a variety of environmental agents. However, adenocarcinoma has rapidly increased in frequency in the United States, possibly in relation to the increased frequency of Barrett esophagus related to changes in dietary habits, and it is now more common than squamous cell carcinoma. In either case, the tumor gradually narrows the lumen of the esophagus, frequently infiltrates the surrounding tissues, and may invade the trachea. Necrosis of the tumor extending between the esophagus and trachea may lead to the formation of an abnormal communication between these two structures called a **tracheoesophageal fistula** (*fistula* = tube). The tumor is often discovered at an advanced stage, requiring esophagectomy, chemotherapy, and radiation.

Food Impaction

Obstruction of the esophagus may be caused by impaction of poorly chewed meat in the distal part of the esophagus. This is sometimes encountered in people who are unable to chew their food properly because they have poor teeth or improperly fitting dentures or who have poor eating habits.

Stricture

A stricture is a narrowing caused by scar tissue. Reflux esophagitis with ulceration and scarring is the most common cause of stricture. Esophageal scarring also may result from accidentally or deliberately swallowing a corrosive chemical that causes necrosis and inflammation. Severe scarring eventually follows. A common cause of esophageal stricture in children is accidental swallowing of commercial lye solutions (used for cleaning clogged drains). Ingestion of other household cleaning agents and disc batteries also are frequent causes.

Tracheoesophageal fistula Abnormal communication between the esophagus and trachea.

Gastritis Inflammation of the stomach.

Diseases of the Stomach

Diseases of the stomach include acute and chronic gastritis, peptic ulcer, carcinoma of the stomach, and gastroenteritis.

GASTRITIS

Inflammation of the stomach is called **gastritis,** and the inflammation may be either acute or chronic. Many patients with gastritis have few symptoms, but some experience abdominal discomfort and nausea. However, acute gastritis may be severe enough to result in life-threatening hemorrhage.

Acute Gastritis

In most cases, acute gastritis is a self-limited inflammation of short duration. However, at times, the acute inflammation may be quite severe and may be complicated by ulceration of the mucosa with bleeding from the ulcerated areas. Patients in whom the acute gastritis is associated with mucosal ulceration often have more pronounced symptoms, and the ulcerated areas may bleed profusely, a condition called acute hemorrhagic gastritis.

There are many causes of acute gastritis, but the most common is related to the use of non-steroidal anti-inflammatory drugs (NSAIDs) such as aspirin, ibuprofen, and naproxen. These drugs are widely used to treat symptoms of arthritis and related musculoskeletal pain problems. The drugs act by inhibiting an enzyme called **cyclooxygenase,** which is required for the synthesis of prostaglandins (potent mediators discussed in the inflammation and repair section). Prostaglandins are produced by many different cells and have many different functions. Those produced by gastric epithelial cells help protect the stomach from the damaging effects of gastric acid by promoting the secretion not only of sodium bicarbonate to counteract the acid but also of mucin to coat and protect the stomach lining. Consequently NSAIDs cause the mucosa to become more vulnerable to injury from acidic gastric juice, which may lead to acute inflammation of the mucosa and in some cases even be followed by mucosal ulceration with bleeding.

There are two forms of cyclooxygenase. One form (COX-1) is constitutive (is always active) and promotes the synthesis of the prostaglandins that protect the gastric mucosa. The other form (COX-2) is involved in the synthesis of the prostaglandins that function as mediators of inflammation and the symptoms associated with infections. COX-2 is not always active but is induced by these inflammatory conditions. NSAIDs such as aspirin, which are available "over the counter," inhibit both forms of the enzyme, suppressing the symptoms of inflammation (fever aches and pains) but also placing the gastric mucosa at risk. Some NSAIDs are more selective for COX-2, reducing the risk to gastric mucosa. Unfortunately, patients treated with some COX-2 inhibitors had a higher risk of heart attacks and strokes than did a comparable group treated with nonselective NSAIDs. Hence, many physicians favor limiting the use of COX-2 selective inhibitors unless their benefits outweigh the possible cardiovascular risks.

Excess ingestion of alcoholic beverages is another common cause of acute gastritis because the alcohol is a gastric irritant and also stimulates gastric acid secretion. In addition, any type of stress (such as burns, surgery, or serious systemic infections) may compromise the circulation to the stomach and contribute to the formation of acute gastritis, erosion of the stomach wall, and, if severe, stress ulcers.

Chronic Gastritis and Its Complications: The Role of *Helicobacter Pylori*

Many cases of chronic gastritis are related to growth (colonization) of a small, curved, gram-negative organism called *Helicobacter pylori* on the surface of the gastric mucosa. This unique organism grows in the layer of mucus covering the epithelial cells lining the stomach, where it can be identified by special bacterial stains, by culture, or by other specialized tests. The organism produces an enzyme called urease, which decomposes urea, a normal by-product of protein metabolism present in small amounts in blood and body fluids. Decomposition of urea yields ammonia, a substance that neutralizes the gastric acid and allows the organism to flourish in an acid environment that would destroy other bacteria. *Helicobacter* also produces enzymes that can break down the layer of protective mucus that covers the epithelial surface. Presumably, the chronic gastritis is caused by the ammonia and other products produced by the organism that damage the gastric mucosa of susceptible individuals.

Colonization of the gastric mucosa by *H. pylori* is very common, and not all people who harbor the organism have chronic gastritis. About 30 percent of people younger than thirty years of age are colonized by *H. pylori*. By age fifty, the proportion increases to about 50 percent and may be as high as 65 percent in people older

Cyclooxygenase Enzyme needed for synthesis of prostaglandins.

than age sixty-five. The spread of the organisms appears to be by mouth-to-mouth contact and also by the fecal–oral route; the organism has been cultured from both dental plaque material and from fecal material.

There are also some uncommon but important long-term harmful effects of *Helicobacter* infection. Chronic gastritis caused by this organism slightly increases the risk of two different gastric tumors: gastric carcinoma and malignant lymphoma arising from lymphocytes in the gastric mucosa (called mucosa-associated lymphoid tissue, MALT). The gastric carcinoma risk occurs because the gastritis often leads to atrophy of the gastric mucosa and causes the gastric epithelium to change into an abnormal intestinal-type epithelium (a process called intestinal metaplasia). It is these cellular changes in the gastric mucosa that predispose to gastric carcinoma. The lymphoma risk probably results because the gastritis overstimulates the mucosa-associated lymphoid tissue, which may lead to unregulated growth of lymphocytes that eventually progresses to gastric lymphoma.

PEPTIC ULCER

Peptic ulcer is a chronic ulcer that usually involves the distal stomach or proximal duodenum (**FIGURE 23-7**). The ulcer results from digestion of the mucosa by acid gastric juice. People who secrete large volumes of acidic gastric juice and who are infected with *H. pylori* are prone to ulcers. The bacteria is present in nearly all patients with duodenal ulcer disease but is not, in itself, sufficient to cause the disease; many people harboring the agent do not develop ulcers. Only about 75 percent of patients with gastric ulcers have *H. pylori* infection, and cases in noninfected patients are likely related to other causes.

The initial event is probably a small, superficial erosion of the gastric or duodenal mucosa. Gastric acid and pepsin begin to digest the deeper tissues, which have been denuded of covering epithelium. Hypersecretion of acid (in part related to inflammation caused by *H. pylori* infection) appear important in this process *H. pylori* is

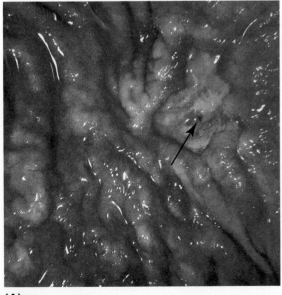

(A)

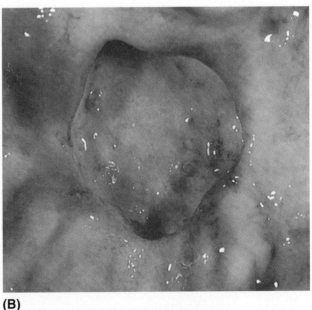

(B)

FIGURE 23-7 Peptic ulcers. **(A)** Gastric ulcer, which eroded a blood vessel in the base of the ulcer (*arrow*) and bled profusely. **(B)** Large chronic duodenal ulcer.

Courtesy of Leonard V. Crowley, MD, Century College.

not generally found in the duodenum (but rather the gastric mucosa), so an indirect role for the organism in stimulating acid secretion seems likely. Attempts at healing in the presence of continuing digestion eventually lead to considerable scarring at the base of the ulcer. Clinically, ulcers produce pain that is usually relieved by ingestion of food or antacids that neutralize the gastric acid.

Peptic ulcer complications include hemorrhage, perforation, and obstruction. An ulcer may erode into a large blood vessel, causing severe hemorrhage, or erode completely through the wall of the stomach or duodenum, causing a perforation through which gastric and duodenal contents leak into the peritoneal cavity, resulting in a generalized inflammation of the peritoneum (peritonitis). Sometimes the scarring that follows healing of a gastric ulcer may be so severe as to cause obstruction of the outlet of the stomach, called the pylorus, preventing the stomach from emptying properly.

Peptic ulcer is generally treated by antacids, which neutralize the excess gastric acid, or by drugs that block the secretion of acid by the gastric epithelial cells (histamine receptor blockers and proton pump inhibitors). Antibiotics are used to eliminate *H. pylori*. **Triple therapy**, using a proton pump inhibitor combined with two antibiotics (clarithromycin and amoxicillin), is successful in up to 90 percent of cases and is often undertaken in the absence of laboratory confirmed bacterial infection.

Triple therapy Treatment of ulcer with proton pump inhibitors combined with two antibiotics.

Norovirus An extremely infectious RNA virus easily spread from person to person and by contaminated food or water.

CARCINOMA OF THE STOMACH

At one time, carcinoma of the stomach was the most common malignant tumor, but the incidence has been decreasing. This may be related to the decreased consumption of smoked and cured meat products with the advent of refrigerators for the preservation of fresh foods. The initial symptom may be only vague, upper abdominal discomfort. Sometimes the first manifestation is an iron deficiency anemia, the result of chronic blood loss from the ulcerated surface of the tumor. Gastric carcinoma is treated by resection of a large part of the stomach together with the surrounding tissues and draining lymph nodes (**FIGURE 23-8**). Unfortunately, a gastric carcinoma is often far advanced and has metastasized by the time it causes symptoms; consequently, long-term survival of patients with stomach carcinoma is relatively poor. Some cases of gastric carcinoma may be restricted to the mucosa or submucosa (termed early gastric cancer). This may be a unique form of the disease and appears to have a much better surgical outcome. Sometimes gastric carcinoma may produce symptoms similar to those of a benign peptic ulcer. The distinction usually can be made by endoscopic techniques (gastroscopy) and, if necessary, via examination of biopsy material.

Diseases of the Small Intestine

Diseases of the intestine can be divided into those that predominantly affect the small bowel or the large (colon) although there is some overlap. Acute viral and bacterial enteritis predominantly affect the small intestine (and in some cases the stomach, so the term gastroenteritis is sometimes used).

ACUTE VIRAL GASTROENTERITIS

Viral gastroenteritis is commonly caused by either rotavirus or **norovirus**, both having RNA genomes. The condition is characterized by an abrupt onset of nausea, vomiting, abdominal cramps, and profuse diarrhea, which may affect only a few people or may occur as an epidemic affecting large numbers of people. Usually, the illness

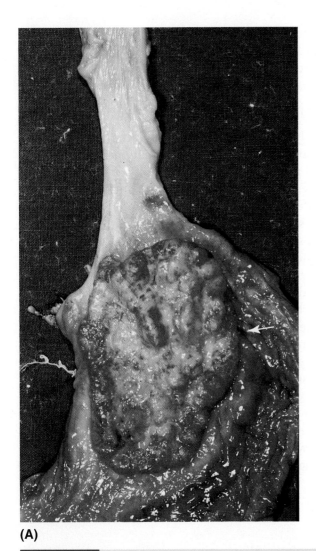

(A)

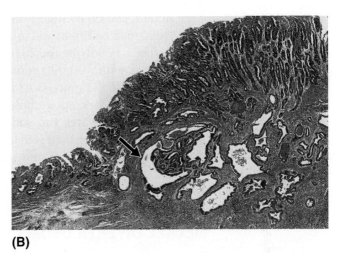

(B)

FIGURE 23-8 Carcinoma of the stomach. **(A)** The stomach has been opened, revealing a large ulcerated neoplasm arising from the gastric mucosa (*arrow*) and extending upward to the gastroesophageal junction. Esophagus is seen in upper part of photograph. **(B)** Photomicrograph of carcinoma of the stomach in the setting of chronic atrophic gastritis. Glands (adenocarcinoma) invading the body of the stomach are highlighted (*arrow*).

(A) Courtesy of Leonard V. Crowley, MD, Century College; (B) Courtesy of Department of Pathology and Laboratory Medicine, University of North Carolina at Chapel Hill.

subsides spontaneously within a few days and no specific treatment is required. Severely affected people may require intravenous fluids to replace depleted body fluids and electrolytes resulting from the diarrhea.

Rotavirus primarily affects infants and young children, most commonly in the winter and spring. It is spread via an oral–fecal route and can contaminate food and surfaces. Outbreaks occur in the day care setting and occasionally as widespread epidemics related to contaminated food or water. An effective oral vaccine is now available.

Norovirus is extremely contagious and is now the leading cause of illness from contaminated food in the United States. Contaminated leaf greens, fresh fruits, and shellfish are the most common sources. The illness is also spread from person to person, stool and vomitus being viral sources. Outbreaks tend to occur in closed places such as day care centers, nursing homes, and on cruise ships. Unlike the case with rotavirus, no vaccine is available and proper sanitary techniques (including frequent hand washing and washing contaminated clothing) is critical for prevention.

Norovirus is resistant to some disinfecting agents, so the use of agents registered to be effective against the virus (such as 5.3 percent chlorine bleach) is important. There are many strains of norovirus, and recurrent infection is possible.

ACUTE BACTERIAL GASTROENTERITIS

Acute bacterial infections are usually caused by known pathogens or their toxins (see the discussions on pathogenic microorganisms and animal parasites) and are predominantly diseases of the small intestine. They are generally of short duration and may subside without specific treatment, or may respond to appropriate antibiotics or other agents. Clinical manifestations include nausea, vomiting, abdominal discomfort, and passage of many loose stools. In severe infections, the bowel mucosa may be ulcerated, and the diarrheal stools may be bloody. Bacterial diarrhea (commonly caused by *Escherichia coli* and *Vibrio* species) are a major cause of death in young children, accounting for more than three-quarters of the deaths of children in developing countries in Africa and Asia.

Cholera, caused by ingestion of the bacteria *Vibrio cholerae* from contaminated water, remains a common and in some regions endemic cause of severe and potentially fatal diarrhea. Following the 2010 earthquake in Haiti, cholera has become a continuing problem, with 700,000 suspected cases and 8,500 deaths to date. The bacteria does not invade the mucosa of the small bowel but rather multiply in the mucous layer where they secrete a cholera toxin that causes the intestinal cells to secrete large amounts of water and sodium ion into the intestinal lumen, which results in profound diarrhea and salt loss leading to dehydration shock and death if untreated. Replacement of lost fluids and salt with oral rehydration fluid consisting of water, salt, and glucose is a simple and highly effective therapy. Antibiotics shorten the course of the disease.

MECKEL DIVERTICULUM

A number of congenital disorders of the small intestine occur. These include atresia and stenosis (complete and partial blockage of the lumen, respectively). The most common is **Meckel diverticulum**, an abnormal retention of the **vitelline duct** (*vitellus* = yolk) that connects the yolk sac to the developing embryo during embryogenesis. Normally, the duct disappears prior to birth and no trace persists. In about 2 percent of people, however, a remnant termed the Meckel diverticulum remains as a small tubular outpouching from the distal ileum (**FIGURE 23-9**). Most Meckel diverticula are asymptomatic, but sometimes the diverticulum becomes infected, causing the same symptoms and complications as an acute appendicitis. If a Meckel diverticulum contains misplaced (ectopic) gastric mucosa, the acidic "gastric juice" secreted by the diverticulum may cause a peptic ulcer of the diverticulum, which is at times complicated by bleeding or perforation. Hence, the surgeon searches for a Meckel diverticulum in cases of suspected appendicitis or other abdominal surgery.

Meckel diverticulum Abnormal retention of vitelline duct as small outpouching.

Vitelline duct Duct connecting the yolk sac to the developing embryo during embryogenesis.

Disturbances of Bowel Function: Food Intolerance

Some patients manifest crampy abdominal pain, abdominal distention, flatulence (excessive gas in the intestinal tract), and frequent loose stools as a result of food intolerance. The two most common types are lactose intolerance and gluten intolerance.

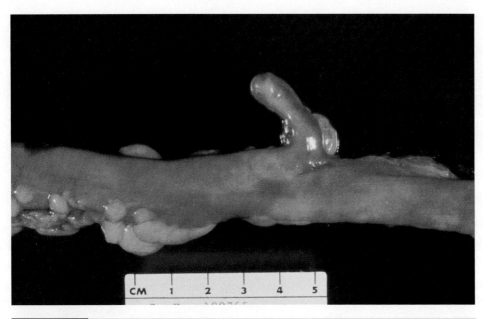

FIGURE 23-9 Meckel diverticulum of ileum.

Courtesy of Leonard V. Crowley, MD, Century College.

LACTOSE INTOLERANCE

Lactose is a disaccharide found in milk and dairy products. During digestion, lactose must be split into its two component monosaccharides, glucose and galactose, before it can be absorbed. This process is accomplished by an enzyme called lactase, which is present on the mucosal surface of the epithelial cells in the small intestine. The enzyme is abundant in infants and young children. In many populations, however, the concentration of lactase gradually declines to very low levels during adolescence and early adult life. However, some populations tend to have persistent levels of lactase into adulthood. The enzyme is deficient in about 20 percent of adult whites, 70 percent of American blacks, 90 percent of American Indians, and almost all Asians. Congenital (inherited) complete deficiency of lactase is a rare autosomal recessive trait found in some Finnish families. It has serious consequences because neonates cannot digest milk.

People in whom lactase is deficient are unable to digest lactose. Consequently, lactose cannot be absorbed and remains within the intestinal lumen, where it raises the osmotic pressure of the intestinal contents. Because of the high intraluminal osmotic pressure, fluid is retained within the intestinal tract instead of being absorbed normally, leading to abdominal discomfort, cramps, and diarrhea. Some of the unabsorbed lactose is fermented by bacteria in the colon, yielding lactic acid and other organic acids that further raise the intraluminal osmotic pressure and contribute to the person's discomfort. The symptoms are related to ingestion of dairy products and abate promptly when intake of dairy products is reduced or discontinued.

GLUTEN INTOLERANCE

Gluten is a general term that refers to a group of similar proteins found in wheat, rye, oats, and barley. The gluten in wheat flour is responsible for imparting the elasticity to bread dough. Some people have a hereditary predisposition to become sensitive to the protein in gluten called **gliadin**. These individuals form antigliadin antibodies and activated gliadin-sensitized T cells, which leads to atrophy of the intestinal villi

Gliadin Protein in gluten causing sensitivity.

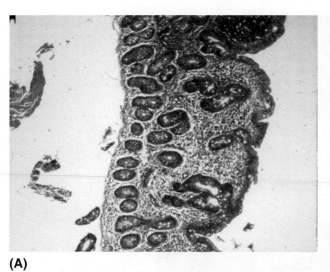
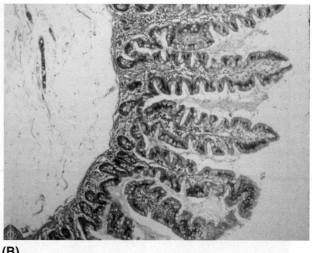

(A) **(B)**

FIGURE 23-10 Low-magnification photomicrographs comparing appearance of atrophic intestinal villi caused by gluten sensitivity **(A)** with normal appearing villi after excluding gluten from the diet for several months **(B)**.

Courtesy of Leonard V. Crowley, MD, Century College.

Gluten sensitive enteropathy (GSE) Damage to intestinal villi caused by ingesting gluten-containing foods by people sensitive to a protein in gluten; characterized by passage of large bulky stools containing a large amount of poorly absorbed fat.

Tissue transglutaminase Human enzyme target of antibodies detected in gluten sensitivity.

Borborygmi Loud bowel sounds.

Irritable bowel syndrome (IBS) Condition characterized by frequent loose stools and excessive amounts of mucus.

in the duodenum and proximal jejunum (**FIGURE 23-10**). As a result, digestion and absorption of fats and other nutrients is impaired. Several different names have been applied to this condition. The most descriptive term is **gluten sensitive enteropathy (GSE)**, but the condition is also known as celiac disease or celiac sprue. Clinically, the condition is characterized by passage of frequent large, bulky stools containing much unabsorbed fat and is associated with weight loss and vitamin deficiencies as a result of the impaired intestinal absorption. GSE has a major genetic component because essentially all patients have two specific separate genes in different parts of the HLA complex. In addition, infection with adenovirus type 12 may be a factor because the virus has a protein similar in structure to alpha-gliaden.

A simple serological test for the presence of antibodies to the human enzyme **tissue transglutaminase** or tests for the presence of antibodies reactive with the endomysium (muscle fiber sheath rich in tissue transglutaminase) have much simplified diagnosis of GSE and reduced the need for biopsy of the small intestinal mucosa to reveal atrophy of the intestinal villi. When indicated, the specimen for biopsy is obtained by a flexible biopsy device with a small capsule on the end that is swallowed by the patient. The device is positioned in the upper jejunum and is manipulated so that a small bit of intestinal mucosa enters the capsule. Then the capsule is closed, cutting off and retaining a piece of mucosa. Treatment by a gluten-free diet promptly cures the condition, and the intestinal villi return to normal in three or four months.

IRRITABLE BOWEL SYNDROME

Some patients exhibit episodes of crampy, abdominal discomfort, loud gurgling bowel sounds (**borborygmi**), and disturbed bowel function. Frequent loose stools sometimes alternate with periods of constipation, and excessive amounts of mucus are secreted by the colonic mucosal glands. These manifestations are frequently quite distressing to the affected individual, but no structural or biochemical abnormalities can be identified to account for the functional disturbances. This condition is often called **irritable bowel syndrome (IBS)**. Other terms for this very common condition are spastic colitis and mucous colitis.

The diagnosis of IBS is one of exclusion. The physician must rule out infections as a result of pathogenic bacteria and intestinal parasites, food intolerance, and various types of chronic enteritis such as Crohn disease and chronic ulcerative colitis.

Treatment consists of measures that reduce emotional tension and improve intestinal motility. Sometimes substances that increase the bulk of the stool provide relief of symptoms.

Inflammatory Diseases of the Bowel

The intestine may be the site of both acute and chronic inflammation. The term **enteritis** (*enteron* = bowel) is used to describe inflammation of any part of the intestinal tract. The term **colitis** denotes inflammation restricted to the colon, and the general term *bowel inflammation* refers to any part of the intestinal tract, either small intestine, colon, or both.

Enteritis Inflammation of the intestinal tract.

Colitis Inflammation restricted to colon.

Crohn disease Chronic enteritis.

APENDICITIS

Appendicitis is the most common inflammatory lesion of the bowel. In many animals, the portion of the bowel represented in humans by the appendix is a large, wide-caliber intestinal segment, similar in appearance to the remainder of the colon. In humans, this segment of bowel is reduced in both size and caliber to the extent that it approaches being a vestigial structure.

The high incidence of acute appendicitis is due primarily to the narrow caliber of the appendix, the base of which often becomes plugged by firm bits of fecal material or in some cases plant seeds or parasitic worms. Because of the obstruction, the secretions normally produced by the epithelial cells lining the appendix drain poorly from the area distal to the blockage. The accumulated secretions create pressure within the appendiceal lumen. This compresses the blood vessels in the mucosa, impairing its viability (**FIGURE 23-11**). Bacteria normally present in the appendix and colon invade the devitalized wall, causing an acute inflammation.

Clinically, appendicitis is characterized by generalized abdominal pain that soon becomes localized to the right lower part (quadrant) of the abdomen. Examination of the abdomen reveals localized tenderness over the appendix when pressure is applied to the abdomen by the fingers of the examiner. Often, the patient also experiences pain when the pressure is released suddenly (rebound tenderness). In addition, there is usually reflex contraction of the abdominal muscles (abdominal rigidity) in response to the underlying inflammation. Laboratory tests reveal that the number of polymorphonuclear leukocytes in the blood also is increased as a result of the infection. Currently, CT examination of the abdominal area and in some cases (particularly in children) ultrasound are highly accurate in establishing a diagnosis, and laparoscopy is rarely needed.

Mild cases of appendicitis may heal spontaneously. More severe inflammation may lead to rupture of the appendix and peritonitis. For this reason, it is essential to identify appendicitis and remove the appendix in any patient in whom appendicitis is suspected.

CHRONIC ENTERITIS

Chronic enteritis is less common and more difficult to treat. The two important types of chronic enteritis are **Crohn disease** and chronic ulcerative colitis. Crohn disease can affect the entire gastrointestinal tract (most commonly the terminal ileum and sometimes the right colon) whereas ulcerative colitis tends to affect the rectum and

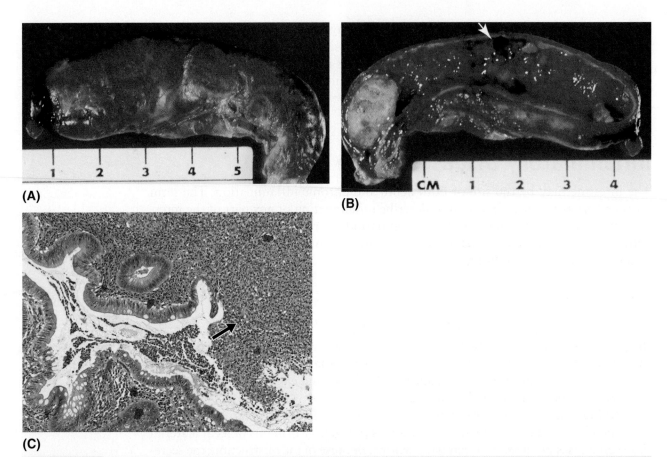

(A)

(B)

(C)

FIGURE 23-11 Acute appendicitis. **(A)** Exterior of appendix is swollen, congested, and covered with inflammatory exudate. **(B)** Appendix bisected to reveal interior. Pus within lumen has been removed. Mucosa is congested and ulcerated (*arrow*). The base of the appendix (*left side*) is plugged by a firm mass of fecal material. **(C)** Photomicrograph of removed appendix. Lumen is filled with inflammatory cells (pus). The wall of the intestine has been destroyed and replaced by an area of inflammatory cells (*arrow*).

(A, B) Courtesy of Leonard V. Crowley, MD, Century College; (C) Courtesy of Department of Pathology and Laboratory Medicine, University of North Carolina at Chapel Hill.

progresses proximally up the colon. Often, the two diseases are grouped together under the general term *chronic inflammatory bowel disease* (IBD). Both diseases tend to be chronic, with periodic flare-ups manifested by cramplike abdominal pain and diarrhea, followed by periods when the disease is inactive. During periods of activity, the affected individuals may also have systemic manifestations, including joint inflammation, eye inflammation, and various types of skin nodules and skin infections. Although the diseases have similarities, there are also significant differences between them.

These two diseases appear to have both genetic and environmental components (see discussion on immunity, hypersensitivity, allergy, and autoimmune diseases). Recent studies have provided further insight into their pathogenesis. Although multiple genes have been associated with susceptibility to each disease, the significance of this remains unclear. It is most likely that multiple factors, both environmental and genetic, work together to trigger the inflammatory response that leads to these diseases, including an impaired immune response, defective barrier epithelium leading to penetration by intestinal bacteria, and the presence of activated T lymphocytes. However, it is uncertain whether the inflammatory reaction that damages the bowel is directed against intestinal bacteria that get into the intestinal wall periodically because epithelial barrier function is defective, or whether it is in part an autoimmune response directed against the patient's own cells because they contain some of the same antigenic determinants (cross-reacting antigens) as those possessed by the intestinal bacteria to which the immune system has responded.

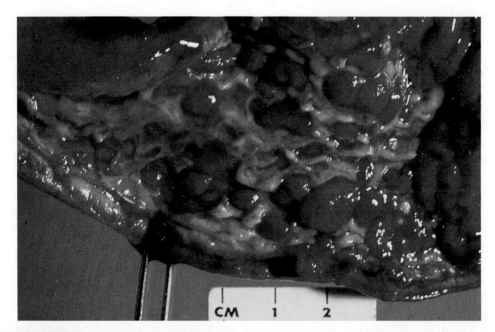

FIGURE 23-12 Crohn disease (regional enteritis). Mucosa is ulcerated and covered by inflammatory exudate.
Courtesy of Leonard V. Crowley, MD, Century College.

CROHN DISEASE

Crohn disease is a chronic inflammation and ulceration of the bowel mucosa with marked thickening and scarring of the entire bowel wall (**FIGURE 23-12**). The inflammation often affects scattered areas of the small bowel (skip lesions), leaving normal intervening segments of bowel between the areas of severe disease. Occasionally, affected individuals have such severe thickening and scarring of an involved segment of bowel that the lumen becomes greatly narrowed or even completely blocked, which impedes passage of bowel contents. Crohn disease was originally called regional ileitis because the inflammatory process is often localized to the distal ileum, but other parts of the small intestine may be involved, and the disease may involve the colon as well.

CHRONIC ULCERATIVE COLITIS

In contrast to Crohn disease, chronic ulcerative colitis targets the colon, not the small intestine. The inflammation is limited to the mucosa, and the bowel wall is not thickened as in Crohn disease. Frequently, the disease begins in the rectal mucosa but may spread progressively until eventually the entire colon is involved. In severe cases, the ulcerated mucosa may bleed profusely, leading to bloody diarrhea, and at times the inflammatory process becomes so extensive that it leads to a perforation of the colon with escape of bowel contents into the peritoneal cavity. Affected people with long-standing disease also may develop carcinoma arising in the diseased regions of the colon or rectum.

TREATMENT OF CHRONIC ENTERITIS

Treatment of inflammatory bowel disease involves symptomatic and supportive measures, including antibiotics and corticosteroids to control disease symptoms during flare-ups and immunosuppressive drugs. Eventually, surgical resection of severely diseased bowel segments may be required in many patients. People with severe and extensive chronic ulcerative colitis may require total removal of the entire colon and rectum, both to control the disease and to eliminate the risk of colon carcinoma, which is prone to occur in patients with long-standing chronic disease.

PSEUDOMEMBRANOUS COLITIS

Some people taking broad-spectrum antibiotics develop mild diarrhea. Others, unfortunately, develop severe bloody diarrhea with abdominal pain, fever, and other systemic manifestations, which may be life-threatening, that are associated with exudative inflammatory plaques on the colonic mucosa (termed pseudomembranes). The multiple ulcerations of the colonic mucosa are covered by masses of fibrin and inflammatory cells. The most common causative agent is the anaerobic spore-forming intestinal bacterium *Clostridium difficile.*

Broad-spectrum antibiotics cause the colitis by changing the intestinal bacterial flora. Most of the normal flora is destroyed, allowing the overgrowth of the more resisitant *C. difficile* organism, which produces two toxins that cause the intestinal inflammation and necrosis.

The diagnosis of antibiotic-associated colitis is most commonly established by detection of the bacterial toxin in the stool. Treatment consists of stopping the inciting antibiotic and giving antibiotics such as metronidazole or vancomycin that inhibit growth of the organism. Treatment should not include drugs that reduce the diarrhea by inhibiting intestinal motility. These drugs prolong the illness by allowing the injurious clostridial toxins to remain in the intestine instead of being eliminated rapidly in the diarrheal stools. The disease may reoccur and in some cases be life-threatening due in part to increased bacterial resistance to antibiotics. In these cases, "fecal transplants" from healthy donors have proved successful as a therapeutic measure for restoring the normal intestinal flora.

Structural Diseases of the Bowel

INTESTINAL OBSTRUCTION

If the normal passage of intestinal contents through the bowel is blocked, the patient is said to have an intestinal obstruction. The site of the blockage may be either the small intestine (high intestinal obstruction) or the colon (low intestinal obstruction). Bowel obstruction is always serious. The severity of the symptoms depends on the location of the obstruction, its completeness, and whether there is interference with the blood supply to the blocked segment of bowel.

Obstruction of the small intestine causes severe, crampy pain as a result of vigorous peristalsis, reflecting the attempt of the intestine to force bowel contents past the site of obstruction. This is associated with vomiting of copious amounts of gastric and upper intestinal secretions, resulting in loss of large quantities of water and electrolytes. As a consequence, the patient becomes dehydrated and develops pronounced fluid and electrolyte disturbances.

Symptoms are much less acute when the distal colon is obstructed. There may be mild, crampy abdominal pain and moderate distention of the abdomen. However, vomiting with associated loss of fluid and electrolytes is not as serious a problem as in high intestinal obstruction. Disturbances of fluid and electrolytes do not develop as rapidly.

The common causes of intestinal obstruction are intestinal adhesions, hernia, tumor, volvulus, intussusception, or neoplastic disease (most commonly carcinoma).

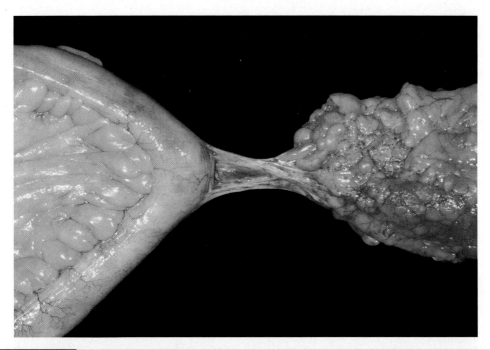

FIGURE 23-13 Fibrous adhesion between loop of small intestine (*left side*) and omentum.
Courtesy of Leonard V. Crowley, MD, Century College.

Adhesions

Adhesive bands of connective tissue (**adhesions**) may form within the abdominal cavity after surgery (**FIGURE 23-13**). Sometimes a loop of bowel becomes kinked, compressed, or twisted by an adhesive band, causing obstruction proximal to the site of the adhesion. This often results from surgical procedures involving the bowel.

Hernia

A **hernia** is a protrusion of a loop of bowel through a small opening, usually in the abdominal wall. The herniated loop pushes the peritoneum ahead of it, forming the hernia sac. Inguinal hernia is quite common in men. A loop of small bowel protrudes through a weak area in the inguinal ring and may descend downward into the scrotum. Umbilical and femoral hernias occur in both sexes. In an umbilical hernia, the loop of bowel protrudes into the umbilicus through a defect in the abdominal wall (**FIGURE 23-14**). In a femoral hernia, a loop of intestine extends under the inguinal ligament along the course of the femoral vessels into the groin. If a herniated loop of bowel can be pushed back into the abdominal cavity, the hernia is said to be reducible. Occasionally, a herniated loop becomes stuck and cannot be reduced. This is called an incarcerated hernia. Sometimes the loop of bowel is so tightly constricted by the margins of the defect that allowed the herniation that the blood supply to the herniated bowel is obstructed, causing necrosis of the protruding segment of bowel. This is called a strangulated hernia and requires prompt surgical intervention.

Volvulus and Intussusception

A **volvulus** is a rotary twisting of the bowel on the fold of peritoneum (the mesentery) that suspends the bowel from the posterior wall of the abdomen. The blood supply to the twisted segment also is impaired because the blood vessels supplying the bowel travel in the mesentery, and they are compressed when the bowel and mesentery become twisted. The sigmoid colon is the usual site (**FIGURE 23-15**).

Adhesions Bands of connective tissue in abdominal cavity after surgery.

Hernia A protrusion of a loop of bowel through a narrow opening, usually in the abdominal wall.

Volvulus Rotary twisting of the bowel.

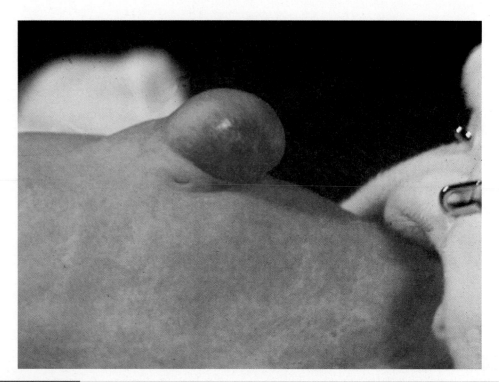

FIGURE 23-14 A large umbilical hernia in an infant.
Courtesy of Leonard V. Crowley, MD, Century College.

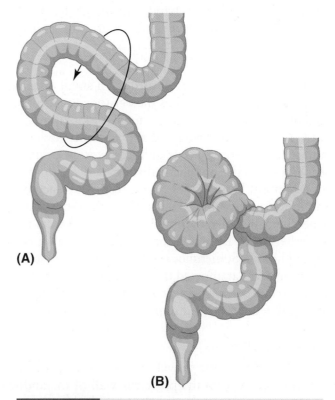

(A)

(B)

FIGURE 23-15 Pathogenesis of volvulus. **(A)** Rotary twist of sigmoid colon on its mesentery. **(B)** Obstruction of colon and interruption of its blood supply caused by volvulus.

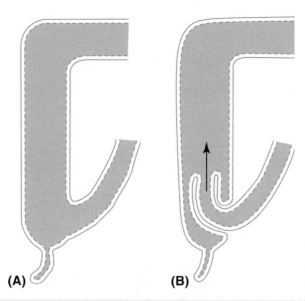

FIGURE 23-16 Pathogenesis of ileocecal intussusception. **(A)** Normal anatomic relationships. **(B)** Vigorous peristalsis carries distal ileum into cecum. *Dashed line* indicates mucosa.

An **intussusception** is a telescoping of one segment of bowel into an adjacent segment. This is a common cause of intestinal obstruction in children and usually results from vigorous peristalsis that telescopes the terminal ileum into the proximal colon through the ileocecal valve (**FIGURE 23-16** and **FIGURE 23-17**). In adults, the condition is usually secondary to a tumor of the bowel that is supported by a narrow stalk. A tumor of this type is often called a pedunculated tumor, the name being derived from the stalk (pedicle) that supports it (*pediculus* = little foot). As the tumor is propelled by a peristaltic wave, the base of the tumor exerts traction on the bowel wall at its site of attachment, causing the proximal segment to telescope into the distal bowel (**FIGURE 23-18** and **FIGURE 23-19**). In children, the cause is most often unknown but may be related to an intestinal infection or, rarely, to a rotavirus vaccine immunization that causes enlargement of gut lymph, which become "caught" in peristalsis and lead to the formation of the intussusception. In children, the use of either an air

Intussusception
Telescoping of a bowel segment into an adjacent segment.

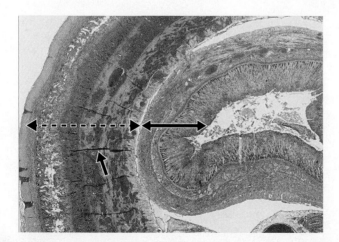

FIGURE 23-17 Photomicrograph of an ileocecal intussusception. *Solid line* indicates invaginated ileum, *dashed line* indicates multiple layers of cecum that are necrotic as a result of compromise of blood supply. An artifactual fold in tissue (*arrow*) occurred during processing.

Courtesy of Department of Pathology and Laboratory Medicine, University of North Carolina at Chapel Hill.

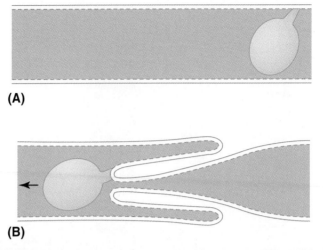

(A)

(B)

FIGURE 23-18 Pathogenesis of intussusception caused by tumor. **(A)** Pedunculated tumor protrudes into lumen of bowel. **(B)** Peristalsis propels tumor and produces traction on its base, causing proximal segment of bowel to be telescoped into distal segment. *Dashed line* indicates mucosa.

or barium enema may lead to unfolding and release of the intussusception. If not relieved, the intussusception can result in bowel infarction (necrosis as a result of compromised blood supply) (Figure 23-17).

MESENTERIC THROMBOSIS

The blood supply to the gastrointestinal tract is derived from several large arteries arising from the aorta. The blood supply to most of the bowel is provided by the superior mesenteric artery. This vessel supplies blood to the entire small intestine and the proximal half of the colon. The arteries supplying the gastrointestinal tract may develop arteriosclerotic changes and become occluded by thrombosis in the

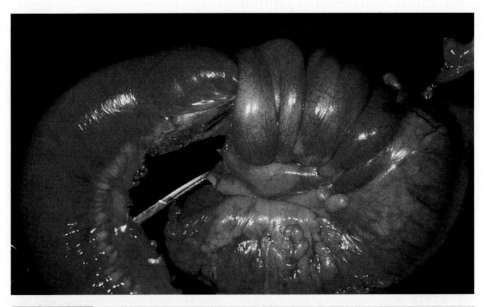

FIGURE 23-19 Intussusception of colon as a result of colon tumor. Midportion of colon is swollen because of telescoping of the proximal segment (*left side*) into distal segment (*right side*).

Courtesy of Leonard V. Crowley, MD, Century College.

same way as many other arteries. Thrombosis of the superior mesenteric artery leads to an extensive infarction of most of the bowel, a medical emergency with a very poor prognosis.

Diseases of the Colon and Anus

Diseases of the colon and anus include diverticulosis, diverticulitis, tumors both benign and malignant, and hemorrhoids.

DIVERTICULOSIS AND DIVERTICULITIS

Outpouchings of the mucosa of the colon often project through weak areas in the muscular wall of the large intestine. These outpouchings are called **diverticula (singular, diverticulum)**, and the condition is called **diverticulosis** (**FIGURE 23-20** and **FIGURE 23-21**). This is an acquired condition, in contrast to a Meckel diverticulum, which is a congenital abnormality (see Figure 23-9). Diverticula, which usually occur in the distal colon, are encountered with increasing frequency in older patients. Highly refined, low-residue diets predispose to diverticula because stools are small and hard and high intraluminal pressure must be generated by peristalsis to propel the stool through the colon. This high intracolonic pressure forces the mucosa through weak areas in the muscular wall. In contrast, people who subsist on high-residue diets have large, bulky stools that can be propelled through the colon easily at low intraluminal pressures, and diverticula occur infrequently among them.

Diverticula/diverticulum An outpouching from an organ, as from the mucosa of the colon, that projects through the muscular wall.

Diverticulosis A condition characterized by outpouchings of the colonic mucosa through weak areas in the muscular wall.

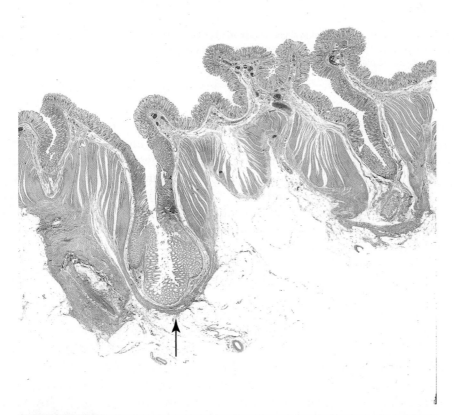

FIGURE 23-20 A low-magnification photomicrograph of colon illustrating diverticula. Mucosa of the colon (*upper part*) protrudes through muscular wall (*arrow*) into the serosa of colon.

Courtesy of Leonard V. Crowley, MD, Century College.

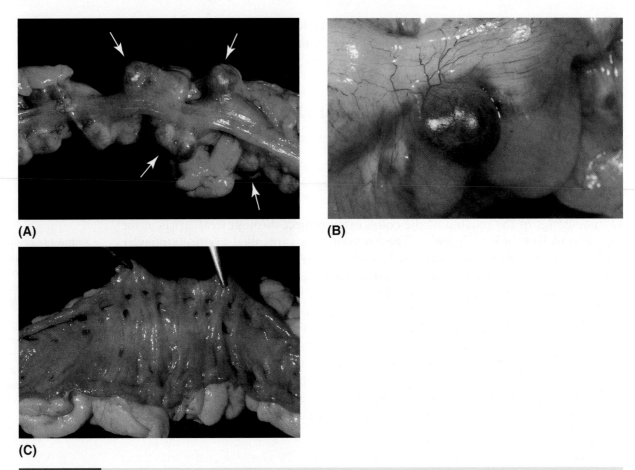

(A)

(B)

(C)

FIGURE 23-21 Diverticulosis of colon. **(A)** Exterior of colon illustrating several diverticula projecting through wall of colon (*arrows*). **(B)** A closer view of diverticulum. **(C)** Interior of colon, illustrating openings of multiple diverticula. Several of the openings are well demonstrated in the mucosa just below the clamps.

Courtesy of Leonard V. Crowley, MD, Century College.

Diverticulitis An inflammation of a diverticulum.

Most diverticula are asymptomatic, but occasionally problems arise. Bits of fecal material may become trapped within these pouches and incite an inflammatory reaction called **diverticulitis**. The inflammation may be followed by considerable scarring. Occasionally, perforation of a diverticulum may occur, leading to an abscess in the pelvis. Sometimes blood vessels in the mucosa of the diverticulum become ulcerated by abrasion from the fecal material, resulting in bleeding. Diverticula attended by such complications as infections, perforation, or bleeding may require surgical resection of the affected segment of bowel.

TUMORS OF THE BOWEL

Tumors of the small intestine are uncommon. Unfortunately, this is not the case for tumors of the colon and rectum. Eight percent of all new cases of cancer as well as 8 percent of all cancer deaths occur as a result of disease in the colon and rectum. It is estimated that 93,000 new cases of colon cancer and almost 50,000 deaths occur yearly as a result of colorectal cancers. Colon cancer (by which we mean colorectal cancer) is a disease of aging with rates accelerating after age fifty. However, due to colonoscopy screening, the incidence of colorectal cancer continues to drop. When colon cancer is detected and confined to the colon, there is a 90-percent five-year survival. When the cancer has spread (metastasized) to distant locations, the five-year survival is a dismal 13 percent. Not only can colonoscopy detect early colon and rectal cancer, but it can prevent cancer from occurring by detecting precancerous lesions termed adenomas (polyps) and removing them before they have a chance to become cancer (adenocarcinoma). The natural history of colorectal cancer may stretch for many years, developing slowly from the first precancerous lesion until it becomes colon cancer. For this reason, colonoscopy need not be undertaken frequently. In the absence of risk factors, screening every ten years is suggested for people over fifty years of age.

The beginnings of colorectal cancer is a complicated story. As is the case with every cancer, colon cancer begins with a mutation in the DNA of a cell, in this case in the colon/rectum. The first gene to be lost is usually *APC*, so named because it is associated with a genetic disease called adenomatous polyposis coli or **familial adenomatous polyposis (FAP)**. People who inherit a germline mutation in the *APC* gene develop FAP, a disease characterized by the presence of hundreds of polyps (adenomas) in the colorectal region (**FIGURE 23-22**). By the age of forty, colorectal cancer is inevitable in FAP patients unless the colon is totally removed. However, the great majority (over 99 percent) of individuals who develop colorectal cancer do not have germline (inherited) mutations in the *APC* gene. Rather, the extraordinary number of dividing cells in the colorectal region develop spontaneous mutations in the *APC* gene as the person ages. Because *APC* is a tumor suppressor gene, it must function normally to control cell growth. Cells begin the pathway to colorectal cancer when both copies of *APC* are lost in the same cell. Patients with FAP are halfway there because they have inherited one defective copy of the gene and need to lose only one copy in a colorectal cell to begin the path to polyp formation and cancer, something that is inevitable. People with sporadic colorectal cancer need "two hits" to begin the process. Hence, sporadic (noninherited) colorectal cancer is not inevitable and is predominantly a disease of aging people. Cells that have lost *APC* have a growth advantage over their normal counterparts. Because they grow rapidly, they are more likely to accumulate many additional mutations that further disregulate their growth. Ultimately loss of the *Tp53* gene, which is important in maintaining DNA integrity, is associated with transformation of the benign adenoma into a malignant adenocarcinoma capable of metastasis to distant sites. This prolonged and stepwise process of carcinogenesis in illustrated in **FIGURE 23-23**.

Carcinoma of the colon may arise anywhere in the large intestine or rectum. Carcinoma arising in the cecum and right half of the colon generally does not cause

Familial adenomatous polyposis (FAP) Genetic disease characterized by many polyps in the colorectal region.

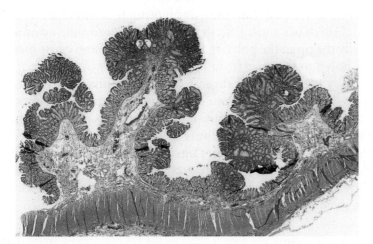

FIGURE 23-22 Photomicrograph of a segment of colon removed from a patient with FAP demonstrating multiple polyps.

Courtesy of Department of Pathology and Laboratory Medicine, University of North Carolina at Chapel Hill.

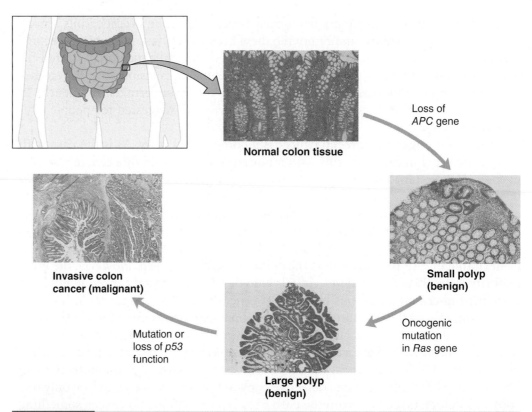

FIGURE 23-23 Stages in the progression of invasive colon cancer. Malignant colon cancer is defined by its ability to invade distant anatomic sites.

Photographs courtesy of Kathleen R. Cho, University of Michigan Medical School.

obstruction of the bowel because the caliber of this portion of the colon is large and the bowel contents are relatively soft. However, the tumor often becomes ulcerated and bleeds, leading to chronic iron deficiency anemia. The patient with a carcinoma of the right half of the colon may consult a physician because of weakness and fatigue caused by the anemia, without experiencing any symptoms referable to the intestinal tract, or the lesion may have been detected by screening the stool for occult (not obvious) blood. Carcinoma of the distal portion of the colon, which has a much smaller caliber than the proximal colon, often causes partial obstruction of the bowel and leads to symptoms of lower intestinal obstruction (**FIGURE 23-24** and **FIGURE 23-25**). Polyps are most often symptom free until they advance into cancer, but occasionally the tip of the polyp may become eroded and cause bleeding. Because removal of a polyp prevents it from becoming cancerous, survey of the bowel by colonoscopy may well prevent cancer. Colonoscopy involves inserting a flexible, tubelike device through the anus into the rectum and colon. The procedure is done under mild sedation and is not painful. The most unpleasant part of the procedure is the bowel cleaning required prior to the test, which involves inducing diarrhea using large volumes of an oral fluid or other agents to flush the bowel. The colonoscope not only allows visualization of the bowel but a stalked (peduculated) polyp can be removed by cutting the narrow stalk. Flat lesions can be cauterized when they cannot be removed.

IMPERFORATE ANUS

Imperforate anus is an uncommon congenital abnormality in which the colon fails to acquire a normal anal opening. It occurs in about 1 in 5,000 live births. There are two

Imperforate anus
Congenital absence of anal opening, often associated with absence of distal rectum as well.

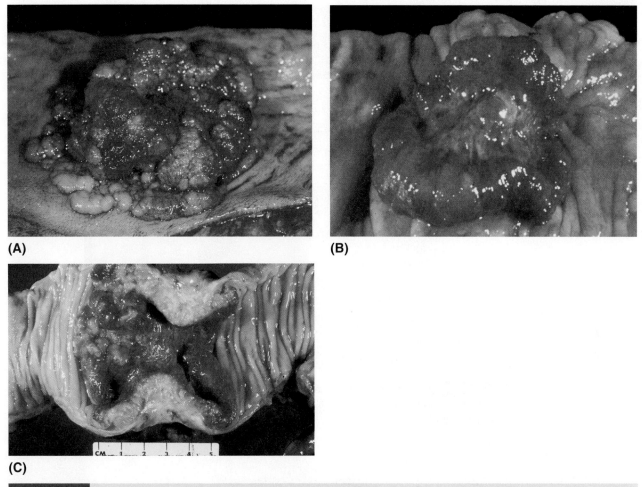

(A)

(B)

(C)

FIGURE 23-24 Stages in the progressive growth of a colon carcinoma. **(A)** Broad-based overgrowth of neoplastic epithelium. No ulceration or invasion of bowel wall. **(B)** Central necrosis within more advanced carcinoma. Tumor invades bowel wall. **(C)** Ulcerated far-advanced colon carcinoma completely encircles the bowel wall, reducing the caliber of the lumen, and extends completely through the bowel wall.

Courtesy of Leonard V. Crowley, MD, Century College.

major types. In one type, the rectum and anus are normally formed and extend to the level of the skin, but no anal orifice is present. Often a small tract (fistula) extends from the blind end of the anal canal to terminate in the urethra, in the vagina, or on the surface of the skin. Usually this type of imperforate anus can be easily treated by excising the tissue covering the anal opening. In the second type of imperforate anus, the entire distal rectum fails to develop, and often there are associated abnormalities of the urogenital tract and skeletal system. Surgical repair of this type of abnormality is much more difficult, and results are less satisfactory.

HEMORRHOIDS

Hemorrhoids are varicosities, structural dilations of the veins of the venous plexus that drains the rectum and anus (**FIGURE 23-26**). Constipation and increased straining during bowel movements predispose to their development as does pregnancy (presumably because of increased abdominal pressure). Internal hemorrhoids, which involve the veins of the lower rectum, may become eroded and bleed, may become thrombosed, or may prolapse through the anus. External hemorrhoids involve the veins of the anal canal and perianal skin. They sometimes become thrombosed, which causes considerable anorectal discomfort.

Hemorrhoids Varicosities of anal and rectal veins.

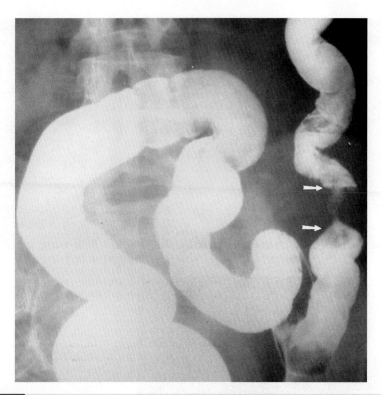

FIGURE 23-25 Colon carcinoma demonstrated by barium enema. The tumor narrows the lumen of the colon, which appears as a filling defect in the column of barium (*arrows*).

Courtesy of Leonard V. Crowley, MD, Century College.

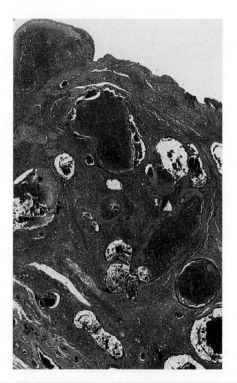

FIGURE 23-26 Photomicrograph of excised protuberant external hemorrhoids. External perianal epithelium is on top. There are many examples of thrombosed and blood engorged vessels with abundant inflammatory cells throughout the tissue.

Courtesy of Department of Pathology and Laboratory Medicine, University of North Carolina at Chapel Hill.

Symptoms of hemorrhoids can often be relieved by a high-fiber diet rich in fruits and vegetables, which promotes large, bulky stools that can be passed without excessive straining. Stool softeners and local application of rectal ointments may also provide temporary relief. Hemorrhoids can be removed surgically if they do not respond to more conservative therapy.

Diagnostic Evaluation of Gastrointestinal Disease

Although the gastrointestinal tract cannot be examined as easily as many other parts of the body, it is possible to visualize the interior of the esophagus, the stomach, the duodenum, and the entire colon by endoscopic procedures using specially designed instruments inserted into the gastrointestinal tract either through the oral cavity or the anus. Recent development of "pill cameras," which transmit an image of the region of the gut they pass through, has made it easier to examine regions of the small intestine formerly difficult or impossible to image visually. (Endoscopy is described in the general concepts of disease in the section on diagnostic procedures.) Endoscopic procedures are generally employed if the patient experiences symptoms suggesting disease of the esophagus, stomach, or colon. Abnormal areas in the mucosa can be visualized, biopsied, and examined histologically.

Areas that cannot be visualized directly can be studied by radiologic examination. Examination of the upper gastrointestinal tract is accomplished by having the patient ingest a radiopaque material (contrast medium), allowing the clinician to visualize the transport of the material through the intestinal tract by x-ray studies. This technique also allows the clinician to visualize the contours of the gastrointestinal mucosa and thereby to identify the location and extent of disease affecting the bowel mucosa, such as ulcer, stricture, tumor, or an area of chronic inflammation. The colon can be studied in a similar manner by instilling radiopaque material into the bowel through the anus to outline the contours of the large intestine. This type of study is called a barium enema (see Figure 23-25).

Eating Disorders

Eating disorders are conditions in which food intake is inappropriate and harmful because it leads to serious health consequences. Excessive food intake leading to obesity, which has many harmful effects on health, is the most prevalent disorder. However, abnormal eating habits associated with anorexia nervosa, bulimia nervosa, and binge eating disorders also pose serious health problems for those affected.

OBESITY

Causes of Obesity

Fat is the storage form of energy. Any caloric intake that exceeds requirements is stored as adipose tissue, and weight is gained. Each excess pound of body weight represents the storage of approximately 3,500 calories. Weight is lost if caloric intake is reduced below the amount required for total daily energy expenditure (TDEE). About 60 percent of TDEE is related to basal metabolic rate (the energy expenditure at rest, including the energy necessary for processes vital for life). Smaller proportions of the TDEE are used to digest food, to store resultant calories, and to regulate thermogenesis in response to the environment. The major adjustable component of TDEE is activity thermogenesis, which is the result of physical movement and deliberate exercise, thus emphasizing the importance of exercise on weight management. Many genetic, environmental, and hormonal factors play a role in regulating body weight by affecting appetite and satiety, thereby controlling food intake, and by influencing the metabolic pathways that convert food into energy or into adipose tissue. Obesity may be caused by a genetic defect, endocrine gland malfunction, hypothyroidism, or adrenal cortical hyperfunction, but these are uncommon situations. Most obese individuals have no detectable genetic, endocrine, or metabolic disturbances. In the majority of cases, obesity is the result of overeating and could be "cured" by reducing food intake. Easy in theory, but often difficult in practice because of behavioral issues not easily amenable to control.

Current data indicate that 60 percent of Americans are overweight. Half of the people in this overweight group are classified as obese, which is defined as 20 percent or more over ideal body weight, or a body mass index of 30 or more. (Body mass index [BMI] is a calculated value based on weight in kilograms divided by the square of height in meters.) The prevalence of obesity has increased about 8 percent in the last decade. About 6 percent of women and 3 percent of men are more than 100 percent over their ideal body weight, which is called morbid obesity.

Health Consequences of Obesity

Overweight people have a higher incidence of diabetes, hypertension, cardiovascular disease, and several other diseases than do people of normal weight. Therefore, being significantly overweight is undesirable, and extreme obesity is a major health hazard. Obese people have a mortality rate almost twice that of normal individuals. The excess fat is harmful to the cardiovascular system because blood volume and cardiac output must increase, there is a tendency to high blood pressure, and elevated blood lipids can predispose to arteriosclerosis.

The high incidence of diabetes in obese people is the result of an impaired ability to utilize insulin efficiently (described in the discussion on pancreas and diabetes mellitus). Musculoskeletal disabilities such as osteoarthritis are frequent because the excess weight places undue stress on the bones, joints, and ligaments. Finally, the obese individual is at a serious disadvantage if an operation is required. The operative procedure carries a higher risk, and postoperative complications are more frequent. Any surgical procedure is technically much more difficult in an obese person, and wound healing is delayed. The adipose tissue, which has a relatively poor blood supply, heals poorly and is also quite vulnerable to infection, resulting in an increased incidence of postoperative wound infections.

Treatment of Obesity

Most overweight people are too heavy because they are eating too much and are not active enough. However, the results of treatment of obesity by dieting have been surprisingly poor, likely because satiety and appetite are controlled by a complex interaction between behavior (and the environment interacting with such) and genetics. Hence, simply saying "eat less, exercise more," although correct, rarely leads to maintained weight loss.

Because of the limited success of treating obesity by diet, various other measures have been proposed. Drugs that suppress appetite have been used, but many of these drugs have undesirable side effects and have had very limited success. As a last resort, massive obesity is sometimes treated by various surgical operations (bariatric surgery). The current surgical procedures produce weight loss primarily by restricting the capacity of the stomach without resorting to drastic restriction of nutrient absorption in the small intestine. They can be performed using standard surgical incisions or by laparoscopy using small abdominal incisions and are often grouped together

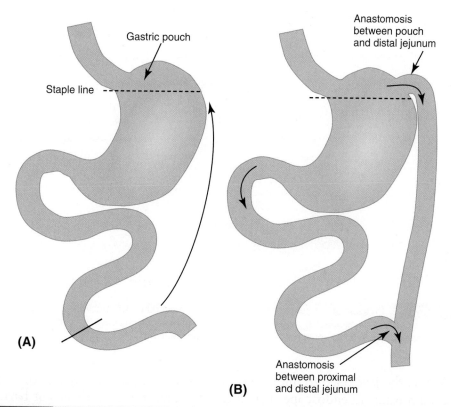

Gastric pouch

Staple line

(A)

Anastomosis
between pouch
and distal jejunum

Anastomosis
between proximal
and distal jejunum

(B)

FIGURE 23-27 Gastric bypass. **(A)** The upper *dashed line* indicates the location of gastric staples placed to create a gastric pouch. The lower *solid line* indicates the site where the jejunum is divided. The *arrow* indicates how the distal segment of jejunum is moved for anastomosis with the gastric pouch. **(B)** Completed bypass illustrating proximal and distal anastomoses. The *arrows* indicate the direction of movement of the gastrointestinal contents.

under the general term of "stomach stapling operations." The best known and most widely used of these procedures is called the Roux-en-Y gastric bypass, named after the man who devised it (Roux) and the Y-shaped connection made between the small bowel loops in the procedure (**FIGURE 23-27**). When the procedure is completed, food from the gastric pouch empties directly into the jejunum. The main part of the stomach no longer receives food. Gastric secretions can drain into the duodenum normally, but the secretions enter the jejunum distal ("downstream") to the segment of jejunum receiving the contents from the gastric pouch. Unfortunately, gastric bypass procedures may lead to late complications in many patients: anemia caused by poor absorption of iron and vitamin B_{12} and weakening of bones (osteoporosis) as a result of inadequate calcium intake and absorption.

Adjustable gastric banding is another laparoscopic procedure to control food intake by placing an inflatable, saline-filled, adjustable gastric band around the upper part of the stomach. The band compresses the stomach to form a small upper gastric pouch that is almost completely separated from the rest of the stomach except for a very small channel that allows food in the upper gastric pouch to empty slowly into the lower part of the stomach. The amount of compression applied to the inflatable band, which controls the rate of gastric emptying, can be adjusted by adding or removing saline through a port placed under the skin of the abdomen. The procedure has the advantage of not requiring a "major redesign" of the gastrointestinal tract, but banding does not lead to as much weight loss as a gastric bypass (**FIGURE 23-28**).

Adjustable gastric banding A method for treating obesity by applying an adjustable gastric band to the stomach to reduce its capacity, thereby promoting weight loss.

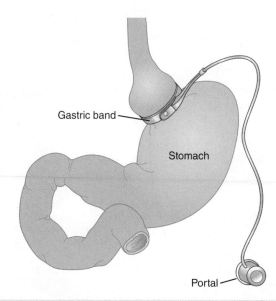

FIGURE 23-28 Principle of the adjustable gastric banding procedure. Adjustable band filled with saline limits the capacity of the stomach by constricting outflow from the stomach above the band. Rate of gastric emptying can be regulated by adding or removing saline from the band.

A recently developed technique uses a plastic liner placed and anchored in the duodenum using an endoscope. The liner acts as an intestinal sheath or barrier to separate consumed nutrients from the gut mucosa. If necessary, the sheath can easily be removed. The technique has shown promise in treating type 2 diabetes complicated by obesity. Large-scale clinical trials are under way in the United States.

ANOREXIA NERVOSA AND BULIMIA NERVOSA

These two conditions are characterized by profound eating disturbances. Although they are separate disorders, there is considerable overlap between the two conditions. Both of these conditions can lead to extreme malnutrition caused by inadequate nutrients, along with associated vitamin and mineral deficiencies. These conditions can lead to serious health consequences, which can be fatal if not adequately treated.

Anorexia Nervosa

In this condition, affected individuals have a false perception of being too fat when they are actually much too thin, and they continue to lose weight by restricting food intake and exercising excessively. The condition occurs much more frequently in women than in men and is more prevalent in Western countries where a slim body is considered ideal and excessive weight is thought to be undesirable. Fashion models, ballet dancers, and other groups in whom a slender body is required are disproportionately represented.

Anorexia nervosa often begins in adolescent girls during puberty as their bodies change along with the distribution of their body fat. Patients perceive themselves as getting fat from overeating and they use dieting and exercise to deal with the perception of being overweight. As their weight loss accelerates, other measures may be taken to reduce weight, such as self-induced vomiting or taking laxatives. The excessive weight loss disrupts many of the body's physiologic processes. Menstrual periods cease, thyroid function declines, fluid and electrolyte disturbances develop, and bones become fragile from loss of calcium (osteoporosis). Extreme emaciation is a life-threatening condition that may lead to death if not treated.

Severe anorexia nervosa is difficult to treat; both medical and psychological problems associated with the condition must be addressed. Medical treatment requires correcting the physiologic disturbances caused by fasting, which may require intravenous fluids and whatever other methods are needed to restore health. Psychological treatment requires the assistance of a psychiatrist or clinical psychologist experienced in dealing with eating disorders. The affected person needs to acquire a more realistic perception of her (or his) own body, needs to understand what may have led to the eating problem, and needs to learn how to adjust eating habits to prevent a recurrence of the condition.

Bulimia Nervosa

This condition is another method of weight control that is characterized by repeated episodes of binge eating (rapidly eating an excessively large amount of food) followed by purging (self-induced vomiting) to counteract the effects of the bingeing, along with guilt and remorse at the inability to control the binge–purge behavior. Purging may be supplemented by taking laxatives to decrease food absorption by promoting rapid passage of digested food through the small intestine. The condition occurs most often in young women. Their body weight may fluctuate in relation to their binge–purge behavior, but they do not become emaciated. Their friends and relatives usually are not aware of their problem because they look normal and carefully conceal their binge–purge behavior.

Bulimia nervosa carries with it some serious health problems. Repeated self-induced vomiting leads to dental problems due to the corrosive effect of gastric acid on tooth enamel. The repeated loss of excess gastric juice may lead to metabolic alkalosis and electrolyte disturbances (see discussion in water, electrolyte, and acid–base balance). One of the most serious effects of self-induced vomiting is a tear in the mucosa of the stomach near the gastroesophageal junction, which can bleed profusely and may be fatal (see Figure 23-7). Treatment involves the same medical and psychological approaches used to deal with anorexia nervosa.

Chronic Malnutrition: Its Causes and Effects

CAUSES OF MALNUTRITION

Malnutrition results when the intake of nutrients is insufficient to supply the body's needs either because there is insufficient food available or the food is not being used efficiently. In developing countries, inadequate food to supply the population may result from crop failure, a natural disaster such as a flood or a drought, poor food distribution, an unstable government, or other causes that have an impact on food production or delivery. Often, infants and children are disproportionately affected because they have a greater need for nutrients to sustain their rapid growth rate during infancy and childhood.

In modern industrialized countries, many cases of chronic malnutrition are caused by diseases that impair food intake, digestion, or absorption or by conditions that increase nutrient and protein requirements, such as an acute illness, a severe burn, or a major surgical procedure. Other people at risk are those living in poverty, the elderly, people who consume alcohol in excess, drug abusers, or those with advanced cancer or eating disorders. Treatment consists of supplying adequate nutrients together with vitamins and minerals before the malnutrition-induced organ damage has progressed to such a degree that response to treatment is unlikely to be successful.

In nonindustrialized countries, global deficiency of caloric intake in infants and children, termed **marasmus**, is not uncommon, particularly in children who have

Marasmus Global deficiency of caloric intake in infants and children.

been weaned. The child will suffer from growth failure and wasting. Immunosuppression occurs accompanied by repeated infections. There is general wasting and loss of subcutaneous fat. **Kwashiorkor** occurs when a diet is sufficient in calories but not in protein, most often in children whose diet consists nearly exclusively of carbohydrate. Severe edema and skin abnormalities occur. The hair takes on a red color. Intestinal changes may interfere with nutrient absorption even when nutrition becomes improved, and diarrhea is likely. However, caloric intake is sufficient, so subcutaneous fat is normal. Under any circumstances extreme emaciation is a life-threatening condition, and loss of over 30 percent of body weight may be fatal.

CASE 23-1

Maddy is a nineteen-year-old first year student in a local community college. She has been in good health until recently except for an occasional sinus infection treated by her local family physician. Her medical history is notable only for an appendectomy at the age of nine years. Recently she noted an increase in weakness and fatigue during midterm week. Her friends began to tease her because she had "noisy tummy" (borborygmus) and tended to pass gas (be flatulent). She noted an increased incidence of diarrhea followed by periods of constipation. Her digestive disturbances were accompanied by moderate abdominal pain, which was relieved by passing gas.

Several of her friends suggested that she might consider "going gluten free," stating that such a diet made them "feel better and think more clearly." Maddy began by restricting her intake of pizza to a gluten-free brand and, feeling better, found it easy to switch to a gluten-free or low-gluten diet because the cafeteria in her college provided these products. She also reduced her intake of milk and dairy products, which also seemed to relieve her symptoms. On a weekend trip she consumed a large amount of double cheese pizza. The restaurant did not have a gluten free product. The next morning she noted a severe recurrence of abdominal discomfort and did poorly on a series of school examinations. Her friends suggested that she had "gluten sensitivity." Maddy developed an annoying itchy rash on her back and buttocks and decided to consult her physician asbout the possibility she might have some type of gluten sensitivity or celiac disease; her friends told her this was very common.

Maddy's physical examination noted the following. She had a mild papulovesicular ("bumps and small blisters") rash that appeared to be receding. Maddy noted she had switched to a new shower gel recently and had gone back to her prior product. Maddy had a slightly protuberant abdomen and increased bowel sounds that the physician attributed to intestinal gas. No weight loss was noted. Her blood count was normal, but she did have borderline anemia. On reviewing Maddy's history of abdominal discomfort associated with her consumption of pizza, the physician suggested a possibility of lactose intolerance producing excessive intestinal gas and suggested Maddy keep a food diary to correlate symptoms with food consumption. Maddy was quite upset at the results of the examination as she (and her friends) believed it was likely she had gluten sensitivity. Her physician suggested two additional blood-based tests useful in diagnosing celiac disease (gluten-senstive enteropathy). One test looked for autoantibodies to a protein associated with celiac disease. The second test assayed for the presence of certain genetic markers on cells (major histocompatibility markers) that occurred in most individuals who have the disease. Maddy was negative in both tests. She continued to maintain that a gluten-free diet made her feel much better and joined a support group for non–celiac gluten sensitivity.

CASE 23-1 (Continued)

Discussion (Pathophysiology)

Celiac disease (gluten sensitive enteropathy) is a complex autoimmune disease associated with the production of an immune response to peptides derived from gluten, a high molecular weight seed storage protein found in grass-related grains such as wheat, rye, and barley. The protein is responsible for the ability of bread dough to become elastic, retain gas produced by leavening agents such as yeast, and rise prior to baking. The use of gluten is widespread in many food products. In celiac disease, the immune system recognizes a soluble component of gluten (gliaden), which has many glutamine amino acid residues clustered at one end of the molecule. Gliaden-derived peptides are transported to the gut where an enzyme (tissue transglutaminase, or TG2) deamidates (removes the side-chain amino group of) certain glutamine residues in the gliaden peptide. In individuals with particular HLA (major histocompatibility) types, the TG2 altered peptides are recognized by CD4+ helper T cells and result in cellular immunity directed toward the altered peptides in the small intestine. This results in the activation of inflammatory pathways leading to immune-mediated damage to the absorptive surface of the small intestine and a variety of malabsorptive and digestive symptoms. A second major component of celiac disease is autoimmune production of antibodies to TG2. Although the exact mechanism remains unclear, gliaden-derived peptides in combination with TG2 induce the formation of antibodies to both gliaden and TG2. These antibodies are likely to contribute to the intestinal damage, but antibodies to TG2 (and in particular IgA antibodies) are most likely to be responsible for the non-gut-related autoimmune disease seen in celiac disease (as TG2 is found in many sites in the body). Hence, celiac disease is associated with a confusing array of symptoms, some of which (diarrhea, malabsorption of fats, flatulence, weight loss, anemia and osteoporosis) are clearly associated with damage to the absorptive capacity of the intestine. Other symptoms (neurologic, hormonal disturbances, and skin disorders such as **dermatitis herpetiformis** consistent with Maddy's rash) may be related (at least in part) to a systemic autoimmune response. (It should be noted that this list of symptoms is by no means exhaustive.)

Discussion (Diagnosis)

Until the early 2000s celiac disease was considered uncommon with a frequency of about 1 in 6,000 people. Diagnosis was costly and invasive, requiring intestinal biopsy and tissue evaluation by a pathologist. However, the development of several relatively easy serological tests that measured antibodies to TG2 defined an increased incidence of the disease to perhaps as high as 1 percent as measured by positivity in these assays. Many "new" cases are diagnosed in women and adults who have symptoms that may be less severe and "nonspecific." The number of seropositive individuals who have celiac disease as defined by intestinal biopsy is also unclear, and the area remains extremely controversial.

What about Maddy? Celiac disease has a very strong genetic component. Well over 90 percent of patients with celiac disease have particular pairs of HLA markers. Tests for these markers are very sensitive (but not very specific) and are excellent for excluding this disease. On this basis alone, Maddy is very unlikely to have celiac disease. The utility of serological testing depends strongly on test specifics. Assuming the best technique was used, sensitivity and specificity are over 90 percent, again arguing that Maddy was unlikely to have celiac disease. However, does this mean Maddy was not sensitive to gluten consumption? In one study, 60 percent of patients with symptoms similar to Maddy's could not be classified as having celiac disease. Maddy's symptoms could have been related to lactose intolerance or irritable bowel disease. Both were hinted at in the case presentation. Maddy's rash could have been related to a shower gel. Because of this uncertainty, which is often a problem with diseases that are solely self-reported, a condition termed **non-celiac**

(continues)

CASE 23-1 (Continued)

gluten sensitivity has been defined (predominantly based on the lack of objective symptoms and laboratory tests). Perhaps this is what Maddy had, perhaps stress contributed to irritable bowel disease, perhaps she was lactose intolerant.

Etiology and pathogenesis

Undefined, fits the diagnostic category non-celiac gluten sensitivity.

Questions

1. The Case notes that HLA testing is very useful in diagnosing potential cases of celiac disease. If someone has the appropriate HLA markers, does this mean the person has the disease?

2. Why was HLA typing unlikely to have been offered to Maddy as an initial test?

3. The Case suggests Maddy might have been lactose intolerant. What characteristics of Maddy's background (deliberately excluded in the Case) might have made this more likely?

4. How could lactose intolerance have been confirmed?

5. Maddy was scrupulous in avoiding gluten-based products, excelled in college, and had much reduced intestinal symptoms. Does this mean she had celiac disease or non-celiac gluten sensitivity?

QUESTIONS FOR REVIEW

1. What is a cleft palate? What is its usual mode of inheritance? How is it treated?

2. What factors affect the development of dental caries? What complications may result from dental caries? What are the causes and possible effects of periodontal disease?

3. What are some of the major causes of esophageal obstruction? What symptoms does esophageal obstruction produce?

4. What is peptic ulcer? In what parts of the gastrointestinal tract are peptic ulcers encountered? What factors contribute to the development of peptic ulcers? What are the complications of a peptic ulcer?

5. What is the difference between Crohn disease and chronic ulcerative colitis? Diverticulosis and diverticulitis?

6. What is a Meckel diverticulum? Where is it located? What clinical manifestations can it produce?

7. What is intestinal obstruction? What symptoms does it produce? What are some of the common causes of intestinal obstruction?

8. What is the pathogenesis of acute appendicitis?

9. What symptoms and physical findings are likely to be encountered in a patient with a carcinoma of the colon? Why?

10. What is an intussusception? How is it caused? What is the difference between volvulus and intussusception?

SUPPLEMENTARY READINGS

Loeffler, A. G., and Hart, M. N., Chapter 14, "Gastrointestinal Tract." 2015. In *Introduction to Human Disease.* 6th ed. Burlington, MA: Jones & Bartlett Learning.
▶ The chapter presents an overview and some additional details on gastrointestinal disease. Any of a number of pathology texts used in undergraduate medical education will provide additional details.

Elrasheid, A. H., et al. 2013. Molecular biology of colorectal cancer: Review of the literature. *American Journal of Molecular Biology* 3:72–80.

Moorcraft, S. Y., et al. 2013. The role of personalized medicine in metastatic colorectal cancer. *Therapeutic Advances in Gastroenterology* 6:381–95.
▶ Two up-to-date review articles on genes related to cancer development and the hereditary types of colon cancer. The second reference discusses therapeutic implications.

Specter, M. 2012. Germs are us. *The New Yorker* (October 22).

The Helicobacter Foundation. Perth, Australia. www.helico.com
▶ The first entry is an enjoyable article on the discovery and scientific background related to *H. pylori* infection. The second entry is for Dr. Barry Marshall's website; he established the relationship of *H. pylori* to gastrointestinal disease. It has an up-to-date reference list and excellent quick reviews.

American Society for Metabolic and Bariatric Surgery. *Bariatric surgery procedures.* http://asmbs.org/patients/bariatric-surgery-procedures

Mayo Clinic. *Obesity diseases and conditions.* http://www.mayoclinic.org/diseases-conditions/obesity/basics/definition/con-20014834

CDC Division of Nutrition, Physical Activity and Obesity. *Overweight and obesity.* http://www.cdc.gov/Obesity/
▶ These three references describe the magnitude of the "obesity epidemic" and the applications and limitations of various surgical procedures used to treat morbid obesity.

Christakis, N. A., and Fowler, J. H. 2007. The spread of obesity in a large social network over 32 years. *New England Journal of Medicine* 357:370–79.

▶ Evaluation of a densely connected social network of 12,067 people assessed repeatedly from 1971 to 2003 as part of the Framingham Heart Study revealed that obesity spreads within social groups, especially among close friends, siblings, and spouses, strongly suggesting that the spread of obesity among spouses, brothers and sisters, close friends, and associates may be influenced by developing shared ideas and concepts about the acceptability of overeating, weight gain, and obesity. Still thought-provoking reading.

Centers for Disease Control and Prevention. *Norovirus.* http://www.cdc.gov/norovirus/

Centers for Disease Control and Prevention. *Rotavirus.* http://www.cdc.gov/rotavirus/

▶ These two CDC websites will tell you everything you need to know about the two viral forms of gastroenteritis. They contain useful and detailed lists of publications, most of which are available online.

Stanley, J. D., et al. 2013. Clostridium difficile infection. *Current Problems in Surgery* 50:302–7.

Rao, K., and Young, V. B. 2015. Fecal microbiota transplantation for the management of Clostridium difficile infection. *Infectious Disease Clinics of North America* 29:109–22.

▶ The first article presents a thorough overview of the area. The second article discusses recent advances in the use of fecal transplantation in cases of the disease. Note that volume 29(1) of *Infectious Disease Clinics of North America* contains many additional current reviews on C. difficile infection.

Spechler, S. J., and Souza, R. F. 2014. Barrett's esophagus. *New England Journal of Medicine* 371:836–45.

▶ An overview of the epidemiology, pathogenesis, diagnosis, and treatment of Barrett's and gastroesophageal reflux syndrome.

Shogilev, D. J., et al. 2014. Diagnosing appendicitis: Evidence-based review of the diagnostic approach in 2014. *Western Journal of Emergency Medicine* 15:859–71.

Segev, L., et al. 2015. Acute appendicitis in the elderly in the twenty-first century. *Journal of Gastrointestinal Surgery* 19(4):730–35.

▶ Diagnosis of appendicitis is a far from settled medical issue. The best approaches for different patient populations are reviewed in these two references.

Aziz, I., Branchi, F., and Sanders, D. S. 2015. The rise and fall of gluten. *Proceedings of the Nutrition Society* 74(3):221–26.

Husby, S., and Murray, J. A. 2014. Diagnosing celiac disease and the potential for serological markers. *Nature Reviews Gastroenterology & Hepatology* 11:655–63.

Meresse, B., Malamut, G., and Cerf-Bensussan, N. 2012. Celiac disease: An immunological jigsaw. *Immunity* 36:907–17.

▶ These three references were the most valuable for use in constructing the Case. The first is an amusing overview that touches on the controversial aspects of celiac disease diagnosis. The second presents a more in-depth analysis of diagnostic technology, and the third details the immunopathology of the disease.

The Endocrine Glands

1. Explain the normal physiologic functions of the pituitary hormones. Name the common endocrine disturbances, and describe the methods of treating each disturbance.

2. Describe the major disturbances of thyroid function and their clinical manifestations, and explain the methods of treatment.

3. Explain the normal physiologic functions of the adrenal cortex and medulla. Name the common endocrine disturbances

resulting from dysfunction, and describe methods of treatment.

4. Define the causes and effects of parathyroid dysfunction, and describe the methods of treatment.

5. Understand the concept of ectopic hormone production by nonendocrine tumors.

6. Explain how stress affects the endocrine system.

Endocrine Functions and Dysfunctions

Endocrine glands secrete their products directly into the bloodstream and exert a regulatory effect on various metabolic functions. The major endocrine glands are the pituitary, thyroid, and parathyroid glands along with the adrenal cortex and medulla. Other organs such as the pancreatic islets and the ovaries and testes also secrete hormones (discussed in presentations on the pancreas and male or female sex organs). In addition, many other groups of specialized cells throughout the body also secrete hormones. Renin and erythropoietin are secreted by the kidneys; the hormones gastrin, secretin, and cholecystokinin are produced by the mucosa of the gastrointestinal tract. By convention, these hormones are considered along with the organs with which they are associated and are not generally regarded as part of the endocrine system (**FIGURE 24-1**).

The amount of hormone synthesized and released into the circulation by an endocrine gland may be regulated directly by the level of hormone circulating in the blood, or indirectly, by the level of a substance under hormonal control, such as the concentration of glucose or sodium in the blood. Mechanisms of this type are called **feedback mechanisms**. Most commonly, an increase in the level of hormone or hormone-regulated substance suppresses further hormone output. This is called a negative feedback mechanism, or feedback inhibition, and is illustrated by the control mechanisms regulating output of pituitary hormones. Tropic hormones secreted by

Feedback mechanisms Biological control using levels of hormones to control further production of substances.

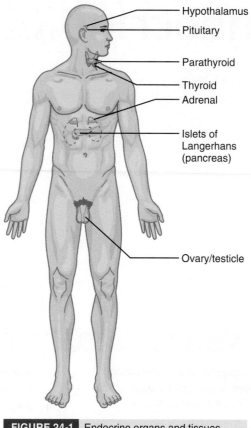

Hypothalamus

Pituitary

Parathyroid

Thyroid

Adrenal

Islets of
Langerhans
(pancreas)

Ovary/testicle

FIGURE 24-1 Endocrine organs and tissues.

the pituitary control the level of secretion of hormones by target endocrine glands. For example, the pituitary will secrete additional thyroid-stimulating hormone in response to low circulating levels of thyroid hormones. Conversely, high levels of thyroid hormone suppress the production of thyroid-stimulating hormone by the pituitary. A disorder of an endocrine gland may consist of either hypersecretion of the gland, manifested as overactivity of the target organ regulated by the gland, or insufficient secretion, resulting in underactivity of the organ controlled by the gland. This may result because of intrinsic abnormalities of the target gland (the thyroid in the example) or because of either a deficit or excess secretion of tropic hormones by the pituitary (**FIGURE 24-2**).

The clinical effects of a disturbance of endocrine gland function are determined by the degree of dysfunction of the gland and by the age and sex of the affected individual. Symptoms of dysfunction range from barely detectable variations from normal to extreme hypofunction or hyperfunction. The age of the person when the endocrine disturbance becomes manifest has a pronounced effect on the clinical features. Some endocrine glands, such as the thyroid gland, affect growth and development as well as metabolic processes; therefore, disturbed function in a child will produce a somewhat different clinical picture from a similar disturbance in an adult. The sex of the individual also influences the effect of disturbed endocrine function because many hormones are concerned with the development and maintenance of sexual function and secondary sexual characteristics. Some endocrine disturbances cause alteration in sexual development in children, whereas the effects are much less pronounced in adults. Overproduction of an inappropriate sex hormone in some endocrine diseases causes masculinization (virilization) of the female or feminization of the male; conversely, overproduction of a sex hormone appropriate to the sex of the individual has little clinical effect.

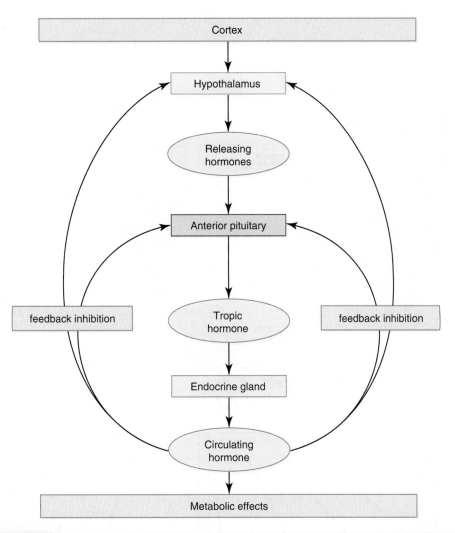

FIGURE 24-2 Normal mechanisms controlling elaboration of tropic hormones by the pituitary gland.

The Pituitary Gland

The pituitary gland is a small, pea-shaped gland suspended by a narrow stalk from the hypothalamus at the base of the brain. The gland, composed of an anterior lobe and a posterior lobe, is located in a small depression within the sphenoid bone, called the pituitary fossa or sella turcica (named because of a supposed resemblance to a Turkish saddle), just behind the optic chiasm. Many mammals also have an intermediate lobe located between the anterior and posterior lobes that produces melanin-stimulating hormone (MSH). However, in humans, the intermediate lobe consists only of a series of small cystic cavities whose function is unclear and is no longer present as a distinct structure (**FIGURE 24-3A** and **FIGURE 24-3B**).

The anterior lobe is composed of cords of epithelial cells containing hormones that are synthesized and stored within the lobe. Anterior lobe cells have been classified on the basis of the staining reaction of their cytoplasmic granules, using routine staining methods. Three cell types were recognized: **eosinophils**, which contain bright-red–staining cytoplasmic granules; **basophils**, which have abundant blue-staining granules in their cytoplasm; and **chromophobe cells**, which contain sparse, poorly stained granules. Currently five different cell types are defined based on the specific hormone each produces as detected using immunological staining procedures. For example,

Eosinophil A cell whose cytoplasm is filled with large, uniform granules that stain intensely red with acid dyes. See also *basophil*.

Basophil A cell that contains numerous variable-sized granules that stain intensely purple with basic dyes. See also *eosinophil*.

Chromophobe cells Anterior lobe pituitary epithelial cells containing sparse, poorly stained granules. See also eosinophil *and* basophil.

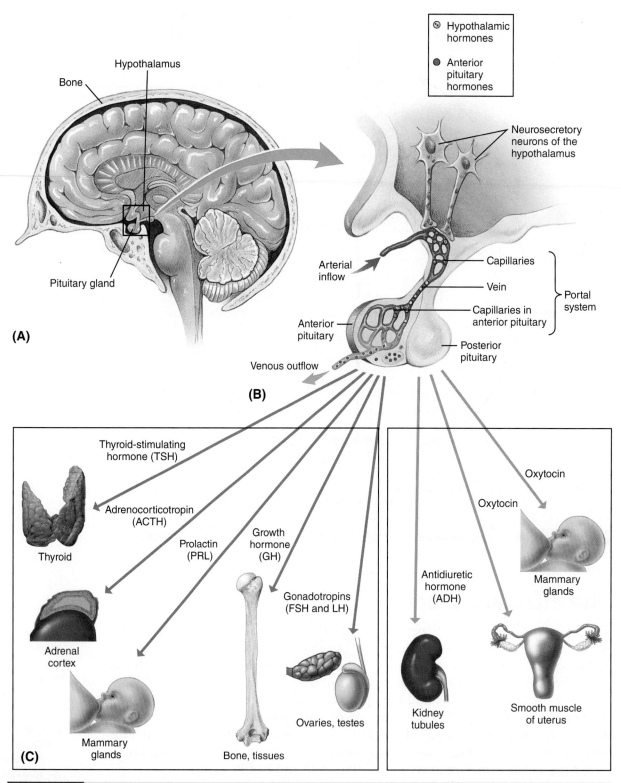

FIGURE 24-3 The pituitary gland. **(A)** Cross section of the brain showing the location of the pituitary and hypothalamus. **(B)** The structure of the pituitary gland. **(C)** Releasing and inhibiting hormone travel via the hypothalamus to the anterior pituitary where they affect tropic hormone secretion as indicated.

TABLE 24-1 Hypothalamic Hormones and Their Targets	
Hypothalamic hormone	**Response of pituitary and target gland**
Thyrotropin-releasing hormone (TRH)	1. Stimulates release of thyroid-stimulating hormone (TSH), which in turn stimulates production and release of thyroid hormone. 2. Stimulates prolactin production and release.
Corticotropin-releasing hormone (CRH)	Stimulates release of adrenocorticotropic hormone (ACTH), which in turn stimulates production and release of adrenal cortical hormones.
Gonadotropin-releasing hormone (GnRH)	Stimulates follicle-stimulating hormone (FSH) and luteinizing hormone (LH), which in turn affect gonadal function.
Growth hormone releasing hormone (GHRH)	Stimulates synthesis of growth hormone, which in turn promotes production of growth factors that promote general tissue growth.
Prolactin inhibitory hormone (Dopamine)	1. Inhibits prolactin release from pituitary gland. 2. Inhibits FSH and LH.
Somatostatin	1. Inhibits secretion and release of growth hormone, which in turn inhibits growth factors that promote general tissue growth. 2. Inhibits TSH.

those cells secreting thyroid-stimulating hormone are called thyrotrophs; the most common cell type is somatotrophs, which secrete growth hormone (somatotropin).

The anterior lobe is connected to the hypothalamus by a special system of blood vessels called a portal system, which begins as capillaries in the hypothalamus and extends down the pituitary stalk to terminate as capillaries around the cells of the anterior lobe. Release of the hormones stored within the cells of the anterior lobe is regulated by hormonal substances called **releasing hormones**, which are synthesized in the hypothalamus and carried to the cells of the anterior lobe in the blood flowing through the portal system. Usually, a hypothalamic releasing hormone activates a single gland, but some releasing hormones affect more than one gland. Other hypothalamic hormones inhibit rather than stimulate specific glands, and the hormone response of the target gland reflects the net effect of the interaction between releasing and inhibiting hormones (**TABLE 24-1**).

The posterior lobe consists of a meshwork of nerve fibers intermixed with modified neuroglial cells and is connected to the hypothalamus by bundles of nerve fibers extending through the pituitary stalk rather than by the portal circulation. The hormones in the posterior lobe are synthesized within the hypothalamus and are then transmitted down the nerve axons in the pituitary stalk to the posterior lobe, where they are stored. They are then released from the posterior lobe in response to nerve impulses transmitted from the hypothalamus down the pituitary stalk.

The hypothalamus, which controls release of hormones from both the anterior and posterior lobes, is in turn under the control of higher cortical centers; consequently, pituitary secretion is to some extent influenced by emotional stimuli such as anxiety, rage, and fear and is also influenced by sensory impulses that enter the nervous system and are in turn relayed to the hypothalamus.

Releasing hormones
Substances causing release of hormones from the anterior pituitary.

Growth hormone (GH) An anterior lobe pituitary hormone that stimulates growth of bone and other body tissues.

Prolactin Hormone produced by the anterior lobe of the pituitary gland that stimulates milk secretion.

Thyroid-stimulating hormone (TSH) Hormone secreted by the anterior lobe of the pituitary; regulates thyroid function.

Adrenocorticotrophic hormone (ACTH) A hormone secreted by the anterior lobe of the pituitary that stimulates the adrenal cortex to manufacture and secrete adrenal cortical hormones.

Follicle-stimulating hormone (FSH) One of the gonadotropic hormones secreted by the anterior lobe of the pituitary, which regulates growth and function of the gonads (ovary and testis).

Luteinizing hormone (LH) One of the gonadotropic hormones secreted by the anterior lobe of the pituitary that regulates growth and function of the gonads (ovary and testis).

Melanin-stimulating hormone (MSH) One of the hormones produced by the pituitary. Causes darkening of the skin.

Antidiuretic hormone (ADH) Posterior lobe pituitary hormone that regulates urine concentration by altering the permeability of the renal collecting tubules.

Oxytocin A hormone that is stored in the posterior lobe of the pituitary gland that causes uterine contractions during labor and ejection of milk from the breast lobules into the larger ducts.

PITUITARY HORMONES

The pituitary gland secretes a total of eight separate hormones, which have multiple functions. Six are produced by the anterior lobe: **growth hormone (GH)**, **prolactin**, **thyroid-stimulating hormone (TSH)**, **adrenocorticotropic hormone (ACTH)**, **follicle-stimulating hormone (FSH)**, and **luteinizing hormone (LH)**. **Melanin-stimulating hormone (MSH)** is sometimes considered as a ninth. Two, **antidiuretic hormone (ADH)** and **oxytocin**, are produced by the posterior lobe. The four anterior lobe hormones, which regulate other endocrine glands, are called tropic hormones (**FIGURE 24-3C**).

Anterior Lobe Hormones

Growth hormone, also called somatotropin, has multiple actions, all concerned with general tissue growth. Growth hormone exerts its growth-promoting effects on tissues indirectly by stimulating the liver to produce a peptide called insulin-like growth factor 1, or somatomedin (*soma* = body + *medin* = mediator of growth). The growth factor enters the circulation and travels throughout the body where it promotes growth of the skeletal system and internal organs. Prolactin stimulates the secretion of milk by the breast, which has been previously stimulated by estrogen and progesterone. TSH, also called thyrotropin, stimulates the thyroid gland to secrete thyroid hormone. ACTH, also called corticotropin, stimulates the adrenal cortex to manufacture and secrete adrenocortical hormones. ACTH exerts its main effect on the adrenal hormones that control carbohydrate metabolism (glucocorticoids), and it is produced from a large precursor molecule that gives rise not only to ACTH but also to MSH as a "by-product" of ACTH synthesis. MSH causes darkening of the skin by stimulating melanocytes, but normally not enough is produced to have any significant effect when output of ACTH is normal. However, darkening of skin may be a result of excess ACTH synthesis. FSH and LH are gonadotropic hormones. They regulate the growth and development of the gonads (ovaries and testes) and control the output of sex hormones, which are responsible for the development of male and female secondary sex characteristics.

Posterior Lobe Hormones

ADH causes the cells of the renal collecting tubules to become more permeable to water so that more water is reabsorbed and a concentrated urine is excreted. Secretion of ADH is regulated by receptors in the hypothalamus, which respond to variations in the osmolarity of the extracellular fluid. If the osmolarity rises, the hypothalamic neurons send impulses to the posterior lobe to stimulate release of ADH. Water is retained instead of being excreted, which dilutes the extracellular fluid and lowers its osmolarity. Conversely, if the extracellular fluids become too dilute, the hypothalamus directs the pituitary to decrease its output of ADH. More water is excreted in the urine, which causes the osmolarity of the body fluids to rise.

Oxytocin stimulates the contraction of the pregnant uterus and causes release of milk from the lactating breast. Oxytocin is secreted in response to stimulation of the nipples during nursing. The sensory nerve impulses are transmitted to the hypothalamus, and the hypothalamic neurons in turn send impulses to the posterior lobe, which causes the release of oxytocin.

PHYSIOLOGIC CONTROL OF PITUITARY HORMONE SECRETION

The level of the various trophic hormones produced by the pituitary is regulated by the level of circulating hormone produced by the target gland (Figure 24-2). Cells in the hypothalamus measure the level of the various hormones in the blood and liberate various releasing and inhibiting hormones that control the release of pituitary hormones into the circulation. Several hormones produced by the hypothalamus and pituitary gland are released in pulses rather than as a continuous output. Many hormone levels also may vary over a twenty-four-hour period (called a diurnal variation). This is most notable for ACTH; the highest levels occur in the early morning, followed by a gradual fall throughout the day. When the concentration of the hormone falls below a certain level, releasing hormones increase and travel by the portal venous system to the pituitary gland, causing release of the tropic hormone. This, in turn, affects the target organ. The level of the hormone produced by the target organ rises until it reaches the upper range of normal. At this point, the high level of circulating hormone "shuts off" further elaboration of tropic hormone. This mechanism maintains a relatively steady hormone output from the target organ and prevents wide fluctuations in hormonal level that might disrupt the smooth functioning of the body's hormone-regulated organ systems. It should be noted that the set point at which a hormone produced by a target gland turns off tropic hormone secretion varies considerably from individual to individual.

Prolactin secretion is regulated by a somewhat different mechanism than the other pituitary hormones. With other hormones, the main effect of hypothalamic releasing hormones is to stimulate secretion. For prolactin, however, the principal control is by an inhibitory substance, the neurotransmitter **dopamine**. Secretion of prolactin would continue unabated if it were not continuously suppressed. Release of prolactin is affected by stimuli from the nipples during nursing. The stimuli are relayed to the hypothalamus, which responds by releasing less dopamine and prolactin secretion increases.

Effects of Abnormalities in the Secretion of Tropic Hormones

Abnormalities in the secretion of tropic hormones may involve either single or multiple hormones and may be manifested as either a hypofunction or an overproduction of pituitary hormone.

PITUITARY HYPOFUNCTION

Sometimes the anterior lobe of the pituitary gland is destroyed by a tumor, neurological injury, cranial radiation therapy, or undergoes necrosis owing to a disturbance of its blood supply as sometimes occurs in the postpartum period (Sheehan syndrome). Rare congenital defects in the development of the pituitary also occur. In this condition, called **panhypopituitarism** (*pan* = multiple + *hypo* = decrease), the anterior lobe fails to secrete any hormones. The functions of the thyroid gland, adrenal glands, and gonads are impaired because tropic hormone stimulation is lost. Pituitary hypofunction can lead to pituitary dwarfism or diabetes insipidus.

Pituitary dwarfism, an isolated deficiency of growth hormone in a child, is characterized by retarded growth and development. In some cases, this is related to mutations in the growth hormone gene, but in most cases the cause is unknown. Normal growth and development can be restored by administering growth hormone produced by recombinant DNA technology. **Diabetes insipidus** is a rare disease usually caused by failure of the posterior lobe of the pituitary gland to secrete antidiuretic hormone (ADH) because of injury, tumor, or some other disease involving the posterior lobe. Because of the lack of ADH, the affected person is unable to absorb water from the renal collecting tubules and excretes a large volume of extremely dilute urine. Large

Dopamine Chemical mediator released by hypothalamic neurons.

Panhypopituitarism Failure of secretion of all anterior lobe pituitary hormones.

Pituitary dwarfism Stunted growth cause by a deficiency of growth hormone in a child.

Diabetes insipidus A condition resulting from a deficiency of antidiuretic hormone, characterized by excretion of a large volume of very dilute urine.

amounts of water must be consumed to compensate for the excessive water loss and to prevent dehydration. In some cases of diabetes insipidus, however, the problem is not with inadequate output of ADH but with an inability of the kidneys to respond to the hormone. This condition is called nephrogenic diabetes insipidus to set it apart from the disease caused by posterior lobe malfunction. Treatment differs depending on the cause of the diabetes insipidus. If the posterior lobe is at fault, treatment consists of supplying ADH. If it is a kidney problem, drugs are given to make the kidney more responsive to ADH.

PITUITARY TUMORS

Many conditions affecting the pituitary gland result from pituitary tumors involving the anterior lobe of the gland, many of which are functional (produce hormone). Tumors that do not produce hormones are called nonfunctional tumors. Although no hormones are produced, a nonfunctional tumor may cause problems because of its location, which is close to the optic chiasm, optic nerves, and other vital structures at the base of the brain. An enlarging tumor may erode the pituitary fossa, encroach on the optic chiasm, and may disrupt the hormone-producing functions of adjacent normal anterior lobe cells that are compressed by the expanding tumor.

Clinical manifestations of a functional tumor are determined by what hormone it makes, how much hormone it produces, the size of the tumor, and the age of the individual. The two most common functional pituitary tumors produce growth hormone and prolactin. Generally, each type of tumor produces a characteristic clinical syndrome. The great majority of pituitary tumors are adenomas; that is, they are benign glandular tumors that do not metastasize but may be associated with significant disease (**FIGURE 24-4**).

Treatment of a pituitary tumor is determined by the type of tumor, the hormones it produces, and the size of the tumor. A small prolactin-secreting adenoma may respond well to drugs that shrink the tumor, or secretion of growth hormone can be suppressed by drugs. In most cases, however, the treatment of a pituitary tumor is surgical removal, occasionally followed by radiation treatment in selected patients.

Because a pituitary tumor is so difficult to approach through the cranial cavity, it is usually resected through the nasal cavity and sphenoid sinus, a procedure called

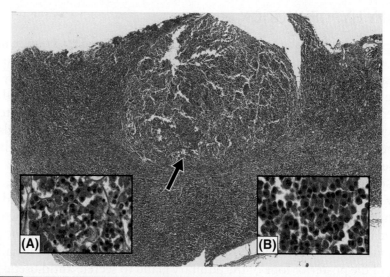

FIGURE 24-4 Pituitary gland showing a small adenoma (*arrow*). **(A)** Normal pituitary tissue showing characteristic multiple cell types. **(B)** Uniform acidophilic cell population of the adenoma.
Courtesy of Department of Pathology and Laboratory Medicine, University of North Carolina at Chapel Hill.

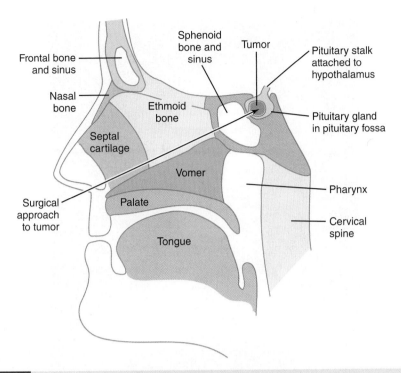

FIGURE 24-5 Transsphenoidal resection of a pituitary tumor.

a transsphenoidal resection (**FIGURE 24-5**). The transsphenoidal method for resecting all types of pituitary tumors involves entering the nasal cavity either directly or through an incision under the upper lip and removing part of the nasal septum. Then the sphenoid sinus is entered, and the anterior part of the pituitary fossa (sella turcica) is opened to expose the pituitary tumor, which is resected. Finally, the nasal incision is repaired.

OVERPRODUCTION OF GROWTH HORMONE

Overproduction of growth hormone in children and adolescents, whose epiphyses have not yet fused, causes excessive growth in the length of bones, and the person becomes too tall. This condition is called **pituitary gigantism**. Some associated coarsening of the facial features usually occurs in response to the effect of growth hormone on the structure of the facial bones.

In adults, excessive growth hormone causes **acromegaly**. Because the epiphyses have fused, there can be no growth in height, but the growth hormone produces thickening and coarsening of bones and generalized enlargement of the viscera. Affected individuals have coarse facial features, large prominent jaws, and large spadelike hands, but they are no taller than normal (**FIGURE 24-6**). The term acromegaly (*acron* = extremity + *megas* = large) describes one prominent feature of the disease. Growth hormone excess is almost always associated with pituitary adenomas. In addition to the hormonal effects, manifestations related to the size and location of the tumor may also occur. As noted previously, surgery is curative.

OVERPRODUCTION OF PROLACTIN

In a nonpregnant woman, excess secretion of prolactin may cause spontaneous secretion of milk from the breasts (**galactorrhea**) and cessation of menstrual periods (**amenorrhea**). Galactorrhea results from the effect of the hormone on breast tissue.

Pituitary gigantism
A condition resulting from excessive secretion of growth hormone in the child.

Acromegaly A condition resulting from excessive secretion of growth hormone in the adult.

Galactorrhea Secretion of milk by breast not associated with pregnancy or normal lactation.

Amenorrhea Absence of menses.

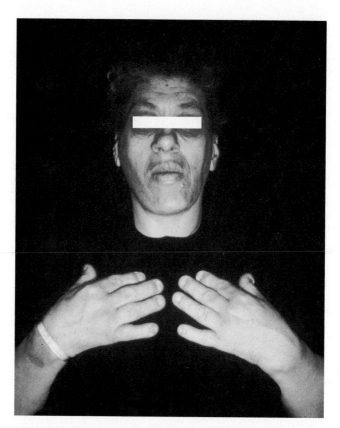

FIGURE 24-6 The appearance of an individual with advanced acromegaly.

Courtesy of Leonard V. Crowley, MD, Century College.

Amenorrhea occurs because high levels of prolactin also inhibit secretion of pituitary gonadotropins FSH and LH, which in turn leads to cessation of ovulation and menstrual cycles. This is sometimes called the amenorrhea-galactorrhea syndrome. In males, overproduction of prolactin is associated with infertility, hypogonadism, and reduced sexual function.

The various causes of the amenorrhea-galactorrhea syndrome are summarized in **FIGURE 24-7**. A prolactin-secreting pituitary adenoma is the most likely possibility. Sometimes the tumor is quite small (called a microadenoma) and causes few symptoms other than those related to the increased prolactin production. Larger tumors may cause enlargement of the pituitary fossa and visual disturbances like those produced by adenomas that secrete growth hormone. A prolactin-secreting pituitary adenoma can be removed surgically, but a small adenoma can often be inhibited by a **dopamine agonist** drug (*agon* = competitor), which is a drug that functions like dopamine, such as bromocriptine or a similar drug that attaches to dopamine receptors on the prolactin-secreting anterior lobe cells. The attachment suppresses output of prolactin, which in turn suppresses the growth and secretion of the prolactin-secreting adenoma.

There are other causes of hyperprolactinemia. Some drugs and medications may at times raise prolactin levels, resulting in amenorrhea and galactorrhea. These include estrogens, antihypertensive drugs, and drugs used to treat mental or emotional problems. Antihypertensive drugs, phenothiazine drugs (used to treat mental illness), and antidepressant drugs raise prolactin levels by depleting dopamine or blocking dopamine receptors in the hypothalamus. Prolactin levels also rise in hypothyroidism, which is related indirectly to reduced thyroid hormone secretion.

Dopamine agonist A drug such as bromocriptine that combines with cell dopamine receptors and causes the same cell response that would be produced by dopamine, such as inhibition of prolactin secretion.

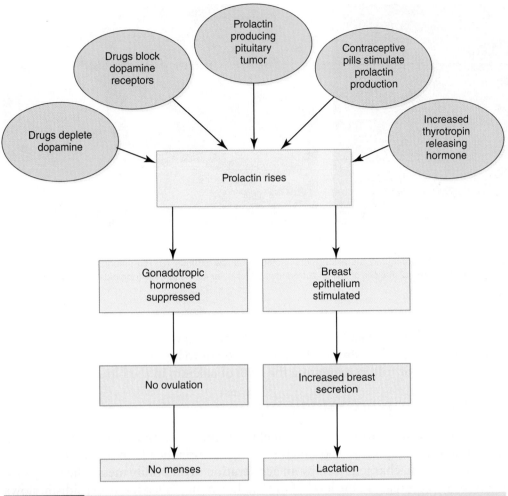

FIGURE 24-7 Factors regulating prolactin secretion and pathogenesis of amenorrhea-galactorrhea syndrome.

The Thyroid Gland

The thyroid gland, consisting of two lateral lobes connected by a narrow isthmus (**FIGURE 24-8A**), is located in the neck overlying the upper part of the trachea and is regulated by pituitary thyroid-stimulating hormone (TSH). The parathyroid glands (most often four in number) are located on its posterior surface.

Histologically, the thyroid gland is composed of multiple minute spherical vesicles called thyroid follicles. Each follicle consists of a central mass of eosinophilic protein material called **colloid**, which contains the protein **thyroglobulin** to which the thyroid hormone is attached. The colloid is surrounded by a layer of cuboidal epithelial cells called follicular cells (**FIGURE 24-8B**). Under the influence of TSH, the follicular cells synthesize two hormones—triiodothyronine (T_3) and thyroxin (T_4)—that regulate the body's metabolic processes and are also required for the normal development of the nervous system. Thyroid hormone is a general term referring to the two metabolic hormones, T_3 and T_4; the numbers indicate the number of iodine atoms attached to the molecules. More than 80 percent of T_3 (the more active hormone) is derived in the circulation from secreted T_4. Most of the thyroid hormone circulates bound to a protein called thyroid-binding globulin and is biologically inactive. The small amount of hormone that circulates unbound to protein is the physiologically active form of the hormone.

Colloid An eosinophilic protein material present within the thyroid follicles.

Thyroglobulin A protein within the colloid of the thyroid follicles which is a precursor of thyroid hormone.

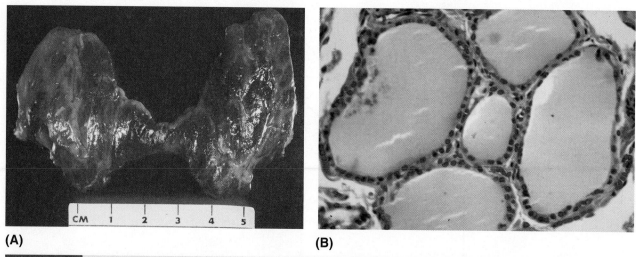

(A)

(B)

FIGURE 24-8 **(A)** Normal thyroid gland, illustrating two lateral lobes connected by narrow isthmus. **(B)** High-magnification photomicrograph of normal thyroid follicles, illustrating central masses of colloid surrounded by follicular epithelial cells (original magnification ×400).

Courtesy of Leonard V. Crowley, MD, Century College.

Calcitonin A hormone that lowers blood calcium, produced by the interfollicular cells of the thyroid gland.

Goiter Any enlargement of the thyroid gland.

Specialized parafollicular cells located between the thyroid follicles elaborate a third hormone called **calcitonin**. This hormone tends to lower blood calcium but plays a relatively minor role in regulating the level of calcium in the blood.

ACTIONS OF THYROID HORMONE

Thyroid hormone controls the rate of metabolic processes and is required for normal growth and development. Too much thyroid hormone leads to a condition called hyperthyroidism, characterized by an acceleration of all bodily metabolic functions. Conversely, a decrease in the level of thyroid hormone, called hypothyroidism, slows metabolic processes.

Clinically, some of the most pronounced effects of excess thyroid hormone are manifested in the cardiovascular and neuromuscular systems. The heart rate is accelerated. Reflexes are hyperactive, and frequently a fine tremor of the muscles is apparent. The hormone also has conspicuous effects on emotional and intellectual functions. Individuals with excess thyroid hormone are hyperactive, emotionally labile, and often quite irritable. They may have difficulty concentrating because mental processes are accelerated excessively.

The effects of thyroid hypofunction are the reverse of those in hyperthyroidism. The hypothyroid individual is slow and lethargic. Bodily metabolic functions are subnormal. Reflexes and speech are slow and sluggish. **TABLE 24-2** summarizes the major clinical effects resulting from abnormal levels of thyroid hormone.

GOITER

An enlargement of the thyroid gland is called a **goiter**. A goiter that does not secrete excess thyroid hormone is called a nontoxic goiter. The gland may be uniformly enlarged, called a diffuse goiter, or multiple nodules of proliferating thyroid tissue may form a nodular goiter. An enlarged gland that produces an excessive amount of hormone and causes symptoms of hyperthyroidism is called a toxic goiter.

The basic cause of both nodular and diffuse nontoxic goiters is an inadequate secretion of thyroid hormone. The reduced hormone output causes the hypothalamus to elaborate releasing hormone, which in turn stimulates the pituitary to liberate more TSH (**FIGURE 24-9**). As a result, the gland enlarges to produce more hormone.

TABLE 24-2	Comparison of Major Effects of Hyperthyroidism and Hypothyroidism	
	Hyperthyroidism	**Hypothyroidism**
Cardiovascular effects	Rapid pulse, increased cardiac output	Slow pulse, reduced cardiac output
Metabolic effects	Increased metabolism, skin hot and flushed, weight loss	Decreased metabolism, cold skin, weight gain
Neuromuscular effects	Tremor, hyperactive reflexes	Weakness, lassitude, sluggish reflexes
Mental, emotional effects	Restlessness, irritability, emotional lability	Mental processes sluggish and retarded, personality placid and phlegmatic
Gastrointestinal effects	Diarrhea	Constipation
General somatic effects	Warm, moist skin	Cold, dry skin

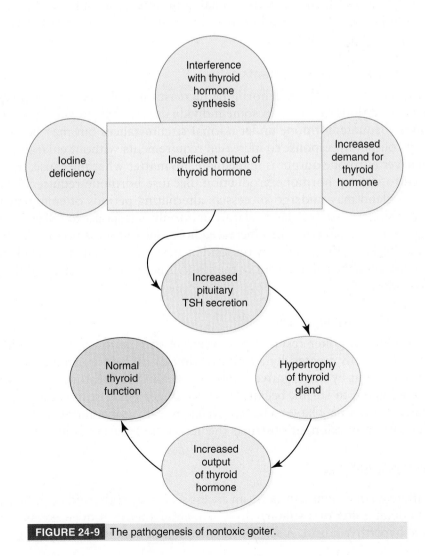

FIGURE 24-9 The pathogenesis of nontoxic goiter.

Three major factors predispose to the development of a nontoxic goiter: iodine deficiency, deficiency of enzymes required for synthesis of thyroid hormone or ingestion of substances that interfere with the function of these enzymes, or increased hormone requirements due to the individual's developmental stage.

Iodine Deficiency

If iodine is deficient in the diet, not enough will be available to produce adequate hormone for the needs of the individual. The enlargement of the gland in response to TSH stimulation is an attempt to extract the meager amount of iodine from the blood more efficiently to make enough hormone. Iodine deficiency is rarely a cause of goiter in the United States because table salt, bread, and many other foods are fortified with iodine. However, it continues to be a problem in some nonindustrialized countries where food sources are naturally low in iodine and salt is not fortified.

Enzyme Deficiency or Impaired Enzyme Function

Goiter more commonly results from a mild deficiency in a glandular enzyme that is required for hormone synthesis; the enzyme-deficient gland is unable to produce sufficient hormone without enlarging. Less commonly, the enzymes are present in normal amounts, but their functions are impaired by ingestion of drugs or other substances that interfere with the action of the enzymes. Even some "natural" foods, such as cabbage and turnips, contain small amounts of substances that interfere with thyroid-hormone synthesis, but these foods are not usually eaten in quantities sufficient to cause difficulty.

Increased Hormone Requirements

Normally, the need for thyroid hormone increases in puberty, during pregnancy, and under conditions of stress. In some individuals, the thyroid gland may be able to produce adequate hormone under normal circumstances but may be unable to increase its output in response to increased requirements without enlarging.

Whenever hormone output is inadequate, no matter what the cause, more TSH is released to step up hormone production. Because hormone requirements often fluctuate, a gland may undergo successive alternating periods of enlargement and reduction in size. At first, the gland enlarges uniformly in response to TSH stimulation, returning to its original size when increased hormone output is no longer required. Eventually, however, the gland may respond in an irregular manner to TSH stimulation. If this occurs, the enlargement of the gland is not uniform and a nodular goiter results (**FIGURE 24-10**).

Treatment of Nontoxic Goiter

Because a nontoxic goiter results from excessive stimulation of the thyroid gland by TSH, it is usually treated by administration of thyroid hormone, which suppresses TSH output by the negative feedback mechanism. Treatment usually causes the enlarged gland to shrink because it is no longer being stimulated by TSH. A large nodular goiter may have to be removed surgically if it compresses the trachea, interferes with respiration, or obstructs the neck veins returning blood to the heart.

HYPERTHYROIDISM

Many different conditions can cause an excess secretion of thyroid hormone. Sometimes a nodular goiter or a solitary thyroid adenoma may produce excess hormone and cause hyperthyroidism. A few other uncommon conditions may also increase

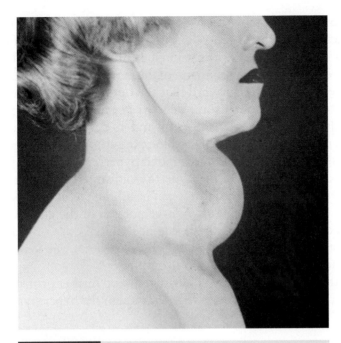

FIGURE 24-10 Large nodular goiter.
Courtesy of Leonard V. Crowley, MD, Century College.

hormone output. However, hyperthyroidism usually is caused by an autoimmune disease in which various autoantibodies target thyroid cells. This condition is usually called either **Graves disease**, after the Irish physician who described the condition, or **exophthalmic goiter**, after a common eye manifestation of the disease. The most important of the antithyroid autoantibodies in this disease is the one that mimics the function of TSH and combines with TSH receptors on thyroid cells, driving the thyroid to secrete excess hormone unresponsive to the inhibitory feedback control mechanism that regulates normal thyroid activity. Indeed, the normal TSH produced by the pituitary gland is suppressed by the excess hormone output, but nevertheless, the autoantibody continues to force the thyroid gland to produce hormone. In most patients, the thyroid gland is diffusely enlarged, but the degree of enlargement is not always marked (**FIGURE 24-11**).

The eye changes that occur in many subjects with Graves disease are also caused by the autoimmune disease. Activated T lymphocytes infiltrate the fat, connective

Graves disease An autoimmune thyroid disease in which autoantibodies resembling thyroid-stimulating hormone stimulate an excessive output of thyroid hormone, causing hyperthyroidism.

Exophthalmic goiter Another term for Graves disease, named for the protrusion of the eyes seen in many patients with this disease.

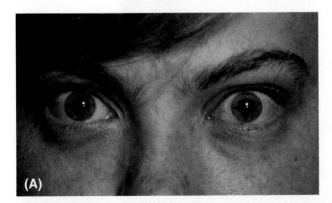
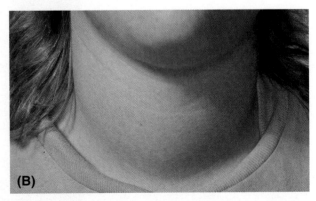

FIGURE 24-11 Graves disease. **(A)** Exophthalmos is characterized by a wide-eyed staring gaze. **(B)** Diffuse swelling of the neck due to goiter.
Courtesy of Dr. Don Schalch, Division of Endocrinology, University of Wisconsin School of Medicine and Public Health.

tissue, and the muscles that move the eyes (extraocular muscles) located in the orbital cavities behind the eyes, which causes inflammation and swelling of the tissues and pushes the eyes forward. The eye protrusion may interfere with the ability of the eyelids to close the eyes and with the function of the extraocular muscles. In severe cases, the eyes may be pushed so far forward that the optic nerves are stretched and may be injured. Fortunately, although some degree of eye protrusion is present in many affected individuals, extreme eye protrusion and its complications are uncommon.

At present, no method is available to block the stimulation of the thyroid gland by the autoantibodies causing the unregulated hypersecretion of thyroid hormone. It is possible, however, to control the hyperthyroidism. Three different methods of treatment can be used. Antithyroid drugs can be administered to block the synthesis of hormone by the hyperactive gland. A large portion of the gland can be removed surgically, reducing the source of the hormone. A large dose of radioactive iodine can be administered to be taken up by the thyroid gland. The irradiation destroys part of the gland and reduces its hormone output.

Successful treatment of hyperthyroidism may stop further protrusion of the eyes, but sometimes the protrusion progresses even though the hyperthyroidism has been controlled.

HYPOTHYROIDISM

Hypothyroidism in the Adult

Myxedema Hypothyroidism in the adult.

Hypothyroidism in the adult is sometimes called **myxedema** (**FIGURE 24-12**) and is manifested by a general slowing of the body's metabolic processes. Frequently, there are localized accumulations of mucinous material in the skin, from which the disease

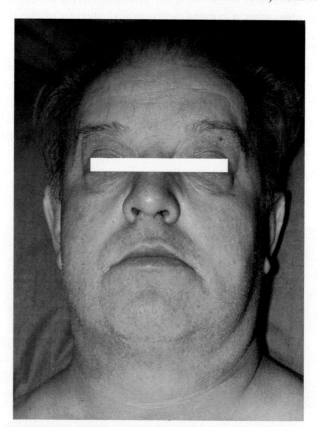

FIGURE 24-12 The appearance of a patient with myxedema.

Courtesy of Leonard V. Crowley, MD, Century College.

received its name (*myx* = mucin + *edema* = swelling). Hypothyroid individuals have low levels of circulating thyroid hormone and high levels of TSH that reflect stimulation of the gland in an unsuccessful attempt to increase hormone output. The condition is treated by supplying the deficient hormone, which results in clinical improvement, return of thyroid hormone level to normal, and a fall in TSH.

Neonatal Hypothyroidism

Hypothyroidism in the newborn infant is called congenital hypothyroidism. This condition may be caused by failure of the thyroid gland to develop or may result from a genetically determined deficiency of enzymes necessary for thyroid hormone synthesis. In the latter condition, the gland undergoes hyperplasia caused by excessive TSH stimulation but is unable to produce adequate hormone because of the enzyme deficiency.

Usually the affected infant appears normal at birth because the mother has supplied the fetus with significant amounts of thyroid hormone, which crossed the placenta to make up for the deficient fetal hormone synthesis. However, as the level of passively transferred maternal thyroid hormone in the newborn infant gradually falls, clinical manifestations of hypothyroidism appear within the first few months after birth. Thyroid hormone not only regulates metabolic processes but is also required for normal growth. The hormone is essential for the normal development of the nervous system, which continues for several months after birth. If neonatal hypothyroidism is recognized and treated promptly, the affected infant will usually grow and develop normally. If the condition remains undetected, the unfortunate infant will remain permanently stunted in growth and mentally retarded. Historically this condition was called **cretinism** and was associated with endemic congenital iodine deficiency. In the United States and Europe, developmental defects in thyroid development or in hormone production are usually responsible. Screening tests for neonatal hypothyroidism are performed routinely on newborn infants to identify neonatal hypothyroidism by detecting the low levels of thyroid hormone and elevated levels of TSH.

CHRONIC THYROIDITIS: HASHIMOTO THYROIDITIS

Acute and chronic inflammation of the thyroid gland caused by a bacterial or viral infection is usually called either acute or chronic thyroiditis, depending on its clinical manifestations and the type of inflammatory cells present. Another thyroid disease in which the gland is infiltrated by lymphocytes is called **chronic thyroiditis** or **Hashimoto thyroiditis** and is not an infection. It is an autoimmune disease in which antithyroid autoantibodies and activated T lymphocytes directed against thyroid antigens attack and destroy the thyroid gland. This is the most common cause of hypothyroidism in adults, and it occurs predominantly in middle-aged women. One of the autoantibodies formed in this disease is directed against TSH receptors on the thyroid cells and destroys the receptors so that TSH is unable to attach to thyroid cells and stimulate the thyroid gland. Consequently, output of thyroid hormone falls as TSH receptor damage progresses. The normal feedback control system that regulates hormone output (Figure 24-2) responds to the low hormone level, and TSH rises as thyroid hormone falls. The behavior of the autoantibody in Hashimoto thyroiditis is quite different from that of the autoantibody in hyperthyroidism (Graves disease). In the first case, the antibody destroys the receptors, causing hypothyroidism; in the second case, the autoantibody stimulates the receptors, causing hyperthyroidism.

The thyroid gland of a person with Hashimoto thyroiditis is usually enlarged by diffuse infiltration of activated T lymphocytes and plasma cells that are destroying the

Cretinism Hypothyroidism in the infant.

Chronic thyroiditis (Hashimoto thyroiditis) An autoimmune disease in which an autoantibody directed against thyroid epithelial cells causes progressive destruction of the thyroid gland, leading to hypothyroidism. Also called Hashimoto thyroiditis.

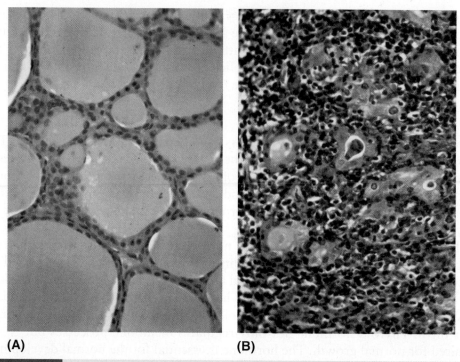

(A) **(B)**

FIGURE 24-13 Low-magnification photomicrographs comparing cellular structure of normal thyroid gland **(A)** with that in chronic thyroiditis **(B)**. Gland is heavily infiltrated by lymphocytes. Follicles are small and lack colloid (original magnification ×100).

Courtesy of Leonard V. Crowley, MD, Century College.

thyroid gland (**FIGURE 24-13**). No specific treatment is available to arrest the relentless progression of the disease, but the hypothyroidism can be treated by administration of thyroid hormone. Both the level of thyroid hormone in the blood and the level of TSH are taken into account to determine how much thyroid hormone to give the patient.

TUMORS OF THE THYROID

The thyroid gives rise to benign adenomas and several different types of carcinoma. Thyroid follicular adenomas are completely encapsulated nodules composed of cells that differ in pattern from the thyroid gland outside the nodule (**FIGURE 24-14**). Thyroid nodules are very common (over 50 percent of the population have them present at autopsy). Although most such nodules are benign, up to 20 percent may be malignancies. Three distinct types of follicular cell derived thyroid carcinoma are recognized: follicular, papillary, and anaplastic.

The most common type, illustrated in **FIGURE 24-15**, is called a papillary carcinoma because the tumor is composed of well-differentiated papillary processes covered by well-differentiated thyroid epithelial cells. It is strongly associated with radiation exposure in children (such as from the Chernobyl disaster or from therapeutic procedures). It has an excellent prognosis in the young, but it may present as aggressive disease in older males. A less common type of tumor is called a follicular carcinoma because the tumor cells form colloid-filled follicles, which resemble normal thyroid tissue. They occur in an older population and, unlike papillary carcinomas, may be associated with metastatic disease. Treatment of both types is by surgical resection of the thyroid gland (thyroidectomy). Partial resection may be undertaken in the case of papillary cancer; however, total resection followed by treatment with radioactive iodine is used in treating follicular cancer.

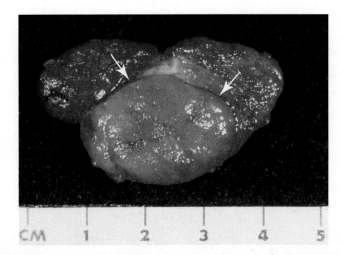

FIGURE 24-14 A benign, well-circumscribed adenoma of the thyroid gland (*arrows*). The surrounding thyroid tissue appears normal.

Courtesy of Leonard V. Crowley, MD, Century College.

Undifferentiated (anaplastic) carcinoma is uncommon and develops in older people. The disease is composed of rapidly growing bizarre tumor cells and has a poor prognosis. Treatment is by means of surgical resection combined with radiation and chemotherapy.

Medullary carcinoma is an uncommon tumor derived from the calcitonin-secreting parafollicular cells of the thyroid with a characteristic histologic pattern in which small cells are embedded in a hyalinized (glasslike) framework containing collagen and a calcitonin precursor (**FIGURE 24-16**). Measurement of calcitonin levels in the blood has been used as a diagnostic test for this type of thyroid cancer because the tumor cells often secrete calcitonin. Although the effect of calcitonin is to lower blood calcium, the excess hormone secretion has no significant effect on blood calcium because the effect of the calcitonin is counteracted by an increased secretion of parathyroid hormone, preventing blood calcium from falling. (The physiologic effects of parathyroid hormone are considered in conjunction with diseases of the parathyroid glands.)

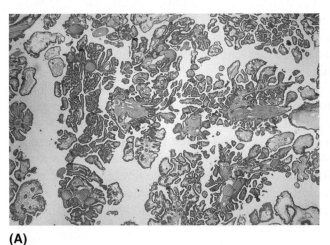

(A)

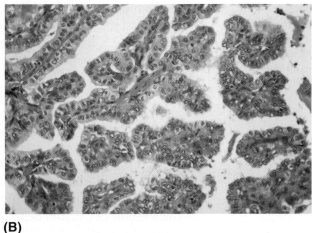

(B)

FIGURE 24-15 Well-differentiated papillary carcinoma of thyroid. **(A)** A low-magnification view illustrating papillary structure (original magnification ×40). **(B)** Higher magnification of papillary processes covered by well-differentiated neoplastic thyroid epithelium (original magnification ×160).

Courtesy of Leonard V. Crowley, MD, Century College.

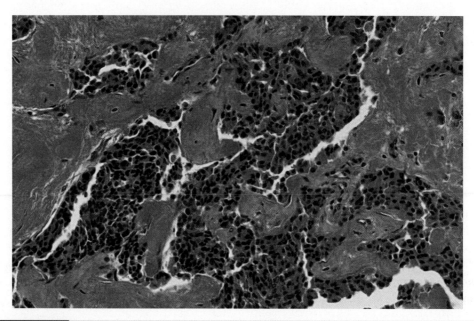

FIGURE 24-16 Medullary thyroid carcinoma. Small, polygonal tumor cells are embedded in a hyalinized collagenous acellular framework.

Courtesy of Department of Pathology and Laboratory Medicine, University of North Carolina at Chapel Hill.

The Parathyroid Glands and Calcium Metabolism

The parathyroid glands are located on the posterior surface of the lateral lobes of the thyroid gland and produce a hormone that regulates the level of calcium in the blood. Although the most common number of glands is four, this may vary from one to more than ten. Usually the blood calcium is in equilibrium with the calcium salts present in bone. Half the blood calcium is present as calcium ions (Ca^{2+}) and is the active form. The other half is bound to blood proteins and is biologically inactive. An adequate concentration of ionized calcium is required for normal cardiac and skeletal muscle contraction, for transmission of nerve impulses, and for coagulation of the blood. A subnormal level of ionized calcium causes increased excitability of nerve and muscle cells, leading to spasm of skeletal muscles, which is called **tetany**. Conversely, a high level of ionized calcium diminishes neuromuscular excitability and leads to generalized muscular weakness.

The parathyroid hormone regulates the level of calcium by regulating the release of calcium from bone, the absorption of calcium from the intestine, and the rate of excretion of calcium by the kidneys. The secretion of parathyroid hormone is regulated by the level of ionized calcium in the blood rather than by a tropic hormone elaborated by the pituitary gland. If the level of ionized calcium in the blood decreases, the parathyroids secrete more hormone. If the ionized calcium level rises, parathyroid hormone secretion declines. Any abnormality in the secretion of parathyroid hormone changes the concentration of ionized calcium in the blood and will eventually alter the amount of calcium deposited in bone.

HYPERPARATHYROIDISM

Primary hyperparathyroidism is a relatively common problem and is usually the result of a hormone-secreting parathyroid adenoma. In response to increased output of

Tetany Spasm of skeletal muscles caused by subnormal level of ionized calcium in the blood or certain bacterial toxins.

hormone, the blood calcium rises (hypercalcemia) and excessive calcium is withdrawn from bone. The bones become excessively fragile and are easily broken.

Excessive amounts of calcium are excreted in the urine (hypercalciuria), sometimes leading to formation of calcium stones within the urinary tract. Occasionally, calcium precipitates out of the blood and becomes deposited in the kidneys, lungs, and other tissues, producing tissue injury and functional impairment. Treatment consists of surgical removal of the tumor. Secondary hyperparathyroidism occurs with chronic renal disease rather than an abnormality of the parathyroids.

HYPOPARATHYROIDISM

Hypoparathyroidism usually results from accidental removal of all parathyroid glands during an operation for a diffuse toxic goiter or a nodular goiter in which most of the thyroid gland is removed. Blood calcium falls precipitously, which leads to increased neuromuscular excitability and tetany. Treatment consists of raising the level of blood calcium by the administration of a high-calcium diet and supplementary vitamin D, which promotes absorption of calcium from the intestinal tract. Congenital and autoimmune-mediated forms of hypoparathyroidism also occur. Patients with congenital DiGeorge syndrome, associated with T cell immunodeficiency and craniofacial defects, also have neonatal hypoparathyroidism in about half of the cases.

The Adrenal Glands

The adrenals are paired glands located above the kidneys. Each adrenal consists of two separate endocrine glands: an inner adrenal medulla surrounded by an outer adrenal cortex. The adrenal cortex may be further divided into three zones (the zona glomerulosa just under the capsule, the zona fasiculata, and the zona reticularis adjacent to the medulla). The two glands secrete different hormones (**FIGURE 24-17**).

THE ADRENAL CORTEX

The adrenal cortex secretes three major classes of steroid hormones: **glucocorticoids**, **mineralocorticoids**, and sex hormones. Different zones of the adrenal cortex differ in their synthetic profile. The zona glomerulosa is responsible for mineralocorticoids; the zona fasiculata produces most of the glucocorticoids (and some sex hormone); the zona reticularis produces most of the sex hormones (and some glucocorticoids).

> **Glucocorticoid** An adrenal cortical hormone that regulates carbohydrate metabolism.
>
> **Mineralocorticoid** Adrenal cortical hormone that regulates salt and water metabolism.

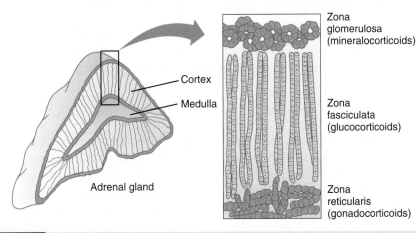

FIGURE 24-17 The adrenal gland.

Glucocorticoids raise the blood glucose by decreasing glucose utilization in many tissues, except the brain, and promote fat breakdown with utilization of fatty acids rather than glucose as an energy source. They inhibit protein synthesis and promote breakdown of body proteins, some of which are converted into glucose by the liver. The net effect is to deplete tissue proteins and raise blood glucose. (The adverse effect of glucocorticoids on wound healing and tissue repair is a result in part of their protein-depleting effects.) Also they act at multiple sites to suppress the inflammatory reaction. (The use of adrenal corticosteroids to treat various types of inflammatory disease is related to the anti-inflammatory property of the glucocorticoids.)

Glucocorticoids are secreted in response to stimulation by adrenocorticotropic hormone (ACTH), and their output is controlled by the same type of negative feedback mechanism that regulates secretion of thyroid hormone. The major glucocorticoid is **cortisol**.

Mineralocorticoids regulate electrolyte and water balance by promoting absorption of sodium and water and excretion of potassium by the renal tubules. The major mineralocorticoid is **aldosterone**, whose secretion is regulated by more than one mechanism. Although ACTH increases aldosterone secretion to some extent, the most potent stimulus for aldosterone secretion is the renin-angiotensin system (see discussion on the urinary system), which responds to a reduction in renal blood flow or blood pressure. The kidneys "interpret" the reduced blood flow and pressure to mean that blood volume is low; aldosterone secretion is then called for to promote retention of sodium and water, thus increasing blood volume.

SEX HORMONES

The adrenal cortex also produces weak androgenic (testosterone-like) steroid hormones in response to ACTH stimulation, which are further metabolized into testosterone and into estrogens by both males and females. In men, the estrogens have little effect because of the much greater testicular production of testosterone. In women, the testosterone is responsible for sex drive but otherwise has little physiologic effect because it is overshadowed by estrogen produced by the ovaries. The additional estrogens made from adrenal androgenic hormones do not add much to the large amount already made by the ovaries. However, in estrogen-deficient postmenopausal women, the estrogens produced from adrenal androgens may be very significant (described in the discussion on the breast). In some diseases, the output of adrenal androgens is greatly increased, which may exert undesirable masculinizing effects.

DISTURBANCES OF ADRENAL CORTICAL FUNCTION

Abnormal adrenal cortical function produces abnormalities in the metabolism of carbohydrates and protein as a result of abnormal glucocorticoid secretion, as well as disturbances of salt and water metabolism caused by disturbed mineralocorticoid secretion.

Addison Disease

Adrenal cortical hypofunction, called **Addison disease**, results from atrophy or destruction of both adrenal glands leading to a deficiency of all of the steroid hormones produced by these glands. In most cases, the disease results from an autoimmune disorder in which destructive autoantibodies directed against adrenal cortical cells and invading cytotoxic lymphocytes destroy the cortex. Less commonly, the adrenal destruction is caused by tuberculosis, histoplasmosis, or metastatic carcinoma involving both adrenal glands.

Cortisol The major glucocorticoid.

Aldosterone A steroid hormone produced by the adrenal cortex that regulates the rate of sodium absorption from the renal tubules.

Addison disease A disease caused by chronic adrenal cortical hypofunction.

As a result of a glucocorticoid deficiency, the blood glucose level is subnormal and may decline during fasting to such a low level that symptoms develop. The body's ability to regulate the content of sodium, potassium, and water in body fluids is disturbed as a result of the mineralocorticoid deficiency. Blood volume and blood pressure fall, as does the concentration of sodium in the blood, and blood potassium rises. The blood volume may become so reduced that the circulation can no longer be maintained efficiently.

People with Addison disease also frequently exhibit increased pigmentation of the skin, which is caused by increased secretion of ACTH, along with MSH, which is produced from the same precursor molecule that gives rise to ACTH. The MSH simulates the melanin-producing cells in the skin and is responsible for the increased skin pigmentation characteristic of Addison disease (**FIGURE 24-18**). ACTH output is regulated by a negative feedback mechanism. In Addison disease, secretion of cortisol is greatly diminished, which causes ACTH to rise in an unsuccessful attempt to increase cortisol output. Treatment of Addison disease consists of administering the deficient corticosteroids.

Cushing Disease and Cushing Syndrome

Adrenal cortical hyperfunction causes a characteristic clinical syndrome, which results from excess production of adrenal corticosteroids. The glucocorticoid excess causes disturbances of carbohydrate, protein, and fat metabolism. The blood glucose rises. Protein synthesis is impaired, and body proteins are broken down, which leads to loss of muscle fibers and muscle weakness. Bones become weaker and more susceptible to fracture (osteoporosis) as the protein breakdown leads to loss of the connective tissue framework of the bones. The amount and distribution of body fat is altered. Fat tends to accumulate on the trunk, and the extremities appear thin and wasted because of muscle atrophy.

The skin becomes thin and bruises easily. Stretch marks (striae) often appear in the skin as fat deposits accumulate in the subcutaneous tissues of the trunk. The face appears full and rounded, which is sometimes called a "moon face." Salt and

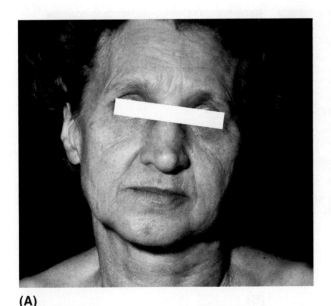 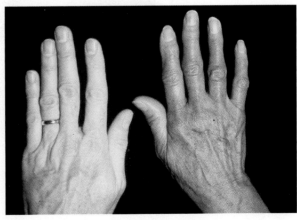

(A) **(B)**

FIGURE 24-18 Patient with Addison disease. **(A)** Appearance of face illustrating increased skin pigmentation. **(B)** Appearance of hand (*right side*) compared with the hand of a normal person.
Courtesy of Leonard V. Crowley, MD, Century College.

water are retained because of the increased output of mineralocorticoids, leading to an increase in blood volume and a rise in blood pressure. Excess adrenal androgens may lead to increased growth of facial and body hair in women.

Corticosteroid excess can result from four different causes: an ACTH-producing tumor of the pituitary gland, which stimulates the adrenal glands to enlarge and produce excess hormone (**Cushing disease**); a corticosteroid–hormone-producing tumor of the adrenal cortex (**adrenal Cushing syndrome**); administration of large amounts of corticosteroid hormone to help suppress the immune response in recipients of organ transplants or patients with autoimmune diseases (exogenous Cushing syndrome); or overproduction of active ACTH by nonendocrine tumors, usually small cell tumors of the lung (ectopic Cushing syndrome). The most common cause of a corticosteroid excess is Cushing disease caused by a small ACTH secreting pituitary adenoma. In all other cases, the term Cushing syndrome is used.

The treatment of this condition depends on the cause. If it is Cushing disease caused by a pituitary microadenoma, the usual method of treatment is transsphenoidal resection of the tumor. Cushing syndrome caused by an adrenal cortical tumor is treated by resection of the adrenal tumor. Successful treatment is followed by regression of the clinical manifestations of the disease (**FIGURE 24-19**).

Overproduction of Aldosterone

Aldosterone promotes absorption of salt and water by the kidneys in exchange for potassium, which is excreted; its secretion is regulated primarily by the renin-angiotensin–aldosterone mechanism described in the discussion on the urinary system. However, sometimes the adrenal cortex gives rise to an aldosterone-secreting adenoma called an aldosteronoma. This condition is termed Conn syndrome. The aldosterone excess produced by the tumor promotes excessive absorption of sodium and excessive excretion of potassium by the kidneys. Because water is absorbed along with the sodium, the blood volume increases along with the sodium concentration, and the blood pressure also rises along with the blood volume. The excessive

Cushing disease Caused by an ACTH-producing tumor of the pituitary gland that stimulates the adrenal glands to enlarge.

Adrenal Cushing syndrome Caused by a corticosteroid hormone-producing tumor of the adrenal cortex.

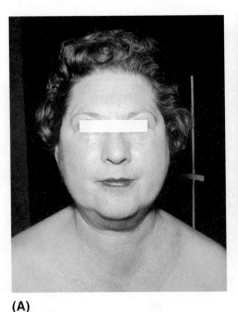 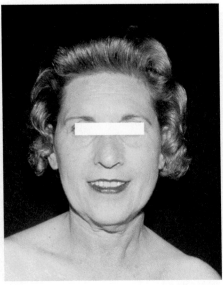

(A)　　　　　　　　　　　**(B)**

FIGURE 24-19 Cushing disease before and after treatment. **(A)** Full, rounded face ("moon face") prior to treatment. **(B)** Normal facial appearance after treatment.

Courtesy of Leonard V. Crowley, MD, Century College.

hormone-induced excretion of potassium lowers blood potassium, which impairs neuromuscular function and leads to muscle weakness. The high aldosterone output exerts a negative feedback effect on renin production by the kidneys, and plasma renin falls.

Although an aldosterone-secreting adenoma is not a common cause of hypertension, it may be suspected by the physician when the hypertension is associated with an elevated plasma sodium and a low plasma potassium. This can be confirmed by additional laboratory studies that reveal an elevated plasma aldosterone and low renin. Treatment consists of identification of the adrenal tumor, often accomplished by CT or MRI examinations, followed by removal of the tumor.

Overproduction of Adrenal Sex Hormones: Congenital Adrenal Hyperplasia

Adrenal gland dysfunction associated with abnormal production of sex hormone is uncommon. This may result from congenital hyperplasia of the adrenal glands or, very rarely, from an adrenal sex hormone–producing tumor.

Congenital adrenal hyperplasia is the result of a congenital deficiency of certain enzymes required for the synthesis of various steroid hormones. In the normal biosynthesis of hormones by the adrenal cortex, cholesterol is initially converted into an intermediate compound (pregnenolone), which is a precursor of the other steroids produced in the adrenal cortex (**FIGURE 24-20**). The chief metabolic pathways are concerned with the conversion of the intermediate compound into aldosterone, the major mineralocorticoid (pathway 1) and into the glucocorticoid cortisol (pathway 2). A third minor metabolic pathway leads to the production of adrenal androgens (pathway 3).

Biosynthesis of hormones in the major pathways (1 and 2) requires a series of additions of hydroxyl groups to the steroid molecules, catalyzed by enzymes called hydroxylases. If certain hydroxylases are absent or deficient, synthesis of aldosterone and cortisol will be impaired. This leads to increased ACTH secretion (because the pituitary interprets the low steroid levels in the blood as a signal to produce more ACTH). ACTH stimulation produces hyperplasia of the adrenal glands and increased synthesis

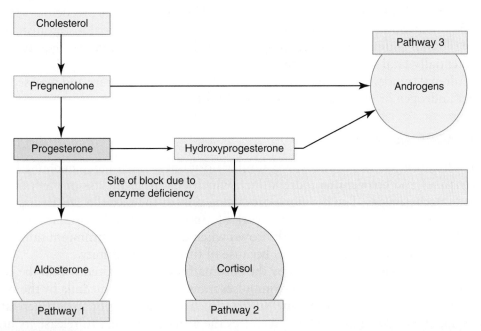

FIGURE 24-20 Biosynthesis of adrenal cortical hormones and the site of enzymatic block leading to overproduction of adrenal androgens.

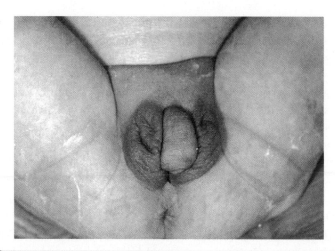

FIGURE 24-21 Masculinization of external genitalia of infant girl. The enlarged clitoris resembles a penis. Vulvar labia are wrinkled and resemble a scrotum.

Courtesy of Leonard V. Crowley, MD, Century College.

of precursor compounds, a condition termed **congenital adrenal hyperplasia (CAH)**. However, because an enzymatic block affects the major pathways of steroid production, biosynthesis is shifted in the direction of androgenic steroids (pathway 3). Consequently, the major steroid output from the adrenals consists of androgenic compounds.

The clinical disorder produced by these enzymatic defects in CAH is often called the adrenogenital syndrome. This syndrome has several clinical varieties depending on which of the hydroxylase enzymes is deficient and the extent of the deficiency. All have the common feature of producing premature sexual development, called precocious puberty. In the female, sexual development is masculine because of the effect of the androgens. The age at which the hormonal effects become manifest depends on the degree of the enzyme deficiency. Congenital virilization, which may be noted at birth (**FIGURE 24-21**), is the most common cause of ambiguous genitalia in neonatal females. If the deficiency is less severe, symptoms may not appear until the child is older. In males, sexual organs are normal but there may be precocious sexual development. Some forms of CAH are also associated with hypoaldosteronism and severe loss of sodium and potassium; the associated dehydration and hypotension is potentially fatal soon after birth.

Adrenal tumors that elaborate sex hormones are extremely rare and may secrete either androgen or estrogen (or sometimes both).

THE ADRENAL MEDULLA

The adrenal medulla produces two similar hormones called **norepinephrine** (nor-adrenaline) and **epinephrine** (adrenaline), which belong to a class of compounds called **catecholamines**. The hormone-producing cells of the medulla are arranged in small groups surrounded by a rich network of capillaries. The cell cytoplasm is filled with fine granules that become dark brown when treated with chromium salts, and the cells are termed chromaffin cells because of this staining affinity.

The catecholamines produced by the chromaffin cells are stored within the cells and are released in response to nerve impulses transmitted to the medulla by the sympathetic nervous system. Any emotional stress such as anger, fear, or anxiety activates the sympathetic nervous system and causes the adrenal medulla to release its hormones. The liberated catecholamines cause a rapid heart rate, rise in blood pressure, and other effects that prepare the individual to cope with the stress of an emergency.

Norepinephrine One of the compounds (catecholamines) secreted by the adrenal medulla.

Epinephrine One of the compounds (catecholamines) secreted by the adrenal medulla.

Catecholamines The adrenal medullary hormones epinephrine and norepinephrine.

TUMORS OF THE ADRENAL MEDULLA

Rarely, a benign tumor called a **pheochromocytoma** arises from the chromaffin cells of the medulla. A pheochromocytoma often secretes large amounts of catecholamines and produces severe effects on the heart and vascular system. The tumor may discharge catecholamines intermittently and induce periodic episodes of high blood pressure and increased heart rate. At times, the blood pressure may rise so severely that a cerebral blood vessel ruptures, causing a cerebral hemorrhage. In other cases, the increased output of catecholamines by the tumor is continuous and causes a sustained high blood pressure. Treatment consists of surgical removal of the tumor. Pheochromocytomas may also occur outside the adrenal gland. In such cases they are called paragangliomas.

> **Pheochromocytoma**
> Catecholamine-secreting tumor of the adrenal medulla.

MULTIPLE ENDOCRINE NEOPLASIA SYNDROME (MEN)

Most pheochromocytomas occur sporadically. However, in some cases pheochromocytomas and other tumors of endocrine glands are associated with autosomal, dominant, inherited diseases associated with mutations of two genes, *MEN-1* and *MEN-2*. MEN-type 1 is associated with pituitary and parathyroid adenomas and islet cell tumors of the pancreas. Almost all patients with MEN-type 2 suffer from medullary thyroid cancer and about half from pheochromocytoma.

HORMONE PRODUCTION BY NONENDOCRINE TUMORS

Sometimes nonendocrine tumors secrete hormones that produce the same clinical manifestations as those of tumors arising from endocrine glands. These hormones are called ectopic hormones (*ecto* = outside) because they are formed outside the endocrine glands, which are the normal sites of hormone production. An ectopic hormone is a protein that is either identical with the true hormone produced by the endocrine gland or has such a close resemblance that it mimics the action of the true hormone. Many different ectopic hormones have been identified, including ACTH, TSH, gonadotropins, ADH, parathyroid hormone, and insulin. Most hormone-producing nonendocrine tumors are malignant and are associated with carcinomas of the lung, pancreas, or kidneys, or by malignant connective-tissue tumors. These effects are often referred to as a paraneoplastic syndrome.

ENDOCRINE FUNCTION OF THE PANCREATIC ISLETS

In addition to manufacturing digestive enzymes, the pancreas functions as an endocrine gland. Scattered throughout the pancreas are more than a million small clusters of cells called the pancreatic islets or islets of Langerhans, which produce three different hormones: insulin, glucagon, and somatostatin. Diseases of the islets are considered in conjunction with diseases of the pancreas (see discussion on the pancreas and diabetes mellitus).

THE GONADS

The gonads have two functions: the production of germ cells, either eggs or sperm, and the production of sex hormones responsible for the development of secondary sexual characteristics. This function is controlled by the gonadotrophic hormones of the pituitary gland.

Occasionally, sex hormone–secreting tumors develop in the ovary or testis. They may secrete sex hormone appropriate to the sex of the individual or, paradoxically, sex hormone characteristic of the opposite sex. No endocrine symptoms result from a tumor that produces the "proper" sex hormone; however, elaboration of the inappropriate sex hormone by the tumor causes masculinization in the female or feminization in the male. Sex hormone–secreting tumors of the gonads are usually benign, and the disorder can be cured by surgical excision.

Stress and the Endocrine System

Homeostasis Maintenance of a steady state by the body's internal control systems.

The maintenance of a steady state by the body's internal control systems (**homeostasis**) is the result of regulatory mechanisms that attempt to maintain the steady state under which the body functions most effectively. In a general sense, stress can be defined as any event that disturbs this stable internal environment. The event may be physical trauma, such as an injury or surgical operation, prolonged exposure to cold, vigorous exercise, pain, or a strong emotional stimulus such as anxiety or fear. Any of these events result in a response that helps the body maintain homeostasis. There are two distinct but overlapping responses to stress, whose use depends on both the intensity and the duration of the stress. The acute, short-term response is mediated by the sympathetic nervous system and the adrenal medulla, and the chronic, longer term response includes the participation of several endocrine glands, with the adrenal cortex playing the major role. Both the acute and the chronic responses are initiated in the hypothalamus, which directs both the autonomic nervous system and many endocrine glands, and the hypothalamus, which in turn receives input from higher cortical centers.

The acute stress response is the well-known fear-fight-flight reaction triggered by the sympathetic nervous system. Norepinephrine released from sympathetic nerve endings, supplemented by norepinephrine and epinephrine released from the adrenal medulla in response to sympathetic nerve impulses, prepares the body to deal with the acute situation. Blood glucose rises as liver glycogen is broken down into glucose and released into the bloodstream. Peripheral vessels constrict, diverting more blood to the brain, heart, and skeletal muscles. The blood pressure rises, and the heart beats more forcefully. All of these systemic effects are of short duration and gradually subside when the stressful event is no longer present.

In contrast, long-term stress of any type, either physical or emotional, initiates a slower but more complex chain of events. Hypothalamic-releasing hormones, acting through the pituitary gland, cause the adrenal cortex to increase its output of cortical hormones; they also increase the output of growth hormone and thyroid hormone while suppressing the output of gonadotropic hormones. Excess cortisol production has pronounced effects on glucose, protein, and fat metabolism, as described earlier in connection with Cushing disease. The cortisol excess also dampens the inflammatory response and reduces the responsiveness of the immune system. In addition, cortisol excess tends to raise blood pressure by making the peripheral arterioles more responsive to the vasoconstrictor effect of norepinephrine released from sympathetic nerve endings. Increased aldosterone output promotes retention of salt and water, which also tends to raise blood pressure by increasing intravascular fluid volume.

The stress-related fall in gonadotropin output impairs gonadal function, which has widespread physiologic effects, and in women may lead to stress-related cessation of menstrual periods. Stress-related amenorrhea has well-defined adverse effects on the skeletal system (described in the discussion on the musculoskeletal system).

The increased output of thyroid hormone speeds up metabolic processes to allow the body to deal more effectively with the stress, as does increased output of growth hormone, which also stimulates the body's metabolic processes.

Unfortunately, chronic stress takes its toll on the body and, over the long term, may predispose to illness. Excessive demands are placed on the cardiovascular system, which may contribute to heart disease, and the chronic corticosteroid excess places undue demand on the vascular system, as well as on other organ systems. Perhaps even more important, the chronic corticosteroid excess may increase our susceptibility to many types of illnesses by reducing our ability to generate an effective inflammatory reaction and by reducing the responsiveness of our immune system.

Stress initiates many physiologic responses that are designed to help protect us from harm, but chronic, unrelieved stress can cause us harm, and stress-relieving activities can help protect us from its long-term injurious effects.

CASE 24-1

Irene is the second child of the Mikros family. She is currently five and a half years old and is the product of an uneventful pregnancy. Her brother Georgio, who is nine years old, has no outstanding health problems although his pediatrician is a bit concerned about his weight gain. His height is appropriate for his age, but he is in the eight-fifth percentile for weight (85 percent of a standard group of children his age weigh less).

The Mikros family always wanted a female child, and Irene's mother Eleni has made an effort to record Irene's development by measuring her height twice a year on a standard growth chart for girls. FIGURE 24-22 is an example of such a chart and has patient height data from age two to the present. Although Irene was a healthy and well-behaved child for the first four years of her life, her mother has become concerned. Irene was always small in stature, being in the twenty-fifth percentile for her age and sex through the fourth year. Irene's pediatrician was reassuring, noting that the child's weight was appropriate for her height and that she was meeting (and in some cases exceeding) her developmental milestones. Eleni has now noted that in Irene's fifth year there has been a marked drop in her rank in height to the fifth percentile. Eleni and her husband are considerably taller than average, so they do not understand Irene's slow gain in stature.

In addition, Irene's parent have noticed that she has begun to have what they call "sinking spells" in the late afternoon when she returns from day care. Although her food intake is normal at day care, she becomes "fussy" and complains of being dizzy. Providing Irene with a predinner snack of fruit and crackers appears to perk her up, so her mother suspects she may have mild hypoglycemia (low blood sugar).

Irene recently caught a gastrointestinal virus at day care and refused all food for twenty-four hours. By morning she was sweating, confused, and lethargic (being hard to arouse). At the pediatrician's urging, her parents brought her to the local pediatric emergency room. On examination, Irene is found to be markedly hypoglycemic and suffering from mild ketonuria (see discussion on the pancreas, along with diabetes and it consequences). She is treated with an intravenous glucose infusion and is asymptomatic within several hours.

Marked metabolic derangement after a twenty-four-hour fast is unusual in a healthy child. Hence, Irene's pediatrician suspects that the child may be suffering from an endocrine disorder that is affecting her growth and refers the Mikros family to a pediatric endocrinologist who is expert in **auxology** (the study of growth and development in children).

Irene's past medical history is significant for what was a continued (but stable) history of small stature with recent marked slowing of her rate of growth (called height velocity). At birth she was not noted to be small for her gestational age. Her mother's pregnancy was uneventful, and there is no family history of endocrine or genetic diseases. Irene's parents are of above average height and reached puberty at average ages. Irene is noted to be well dressed and comes from a family that does not have financial problems. Although clearly small for her age, she is well proportioned, has no obvious signs of developmental disease, and has normal **facies** (facial appearance that, when abnormal, can provide clues to possible congenital disease). Irene shows normal to accelerated developmental signs.

The pediatric endocrinologist orders a karyotype analysis and a battery of tests for the level of pituitary and other hormones. This includes measurement of the level of growth

(continues)

CASE 24-1 (Continued)

hormone, IGF-1 (insulin-like growth factor 1), thyrotropin, and ACTH. The pediatrician also orders an MRI study of the brain with emphasis of the region of the sella. Although results indicate a low level of growth hormone and markedly reduced levels of IGF-1, no other hormonal abnormalities are noted. Irene's karyotype reveals a normal female chromosomal complement. Her brain MRI discloses no abnormalities. The pediatric endocrinologist diagnoses isolated growth hormone deficiency of potentially genetic origin, most likely autosomal recessive in nature, and offers the Mikros family the opportunity for extensive molecular testing and further genetic counseling, an offer that is deferred.

Irene is started on subcutaneous recombinant growth hormone treatment. She is taught to dose herself three times weekly using an automated injector "pen." After four weeks of therapy, her IGF-1 level is near normal, and she achieves a normal height velocity. Ongoing monitoring every six months is indicated to measure her continuing growth and development. With continued treatment, it is hoped she will have a normal puberty and attain an adult height consistent with that predicted from the height of her parents (the midparental height, which can be easily calculated based on parental heights and the child's sex).

Discussion

The factors that control the rate of growth in developing children and eventual adult height are exceedingly complex and depend on both environmental factors and multiple genetic determinants. Clearly, expected adult height (target height) is highly dependent on parental height and can be calculated. Thus, a child of two short parents might be expected to fall below the age average for height but ultimately reach his or her target height predicted by that of the parents. When evidence that the target height will be reached and that bone growth is normal, such a short child is defined as having familial short stature (FSS). These cases generally need no therapy although in severe cases of FSS growth hormone therapy may be undertaken. A variant of FSS is constitutional delay of growth and puberty (CDGP). In CDGP, bone development is delayed compared to chronological age, but the growth rate is appropriate if compared to bone age rather than chronological age. These individuals are often "late bloomers" with delayed puberty, but they eventually reach their target height. These patients are not considered pathological, and other organic defects affecting growth would not be expected. However, a variety of chronic disease states can cause a pathological failure of bone growth. The list is long and includes infectious disease such as recurrent ear infections and diseases associated with immunodeficiency. Chronic inflammatory disease, such as Crohn disease with gastrointestinal symptoms, juvenile idiopathic arthritis, and severe asthma are all associated with growth delay and failure. Prolonged use of glucocorticoids (perhaps as part of asthma therapy) is also associated with growth defects.

Having ruled these out (as was the case with the Mikros family), endocrine disease must be considered (either congenital or acquired) as well as other nonendocrine genetic diseases associated with growth failure. For example, Turner syndrome (discussed with congenital and hereditary disease) is characterized by an XO karyotype and has symptoms of recognizable abnormalities such as disproportionate growth, skeletal and cardiovascular abnormalities, and marked short stature. Turner syndrome is not rare (about 1 in 2,000 female births) and varies in severity of symptoms. For this reason, the establishment of a normal female karyotype in Irene was a reasonable diagnostic approach. Many other nonendocrine syndromes are associated with short stature, one example being **achondroplasia**, the failure of bone ossification associated with short limb dwarfism. These syndromes are almost always recognizable in a thorough physical examination, and Irene had no evidence of such.

The low growth hormone (GH) level in Irene in the presence of normal levels of other pituitary hormones suggests an isolated defect in growth hormone synthesis or release. This is an important finding as about 25 percent of GH deficiency is associated with an organic (nongenetic) etiology. The two most common of these are tumors of the central

Achondroplasia The failure of bone ossification associated with short limb dwarfism.

CASE 24-1 *(Continued)*

nervous system (notably craniopharyngioma, a tumor derived from the sellar region that may damage or destroy the pituitary). Developmental defects of the pituitary (some of which are of known genetic origin) can result in a missing, malformed, or hypoplastic pituitary that does not synthesize a normal array of hormones. An isolated defect in GH would not be expected from this, and the normal brain imaging study in Irene rules out a tumor or maldevelopment of the pituitary.

Unfortunately, GH is difficult to measure in the laboratory. The hormone is released in pulses, generally during the evening, and blood levels vary markedly with time. Because growth hormone stimulates the release of IGF-1 (which mediates most or all of the biological effects of GH), IGF-1 is commonly used as a surrogate marker for GH because it is easier to assay and its level correlates with the average level of GH secreted. Hypoglycemia in newborns is associated with GH deficiency in about 20 percent of severe cases. Hypoglycemic events also may occur in fasting children with low GH levels. The mechanism is complex but may be related to low liver glycogen and decreased glucose production related to low IGF-1 levels.

The frequency of mutations in the GH gene is poorly defined, but it is certain that a percentage of cases of isolated GH deficiency (i.e., in the absence of other pituitary hormonal defects) is related to mutations in GH (and in about 10 percent of cases to a mutation in the hypothalamic receptor that binds the growth hormone releasing hormone). Irene has no evidence of any other disease process, suggesting that she does, in fact, have a defect in the GH gene, which is presumed to be recessive as neither parent is affected. Type IA growth hormone mutations result in total absence of GH synthesis and in severe growth retardation by the age of six months. Type IB disease is associated with low but detectable levels of GH and a milder form of growth retardation that may become obvious with time. The relatively sudden slowing of Irene's rate of growth at age four is suggestive of Type IB GH deficiency disease, but further molecular analysis would be required for confirmation. The successful use of recombinant growth hormone in Irene's case does confirm the relationship between her low GH (and IGF-1) and her slow rate of growth.

Questions (and Some Things to Try)

1. Although not specifically stated, the Mikros family is of Greek origin. Why might ethnic background have been important in this case? The physician neglected to ask an important question in obtaining family history. Do you know what that question is and why it is important?

2. The pattern of Irene's increase in stature is sometimes called "line crossing" and is considered to be a very important observation in the investigation of a child's development. Why is this term used, and why is it important? (Hint: plot Irene's data on the appropriate growth chart.)

3. Many families keep data on children's height with time. If your data is available, plot your height on a growth chart and observe the pattern of development. (The reference by Rogol and Hayden explains how to calculate target height, and calculators to establish **midparental height** are available on the web.) Calculate your target height (midparental height) and observe whether it works in your case.

4. Human growth hormone was originally prepared from cadaveric pituitary glands. This material was used from the late 1950s until the mid-1980s when it was suddenly withdrawn from the market until recombinant growth hormone became available in 2005. What prompted the withdrawal? What are the risks of using human material in therapeutic agents?

5. Human growth hormone is a carefully regulated substance because of widespread off-label use and misuse. Currently how is growth hormone being used by adults in settings other than to treat growth deficiency? Do you believe this is inappropriate and why?

2 to 20 years: Girls
Stature-for-age and Weight-for-age percentiles

NAME _____

RECORD # _____

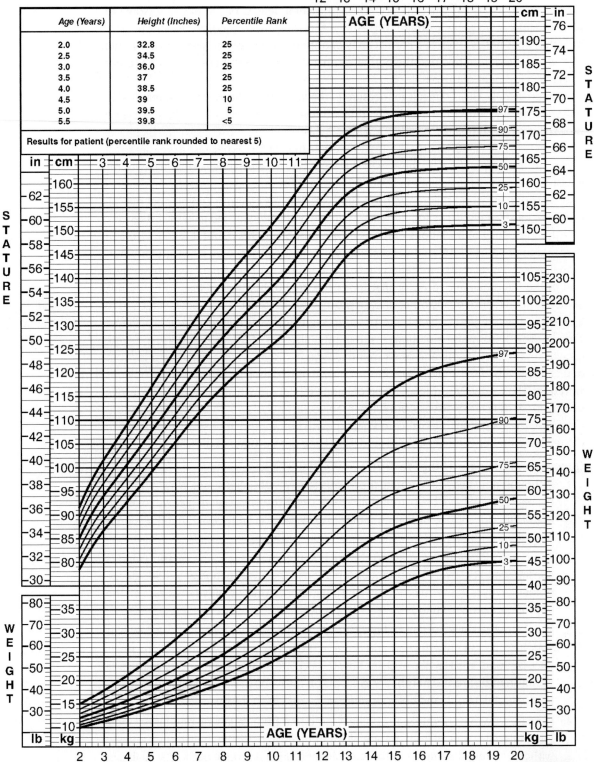

Age (Years)	Height (Inches)	Percentile Rank
2.0	32.8	25
2.5	34.5	25
3.0	36.0	25
3.5	37	25
4.0	38.5	25
4.5	39	10
5.0	39.5	5
5.5	39.8	<5

Results for patient (percentile rank rounded to nearest 5)

Published May 30, 2000 (modified 11/21/00).
SOURCE: Developed by the National Center for Health Statistics in collaboration with
the National Center for Chronic Disease Prevention and Health Promotion (2000).
http://www.cdc.gov/growthcharts

CDC
SAFER • HEALTHIER • PEOPLE™

FIGURE 24-22 Standard growth chart for girls age two to twenty years. Data for Irene Mikros is included for years two to five and a half. (Available from the Centers for Disease Control at www.cdc.gov/growthcharts)

Growth chart is published by the CDC http://www.cdc.gov/growthcharts.

QUESTIONS FOR REVIEW

1. What are the major hormones produced by the pituitary gland? What factors regulate secretion of pituitary hormones?

2. What is the effect of overproduction of growth hormone?

3. What factors regulate the rate of production of thyroid hormone? What are the major effects of an abnormal output of thyroid hormone? What is the difference between cretinism and myxedema?

4. Why does the thyroid gland become enlarged as a result of iodine deficiency?

5. What is the difference between Cushing disease and Cushing syndrome?

6. What are the main classes of hormones elaborated by the adrenal cortex? What diseases result from adrenal cortical dysfunction?

7. What factors regulate the output of parathyroid hormone? What are the possible effects of parathyroid dysfunction?

8. What factors regulate the release of prolactin? What are the clinical effects of hyperprolactinemia? What are the causes of hyperprolactinemia?

9. What is Addison disease? What is the cause of the skin pigmentation?

SUPPLEMENTARY READINGS

Hammett-Stabler, C. A., and Maygarden, S. J., Chapter 15, "Pathology of the Endocrine System." 2015. In *Pathology: A Modern Case Study*, edited by H. M. Reisner New York, NY: McGraw Hill Lange.

Hamett-Stabler, C. A., Chapter 6, "Clinical Practice: Laboratory Medicine and Patient Care." 2015. In *Pathology: A Modern Case Study*, edited by H. M. Reisner. New York, NY: McGraw Hill Lange.

▶ Endocrinology is an exceedingly complex area that is heavily dependent on clinical laboratory medicine for diagnosis. These two chapters are aimed at undergraduate medical students and provide a brief and targeted presentation toward understanding clinical case presentations. The first chapter includes brief reviews of the physiology of endocrine hormones. The second chapter provides a good overview of how laboratory medicine affects patient care. This is particularly pertinent in the evaluation of endocrine disease.

Dong, Y. H., and Fu, D. G. 2014. Autoimmune thyroid disease: Mechanism, genetics and current knowledge. *European Review for Medical and Pharmacological Science* 18:3611–18.

Vigneri, R., Malandrino, P., and Paoli, V. 2015. The changing epidemiology of thyroid cancer. *Current Opinion in Oncology* 27:1–7.

Tuttle, R. M., Vaisman, F., and Tronko, M. D. 2011. Clinical presentation and clinical outcomes in Cernobyl-related paediatric thyroid cancers: What do we know now? What can we expect in the future? *Clinical Oncology* 23:268–75.

Kamiya, K., et al. 2015. Long-term effects of radiation exposure on health. *The Lancet* 386:469–78.

▶ The first entry presents a recent overview of autoimmune disease in the thyroid and is of relevance to other endocrine organs. The second and third entries are concerned with changes in the epidemiology of thyroid cancer and the relation of such to potential environmental agents (such a radiation). The fourth entry provides an excellent overview of the biological effects of radiation. Although not specific to endocrine disease, it is a first-rate primer to the subject.

Drougat, L., et al. 2015. Novel insights into the genetics and pathophysiology of adrenocortical tumors. *Front Endocrinology* (Lausanne) (Epub June 9).

▶ This article reviews our current understanding of the molecular pathogenesis of adrenocortical adenomas and carcinomas.

Capatina, C., and Wass, J. A. H. 2015. 60 years of neuroendocrinology: Acromegaly. *Journal of Endocrinology* 226:T141–T160.

▶ The Case in this chapter delves into the complexities of growth hormone deficiency. This is an overview of diseases associated with growth hormone excess.

Gold, P. W. 2015. The organization of the stress system and its dysregulation in depressive illness. *Molecular Psychiatry* 20:32–47.

▶ The role of stress in endocrine disease is sometimes underemphasized. This is an expert review of the mechanisms by which stress can affect homeostatic mechanisms and produce disease.

Ergun-Longmire, B., and Wajnrajch, M. 2010. *Growth and growth disorders*. http://www.ncbi.nlm.nih.go2013. An Endotext v/books/NBK279142/

Rogol, A. D., and Hayden, G. F. 2014. Etiologies and early diagnosis of short stature and growth failure in children and adolescents. *Journal of Pediatrics* 164:S1–S14.

Kotch, J. B. 2013. *Maternal and Child Health*. 3rd ed. Burlington, MA: Jones & Bartlett Learning.

▶ The first two articles were the major resources used in the Case construction and present an overview of short stature and growth hormone deficiency. The first entry is notable as an example of a series of freely available review texts produced by Endotext (www.endotext.org) in the field of endocrinology. The third entry is a classic text that goes into detail on developmental stages in children and their evaluation.

The Nervous System

1. Describe the normal structure and basic functions of the brain, meninges, and cerebrospinal fluid.

2. Define muscle tone and voluntary motor activity, and relate these concepts to the two forms of muscle paralysis.

3. Explain the pathogenesis and clinical manifestations of closure defects of the central nervous system. Name the techniques used for prenatal diagnosis.

4. Describe the pathogenesis and manifestations of hydrocephalus, and relate them to treatment measures.

5. Describe the pathogenesis and manifestations of rabies.

6. Name the causes, manifestations, and treatment of transient ischemic attacks.

7. Differentiate the principal types of stroke in regard to pathogenesis, prognosis, and treatment.

8. Describe the pathogenesis, manifestations, and treatment of congenital cerebral aneurysms.

9. Name the types of tumors that affect the central nervous system, and explain their origin, pathogenesis, clinical manifestations, and treatment.

10. Explain the pathogenesis, major clinical manifestations, and general principles of treatment of Parkinson disease, meningitis, multiple sclerosis, and Guillain-Barré syndrome.

Structure and Function

The central nervous system (CNS) consists of the brain, the brain stem, the cerebellum, and the spinal cord, all surrounded by several membranes called **meninges**. The membranes include the **dura**, a firm, fibrous outer membrane; the **pia**, a thin inner membrane that adheres to the surface of the brain and spinal cord; and the **arachnoid**, the middle membrane, interposed between the pia and dura. The space between the arachnoid and the underlying pia is called the **subarachnoid space**, which contains cerebrospinal fluid (CSF) together with fine strands of arachnoidal connective tissue that extend through the space and attach to the tips of the gyri (convolutions on the surface of the cerebral hemispheres separated by the sulci, the intervening spaces).

The brain contains four interconnected cavities called **ventricles**. Arterial blood is supplied to the brain by large blood vessels entering the base of the skull that join to form a circle of vessels (the circle of Willis) at the base of the brain. Branches from the circle extend outward to supply all parts of the brain. Venous blood is returned from the brain into large venous sinuses in the dura, which eventually drain into the jugular veins (**FIGURE 25-1**).

Meninges The membranes covering the brain and spinal cord.

Dura The outer covering of the brain and spinal cord.

Pia The innermost of the three membranes covering the brain and spinal cord.

Arachnoid The middle of the three meninges that cover the brain.

Subarachnoid space The space between the arachnoid and the pia, containing large blood vessels supplying the brain.

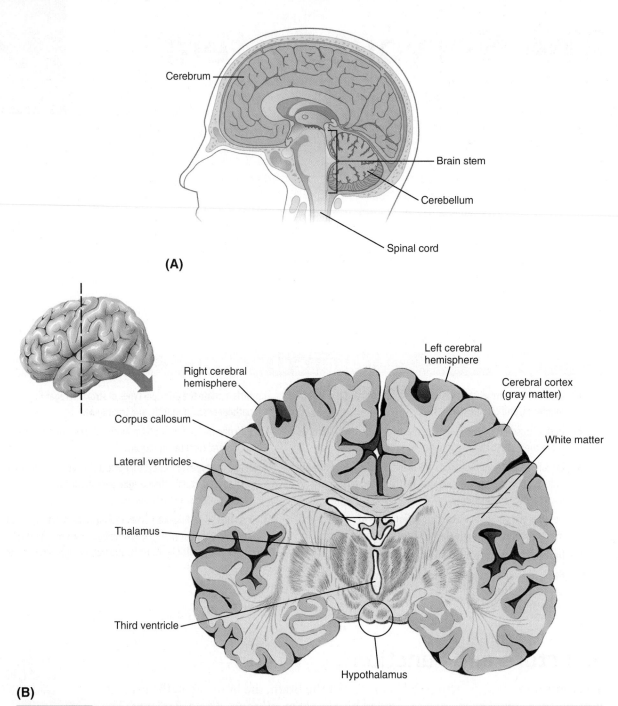

FIGURE 25-1 **(A)** Parts of the central nervous system. **(B)** Structures of the brain. A cross section through the brain showing gray and white matter of the cortex, ventricles, and deeper structures.

Ventricle A small cavity, especially one in the brain or heart. *Ventricles of brain:* The hollow cavities in the brain. *Ventricles of heart:* The muscular chambers that receive blood from the atria and pump the blood into the aorta *(left ventricle)* or pulmonary artery *(right ventricle).*

The brain and spinal cord, surrounded by cerebrospinal fluid (CSF), are encased within protective bony structures: the cranium and the vertebral column. The bony case protects the soft and rather fragile nervous tissue; the cerebrospinal fluid acts as a hydrostatic cushion to insulate the brain from shocks and blows. Because the brain and surrounding cerebrospinal fluid form a closed system within the skull, changes in the volume of either brain tissue or CSF are poorly tolerated. Increases in the volume of either will cause injury to the substance of the brain, leading to death if not relieved (**FIGURE 25-2**).

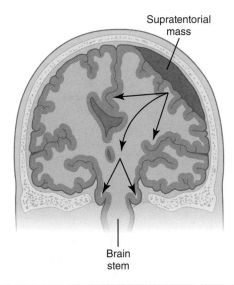

Supratentorial
mass

Brain
stem

FIGURE 25-2 Forces resulting from increased intracranial pressure pushing the brain into the foramen magnum (the hole in the base of the skull through which the spinal cord passes). This results in injury to vital brain structures including the brain stem and, ultimately, to death.

The nerve tissue of the brain and spinal cord is composed of nerve cells called **neurons** with supporting and protective cells called **neuroglia**. Taken together the neurons and neuroglial cells form the **neuropil**, the substance of the CNS. Grossly, the neuropil is divided into the **gray matter**, which is more centrally located in the brain and contains the neuronal cell bodies and the supportive glial cells (**astrocytes**), which support the neurons and play a role in the response of the CNS to injury, and **microglia**, which are macrophage-like mononuclear phagocytes localize at the site of CNS injury. The **white matter** of the CNS is located externally to the gray matter and consists predominantly of the portions of the neurons **axons** that conduct impulses away from the neuronal cell body. Most nerve axons are covered by a fatty insulating myelin sheath produced and maintained by specialized glial cells, the oligodendrocytes, also found in the white matter along with other microglial cells. When a nerve fiber leaves the central nervous system, **Schwann cells**, with the same function as oligodendrocytes in the CNS, produce the myelin that insulates the fiber.

Each individual neuron consists of a central body and one or more long processes extending from the cell body to transmit the impulses. Standard terminology calls a process that transmits impulses toward the cell body a **dendrite** and one conducting impulses away from the cell body an axon. The term "nerve fiber" may also be used when describing nerve cell processes because it can be applied to any nerve process without regard to its direction of impulse transmission.

Neurons are frequently arranged in chains. Although the neurons interconnect with other neurons to transmit impulses, they are not in direct contact with one another. Instead, they are separated by minute gaps called **synapses**. The transmission of a nerve impulse across a synapse uses a chemical neurotransmitter that is released from the end of an axon and activates receptors on the dendrite or cell body of the adjacent neuron. Some of the more important neurotransmitters are acetylcholine, norepinephrine, and dopamine, which is closely related to norepinephrine. A nerve that transmits impulses into the nervous system is called a sensory nerve or afferent nerve (*ad* = to + *ferre* = carry). A motor nerve or efferent nerve (*e* = away) conducts impulses from the brain or spinal cord to muscle.

The nervous system may be regarded as a switchboard, receiving sensory impulses and relaying this information to brain and spinal cord centers concerned with

Neuron A nerve cell, including the nerve cell body and its processes.

Neuroglia Supporting cells of tissue of the nervous system.

Neuropil Substance of the CNS; divided into gray matter and white matter.

Gray matter Centrally located part of the brain containing the neuronal cell bodies and the supportive glial cells.

Astrocytes Supportive cells of the brain.

Microglia Macrophage-like mononuclear phagocytes.

White matter Area of the CNS located externally to the gray matter consisting predominantly of the portions of the neurons that conduct impulses away from the axons.

Axon the portion of the neurons that conducts impulses away from the neuronal cell body.

Schwann cells Cells making myelin for nerve fibers outside the CNS.

Dendrite Nerve process conducting impulses toward the cell body.

Synapse Gap between connecting neurons.

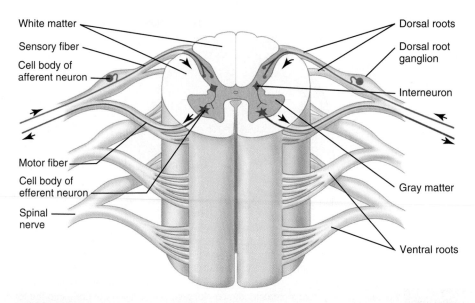

White matter
Sensory fiber
Cell body of afferent neuron
Motor fiber
Cell body of efferent neuron
Spinal nerve

Dorsal roots
Dorsal root ganglion
Interneuron
Gray matter
Ventral roots

FIGURE 25-3 The spinal cord and dorsal root ganglia spinal nerves are attached to the spinal cord by two roots, the dorsal and ventral roots. The dorsal root carries sensory information into the spinal cord. The ventral root carries information out of the spinal cord. Spinal nerves often contain both sensory and motor fibers. Dorsal root ganglia contain the cell bodies of multiple sensory neurons.

Cerebral cortex Receives sensory input and initiates voluntary motor activity.

Cerebellum Part of brain regulating muscle tone, coordination, posture, and balance.

Brain Stem The brain stem is the elongated central portion of the brain connecting the cerebral hemispheres with the spinal cord. It controls the flow of messages to the rest of the body and is critical for autonomic functions such as breathing.

perception of sensation and with motor activity. The **cerebral cortex** receives sensory input and initiates voluntary motor activity. In the depths of each cerebral hemisphere are masses of gray matter: the thalami and the basal ganglia (basal nuclei). The paired thalami, which form the lateral walls of the third ventricle, function as relay stations that receive sensory impulses from lower levels and transmit them to the cortex.

The **brain stem** contains neurons that are involved in multiple functions not under direct cortical control; it also carries the bundles of nerve fibers that pass to higher and lower levels within the central nervous system. The **cerebellum** regulates muscle tone, coordination, posture, and balance (Figure 25-1).

The spinal cord is the continuation of the brain stem. Its central gray matter receives sensory input from spinal nerves entering the cord, and motor neurons exit from the cord to innervate muscles. Spinal sensory and motor neurons are involved in many reflex functions not under cortical control, but spinal motor neurons are also activated by motor impulses originating from cortical neurons. The spinal motor neurons in turn discharge impulses to the skeletal muscles that they supply, causing them to contract (**FIGURE 25-3**).

The fiber tracts conveying sensory impulses to the cortex and those conveying motor impulses from the cortex cross within the brain stem to the opposite side as they transmit impulses to their destination. Consequently, the right hemisphere registers sensation from the left half of the body and innervates the muscles on the left side. Conversely, the left hemisphere receives sensation from the right side of the body and activates muscles on the right side.

Interaction of Nervous System with Muscles

A skeletal muscle contracts in response to impulses discharged from lower motor neurons, motor neurons in the spinal cord, or from corresponding neurons of the cranial nerves in the brain stem. Voluntary motor activity, controlled by nerve impulses originating in motor neurons in the cerebral cortex (sometimes called upper motor neurons) is managed by two separate motor systems: the pyramidal system, which controls voluntary motor functions, and the extrapyramidal system, which regulates muscle groups concerned primarily with balance, posture, and coordination.

The pyramidal system and the extrapyramidal system function together as a single system under cortical control to produce the smooth integrated functions of muscle groups involved in voluntary motor activity. Malfunction of the extrapyramidal system leads to loss of coordinated motor functions. The muscles do not function smoothly, and the malfunction also gives rise to abnormal uncontrollable muscular movements (ataxia).

Muscle tone refers to the firmness of a muscle and its resistance to stretching. A muscle lacking tone is limp and offers no resistance when stretched. Conversely, a muscle with excess tone is firm, resists stretching, and is said to be **spastic**. Muscle tone results from the reflex contraction of muscle in response to stretching. Specialized receptors located in the muscle are activated, and afferent impulses are conveyed to the lower motor neuron, causing reflex discharge of motor impulses that stimulate the muscle to contract and resist the stretching force. Muscle tone is also influenced by impulses discharged from higher centers in the nervous system, which vary the responsiveness of the stretch receptors when stimulated.

Muscle tone The slight contractility (tension) present in resting muscles.

Spastic Muscle with excess tone that resists stretching.

Neural tube The ectodermal tube formed in the embryo that gives rise to the brain and spinal cord.

Muscle Paralysis

A muscle that is no longer subject to voluntary control is said to be paralyzed. There are two different types of paralysis: flaccid paralysis, caused by disease of the lower motor neurons or their fibers; and spastic paralysis, which results from disease affecting the cortical motor neurons or their fibers. Spastic paralysis occurs more frequently than flaccid paralysis because cortical neurons are more often damaged by disease than are spinal motor neurons.

FLACCID PARALYSIS

If the lower motor neuron in the spinal cord is destroyed by a disease such as poliomyelitis or if the peripheral nerve supplying the muscle (which contains the nerve fibers of the spinal neurons) is interrupted, the reflex arc responsible for muscle tone is interrupted or abolished because the muscle is deprived of its innervation. The muscle becomes limp and undergoes severe atrophy.

SPASTIC PARALYSIS

If cortical motor neurons or their fibers that travel in the motor pathways are interrupted, as in a stroke, voluntary control of the muscles supplied by the affected neurons is lost because the pyramidal tract pathway is interrupted. However, because the reflex arc that maintains muscle tone is not disturbed and the muscle retains its innervation, significant atrophy of the muscle does not occur. Generally, muscle tone is increased because extrapyramidal motor impulses descending from the cortex tend to inhibit muscle tone, and this inhibitory effect is lost after an upper motor neuron injury.

Development of the Nervous System

In the embryo, the central nervous system first appears as a thickened band of surface cells (ectoderm) called the neural plate. Its lateral margins become elevated to form neural folds, which fuse to form a hollow tube called the **neural tube**. Fusion

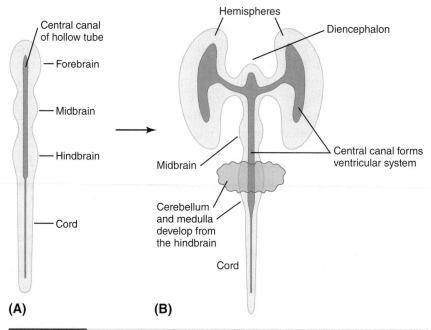

FIGURE 25-4 Early development of the nervous system. **(A)** Formation of the neural ventricular system. **(B)** Cerebral hemispheres grow from the forebrain, and the central region becomes the diencephalon.

begins in the middle of the developing tube and progresses toward both ends until a completely closed tube is formed by the end of the fourth week of embryonic development. Three expansions, called the forebrain, midbrain, and hindbrain, develop from one end of the neural tube (**FIGURE 25-4**). The other end remains narrow and becomes the spinal cord. The cerebral hemispheres develop as lateral outgrowths from the forebrain. The hindbrain forms the medulla and cerebellum.

Neural Tube Defects

Failure of either end of the neural tube to close properly leads to serious congenital malformations called neural tube defects that involve the nervous system and the surrounding tissues as well. A closure defect involving the end of the tube destined to form the cerebral hemispheres (the cephalic end) leads to **anencephaly** (*ana* = without + *encephalon* = brain). If the opposite end of the tube (the caudal end) is involved, **spina bifida** results. These are the two most common congenital malformations of the nervous system with a combined incidence of about 5.5 per 10,000 births in the United States and even higher rates in some other countries. The malformations follow a multifactorial pattern of inheritance (see discussion on congenital and hereditary diseases) and tend to recur in subsequent pregnancies. If parents have already given birth to an offspring with a neural tube defect, the risk of recurrence in a subsequent pregnancy is approximately 1 in 20. The risk is 1 in 10 when the parents have had two affected infants.

A deficiency of folic acid during the early part of pregnancy when the neural tube is forming plays an important role in causing neural tube defects. Intake of 0.4 mg (400 mcg) of folic acid daily beginning before conception and during the early part of pregnancy can reduce by one-half the frequency of neural tube defects. However, consumption of folic acid will not eliminate the problem; a woman who has previously given birth to an infant with a neural tube defect still has a greater than normal risk of having an infant with a neural tube defect in a subsequent pregnancy.

Anencephaly A congenital malformation: absence of brain, cranial vault, and scalp as a result of defective closure of the neural tube.

Spina bifida Incomplete closure of vertebral arches over the spinal cord, sometimes associated with protrusion of meninges and neural tissue through the defect (cystic spina bifida).

ANENCEPHALY

Anencephaly occurs most commonly in female infants and is incompatible with postnatal life. Because the cephalic end of the neural tube fails to close, the exposed neural tissue undergoes secondary degenerative changes that convert it into a mass of vascular connective tissue intermixed with masses of degenerated brain and choroid plexus. The anencephalic infant has a striking appearance (**FIGURE 25-5**). The brain is absent, as are the soft tissues of the scalp and the bones making up the vertex of the skull. The exposed base of the skull is covered only by a vascular membrane. The base of the cranial cavity is abnormally formed, and the orbits are shallow, causing the eyes to bulge outward. The trunk is short, the shoulders are broad, and the neck is not normal; the head arises directly from the trunk and cannot be flexed.

Often the closure defect affects not only the brain but also the part of the neural tube that forms the upper part of the spinal cord. When this occurs, the vertebral arches are absent, as well as the vertex of the skull, and the unclosed spinal cord lies exposed within the wide-open spinal canal, a condition referred to as **rachischisis**.

SPINA BIFIDA

Malformations of the opposite (caudal) end of the neural tube and related vertebral arches are generally considered together as spina bifida, which literally means split spine and refers to the characteristic failure of fusion of the vertebral arches common to all types of spina bifida (**FIGURE 25-6**). Occult spina bifida refers to failure of fusion of vertebral arches in the lower lumbar region, which occurs as an isolated abnormality (**FIGURE 25-6A**), but it produces no clinical symptoms. The more severe types of spina bifida are characterized by a saclike protrusion of meninges or meninges and nerve tissue through the defect in the vertebral arches. The malformation is called a **meningocele** if the protrusion consists only of meninges (**FIGURE 25-6B**) and

> **Rachischisis** Unclosed spinal cord lies exposed within the wide-open spinal canal.
>
> **Meningocele** A protrusion of meninges through a defect in the spinal vertebral arches.

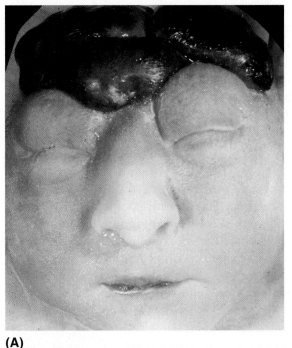 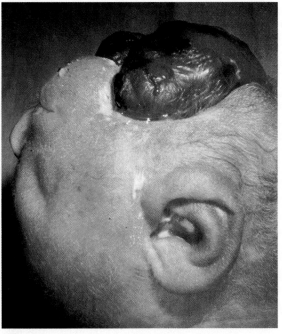

(A) **(B)**

FIGURE 25-5 Characteristic appearance of anencephalic infant. Most of brain, top of skull, and scalp are absent. Maldevelopment of skull causes protrusion of eyes. **(A)** Frontal view. **(B)** Lateral view.

Courtesy of Leonard V. Crowley, MD, Century College.

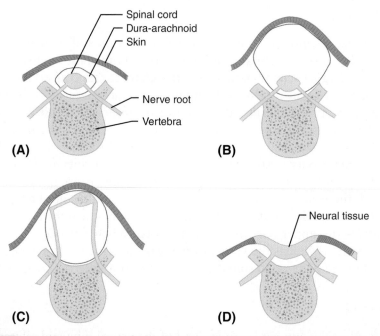

FIGURE 25-6 Various types of spina bifida. **(A)** Occult spina bifida. Failure of formation of vertebral arches. No protrusion of meninges. **(B)** Meningocele. Meninges protrude through defect in the vertebral arches. Cord and nerve trunks are not present in the sac. **(C)** Meningomyelocele. Protrusion of both meninges and nerve tissue. The spinal cord and nerve trunks are frequently incorporated into the wall of the sac. **(D)** Failure of the neural tube to form and separate from the surface ectoderm. The neural tissue is continuous with the adjacent skin.

Meningomyelocele
A type of spina bifida characterized by protrusion of meninges and cord through the defect in the vertebral arches.

is called a **meningomyelocele** (*myelo* = cord) if parts of the spinal cord or nerve roots also are included in the sac (**FIGURE 25-6C**).

In meningomyelocele, there is often a severe neurologic deficit below the level of the sac because the nerve tissue is incorporated into the wall of the sac and is disorganized so that the conduction of nerve impulses is impaired or completely interrupted. In the most severe (and fortunately rare) form of spina bifida, the caudal end of the neural tube completely fails to close. The distal end of the spinal cord is represented by a flattened mass of nerve tissue that is continuous with the adjacent skin (**FIGURE 25-6D**). The larger meningomyelocele sacs often are covered not by skin but merely by a thin, easily ruptured membrane composed only of meninges (**FIGURE 25-7**).

Treatment of Spina Bifida

Occult spina bifida is asymptomatic, and no treatment is required. A meningocele usually can be repaired without difficulty with satisfactory results by excising the sac and closing the spinal dura because the meninges are the only component involved in the defect. Unfortunately, a large meningomyelocele is much more difficult to treat, with much less satisfactory results. The condition may be complicated by hydrocephalus. Because spinal cord and nerve roots are often incorporated in the sac, there is frequently some loss of sensation and motor power in the lower extremities. Bowel and bladder function also may be impaired, leading to stasis of urine in the bladder predisposing to urinary tract infections.

PRENATAL DETECTION OF NEURAL TUBE DEFECTS

It is usually possible to identify a fetus with a neural tube defect prior to birth. An elevated concentration of alpha fetoprotein (AFP) detected on a routine screening

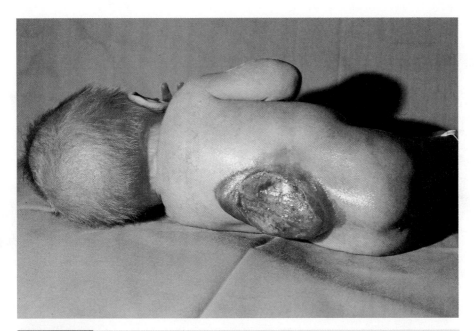

FIGURE 25-7 Large thoracic meningomyelocele covered only by a thin membrane. This condition is associated with neurologic disturbances resulting from incorporation of neural tissue into the wall of the sac.

Courtesy of Leonard V. Crowley, MD, Century College.

test of maternal blood may suggest the possibility of a neural tube defect. This can be confirmed by an ultrasound examination of the fetus at about sixteen-weeks' gestation, as described in the discussion on congenital and hereditary diseases.

Alpha fetoprotein, produced in the fetal liver beginning early in pregnancy, can be readily detected in the fetal blood. Normally, a small amount of AFP diffuses from the fetal blood into the amnionic fluid and into the mother's blood. High amnionic fluid AFP levels are encountered when the fetus is anencephalic or has a cystic spina bifida because of direct diffusion through the neural tube defect into the amniotic fluid. Consequently, AFP levels are much higher in these cases than in a normal pregnancy.

Hydrocephalus

Cerebrospinal fluid serves as a protective cushion around the brain and spinal cord. The fluid, secreted by the choroid plexuses of the ventricles, flows from the lateral ventricles into the third ventricle, through the cerebral aqueduct (aqueduct of Sylvius) into the fourth ventricle, and then out into the subarachnoid space through three small openings in the roof of the fourth ventricle. The fluid circulates around the cord and over the convexity of the brain and is resorbed into the large venous sinuses in the dura. Secretion of cerebrospinal fluid continues even if the flow of fluid through the ventricular system is blocked. Obstruction to the normal circulation of spinal fluid distends the ventricles proximal to the site of obstruction, with associated compression atrophy of brain tissue around the dilated ventricles (**FIGURE 25-8**). When the blockage occurs within the ventricular system, the condition is termed obstructive (or noncommunicating) **hydrocephalus**, which may be congenital or acquired. Blockage of CSF flow after the ventricular system is called communicating hydrocephalus. In these cases all the ventricles dilate; this is generally an acquired defect.

Hydrocephalus Dilatation of the cerebral ventricular system caused by pressure arising from accumulation of cerebrospinal fluid within the ventricles.

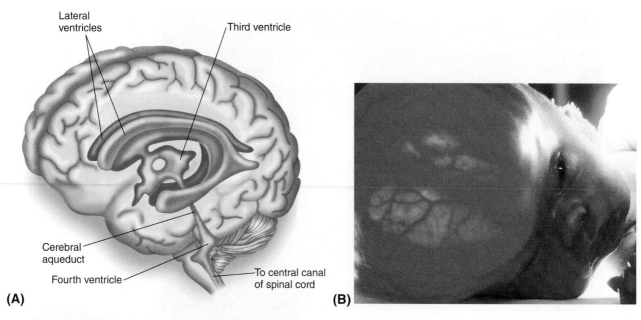

Lateral
ventricles

Third ventricle

Cerebral
aqueduct

Fourth ventricle

To central canal
of spinal cord

(A)

(B)

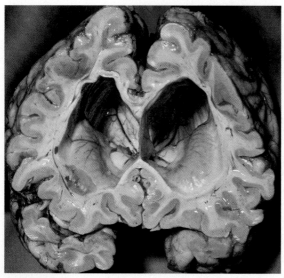

(C)

FIGURE 25-8 **(A)** The brain contains four ventricles, which are filled with cerebrospinal fluid. Hydrocephalus can result from blockage of the cerebral aqueduct of Sylvius and **(B)** cause CSF to build up, thinning the cortex and causing severe brain damage. **(C)** Coronal section of brain revealing marked dilatation of ventricles in patient with congenital hydrocephalus.

© SIU/Visuals Unlimited; Courtesy of Leonard V. Crowley, MD, Century College.

Arnold Chiari malformation
Congenital condition with
spinal cord defects and
compression of the brain
stem and cerebellum
downward.

Congenital Hydrocephalus

Congenital hydrocephalus, usually caused by a congenital abnormality in the ventricular system, is most commonly either a congenital obstruction, an abnormal formation of the cerebral aqueduct of Sylvius (the narrow channel connecting the third and fourth ventricles), or failure of the openings in the roof and lateral walls of the fourth ventricle to form normally; the obstruction blocks escape of cerebrospinal fluid into the subarachnoid space. An aqueduct obstruction leads to distention of the lateral and third ventricles. An obstruction of the outlet channels in the fourth ventricle leads to distention of all four ventricles. A complex congenital condition termed the **Arnold Chiari malformation** results in spinal cord defects (including meningiomyelocoele) and compression of the brain stem and cerebellum downward, sometimes causing a kinking of the lower medulla. The structural defect leads to stenosis of the aqueduct and hydrocephalus. Because in congenital defects the distention can develop before the skull bones have fused, the head may enlarge greatly; the brain undergoes pronounced atrophy secondary to compression by the dilated ventricles. If hydrocephalus develops in the fetus prior to birth, the head may become so large that it is unable to enter the maternal pelvis during labor. More often, the hydrocephalus develops insidiously after birth, depending on the severity of the defect.

Acquired Hydrocephalus

Acquired hydrocephalus is most commonly caused by obstruction of the circulation of the cerebrospinal fluid in the region of the fourth ventricle by fibrous adhesions, which sometimes form after a bacterial infection of the meninges (**meningitis**) and block the outflow of fluid from the fourth ventricle, or by blockage of the ventricular system secondary to a brain tumor. Acquired hydrocephalus develops after the skull bones fuse, so the skull cannot enlarge as in the congenital form of hydrocephalus.

Treatment of Hydrocephalus

Hydrocephalus can often be treated successfully by a shunting procedure in which a plastic tube inserted into one of the dilated ventricles can reroute the fluid into another part of the body where it can be absorbed. The fluid can be shunted into either the right atrium via the jugular vein (ventriculoatrial shunt) or into the peritoneal cavity (ventriculoperitoneal shunt). Whatever type of shunt is used, a one-way valve is incorporated in the tube to prevent any reflux of blood or peritoneal fluid into the ventricles.

> **Meningitis** Inflammation of the meninges.
>
> **Concussion** A temporary loss of consciousness caused by a head injury without any memory of the events that occurred shortly before or after the head injury.
>
> **Contusion** Severe force injury resulting in detectable damage to brain tissue.

Cerebral Injury

The brain is well protected from moderate trauma but may be injured by a blow to the head that jars the brain within its protective cranial cavity. The mildest form of head injury is called a **concussion**, which may be caused by any force injury that causes a temporary loss of consciousness such as might occur in contact sports such as football or boxing. A concussion usually is characterized by temporary loss of consciousness without any memory of the events that occurred shortly before and after the head injury (amnesia). The concussion may be associated with a headache, temporary disorientation, and confusion but does not result in any neuropathology detected grossly. However, repeated head injuries related to football, boxing, or other contact sports may lead to permanently impaired cerebral function associated with axonal damage.

More severe force injuries are called **contusions**, and they can result in detectable (and sometimes permanent) damage to brain tissue and are the equivalent to bruising in other tissues. If sufficiently severe, a blow may injure the brain and fracture the skull (**FIGURE 25-9**). Force injury to the brain may be manifested by loss of consciousness and various neurologic disturbances depending on the severity and nature of the insult. The injured brain becomes swollen and often shows evidence of pinpoint hemorrhages caused by disruption of small intracerebral blood vessels, resulting in increased intracranial pressure that may be life-threatening. Usually the brain injury is located immediately adjacent to the site of the blow (a coup injury), but sometimes the brain injury is caused by violent contact of the displaced brain against the cranial cavity on the side opposite the injury. For example, the force of a blow to the back of the head may displace the brain forward, injuring the front of the brain where it strikes against the front of the bony cranial cavity (a contrecoup injury) (**FIGURE 25-10**).

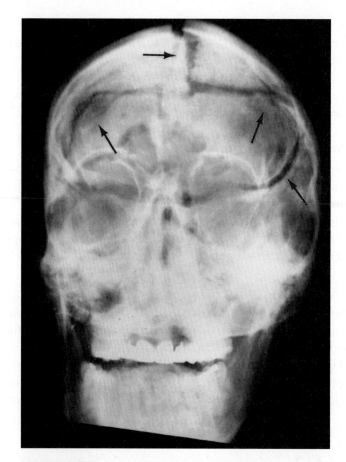

FIGURE 25-9 Skull x-ray illustrating large skull fracture (*arrows*) associated with extensive injury to underlying brain.

Courtesy of Leonard V. Crowley, MD, Century College.

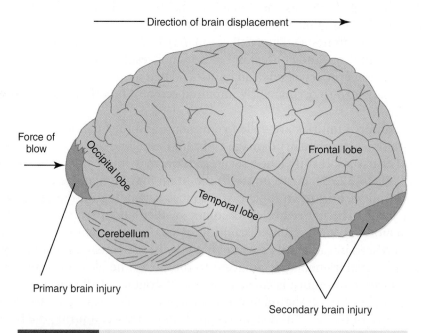

FIGURE 25-10 Mechanism of injury to frontal and temporal poles of brain caused by a blow to the back of the head.

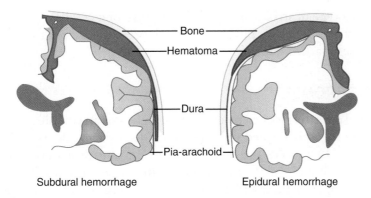

FIGURE 25-11 Comparative locations of epidural and subdural hemorrhages.

Sometimes, a head injury tears blood vessels located between the cranial bones and the dura, or under the dura. The escaping blood may accumulate in any of several locations, depending on which vessels have been damaged: epidural hemorrhage (between the outer layer of dura and the cranial bones), subdural hemorrhage (between the dura and the arachnoid), or subarachnoid hemorrhage (between the arachnoid and the pia) (**FIGURE 25-11**).

Epidural hematomas are most often associated with skull fractures that damage the middle meningeal arteries that lie in grooves in the bone of the skull. If torn, blood from the meningeal artery rapidly fills the epidural space and continues to expand. The hematoma, if not removed, will compress the brain within the unyielding skull, leading to irreversible brain damage and death within a day or two. Subdural hematomas tend to enlarge more slowly because the source of bleeding is from veins. The condition may become chronic with healing within the hematoma followed by occasional rebleeding. The hematoma may ultimately be resorbed and heal, calcify, or continue to expand. Although serious symptoms may be delayed by even months from the occurrence of the injury, seizures, weakness, and lethal brain damage may ultimately occur. In a subarachnoid hemorrhage, the blood often mixes with the cerebrospinal fluid and spreads diffusely through the subarachnoid space. Subarachnoid hemorrhages may occur as a result of trauma but often are a result of rupture of congenital aneurysms (berry aneurysms), outpouchings that occur in the base of the brain in the vasculature of the circle of Willis.

Stroke

A **stroke**, also called a **cerebrovascular accident (CVA)**, designates any injury to brain tissue resulting from disturbance of blood supply to the brain and encompasses three conditions: cerebral thrombosis, cerebral embolism, and cerebral hemorrhage. A **cerebral thrombosis**, as indicated by the name, results from thrombosis of a cerebral artery narrowed by arteriosclerosis and is the cause of most strokes. Strokes are the third leading cause of death in the United States.

A **cerebral embolus**, which occurs less frequently than a cerebral thrombosis, is caused by blockage of a cerebral artery by a fragment of a blood clot dislodged from the surface of an ulcerated atherosclerotic plaque in the carotid artery or from a blood clot that formed within the heart and subsequently carried to the brain. Three cardiac conditions predispose to cerebral emboli: (1) a mural thrombus that forms on the wall of the left ventricle adjacent to a healing myocardial infarct, (2) a thrombus that forms on the rough surface of a diseased mitral or aortic valve, and (3) a small thrombus in a left atrium demonstrating fibrillation. A **cerebral hemorrhage**,

Stroke/cerebrovascular accident (CVA) An injury to the brain resulting in a disturbance of cerebral blood flow caused by a cerebral thrombosis, cerebral embolism, or cerebral hemorrhage.

Cerebral thrombosis A stroke caused by thrombosis of an arteriosclerotic cerebral artery.

Cerebral embolus A stroke caused by blockage of a cerebral artery by a blood clot that had formed elsewhere in the circulatory system and was transported in the bloodstream to the brain.

Cerebral hemorrhage A stroke caused by rupture of a cerebral artery, usually in a person with hypertension, that allows blood to escape under high pressure into the brain.

the most serious type of stroke, is caused by rupture of a cerebral artery most often in a person with hypertension. Blood under high pressure escapes from the ruptured vessel and causes marked damage to the brain.

CEREBRAL THROMBI

When a cerebral artery is blocked by either a thrombus or an embolus, the brain tissue in the distribution of the blocked vessel becomes necrotic and degenerates, a **cerebral infarct** (**FIGURE 25-12** and **FIGURE 25-13**). The myelin sheath material breaks down, and the debris resulting from the necrosis of brain tissue is eventually cleaned up by phagocytes, leaving a cystic cavity. Because the end stage of a brain infarct is cystic, in contrast to the appearance of infarcts in other tissues, the term **encephalomalacia** (*encephalon* = brain + *malacia* = softening) is sometimes used to describe this kind of lesion (**FIGURE 25-14**).

Although most thrombotic cerebral infarcts are not associated with bleeding, a small amount of blood can leak into the degenerated brain tissue from adjacent damaged cerebral blood vessels, as illustrated in Figure 25-13. Bleeding is more common in embolic infarcts because the "plugged" vessel tends to leak beyond the point of blockage. This type of infarct is sometimes called a hemorrhagic infarct, but the term should not be confused with a cerebral hemorrhage, which is a large hemorrhage within the brain resulting from a ruptured cerebral artery, a very different and much more serious condition.

Some patients who have had a cerebral thrombosis may benefit from the same type of thrombolytic drugs used to dissolve blood clots in coronary arteries (see discussion on the diseases of blood circulation). Unfortunately, flow through a blocked cerebral artery must be restored almost immediately or permanent brain damage occurs; also sometimes the thrombolytic drug treatment may be complicated by hemorrhage within the damaged brain tissue.

Cerebral infarct Brain tissue that became necrotic after a stroke.

Encephalomalacia Cystic lesion of degenerated brain tissue as a result of obstruction of cerebral blood supply. Same as cerebral infarct.

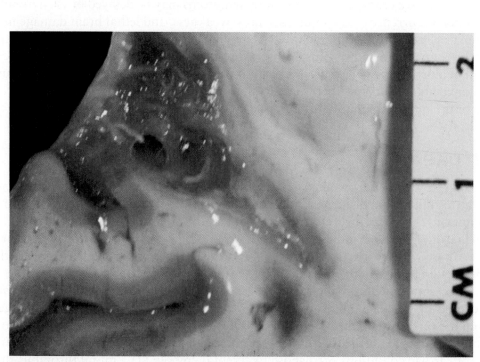

FIGURE 25-12 A small, older infarct of the cerebral cortex that is undergoing cystic breakdown (encephalomalacia).

Courtesy of Leonard V. Crowley, MD, Century College.

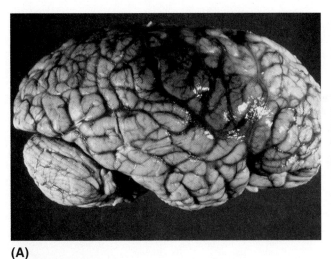
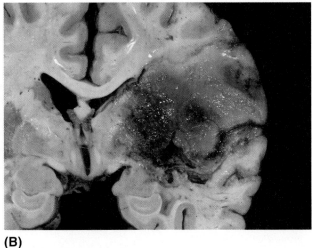

FIGURE 25-13 Large recent infarct of right cerebral hemisphere caused by thrombosis of middle cerebral artery. **(A)** External surface of brain illustrating the swollen, dark, infarcted area in the right hemisphere. **(B)** Coronal section through hemispheres at level of basal ganglia. Cerebral tissue is necrotic and discolored and involves a large part of the hemisphere.

Courtesy of Leonard V. Crowley, MD, Century College.

STROKE CAUSED BY ARTERIOSCLEROSIS OF EXTRACRANIAL ARTERIES

A stroke also may be caused by arteriosclerosis (specifically atherosclerosis) of one of the major arteries arising from the aorta to supply the brain. A commonly affected site is at the origin of the internal carotid artery in the neck, where atheromatous plaques may narrow the lumen and reduce cerebral blood flow. The plaques may become ulcerated, with thrombi forming on the roughened surfaces. Bits of atherosclerotic debris or thrombus material may break loose from the plaque and be carried into the intracerebral circulation, where they may block small cerebral arteries and cause

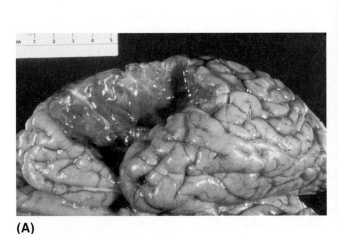
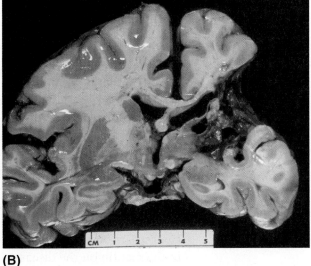

FIGURE 25-14 A large old infarct in the left hemisphere sustained several years previously, which caused paralysis of the right side of the body and loss of speech. **(A)** External surface of the brain, illustrating the large defect in the left hemisphere at the site of the old infarct. **(B)** Coronal section through the hemisphere revealing complete loss of cerebral tissue at the site of the old infarct, leaving only a few strands of glial tissue.

Courtesy of Leonard V. Crowley, MD, Century College.

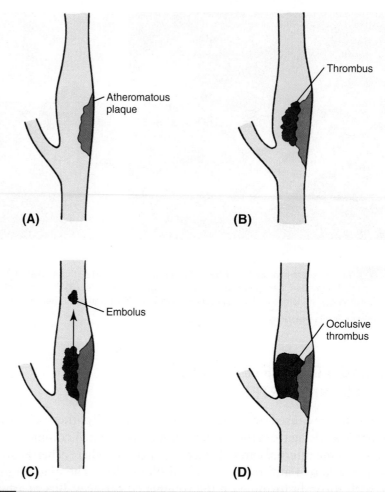

FIGURE 25-15 Effects of atherosclerosis of carotid artery in neck. **(A)** Atherosclerotic plaque narrows lumen, and surface frequently becomes ulcerated. **(B)** Formation of thrombus on ulcerated surface of plaque, further narrowing vessel. **(C)** Thrombus material dislodged from plaque to form emboli, which are carried to the brain. **(D)** Complete occlusion of artery by thrombus. (R. Escourolle J. and Poirier. 1977. *Manuel élémentaire de neuropathology*. Paris: Masson S. A. English translation: Philadelphia: W. B. Saunders, 1978.)

Data from Escourolle and Poirier: Manuel elementaire de neuropathology. Masson S. A., Paris, 1977. English translation: W. B. Saunders, Philadelphia, 1978.

embolic strokes. A 50-percent reduction in the lumen of the artery corresponds to a 75-percent reduction in the cross-section area of the lumen and is associated with a large reduction in flow rate through the artery. Rarely, the internal carotid artery may become completely blocked by a thrombus that has formed on the roughened surface of the artery, leading to a large cerebral infarction. **FIGURE 25-15** illustrates the possible effects of atherosclerosis of the internal carotid artery in the neck. Ultrasound analysis of blood flow in the carotid artery (duplex carotid ultrasound) is used to diagnosis the degree of blockage of the carotid. Atherosclerotic plaques that occlude the carotid artery and impede cerebral blood flow can be removed surgically using a procedure called a carotid endarterectomy (*endo* = within + artery + *tome* = incision). Other less invasive methods include the same type of balloon angioplasty and stent insertion procedures that are used to treat coronary artery plaques (discussed in the section on the diseases of blood circulation).

CEREBRAL HEMORRHAGE

A cerebral hemorrhage is a much more serious type of stroke most often found in people who have high blood pressure. Blood from the ruptured vessel escapes into

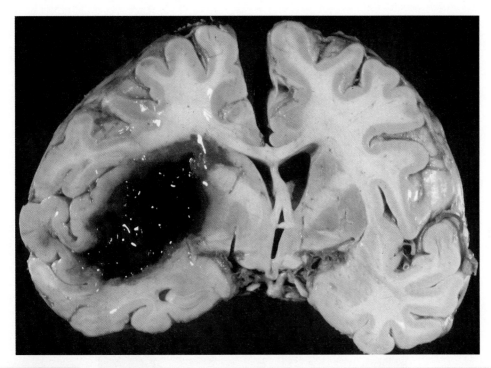

FIGURE 25-16 Coronal section of brain illustrating large cerebral hemorrhage that has compressed and displaced the cerebral ventricles.

Courtesy of Leonard V. Crowley, MD, Century College.

the brain under high pressure and causes extensive damage to brain tissue. A large cerebral hemorrhage is frequently fatal (**FIGURE 25-16**).

It is possible to distinguish a cerebral infarct (caused by a thrombosis) from a cerebral hemorrhage using either CT or MRI scans. In a CT image, cerebral hemorrhage appears as a dense area within the brain because blood is denser than normal brain tissue (**FIGURE 25-17**). However, an infarct may be somewhat less dense and difficult to detect. MRI scans have particular utility in the early diagnosis of cerebral infarcts and are much more sensitive than CT scans.

MANIFESTATIONS OF STROKE

The clinical effects of a stroke depend on the location of the brain damage and the amount of brain tissue injured. Small infarcts may cause little functional disturbance and are usually followed by prompt recovery with little or no residual disability. Unfortunately, many strokes resulting from occlusions of the middle cerebral artery or one of its major branches or from a hemorrhage in a part of the brain supplied by the artery cause major damage including partial paralysis by disrupting the nerve fibers that carry impulses to the spinal motor neurons and motor neurons of the cranial nerves (lower motor neurons). Nerve fibers carrying sensory impulses to the cortex are often damaged as well, leading to various sensory disturbances.

Sensory and motor fiber tracts cross in the brain stem as they ascend or descend; so the motor neurons from the right cerebral hemisphere supply the left side of the body, and sensory impulses received by this hemisphere come from the left side of the body. Conversely, the left hemisphere controls the right half of the body and receives sensory input from the right side. Consequently, a stroke involving one cerebral hemisphere often leads to weakness or paralysis on the opposite side, called **hemiplegia** (*hemi* = half + *plege* = stroke) or hemiparesis (*paresis* = weakness), with

Hemiplegia Paralysis of one side of the body.

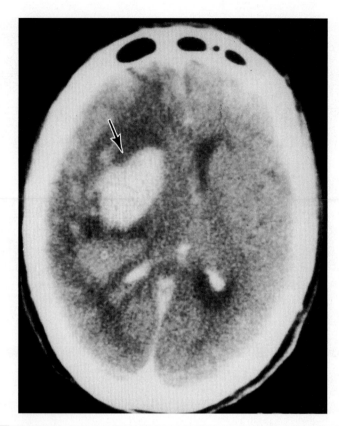

FIGURE 25-17 A computed tomography (CT) scan of a patient with cerebral hemorrhage (*arrow*), which appears white because blood is denser than brain tissue.

Courtesy of Leonard V. Crowley, MD, Century College.

some sensory impairment on the paralyzed side as well. Speech also may be affected, but usually the affected individual does not lose consciousness.

REHABILITATION OF THE STROKE PATIENT

Many patients who suffer a major stroke are partially paralyzed, and may have speech impairment as well. Rehabilitation, which is begun as soon as possible, helps the patient achieve several goals: regain the ability to walk, relearn self-care activities, prevent stiffness and limitation of motion in the joints of the paralyzed limbs, and make an emotional adjustment to the disability. These goals are achieved primarily by a program of exercises and relearning. If speech is impaired, speech therapy also is started. Many patients can learn to walk again, although in some cases a leg brace and cane may be required. It is more difficult to regain useful function in a paralyzed upper limb.

Other Types of Neurologic Dysfunction

TRANSIENT ISCHEMIC ATTACK

Transient ischemic attack Temporary cerebral dysfunction as a result of transient obstruction of a cerebral vessel by a bit of atheromatous debris or blood clot, usually embolized from an arteriosclerotic plaque in the carotid artery.

Transient ischemic attack (TIA) refers to brief episodes of neurologic dysfunction, such as temporary paralysis of an arm or leg, loss of speech, or disturbances of vision. The episodes, which tend to occur in older people, often last only a few minutes to a few hours and clear completely. They are usually caused by bits of thrombus or arteriosclerotic debris that break loose from an ulcerated plaque in the internal carotid artery and obstruct a small cerebral artery. The episodes are brief because the obstructing debris or small clot becomes fragmented and dissolved, and the circulation through the blocked vessel is restored before permanent damage to brain tissue occurs.

About one-third of patients with transient ischemic attacks eventually suffer a major stroke within five years (most often within a month of the initial event), but the majority experience no further difficulties. Treatment consists either of surgical resection of the ulcerated plaque in the carotid artery by means of a carotid endarterectomy or administration of drugs that decrease the likelihood that thrombi will form on the ulcerated plaques, thereby reducing the risk of embolization.

MULTI-INFARCT VASCULAR DEMENTIA

Not all cerebral infarcts result in paralysis. In people with vascular disease caused by hypertension, diabetes, or abnormal blood lipids, the smaller cerebral blood vessels are affected as well as the large cerebral arteries. Those affected may have repeated small strokes caused by blockage of smaller cerebral blood vessels that damage brain tissue but may not affect motor neurons or lead to muscle paralysis. Each additional small stroke further compromises cerebral function. Eventually the cumulative brain damage causes dementia similar to that seen in Alzheimer disease. The condition is called **vascular dementia** or **multi-infarct dementia** and is the most common cause of dementia after Alzheimer disease. Diagnosis of vascular dementia is made by computed tomography (CT) or magnetic resonance imaging (MRI) studies that reveal the marked brain damage caused by multiple small strokes. Progression of vascular dementia can be slowed or even prevented by treating the conditions that predispose to the cerebral vascular disease.

In addition to multi-infarct dementia, dementia can result from additional diseases that damage small vessels of the brain. Disease of the white matter (Binswanger disease) results from degenerative changes in small arteries and larger vessels. The deposition of an abnormal insoluble protein (amyloid) in cerebral vessels leads to cerebral amyloid angiopathy. The affected vessels are prone to repeated cerebral hemorrhages that can result in dementia.

Vascular dementia/ multi-infarct dementia Compromise of cerebral function caused by blockage of small cerebral blood vessels.

Aneurysm A dilatation of a structure, such as the aorta, a cerebral artery, or a part of the ventricular wall.

CEREBRAL ANEURYSM

Occasionally, **aneurysms** occur in the large cerebral arteries at the base of the brain. The most common type, a congenital cerebral aneurysm, results from a congenital defect in the elastic and muscular tissue of the vessel wall, usually at the point where the artery branches. Because of the congenital weakness, the lining of the arterial wall (intima) eventually protrudes through the defect at the point of branching, leading to the formation of a saclike outpouching (**FIGURE 25-18**).

Although the weakness of the vessel wall is congenital, the actual aneurysm does not develop until young adulthood or middle age. People with congenital polycystic kidney disease (see discussion on the urinary system) are prone to develop aneurysms of this type. Congenital aneurysms are hazardous because they may rupture, producing severe and often fatal hemorrhage within the cranial cavity (**FIGURE 25-19**). Individuals with high blood pressure are especially prone to this complication. The initial symptoms of a ruptured aneurysm are severe headache and a stiff neck. The headache results from the increased intracranial pressure caused by the sudden escape of blood into the subarachnoid space. The stiff neck occurs because the escaping blood irritates the meninges, setting off reflex contraction of the neck muscles. The location of the aneurysm can be determined by a cerebral angiogram. Radiopaque material (contrast medium) is injected into the arteries supplying the brain and fills the aneurysm sac, defining both its size and position (**FIGURE 25-20**).

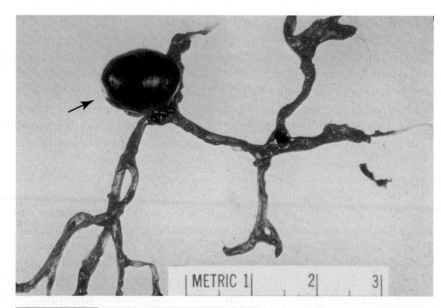

FIGURE 25-18 Dissection of vessels from the brain of a person with large congenital cerebral aneurysm.

Courtesy of Leonard V. Crowley, MD, Century College.

Treatment usually consists of occluding (closing off) the aneurysm by applying a small metal clip to the narrow neck of the sac at its attachment to the arterial wall. Another approach involves filling the aneurysm sac with coils of material to stop

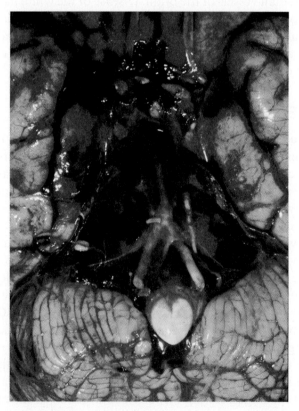

FIGURE 25-19 Undersurface of brain, illustrating subarachnoid hemorrhage secondary to ruptured cerebral aneurysm.

Courtesy of Leonard V. Crowley, MD, Century College.

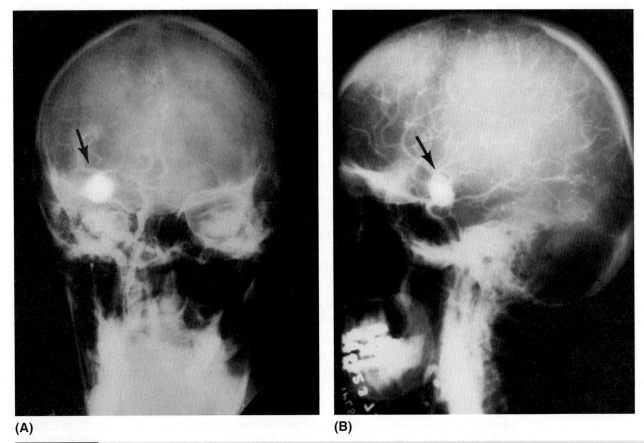

(A)　　　　　　　　　　　　　　　　　**(B)**

FIGURE 25-20　A cerebral aneurysm (*arrow*) demonstrated by an angiogram. **(A)** Front view. **(B)** Side view.
Courtesy of Leonard V. Crowley, MD, Century College.

blood from filling the aneurysm. To perform the coiling procedure, a catheter is inserted into the femoral artery, advanced through the aorta into the carotid artery, and then advanced to the base of the aneurysm. Then, multiple coils of material are passed through the catheter into the aneurysm to completely fill the aneurysm sac.

Infections of the Nervous System

Many different organisms can infect the nervous system, including bacteria, viruses, and fungi. An infection that predominantly affects the meninges surrounding the brain and spinal cord is called a **meningitis**. An infection of the brain tissue is called an **encephalitis**. If both brain and meninges are affected, the term meningoencephalitis is often used. An infection of the spinal cord is called a **myelitis**.

The manifestations of an infection of the central nervous system are those of any systemic infection: elevated temperature and other nonspecific symptoms. In addition, there are manifestations of meningeal irritation, consisting of a headache and a stiff neck. Involvement of brain tissue is associated with alteration of consciousness and neurologic symptoms resulting from dysfunction of localized areas within the brain.

Diagnosis of a central nervous system infection is established by examination of the spinal fluid, which contains a large number of leukocytes and an elevated protein concentration if infection is present. In bacterial infections, the leukocytes are primarily neutrophils, whereas lymphocytes predominate in viral infections. In bacterial and fungus infections, the organism responsible for the infection can often be identified in stained smears prepared from the spinal fluid and by culture of the spinal fluid.

Meningitis Inflammation of the meninges.

Encephalitis An inflammation of the brain.

Myelitis An inflammation of the spinal cord.

MENINGITIS CAUSED BY BACTERIA AND FUNGI

Two organisms are responsible for most cases of bacterial meningitis: the meningococcus (*Neisseria meningiditis*) and the pneumococcus (*Streptococcus pneumoniae*). Until recently, a third organism, *Haemophilus influenzae*, was a common cause of meningitis in children. Infants and children are now routinely immunized against this organism, so *Haemophilus influenzae* meningitis, as well as other infections caused by this organism, occur much less frequently than in the past.

The use of a vaccine that prevents many (but not all) strains of meningococcus has reduced the incidence of this disease in many parts of the world. Because meningococcal infections occur primarily in young adults and often become epidemic where people live in close quarters, such as college dormitories and army camps, mandatory vaccination for these individuals is becoming frequent. If an individual does develops meningococcal meningitis, people who have had close contact with the infected individual are treated with prophylactic antibiotics. In contrast, pneumococcal meningitis occurs sporadically in older adults, but it is not transmitted from person to person as is meningococcal meningitis. Consequently, people who have had contact with an individual who develops pneumococcal meningitis do not require antibiotic prophylaxis, and communitywide immunizations are not required. Other bacteria may occasionally cause meningitis, especially in neonates, where *E. coli* is a common causative agent, or in people whose immunologic defenses have been weakened by disease or immunosuppressive therapy or under conditions in which bacteria are introduced directly into the nervous system.

Bacterial meningitis is often preceded by a mild upper-respiratory infection, during which small numbers of bacteria gain access to the bloodstream. They are carried to the meninges, where they localize and initiate an acute infection (**FIGURE 25-21**). Occasionally, the pathogens may spread directly to the meninges from a sinus or

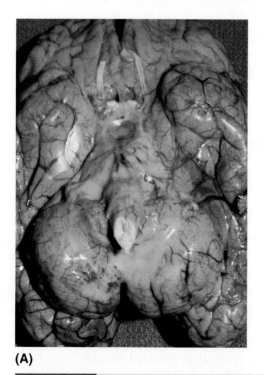

(A)

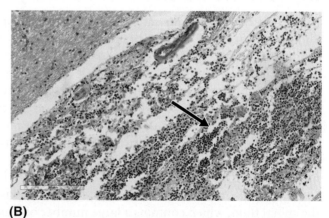

(B)

FIGURE 25-21 **(A)** Bacterial meningitis, illustrating purulent exudate in the meninges. Exudate is most noticeable over the pons (*middle*) and cerebellum. **(B)** Microscopic view of bacterial meningitis showing purulent exudate containing neutrophils (*arrow*) in the arachnoid space.

(A) Courtesy of Leonard V. Crowley, MD, Century College; (B) Courtesy of Department of Pathology and Laboratory Medicine, University of North Carolina at Chapel Hill.

middle-ear infection, or may be introduced into the nervous system directly from a serious head injury such as a gunshot wound or severe skull fracture.

Meningitis caused by the tubercle bacillus or pathogenic fungi is uncommon and tends to be chronic rather than acute. Both tuberculous meningitis and fungal meningitis result from the spread of organisms from a primary infection in the lung (see discussion on the respiratory system). Many cases of fungal meningitis develop in immunocompromised individuals. The most common type of fungal meningitis is caused by the *Cryptococcus neoformans* (see discussion on pathogenic microorganisms). Disease may also occur in immunocompetent individuals after exposure to excreta from birds who are a major host for the fungus. Several other fungal pathogens, including *Coccidiodes immitis* (found predominantly in the San Joaquin Valley of California and other locations in the Southwest), and *Histoplasma capsulatum* (found in areas surrounding the Mississippi basin) may occasionally result in pulmonary disease that spreads to the brain. Bacterial and fungal infections are treated with appropriate antibiotics.

VIRAL INFECTIONS

Many viruses can infect the nervous system, including rabies, the measles and mumps viruses, various intestinal and respiratory viruses (enteroviruses), the herpes simplex virus, cytomegalovirus, poliomyelitis virus, and an important group of viruses called arboviruses, which are zoonoses spread from an animal host in which the virus is transmitted to humans by insects.

Manifestations of Nervous System Virus Infection

A viral infection may affect either the meninges (meningitis) or the brain tissue (encephalitis). A viral infection restricted to the meninges is often called aseptic meningitis to distinguish it from suppurative (pus-producing) meningitis caused by pathogenic bacteria. The affected individual has an elevated temperature, headache, and a stiff neck but does not usually appear seriously ill and recovers completely. Viral encephalitis is a much more serious infection. Affected patients are often very sick and exhibit various neurologic disturbances, such as confusion, disorientation, coma, cranial nerve dysfunction, weakness, and paralysis. Some cases are fatal (such as rabies), and patients who recover may be left with some permanent neurologic disability. Unfortunately, there is no specific treatment for most cases of viral encephalitis. However, some antiviral drugs may be effective in herpes simplex encephalitis if administered early in the course of the disease (antiviral drugs are considered in the pathogenic microorganisms discussion).

Rabies

Rabies encephalitis is an invariably fatal disease caused by an RNA virus transmitted from infected animals to humans via virally contaminated saliva introduced in bites or other forms of contact. Currently, the few cases of rabies seen in the United States are a result of contact with rabid bats. Bat bites may be painless and hence the infected individual may be unaware of exposure. Although companion animals are routinely immunized, rabies is common in wild populations of wolves, foxes, skunks, and raccoons and may also occasionally occur in some domestic animals. Although fatal rabies is rare in the United States, it is endemic in many parts of the world with more than 50,000 annual deaths. The rabies virus is carried from the site of infection via peripheral nerves upward through the spinal cord and brain, resulting in destruction of the brain stem and generalized encephalopathy. The virus may take from ten days to several months to reach the brain, so symptoms may occur remote in time from the initial injury. Postexposure vaccination and treatment with hyperimmune antirabies globulin (from immune donors) is absolutely critical for survival because death is inevitable once symptoms occur. Individuals who have occupational exposure to potentially rabid animals, such as veterinarians, are preimmunized to the agent.

Arbovirus Infections

Arbovirus is responsible for many cases of meningitis and encephalitis. The viruses infect birds and animals as well as humans and are transmitted by mosquitoes. The term **arbovirus** is a contraction of the words **arthropod-borne virus**. Several different types of arboviral encephalitis are recognized, and they are named for the location where they were first characterized. In the United States, western equine encephalitis occurs primarily in the West, and eastern equine encephalitis in the eastern part of the county. As the names imply, the viruses also cause encephalitis in horses (*equus* = horse). Two other types of encephalitis, St. Louis encephalitis and California encephalitis, are not limited to the area implied by their names but are quite widely distributed. Encephalitis caused by various other arboviruses occur in other countries, but until recently "foreign" arbovirus infections were uncommon in the United States and Canada. Unfortunately, this situation changed with the arrival of the **West Nile virus** in the United States in 1999; the first case was identified in a person living in the New York City area. The virus also became established in many wild birds at about the same time. Zika virus, an arbovirus related to that causing West Nile and an Asiatic form of encephalitis is currently spreading through South, Central and limited areas of North America. Infection of pregnant women is associated with extremely serious defects in brain development in the fetus.

West Nile Virus Infections

Since the first U.S. case was identified in 1999, the virus has spread rapidly through the United States, as well as into Canada and Mexico, and has caused the largest outbreak of arbovirus infections ever recorded in the Western Hemisphere. The West Nile virus infects many species of wild birds, horses, and other animals, as well as people, and can be transmitted by many species of mosquitoes. The virus has also been transmitted by transfusion of blood from blood donors infected with the virus and by organ transplants. These routes of transmission are no longer possible because all blood collected for transfusion and all organ transplants are screened to exclude West Nile virus infections today. The virus also can be transmitted across the placenta from a pregnant, virus-infected mother to her infant and in breast milk from an infected mother to a nursing infant.

Although most people infected with West Nile virus have no symptoms of infection and develop immunity, about 20 percent of infected individuals develop a fever and neurologic manifestations that can vary from mild aseptic meningitis to severe and fatal encephalitis in about 1 percent or fewer cases. Some affected individuals have developed a poliomyelitis-like flaccid paralysis. No vaccine is available to immunize against the virus, and no antiviral therapy is available to treat the disease. However, simple precautions such as the use of insect repellents and protective clothing are effective barriers to mosquitoes.

POLIOMYELITIS

Poliomyelitis was formerly a very important and serious disease that caused much disability and many deaths. The virus enters the body through the gastrointestinal tract, localizing in the gray matter of the spinal cord and sometimes also in the cell bodies of cranial nerves in the brain stem. Destruction of motor neurons leads to

Arthropod-borne virus/ arbovirus An infectious nucleic acid particle (virus) transmitted by mosquitoes.

West Nile virus An arbovirus that infects birds, animals, and humans.

paralysis of the muscles supplied by the affected neurons. The name of the disease refers to the affinity of the virus for the gray matter of the spinal cord (*polios* = gray). Fortunately, widespread immunization has eliminated this disease in the developed countries of the world, and an extensive immunization effort directed toward people at risk in developing countries may soon lead to worldwide elimination of poliomyelitis. The disease may soon join smallpox as another disease that has been completely eradicated by an effective immunization program.

The Post-Polio Syndrome

Between 25 and 40 percent of individuals who survived paralytic poliomyelitis begin to experience slowly progressive muscular atrophy, weakness, and muscle fatigue, beginning many years after the original episode of acute poliomyelitis from which they had recovered. This late-onset muscle weakness and muscle atrophy have been called the post-polio syndrome. The weakness usually involves muscles or muscle groups that had been affected during the original bout of poliomyelitis and from which the individual had made a partial or apparent complete recovery. The exact cause of the post-polio syndrome is unknown. One likely explanation is that overuse of the reinnervated muscles, which compensated for the initial effects of the disease for many years, eventually caused the overworked neurons to fail, leading to weakness and atrophy of the involved muscles as they gradually lost their nerve supply. Unfortunately, no specific treatment can restore function to the muscles that have become weak and atrophic. A program of mild exercise that does not overstress the muscles may be helpful, and measures to improve pulmonary function may be required if respiratory muscles are affected.

NEUROLOGIC MANIFESTATIONS OF HUMAN IMMUNODEFICIENCY VIRUS INFECTIONS

The nervous system is often involved in people infected with the human immunodeficiency virus (HIV, described in the discussion on communicable diseases). Neurologic manifestations fall into three large categories: direct infections by virus, indirect infections by opportunistic pathogens, or AIDS-related tumors of the nervous system (discussed with tumors of the nervous system).

HIV-infected monocytes can transport the virus into the brain, where it can injure the nervous system. In some patients, the infection may be manifested as an acute viral meningitis occurring soon after the initial infection with the AIDS virus. In others, the infection causes a more chronic progressive degeneration of the brain with symptoms similar to those of Alzheimer disease (AIDS-related dementia or AIDS encephalopathy [*encephalon* = brain + *pathy* = disease]). Polyneuritis involving either cranial or spinal nerves also may occur in some patients as a result of infection by the virus. The immunosuppressive effect of AIDS is associated with infection by many of the opportunistic viruses, bacteria, fungi, and parasites, which can cause a primary infection of the nervous system. Some of the more common opportunistic infections are those caused by the herpes virus, cytomegalovirus, the fungus *Cryptococcus neoformans* (see discussion on pathogenic microorganisms), and the protozoan parasite *Toxoplasma gondii* (see discussion on animal parasites) (**FIGURE 25-22**).

MANIFESTATIONS OF PRION INFECTION

Prions (a contracted form of proteinaceous infectious particles) are abnormal forms of specific proteins. The infectious agent is unusually resistant to inactivation by heat or many disinfectants or ultraviolet light, but it can be destroyed by autoclaving or by household bleach. The normal form of the protein (the "good prion," designated PrP^C)

Prion A protein infectious particle responsible for Creutzfeldt-Jakob disease and some other degenerative diseases of the nervous system such as Kuru.

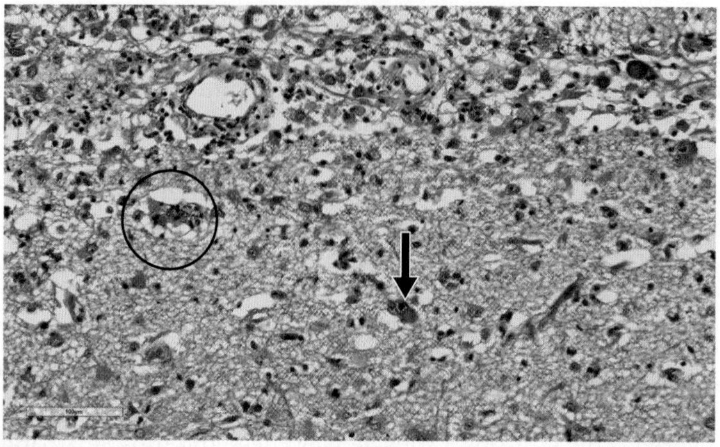

FIGURE 25-22 Cytomegalovirus encephalitis in an AIDS patient. Neural cell demonstrates characteristic "owl eye" nuclear viral inclusion of CMV virus (*arrow*). Multinucleated giant cell characteristic of AIDS virus encephalitis is also present (*circle*).

Courtesy of Department of Pathology and Laboratory Medicine, University of North Carolina at Chapel Hill.

is found in the cell membranes of neurons and in some other tissues. The abnormal form of the protein (the "bad prion," designated PrP^{SC}) is identical except for the way the protein is folded, which causes the protein to have a different configuration (conformation) when viewed in three dimensions. The abnormal prion is able to function as an infectious agent because of its ability to convert normal prions into abnormal forms (i.e., it acts like a catalyst). As progressively more prion proteins are converted into abnormal forms, a self-perpetuating chain reaction occurs as the newly formed abnormal prions convert more normal prions. As the abnormal prion proteins continue to accumulate, they disrupt the functions of the brain cells, which leads to the characteristic clinical and histologic manifestations of Creutzfeldt-Jakob (CJD) disease and several other uncommon conditions.

CREUTZFELDT-JAKOB DISEASE

Sporadic Creutzfeldt-Jakob disease accounts for about 75 percent of cases. The disease occurs in older adults by an unknown mechanism as the *PRNP* gene (which produces the PrP protein) shows no mutations. However, certain inherited variants (polymorphisms) of *PRNP* found in the population are associated with susceptibility to sporadic CJD. Sporadic CJD is found worldwide and is uncommon (about 1 case per million). Some cases of CJD have been **iatrogenic**, the result of the use of material derived from CJD patients (pituitary growth hormone or dura mater used in grafting procedures) or very rare surgical transmission. Careful monitoring and the use of recombinant growth hormone has eliminated this risk. Kuru, the first human prion disease to be characterized, was transmitted by ritual cannibalism practiced by the Fore people of New Guinea and is now extinct.

Inherited (familial) CJD is associated with mutations in *PRNP* located on the short arm of chromosome 20 and is responsible for 15 to 20 percent of cases. Although we do not yet know the function of the protein coded by the normal gene, we know that certain mutations of the gene are associated with a high probability of forming the abnormal prion protein that is responsible for Creutzfeldt-Jakob disease. Certain mutations in this protein are responsible for other rare prion-related diseases (fatal familial insomnia and Gerstmann-Sträussler-Scheinker disease).

Clinically, Creutzfeldt-Jakob disease is characterized by rapidly progressive mental deterioration (dementia) associated with neurologic disturbances in individuals

Iatrogenic Disease resulting from a medical intervention.

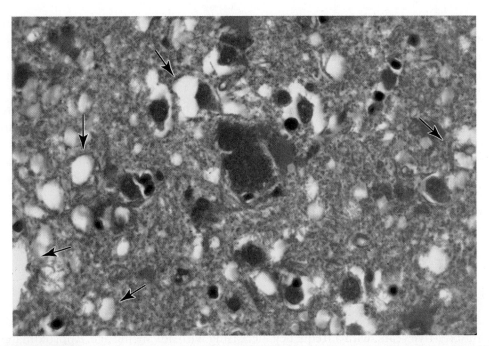

FIGURE 25-23 A photomicrograph of cerebral tissue from a patient with Creutzfeldt-Jakob disease illustrating multiple small vacuoles throughout the cortex (*arrows*) with loss of neurons and proliferation of astrocytes but no inflammatory reaction. The clump of eosinophilic material in the center of the photomicrograph is an aggregate of abnormal prion protein (original magnification ×400).

Courtesy of Leonard V. Crowley, MD, Century College.

with an average age of sixty-five. The disease is usually fatal within six months after the onset of symptoms. Histologically, the brains of affected individuals contain a large number of vacuoles within the neurons, which causes the affected brain tissue to have a spongy appearance, hence the disease is referred to as a spongiform encephalopathy. The affected neurons degenerate, and astrocytes proliferate in response to the neuron loss; however, there is no inflammatory reaction (**FIGURE 25-23**). Unfortunately, no treatment is available for this devastating disease.

MAD COW DISEASE

A somewhat similar prion disease occurs in animals and can be transmitted between animals of the same or in some cases different species by feeding animal tissues from infected animals to healthy animals. One such disease occurs in cattle. Bovine spongiform encephalopathy, or mad cow disease, is associated with a form of Creutzfeldt-Jakob disease (variant Creutzfeldt-Jakob disease vCJD) found in humans that is characterized by an earlier onset of illness (average age about twenty-five), a longer course, and a different clinical course (behavioral and sensory changes) from that of sporadic CJD.

In 1985, several dairy cows in the United Kingdom were diagnosed with bovine spongiform encephalopathy, or mad cow disease, because of the bizarre behavior of the infected animals. During subsequent years, the number of infected cows increased to more than 170,000. This epidemic was traced to cattle feed that had been mixed with protein-rich tissues obtained from sheep that had been infected with another prion disease, scrapie (as well as tissue from discarded sick cattle). After this feeding practice was discontinued, the frequency of the cattle disease declined. Use of animal tissues in animal feed is banned in both Britain and the United States today.

The disease in cattle was followed several years later by cases of vCJD. This variant disease was contracted from eating meat from infected cows, and many people were concerned that more cases would be found because there was a lag time between consumption of infected beef and onset of clinical manifestations. Such an increase in new cases has not materialized. A total of about 225 cases of vCJD were reported as of 2011, most of which were in the UK. Four cases have been reported in the United States. Two of the cases were associated with ingestion of infected beef in England; the other two cases were possibly related to the ingestion of infected beef from Saudi Arabia. There is some concern about possible transmission of a prion-based disease to humans from the ingestion of squirrels and from deer infected with prion-based cervid wasting disease, which is common is some parts of the United States, but there is no hard evidence for human transmission at present.

Other Diseases of the Nervous System

ALZHEIMER DISEASE

Alzheimer disease is a chronic progressive disease that primarily affects people older than sixty-five years, with a frequency increasing with advancing age. Approximately 1 percent of people between the ages of sixty and sixty-four have the disease, increasing to almost 40 percent in people older than age eighty-five. The disease is characterized by progressive failure of recent memory, followed by difficulties in thinking, reasoning, and judgment; it is often associated with emotional disturbances such as depression, anxiety, and irritability. Alzheimer disease is the most common cause of dementia in elderly people. The disease is preceded by about six years of declining cerebral function before Alzheimer disease is diagnosed. The course of the disease differs among individuals but usually is fatal in six to eight years, although some of those affected survive more than ten years. Currently about five million people suffer from Alzheimer disease in the United States. Most Alzheimer cases are sporadic, but 5 to 10 percent of cases are associated with inherited autosomal dominant disease.

The brains of affected patients exhibit progressive loss of neurons with atrophy of cerebral cortex and compensatory ventricular enlargement (hydrocephalus ex vacuo). Two characteristic histologic changes characterize the disease: neurofibrillary tangles and neuritic (senile or Aβ amyloid) plaques. Neurofibrillary tangles result from degenerative changes affecting the thin, delicate, wirelike neurofilaments located within the cytoplasm of the neurons. They become converted into thick, tangled, insoluble masses encircling the nuclei of nerve cells and are demonstrated by special stains containing silver compounds (**FIGURE 25-24A**). Neurofibrillary tangles are mostly composed of a protein termed tau, which in Alzheimer disease is hyperphosphorylated (i.e., has an excessive number of phosphorus groups added to it after it is synthesized). Tau is associated with the pathogenesis of Alzheimer disease but is also found in other degenerative neurological diseases (termed tauopathies).

Neuritic plaques are masses of broken, thickened, nerve filaments that stain intensely with silver-containing stains and that surround a core of acellular protein material, called amyloid protein, with distinct staining properties (**FIGURE 25-24B**). In general, there is a correlation between the degree of intellectual deterioration and the severity of the histopathologic changes. The brains of patients with advanced Alzheimer disease contain large numbers of neuritic plaques and neurofibrillary tangles, whereas those with mild disease have less striking changes.

The Aβ amyloid protein found in neuritic plaque is produced from a membrane protein of unknown function termed APP. APP is cleaved from cells by specific proteases following two different pathways, one of which results in the formation of Aβ

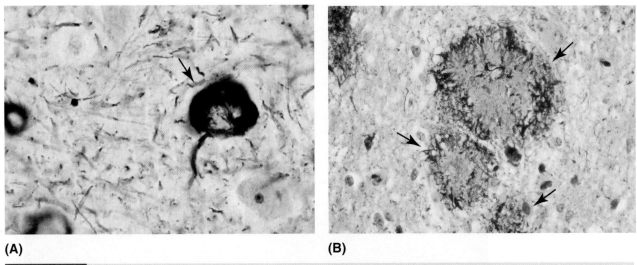

(A) **(B)**

FIGURE 25-24 Alzheimer disease. **(A)** Thickened neurofilaments encircle and obscure the nucleus of nerve cells (*arrow*), forming a neurofibrillary tangle (silver stain, original magnification ×400). **(B)** Three neuritic plaques (*arrows*) composed of broken masses of thickened neurofilaments (silver stain, original magnification ×100).

Courtesy of Leonard V. Crowley, MD, Century College.

amyloid (the amyloidgenic pathway). The other pathway produces a soluble protein that is not associated with disease (the nonamyloidgenic pathway). Familial forms of Alzheimer disease can result from mutations in the *APP* gene or the proteases that cleave the protein and further the amyloidgenic pathway. The *APP* protein gene is found on chromosome 21. People with Down syndrome have three chromosome 21s and produce a higher than normal level of APP. Early onset Alzheimer is extremely common in these individuals, presumably because of the excess of APP. The mechanism for production of Aβ amyloid protein and neuritic plaque in sporadic Alzheimer disease remains a mystery.

The diagnosis of Alzheimer disease is made by excluding other conditions that can impair brain function, such as chronic infections of the nervous system or multiple strokes. Recently specialized forms of MRI imaging and PET scans have become available that are highly predictive of the presence of the disease. Unfortunately, no specific treatment can arrest the relentless progression of the disease, although some drugs may be useful to improve cerebral function temporarily. One group of drugs (cholinesterase inhibitors) prolongs the activity of the acetylcholine in the brain by inhibiting the enzyme (cholinesterase) that breaks down acetylcholine, and other drugs may be helpful to improve the affected person's quality of life. A second drug (mematine), which inhibits a particular class of nerve cells in the brain that use glutamate to transmit impulses, has become available for treatment of moderate to severe Alzheimer. More drugs are being investigated, but no prevention or cure is yet available despite intensive research efforts.

MULTIPLE SCLEROSIS

Multiple sclerosis (MS) is a chronic progressive autoimmune disease characterized by the development of focal areas of degeneration of the myelin sheaths of the nerve fibers in the brain and spinal cord. The lesions develop in a random manner throughout the brain and spinal cord. The areas of demyelination eventually heal by forming masses of glial scar tissue (**FIGURE 25-25**). The name of the disease is derived from the characteristic multiple areas of involvement that heal by sclerosis (another name for scarring). The glial scarring in this disease is produced by a type of neuroglial cell called an **astrocyte** and differs somewhat from the usual fibrous scar produced by

Multiple sclerosis (MS) Chronic disease characterized by focal areas of demyelination in the central nervous system, followed by glial scarring.

Astrocyte A large stellate cell having highly branched processes. Forms the structural framework of the nervous system. One of the neuroglial cells.

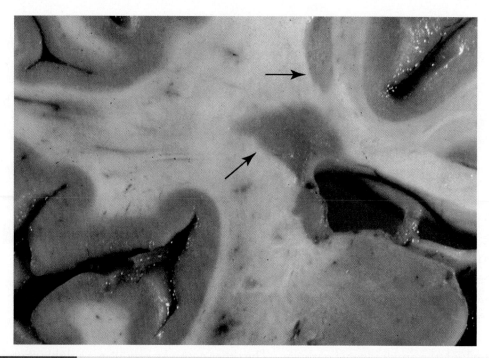

FIGURE 25-25 Coronal section of brain illustrating areas of glial scarring (*arrows*) adjacent to ventricle in multiple sclerosis. The demyelinated areas appear much darker than the adjacent normal white matter because of loss of myelin.

Courtesy of Leonard V. Crowley, MD, Century College.

connective tissue cells. The discrete areas of myelin loss with glial scarring are called multiple sclerosis plaques and are readily demonstrated within the nervous systems of affected individuals by means of magnetic resonance imaging (MRI, described in the discussion on general concepts of disease, principles of diagnosis). This diagnostic procedure is extremely useful for evaluating patients with neurologic disease in whom multiple sclerosis is suspected (**FIGURE 25-26**).

Multiple sclerosis is a disease of young adults. The onset of symptoms before the age of fifteen or after the age of forty is rare. Clinically, the disease is characterized by periodic episodes of acute neurologic disturbances, the nature depending on the location of the demyelination. Each episode is followed by a period of recovery and remission. The course of the disease is prolonged and quite unpredictable, with repeated acute episodes followed by remissions extending over many years. Eventually, the neurologic disabilities become permanent as a consequence of multiple areas of glial scarring, which impair conduction of nerve impulses in the brain and spinal cord. No specific treatment can arrest the progression of the disease. A number of measures, however, are available to relieve symptoms and minimize the neurologic disabilities. Corticosteroids and a variety of more potent anti-inflammatory and immunosuppressive agents are used to suppress the autoimmune response and to shorten the recovery from an acute episode.

Much evidence indicates that multiple sclerosis is an autoimmune disease, possibly initiated by a viral infection in a genetically predisposed individual that stimulates an abnormal immune response. Activated T lymphocytes and monocytes target myelin proteins and destroy the myelin insulation, and autoantibodies to myelin-related proteins are found in the cerebrospinal fluid.

Although at one time the incidence was thought to be low in tropical areas, and considerably higher in temperate zones, this theory is now questioned as some populations living at high latitudes do not have an increased incidence of MS. There

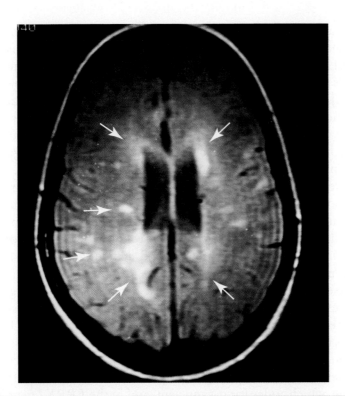

FIGURE 25-26 Multiple sclerosis demonstrated by MRI. The ventricular system is well demonstrated (*center*). Dense white areas adjacent to posterior horns of the ventricles and scattered throughout the brain lateral to the ventricles (*arrows*) are multiple sclerosis plaques.

Courtesy of Leonard V. Crowley, MD, Century College.

is a possible association with low vitamin D levels (as might occur at high latitudes) because high vitamin D levels are felt to be immunoprotective, but this remains speculative. There is also a genetic susceptibility to multiple sclerosis that appears to be related to multiple genes, including genes that code for the individual's HLA antigens. (The relationship of HLA antigens to disease susceptibility is presented in the immunology discussion.) As an example, a specific HLA antigen designated HLA-DRB1 is present in 60 percent of patients with multiple sclerosis but in only about 25 percent of those in a control group. The incidence of multiple sclerosis is higher than usual in people with a family history of the disease, probably because family members may share some of the same HLA and other susceptibility genes with the affected individual. Monozygotic twins show a 25-percent rate of concordance in having the disease, further supporting a role for genetics in susceptibility.

PARKINSON DISEASE

Parkinson disease, a chronic disabling disease that occurs in about 1 percent of individuals over sixty years of age, is characterized by rigidity of voluntary muscles and tremor of fingers and extremities resulting from a progressive loss of neurons in the substantia nigra of the midbrain. The axons of these neurons synapse with neurons in the basal ganglia, where they release the neurotransmitter dopamine, one of the important connections of the extrapyramidal motor system. As a result of the progressive neuron loss in the substantia nigra, fewer fibers are available to release dopamine in the basal ganglia, allowing the concentration of dopamine in the basal ganglia to fall. The muscular rigidity, increased muscle tone, and abnormal repetitive involuntary movements, which are common manifestations of the disease, result from the deranged function of the extrapyramidal system.

Parkinson disease
A chronic disease of the central nervous system characterized by rigidity and tremor, caused by deceased concentration of dopamine in the central nervous system.

As is the case with Alzheimer disease, an accumulation of abnormal proteins within neurons is a characteristic of Parkinson disease. For this reason, both Alzheimer and Parkinson diseases as well as Huntington disease and amyotrophic lateral sclerosis are sometimes termed **neurodegenerative proteinopathies**. Some would also include CJD in this group. In most cases, the cause of the particular disease is unknown (although there are uncommon inherited forms). There is some evidence that proteinopathies may show cell-to-cell transmission of the misfolded abnormal proteins, which act as "infectious agents" spreading within neural tissue of the disease host and leading to additional neuronal injury and death. Parkinson disease is characterized by the presence of **Lewy bodies**, damaged neurites containing intracellular inclusions that are rich in aggregates of α-synuclein, a neuronal protein of uncertain function. Although Parkinson disease starts in the dopaminergic neurons of the midbrain, the disease (as characterized by the presence of Lewy bodies) spreads with time to higher cortical areas and dementia begins to accompany the early motor symptoms.

In most cases, the cause of Parkinson disease is unknown although there is some evidence that exposure to pesticides and herbicides increase the risk of disease by 80 percent. The use of the illicit drug MPTP also leads to a specific loss of dopaminergic neurons because of damage to mitochondrial proteins in those cells, resulting in a disease essentially identical to Parkinson. About 10 percent of cases are genetic in origin and tend to occur in younger people with increased severity. Mutations in the *SNCA* gene, which codes for α-synuclein, and in the *LRRK2* gene, which results in increased autophagy of mitochondria in neurites and leads to changes in neurite structure, are both associated with autosomal dominant disease as are a number of additional gene mutations.

The manifestations of Parkinson disease can be relieved by a drug called L-dopa, which is converted within the brain into dopamine and raises the concentration of dopamine in the basal ganglia, thereby supplying the neurotransmitter that is deficient. Various other drugs also have been used successfully to control the manifestations of Parkinson disease, including a class of drugs called monoamine-oxidase-B (MAO-B) inhibitors. Drugs that potentiate the activity of dopamine (dopamine agonists) are also used. Drug therapy is usually successful for about five years. Some surgical procedures also are available to reduce the tremors associated with the disease when they are not controlled adequately by drugs. In such cases electrodes may be implanted into specific areas of the brain. Electrical stimulation of the electrodes (using an implanted electronic device often located at the collarbone) improves motor function and reduces tremors in the patient. This technique has supplanted previously used surgical destruction of selected brain areas.

Treatment, however, does not arrest the progressive neuron loss in the substantia nigra, nor does it stop the progression of the disease. Attempts to transplant dopamine producing cells into the brain of affected patients have largely been abandoned because these treatments had little effect. It is of interest that Lewy bodies were found in the engrafted normal tissue supporting cell-to-cell transmission of the disease.

HUNTINGTON DISEASE

This is an uncommon but relatively well-known hereditary autosomal dominant disease characterized by progressive mental deterioration associated with abnormal jerky and writhing movements. The first manifestations in affected individuals occur between thirty and fifty years of age. The disease progresses slowly and is usually fatal within fifteen to twenty years. Huntington disease causes progressive atrophy

Neurodegenerative proteinopathies General classification of diseases caused by misfolded abnormal proteins resulting in neural disease.

Lewy bodies Damanged neurites characteristic of Parkinson disease.

of groups of neurons called basal ganglia, which are located deep within the cerebral hemispheres. These structures are part of the extrapyramidal motor system, which regulates smooth and coordinated muscle movements, and damage to the system gives rise to the abnormal movements characteristic of the disease. The cerebral cortex is also affected, which eventually leads to dementia as the disease progresses. CT scans of affected patients demonstrate the cortical and basal ganglia atrophy characteristic of the disease.

The normal gene (*HD*) located on chromosome 4 contains from six to forty or more repeating groups of three nucleotides: cytosine, adenine, and guanine. These are called CAG triplet repeating sequences (coding for glutamine), or simply "repeats." People with Huntington disease have a larger number of repeats (generally thirty-six or more), and the greater the number, the earlier the onset of the disease. This is another disease in which an increased number of triplet repeats disrupts gene function and leads to disease (see discussion on congenital and hereditary diseases). As in the fragile X syndrome, the number of repeats increases during gametogenesis, so the number of repeating sequences in the gene transmitted to the child may be greater than the number in the parent's gene, depending on which parent transmits the gene. In Huntington disease, however, the expansion of triplet repeats increases during spermatogenesis (rather than during oogenesis, as occurs in the fragile X syndrome), so the gene with expanded repeats comes from the affected father instead of the mother.

Although there is no way to arrest the progression of the disease, drugs are available to help control some of its manifestations. Children of people with Huntington disease are offered genetic counseling and should be advised that they can be tested to determine whether they carry the abnormal gene. However, not all of the children of affected individuals want this information. Some prefer living with an uncertain future rather than being tested and possibly learning that they carry the abnormal gene and are destined to acquire the disease.

Spinocerebellar Degenerative Disease

A group of more than twenty-five diseases of genetic origin result in symptoms of cerebellar disturbance (ataxia, loss of control of body movements) as well as deficits in sensory and motor function as a result of neuronal death in corticospinal tracts and peripheral nerves. The **spinocerebellar ataxias (SCA)**, which are given numeric designations (SCA1, SCA2, etc.), have different modes of inheritance as well as different patterns of neuronal damage. Most SCAs are first noted in early middle age and result in a gradual loss of control of body movement over a period of years. The most common SCA, affecting 1 to 2 per 100,000 people, is **Freidreich ataxia (FA)**, which is distinctive in that it has an autosomal recessive pattern of inheritance of an excess of trinucleotide (GAA) repeats in the *frataxan* gene, resulting in a decrease in levels of this mitochondrial protein. Alleles that result in disease generally have between 600 and 900 repeats (normal alleles have 30 or fewer). Characteristically, FA becomes evident at about thirteen years of age and is followed by loss of the ability to move over the next fifteen years. Most individuals die by age forty-five.

> Spinocerebellar ataxia (SCA) Cerebellar disturbances resulting in loss of control of body movements. Most common is Freidreich ataxia.

Motor Neuron Degenerative Disease (ALS)

One of the best known of the neuronal degenerative diseases is amyotrophic lateral sclerosis, better known as Lou Gehrig disease. The disease affects both upper motor neurons projecting into the corticospinal tracts and the lower motor neurons in the brain stem and spinal cord. The loss of lower motor neuron function leads to weakness and eventual flaccid paralysis of muscles. The degeneration of the cortical neurons is followed by secondary degeneration of the corticospinal tracts that descend to synapse with the lower motor neurons in the spinal cord. The disease is relentlessly progressive with muscle atrophy and contractions leading to total disability (often without loss of intellectual capacity). Death results from respiratory failure often two to three years after diagnosis. About 10 percent of ALS cases are clearly familial and at least 10 percent of sporadic cases carry a mutation. Mutations in at least nine genes have been associated with inherited ALS. The most common mutated gene (*C9orf72*) results in the formation of RNA foci in neurons that are transcribed into abnormal polypeptides. Many of the mutations result in the formation of abnormal protein aggregates in neurons and also may result in abnormal RNA processing. The disease may be characterized as a proteinopathy, but the reason for neuronal death is uncertain.

Tumors of the Nervous System

Tumors of the nervous system may arise from three sites: peripheral nerves, meninges, or in the cells of the brain and spinal cord. In addition, the brain is a common location for metastases that arise from malignancies in other organs. Metastatic tumors of the CNS are considerably more frequent than primary tumors.

PERIPHERAL NERVE TUMORS

Tumors of peripheral nerves, cranial nerves, and spinal roots derive from the Schwann cells that invest the nerve fibers and are called **Schwannomas**. These tumors may be solitary or multiple, benign or (rarely) malignant. Most form discrete, well-circumscribed nodules attached to larger nerve trunks and usually can be dissected easily from the adjacent nerve (see discussion on neoplastic disease).

Sometimes a Schwannoma arises from one of the cranial nerves at the base of the brain or from one of the spinal nerves within the spinal canal. A tumor in either of these locations is much more difficult to remove. One of the more common locations for an intracerebral neuroma is the vestibulocochlear nerve (cranial nerve VIII), which is often called by its older name of acoustic nerve. The tumor arising from this nerve is usually called an acoustic Schwannoma. Frequently, the tumor compresses the adjacent brain and the nearby cranial nerves as it grows and may also erode the adjacent temporal bone. Clinically, the tumor causes ringing in the ear (tinnitus) on the affected side. Compression of the nerve causes partial hearing loss on the affected side, and symptoms related to pressure on the adjacent cranial nerves and the brain stem also may be present. Although the tumor is benign, its inaccessibility makes surgical removal difficult.

Neurofibromas are distinct from Schwannomas in that they contain neoplastic Schwann cells, fibroblasts, and other neural associated cells. Multiple neurofibromas are associated with the autosomal dominant disease neurofibromatosis type 1 (NF-1) or **von Recklinghausen disease**. These tumors can be disfiguring and become a malignant neurofibrosarcoma about 5 percent of the time. Multiple café au lait spots, light brown pigment patches on the skin, occur in almost all affected individuals. There is no specific treatment for this disease. Large tumors that encroach on vital organs or are cosmetically disfiguring must be removed surgically. A Schwann cell sarcoma is treated by wide surgical excision, in the same way as is any malignant tumor. Single neurofibomas that occur sporadically are not related to NF-1 and do not become sarcomatous.

Schwannomas Tumor of peripheral nerves deriving from the Schwann cells.

Neurofibromas Tumors that contain neoplastic Schwann cells and other cells; von Recklinghausen disease is an example.

TUMORS OF THE BRAIN

Primary brain tumors may arise from the meninges, from the glial supporting tissues of the brain, from the cells lining the ventricular system, or (rarely) from other tissues such as the blood vessels within the brain. Schwannomas may also arise from the cranial nerves. Tumors do not develop from neurons because adult nerve cells are no longer capable of cell division.

A tumor of meninges is called a **meningioma**. This is a well-circumscribed benign tumor arising from cells in the middle layer of the arachnoid and is firmly adherent to the dura. The tumor causes symptoms as a result of compression of the underlying brain and can be removed successfully if it is located in an accessible location because the tumors are not invasive. The tumors have a distinctive whorled or lamellar pattern when microscopically examined (**FIGURE 25-27**).

Any tumor of neuroglial origin is called a **glioma**. These tumors are further classified according to the type of glial supporting cell from which the neoplasm arises. The most common type arises from astrocytes (**astrocytoma**). A special name, glioblastoma multiforme, is applied to a highly undifferentiated, rapidly growing astrocytoma (**FIGURE 25-28**). The name describes the primitive appearance of the neoplastic astrocytes (*blast* = primitive cell) and their great variability in shape and appearance (*multiform* = having many shapes). Gliomas arise less frequently from other supporting cells. Most astrocytomas are diffuse; they are highly malignant and readily infiltrate the brain tissue. Because they cannot be totally removed surgically, treatment combines radio- and chemotherapy, and prolonged survival is rare. Circumscribed astrocytomas are generally found in young patients and are expansile but do not invade the body of the brain. They often can be totally resected and, if so, have a good prognosis. Oligodendromas arise from oligodendrocytes. Like most astrocytomas they are highly invasive, but prognosis is much better for patients with this type of tumor.

Two other types of tumors are often considered along with the gliomas. One is an uncommon malignant tumor arising from primitive cells in the cerebellum of young children (medulloblastoma). The tumor is malignant but also extremely radiation sensitive. The second is a tumor arising from the cells lining the ventricular system. These cells are called ependymal cells, and the tumor is called an ependymoma. Although some tumors can be totally resected, the tumors may spread broadly through the CSF.

Primary lymphomas also may arise within the central nervous system and are relatively common in patients who are immunosuppressed, posttransplantation, or

Meningioma A benign tumor arising from the meninges.

Glioma Any brain tumor arising from glial (supporting) cells of the brain.

Astrocytoma Neuroglial tumor arising from astrocytes; most common type.

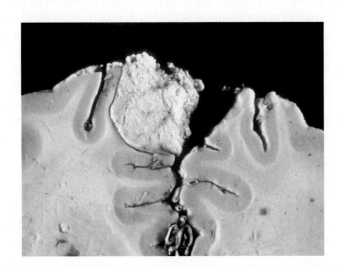

FIGURE 25-27 Meningioma arising from the dura, with displacement but no infiltration of the brain.

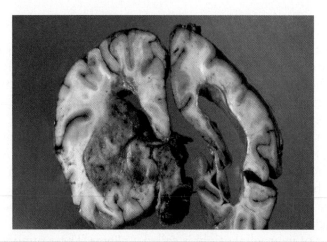

FIGURE 25-28 Glioblastoma. A large pink, tan, and hemorrhagic mass is infiltrating the left side of the brain. It is displacing the midline to the right and impeding the outflow of the ventricle. The right ventricle is greatly dilated, and the remainder of the tissue on the right is markedly atrophic due to the resultant hydrocephalus.

have an AIDS infection. These tumors do not often spread outside the nervous system. Interestingly, lymphomas arising outside the CNS generally do not invade the body of the brain but may be found in the CSF.

Primary central nervous system tumors do not normally spread outside the nervous system, but many carry a poor prognosis because they often lie deep within the brain and are infiltrative. Treatment consists of surgical resection of as much of the tumor as possible. In selected cases, surgery is followed by radiation and sometimes by anticancer chemotherapy as well.

The symptoms of a brain tumor depend on the size and location of the neoplasm. Headache is a common initial manifestation because the increased volume within the cranial cavity caused by the tumor raises the intracranial pressure. Growth of the tumor also disrupts nerve cells and fiber tracts within the brain, leading to various neurologic disturbances including seizures.

Peripheral Nerve Disorders

Demyelinating neuropathy Axon sparing demyelinating disease.

Polyneuropathies An inflammation of multiple nerves.

Peripheral nerves and nerve roots may develop **demyelinating neuropathies** in which the axon is spared (much as is the case in demyelinating disease of the CNS). In such cases remyelination will occur to some degree as Schwann cells (and their precursors) proliferate. Neuronopathies affect the nerve body itself and result in varying degrees of secondary axon degeneration. Clinical manifestations depend on the degree of nerve degeneration and on which nerves are affected. Involvement of a single nerve is usually secondary to injury or external compression. Involvement of multiple nerves, called **polyneuropathies** or sometimes peripheral neuritis, is usually a manifestation of any of a large number of systemic diseases of inflammatory, infectious, or other etiologies.

POLYNEUROPATHIES (PERIPHERAL NEURITIS)

Polyneuropathy, also called peripheral neuritis, is characterized by progressive muscular weakness, numbness and tingling, tenderness, and pain in the parts of the body supplied by the peripheral nerves (called the distribution of the nerves). Often, the muscles supplied by the involved nerves also exhibit some degree of atrophy. Usually, the neural damage is axonal and the weakness and sensory disturbances affect the distal parts of the limbs, whereas strength and sensation remain relatively normal in the proximal parts of the extremities. This "glove and stocking" pattern of sensory and motor dysfunction is quite characteristic of polyneuritis. Most cases result from systemic diseases such as long-standing diabetes or autoimmune diseases or from occupational exposure to toxic drugs, heavy metals, or industrial compounds. Alcoholism is another common cause of peripheral neuritis, which is probably related to a coexisting deficiency of B vitamins. Treatment of the underlying disease may produce some symptomatic improvement.

GUILLAIN-BARRÉ SYNDROME

A special type of autoimmune inflammatory demyelinating polyneuropathy with characteristic clinical manifestations is the Guillain-Barré syndrome. The disease is characterized by widespread patchy demyelination of nerves and nerve roots with mild inflammatory changes and sometimes by axon degeneration as well. Onset is usually a few weeks after a mild influenza-like respiratory or other infection or (much less frequently) following immunizations. The illness appears to be a type of autoimmune reaction to myelin or other neuronal components that is triggered by the preceding infection or immunization.

Clinically, the disease is characterized by muscular weakness that usually begins in the legs and often spreads rapidly to affect the muscles of the trunk and upper extremities. Sensory disturbances are infrequent. Severe respiratory distress may occur if the nerves supplying the intercostal muscles are involved. The muscular weakness generally progresses for one to two weeks, remains stationary for a time, and then gradually improves. The patient usually recovers rapidly if the nerve injury is limited to demyelination. However, several percent of patients will die of respiratory and cardiac failure even with supportive care; many who survive will suffer some degree of long-term disability. Replacement of patient plasma (plasmapheresis) may be beneficial because it removes damaging autoantibodies. Intravenous immunoglobulin, thought to have an anti-inflammatory effect, is also used in therapy.

PERIPHERAL NERVE INJURY

A peripheral nerve may be damaged in association with a deep laceration, a fracture, or a crushing injury. A common cause of a more chronic type of nerve injury is external compression by a fibrous band or ligament. This condition is often called a nerve-entrapment neuropathy. The median nerve that supplies sensory and motor fibers to the hand is often involved in a condition called carpal tunnel syndrome. The nerve is usually compressed on the anterior surface of the wrist, within the confined space between the wrist bones and the overlying ligaments that cross the wrist joint and stabilize the positions of the flexor tendons. The nerve compression causes pain and paresthesias (abnormal sensations such as burning, numbness, and tingling) in the index and middle fingers, together with decreased sensation in the part of the hand supplied by the nerve. The small muscles of the hand at the base of the thumb, which are supplied by the nerve, may also undergo atrophy. Sometimes symptoms can be relieved by conservative measures such as injecting a corticosteroid mixed with a local anesthetic into the confined space (called the carpal tunnel) in which the nerve is compressed. In many cases, however, it is necessary to relieve the compression surgically by resecting the part of the ligament that compresses the nerve.

Guillain-Barré syndrome A type of polyneuritis resulting from an autoimmune reaction to myelin.

Carpal tunnel syndrome Condition resulting from nerves in the hand being compressed on the anterior surface of the wrist.

Paresthesia An abnormal sensation, such as burning, prickling, or numbness.

CASE 25-1

Estrella, an eighteen-month-old female child who lives in a small North Carolina town, is the only child in the family. Estrella's mother states she was born at home in the United States but no documentation is available. Her parents are undocumented Mexican agricultural workers who also do home cleaning and repairs during the winter. Although Estrella has apparently not received pediatric medical care, her mother states that in the past she has always eaten well and been healthy. Estrella has been brought to a community free medical clinic by her parents. Her mother states that on the previous day Estrella was irritable and turned away from bright light (had photophobia). She was unwilling to eat, vomited, and felt very warm. This morning Estrella had a convulsion and became lethargic (did not move much). Her parents became very concerned, prompting the visit to the clinic. The clinic was staffed by a physician's assistant (PA), Jill.

Jill notes that Estrella's height and weight are age appropriate, but her developmental stage is difficult to assess as she is in distress and poorly responsive. On examination, Jill noted that the child was lethargic but could be aroused. She had a fever of 103° F. She cried when her head was turned and appeared to have a stiff neck (nuchal rigidity). Although the "soft spot" on her skull (anterior fontanelle) was almost closed, there appeared to be some bulging of the brain tissue. Jill thought a petechial rash consisting of pinpointlike purple spots was beginning to appear. Jill is concerned about possible signs of a neurological disease (and specifically bacterial meningitis; infection of the meningeal layer of the brain), and these concerns are exacerbated by Estrella's socioeconomic background. To confirm Jill's suspicion, a lumbar puncture was required. Jill was inexperienced (and there are some risks to the patient), so the test was deferred until Estrella could be transferred to the pediatric infectious disease division of a regional hospital.

At the hospital, CSF obtained by lumbar puncture had elevated protein, reduced glucose, and neutrophils were detected (15 cells per microliter of CSF). Estrella also had an elevated neutrophil count in her blood. The gram-negative diplococcus detected in her CSF was determined to be *Neisseria meningitides*, confirming a diagnosis of neisserial meningitis. Estrella was admitted to the pediatric ICU where she demonstrated signs of shock and was given IV fluids. She was immediately started on IV antibiotics (initially vancomycin and cefotaxime), which were continued for ten days, after which she was discharged. Estrella's household contacts (parents) and children in her nursery were treated with prophylactic antibiotics.

Discussion

The classic symptoms of bacterial meningitis are demonstrated in the case; fever, meningeal signs (neck rigidity), bulging fontanelle, photophobia, convulsions, and (had Estrella been able to express herself) undoubtedly headache. Examination of the CSF demonstrated the signs of bacterial meningitis, reduced glucose (said to be related to bacterial consumption), and increased protein (as a result of acute inflammatory changes in the meningeal vasculature). In addition, an elevated blood neutrophil count was indicative of bacterial infection. Detection of gram-negative diplococci in the CSF (and subsequent confirmation by culture) confirmed the organism to be Neisseria, which tends to cause a very rapidly progressive (and potentially lethal) disease. The bacteria colonizes the respiratory system but can spread via the blood in nonimmune individuals. A bacterial endotoxin can result in DIC (see discussion in abnormalities of blood coagulation), a disastrous complication with a very high likelihood of death (or disability if the patient survives). The petechial rash is an indicator of DIC that results from platelet consumption, activation of the coagulation system, and capillary bleeding. Luckily for Estrella, the rash noted by Jill was not related to the disease. Rapid antibiotic therapy is life-saving, and the disease can be spread to contacts

CASE 25-1 (Continued)

(hence, the use of prophylactic antibiotics in contacts). A vaccine is available but not generally used as it has limited effectiveness in young children and is effective only against certain Neisserial strains. The vaccine is used in certain epidemic areas and in individuals who are housed in crowded circumstances (such as students in college dormitories) where it may be required. Another bacterial meningitis caused by *Haemophilus influenzae* group B (HiB) was formerly quite common in children under the age of five. Incidence of this infection has sharply declined because of highly effective nearly universal childhood vaccination. Jill was concerned because she felt it unlikely that Estrella had been vaccinated for this bacteria (and she suspected it might be the causative agent).

Etiology and Pathogenesis

Bacterial infection with *Neisseria meningitides* and subsequent meningitis.

Questions

1. Jill had several specific concerns about Estrella's disease based on socioeconomic background. How would those concerns affect a potential diagnosis?

2. Jill's parents were agricultural (field) workers who lived in substandard housing. What additional etiologies might be suggested in an acutely sick child who came from such a background?

3. Assume that Estrella did, in fact, demonstrate DIC. What additional symptoms would she demonstrate? What laboratory tests might have been used to detect and monitor for DIC?

4. Under what circumstances might it be reasonable to require HiB immunization? Have you personally been immunized, and if so, why?

5. Several simple clinical tests can be used to demonstrate signs of meningeal disease. What are they, and how are they performed? (*Hint:* investigate Brudzinski's sign.)

QUESTIONS FOR REVIEW

1. Briefly describe the organization of the central nervous system. Describe the function and circulation of cerebrospinal fluid. What is meant by the following terms: *upper motor neuron lesion*, *lower motor neuron lesion*, *flaccid paralysis*, and *spastic paralysis*?

2. What are some of the possible effects of a severe blow to the head?

3. What is a stroke? What are the common causes of a stroke? What is a congenital aneurysm of the circle of Willis?

4. What are the common causes of hydrocephalus? How does a brain tumor cause hydrocephalus?

5. What is a neural tube defect? How can it be recognized before birth?

6. What is meant by the following terms: *arachnoid*, *subdural hemorrhage*, *anencephaly*, and *meningioma*?

7. What is a transient ischemic attack? How is it treated?

8. Describe the common tumors of the nervous system. What are their clinical manifestations?

9. What is the difference between a polyneuritis (peripheral neuritis) and Guillain Barré syndrome?

10. Compare Creutzfeldt-Jakob disease and Alzheimer disease.

SUPPLEMENTARY READINGS

Moini, J., Chapter 9, "Nervous System." 2012. In *Anatomy and Physiology for Health Professionals*. Burlington MA: Jones & Bartlett Learning.

Loeffler, A. G., and Hart, M. N., Chapter 23, "Central Nervous System." 2015. In *Introduction to Human Disease: Pathophysiology for Health Professionals*. 6th ed. Burlington MA: Jones & Bartlett Learning.

Fuller, G. N., Goodman, J. C., and Bouldin, T. W., Chapter 28, "The Nervous System." 2014. In *Essentials of Rubin's Pathology*, 6th ed., edited by E. Rubin and H. M. Reisner. Philadelphia, PA: Wolters Kluwer Lippincott.

▶ The area of neurobiology is complex and no one text can do it justice. The first entry presents additional structural details of the nervous system in general and the CNS specifically. The illustrations are excellent. The second selection contains further information on the pathology of CNS disease. The third entry is a standard reference for the pathology of human organ systems written at a level appropriate for undergraduate medical school students. The chapter on the nervous system presents a more detailed view of the pathology of neurological disease.

Copp, A. J., and Greene, N. D. E. 2013. Neural tube defects—Disorders of neurulation and related embryonic processes. *Wiley Interdisciplinary Reviews: Developmental Biology* 2:213–27.

Chitayat, D., et al. 2015. Folic acid supplementation for pregnant women and those planning pregnancy—2015 update. *Journal of Clinical Pharmacology* (ePub November 5).

▶ The first article provides additional details of the process of neurulation and defects that lead to open neural tubes. The article is strong on descriptions of animal models of human disease. The second article is a recent update on the role of folic acid supplementation in the prevention of neural tube defects.

Brown, P. B., et al. 2012. Iatrogenic Creutzfeldt-Jakob disease, final assessment. *Emerging Infectious Diseases* 18:901.

Head, M. W. 2013. Human prion disease: Molecular cellular and population biology. *Neuropathology* 33:221–36.

Lee, J., et al. 2015. Review: Laboratory diagnosis and surveillance of Creutzfeldt-Jakob disease. *Journal of Medical Virology* 87:175–86.

▶ Taken together these three readings provide a current overview of the state of knowledge of prion-based disease (Creutzfeldt-Jakob and variant Creutzfeldt-Jakob disease in particular). Although not a topic of current public concern, careful surveillance (as noted in the third entry) is still a major public health necessity.

Centers for Disease Control and Prevention. *Stroke*. http://www.cdc.gov/stroke

American Heart Association. *Stroke*. http://www.heart.org/HEARTORG/CPRAandECC/HealthcareTraining/Stroke_UCM_001284_SubHomePage.jsp
> ▶ The CDC entry is a useful portal to a large source of material on stroke risk and prevention. An excellent starting point for additional detailed information. The American Heart Association provides a continuing education course designed for in and out of hospital personnel, but it is also a highly useful guide to the diagnosis and rapid therapy of stroke.

Beadell, N. C., Bazan, T., and Lutsep, H. 2015. The year embolectomy won: A review of five trials assessing the efficacy of mechanical intervention in acute stroke. *Current Cardiology Reports* 17:102–12.
> ▶ An interesting review of therapy for stroke comparing drug and surgical/endarterial approaches.

Alzheimer Disease

Reitz, C., and Mayeux, R. 2014. Alzheimer disease: Epidemiological, diagnostic criteria, risk factors and biomarkers. *Biochemical Pharmacology* 88:640–51.

Risacher, S. L., and Saykin, A. J. 2013. Neuroimaging biomarkers of neurodegenerative diseases and dementia. *Seminars in Neurology* 33:386–416.
> ▶ The second reading on Alzheimer disease discusses new diagnostic modalities using neuroimaging applicable to Alzheimer as well as other neurodegenerative conditions.

Parkinson Disease

Irwin, D. J., Lee, VM-Y., and Trojanski, J. Q. 2013. Parkinson's disease dementia: Convergence of alpha-synuclein, tau and amyloid-beta pathologies. *Nature* 14:628.

Lashuel, H. A., Overk, C. R., Queslati, A., and Masliah, E. 2013. The many faces of alpha-synuclein: From structure and toxicity to therapeutic target. *Nature* 14:38.

Huntington Disease

Ross, C. A., Aylward, E. H., Wild, E. J., et al. 2014. Huntington disease: Natural history, biomarkers and prospects for therapeutics. *Nature* 10:204.

Bordelon, Y. M. 2013. Clinical neurogenetics: Huntington disease. *Neurologic Clinics* 31:1085–94.

Multiple Sclerosis

Ellwardt, E., and Zipp, F. 2014. Molecular mechanisms linking neuroinflammation and neurodegeneration in MS. *Experimental Neurology* 262:8–17.

Amyotrophic Lateral Sclerosis

Robberecht, W., and Philips, T. 2013. The changing scene of amyotrophic lateral sclerosis. *Nature* 14:248–64.

Renton, A. E., Chio, A., and Traynor, B. J. 2014. State of play in amyotrophic lateral sclerosis genetics. *Nature Neuroscience* 17(1):17–23.

Freidreich Ataxia

Gonzalez Cabo, P., and Palau, F. 2013. Mitochondrial pathophysiology in Friedreich's ataxia. *Journal of Neurochemistry* 126(suppl. 1):53–64.
> ▶ The previous sets of readings on specific diseases highlight recent advances in the pathophysiology of degenerative neural disease. Many of the reviews highlight the role of proteinopathies in the pathogenesis of degeneration.

Weiss, T., Weller, M., and Roth, P. 2015. Immunotherapy for glioblastoma: Concepts and challenges. *Current Opinion* 6:639–46.

Levin, V. A., Tonge, R. J., Gallo, J. M., et al. 2015. CNS Anticancer Drug Discovery and Development Conference White Paper. *Neuro-Oncology* 17(suppl. 6):vi1–vi26.
> ▶ These two readings review the current state of the art in the treatment of brain cancer.

Muller, M. L., et al. *Pediatric Bacterial Meningitis*. http://emedicine.medscape.com/article/961497_overview
> ▶ A useful review that was used in the Case construction.

The Musculoskeletal System

LEARNING OBJECTIVES

1. Describe the maturation process of bone.
2. Describe the process of bone remodeling.
3. List the major types of arthritis. Describe their pathogenesis and clinical manifestations, and explain the methods of treatment.
4. Describe the metabolic problems leading to gout.
5. Describe the process that occurs to repair a bone fracture.
6. Describe the causes and effects of osteoporosis, and name the methods of treatment.

7. Describe the manifestations, complications, and treatment of scoliosis.
8. Describe the structure of the intervertebral disks, and explain their function. Describe the clinical manifestations of a herniated disk.
9. Compare the pathogenesis and clinical manifestations of muscular atrophy and muscular dystrophy. Name and describe the common types of each.
10. Describe the pathogenesis, manifestations, and treatment of myasthenia gravis.

Structure and Function of the Skeletal System

The skeleton is the rigid supporting structure of the body with all bones having the same basic structure. Bones are composed of an outer layer of compact bone (**cortical bone**) and an inner, spongy layer of bone (**cancellous bone**) arranged in a loose, meshed latticework of thin strands called bone **trabeculae**. The spaces between the trabeculae contain the bone marrow, which consists of fat and blood-forming tissue. Cortical bone provides for mechanical strength and makes up the majority of the skeleton. Cancellous bone contains a high number of bone cells and is responsible for changes in bone growth and structure.

Individual bones vary in size and appearance. They may be long, short, flat, or irregular in shape. The typical long bone, such as is found in the upper and lower limbs, has a tubular shape with expanded ends. The shaft is the long cylindrical part, and the expanded ends of the shaft are called the **epiphyses**. The center of the shaft is hollowed out to form the marrow cavity, which is filled with fat and bone marrow. This type of construction provides considerable strength without excessive weight. The parts of a typical long bone are referred to by specific terms. The ends of the bone, which are in contact with (articulate with) other bones, are the epiphysis, which extends from the cartilage component of the joint (articular cartilage) to the

Cortical bone Outer layer of compact bone.

Cancellous bone Inner, spongy layer of bone.

Trabeculae Thin strands of bone lattice work.

Epiphyses The end part of a long bone, initially growing separately from the shaft.

epiphyseal plate (composed of cartilage in children and critical to the ossification of and growth in length of the long bones). The **diaphysis** is the elongated central region of the shaft of the bone that blends into the more fluted region below the epiphyseal plate, the **metaphysis**. The metaphysis contains the cancellous bone and the active bone marrow (**FIGURE 26-1**and **FIGURE 26-2**).

Bone, a specialized type of connective tissue composed of a dense connective tissue framework composed mostly of type I collagen, becomes impregnated with calcium phosphate salts (hydroxyapatite) along with smaller amounts of calcium carbonate and other minerals. Calcium salts in bone and calcium ions in the blood and body fluid are continuously interchanged. Three different types of cells are found in bone: **osteoblasts**, **osteocytes**, and **osteoclasts**. Osteoblasts are the active bone-forming cells that produce the collagenous bone matrix. They secrete an enzyme, alkaline phosphatase, that promotes deposition of calcium phosphate salts in the bone matrix

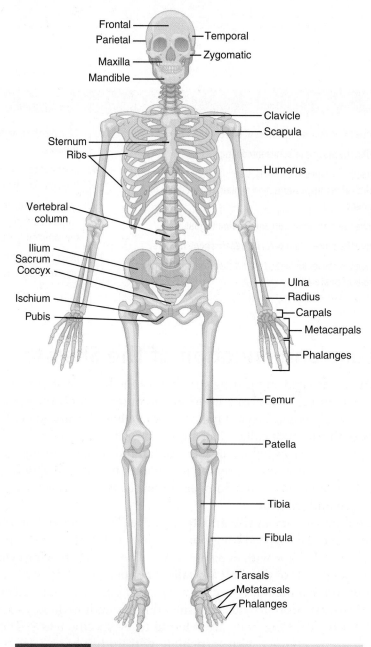

FIGURE 26-1 Major bones and joints of the body.

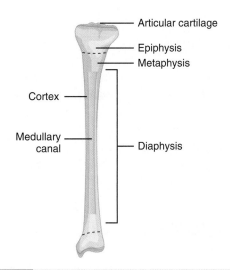

FIGURE 26-2 Structure of a long bone. The tibia is illustrated here.

to calcify the bone. As the bone matrix is formed and calcified, the osteoblasts become incorporated within the bone and become transformed into relatively inactive mature bone cells called osteocytes. Osteoclasts, multinucleated cells related to macrophages, are concerned with bone resorption. They remove the bone matrix by phagocytosis, dissolve the bone salts, and release the calcium and phosphate ions into the circulation (**FIGURE 26-3**).

In general, the strength and thickness of the bones depend on the activities of the individual. A person accustomed to strenuous physical labor has thicker, heavier bones than one who is normally engaged in light, sedentary activities. If an extremity is immobilized and is not allowed to bear weight, as after a fracture, the immobilized bone undergoes significant thinning and decalcification, called **disuse atrophy**.

The bones of the skeleton are connected by joints. Synovial joints are moveable whereas synarthroses are relatively fixed. In fibrous fixed joints (a **syndesmosis**) such as occurs between the bones of the skull, the bones are firmly joined by fibrous tissue to form a firm union called a suture line. In a cartilaginous joint (a **synchondrosis**),

Disuse atrophy Thinning and decalcification of bone due to lack of weight-bearing.

Syndesmosis A fixed joint joined by fibrous connective tissue.

Synchrondrosis Cartilaginous joint.

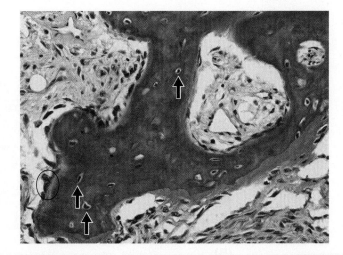

FIGURE 26-3 Bone repair at the site of a fracture. Examples of osteoblasts (*arrows*). The cells are surrounded by halos of matrix not yet calcified. Example of osteoclasts (*circle*), multinucleated cells remodeling surface of bone spicule. Osteocytes (not shown) appear similar to osteoblasts but are embedded in bone matrix and are not surrounded by a clear halo.

Courtesy of Department of Pathology and Laboratory Medicine, University of North Carolina at Chapel Hill.

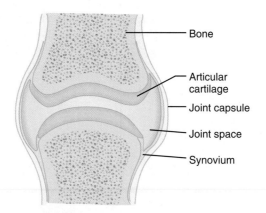

FIGURE 26-4 Structure of a typical movable joint.

such as occurs between adjacent vertebral bodies in the spine and between the pubic bones of the pelvis (symphysis pubis), the ends of the bones are joined by cartilage but there is no joint cavity or synovium. Joints of this type have very little mobility.

A **synovial joint** is a movable joint in which the ends of the bones that move against one another are covered by smooth hyaline cartilage, the articular cartilage (*articulare* = to connect). The ends of the bones are held together by dense fibrous bands (ligaments). The joint capsule is lined by a thin synovial membrane (the synovium), which secretes a small amount of mucinous fluid to lubricate the joint. **FIGURE 26-4** illustrates the structure of a typical movable joint. **FIGURE 26-5** illustrates the histologic appearance of the articular cartilage and underlying bone and the appearance of a

Synovial joint Moveable joint.

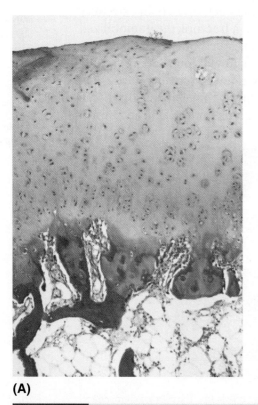

(A)

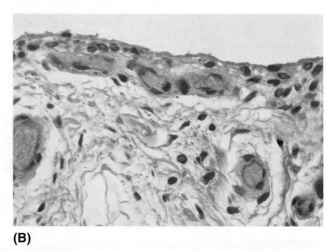

(B)

FIGURE 26-5 **(A)** A low-magnification photomicrograph of cellular structure of normal articular surface, illustrating articular cartilage (*top*), junction of bone and cartilage (*middle*), and normal bone with fatty bone marrow (*bottom*) (original magnification ×40). **(B)** Normal synovium composed of synovial cells (*top*) covering loose connective tissue.

Courtesy of Leonard V. Crowley, MD, Century College.

normal synovium. In joint disease, the structures may be altered by inflammation (inflammatory arthritis) or degeneration (noninflammatory arthritis), leading to derangement in the functions of the joints.

BONE FORMATION

The two types of bone formation are fundamentally similar. In **intramembranous bone formation**, the embryonic connective tissue cells (mesodermal cells) are transformed directly into bone-forming cells (osteoblasts). The osteoblasts secrete a collagenous material called osteoid, which then becomes calcified to form bone. The bones of the vertex of the skull, the facial bones, and a few other bones are formed in this manner. Most of the skeletal system, however, is formed by a process called **endochondral bone formation** (*endo* = within + *chondral* = cartilage). In endochondral bone formation, the mesodermal cells differentiate first into cartilage cells, and the bones are formed initially as cartilagenous precursors. The cartilage is then absorbed and replaced by bone. Conversion of cartilage into bone is accomplished by vascular bone-forming mesoderm, which invades the cartilage.

Bones that have been preformed in cartilage undergo ossification at specific times throughout fetal and postnatal life. In the long bones, ossification begins first in the shaft diaphysis (primary ossification) and continues toward the ends of the bone; later, centers of ossification form at the ends (epiphyses) of the bone (secondary ossification). The actively growing zone of cartilage between the shaft and the epiphysis of a long bone is called the epiphyseal plate (**FIGURE 26-6**).

> **Intramembranous bone formation** Direct formation of bone by osteoblasts without prior formation of a cartilage model.

> **Endochondral bone formation** Formation of bone, first as a cartilage model that is then reabsorbed and converted into bone.

BONE GROWTH AND REMODELING

Bone grows in both length and thickness and is continually remodeled as it grows by absorption of bone in some areas and formation of new bone in others. Bone

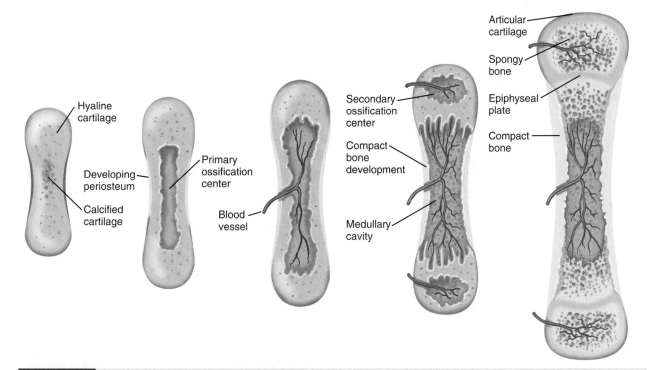

FIGURE 26-6 The major stages in the development of endochondrial bone.

Data from Shier, D.N., Butler, J.L., and Lewis, R. Hole's Essentials of Human Anatomy & Physiology, Tenth Edition. McGraw Hill Higher Education, 2009.

Periosteum The tough, fibrous membrane that covers a bone, except for its articular surfaces.

Rickets Impaired calcification of bone in a growing child caused by vitamin D deficiency, which leads to bowing of leg bones when weight-bearing is attempted.

Osteomalacia Impaired calcification of bone in an adult caused by vitamin D deficiency, which also contributes to bone loss caused by osteoporosis.

grows thicker by adding newly formed bone produced by the **periosteum** (a layer of specialized connective tissue cells surrounding the bone) to its external surface. The periosteal cells differentiate into osteoblasts, which in turn produce bone. Growth in the length of bone is the result of proliferation of cartilage at the epiphyseal plate, which is converted into bone. Growth in bone length continues into adolescence. Eventually, epiphyseal growth ceases, and the cartilagenous epiphyseal plate becomes converted into bone (closure of the epiphyses). Thereafter, no further growth in length of bone is possible.

Bone breakdown and replacement by newly formed bone occurs continuously. Bone remodeling occurs during bone growth in childhood and adolescence, during repair of bone fractures, when required to increase bone strength in response to greater weight-bearing requirements, and even in association with normal weight bearing. Often, microscopic breaks occur in bone structure resulting from the stresses of daily weight bearing, which are repaired or replaced by newly formed bone. Many other factors influence bone remodeling, including calcium, vitamin D, parathyroid hormone, and steroid hormones. Normally, bone breakdown and replacement occur concurrently so the strength and density of the skeletal system are not compromised. However, if bone loss exceeds replacement, the bone density falls and the bones become more susceptible to fractures.

Normal bone growth and maturation require vitamin D, obtained by exposure of the skin to sunlight, or from the diet in vitamin D–fortified milk and other foods. Calcium and phosphate are also needed to calcify the bone as it is formed; the parathyroid glands regulate the level of blood calcium and must function normally (see discussion on the endocrine glands).

BONE GROWTH DISTURBANCES CAUSED BY VITAMIN D DEFICIENCY: RICKETS AND OSTEOMALACIA

Rickets and osteomalacia refer to defects in bone mineralization in children and adults, respectively. Children lacking adequate vitamin D develop **rickets**, now an uncommon disease in industrialized countries as most children receive vitamin D supplements. If vitamin D is insufficient, calcium is not absorbed normally from the intestinal tract, and the blood calcium tends to fall. The parathyroid glands respond to the low calcium by increasing the secretion of parathyroid hormone, which raises blood calcium but also causes the level of phosphate in the blood to fall. As a result, the deposition of calcium phosphate in the bone matrix is impaired because there is not enough phosphate available to combine with calcium, so the bone matrix is not adequately calcified. Osteoid is formed in excess at the epiphyseal ends of the growing bones, but lacks strength because it is so poorly calcified. Consequently, the weakened bones tend to become bowed when weight bearing is attempted. Treatment consists of supplying vitamin D along with additional calcium and phosphate. **Osteomalacia** in adults is caused by defective intestinal absorption of vitamin D and calcium as a result of small intestine disease or liver disease than reduces dietary intake of vitamin D. The reduced absorption is caused by diminished bile production (and hence reduced intestinal uptake of fat soluble vitamin D).

Rickets also can be caused by congenital autosomal recessive diseases that cause deranged vitamin D metabolism or a lack of a functional vitamin D cellular receptor (vitamin D dependent rickets types I and II, respectively). However, the most common type of inherited rickets is X-linked hypophosphatemia (vitamin D resistant rickets), which results from impaired phosphate uptake.

Congenital Malformations of the Skeletal System

ABNORMAL BONE FORMATION

The two most important genetically determined diseases of the skeletal system that result from abnormal bone formation are achondroplasia and osteogenesis imperfecta. In **achondroplasia**, endochondral bone formation is faulty. The abnormality, which is transmitted as a Mendelian dominant trait and is the most common form of short limbed dwarfism, is characterized by disturbed endochondral bone formation at the epiphyseal lines of the long bones, resulting in short thick bones. The disturbance impairs growth of the extremities, causing a type of dwarfism in which the limbs are disproportionately short in relation to the trunk (achondroplastic dwarfism). The head is also abnormally formed because of disturbed endochondral ossification of the bones forming the base of the skull, and there is usually also an exaggerated curvature (lordosis) of the lumbar spine (**FIGURE 26-7**). Affected individuals have normal life spans and mentation.

Osteogenesis imperfecta (meaning literally "imperfect bone formation") is characterized by the formation of very thin and delicate bones that are easily broken under very minimal stress. In the most severe cases, the infant is born with multiple fractures. Some fractures occur before birth, having been sustained as a result of the very minor stresses resulting from the movements of the fetus within the uterus; other fractures occur during delivery. The intrauterine fractures of the extremities usually

Achondroplasia
A congenital disturbance of endochondral bone formation that causes a type of dwarfism.

Osteogenesis imperfecta
A congenital disturbance of bone formation characterized by excessively thin and delicate bones that are easily broken.

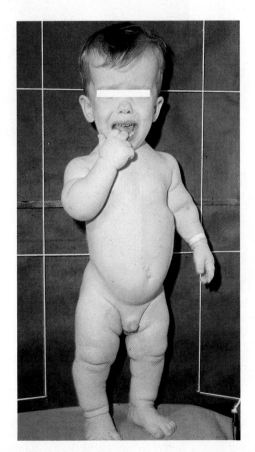

FIGURE 26-7 Characteristic appearance of child with achondroplasia, illustrating the relatively large head and disproportionate shortening of the extremities.

Courtesy of Leonard V. Crowley, MD, Century College.

heal in poor alignment, causing the limbs to appear bent and disproportionately short (**FIGURE 26-8**). In milder forms of the disease, the abnormal fragility of the bone may not become apparent until childhood or adolescence.

The types of osteogenesis imperfecta differ in severity, ranging from mild to lethal, and differ in the age of onset and method of transmission. The disease results from a mutation of a gene concerned with producing type 1 collagen. The newly formed bone is easily broken under very minimal stress in people who do not make enough type 1 collagen or who make such poor quality collagen that the bones cannot withstand normal stress. Other connective tissues containing type 1 collagen, such

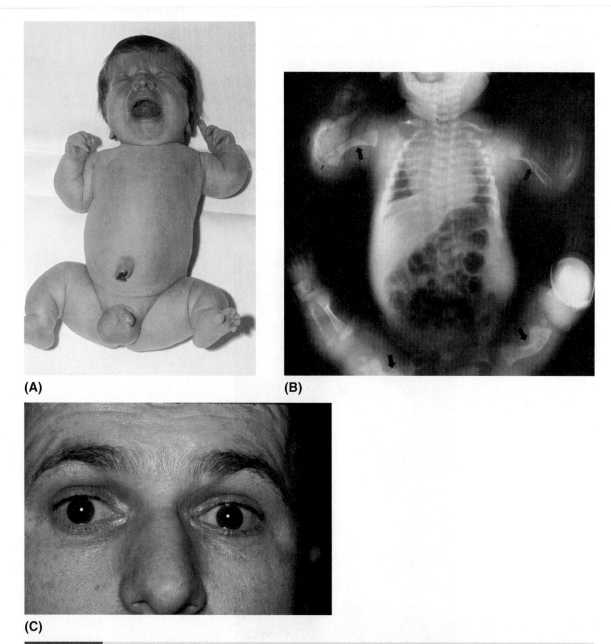

(A)

(B)

(C)

FIGURE 26-8 Severe form of osteogenesis imperfecta. **(A)** Shortening and bowing of the limbs resulting from multiple intrauterine fractures that have healed in poor alignment. **(B)** X-ray film showing multiple fractures of ribs and limb bones, some showing poor alignment and evidence of healing. *Arrows* indicate the location of four fractures. **(C)** Blue sclerae of a person with osteogenesis imperfecta. The thin sclerae allow the black choroid layers to show through the sclerae, which changes the scleral color from white to blue or blue-gray.

Courtesy of Leonard V. Crowley, MD, Century College.

as ligaments and tendons, are not as strong as they should be, leading to excessive joint mobility. Even the connective tissue in the sclerae (the white outer layers of the eyes posterior to the corneas) is often affected. Because the sclerae are thinner than normal, the black pigmented choroid layers in the eyes under the sclerae show through the thin sclerae. As a result, the sclerae appear blue or blue-gray instead of white (**FIGURE 26-8C**).

The characteristic features of osteogenesis imperfecta vary greatly from person to person even within the same family. The diagnosis of the disease is based on the clinical features and family history of the disease and genetic testing. Affected individuals are encouraged to lead as normal a life as possible. Exercise to maintain muscle strength is best achieved by swimming and other in-water activities to minimize the risk of exercise-induced fractures. Affected individuals may obtain limited benefit from some of the same drugs used to treat older adults with thinning bones caused by osteoporosis.

MALFORMATION OF FINGERS AND TOES

Abnormalities of the fingers and toes are relatively common and, generally, can be corrected surgically. The fingers and toes may fail to separate normally during development (syndactyly), leading to the formation of spadelike hands and feet (**FIGURE 26-9A**), a very common defect occurring in about 1 in 2,500 births. It may be simple (not involving the bones) or complex (involving the bones and/or nails). Syndactyly is often part of a number of syndromes that show additional and far more serious effects. In other instances, extra digits are formed (polydactyly, **FIGURE 26-9B**), sometimes in combination with syndactyly.

CONGENITAL CLUBFOOT (TALIPES)

Clubfoot is a relatively common congenital abnormality, having an incidence of about 1 in 1,000 infants. Most cases are of unknown cause and may have a multifactorial pattern of inheritance. The malformation is characterized by an abnormal position of the foot that prevents normal weight-bearing; the affected individual tends to walk on the ankle rather than on the sole of the foot (*talus* = ankle + *pes* = foot). **FIGURE 26-10** illustrates the most common type of clubfoot deformity, talipes equinovarus, in which the foot is turned inward at the ankle (varus position) and

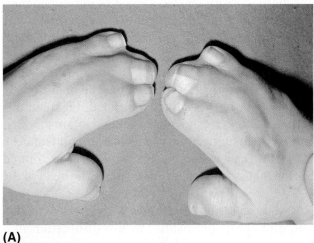
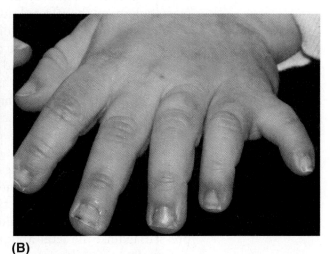

(A) (B)

FIGURE 26-9 Common malformations of fingers. **(A)** Failure of separation of fingers. **(B)** Extra fingers.

Courtesy of Leonard V. Crowley, MD, Century College.

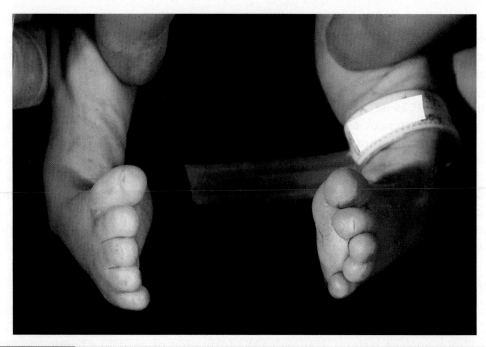

FIGURE 26-10 Common type of congenital clubfoot (*talipes equinovarus*) in newborn infant.
Courtesy of Leonard V. Crowley, MD, Century College.

fixed in tiptoe (equinus) position. Less commonly, the foot is rotated outward (valgus position) and fixed so that the weight is born on the heel (calcaneus position). Any intrauterine fetal position that causes the foot to assume an abnormal position may cause the foot to develop abnormally if the fetus is genetically predisposed to this malformation. Talipes is treated by manipulating the foot into a normal position and maintaining the corrected position with casts or splints; surgical release of the malrotated limb may be required in some cases.

CONGENITAL DISLOCATION OF THE HIP

Congenital dislocation of the hip has an incidence of about 1 in 1,500 infants, occurring most commonly in females. In this malformation, the hip-joint socket (acetabulum) on the affected side is shallow, its upper rim is less well developed than normal, and the ligaments holding the head of the femur in the socket are relatively lax. As a consequence, the head of the femur fails to maintain its normal position and becomes displaced upward and backward out of the shallow socket (**FIGURE 26-11**). Like clubfoot, congenital hip dislocation results from the interaction of genetic factors in conjunction with an abnormal intrauterine fetal position. The depth of the hip socket and the laxity of the ligaments are genetically determined. Ligamentous laxity is also related to the sex of the infant, being greater in female infants (which accounts for the more frequent occurrence of congenital hip dislocation in females). If, in addition, the fetus assumes a position that causes the foot and leg to be rotated externally, the thigh also is rotated externally, which tends to displace the head of the femur out of its socket. Some types of breech positions (fetal buttocks rather than head in the lower part of the uterus and the lower extremities with knees extended pressed against the fetal abdomen and chest) predispose to hip dislocation in a genetically susceptible infant.

Congenital dislocation of the hip can frequently be treated effectively by manipulating the displaced femoral head into the acetabulum and maintaining the head

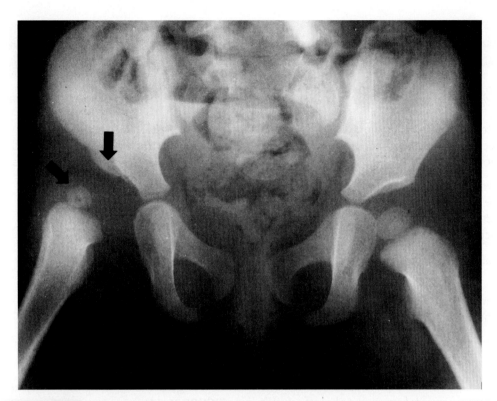

FIGURE 26-11 A congenital dislocation of the right hip in an eighteen-month-old child. Radiograph shows that right hip socket (*left*) is shallow, and its upper end (*upper arrow*) is less well developed than normal, permitting the head of the femur (*lower arrow*) to be displaced upward out of the hip-joint socket. The dislocated head is also less well developed than normal.

Courtesy of Leonard V. Crowley, MD, Century College.

within the socket by means of some device that maintains the leg and thigh in proper position, such as a splint or plaster cast.

Arthritis

Arthritis is one of the most common and disabling diseases of the skeletal system. Although there are many different kinds of arthritis, the three most common in adults are rheumatoid arthritis, osteoarthritis, and gout. **TABLE 26-1** compares the major features of these conditions.

RHEUMATOID ARTHRITIS

Rheumatoid arthritis (RA) is a systemic disease affecting the connective tissues throughout the body, but the most pronounced clinical manifestations are in the joints. Clinically, the disease is a chronic, disabling, and often deforming arthritis affecting several joints. RA is encountered most frequently in young and middle-aged women, usually affecting the small joints of the hands and feet. In the joints, the arthritis is seen as a chronic inflammation and thickening of the synovial membrane. The inflammatory tissue extends over the surface of the articular cartilage, destroying the cartilage (**FIGURE 26-12**). The severe damage to the articular surfaces makes the joint unstable; this in turn leads to deviation or displacement of the bones owing to the pull of the surrounding ligaments and tendons (**FIGURE 26-13**). Fibrous adhesions often develop within the joint, and the ends of the adjacent bones may become completely

Rheumatoid arthritis (RA) A systemic disease primarily affecting the synovium with major manifestations in the small joints.

TABLE 26-1   Comparison of Major Features of Common Types of Arthritis

	Rheumatoid arthritis	Osteoarthritis	Gout
Age and sex of usual patient	Young and middle-aged, female	Adult, older persons, both sexes	Middle-aged, male
Major characteristic	Systemic disease with major effects in joints; causes chronic synovitis	"Wear and tear" degeneration of articular cartilage	Disturbance of purine metabolism; acute episodes caused by crystals of uric acid in joints
Secondary effects of disease	Ingrowth of inflammatory tissue over cartilage destroys cartilage, leads to destruction of joint space; deformities common	Overgrowth of bone; thickening of periarticular soft tissues	Deposits of uric acid in joints with damage to joints (gouty arthritis); soft tissue tophi
Joints usually affected	Small joints of hands and feet	Major weight-bearing joints	Small joints; joint at base of great toe often affected
Special features	Autoantibody against gamma globulin (rheumatoid factor)	No systemic symptoms or biochemical abnormalities	High blood level of uric acid

fused. The end result of these various structural derangements is severe disability and conspicuous deformity of the affected joints (**FIGURE 26-14**).

The ability to produce self-reactive antibodies (autoantibodies) to modified proteins is critical to the pathogenesis of rheumatoid arthritis. Arginine residues in proteins found in the lung and synovial tissue can be converted to citrulline (i.e., are deaminated) as a result of a number environmental factors, including smoking and certain infectious agents. Up to two-thirds of patients with RA have antibodies that react with citrullinated peptides (CP), and virtually all individuals with anti-CP antibodies develop RA. In fact, these antibodies may be found as a precursor to clinically evident disease. For this reason, anti-CP antibodies are an excellent serological

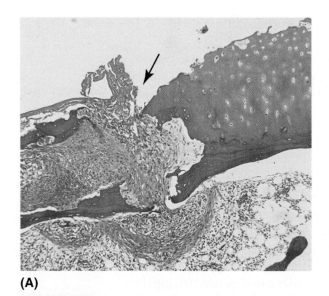

(A)

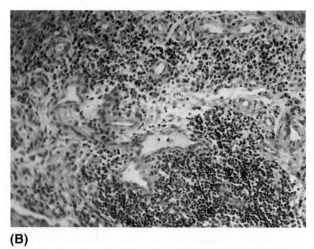

(B)

FIGURE 26-12 Rheumatoid arthritis. **(A)** Low-magnification photomicrograph illustrating destruction of articular cartilage by inflammatory reaction (*arrow*) extending from synovial surface (original magnification ×25). **(B)** Photomicrograph of chronic inflammatory reaction in synovium (original magnification ×100).

Courtesy of Leonard V. Crowley, MD, Century College.

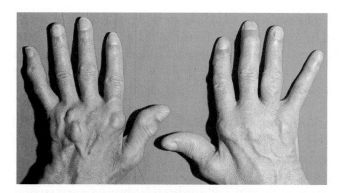

FIGURE 26-13 Rheumatoid arthritis. Early manifestations, illustrating swelling of knuckle joints (metacarpophalangeal joints) as a result of inflammation and ulnar deviation of fingers.

Courtesy of Leonard V. Crowley, MD, Century College.

test for RA. Additionally, the blood and synovial tissues of patients with rheumatoid arthritis often contains a substance called rheumatoid factor (RF), an autoantibody of the IgM class produced by B lymphocytes, that is directed against the individual's own IgG. Although RF is present in many cases of RA (particularly when the disease is severe), it is not specific for the condition and is found in other autoimmune diseases and chronic infections where the formation of antibody-antigen complexes is likely to occur. Perhaps the abovementioned anti-CP antibodies reacting with self-peptides provoke the formation of RF antibodies. Immune complexes, including those composed RF and IgG (and possibly anti-CP and self-peptides), form within the joints, which activates complement and attracts inflammatory cells that damage the joints. The lymphocytes and macrophages (activated monocytes) in the synovial tissues also contribute to joint damage by secreting various injurious cytokines, including tumor necrosis factor and interleukin-1 (see discussion on immunity, hypersensitivity, allergy,

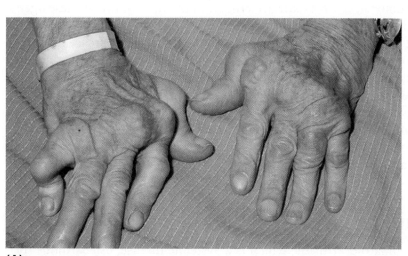

(A)

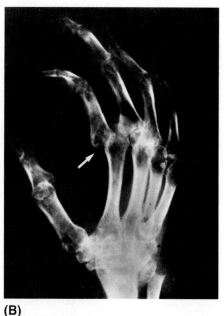

(B)

FIGURE 26-14 **(A)** Advanced joint deformities caused by rheumatoid arthritis. **(B)** Radiograph illustrating destruction of articular surfaces and anterior dislocation of base of index finger (*arrow*) as a result of joint instability.

Courtesy of Leonard V. Crowley, MD, Century College.

and autoimmune diseases). Much of the joint damage characteristic of rheumatoid arthritis is caused by tumor necrosis factor, which is a very destructive cytokine. Some RA patients also may demonstrate disease outside of joints, including dry mucosa (sicca syndrome), pericarditis, fatigue, and low-grade fevers. Because of the systemic nature of the disease and the presence of autoantibodies, rheumatoid arthritis is classified as one of the autoimmune diseases.

As with some other autoimmune diseases, a genetic susceptibility to rheumatoid arthritis is related to the individual's HLA antigens. About half of the people with rheumatoid arthritis have the HLA antigen HLA-DR4, which is present in only about 20 percent of a control group; this is considered a highly significant association. Patients with anti-CP antibodies show a very strong association to a particular set of HLA antigens (called the HLA-DRB1 shared epitope alleles), presumably because those particular alleles are required for the immune recognition of CP-peptides (see discussion on immunity, hypersensitivity, allergy, and autoimmune diseases).

Rheumatoid arthritis tends to fluctuate in severity. Periods in which the disease is active may alternate with periods in which it is inactive. Although there is no cure for rheumatoid arthritis, a number of measures can be used to control the disease and minimize its attending disability and deformity.

Treatment of Rheumatoid Arthritis

The primary objectives of treatment are reduction of joint inflammation and pain, maximal preservation of joint function, and prevention of joint deformity. Treatment consists of rest periods for several hours every day while the disease is active, use of splints to support inflamed joints and reduce deformities caused by muscle spasm, and use of crutches and braces to aid weight-bearing. The affected joints are exercised gently to preserve joint mobility and muscle strength.

Anti-inflammatory drugs such as aspirin and corticosteroids are prescribed to reduce inflammation within the joints early in the course of the disease to offer immediate relief. Disease-modifying antirheumatic drugs (DMARDS) slow the progression of the disease but often take several weeks or months to exert an effect, and all have some toxicity. Methotrexate (a cytotoxic immunosuppressive drug) is often used in combination with other drugs. Newer biological agents most commonly directed against tumor necrosis factor are critical in therapy. Many of these agents are monoclonal antibodies directed either against TNF or components of the immune system important in the inflammatory response. However, tumor necrosis factor also plays a role in protecting us from infections, so blocking its effect increases the infection risk, which can lead to potentially serious complications. For example, patients who had been previously infected with the tubercle bacillus and have latent inactive infections can develop active pulmonary tuberculosis.

If severe joint deformities develop, surgical procedures can be performed to improve joint function. These measures include excision of thickened inflamed synovium, surgical correction of joint dislocations, or even complete reconstruction of damaged joints.

OSTEOARTHRITIS

Osteoarthritis A "wear and tear" degeneration of the major weight-bearing joints.

In contrast to rheumatoid arthritis, which is a systemic disease, **osteoarthritis** (primary osteroarthritis) is a result of "wear and tear" degeneration of one or more of the major weight-bearing joints (*osteo* = bone + *arthro* = joint + *itis* = inflammation). The disease is seen in older adults and may be considered a manifestation of the normal aging process. The primary change in osteoarthritis is degeneration of

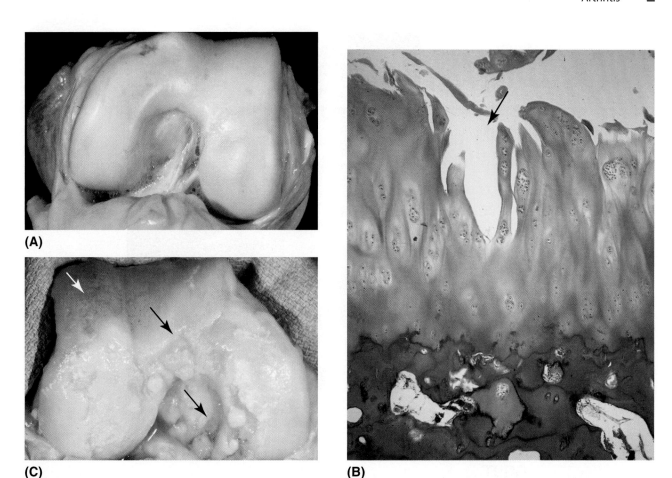

FIGURE 26-15 **(A)** Knee joint, illustrating smooth articular surface of femoral condyles. **(B)** Early histologic changes of osteoarthritis, illustrating splitting and fragmentation of articular cartilage (*arrow*) (original magnification ×160). Compare with normal articular cartilage in Figure 26-5A. **(C)** Advanced osteoarthritis, illustrating loss of articular cartilage (*white arrow*) and nodular overgrowth of bone (*black arrows*).

Courtesy of Leonard V. Crowley, MD, Century College.

the articular cartilage, leading to roughening of the articular surfaces of the bones (**FIGURE 26-15**). As a consequence, the bones grate against one another when the joint moves instead of gliding smoothly. Degeneration of the cartilage sometimes leaves large areas of underlying bone exposed. Secondary overgrowth of bone frequently occurs in response to the trauma of weight-bearing (**FIGURE 26-16**), and some thickening of the synovium and adjacent soft tissues is also common. Osteoarthritis (secondary osteoarthritis) may also result from a defect in bone and joints not related to aging and "wear and tear" but rather to an intrinsic defect that may be genetic in origin or relate to trauma or metabolic defects.

Clinically, people with osteoarthritis experience stiffness, creaking, and some pain on motion of the joints, but disability is usually not severe, and the joints are not destroyed. However, occasionally patients may experience considerable pain and disability from advanced arthritis affecting one or both hip joints. In these cases, it is possible to remove the affected femoral head and articular surface of the hip bone surgically and to replace them with an artificial hip joint. The procedure is called a total hip joint replacement (**FIGURE 26-17**). Similar types of joint replacement procedures have been performed on the knee joint and some other joints as well. Joint replacement operations can provide excellent pain relief and greatly improved joint function in many patients.

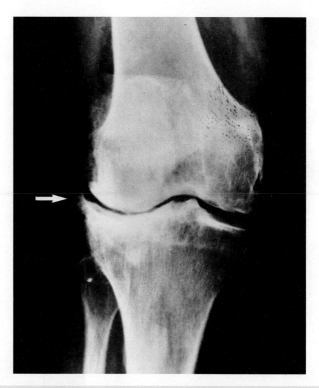

FIGURE 26-16 Osteoarthritis. Radiograph illustrates increased bone density of femoral condyle (*left side*) and adjacent tibia, with overgrowth of bone at margin of tibia (*arrow*).

GOUT

Gout is a clinical syndrome associated with an elevated level of uric acid in the blood and body fluids (hyperuricemia), leading to precipitation of uric acid as sodium urate crystals in joints and other tissues. However, relatively few people with hyperuricemia

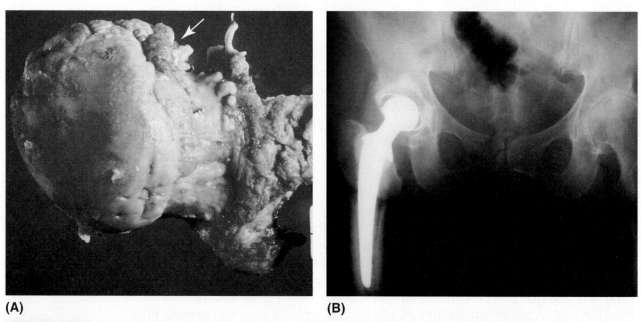

(A)　　　　　　　　　　　　　　　　　　　　　**(B)**

FIGURE 26-17 **(A)** Femoral head that was removed surgically and replaced by an artificial hip joint. Note the irregularity of head and the overgrowth of bone at the margin of the femoral head (*arrow*). **(B)** X-ray illustrating total hip replacement.

Courtesy of Leonard V. Crowley, MD, Century College.

develop gout. In most patients, the condition is caused by a metabolic disorder of purine metabolism, which leads to an overproduction of uric acid, an inadequate excretion of uric acid, or a combination of both. This condition is sometimes called **primary gout** to distinguish it from the much less common **secondary gout** in which the elevated uric acid is secondary to some other disease or condition.

Primary Gout

Purines are double-ring nitrogen compounds used to form the nucleotides adenine and guanine. Along with the pyrimidine nucleotides, they make up the large DNA molecules within the nuclei of our cells. Although our body can produce purines from nonpurine precursor substances, most of the purines that we use to make nucleo-proteins for new cells are salvaged (recycled) from our own worn-out cells when the cells are broken down. The purines that are not salvaged and recycled are converted into the end-product uric acid, which is excreted in the urine. Because uric acid is not very soluble in body fluids, any significant elevation may lead to precipitation of the uric acid in joints and other tissues.

Clinically, the person afflicted with gout experiences periodic episodes of extremely painful acute arthritis, usually involving initially only a single joint, often the joint at the base of the great toe (**FIGURE 26-18A**). The disease is almost completely limited to men. The acute episodes are caused by crystallization of uric acid within the joint, which incites an intense inflammatory reaction. Gradually the symptoms of an acute attack subside, and joint function returns to normal until the next attack. If the disease is not treated, however, the attacks last longer, occur more frequently, and may involve several joints. Eventually, lumpy masses called gouty tophi are deposited in the soft tissues around the joints (**FIGURE 26-18B**) and in other locations. The tophi consist of large masses of urate surrounded by macrophages, multinucleated giant cells, and fibrous tissue. When viewed under polarized light, the needlelike urate crystals have a characteristic appearance diagnostic of gout (**FIGURE 26-19**). In untreated patients, masses of urate crystals deposited in and around the articular surfaces of the joints damage the joint surfaces and adjacent bone; this is called gouty arthritis (**FIGURE 26-20**).

In some people with gout, the disease also targets the kidneys and urinary tract. These people may develop uric acid kidney stones. The uric acid also may precipitate from the tubular filtrate within the kidney tubules, which blocks the tubules, damages

Primary gout A metabolic disease caused by overproduction of uric acid, reduced excretion of uric acid, or a combination of both factors. Clinical manifestations are related to precipitation of uric acid in joints, kidneys, and other sites.

Secondary gout Elevated uric acid and clinical manifestations of gout not caused by the metabolic disease primary gout, but instead caused by some other disease that raises the blood uric acid excessively, such as kidney failure or excessive breakdown of white blood cells in patients with leukemia.

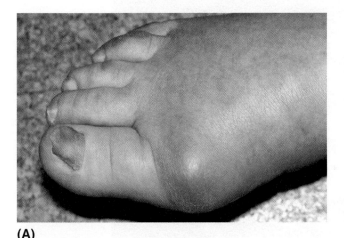

(A)

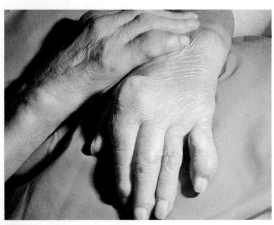

(B)

FIGURE 26-18 **(A)** Acute gout affecting right great toe. **(B)** Deformities of hands caused by accumulation of uric acid crystals (tophi) in and around finger joints.

(A) © Dr. Allan Harris/Phototake; (B) Courtesy of Leonard V. Crowley, MD, Century College.

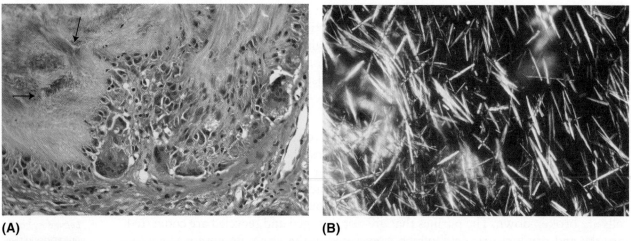

(A)   **(B)**

FIGURE 26-19   **(A)** Margin of tophus illustrating mass of urate crystals (*arrows*) and adjacent zone of macrophages, multinucleated giant cells, and fibrous tissue formed in response to crystal deposits (original magnification ×250). **(B)** Characteristic histologic appearance of needlelike sodium urate crystals from tophus viewed under polarized light (original magnification ×400).

Courtesy of Leonard V. Crowley, MD, Century College.

the kidneys, and impairs renal function. This condition is called urate nephropathy and is described in the discussion on the urinary system.

Gout is treated by administering drugs that reduce the concentration of uric acid in the blood by interfering with the formation of uric acid within the body, or by promoting the excretion of uric acid by the kidneys. Patients are usually advised to avoid foods rich in nucleoproteins, such as liver, kidney, and pancreas, because they tend to raise uric acid levels. Heavy intake of alcohol also should be avoided because alcohol indirectly impairs excretion of uric acid by the renal tubules, causing the blood uric acid level to rise.

Patients also are advised to drink lots of fluids to maintain a high urine volume so the urine is less concentrated, reducing the likelihood of kidney stones forming or of developing urate nephropathy. Several drugs, including colchicine and allopurinol (which inhibits a key enzyme in the synthesis of urea from degraded nucleic acids), are used to help prevent and alleviate attacks.

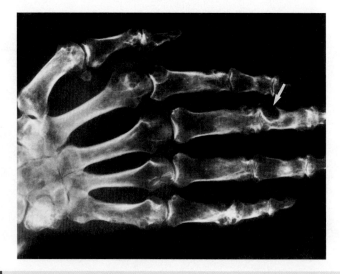

FIGURE 26-20   Radiograph of right hand of patient with gouty arthritis illustrating area of bone destruction (*arrow*) caused by masses of uric acid crystals.

Courtesy of Leonard V. Crowley, MD, Century College.

Secondary Gout

Other conditions also may raise blood uric acid, and at times, the level may be so high that the uric acid precipitates from the blood and produces the same manifestations as gout caused by the metabolic disorder of purine metabolism. The hyperuricemia results either from inadequate renal excretion of uric acid or from excessive nucleoprotein breakdown. This condition is often called secondary gout because the elevated uric acid is secondary to some other disease. Patients with kidney failure may have high blood uric acid because the diseased kidneys are unable to excrete the uric acid efficiently, and some diuretics also may impair renal uric acid excretion. Hyperuricemia may be a problem in leukemia when patients have a greatly increased number of white blood cells, especially after treatment with drugs that destroy the leukemic cells and release large amounts of nucleoprotein from the disrupted cells. The breakdown of the nucleoprotein yields a large amount of uric acid derived from the purine-containing nucleotides in the nucleoprotein. In these conditions, there is no underlying metabolic defect in purine metabolism. The use of a number of drugs (including some diuretics) may result in gout.

Fracture of Bone

A fracture is a break in bone. In a simple fracture, the bone is broken into only two pieces. The term comminuted fracture is used when the bone is shattered into several pieces. A compound fracture is one in which the overlying skin has been broken. A compound fracture is more serious than the other types because of the possibility that bacteria may invade the fracture site and cause a secondary infection of bone (osteomyelitis).

After a fracture, the ends of the broken bone may remain aligned, or may be displaced out of position (**FIGURE 26-21**). "Reduction of a fracture" refers to realigning

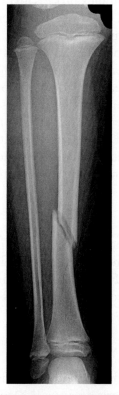

FIGURE 26-21 Displaced fracture of the tibia. Treatment by reduction of fracture and plaster cast.

Courtesy of Dr. Kirkland W. Davis, MD, Department of Radiology, University of Wisconsim School of Medicine and Public Health.

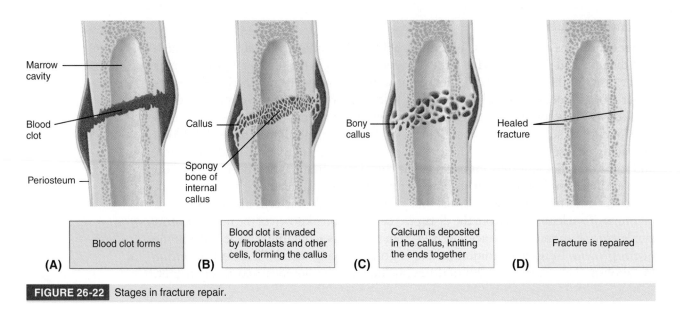

Marrow cavity

Blood clot

Periosteum

Callus

Spongy bone of internal callus

Bony callus

Healed fracture

Blood clot forms	Blood clot is invaded by fibroblasts and other cells, forming the callus	Calcium is deposited in the callus, knitting the ends together	Fracture is repaired
(A)	**(B)**	**(C)**	**(D)**

FIGURE 26-22 Stages in fracture repair.

the ends of the broken bone so that the bone will heal in its normal anatomic position. Sometimes this can be accomplished by manipulating the injured extremity to realign the ends of the bone and then immobilizing it in a plaster cast. However, a surgical operation must sometimes be performed to reduce the fracture and hold it in position by means of a metal plate and screws or a similar device (an open reduction). Sometimes a bone may become so weakened by disease, such as metastatic tumor, that it breaks after minimal stress (e.g., coughing or sneezing). A fracture of this type through a diseased area in bone is called a pathologic fracture.

The healing of fractures is a complex process involving several steps (**FIGURE 26-22**). Initially, within a few days of the fracture, bone necrosis occurs at the site of injury due to the disruption of blood supply to the bone. After about a week, reparative bone (woven bone) begins to appear at the margins of the injury. This is equivalent to the granulation tissue that forms during healing in other tissues. Ultimately a **callus** containing newly synthesized bone (derived from stem cells in connective tissue and bone marrow) and newly formed blood vessels will join the two injure bones. This is the reparative phase. Once the fracture has been bridged, a slow process of remodeling of the newly formed bone occurs based on the stress and mechanical force to which the site of injury is subject. This remodeling phase may continue for years (even after the bone is strong enough to function properly).

Infection of Bone

Osteomyelitis is an infection of bone and adjacent marrow cavity (*osteo* = bone + *myelos* = marrow + *itis* = inflammation) that is usually the result of staphylococci or various gram-negative bacteria. The infecting organisms gain access to bone from a distant site by way of the bloodstream (hematogenous osteomyelitis) or are implanted directly in the bone from various causes.

HEMATOGENOUS OSTEOMYELITIS

Hematogenous osteomyelitis is more common in children than in adults but also occurs in adult IV drug abusers. The bacteria are usually carried to the bone from a skin infection, such as a boil, from a kidney infection, or from some other distant site. In children, the organisms tend to lodge in the growing end of the bone on the diaphyseal side of the epiphyseal plate, where they proliferate and incite an acute inflammation. Local

Callus Newly synthesized bone repairing break.

Osteomyelitis An inflammation of bone.

injury to bone near its very vascular growing end seems to favor localization of bacteria in the bone, probably because a small hemorrhage forms secondary to the injury, and the collection of blood provides conditions favorable for the growth of bacteria.

Once the infection is established, it tends to spread through the bone. In children, the epiphyseal plate cartilage generally prevents the infection from spreading into the adjacent joint. The infection may spread through the cortex, however, and pus may accumulate under the periosteum, stripping the periosteum away from the underlying cortex. Because much of the blood supply to the cortex comes from the periosteum, the part of the cortex deprived of its blood supply may undergo necrosis. Spread of the infection within the bone may also compress blood vessels that nourish bone, thereby further compromising the blood supply to the infected bone. In adults, in whom hematogenous osteomyelitis is less frequent, the periosteum is more firmly applied to the cortex than it is in children, tending to prevent pus from accumulating under the periosteum. However, the infection may instead spread to the end of the bone and break into the joint, causing a secondary infection in the adjacent joint. This condition is called septic arthritis.

New bone formation proceeds concurrently with the inflammatory process, as the body attempts to repair the damage and localize the infection. Initial x-rays taken soon after the onset of the infection may show only swelling of the soft tissues surrounding the bone but no radiologic abnormalities in the affected bone at the site of infection. After the infection has been present for a time, however, evidence of bone destruction and new bone formation can be seen in the x-ray films.

Hematogenous osteomyelitis sometimes occurs in adults. Intravenous drug abusers are at risk because they often inject drugs with unclean needles and syringes that are contaminated with bacteria. Although hematogenous osteomyelitis may affect any bone, the infection frequently localizes in the vertebral bodies rather than in the long bones, probably because the stresses and trauma associated with weight-bearing predispose to localization in the spine.

OSTEOMYELITIS AS A RESULT OF DIRECT IMPLANTATION OF BACTERIA

Various conditions may expose bone to direct infection, including compound fractures, gunshot wounds, or other severe injuries affecting bone. Various surgical procedures performed on bone, such as open reduction and internal fixation of fractures or total joint replacement, may also be complicated by osteomyelitis (**FIGURE 26-23**). Chronic ulcers of the feet, which sometimes develop in diabetic patients, may expose the small bones of the feet to chronic infection.

CLINICAL MANIFESTATIONS AND TREATMENT

Osteomyelitis is usually manifested as an acute febrile illness associated with localized pain, tenderness, and swelling over the affected bone. Sometimes, however, the inflammation is manifested only as chronic pain and localized tenderness over the affected bone. X-rays taken after the inflammation is well established show characteristic changes.

Osteomyelitis is treated by a prolonged course of antibiotic therapy. In some patients, the infection may become chronic and may recur periodically. Chronic osteomyelitis is much more difficult to treat. In addition to intensive antibiotic treatment, surgical procedures may be required to remove infected degenerated bone and drain collections of pus in the bone.

Pathogenic fungi, tubercle bacilli, and various unusual opportunistic organisms may at times cause osteomyelitis, especially in immunocompromised adults. The

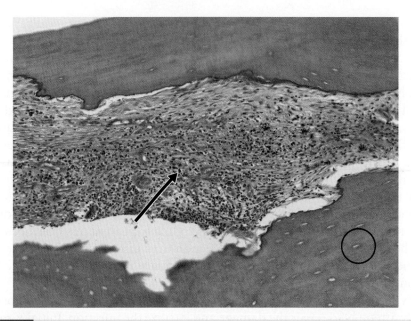

FIGURE 26-23 Chronic osteomyelitis in an amputated limb stump. The bone is necrotic. Note the empty lacunae, which formerly contained osteocytes (*circled*). A large area of chronic inflammation showing both mononuclear and multinucleated cells is present (*arrow*).

Courtesy of Department of Pathology and Laboratory Medicine, University of North Carolina at Chapel Hill.

infections are treated by appropriate antibiotics supplemented by various surgical procedures, if needed.

Tumors of Bone

Benign neoplasms and cystic lesions of bone are relatively common. **Nonossifying fibroma**, a defect in the cortical bone of children, may be found in up to a quarter of the long bones of children during the first decade of life. These defects may not be true neoplasms, and they tend to regress with time. Although malignant tumors of the bone are uncommon and are most frequently metastases from other sites, primary bone tumors are important because they tend to occur in youths and are often fatal if not appropriately treated. Malignant bone tumors most frequently are found in the long tubular bones, the distal femur and proximal tibia. The most common of the primary bone tumors, **osteosarcoma** (**osteogenic sarcoma**), is most prevalent in males in the second decade. The tumor most commonly occurs near the knee and is characterized by the destruction of normal bone and the production of new (woven) bone by malignant osteoblast-like cells. The disease is first noted because of pain and swelling (sometimes mistaken as the result of injury). There is a very characteristic radiographic pattern termed the Codman triangle that consists of newly formed bone extending toward and raising the periosteum (the connective tissue outer surface of the bone) (**FIGURE 26-24**). There is about a 70 percent five-year survival rate when surgery (designed to spare the limb) and chemotherapy are combined. Formerly, rapid limb amputation was considered necessary to prevent metastatic disease.

The second most common primary tumor of bone is **chondrosarcoma** (**FIGURE 26-25**). Unlike osteosarcoma, the tumor is most likely to occur in the fourth to sixth decade. This cartilaginous tumor most frequently derives from the medulla of bone, but there are many variants with very different prognosis depending on tumor grade.

Bone is often affected by metastatic tumors. Carcinoma of breast or prostate, as well as many other tumors, frequently metastasize to bone.

Nonossifying fibroma Defect in the cortical bone of children.

Osteosarcoma/osteogenic sarcoma Primary bone tumor.

Chondrosarcoma Primary bone tumor occurring later in life.

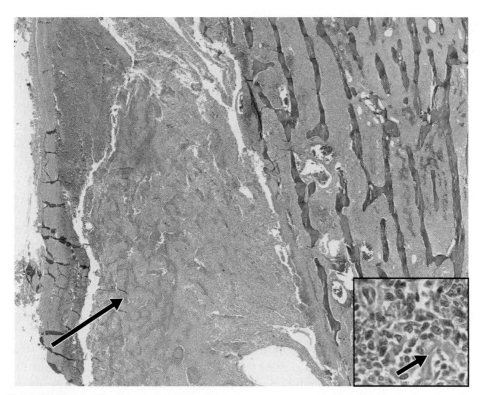

FIGURE 26-24 Osteosarcoma (microscopic view). There is a mass of tumor under the bone surface (*arrow*) and invading into the body of the bone. High power view (*inset*) shows osteosarcoma cells and the small bone spicules they synthesize (*arrow*).

Courtesy of Department of Pathology and Laboratory Medicine, University of North Carolina at Chapel Hill.

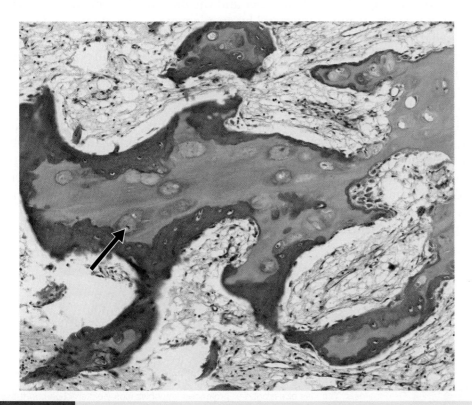

FIGURE 26-25 Chondrosarcoma (microscopic view). Neoplastic chondrocytes with bizarre nuclei are present in the cartilaginous matrix (*arrow*).

Courtesy of Department of Pathology and Laboratory Medicine, University of North Carolina at Chapel Hill.

Metabolic Bone Disease: Osteoporosis

Osteoporosis Generalized thinning and demineralization of bone that tends to occur in postmenopausal women.

Osteoporosis, literally meaning "porous bones," is a generalized thinning and demineralization of the entire skeletal system. It is the most common metabolic bone disease in the United States. Most cases are found in postmenopausal women, beginning in their fifties, and a significant degree of osteoporosis is said to be present in approximately one-fourth of all women in their sixties. Osteoporosis develops whenever bone resorption exceeds bone production. The incidence is high in postmenopausal women because the loss of ovarian function results in estrogen deficiency. Estrogen inhibits bone resorption, and the loss of estrogen accelerates the rate, which results in slowly progressive thinning of the bones. Osteoporosis also develops in older men, but it occurs at a much later age and is usually less severe than in women.

The osteoporotic bones are quite fragile and susceptible to fracture (**FIGURE 26-26**). Fractures of vertebral bodies are frequent, either from the stress of weight-bearing or after minor exertion. These fractures produce back pain and tenderness and are often characterized by collapse of the anterior portions of the vertebral bodies (compression fractures). Collapse of vertebral bodies may compress the spinal nerve roots passing through the intervertebral foramina, causing pain to radiate along the course of the compressed nerve.

Maximum bone density is attained in young adults, and then slowly but steadily declines as the person ages. The greater the bone density as a young adult, the longer it will take before there is enough bone loss to increase the risk of fractures. To use an analogy, bone density is like a savings account at a bank where money is deposited for retirement. The more money accumulated, the longer it takes before the savings account is depleted.

Bone loss can be retarded by regular weight-bearing exercises that help maintain bone density, by a high-calcium diet and calcium supplements if necessary to assure an adequate calcium intake, and by an adequate intake of vitamin D, which is required to promote calcium absorption from the intestine and incorporation into bone. Estrogens are no longer recommended to retard bone loss in postmenopausal women because of the long-term risks associated with estrogen use.

Once marked osteoporosis has developed and fractures occur, it is difficult to restore bone density. A number of drugs are available to restore bone density. Each has advantages and disadvantages. Bisphosphonate drugs, which are usually taken orally, are the first line agents recommended to treat osteoporosis. They act primarily by inhibiting bone resorption by osteoclasts. Over time bisphosphonate drugs also may decrease bone turnover to such a degree that the skeleton has insufficient bone density to maintain skeletal strength, resulting in fractures. This is a particular concern with the most potent agents. Necrosis of the bones of the jaw may occur spontaneously or after dental procedures when using these drugs.

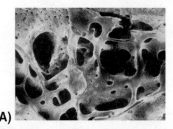 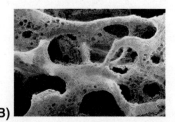

(A) **(B)**

FIGURE 26-26 Osteoporosis. The loss of estrogen or prolonged immobilization weakens bone. In these situations the bone is dissolved and becomes brittle and easily breakable. **(A)** Normal bone. **(B)** Bone weakened by osteoporosis.

(A) © Photo Insolite Realite/ Science Source, Inc.; (B) © Professor Pietro M. Motta/Science Source, Inc.

Selective estrogen receptor modulators (SERM), such as raloxifene, function as estrogen-like drugs taken orally and inhibit bone resorption, like estrogens, but do not have the adverse effects of estrogen on the breast and uterus. Calcitonin, a nasal spray containing a hormone produced by thyroid cells, inhibits the osteoclasts that breakdown bone but may be associated with an increased risk of cancer. Parathyroid hormonelike drugs used in daily injections increase bone density by stimulating osteoblasts, but the amount used is not enough to stimulate osteoclasts.

Significant loss of bone density also may occur in women athletes who engage in prolonged, intense physical activity, such as runners and gymnasts. The high level of physical activity triggers the hypothalamus and pituitary gland to increase adrenal corticosteroid output as an adaptation to the exercise-induced stress. This event, however, also is associated with a fall in the pituitary gonadotropic hormones that stimulate ovarian function. The ovaries, no longer adequately stimulated by pituitary gonadotropins, fail to produce adequate estrogen, which leads to cessation of menses, called exercise-induced amenorrhea. In addition, the estrogen-deficient athlete is at risk of the same type of estrogen-deficiency osteoporosis that develops in postmenopausal women and is subject to the same osteoporosis-related complications.

Osteoporosis related to exercise-induced amenorrhea can be prevented by reducing the level of physical activity enough to reestablish normal menstrual cycles. Alternatively, the athlete who elects to continue the same level of exercise can reduce her risk of osteoporosis by taking supplementary estrogen and progesterone hormones to replace the missing ovarian hormones and by taking calcium supplements.

New x-ray and radioisotope methods are now available that make a quantitative assessment of a patient's bone density and compare the results with normal ranges established for people of the same age and sex. Bone mineral density measurement of the wrist using dual-energy x-ray absorptiometry (DXA) is recommended for all women over the age of sixty-five and for men over the age of seventy. Those patients whose bones are losing mineral content to a greater extent or more rapidly than normal are at high risk of fractures and other complications related to osteoporosis. They should be treated vigorously in an attempt to retard further bone demineralization.

Osteonecrosis (Avascular Necrosis)

Occasionally, the growing cartilaginous ends of bone (epiphyses) undergo necrosis and degeneration, owing to interference with the blood supply to the epiphysis. Although the disease can occur at any age, **avascular necrosis** is most common between the ages of thirty and fifty years. Sometimes it follows an injury or is associated with excessive alcohol use or high-dose corticosteroid therapy, but in most cases the reason for the vascular disturbance is unknown. Common sites of avascular necrosis are the femoral head (**FIGURE 26-27**), the tibial tubercle, the articular surface of the femoral condyle, and occasionally the small bones of the ankle and foot. Symptoms consist of pain and disability related to motion of the affected joint. Avascular necrosis may also occur in adults if the blood supply to a bone is interrupted for any reason, as, for example, if the circulation to the femoral head is disrupted as a result of a hip fracture or dislocation.

Avascular necrosis Bone necrosis caused by interruption of its blood supply.

Structure and Function of the Spine

The vertebral column forms the central axis of the body. It consists of a series of vertebrae joined by intervertebral disks and fibrous ligaments. The vertebral column has four curves. The cervical and lumbar curves arch forward. Those in the thoracic and sacral regions bend in the opposite direction (**FIGURE 26-28A**).

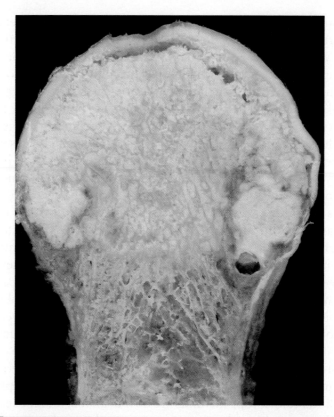

FIGURE 26-27 Avascular necrosis of femoral head. Articular cartilage has separated from the underlying bone, which appears dense and lacks a normal structural pattern. In contrast, bone of the femoral neck (*lower area*) appears normal. Treated by removal of femoral head and replacement with artificial hip joint.
Courtesy of Leonard V. Crowley, MD, Century College.

A typical vertebra has a large cylindrical body and a bony arch that encloses the spinal canal and protects the spinal cord. The parts of the arch that extend posteriorly from the body are called the pedicles, and the parts that roof the spinal canal are called the laminae (singular, lamina). A single midline spinous process projects posteriorly from the bony arch, and paired transverse processes extend laterally. Each vertebra also has two superior articular processes and two inferior articular processes. The superior processes articulate with the inferior processes of the vertebra above, and the inferior processes articulate with the superior processes of the vertebra below. The articulations form synovial joints that contribute to the mobility of the spine (**FIGURE 26-28B**).

When the vertebrae are viewed from the side, the superior and inferior margins of the vertebral pedicles appear concave. The spaces between the concave surfaces of the pedicles of adjacent vertebrae form oval openings called intervertebral foramina (singular, foramen), through which the spinal nerves leave the spinal canal (**FIGURE 26-28C**).

The **intervertebral disks**, interposed between adjacent vertebral bodies, consist of a peripheral fibrous ring, the annulus fibrosus, and a soft central nucleus pulposus. The **annulus fibrosus** ("fibrous ring") is structured as a ring of interlacing connective tissue bundles firmly adherent to adjacent vertebral bodies. Longitudinal bands of connective tissue, called the anterior and posterior longitudinal ligaments, run the entire length of the vertebral column to reinforce the annulus. The **nucleus pulposus** ("pulpy nucleus") consists of a gelatinous material containing a carbohydrate substance called a mucopolysaccharide and is about 80 percent water. Because of its very high water content, it is relatively incompressible.

Intervertebral disk
A fibrocartilaginous joint between adjacent vertebral bodies.

Annulus fibrosus The dense peripheral ring of fibrocartilage making up the intervertebral disk.

Nucleus pulposus The soft elastic center of the intervertebral disk.

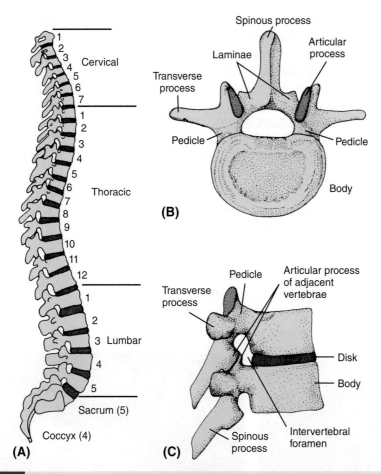

FIGURE 26-28 **(A)** Side view of vertebral column illustrating normal curves. Vertebrae are numbered. **(B)** Structure of typical vertebra viewed from above. The vertebral arch extends posteriorly from the vertebral body. The spinous process projects posteriorly from the arch, and the transverse processes project laterally. The articular processes of adjacent vertebrae articulate with each other by means of small synovial joints. **(C)** Side view of two vertebrae, illustrating the intervertebral disk, articular processes, and intervertebral foramen.

The position of the nucleus pulposus within the disk changes slightly during flexion and extension of the spine. During flexion, as when one bends forward to pick up an object on the ground, compression forces are concentrated on the anterior parts of the vertebral bodies and cause the nucleus to shift slightly posteriorly, moving away from the compressing force. Conversely, when compression forces are concentrated on the posterior part of the vertebral bodies during extension, the nucleus pulposus tends to shift anteriorly. Slight lateral movements of the nucleus also occur during lateral flexion of the spine. The intervertebral disks function somewhat like shock absorbers. Pressure applied to the disks is distributed evenly around the annulus by the soft nucleus pulposus, absorbing the forces of compression to some extent and preventing direct impact between adjacent vertebral bodies.

SCOLIOSIS

Scoliosis, an abnormal lateral curvature of the spine, is a common abnormality estimated to occur in about 4 percent of people. A small percentage of cases result from a congenital abnormality of a spinal vertebra that disturbs the normal vertical alignment of the spinal vertebrae, or results from a neurologic problem that disturbs the innervation of the muscles that maintain the spinal vertebrae in proper position.

The majority of cases, however, occur during the growth spurt just prior to puberty for unknown reasons (idiopathic scoliosis).

The spinal curvatures lead to an asymmetry of the trunk, so one shoulder is higher than the other, and the pelvis is tilted so that one iliac crest is higher than its counterpart on the opposite side. Some degree of rotation of the vertebrae accompanies the curvatures, which may lead to some asymmetry of the ribs that attach to the thoracic vertebrae (**FIGURE 26-29A**). Posterior protrusion of the ribs on one side of the thorax may cause a noticeable humplike deformity.

Scoliosis can be identified by careful examination of the spine while the teenager is standing upright and while bending forward, as when touching the toes. If scoliosis is identified, x-rays are taken to measure the extent of the curvature. A small curvature may not require treatment, but the adolescent needs to be checked periodically because some curves may get worse as the adolescent grows. Usually, a curvature does not progress after the teenager stops growing, but a marked curvature may continue to get worse even after growth stops. Severe degrees of scoliosis may cause significant disability. A marked thoracic curvature greatly reduces the size of the thorax, which interferes with lung function (**FIGURE 26-29B**).

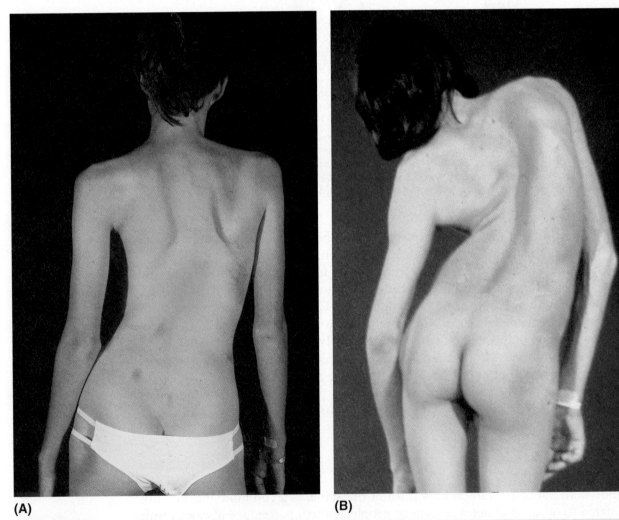

(A)　　　　　　　　　　　　　　　　　　　　**(B)**

FIGURE 26-29 Scoliosis. **(A)** Moderate scoliosis. **(B)** Severe scoliosis, which caused marked asymmetry of the trunk and greatly reduced the size of the thoracic cavities, interfering with pulmonary function.

Courtesy of Leonard V. Crowley, MD, Century College.

Treatment depends on the degree of curvature. Slight curves may not require treatment. A growing teenager with a curvature that is getting worse is treated by means of a spinal brace to help maintain the normal position of the spine and stop the progression of the curvature. A marked scoliosis may require surgical treatment, and various surgical procedures are used to stabilize the spine and correct the curvature.

INTERVERTEBRAL DISK DISEASE

With age, the intervertebral disks undergo a progressive wear-and-tear degeneration of both the nucleus and the annulus. The nucleus becomes more dense because its water content is reduced, and the annulus becomes weakened and thinned. When marked compression force is applied to the anterior part of the disk during flexion of the spine, the nucleus is forced posteriorly against the weakened annulus, and part of the nucleus may be forced into the spinal canal through a weak area or tear in the annulus (**FIGURE 26-30**). Most often, a disk protrusion occurs in the lumbosacral region because this is the part of the vertebral column where the disks are subject to the greatest mechanical compression during lifting. The disk usually protrudes in a posterolateral direction because the dense posterior longitudinal ligament reinforces the annulus in the midline, preventing a direct posterior protrusion.

Symptoms of disk protrusion (disk herniation or "slipped disk") in the lumbosacral region, consist of sudden onset of acute back pain after an episode of lifting. Frequently, the pain is also felt in the leg and thigh on the side of the protrusion because the extruded disk material often impinges on lumbosacral nerve roots, causing pain to radiate along the course of the nerve compressed by the protruded nucleus pulposus. When nerve compression is severe, numbness of the inner thighs, back of legs, and around the anus may occur (saddle anesthesia). If the lowest region of the cord nerve roots (the cauda equina) is compressed, loss of bladder and bowel function may occur, necessitating immediate surgical intervention. Treatment consists of bed rest and measures to minimize pain and disability, such as administration of aspirin or other pain-relieving medications, local application of heat, and use of muscle-relaxing drugs to relieve spasm of the back muscles that occurs after a disk protrusion and contributes to the disability. In some cases, local injection of cortisone may provide relief. Protruded disk material may be resorbed, and the tear in the annulus may be repaired by fibrous tissue. As noted, however, surgical removal of the protruded disk material may be required.

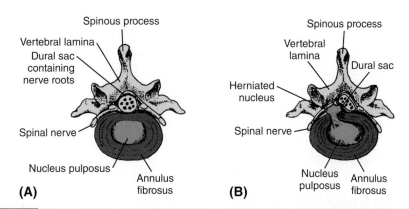

(A)   **(B)**

FIGURE 26-30   Cross section through the lumbar spine at the level of the intervertebral disk. **(A)** Normal relationships of intervertebral disk to spinal canal, dura, and spinal nerves. **(B)** Posterior protrusion of nucleus pulposus, impinging on dural sac and spinal nerve, exiting through the intervertebral foramen.

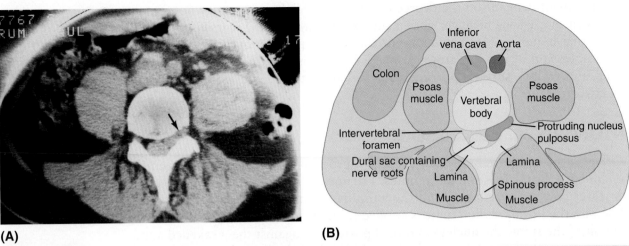

FIGURE 26-31 Demonstration of herniated nucleus pulposus ("slipped disk"). **(A)** CT scan of lumbar region. Protruding nucleus pulposus (*arrow*) is located adjacent to the dural sac and fills intervertebral foramen (*arrow*). Compare with appearance of normal intervertebral foramen on opposite side. **(B)** Schematic of anatomic structures and lesion as demonstrated on a CT scan.

Courtesy of Leonard V. Crowley, MD, Century College.

The protrusion of the disk material into the spinal canal can be demonstrated by CT and MRI scans, noninvasive radiologic examinations described in the discussion on general concepts of disease, principles of diagnosis (**FIGURE 26-31**).

Structure and Function of the Thorax

The skeleton of the chest wall (thorax) consists of the thoracic spine posteriorly, the sternum anteriorly, and the ribs with their costal cartilages that connect them. The upper part of the sternum is called the manubrium, to which the first ribs attach by their costal cartilages. The body of the sternum is attached to the manubrium by a movable joint that acts as a hinge, allowing the sternal body to angle forward and the attached ribs to become more horizontal as the diaphragm descends during inspiration. The ribs articulate posteriorly with the thoracic vertebrae, and all except ribs 11 and 12 also attach to the sternum anteriorly by their costal cartilages. Below the sternal body is the small attached xiphoid process, which moves with the sternal body. The costal cartilages of ribs 3 through 5 attach to the body of the sternum so that the anterior surfaces of the costal cartilages and the body of the sternum form a uniform, relatively flat surface that is characteristic of the anterior surface of the chest wall. Ribs 6 and 7 attach to the lower part of the sternal body and xiphoid process.

The ribs protect the lungs, and the sternum protects the heart, which is located in the mediastinum (the region between the lungs). However, the space available to the heart in the mediastinum is limited anteriorly by the sternum, and posteriorly by the vertebral bodies of the thoracic spine. Consequently, part of the left ventricle must project into the left pleural cavity to obtain additional space, which reduces slightly the space for expansion of the left lung during inspiration when compared to the size of the right pleural cavity.

CHEST WALL ABNORMALITIES

Chest wall abnormalities result from abnormal growth and attachment of the rib cartilages to the body of the sternum, which changes the position of the sternum. In the most common and important condition, the lower part of the sternum is displaced posteriorly, which is called **pectus excavatum** (*pectus* = chest 1 *excavatum* = hollowed out), sometimes called a "funnel chest." An anterior sternal protrusion, pectus carinatum (*carina* = prow of a ship), is much less frequent, and it is sometimes called a "pigeon breast" because it resembles the anterior protrusion of the sternum in a bird.

Pectus Excavatum

In this condition, the lower two-thirds of the sternum is displaced posteriorly along with the lower costal cartilages, which curve inward to form a broad midline chest depression with the deepest depression in the lowest part of the sternum just above the xiphoid process. The posterior displacement of the sternum appears to be caused by excessive unbalanced growth of the lower costal cartilages 3 through 5, which pushes the sternum posteriorly. The sternal displacement also affects the position of the ribs, which may lead to some asymmetry of the thorax manifested as slight scoliosis. The manubrium and the attached first and second costal cartilages are unaffected. The abnormality usually becomes apparent soon after birth, progresses during childhood, and becomes even more pronounced during the rapid skeletal growth phase associated with adolescence but does not progress after skeletal growth ceases.

Pectus excavatum (PE) is a relatively common abnormality that occurs in about 1 in 300 to 400 white males, and less often in white females and other ethnic groups. About 40 percent of affected individuals also have family members with PE, but the genetic basis has not yet been established.

Clinical Effects of Pectus Excavatum

A relatively minor posterior sternal depression may not encroach to a significant extent on the heart or the adjacent pleural cavities, but it can be a psychological problem to a teenager concerned about his or her body image. This is of particular concern in adolescent females because the condition results in breast asymmetry. Most cases of pectus excavatum show no functional defects. However, a marked posterior sternal depression can compromise both cardiac and pulmonary function, and exercise tolerance may be compromised, particularly with aging.

Treatment of Pectus Excavatum

Only a major degree of sternal depression is treated surgically, so it is important to document the severity of the deformity. X-ray or CT examinations can be used to determine the extent of the posterior sternal displacement, and other studies can assess its effects on cardiac and pulmonary function. Only marked posterior sternal displacement is considered for surgical repair, especially if cardiac and pulmonary function studies are abnormal.

Minimally invasive surgery is performed in which a long, curved metal bar is inserted through a small lateral chest incision with the concave surface of the bar positioned anteriorly. Then the bar is passed through the chest behind the sternum. When properly positioned, the bar is turned ("flipped") so that the convex surface of the bar is directed anteriorly, which pushes the sternum anteriorly along with the attached ribs. The bar is left in place for two to four years and then removed. The goal is to maintain the chest bar in place until the bones and joints reshape to the new chest position and the chest muscles are able to help maintain the new chest position.

Pectus Carinatum

A less common chest wall abnormality is called pectus carinatum because of the anterior, ridgelike projection of the sternum that has been compared to the prow of

> **Pectus excavatum**
> Posterior displacement of the sternum caused by excessive growth of costal cartilages, which reduce the size of the retrosternal space available for the heart within the mediastinum.

a ship (*carina* = ship's prow). Another commonly used term is "pigeon breast" from its resemblance to a bird's sternum. Although the abnormality may be a concern to the individual, usually there are no associated disturbances of cardiac or pulmonary function. Braces worn by the patient have been used to push the sternum back into a more normal position, but they are not very effective. Surgical reconstruction of the chest wall can be performed if desired.

Connective Tissue Disease

The two important types of connective tissue are the widely distributed collagen fibers that provide strength but lack flexibility, and elastic tissue fibers that can stretch and return to their former shape when the stretching force ceases. Elastic fibers are abundant in blood vessels, where their elasticity permits the aorta and its branches to stretch and recoil in response to the blood pumped into the vessels during ventricular systole, and are present in many other tissues along with collagen fibers, where they perform various "stretchability" functions including the skin and subcutaneous tissues, and in the eyes where they attach the lens to the ciliary body in the correct position required for normal vision. Connective tissue fibers are constructed from a precursor protein called fibrillin. A mutation of the gene coding for fibrillin (*FBN1*) gives rise to a group of abnormalities grouped together as a relatively common disease called **Marfan syndrome** (**FIGURE 26-32**).

Its incidence is about 1 in 5,000 people, and the condition usually is transmitted as a dominant trait. Less often, the disease results from a new spontaneous *FBN1* gene mutation in the affected person. When the mutation is transmitted from a parent, its severity may differ among affected individuals in the same family. The gene mutation leads to excessive growth in height; excessively long, thin fingers and toes with excessive joint flexibility; and various chest wall abnormalities, usually pectus excavatum. The fibers that hold the lens in correct position behind the iris may not be able to maintain the lens in proper position, which leads to visual disturbances. However, the most serious complication of Marfan syndrome involves the cardiovascular system, which is caused by defective elastic fibers in the aorta. As a result, the aorta gradually dilates because the defective elastic fibers in the aortic wall are unable to maintain the normal shape of the aorta. Excessive dilation of the aorta may lead to a dissecting aneurysm of the aorta and its complications (described in the discussion on the cardiovascular system). If the excessive dilation occurs in the ascending aorta, the cusps of the aortic valve, which are attached to the dilated aorta, are unable to fit closely together in diastole to close the aortic valve, which leads to aortic valve insufficiency. Mitral valve defects also occur. There is no specific treatment for the

Marfan syndrome
A hereditary connective tissue disease characterized by excessive joint flexibility along with various skeletal and cardiovascular abnormalities.

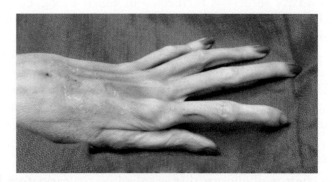

FIGURE 26-32 Marfan syndrome. This disorder used to be called arachnodactyly, literally "spider fingers."

disease, although some antihypertensive agents may retard the rate of aortic dilation and reduce the risk of a dissecting aneurysm. Surgical procedures such as the use of prosthetic grafts are also available to treat the complications caused by dilation of the aorta, and prosthetic valves may be necessary to correct disturbed valve functions. Annual ultrasound examinations are recommended to monitor the progression of the aortic dilation, which may require eventual surgical repair to reduce the risk of a dissecting aneurysm or rupture of the aorta. Pectus excavatum often occurs in Marfan syndrome. In one series of cases, one-third of a group of patients treated for pectus excavatum were later considered to have Marfan syndrome.

Structure and Function of Skeletal Muscle

Muscle cells are highly specialized contractile cells. Three different types of muscle are recognized: smooth muscle, skeletal muscle, and cardiac muscle. Smooth muscle is found in the walls of the gastrointestinal tract, biliary tract, urogenital system, respiratory tract, and blood vessels. Skeletal muscle is attached to the skeleton by tendons and ligaments; it functions in voluntary muscular activity. Cardiac muscle closely resembles skeletal muscle but has certain special features related to its function of producing rhythmic contractions of the heart. Lesions of smooth muscles are rare, and disorders of cardiac muscle are considered in the discussion on the cardiovascular system.

CONTRACTION OF SKELETAL MUSCLE

Skeletal muscles are long, straplike fibers that measure as much as 30 cm in length. The cytoplasm (sarcoplasm) contains multiple nuclei located just beneath the cell membrane (sarcolemma). Filling the cytoplasm are long threadlike myofibrils composed of the contractile myofilaments actin and myosin. The cytoplasm also contains many energy-rich organic compounds, ions, and enzymes required for the metabolic activity of the muscle cell (**FIGURE 26-33**).

Muscle cells contract in response to motor nerve impulses conveyed to the muscle. The area of communication between the nerve endings and the muscle cell is called the neuromuscular junction, or **motor end plate**. The actual stimulation of the muscle cell is the result of a chemical called **acetylcholine**, which is released from the nerve endings at the neuromuscular junction and interacts with acetylcholine receptors on the surface of the muscle fibers. The chemical mediator acetylcholine initiates the biochemical chain of events that causes the actin and myosin filaments to slide together, which leads to shortening of the muscle fiber. The duration of the chemical mediator is quite brief because this substance is rapidly broken down by the enzyme cholinesterase, which is present at the neuromuscular junction.

FACTORS AFFECTING MUSCULAR STRUCTURE AND FUNCTION

The normal structural and functional integrity of skeletal muscle depends on an intact nerve supply, normal transmission of impulses across the myoneural junction, and normal metabolic processes within the muscle cell. As considered in the discussion on the nervous system, skeletal muscles that are not used or muscles deprived of their nerve supply undergo marked **atrophy** (**FIGURE 26-34**). Conversely, when additional work is required of the muscles, they undergo hypertrophy in response to the increased demands.

Muscle cells contain a highly complex metabolic machinery capable of translating nerve impulses into muscle contractions. Any disturbance in the metabolism of

Motor end plate Neuromuscular junction between nerve and muscle.

Acetylcholine A chemical secreted by nerve endings that activates neurons or muscle cells.

Atrophy Wasting of tissue due to underuse; typically due to the degeneration of cells.

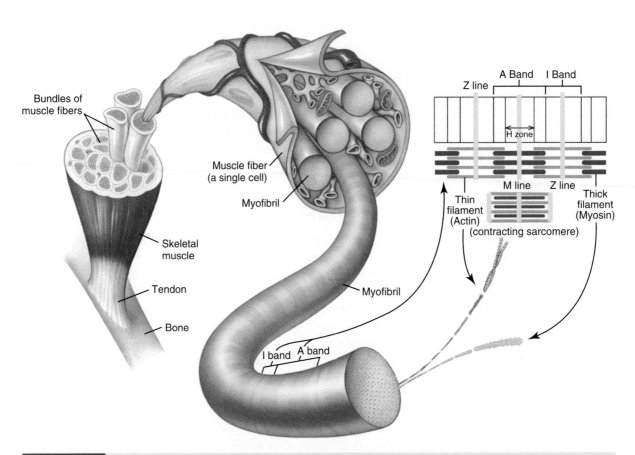

FIGURE 26-33 Structure of the skeletal muscle fiber. Molecular details of the contractile apparatus are shown on the left of the figure.

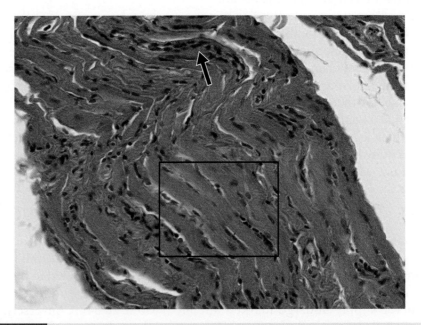

FIGURE 26-34 Muscle atrophy as a result of denervation (microscopic view). Necrotic muscle fibers being phagocytozed by macrophages, called lengthwise segmental necrosis (*arrow*). Area of necrotic muscle fibers that are anucleate and pale (*box*).

Courtesy of Department of Pathology and Laboratory Medicine, University of North Carolina at Chapel Hill.

the muscle cell leads to a disturbance in the function of the cell. The intracellular metabolic processes are also influenced by the endocrine glands that regulate the rate of metabolism within the muscle cell and affect the concentration of the various ions required for normal muscle contraction.

Diseases of skeletal muscle are uncommon. The principal disorders consist of inflammatory lesions, muscular atrophy, degeneration (dystrophy) of muscle, and disturbance of impulse conduction at the neuromuscular junction.

Inflammation of Muscle (Myositis)

LOCALIZED MYOSITIS

Small areas of inflammation in skeletal muscle are encountered in many systemic diseases and have no major clinical significance. Inflammation of muscle also may follow injury or muscular overexertion. The inflammation is secondary to necrosis and disruption of muscle cells and is associated with swelling and tenderness of the affected muscle. The inflammation gradually subsides as the muscle injury heals.

GENERALIZED MYOSITIS

Generalized inflammations of skeletal muscle (inflammatory myopathy) are uncommon but serious systemic diseases believed to be of autoimmune etiology. They are characterized by widespread degeneration and inflammation of skeletal muscle and associated progressive weakness of muscles and, ultimately, muscle wasting. Dermatomyositis, a type of inflammatory myopathy associated with swelling and inflammation of the skin, affects both children and adults and is associated with autoimmune damage to capillaries and small vessels (microangiopathy) as a result of deposition of immune complexes in vessel walls (see discussion on immunity, hypersensitivity, allergy, and autoimmune diseases). This results in ischemic damage to the muscle. Unlike dematomyositis, polymyositis is limited to adults and is associated with T cell–mediated damage to muscles although autoantibodies are also present and of unknown significance. Polymyositis is often associated with systemic disease of connective tissue of multiple organs, particularly the lung. Both forms of inflammatory myositis respond to corticosteroid therapy (**FIGURE 26-35**).

> **Myositis** Inflammation of muscle.

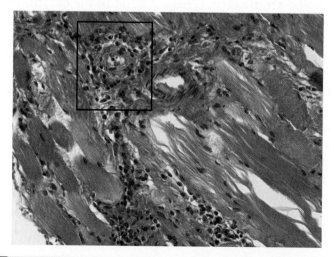

FIGURE 26-35 Dermatomyositis demonstrating perivascular inflammation (*box*). Microscopic view.
Courtesy of Department of Pathology and Laboratory Medicine, University of North Carolina at Chapel Hill.

Muscular Dystrophy

The muscular dystrophies are a group of relatively rare diseases characterized by progressive degeneration of skeletal muscle not primarily associated with inflammation. The muscle tissue shows necrosis and concomitant attempts at regeneration. Ultimately, muscle is replaced by fibrosis and fatty tissue. Many of the dystrophies are hereditary. Various clinical syndromes are recognized, depending on the muscle groups affected, the patterns of inheritance, and the rate of progression of the disease. In general, the diseases are characterized by progressive muscular weakness and gradually increasing disability, eventually terminating in death from paralysis of the respiratory muscles or superimposed respiratory infection.

In the muscular dystrophies, the nerve supply to the muscles is unaffected. The basic disturbance is an abnormality in the muscle fibers that causes them to degenerate. The most common and severe type is called Duchenne muscular dystrophy, and a milder form of muscular dystrophy is called Becker muscular dystrophy. Both forms result from the mutation of a large gene on the X chromosome, and the disease is transmitted as an X-linked trait to male children of women who carry the defective gene. The normal gene codes for a muscle protein called dystrophin, which is located on the inner surface of the sarcolemma; it plays a role in maintaining the structure and functions of the muscle fibers by aiding in connecting the muscle cell membrane to the external extracellular matrix.

As a result of the gene mutation, the absent or defective dystrophin is responsible for the manifestations of the disease, which appears first during early childhood and progress rapidly, leading to death in late adolescence or early adulthood. The muscles primarily affected are those of the lower extremities, trunk, hips, and shoulder girdle. Often, the extent of atrophy is visibly masked because the muscles are infiltrated by fat and fibrous tissue as they atrophy. The fat infiltration may at times be so extreme that the affected muscles appear hypertrophied, leading to the paradox of profound muscular weakness in an individual whose muscles appear (but are not) very well developed (**FIGURE 26-36**).

The less-severe Becker muscular dystrophy also is caused by a mutation of the same dystrophin-producing gene that causes Duchenne muscular dystrophy. Dystrophin is produced by the mutated gene but is either abnormal or produced in insufficient amounts. In both diseases, the muscle enzyme creatine kinase (CK) leaks from the abnormal muscle fibers, resulting in high levels of the enzyme in the blood of those who are affected. (This is similar to the enzyme that leaks from the heart muscle when the muscle is damaged, as described in the discussion on the cardiovascular system.) The diagnosis of muscular dystrophy is made on the basis of the clinical features together with the very high CK blood concentration. Genetic testing reveals the gene mutation, and muscle biopsies reveal absence of dystrophin in Duchenne dystrophy and an abnormal or reduced amount of dystrophin in Becker dystrophy.

Although the various types of muscular atrophy and muscular dystrophy are uncommon, they are of major concern, not only to the patient but to the family, because of the hereditary nature of many of these illnesses. Unfortunately, there is no way at present to arrest the relentless progression of the disease. Gene therapy to eventually allow insertion of replacement genes in muscle fibers to code for the synthesis of the missing or defective dystrophin is being actively investigated but has not yet been successful.

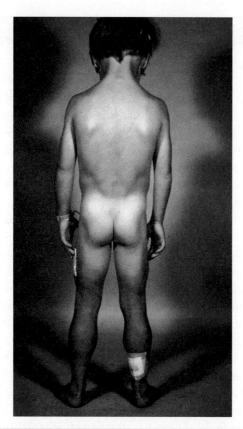

FIGURE 26-36 Duchenne muscular dystrophy. Note the "pseudohypertrophy" of the calves.

MYASTHENIA GRAVIS

Myasthenia gravis is a chronic disease characterized by abnormal fatigability of the voluntary muscles as a result of an abnormality at the neuromuscular junction. Fatigue develops rapidly when the muscles are used and subsides when they are rested. Often, the dysfunction is most conspicuous in the small muscles of the face and in the muscles concerned with eye movement (extraocular muscles). Myasthenia gravis appears to be an autoimmune disease. The blood of affected patients contains an autoantibody directed against acetylcholine receptors on the surface of the muscle fibers at the neuromuscular junction. The manifestations of the disease occur because the antibody damages and greatly reduces the number of receptors available to interact with the acetylcholine liberated from motor nerve endings.

Symptoms can be relieved by drugs that inhibit the action of the enzyme cholinesterase. This prolongs the action of the chemical mediator acetylcholine so that it can continue to stimulate the reduced numbers of receptors for a longer time. Many patients with myasthenia gravis have either a tumor or a benign hyperplasia of the thymus gland that plays a role in the progression of the disease. Patients with hyperplasia or a tumor of the thymus gland sometimes are improved by removal of the thymus.

> **Myasthenia gravis**
> An autoimmune disease characterized by abnormal fatigability of muscle and caused by an autoantibody that damages the acetylcholine receptors at the neuromuscular junction.

CASE 26-1

Charles was the first child in the family. When he was four years old, his parents became concerned about his unusual way of walking (gait). He appeared to "waddle." When Charles attempted to stand, he first got onto his knees and pushed himself up (Gower sign). He also seemed to occasionally walk on his toes. Concerned, his parents brought Charles to Dr. Jane, their pediatrician. Dr. Jane questioned Charles's mother Annie about her family history and, in particular, if any of her male relatives had muscle problems. Annie said that she was an adoptee and had no knowledge of her biological parents. Dr. Jane asked Annie if she had any unusual muscle weakness or had been diagnosed with any other medical problems. Annie said she had been in good health for the past several years. Dr. Jane noted that all of Charles's motor milestones were markedly delayed. She sent a sample of Charles's blood for a determination of creatinine kinase level (found to be abnormally high). Suspecting that Charles had a dystrophic muscle disease, most likely muscular dystrophy, she referred Charles to a specialist in muscular diseases. The neuromuscular specialist obtained a muscle biopsy from Charles and ordered molecular analysis of his *DMD* gene.

Analysis of the muscle biopsy revealed a mixture of degenerating and regenerating fibers characteristic of a muscular dystrophy. Further analysis showed that Charles did have dystrophin, the protein product of the *DMD* gene present, but in reduced amount (about 50 percent of normal). However, the dystrophin did not have a normal structure; it was shorter than the normal protein. The specialist explained to Charles's parents that there are two types of muscular dystrophy that differ in severity and age of onset, but both are related to a mutation in the same *DMD* gene found on the X chromosome. Both are expressed in males, but females carry the disease and are sometimes affected. Duchenne muscular dystrophy (DMD) is the more common (about 1 in 3,000 live male births). The disease usually shows up (presents) between three and five years of age and progresses with increased weakness for six to seven years. The children become wheelchair bound and die of pulmonary and cardiac failure, usually in their early twenties. There is no current therapy, but corticosteroids delay the course of the disease by one to two years. Becker muscular dystrophy (BMD) is a less severe form of the disease. It is far less common (about 1 in 30,000 male births) and is very variable. Although sometimes symptoms may be found in a child of Charles's age, the disease usually is not diagnosed until a child is eleven or twelve years old. Most often BMD patients continue to walk until the late twenties and, on the average, live until the fifth decade of life, usually dying from cardiac failure. Charles's parents ask, "What about our son. Does he have DMD or BMD?" To answer, the specialist explains, he will have to do additional studies of the defect in Charles's *DMD* gene.

Discussion

Given the age of onset of the disease in Charles, DMD is most likely. However, the presence of a significant amount of dystrophin argues toward BMD. Mutations that result in very little or no dystrophin result in DMD. However, mutations in which a reduced amount of a "short" DMD molecule is made may function to some degree, but not always.

Why is this? Dystrophin is necessary to provide a stable structure in the muscle cell. The *DMD* gene is the largest gene found to date and takes up about 2 percent of the X chromosome. The protein dystrophin forms a "dumbbell" with two spherical areas (the amino and carboxy termini of the molecules) connected by a central rodlike domain. The protein bridges the contractile actin fibers in the muscle cell to the connective tissue on the outside of the muscle cell. The spherical areas on the ends of the molecule are the "connectors" to the actin and exterior connective tissue. The rodlike area links the two connectors. Many BMD patients have an "in-frame" mutation that deletes part of the central rodlike domain. The molecule is shorter (as was the case for Charles) but still has some ability to function as a bridge. Unfortunately, in Charles's case, the mutation was "in-frame"

CASE 26-1 (Continued)

and deleted part of the central rod but also deleted an important part of the carboxy terminal part of the molecule, which is necessary for it to connect to the extracellular matrix. (Note that this is a much simplified picture of the actual molecule.) Although Charles made a short dystrophin molecule, often characteristic of BMD, the molecule had no function in his muscle cells, meaning that Charles had DMD.

Etiology and Pathogenesis

Duchenne muscular dystrophy resulting from an in-frame mutation producing a nonfunctional dystrophin protein.

Questions

1. Why did the pediatrician start by asking Annie if she had male relatives with muscle problems? Would such problems be expected on the maternal or paternal part of the family? Review sex-linked inheritance. Do you think Annie might show symptoms as she ages?

2. The case uses the term "in-frame mutation." What is an in-frame mutation? Why are out-of-frame or truncating mutations more likely to result in DMD rather than BMD?

3. Predict the future; that is, make a prognosis. What are some potential approaches to therapy for DMD?

4. Often patients diagnosed with a particular disease show variability in severity and age of onset compared to others with the disease. What are some potential reasons?

QUESTIONS FOR REVIEW

1. Describe the structure of the typical movable joint.

2. Describe the structure and function of the spine.

3. Describe the structure and function of the thorax.

4. What is the difference between a simple fracture and a compound fracture? What are the complications of a compound fracture? What is a comminuted fracture? A pathologic fracture?

5. What is a "slipped disk"? Why does it occur? Why does it sometimes produce pain radiating down the leg? How is it treated?

6. What is rheumatoid arthritis? What is its relationship to the immune system? How is it treated?

7. What are the types of muscle cells?

8. What is meant by the following terms: *neuromuscular junction, acetylcholine,* and *myositis?*

9. What is the difference between muscular atrophy and muscular dystrophy? What are the most common types of atrophic disease of the muscles? Of dystrophic disease?

SUPPLEMENTARY READINGS

Fritchie, K., Chapter 18, "Soft Tissue and Bone Pathology," and Lee, E. T., and Chahin, N. Chapter 19, "Neuromuscular Pathology." 2015. In *Pathology: A Modern Case Study*, edited by H. M. Reisner. New York, NY: Lange McGraw Hill.
  ▶ Rheumatology, orthopedics, neurology, and neurosurgery all intersect in the study of diseases of the bone, muscle, and connective tissue. These two chapters are suggested as an advanced introduction to the etiology and pathogenesis of these diseases. The indicated source is rich in illustrations and brief case studies.

Baum, R., and Gravallese, E. M. 2014. Impact of inflammation on the osteoblast in rheumatic disease. *Current Osteoporosis Reports* 12:9–16.
  ▶ Bone is continually remodeled based on stress. Inflammation disturbs the balance between osteoclasts and osteoblasts. This review looks at the mechanisms that maintain and disturb the balance between bone growth and degradation.

Harrington, J., and Sochett, E. 2015. The child with multiple fractures, what next? *Pediatric Clinics of North America* 62:841–55.

Shaker, J. L., et al. 2015. Recent developments in osteogenesis imperfecta. *F1000Research* (ePub September 7). doi: 10.12688/f1000research.6398.1
  ▶ An introduction to an all too common pediatric problem. The first entry explores the implications for potential child abuse. The second entry is a recent review of genetic conditions responsible for brittle bones and multiple fractures.

National Institutes of Health, Office of Dietary Supplements. *Vitamin D fact sheet for health professionals.* https://ods.od.nih.gov/factsheets/VitaminD-HealthProfessional/
  ▶ An excellent resource for information on the function of Vitamin D and appropriate vitamin D supplementation. This is an area rife with misinformation. This resource provides a wealth of current trustworthy information.

National Institutes of Health, Osteoporosis and Related Bone Diseases, National Resource Center. *Bone mass measurement: What the numbers mean.* http://www.niams.nih.gov/Health_Info/Bone/Bone_Health/bone_mass_measure

National Institutes of Health, Osteoporosis and Related Bone Diseases, National Resource Center. *Osteoporosis.* http://www.niams.nih.gov/Health_Info/Bone/Osteoporosis/
  ▶ These two resources serve as a gateway to a wealth of material on the structure of bone (bone basics) and diseases of bone, including osteogenesis imperfecta, osteoporosis, and Paget disease (not discussed in the text). An excellent first place to look for additional trustworthy information in the area. The second entry provides extensive information on all aspects of osteoporosis.

Mankia, K., and Emery, P. 2015. Is localized autoimmunity the trigger for rheumatoid arthritis? Unravelling new targets for prevention. *Discovery Medicine* 20:129–35.

▶ An overview of recent concepts of the etiology and pathogenesis of rheumatoid arthritis.

U.S. National Library of Medicine. MedlinePlus. *Arthritis.* https://www.nlm.nih.gov/medlineplus/arthritis.html

▶ A portal for additional information on all aspects of arthritic disease.

Sivera, F., et al. 2014. Diagnostic value of clinical, laboratory, and imaging findings in patients with a clinical suspicion of gout: A systemic literature review. *Journal of Rheumatology: The Supplement* 92:3–8.

▶ The diagnosis of gouty arthritis may seem trivial, but it presents surprising difficulties. An interesting review of the literature that asks which combination of diagnostic criteria are most useful.

Falzararano, M. F., et al. 2015. Duchenne muscular dystrophy: From diagnosis to therapy. *Molecules* 20:18168–84.

Wicklund, M. P. 2013. The muscular dystrophies. *Continuum* 19:1535–70.

▶ Duchenne muscular dystrophy is at the center of numerous attempts to provide gene-based therapy. The first entry is a recent review of these attempts as well as a good overview of diagnosis. The second entry was used in part in the Case construction. It reviews not only the more common muscular dystrophies but also several less common but distinctive conditions.

Glossary

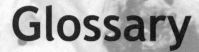

ABO hemolytic disease A mild hemolytic disease in group A or B infants or group O mothers as a result of maternal anti-A and anti-B antibodies.

Abruption Partial detachment of the placenta.

Abscess A localized accumulation of pus in tissues.

Acalasia/cardiospasm Inability of the sphincter to remain relaxed.

Acalculous cholecystitis Results from infection, prolonged fasting, or trauma.

Acetylcholine A chemical secreted by nerve endings that activates neurons or muscle cells.

Achondroplasia A congenital disturbance of endochondral bone formation that causes a type of dwarfism. The failure of bone ossification associated with short limb dwarfism.

Acini/acinar Small lobules of glands composed of a cavity surrounded by secretory cells/having properties of acini.

Acquired immune deficiency syndrome (AIDS) An infection caused by the human immunodeficiency virus. The virus attacks and destroys helper T lymphocytes, which compromises cell-mediated immunity, leading to increased susceptibility to infection and some tumors.

Acromegaly A condition resulting from excessive secretion of growth hormone in the adult.

Acrosome Previously the sperm golgi apparatus; contains enzymes necessary for penetration of the ovum.

Actin Contractile protein that cause muscles to shorten.

Actin microfilament One type of cell framework filament.

Actinic keratosis A precancerous warty proliferation of squamous epithelial cells in sun-damaged skin of older persons.

Activated neutrophil Neutrophil stimulated by various substances resulting in degranulation.

Active immunization Exposing a person to a noninfectious pathogen to provoke an immune response.

Active transport Transfer of materials against a concentration gradient that is necessary to a maintain proper concentration of intracellular and extracellular ions.

Acute calculous cholecystitis Mucosal injury from concentrated bile within gallbladder.

Acute coronary syndromes (ACS) A classification of patients with coronary artery disease complaining of chest pain into one of three separate groups (unstable angina, non-ST elevation myocardial infarction, and ST elevation myocardial infarction) based on ECG and cardiac enzyme tests, used to assess prognosis and guide treatment.

Acute hemorrhagic pancreatitis Severe pancreatic inflammation with necrosis of pancreatic ducts and release of pancreatic enzymes that damage the pancreas.

Acute inflammation Earliest phase of the inflammatory response.

Acute kidney injury/AKI Injury to any part of the kidney. May also be defined as prerenal or postrenal.

Acute phase proteins Proteins produced by the liver in response to inflammation.

Adaptive immunity Immune response that can change based on intruding molecules; has the ability to respond to almost any foreign molecule.

Addison disease A disease caused by chronic adrenal cortical hypofunction.

Adenosine triphosphate (ATP) A high-energy phosphate compound that liberates energy to power numerous cellular metabolic processes.

Adhesions Bands of fibrous tissue that form subsequent to an inflammation and bind adjacent tissues together. Also, bands of connective tissue in abdominal cavity after surgery.

Adipose tissue Loose, fibrous tissue containing fat cells.

Adjustable gastric banding A method for treating obesity by applying an adjustable gastric band to the stomach to reduce its capacity, thereby promoting weight loss.

Adjuvant Substance that enhances an immune response.

Adjuvant chemotherapy Anticancer chemotherapy administered before or after surgical resection of a tumor in an attempt to destroy any small, undetected foci of metastatic tumor before they become clinically detectable.

Adrenal corticosteroid hormones/steroids Chemicals that suppress the inflammatory process.

Adrenal Cushing syndrome Caused by a corticosteroid hormone-producing tumor of the adrenal cortex.

Adrenocorticotrophic hormone (ACTH) A hormone secreted by the anterior lobe of the pituitary that stimulates the adrenal cortex to manufacture and secrete adrenal cortical hormones.

Adult polycystic kidney disease Autosomal dominant disease characterized by the formation of multiple cysts throughout both kidneys.

Adult respiratory distress syndrome (ARDS)/diffuse alveolar damage (DAD) Result of process disturbing the alveolar capillary permeability barrier.

Aerobic organisms Microbes that grow best in the presence of oxygen.

Affinity maturation Improvement in ability to bind antigen by immunoglobulin resulting from somatic mutations.

Akinetic/hypokinetic Lacking or showing reduced contraction.

Albumin Blood protein providing colloid osmotic pressure in blood.

Albumin to creatinine ratio (ACR) Measurement of urine albumin levels compared to amount of creatinine.

Alcoholic liver disease Injury associated with excessive amounts of alcohol.

Alcoholic steatosis Condition of abnormal intracellular accumulation of lipid in the liver following ingestion of quantities of ethanol.

Aldosterone A steroid hormone produced by the adrenal cortex that regulates the rate of sodium absorption from the renal tubules.

Alkylating agent An anticancer drug that disrupts cell function by binding DNA chains together so they cannot separate.

Allele One of several related forms of a single gene.

Allogeneic/syngeneic/autologous Terms used to classify the relationship of donor cells to the patient, not from self/from an identical twin/from self.

Alpha fetoprotein (AFP) Protein produced by fetal liver early in gestation. Sometimes produced by tumor cells. Level is elevated in amnionic fluid when fetus has neural tube defect.

Alveoli/alveolus One of the terminal air sacs of the lung.

Ameloblasts Epithelial derived cells that form the tooth enamel.

Amenorrhea Absence of menses.

Amniocentesis Direct sampling of amniotic fluid.

Amnionic sac The fluid-filled sac surrounding the embryo. One of the fetal membranes.

Ampulla of Vater Common channel through the pancreas.

Anaerobic organisms Microbes that grow best in the absence of oxygen.

Anaphylactoid reaction Immune response resembling an anaphylactic reaction but by direct action on mast cells or by activating complement.

Anaphylaxis A widespread systemic hypersensitive reaction.

Anaplastic cell Type of tumor cell whose structure is so deranged as to make identification of origin difficult.

Anasarca Widespread edema.

Anastomosis A communication between two blood vessels or other tubular structures. Also refers to a surgical connection of two hollow tubular structures, such as the divided ends of the intestine or a blood vessel (surgical anastomosis).

Anemia A decrease in hemoglobin or red cells or both.

Anencephaly A congenital malformation: absence of brain, cranial vault, and scalp as a result of defective closure of the neural tube.

Anergy Continued nonresponsiveness of T cells to a host or foreign antigen.

Aneuploidy Condition denoting abnormal number of chromosomes.

Aneurysm A dilatation of a structure, such as the aorta, a cerebral artery, or a part of the ventricular wall. Outpouching of walls of blood vessels.

Angiogenesis Ability to stimulate the formation of new blood vessels.

Anicteric hepatitis Symptoms of hepatitis without appearance of jaundice.

Anions Negatively charged ions in electrolytes.

Annulus fibrosus The dense peripheral ring of fibrocartilage making up the intervertebral disk.

Anthracosis Carbon pigment deposited in the connective tissue around the individual lobules of lung.

Antibody Immunoglobulin molecule that can recognize a foreign substance.

Antibody-dependent cellular cytotoxicity (ADCC) Recognition and destruction of cells coated with antibody.

Anticodon Code complementary to the codon on the mRNA, which allows the correct amino acid to be deposited by the tRNA.

Antidiuretic hormone (ADH) Posterior lobe pituitary hormone that regulates urine concentration by altering the permeability of the renal collecting tubules.

Antigen Foreign substance.

Antigen presenting cell (APC) Cell that displays the foreign material.

Antigenic determinants/epitopes Number of antigenic sites on a single molecule.

Antimetabolite A substance that competes with or replaces another substance (metabolite) required for cell.

Anuric The absence of urine formation.

Aortic valve Semilunar valve surrounding the orifices of the aorta.

Aplastic anemia Lack of mature blood cells and platelets caused by stem cell damage.

Apoptosis Programmed cell death that does not provoke a host protective response; occurs after a cell has lived its normal life span.

Appendicolith A calcified stone in the appendix.

Arachnoid The middle of the three meninges that cover the brain.

Arnold Chiari malformation Congenital condition with spinal cord defects and compression of the brain stem and cerebellum downward.

Aromatase inhibitor A drug that inhibits the conversion of adrenal androgenic steroids to estrogens, used as postresection adjuvant therapy to treat postmenopausal women with estrogen-positive breast carcinoma.

Arrhythmia An irregularity of the heartbeat.

Arthropod Invertebrate animal with jointed limbs and segmented body, such as insect and spider. Important arthropods that parasitize humans include the crab louse and the organism causing scabies.

Arthropod-borne virus/arbovirus An infectious nucleic acid particle (virus) transmitted by mosquitoes.

Asbestosis A type of pneumoconiosis caused by inhalation of asbestos fibers.

Ascites Fluid accumulating in body cavities due to low albumin. Swelling of abdominal area and legs caused by excess extracellular fluid.

Astrocyte A large stellate cell having highly branched processes. Forms the structural framework of the nervous system. One of the neuroglial cells.

Astrocytes Supportive cells of the brain.

Astrocytoma Neuroglial tumor arising from astrocytes; most common type.

Asymptomatic Disease without symptoms.

Atelectasis Collapse of the lung, either caused by bronchial obstruction (obstructive atelectasis) or external compression (compression atelectasis).

Atheroma Formation of plaque with a necrotic core rich in lipids.

Atherosclerosis Formation of lipid-rich plaques in large and medium arteries.

Atrium/atria Upper chambers of the heart.

Atrioventricular (AV) valve The flaplike heart valve located between the atrium and the ventricle.

Atrophy Reduction in size of cells or organs in response to diminished function. Wasting of tissue due to underuse; typically due to the degeneration of cells.

Attack complex Group of complement molecules that destroys the target micro-organism or abnormal cell.

Autoantibody An antibody formed against the host's own cells or tissue components.

Autocrine Cytokine that enhances the response of T cells to itself. Also, self-acting loop in cancer responsible for uncontrolled growth.

Autoimmune disease A disease associated with formation of cell-mediated or humoral immunity against the subject's own cells or tissue components.

Autoimmunity Immunological activity against self antigen markers.

Autophagy Process by which cellular organelles are degraded and recycled by the cells.

Autosomal chromosomes Chromosomes other than sex chromosomes. A human has 22 pairs of autosomes.

Avascular necrosis Bone necrosis caused by interruption of its blood supply.

Axon Portion of neuron that conducts impulses away from the cell body.

B lymphocyte/B cell A lymphocyte that differentiates into plasma cells and is associated with humoral immunity.

Bacillus Rod-shaped bacteria.

Barr body The inactivated X chromosome attached to the nuclear membrane in the female. Sex chromatin body.

Barrett esophagus Squamous lining changes to a more acid-resistant columnar mucosa.

Basal-like tumors Type of breast cancer cell demonstrating a specific gene expression profile.

Basophil A cell that contains numerous variable-sized granules that stain intensely purple with basic dyes. See also eosinophil.

Bell-clapper defect Anatomic abnormality responsible for increased testicular mobility.

Benign Neoplasms that do not spread to sites distant from their origin.

Bile A secretion of the liver containing bile salts, cholesterol, and other substances.

Bile canaliculi Small terminal bile channels located between liver cords.

Bile salts Derivatives of bile acids present in bile that act as emulsifiers to promote fat digestion and absorption.

Biliary cirrhosis Diffuse liver cell damage and scarring with distortion of liver cell structure and function (cirrhosis) caused by obstruction of bile ducts. Liver damage of the epithelium of the bile ducts.

Biliary colic Abdominal pain that results when a gallstone enters the biliary duct system.

Bilirubin One of the bile pigments derived from the breakdown of hemoglobin.

Bioinformatics Massive databases used for the study of the human genome.

Biopsy Removal of a small sample of tissue for examination and diagnosis by a pathologist.

Blastocyst A stage of development of the fertilized ovum (zygote) in which a central cavity forms within the cluster of developing cells.

Blastomycosis A systemic fungus infection caused by the fungus *Blastomyces dermatiditis*.

Bleeding time Time needed for a small standardized skin incision to stop bleeding.

Blood agar plates Bacteria media incorporating red blood cells.

Body stalk The structure connecting the embryo to the chorion. Eventually develops into the umbilical cord.

Borborygmi Loud bowel sounds.

Botulism Food poisoning caused by ingestion of a neurotoxin produced by an anaerobic spore-forming bacillus *Clostridium botulinum* growing in improperly canned or preserved food.

Bowman's capsule The cuplike expanded end of the nephron that surrounds the tuft of glomerular capillaries.

Bradykinin A chemical mediator of inflammation derived from components in the blood plasma.

Brain Stem The brain stem is the elongated central portion of the brain connecting the cerebral hemispheres with the spinal cord. It controls the flow of messages to the rest of the body and is critical for autonomic functions such as breathing.

Breast conserving surgery Surgery designed to remove the minimal amount of breast tissue.

Bronchi/bronchus One of the large subdivisions of the trachea.

Bronchiectasis Dilatation of bronchi caused by weakening of their walls as a result of infection.

Bronchiole One of the small terminal subdivisions of the branched bronchial tree.

Buccal plate Specialized attachment organ of hookworms.

Budd Chiari syndrome/postsinusoidal portal hypertension Hypertension resulting from thrombosis of the hepatic vein.

Calcitonin A hormone that lowers blood calcium, produced by the interfollicular cells of the thyroid gland.

Calculi Stones formed within the body, as in the kidney or gallbladder.

Callus Newly synthesized bone repairing break.

Cancellous bone Inner, spongy layer of bone.

Canker sores Inflammatory disease of the oral cavity.

Capacitation Process in which the surface of the sperm is altered.

Capsid The protein covering the central nucleic acid core of a virus. Protein coat of the HIV virus.

Capsomere One of the subunits that make up the protein shell (capsid) of a virus.

Capsular epithelium Outer layer of cells of Bowman's capsule. It is also termed the parietal layer of Bowman's capsule.

Carcinoembryonic antigen (CEA) A tumor-associated antigen that resembles the antigen secreted by the cells of the fetal gastrointestinal tract.

Carcinogenesis Development of cancer.

Carcinoma A malignant tumor derived from epithelial cells.

Carcinoma in situ Neoplasm occupying full thickness of the epithelium.

Cardiac arrest Complete cessation of cardiac activity.

Cardiac muscle Muscle found only in the heart; has features of both striated and smooth muscle.

Cardiac tamponade Accumulation of blood adjacent to the heart due to blood leaking through ruptured heart muscle and compressing the heart, preventing normal cardiac function.

Cardinal signs of inflammation Heat, swelling, redness, and pain observed at site of injury.

Caries Tooth decay.

Carpal tunnel syndrome Condition resulting from nerves in the hand being compressed on the anterior surface of the wrist.

Cartilage A type of supporting tissue in which cells are dispersed in a dense matrix.

Caseous Necrotic center of nodule characteristic of tuberculosis.

Catecholamines The adrenal medullary hormones epinephrine and norepinephrine.

Cations Positively charged ions in electrolytes.

Cavity (dental) A loss of tooth structure caused by the combined action of mouth bacteria and organic acids derived from bacterial fermentation of retained food particles.

CCR5 co-receptor antagonists Drugs that prevent the CCR5 receptor on CD4 T cells from interacting with an HIV protein.

Cell The basic structural and functional unit of the body.

Cell-mediated defense mechanism The defense against foreign antigens provided by a population of T lymphocytes that can attach and destroy the foreign antigens.

Cell-mediated immunity Immunity associated with population of sensitized lymphocytes.

Cellular component Circulating blood cell part of acute inflammation.

Cellulitis An acute spreading inflammation affecting the skin or deeper tissues.

Cementum Bonelike tissue covering the root of the tooth.

Central tolerance Part of the development of cellular and humoral immunity; cells reacting against self-antigen are removed during development.

Central zone Part of the prostate that surrounds the ejaculatory ducts.

Centrioles Short, cylindrical structures located adjacent to the nucleus that participate in the formation of spindle fibers during cell division.

Centromere/centriole The structure that joins each pair of chromatids formed by chromosome duplication.

Cerebellum Part of brain regulating muscle tone, coordination, posture, and balance.

Cerebral cortex Receives sensory input and initiates voluntary motor activity.

Cerebral embolus A stroke caused by blockage of a cerebral artery by a blood clot that had formed elsewhere in the circulatory system and was transported in the bloodstream to the brain.

Cerebral hemorrhage A stroke caused by rupture of a cerebral artery, usually in a person with hypertension, that allows blood to escape under high pressure into the brain.

Cerebral infarct Brain tissue that became necrotic after a stroke.

Cerebral thrombosis A stroke caused by thrombosis of an arteriosclerotic cerebral artery.

Cervical intraepithelial neoplasia (CIN) Precancerous condition characterized by cervical dysplasia in mucosa of cervix.

CGG repeats Expansion of cytosine-guanine-guanine repeating sequences; defect responsible for fragile X syndrome.

Chancre Small ulcer at site of syphilis inoculation.

Chemical mediators of inflammation Messenger molecule that acts on blood vessels, inflammatory cells, or other cells to contribute to an inflammatory response.

Chemotaxis Process of active movement of inflammatory cells to the site of the injury.

Cholecystitis Inflammation of the gallbladder.

Cholelithiasis Formation of gallstones.

Cholestasis Decreased bile flow and bile stasis.

Cholesterol A complex lipid (sterol) containing several ring structures.

Chondrosarcoma Primary bone tumor occurring later in life.

Chordae tendineae Bands of fibrous tissue connecting the margins of the valves to papillary muscles.

Choriocarcinoma A malignant proliferation of trophoblastic tissue.

Chorion The layer of trophoblast and associated mesoderm that surrounds the developing embryo.

Chorionic vesicle The chorion with its villi and enclosed amnion, yolk sac, and developing embryo.

Chorionic villi examination Sampling of fetal derived placental cells.

Chorionic villi Fingerlike columns of cells extending from the chorion that anchor the chorionic vesicle in the endometrium.

Chromatid One of two newly formed chromosomes held together by the centromere.

Chromatin Tightly wound DNA in the nucleus; formed in part from nucleosomes.

Chromophobe cells Anterior lobe pituitary epithelial cells containing sparse, poorly stained granules. See also eosinophil *and* basophil.

Chromosomal mosaics Individual with both normal cells and cells having a chromosomal abnormality.

Chromosome deletion Loss of part of a chromosome during meiosis.

Chromosome Cell structure organizing the molecules of DNA. Individual structural units of DNA which are best seen in dividing cells.

Chronic cholecystitis Ongoing irritation of the gallbladder by repeated bouts of acute disease.

Chronic granulomatous disease Disease caused by lack of oxidative killing of pathogens.

Chronic inflammation Cellular reaction leading to repair.

Chronic obstructive pulmonary disease (COPD) Combination of emphysema and chronic bronchitis.

Chronic thyroiditis An autoimmune disease in which an autoantibody directed against thyroid epithelial cells causes progressive destruction of the thyroid gland, leading to hypothyroidism. Also called Hashimoto thyroiditis.

Cilia Specialized hairlike processes on cells.

Cirrhosis of the liver A disease characterized by diffuse intrahepatic scarring and circulatory disturbance within the liver.

Class switch A change in the immunoglobulin constant region using the same variable region.

Clear cell carcinoma Glycogen-rich tumors similar to endometroid carcinoma.

Cleft lip Defect in the upper lip of variable degree, as a result of a developmental disturbance.

Cleft palate Defect in hard palate allowing communication between oral cavity and nasal cavity as a result of a developmental disturbance.

Clinician Physician having direct contact with patients.

Clonal Derived from a single cell.

Clonal expansion Proliferation of a population from a single cell.

Coarctation Localized narrowing of the proximal aorta.

Coccidioidomycosis A disease caused by the pathogenic fungus *Coccidioides immitis*.

Coccus Spherical bacteria.

Codominant gene Products of both genes are expressed in the heterozygous state.

Codon Triplet of bases coding for one piece of information or for one amino acid.

Colitis Inflammation restricted to colon.

Collagen Main constituent of fibrous proteins in the human.

Collagen fibers Fibers that are strong but do not stretch.

Collateral circulation An accessory circulation capable of delivering blood to a tissue when the main circulation is blocked, as by a thrombus or embolus.

Colloid An eosinophilic protein material present within the thyroid follicles.

Colonoscopy Examination of the colon with an endoscopic procedure.

Colposcope A binocular magnifying instrument used to view the cervix and endocervical canal.

Columnar cells Tall, narrow cells.

Communicable disease A disease transmitted from person to person.

Complement Group of proteins interact to produce by-products, some of which act as mediators of inflammation.

Complementary The relationship between the base sequence of the two strands in a DNA molecule. During DNA replication, either strand can make an exact copy of the other. Complementary DNA strands bind to each other by base pairing.

Computed tomographic (CT) scan An x-ray technique producing detailed cross-sectional images of the body by means of x-ray tube and detectors connected to a computer. Sometimes called a CAT scan.

Concussion A temporary loss of consciousness caused by a head injury without any memory of the events that occurred shortly before or after the head injury.

Condyloma A warty tumorlike overgrowth in the squamous epithelium of the anorectal or genital tract, caused by a virus that is spread by sexual contact.

Congenital Present at birth.

Conjoined twins Identical twins that are joined to one another and often share organs in common. Siamese twins.

Conjugated bilirubin A more soluble form of bilirubin produced by the addition of two molecules of glucuronic acid to the bilirubin molecule.

Consumption coagulopathy See disseminated intravascular coagulation.

Contusion Severe force injury resulting in detectable damage to brain tissue.

Corona radiata Crownlike structure composed of layers of granulosa cells.

Coronary thrombosis Thrombus formation on the surface of a plaque blocking the coronary artery.

Cortex Outer part of the kidney.

Cortical bone Outer layer of compact bone.

Cortisol The major glucocorticoid.

Costimulator molecules Additional molecules on the surface of the T cell and APC needed for the immune response.

Councilman/apoptotic bodies Cell shrinkage/apoptotic cell death in inflammation of the liver.

Crab louse A parasite of the pubic area; causes intense itching.

C-reactive protein An acute-phase reactant associated with inflammation.

Creatinine clearance test A test of renal function that measures the ability of kidneys to remove (clear) a substance from the blood and excrete it in the urine.

Crescentic glomerulonephritis Form of glomerulonephritis in which Bowman's space (surrounding the glomerular capillary tuft) becomes filled with proliferating cells derived from the parietal epithelium of Bowman's capsule.

Cretinism Hypothyroidism in the infant.

Crigler-Najjar syndrome Lack of UGT, which causes a severe disease of early childhood.

Crohn disease Chronic enteritis.

Cuboidal cells Cube-shaped cells.

Cushing disease Caused by an ACTH-producing tumor of the pituitary gland that stimulates the adrenal glands to enlarge.

Cyanosis Blue skin color caused by low oxygen content of arterial blood.

Cyclooxygenase Enzyme needed for synthesis of prostaglandins.

Cystic fibrosis Autosomal recessive disease caused by a defective sodium ion transporter gene.

Cystitis/pyelonephritis Urinary tract infections affecting only the bladder or upper urinary tract.

Cytokine Small protein released by cells that modulate the production of mediators of inflammation. A general term for any protein secreted by cells that functions as an intercellular messenger and influences cells of the immune system. Cytokines are secreted by macrophages and monocytes (monokines), lymphocytes (lymphokines), and other cells.

Cytomegalovirus One of the herpes viruses. Causes an infectious mononucleosis-like syndrome in adults; may cause congenital malformation in fetus.

Cytoskeleton Protein tubules and filaments that form the structural framework of cells.

Cytotoxic Causing cell death.

Damage associated molecular patterns (DAMPs) Molecules that can initiate and perpetuate immune response in the noninfectious inflammatory response.

Daughter cell A cell resulting from division of a single cell (called the parent cell).

Debrides Removes dead, infected, and excess granulation tissue from the wound bed.

Decidua The endometrium of pregnancy.

Definitive host Residence of mature form of a parasite.

Degenerate code Condition in which each amino acid has many different codons.

Delayed hypersensitivity A state of abnormal reactivity to a foreign material that takes time to develop.

Demyelinating neuropathy Axon sparing demyelinating disease.

Dendrite Nerve process conducting impulses toward the cell body.

Dental plaque Masses of bacteria, bacterial products, and salivary proteins adherent to teeth, which predispose to tooth decay.

Dentine Bony structure of the tooth.

Deoxyribonucleic acid (DNA) The nucleic acid present in the chromosomes of the nuclei of cells that carries genetic information.

Dermatophyte A fungus that causes a superficial infection of the skin.

Desensitization Treatment for allergy that induces the formation of IgG antibodies.

Diabetes insipidus A condition resulting from a deficiency of antidiuretic hormone, characterized by excretion of a large volume of very dilute urine.

Diabetes mellitus A metabolic disease characterized by hyperglycemia and caused by insufficient insulin secretion or inefficient utilization of insulin.

Diabetic glomerulosclerosis Diffuse and nodular thickening of glomerular basement membranes, a common occurrence in patients with long-standing diabetes mellitus.

Diabetic ketosis A disturbance of the body's acid–base balance (acidosis) caused by an inability to utilize glucose, which requires the body to use fat as an energy source. Fat metabolism generates excessive amounts of acid ketone bodies, which disrupts the normal alkalinity of body fluids.

Diagnosis The determination of the nature and cause of a patient's illness.

Diaphysis Enlongated central region of the bone shaft.

Diastole Ventricular relaxation.

Diastolic heart failure Heart failure caused by inadequate filling of the ventricles during diastole, in contrast to systolic heart failure in which ejection of blood from the ventricles during systole is inadequate.

Differential diagnosis Consideration of the different diseases possible given the patient's symptoms.

Dilatation and curettage (D&C) Procedure involving scraping the lining of the uterus; used to treat irregular bleeding.

Diploid Cell containing 2N (pairs) of each chromosome.

Disease Any disturbance of the structure or function of the body.

Disseminated intravascular coagulation (DIC) A disturbance of blood coagulation as a result of the uncontrolled activation of the coagulation mechanism.

Disuse atrophy Thinning and decalcification of bone due to lack of weight-bearing.

Diverticula/diverticulum An outpouching from an organ, as from the mucosa of the colon, that projects through the muscular wall.

Diverticulitis An inflammation of a diverticulum.

Diverticulosis A condition characterized by outpouchings of the colonic mucosa through weak areas in the muscular wall.

DNA Deoxyribonucleaic acid (DNA) is the molecule carrying the coding information for genes.

DNA repair gene Gene that normally functions to repair DNA.

Dominant gene A gene that expresses a trait in the heterozygous state.

Dopamine Chemical mediator released by hypothalamic neurons.

Dopamine agonist A drug such as bromocriptine that combines with cell dopamine receptors and causes the same cell response that would be produced by dopamine, such as inhibition of prolactin secretion.

Dorsal Front surface.

Dosage effects Differing amounts of gene product in the heterozygous and homozygous states.

Double Y syndrome The presence of an extra Y chromosome in the male.

Down syndrome Condition resulting from trisomy of chromosome 21.

Ductal carcinoma in situ (DCIS) The precursor lesion to most breast cancer.

Ductal carcinoma Tumor arising from the epithelium of the ducts.

Ductus arteriosus A fetal artery connecting the pulmonary artery with the aorta that permits pressure determined blood flow from pulmonary artery into the aorta, bypassing blood flow to the nonfunctional fetal lungs.

Dura The outer covering of the brain and spinal cord.

Dysmenorrhea Painful menstruation.

Dysphagia Difficulty swallowing.

Dysplasia Abnormal maturation of cells. Localized areas of dysregulated growth.

Ecchymosis Bruise.

Echocardiogram An examinination of the cardiovascular system using ultrasound. A record obtained from an ultrasound examination of the heart and related blood vessels; used to assist in the diagnosis of cardiovascular disease.

Eclampsia One or more convulsions in a pregnant woman with preeclampsia.

Ectoderm The outer germ layer in the embryo that gives rise to specific organs and tissues.

Ectopic pregnancy A pregnancy outside the endometrial cavity.

Edema Accumulation of an excess of fluid in the interstitial tissues.

Edematous Filled with fluid.

Effector T cell Cell active in host defense.

Eisenmenger syndrome Blood shunts between the atria in the opposite direction of normal.

Ejection fraction Percentage of the ventricular volume ejected during systole.

Elastic cartilage Contains elastic fibers.

Elastic fibers Fibers made of elastin that stretch.

Elastin Component of elastic fibers.

Electrocardiogram (ECG) A technique for measuring the serial changes in the electrical activity of the heart during the various phases of the cardiac cycle. (Often called ECG or EKG.)

Electrocardiogram (ECG)/electroencephalogram (EEG)/electromyogram (EMG) Tests using the electrical impulses of the body to measure activity in the heart, brain, and nervous systems.

Electrolytes Dissolved mineral salts.

Embolism A condition in which a plug composed of a detached clot, mass of bacteria, or other foreign material (embolus) occludes a blood vessel.

Embryo The developing human organism from the third to the seventh weeks of gestation.

Embryonal carcinoma A malignant testicular tumor in which the malignant cells have features resembling rapidly growing trophoblastic tissue.

Emigration Cells move through walls of blood vessels.

Emphysema Disease in which the air spaces in the lung are enlarged and their walls destroyed.

Encephalitis An inflammation of the brain.

Encephalomalacia Cystic lesion of degenerated brain tissue as a result of obstruction of cerebral blood supply. Same as cerebral infarct.

Endemic disease A communicable disease in which small numbers of cases are continually present in a population.

Endochondral bone formation Formation of bone, first as a cartilage model that is then reabsorbed and converted into bone.

Endocrine Cell to cell communication by direct contact through soluble mediators acting across a distance between cells.

Endocrine glands A gland that discharges its secretions directly into the bloodstream, in contrast to an exocrine gland that discharges its secretion through a duct onto a mucosal surface.

Endometrial cyst An ovarian cyst lined by endometrium and filled with old blood and debris. A manifestation of endometriosis.

Endometrioid tumor Tumor epithelium resembles endometrium.

Endometriosis Presence of endometrial tissue in abnormal locations, such as in the ovary or pelvis.

Endoplasmic reticulum A mass of hollow tubular channels within the cytoplasm of the cell, frequently bordered by ribosomes.

Endoscopy An examination of the interior of the body by means of various lighted tubular instruments. Method may also be used to obtain tissue samples.

Endometrial intraepithelial neoplasia (EIN) Result of long-term nonatypical endometrial hyperplasia; a precursor lesion to cancer.

Endothelium The internal lining of blood vessels and interior of the heart.

Enteritis Inflammation of the intestinal tract.

Endoderm The inner germ layer of the embryo that gives rise to specific organs and tissues.

Enzymatic fat necrosis See fat necrosis.

Eosinophil A cell whose cytoplasm is filled with large, uniform granules that stain intensely red with acid dyes. See also *basophil*.

Epicardium/myocardium/endocardium Three layers of the heart moving from outside in.

Epidemic disease A communicable disease affecting concurrently large numbers of people in a population.

Epinephrine One of the compounds (catecholamines) secreted by the adrenal medulla.

Epiphyseal plate Cartilagenous end of ephiphyses critical to ossification of the long bone.

Epiphyses The end part of a long bone, initially growing separately from the shaft.

Epispadias Opening of the urethra on the dorsum of the penis.

Epistaxis Severe spontaneous nosebleed.

Epitheliod marcophages Appearance of macrophages around the tubercle bacillus.

Epstein-Barr (EB) virus A virus that causes infectious mononucleosis.

Erythrocyte Red cell.

Erythrocyte sedimentation rate (ESR) A laboratory test to measure the speed red cells settle out of the blood; used to detect inflammation.

Erythroplakia Depressed red lesions on the oral mucosa.

Erythropoietin A humoral substance made by the kidneys that regulates hematopoiesis.

Eschar Scab.

Esophageal varices Thin-walled vessels that can rupture.

Essential hypertension High blood pressure with no identifiable cause.

Estrogen receptors (ER)/progesterone receptors (PR) Breast cell surface receptors.

Etiology The cause, especially the cause of a disease.

Evidence-based medicine Definition of treatment plan, risks/benefits/costs based on prior rigorous investigation.

Exchange transfusion Partial replacement of blood of infant with hemolytic disease by blood lacking the antigen responsible for hemolytic disease, as when transfusing Rh negative blood to an Rh positive infant. Performed to reduce intensity of hemolytic jaundice.

Exocrine glands A gland that discharges its secretions through a duct onto a mucosal surface, in contrast to an endocrine gland that delivers its secretions directly into the bloodstream.

Exome The set of all expressed genes.

Exon The part of a chromosomal DNA chain that codes for a specific protein or enzyme.

Exophthalmic goiter Another term for Graves disease, named for the protrusion of the eyes seen in many patients with this disease.

Exophytic Outward growing mass of tissue protruding from the wound.

Expression vector A set of DNA sequences necessary for the expression of a foreign gene in an organism. Often engineered to promote high levels of production of the gene product.

Extravasation Leakage of plasma from dilated vessels.

Extrinsic pathway Clotting process needing substances outside the vascular system for activation.

Exudate The fluid, leukocytes, and debris that accumulate as a result of an inflammation.

False negative Negative test result which should be positive.

False positive Positive test result which should be negative.

Familial adenomatous polyposis (FAP) Genetic disease characterized by many polyps in the colorectal region.

Fat necrosis A sterile form of inflammation that occurs after trauma (or other damage) to areas of the body rich in lipid.

Fatty casts Aggregated lipids that maintain the cylindrical shape of the tubule.

Fatty streak lesions Early sign of atherosclerosis as elongated flat accumulations of foam cells.

Favism Condition in which ingestion of fava beans can result in red cell hemolysis.

Fc receptor Cell surface receptor for the constant region of the immunoglobulin molecule.

Feedback mechanisms Biological control using levels of hormones to control further production of substances.

Fertilization Penetration of the ovum by the sperm.

Fetal alcohol syndrome Developmental abnormalities related to heavy alcohol consumption during pregnancy.

Fetal deformation Misshapen fetus caused by compression or mispositioning during fetal development.

Fetal disruptions Congenital abnormality caused by physical disruption of the fetus.

Fetal hemoglobin A type of hemoglobin containing two alpha and two gamma chains that is able to take up and release oxygen at much lower PO_2 (oxygen partial pressure) than in adult hemoglobin.

Fetus The unborn offspring after eight weeks' gestation.

Fibrin The meshwork of protein threads that form during the clotting of blood.

Fibrinogen Blood protein forming a key element in clotting. A precursor in plasma converted into fibrin by thrombin during blood coagulation. An acute-phase protein important in blood coagulation.

Fibrinolytic system Process of breaking down clots.

Fibrinous Fibrin-rich exudate.

Fibrocartilage Contains many dense collagen bundles.

Fibrocystic change (FCC) Common benign cystic change in breast tissue.

Fibromas Benign tumor arising from the fibrous connective tissue of the ovary.

Fibrosis Scar formation.

Fibrous framework Layer of dense fibrous tissue located between the atria and the ventricles.

Fine needle aspiration Sampling fluid and cells from a surface accessible lesion.

Flagellum/flagella A whiplike process that propels an organism or sperm.

Fluorescent probes Artificial pieces of DNA labeled with a dye.

Foamy macrophages Macrophages carrying lipids.

Focal segmental glomerulosclerosis (FSGS) Scar tissue in the filtering unit of the kidney.

Follicle B cell rich area of the lymph node.

Follicle-stimulating hormone (FSH) One of the gonadotropic hormones secreted by the anterior lobe of the pituitary, which regulates growth and function of the gonads (ovary and testis).

Fomite Contaminated inanimate object that can transmit disease.

Foramen ovale An opening in the atrial septum covered by a one-way flap valve regulated by pressure differences between the atria, permitting blood flow from right to left atrium but not in the opposite direction, thereby bypassing blood flow from right cardiac chambers to the nonfunctional fetal lungs.

Fragile X syndrome Condition resulting from defects in a gene on the X chromosome associated with mental retardation.

Frozen section A method of rapid diagnosis of tumors used by the pathologist; tissue is frozen solid, cut into thin sections, stained, and examined microscopically.

Full mutation Large number of CGG repeats resulting in detectable disease.

Galactorrhea Secretion of milk by breast not associated with pregnancy or normal lactation.

Gametes Reproductive cells, eggs, and sperm, each containing 23 chromosomes, which unite during fertilization to form a zygote containing 46 chromosomes.

Gametogenesis The development of mature eggs and sperm from precursor cells.

Gangrene Tissue death caused by bacterial infection or lack of blood circulation.

Gastritis Inflammation of the stomach.

Gastroesophageal/cardiac sphincter Lower esophageal sphincter.

GB virus C Once called hepatitis G virus; does not cause clinical disease in humans.

Gene amplification Generation of multiple copies of a gene, increasing gene activity.

Gene expression profile List of proteins synthesized by breast cancer cells.

Gene mutation Change in gene structure.

Gene therapy Introduction of genes into cells with the object of curing diseases associated with the deficiency of a protein related to a genetic mutation.

Genetic anticipation Tendency for a mutation to become worse with each generation.

Genetic code The information carried by DNA molecules in chromosomes. The DNA basis of the phenotype/genotype.

Genetic mosaic Different cell populations having different genotypes in a single organism.

Genetic probes Preparations of nucleic acid devised to identify specific sequences in bacteria.

Genome The total of all the genes contained in a cell's chromosomes.

Genomewide association studies (GWAS) Process using tests of many SNPs to identify genes associated with particular diseases or traits.

Genomics Bioinformatic techniques applied to studies of human genome.

Genotype DNA/chromosome basis of inherited traits in an individual.

Germ disk A three-layered cluster of cells that will eventually give rise to an embryo.

Germ layers The three layers of cells derived from the inner cell mass; each layer is destined to form specific organs and tissues in the embryo.

Germinal center Site in lymph node where selection for strong binding B cells occurs.

Gestation Duration of pregnancy from fertilization to delivery.

Gestational diabetes Diabetes during pregnancy. Elevated blood glucose caused by insulin resistance resulting from elevated hormones related to the pregnancy. Blood glucose returns to normal postpartum, but the woman has increased risk of diabetes later in life.

Gestational trophoblast disease A general term for all diseases characterized by abnormal trophoblast proliferation. Includes both hydatidiform mole and choriocarcinoma.

Ghon complexes Inactive tubercular lesions.

Gilbert syndrome Common inherited condition related to a mild lack of uridine diphosphate-glucuronyl transferase (UGT).

Gingivitis Gum inflammation.

Glia cells/neuroglia Supporting cells of tissue of the nervous system.

Gliadin Protein in gluten causing sensitivity.

Glioma Any brain tumor arising from glial (supporting) cells of the brain.

Globins Protein with globin fold, a series of eight alpha helical segments. Part of hemoglobin.

Glomerular epithelium Layer of Bowman cells closely applied to the capillaries. It is also termed the visceral layer of Bowman's capsule.

Glomerular filtration rate (GFR) Measure of the volume of body fluid cleared by the kidneys per unit of time.

Glomerulonephritis An inflammation of the glomeruli caused by either antigen—antibody complexes trapped in the glomeruli or by antiglomerular basement membrane antibodies.

Glucocorticoid An adrenal cortical hormone that regulates carbohydrate metabolism.

Gluten sensitive enteropathy (GSE) Damage to intestinal villi caused by ingesting gluten-containing foods by people sensitive to a protein in gluten; characterized by passage of large bulky stools containing a large amount of poorly absorbed fat.

Glycated hemoglobin test/hemoglobin A1c test A test that measures the amount of glucose permanently attached to hemoglobin, which is higher than normal in many people with diabetes.

Glycosaminoglycans (GAGs) Long, unbranched polysaccharides making up the ground substance.

Goiter Any enlargement of the thyroid gland.

Golgi apparatus A group of membrane-lined sacs found in the cytoplasm of the cell near the nucleus; functions with the endoplasmic reticulum to synthesize and package secretory granules.

Gonad A general term referring to either the ovary or the testis.

Gout A disorder of nucleoprotein metabolism characterized by elevated uric acid and deposition of uric acid in and around joints.

Grade Term describing how closely the neoplasm resembles host tissue.

Graft versus host disease Condition where a graft of immunologically active cells mounts a response to the host.

Gram stain Staining process used to identify bacteria.

Granulation tissue Normal part of the healing process.

Granulocytes Collective name for neutrophils, eosinophils, and basophils.

Granulosa cell tumor-thecoma An estrogen-producing ovarian tumor arising from the estrogen-producing granulose cell of an ovarian follicle.

Granulosa cells Cells lining the ovarian follicles.

Graves disease An autoimmune thyroid disease in which autoantibodies resembling thyroid-stimulating hormone stimulate an excessive output of thyroid hormone, causing hyperthyroidism.

Gray matter Centrally located part of the brain containing the neuronal cell bodies and the supportive glial cells.

Gross examination Study of diseased organ with the naked eye.

Ground substance Matrix in which the fibers are embedded.

Growth factor A soluble growth promoting substance produced by cells that attaches to receptors on the cell membrane of other cells, which activates the receptors and initiates events leading to growth or division of the target cells.

Growth hormone (GH) An anterior lobe pituitary hormone that stimulates growth of bone and other body tissues; also known as somatotropin.

Guillain-Barré syndrome A type of polyneuritis resulting from an autoimmune reaction to myelin.

Gynecomastia Excessive development of the male breast.

Haploid Cell containing 1N of each chromosome, a gamete.

Hashimoto thyroiditis Another name for chronic thyroiditis.

Hayflick limit Fixed number of cell divisions possible for a normal cell.

Heavy chains (H chains) Longer of two types of chains making up an immunoglobulin molecule.

Hemarthrosis Arthritic condition caused by bleeding into the joint; hematoma within joint.

Hematemesis Bloody vomit.

Hematoma Accumulation of blood within tissue.

Hematopathologist Pathologist who specializes in the study of blood forming tissue.

Hematopoietic tissue Tissue that forms the blood.

Hemiplegia Paralysis of one side of the body.

Hemizygous A term applied to genes located on the X chromosome in the male.

Hemochromatosis An autosomal recessive genetic disease characterized by excessive iron absorption, leading to accumulation of excessive amounts of iron in the body, causing organ damage.

Hemoglobin An oxygen transport protein within red cells composed of an iron-porphyrin complex (heme) combined with a protein chain (globin).

Hemolysis Hemoglobin leakage from red cells caused by damaged cell membranes. Also, destruction of blood cells around bacterial colonies.

Hemopericardium Hematoma between the heart and its pericardial lining.

Hemophilia A Bleeding disease caused by lack of active F.VIII.

Hemophilia B Bleeding disease caused by lack of active F.IX.

Hemorrhage Release of blood into surrounding tissue.

Hemorrhagic exudate Red-cell-rich inflammatory fluid.

Hemorrhagic diathesis Variety of clinical disorders in which small injuries lead to unusual bleeding.

Hemorrhoids Dilated veins around the rectum; varicosities of anal and rectal veins.

Hemostasis Process of blood clotting.

Hemothorax Hematoma within the chest.

Heparin An anticoagulant obtained from the liver.

Hepatitis Inflammation of the liver.

Hepatitis B core antigen (HBcAg) The antigen contained in the core of the hepatitis B virus.

Hepatitis B surface antigen (HBsAg) The coating of the hepatitis B virus that is also found in great excess in the blood of infected patients.

Hepatitis e antigen (HBeAg) Antigen associated with active hepatitis B virus proliferation.

Hepatocellular carcinoma (HCC) Most common liver cancer.

Hepcidin Protein synthesized by the liver that blocks dietary iron uptake; part of the control mechanism for iron metabolism.

Hereditary or genetic disease Condition resulting from a chromosome abnormality or defective expression of a gene.

Hereditary spherocytosis/ hereditary elliptocytosis Cause of abnormally shaped red cells, either spherical or elliptical.

Hernia A protrusion of a loop of bowel through a narrow opening, usually in the abdominal wall.

Herpes zoster A skin rash caused by reactivation of the varicella-zoster virus that caused chicken pox.

Heterochromatin Small dense mass of condensed chromatin appearing in inactivated X chromosomes.

Heterodimer T cell receptor formed from an alpha and beta chain.

Heterophile antibodies Antibodies that react with substances unrelated to the immunizing antigen.

Heterozygous Presence of two different alleles at given gene loci on the homologous pair of chromosomes.

High-density lipoprotein (HDL) Plasma protein molecule carrying cholesterol away from the tissue.

Hilus Region of kidney where blood vessels enter.

Histamine Chemical released by mast cells.

Histocompatibility (HLA) Genetic locus controlling self-recognition.

Histologic examination Study of disease using a microscope to examine tissue.

Histone Nuclear proteins forming the nucleosome.

Histoplasmosis An infection caused by the fungus *Histoplasma capsulatum*.

HIV entry inhibitors/fusion inhibitors Drugs that block the binding entry and fusion of HIV with the target cell.

HIV integrase Viral enzyme allowing the viral genes to direct the synthesis and assembly of more virus.

HIV protease Enzyme that cuts and assembles the virus protein.

HLA system The genes of the histocompatibility complex and the antigens that they determine on the surface of cells.

Hodgkin's disease A form of lymphoma that occurs in young adults with Reed-Sternberg cells mixed with other cell types.

Homeostasis Maintenance of a steady state by the body's internal control systems.

Homocysteine/homocysteinemia Sulfur containing amino acid/excessive levels of homocysteine.

Homologous chromosomes A matched pair of chromosomes, one derived from each parent.

Homozygous Presence of the same alleles at a given gene loci on the chromosome pair.

Host Individual infected with a disease-producing organism.

Human chorionic gonadotropin (hCG) A hormone made by the placenta in pregnancy that has actions similar to pituitary gonadotropins. The same hormone is made by neoplastic cells in some types of malignant testicular tumors.

Human chorionic somatomammotropin (HCS) One of the hormones produced by the placenta that has properties similar to pituitary growth hormone. Also called human placental lactogen.

Human epidermal growth factor receptor 2 (HER-2) Breast cell surface receptor.

Human papillomavirus (HPV) A virus that stimulates epithelial cell proliferation. Causes warts and genital tract condylomas.

Humoral immunity Immunity associated with formation of antibodies produced by plasma cells.

Hyaline cartilage Most common type of cartilage; contains only a few fine collagen fibers.

Hydatidiform mole A neoplastic proliferation of trophoblast associated with the formation of large cystic villi.

Hydrocele An accumulation of excess fluid within the tunica vaginalis of the testis.

Hydrocephalus Dilatation of the cerebral ventricular system caused by pressure arising from accumulation of cerebrospinal fluid within the ventricles.

Hydronephrosis A dilatation of the urinary drainage tract proximal to the site of an obstruction.

Hydropic swelling Cell swelling as a result of excessive water uptake by a cell. Associated with failure of active transport of ions.

Hydrops fetalis Fatal condition occurring in a fetus with no functional hemoglobin alpha chain genes.

Hydrothorax Accumulation of fluid in the pleural cavity.

Hydroureter A dilatation of the ureter secondary to obstruction of the urinary drainage system, often associated with coexisting dilatation of the renal pelvis and calyces (hydronephrosis).

Hygiene hypothesis Theory that lack of early childhood exposure to infectious agents, symbiotic microorganisms (such as the gut flora or probiotics), and parasites increases susceptibility to allergic diseases by suppressing the natural development of the immune system.

Hyperbilirubinemia High levels of unconjugated bilirubin in the newborn.

Hypercholesterolemia Elevated blood cholesterol.

Hyperemia Increased blood flow through vessels.

Hyperglycemia Excessively high blood glucose concentration.

Hyperlipidemia Elevated blood lipids.

Hyperemesis gravidum Excess vomiting associated with pregnancy.

Hyperosmolar coma Coma resulting from neurologic dysfunction caused by hyperosmolarity of body fluids as a consequence of severe hyperglycemia.

Hyperplasia An increase in the number of cells.

Hypersensitivity reaction A state of abnormal reactivity to a foreign material.

Hypertension Excessively high systemic blood pressure.

Hypertonic solution A solution having a greater osmolarity than body fluids, which causes cells to shrink in such a solution because water moves by osmosis from the cells into the hypertonic solution.

Hypertrophy An enlargement or overgrowth of an organ caused by an increase in the size of its constituent cells.

Hyphae Filamentous branching structures formed by fungi.

Hypochromic Pale red cell color due to reduced hemoglobin content.

Hypoglycemia Lower than normal concentration of glucose in the blood.

Hyponatremia Lower concentration of sodium ions in extracellular fluid as it becomes diluted.

Hypospadias A congenital abnormality of penile development.

Hypotension Abnormally low blood pressure.

Hypotonic solution A solution having a lower osmolarity than body fluids, causing cells in the solution to swell because water moves by osmosis from the hypotonic solution into the cells.

Iatrogenic Disease resulting from a medical intervention.

Idiopathic Disease of unknown origin.

IgE Immunoglobulin molecule with the E heavy chain type.

Iliac crest Area of hip bone in abdomen.

Immune complex Combination of antibody and antigen forming a lattice.

Immune memory Enhancement of immune response upon secondary encounter with antigen in adaptive immunity.

Immunogen Antigen that can provoke an adaptive immune response as well as bind to antigen receptors.

Immunoglobulins Class of proteins including antibodies.

Immunological techniques Techniques using antibody or antigen preparations, usually with chemical labels.

Immunologist Person who studies the immune response.

Immunopathologist Physician who studies the immune response associated with disease or who uses immunological-based testing tools.

Immunotherapy Treatment given to retard growth of a disseminated malignant tumor by stimulating the body's own immune defenses.

Imperforate anus Congenital absence of anal opening, often associated with absence of distal rectum as well.

Inborn errors of metabolism Genetically determined enzyme defects.

Inbreeding Mating between closely related individuals.

Inclusion bodies Spherical structures in the nucleus or cytoplasm of virus-infected cells or intracytoplasmic clusters of organisms such as Chlamydiae within a cell.

Infarct Necrosis of tissue caused by interruption of its blood supply.

Infarction Impaired blood supply to tissue.

Infection Inflammation caused by a disease-producing organism.

Infectious mononucleosis A common viral disease, the most common cause of benign lymphocytosis.

Inflammation An early defensive reaction by the body to insult.

Innate immunity Preprogramed immune response; a quick response to a predetermined array of chemical signals.

Inner cell mass A group of cells derived from the fertilized ovum that is destined to form the embryo.

Insulin reaction/insulin shock Condition in which there is too much insulin in the blood.

Insulin resistance Condition when target tissues are relatively insensitive to the action of insulin.

Integrase inhibitors Drugs that block the enzyme responsible for inserting the HIV viral DNA into the cell DNA.

Interferon A broad-spectrum antiviral agent manufactured by various cells in the body.

Interferon alpha A broad-spectrum antiviral agent manufactured by various cells in the body.

Interleukin A lymphokine that stimulates growth of lymphocytes.

Interleukin-1 (IL-1) Pro-inflammatory cytokine.

Interleukin-2 (IL-2) A lymphokine that stimulates growth of lymphocytes.

Intermediate filaments Small, tough filaments of high tensile strength within the cell cytoplasm.

Intermediate host Place of residence of an immature form of a parasite.

Interstitial pneumonia Characterized by thickening of supporting tissues between the air sacs of the lungs.

Intervertebral disk A fibrocartilaginous joint between adjacent vertebral bodies.

Intramembranous bone formation Direct formation of bone by osteoblasts without prior formation of a cartilage model.

Intraoperative During surgery.

Intrinsic pathway Clotting process needing only substances within the blood vessels.

Intron A noncoding part of a chromosomal DNA chain.

Intussusception Telescoping of a bowel segment into an adjacent segment.

Invasive Test requiring a physical invasion of the body. Also, a tumor type that infiltrates host tissue.

Invasive hydatidiform mole An aggressive hydatidiform mole that invades the uterine wall.

Irritable bowel syndrome (IBS) Condition characterized by frequent loose stools and excessive amounts of mucus.

Islets of Langerhans Cluster of endocrine cells in the pancreas.

Isotonic solution A solution having essentially the same osmolarity as body fluids so that cells neither shrink nor swell when exposed to the solution.

Jaundice Yellow discoloration of skin and white of eyes resulting from an accumulation of bilirubin in the body.

Juxtacrine Cell to cell communication by direct contact.

Juxtaglomerular apparatus A specialized group of cells at the vascular pole of the glomerulus that regulates blood flow through the glomerulus of the kidneys.

Karyotype Chromosomes from a single cell arranged in pairs in descending order according to size of the chromosomes and the positions of the centromeres used to visualize the chromosome composition of an individual.

Keratin An insoluble sulfur-containing protein that is the principal constituent of the hair and nails.

Keratin filament Type of filament in epithelial cells.

Keratinization Accumulation of a fibrous protein called keratin inside cells.

Kernicterus/bilirubin encephalopathy Condition caused by high levels of unconjugated bilirubin in the infant.

Ketone bodies Various derivatives of acetyl-CoA, resulting from excessive mobilization of fat as an energy source.

Ketosis Results from overproduction of products of fat metabolism.

Klinefelter syndrome A congenital syndrome caused by an extra X chromosome in the male.

Labile cell population Cells that divides continually.

Laboratory medicine Study of the composition of body fluids to diagnose disease.

Laceration An irregular jagged wound.

Lamin filament Type of filament involved in nuclear structure in all cells.

Laparoscope A long tubular telescope-like instrument passed through the abdominal wall to examine structures within the peritoneal cavity.

Latent A viral infection producing no symptoms.

Latent autoimmune diabetes of adults (LADA) Subtype of type 1 diabetes first appearing in adults.

Latent tuberculosis Arrested tuberculosis infection containing viable organisms.

Lecithin A phosphorus-containing lipid (phospholipid) having detergent properties similar to bile salts.

Legionnaires' disease A type of pneumonia caused by an airborne bacterium called *Legionella pneumophila*.

Leiomyomas Benign, smooth muscle tumors.

Lesion Any structural abnormality or pathologic change.

Leukemia A neoplasm of hematopoietic tissue; a neoplastic proliferation of leukocytes.

Leukocyte Collective term for white cells.

Leukopenia An abnormally small number of leukocytes in the peripheral blood.

Leukoplakia White lesions on the mucosa of the oral cavity. A white patch of hyperplastic and usually atypical squamous epithelium on the oral mucosa or genital tract mucosa.

Peroxisome A cytoplasmic organelle containing various enzymes, including those that decompose potentially toxic compounds through the production of hydrogen peroxide.

Petechia/ecchymoses Small pinpoint hemorrhage or larger hemorrhage caused by decreased platelets, abnormal platelet function, or capillary defect.

Petechia/petechiae Small hemorrhages. A small pinpoint hemorrhage caused by decreased platelets, abnormal platelet function, or capillary defect.

Phagocytic Engulf injurious agents into the cell.

Phagocytic vacuole Membrane-lined vacuole used to contain the foreign material.

Phagocytosis Process by which cell engulfs foreign material. Ingestion of particulate foreign material by cells.

Phenotype Collection of inherited/phenotypic traits detectable in an individual. Appearance of individual as opposed to genes present.

Phenotypic traits Characteristics apparent in the individual.

Phenylketonuria Autosomal recessive disease caused by the inability to convert phenylalanine to tyrosine.

Pheochromocytoma Catecholamine-secreting tumor of the adrenal medulla.

Philadelphia chromosome Chromosome translocation common in neoplastic cells of chronic myelogenous leukemia.

Phimosis The inability to retract the foreskin in newborn males.

Phlebitis Inflammation of a vein.

Phocomelia Reduction of bones of the extremities.

Phototherapy Fluorescent light treatment of jaundiced babies to reduce the concentration of unconjugated bilirubin in their blood.

Physiological adaptive change Cell or organ response to changing conditions.

Pia The innermost of the three membranes covering the brain and spinal cord.

Pinocytosis Process similar to phagocytosis but for the ingestion of water.

Pinworm A small parasitic worm infecting humans. Lives in lower bowel and causes perianal pruritus.

Pituitary dwarfism Stunted growth cause by a deficiency of growth hormone in a child.

Pituitary gigantism A condition resulting from excessive secretion of growth hormone in the child.

Pituitary gonadotrophic hormones Hormones controlling cyclic ovulation.

Placenta Flat, disk-shaped structure that maintains the developing organism within the uterus.

Placenta previa Attachment of the placenta in the uterus such that it partially or completely covers the cervix.

Plasma oncotic pressure Concentration of the plasma proteins in blood.

Plasmin Blood enzyme that degrades blood plasma proteins including fibrin clots.

Plasminogen Precursor compound of plasmin in the blood.

Platelet A component of the blood; a roughly circular or oval disk concerned with blood coagulation; blood cells that adhere to collagen and mediate blood coagulation.

Platelet activation Release of active clotting components after adhesion of platelets.

Platelet agonists Substances promoting platelet function.

Pleura The mesothelial covering of the lung (visceral pleura) and chest wall (parietal pleura).

Pluripotential hemopoietic stem cell Precursor for all blood cells.

Pneumoconiosis An occupational lung disease caused by inhalation of injurious substances such as rock dust.

Pneumonia Inflammation of the lung.

Pneumothorax Accumulation of air in the pleural cavity.

Podocytes Cells with highly branched cytoplasmic processes covering the glomerular capillaries of the kidneys.

Point-of-care test Laboratory test that can be performed at the patient's bedside or in the physician's office.

Polar body Structure extruded during the meiosis of the oocyte. Contains discarded chromosomes and a small amount of cytoplasm.

Polyclonal antibodies Humoral response consisting of antibodies produced by a number of clones of B cells.

Polycystic ovary syndrome (PCOS) Common endocrine disorder and common cause of anovulatory infertility; associated with obesity, diabetes, and hirsutism.

Polycythemia Increased number of red cells and hemoglobin above normal levels. May be caused by some types of chronic heart or lung disease (secondary polycythemia) or to marrow erythroid hyperplasia of unknown causes (primary polycythemia).

Polyhydramnios An excess of amnionic fluid.

Polymerase chain reaction (PCR) Technology used to amplify streatches of DNA.

Polymorphism Collection of alleles for a single gene.

Polymorphonuclear neutrophils (PMN) A leukocyte having a multilobed nucleus whose cytoplasm is filled with fine granules.

Polyneuropathies An inflammation of multiple nerves.

Polyp/papilloma Wart-like benign tumor often associated with viral infection.

Porins Unique proteins on bacteria outer membrane contributing to resistance to antimicrobial agents.

Portacaval shunt Surgically created anastomosis between the portal vein and the vena cava, performed to lower portal pressure in the treatment of esophageal varices.

Portal hypertension Characterized by increased resistance to blood outflow and impaired liver function,

Portal tract/triad Branch of hepatic artery, portal vein, and bile duct located at periphery of liver lobule.

Positive/negative selection Immature T lymphocytes must bind to self HLA molecules to remain positively selected; T lymphocytes with strong binding to self are removed (negative selection).

Positron emission tomography (PET scan) Imaging using positron emitting radiolabels.

Posterior urethral valves (PUV) Most frequent developmental abnormality in the lower urinary tract of males.

Precancerous Area of dysplasia in early stages of cancer development.

Prediabetes Higher than normal blood glucose but not high enough to establish diagnosis of diabetes.

Preeclampsia A pregnancy-related complication characterized by hypertension and proteinuria that usually occurs after the twentieth week of gestation, thought to be caused by placental dysfunction.

Premutation Condition in carriers of fragile X; relatively few repeats.

Presinusoidal portal hypertension Portal hypertension resulting from occlusions in portal vein.

Primary gout A metabolic disease caused by overproduction of uric acid, reduced excretion of uric acid, or a combination of both factors. Clinical manifestations are related to precipitation of uric acid in joints, kidneys, and other sites.

Primary hemostasis Part of hemostatic process that is mostly platelet dependent.

Primary hemostatic plug Mass of aggregated platelets at site of injury.

Primary lymphoid organs Bone marrow and thymus.

Primary response Initial response to foreign substance.

Primary site Tissue of origin for neoplasm.

Primary tuberculosis Initial infection of tuberculosis.

Primary union Form of healing of a sutured wound.

Prion A protein infectious particle responsible for Creutzfeldt-Jakob disease and some other degenerative diseases of the nervous system such as Kuru.

Proerythroblast Precursor cells in the bone marrow that give rise to red blood cells.

Progenitor cell Precursor of red cells, nonlymphoid white cells, and platelets.

Progerias Diseases characterized by dramatic and premature aging.

Prognosis The probable outcome of a disease or disorder, the outlook for recovery.

Progressive primary tuberculosis Initial tubercular infection that does not go into remission.

Prolactin Hormone produced by the anterior lobe of the pituitary gland that stimulates milk secretion.

Proliferative phase Growth of endometrial cells lining the uterus.

Promotor Substance needed to stimulate growth of cells after contact with carcinogen.

Prostaglandin A series of derivatives of archidonic acid that have widespread physiologic effects.

Prostatic-specific antigen (PSA) An antigen produced by prostatic epithelial cells that is often found in higher-than-normal concentrations in the blood of patients with prostatic cancer and other diseases of the prostate.

Protease inhibitors Drugs used to treat HIV infection that block the enzyme that cuts the viral protein into segments and assembles them around the viral RNA to form the infectious virus particle. As a result, the virus particle is improperly constructed and is not infectious.

Proteoglycans/mucoproteins Extremely large molecules in connective tissue.

Prothrombin time (PT) test A test that detects defects in extrinsic coagulation and used to monitor warfarin-like therapy.

Prothrombin Clotting factor activated by factor X to release thrombin/F.IIa.

Proto-oncogenes A gene promoting cell growth, differentiation or mitotic activity associated with neoplasia.

Protozoa Simple one-celled animal parasites, such as the plasmodium causing malaria.

Proud flesh Growth of excessive granulation tissue that can gape above the wound.

Pseudoautosomal genes Genes carried on the X chromosome not subject to random X inactivation.

Public health Area of medicine concerned with the health of populations.

Pulmonary angiogram Test that directly visualizes the pulmonary artery and its branches.

Pulmonary congestion Pooling of blood in the lungs.

Pulmonary valve Semilunar valve surrounding the orifices of the pulmonary artery.

Pulpitis Inflammation of the dental pulp.

Purpura Skin or mucous membrane bleeding; larger hemorrhages in the skin.

Purulent Neutrophil-rich exudate, also called pus.

Rachischisis Unclosed spinal cord lies exposed within the wide-open spinal canal.

Radiograph/x-ray An image taken with x-rays.

Radiologist Physician expert in the use and analysis of imaging techniques and results.

Reactive oxygen species (ROS) Harmful chemicals either environmental or self-produced that can damage cells.

Receptor molecules/Pattern/Pathogen Recognition Receptors (PRRs) Receptors on cells recognizing molecular markers of disease causing microorganism.

Receptor Cell surface signal receiver.

Recessive gene A gene that expresses a trait only when present in the homozygous state.

Recombinant DNA technology/genetic engineering/gene splicing Methods for combining a gene from one organism, such as a gene specifying insulin synthesis, with genes from another organism, such as a bacterium.

Recombination/crossover Interchange of genetic material between homologous chromosomes during synapse and meiosis. Recombination between genes can be observed.

Reduction division Process occurring in meiosis reducing the 2N pairs of chromosomes to 1N.

Reflux esophagitis Inflammation of the lining of the esophagus caused by reflux of acidic gastric secretions through an incompetent lower gastroesophageal sphincter.

Regulatory T cells Cells specific for self-antigens that block the activation of autoreactive T cells.

Regurgitation Backward flow of blood because valve does not close properly.

Relapse Return of cancer cells after a period of remission.

Releasing hormones Substances causing release of hormones from anterior pituitary.

Remission Patient appears to be completely recovered from neoplastic disease with no cancer cells present.

Renal pelvis/major calyces Expanded upper end of the ureter and divisions of the renal pelvis.

Renin A humoral substance secreted by the kidneys in response to a fall in blood pressure, blood volume, or sodium concentration.

Resolution Regression of an inflammatory process without significant tissue destruction and with return of the tissues to normal.

Respiratory acidosis A disturbance in the body's acid–base balance in which the pH of the extracellular fluids is shifted toward the acidic side of normal.

Respiratory alkalosis A disturbance in the body's acid–base balance in which the pH of the extracellular fluids is shifted toward the alkaline side of normal.

Respiratory unit A functional unit of the lung consisting of a cluster of respiratory bronchioles, alveolar ducts, and alveoli derived from a single terminal bronchiole. Another term for acinus.

Reticular tissue A special type of connective tissue characterized by fine reticulin fibers.

Reticulin fibers Very thin fibers made of collagen.

Reticulocytes A young red blood cell identified by special staining techniques.

Retrovirus Class of RNA viruses including HIV.

Reverse transcriptase Enzyme included within the genome of the HIV virus necessary for viral replication.

Reye's syndrome Acute illness following mild viral infection in children, characterized by brain swelling associated with aspirin consumption.

Rheumatic fever A disease caused by hypersensitivity to antigens of the beta streptococcus, characterized by fever, joint pains, and inflammation of heart valves and muscle. Inflammatory disease that occurs following a *Streptococcus pyogenes* infection that can involve the heart, joints, skin, and brain.

Rheumatoid arthritis (RA) A systemic disease primarily affecting the synovium with major manifestations in the small joints.

Ribonucleic acid (RNA) A type of nucleic acid contained in the nucleoli of cells. A component of messenger, transfer, and ribosomal RNA.

Ribosome A small cytoplasmic organelle that serves as the site of protein synthesis. Ribosomes are usually attached to the endoplasmic reticulum but may be free in the cytoplasm.

Rickets Impaired calcification of bone in a growing child caused by vitamin D deficiency, which leads to bowing of leg bones when weight-bearing is attempted.

Rocky Mountain spotted fever Disease caused by rickettsial infection of endothelial cells.

Root canal Replacement of tooth root canal with a filling material.

Rough endoplasmic reticulum (RER) Cell structure containing ribosomes and synthesizing protein.

Salpingitis Inflammation of the fallopian tubes.

Sarcoma A malignant tumor arising from connective and supporting tissues.

Schistocytes Fragmented red cells.

Schwann cells Cells making myelin for nerve fibers outside the CNS.

Schwannomas Tumor of peripheral nerves deriving from the Schwann cells.

Screening Examining a large asymptomatic population for signs of future disease.

Secondary gout Elevated uric acid and clinical manifestations of gout not caused by the metabolic disease primary gout, but instead caused by some other disease that raises the blood uric acid excessively, such as kidney failure or excessive breakdown of white blood cells in patients with leukemia.

Secondary hemostatic plug Formation of mature thrombus along with fibrin.

Secondary hemostatis Process involving plasma coagulation factors.

Secondary lymphoid organs Lymph nodes, spleen bone marrow, and mucosal-associated lymphoid tissue.

Secondary response Rapid response, part of immune memory.

Secondary site Site of tumor following metastic growth.

Secondary union Form of healing of a large unsutured wound.

Self-tolerance Selection process to remove ability to recognize self.

Semiconservative replication Production of duplicating DNA strands using complementary strands as a guide.

Semilunar valve The cup-shaped valve located between the ventricles and the aorta or pulmonary artery.

Seminoma One type of malignant tumor of the testis.

Sensitivity Classification of diagnostic tests in regard to percentage of patients classified as positive by a test who do have the disease.

Sentinel lymph node The lymph node in a group of lymph nodes that is located closest to a malignant tumor, which is examined to determine whether the tumor has spread to the node. If the sentinel node is not involved, additional lymph node dissection is not required.

Septicemia An infection in which large numbers of pathogenic bacteria are present in the bloodstream.

Seropositive Having antibodies to a pathogen.

Serotonin A vasoconstrictor mediator of inflammation released from platelets.

Serotype Immunologically detected pathogen strains.

Serous Fluid-rich exudate.

Serous tumor Ovarian tumor resembling cells in the fallopian tube.

Sex chromosomes The X and Y chromosomes that determine genetic sex. A human has 1 pair of sex chromosomes.

Sex-linked gene Gene present on the X or Y chromosome.

Sex-linked trait Product of gene present on X or Y chromosome.

Shingles Another name for herpes zoster.

Shock A general term for any condition leading to such a marked fall of blood pressure that body tissues do not receive an adequate amount of oxygen, most often caused by acute blood loss or severe infection (sepsis).

Shock wave lithotripsy A method for removing stones from the urinary tract by breaking them into small bits that can be excreted in the urine.

Sickle cell anemia Condition in individuals homozygous for the sickle hemoglobin gene.

Sickle cell trait Condition in individuals heterozygous for the sickle hemoglobin gene.

Sickle hemoglobin An abnormal hemoglobin that crystallizes under reduced oxygen tension causing red cells to change shape.

Signs Physical findings of disease.

Silicosis A type of occupational lung disease caused by inhalation of silica-rich rock dust.

Simple mastectomy/radical mastectomy Surgery to remove the breast and sometimes underlying tissue. May be simple mastectomy (only breast tissue) or radical mastectomy (breast and underlying tissue).

Single nucleotide polymorphisms (SNPs) Minor variations in the nucleotides contained in the individual genes of different individuals.

Sinusoid The modified blood vessel between the sheets of hepatocytes, forming the bulk of the liver.

Smooth endoplasmic reticulum (SER) Cell structure containing enzymes and synthesizing lipids.

Smooth muscle Muscle that functions automatically.

Solid Tumor type that is embedded in host tissue.

Somatic recombination Process during which gene segments are spliced together to form a mature antigen receptor molecule.

Somatostatin Hormone produced by the delta cells of the pancreas.

Spastic Muscle with excess tone that resists stretching.

Specific treatment Treatment of underlying cause of disease.

Specificity Classification of diagnostic tests in regard to the percentage of patients without the disease who are classified as negative by the test.

Spermatids Germ cells in a late stage of sperm development just before complete maturation to form mature sperm. *Spermatogonia* and *spermatocytes* are terms for an earlier stage.

Spermatocytes Precursor cells to sperm formed by mitotic division of spermatogonia.

Spermatogonia Precursor cells of sperm.

Spina bifida Incomplete closure of vertebral arches over the spinal cord, sometimes associated with protrusion of meninges and neural tissue through the defect (cystic spina bifida).

Spindle fibers The structure critical for proper alignment and separation of chromosomes during mitosis and meiosis.

Spinocerebellar ataxia (SCA) Cerebellar disturbances resulting in loss of control of body movements. Most common is Freidreich ataxia.

Splenorenal shunt Surgically created anastomosis between splenic vein and renal vein, performed to lower portal pressure in the treatment of esophageal varices.

Spores A highly resistant spherical structure produced by some bacteria to assure survival under adverse conditions.

Squamous cells Flat, platelike cells.

Squamous intraepithelial lesions (SIL) Precancerous results of infection with some HPV serotypes.

Stabile Population of cells that show little cell division.

Stable angina Temporary chest pain during stress or exertion caused by partial chronic blockage of the coronary vasculature.

Statins Drug agents effective against development of atherosclerosis.

Steatosis Abnormal storage of fat in the liver. Can result from alcoholic damage or some other cause.

Stem cells A self-renewing pool of cells that normally give rise to mature differentiated progeny.

Stenosis Narrowing of a valve orifice.

Stent Short tube often made of expandable metal mesh used to hold the blood vessel open.

Stillbirth Spontaneous abortion after twenty weeks' gestation.

Stomatitis Inflammation of the oral cavity.

Striated muscle Muscle that moves the skeleton; under voluntary control.

Stroke/cerebrovascular accident (CVA) An injury to the brain resulting in a disturbance of cerebral blood flow caused by a cerebral thrombosis, cerebral embolism, or cerebral hemorrhage.

Stroma The tissue that forms the framework of an organ.

Subarachnoid space The space between the arachnoid and the pia, containing large blood vessels supplying the brain.

Subclinical hepatitis Liver inflammation resulting in few symptoms.

Sudden infant death syndrome (SIDS) Unexplained death of child under the age of one year.

Superantigens Toxins produced by Staphylococcus aureus in toxic shock that cause widespread activation of T cells and release of cytokines.

Surfactant A lipid material secreted by Type II pneumocytes that facilitates respiration by decreasing the surface tension of the fluid lining the pulmonary alveoli.

Sweat test Diagnostic test for cystic fibrosis.

Symptomatic treatment Treatment of symptoms rather than underlying cause of disease.

Symptoms Subjective manifestations of disease.

Synapse Pairing of homologous chromosomes in meiosis. Also, gap between connecting neurons.

Synchrondrosis Cartilaginous joint.

Syndesmosis Fixed joint joined by fibrous connective tissue.

Syndrome Defect characterized by a common set of abnormalities related to a single cause.

Synovial joint Moveable joint.

Systolic heart failure Heart failure caused by inadequate ejection of blood from the ventricles during systole, in contrast to diastolic heart failure in which filling of the ventricles in diastole is inadequate.

T cell A type of lymphocyte associated with cell-mediated immunity.

T cell help Requirement of a T cell to present antigen for a B cell humoral response.

T cell independent/T cell dependent Whether T cells are needed or not needed for a response from B cells.

T cell receptor Antigen recognition molecule.

Tay-Sachs disease Autosomal recessive disease caused by the absence of lysosomal enzyme hexosaminidase A.

Teratocarcinomas/malignant teratomas A malignant testicular tumor composed of many different types of malignant tissues.

Teratoma A tumor of mixed cell components.

Terminal duct lobular unit (TDLU) Lobe of female breast including the cluster of milk gland ducts and stromal tissue.

Tetany Spasm of skeletal muscles caused by subnormal level of ionized calcium in the blood or certain bacterial toxins.

Thrombin time test A laboratory test measurement that determines the concentration of fibrinogen in the blood by determining the clotting time of the blood plasma after addition of thrombin.

Thrombin A coagulation factor formed by activation of prothrombin in the process of blood coagulation.

Thrombocytopenia A deficiency of platelets.

Thrombosis The pathologic activation of hemostasis under inappropriate conditions. The formation of blood clots (thrombi) within the vascular system.

Thrombotic stroke Reduction in blood flow in brain due to thrombus.

Thrombus Clot.

Thrush Superficial infection of mouth caused by *Candida albicans*.

Thyroglobulin A protein within the colloid of the thyroid follicles which is a precursor of thyroid hormone.

Thyroid-stimulating hormone (TSH) Hormone secreted by the anterior lobe of the pituitary; regulates thyroid function.

Tissue A group of similar cells joined to perform a specific function.

Tissue factor Protein that is a trigger for extrinsic coagulation.

Tissue transglutaminase Human enzyme target of antibodies detected in gluten sensitivity.

Tonicity Measure of ionic concentration determined only by solutes that cannot cross the membrane.

TORCH complex Mnemonic for organisms causing maternal infections injurious to the developing fetus.

Toxic shock syndrome (TSS) Disease characterized by elevated temperature, vomiting and diarrhea, muscular aches, and a fall in blood pressure.

Toxoplasma gondii A small intracellular parasite of birds, animals, and humans. Causes the disease toxoplasmosis.

Trabeculae Thin strands of bone lattice work.

Tracheoesophageal fistula Abnormal communication between the esophagus and trachea.

Transcription Process of copying information from DNA to mRNA.

Transfer RNA (tRNA) RNA molecule that "picks up" appropriate amino acid to build the gene product.

Transient ischemic attack (TIA) Temporary cerebral dysfunction as a result of transient obstruction of a cerebral vessel by a bit of atheromatous debris or blood clot, usually embolized from an arteriosclerotic plaque in the carotid artery.

Transition zone Area of cervix where the columnar music producing epithelial cells meet the squamous epithelial cells. Also, part of the prostate that surrounds the urethra.

Transitional cell tumor/Brenner tumor Benign tumor containing nests of urothelial-like cells.

Transjugular intrahepatic portosystemic shunt A nonsurgical method used to lower portal vein pressure in a person with cirrhosis by connecting an intrahepatic branch of the portal vein to a hepatic vein branch.

Translation Process of building a gene product using information from the mRNA.

Translocation A transfer of a piece of one chromosome to a nonhomologous chromosome.

Trauma Injury caused by a physical extrinsic agent.

Treponema pallidum The spiral organism causing syphilis.

Tricuspid valve AV valve separating the right atrium and ventricle.

Triglycerides Lipids used to store excess calories in fat cells.

Trigone Triangular area at the base of the bladder.

Triple therapy Treatment of ulcer with proton pump inhibitors combined with two antibiotics.

Triple X syndrome Presence of one or more extra X chromosomes.

Triple-negative Breast cancer cell lacking ER, PR, and HER-2.

Trisomy The presence of an extra chromosome within a cell; having three of a given chromosome instead of the usual pair.

Trophoblast Cell derived from the fertilized ovum that gives rise to the fetal membranes and contributes to the formation of the placenta.

Trophozoite Active, motile vegetative phase of a parasite.

Tumor A benign or malignant overgrowth of tissues that serves no normal function which is no longer under homeostatic control.

Tumor necrosis factor alpha (TNFα) Pro-inflammatory cytokine.

Tumor suppressor gene Gene that normally functions to suppress abnormal cell growth.

Tumor-associated antigen An antigen associated with growing tumor cells that serves as an indicator of tumor growth in the body.

Turner syndrome A congenital syndrome usually caused by absence of one X chromosome in the female.

Type 1 diabetes mellitus (T1DM) Diabetes resulting from a deficit in insulin production.

Type 2 diabetes mellitus (T2DM) Diabetes resulting from the resistance of target tissue to the effect of insulin with a compensatory oversecretion by the pancreas.

Type I membranoproliferative glomerulonephritis A more severe form of glomerulonephritis associated with infections of the heart, bone, and chronic hepatitis C.

Type I pneumocytes/type II pneumocytes Cells lining the alveoli.

Tyrosine kinase Enzyme that produces multiple effects concerned with cell growth and cell division by phosphorylation of tyrosine residues in a protein.

Unstable angina Angina of prolonged duration resistant to therapy.

Urea Normal by-product of protein metabolism excreted in the urine.

Uremia An excess of urea and other waste products in the blood, resulting from renal failure.

Urinalysis A commonly performed chemical and microscopic analysis of the urine.

Variable region Region on the immunoglobulin molecule specific for a particular pathogen. Amino-terminal end of the immunoglobulin chain; part that recognizes antigen.

Varicocele Varicose veins that develop within the spermatic cord veins.

Varicosities Excessive tortuosity and dilation of blood vessels.

Vascular claudication Severe cramping leg pain due to atherosclerosis of arteries in leg.

Vascular dementia/multi-infarct dementia Compromise of cerebral function caused by blockage of small cerebral blood vessels.

Vascular pole Site where the afferent arteriole enters the glomerulus and the efferent arteriole exits.

Vasodilator A substance that dilates blood vessels.

Vaso-occlusive crisis Serious consequence of sickle cell anemia characterized by severe pain when blood vessels are blocked by sickled cells.

Vectors Transmission agent of parasite; may be insects or other animals.

Velamentous insertion of umbilical cord Attachment of the umbilical cord to the fetal membranes rather than to the placenta.

Ventilation/perfusion scan (V/Q scan) Procedure used to detect a pulmonary embolus.

Ventricle A small cavity, especially one in the brain or heart. *Ventricles of brain:* The hollow cavities in the brain. *Ventricles of heart:* The muscular chambers that receive blood from the atria and pump the blood into the aorta *(left ventricle)* or pulmonary artery *(right ventricle).*

Ventricular systole Period of ventricular contraction.

Vesicoureteral reflux Retrograde flow of urine from the bladder into the ureter during voiding.

Vimentin filament Type of filament in connective and muscle cells.

Viremia Presence of large numbers of viral particles.

Virtual colonoscopy A high resolution contrast CT image of the colon. May be substituted for colonoscopy in special cases.

Virulence/virulent Ability of an organism to cause disease.

Virulence factors Elements of microbe that cause disease.

Vital capacity The maximum volume of air that can be forcefully expelled after a maximum inspiration.

Vitelline duct Duct connecting the yolk sac to the developing embryo during embryogenesis.

Volvulus Rotary twisting of the bowel.

von Willebrand Factor (vWF) A large protein that acts to adhere platelets to collagen.

Vulvar intraepithelial neoplasia (VIN) Cancer of the vulva.

Well-circumscribed Tumor with a clear border.

West Nile virus An arbovirus that infects birds, animals, and humans.

White cell count Count of number and type of while cells present in the blood. A test for inflammation.

White matter Area of the CNS located externally to the gray matter consisting predominantly of the portions of the neurons that conduct impulses away from the axons.

Xerostoma Dry mouth which is lacking in saliva.

Yolk sac A sac formed adjacent to the germ disk that will form the gastrointestinal tract and other important structures in the embryo.

Zenker diverticulum Outpouching in the upper portion of the esophagus.

Zona pellucida A layer of acellular material surrounding the ovum.

Zygote The fertilized ovum.

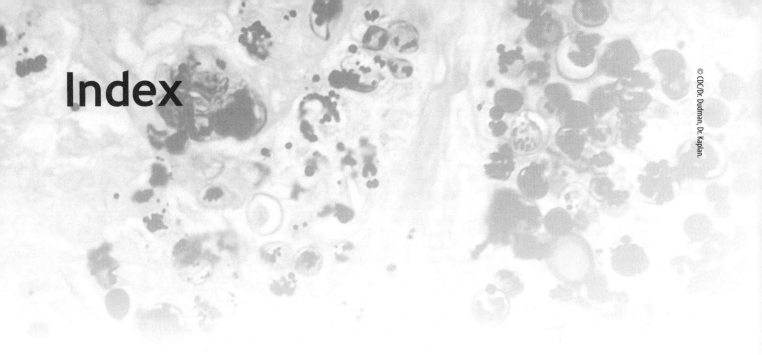

Index

Note: Page numbers followed by *f*, *t*, and *c* denote figures, tables, and cases, respectively.